A G Millard
B. Eng Sc. M.I.S.O
A. Ind Sc. Studies

BLACK'S MEDICAL DICTIONARY

BLACK'S MEDICAL DICTIONARY

Edited by C. W. H. Havard, MA, DM, FRCP

Thirty-sixth edition

A & C BLACK • LONDON

36th edition published by
A & C Black (Publishers) Limited
35 Bedford Row, London WC1R 4JH

ISBN 0-7136-3208-9

A CIP catalogue record for this book
is available from the British Library

In its earlier editions *Black's Medical Dictionary* was edited by:
J. D. Comrie, MD—first to seventeenth editions, 1906–42
H. A. Clegg, FRCP—eighteenth edition, 1944
W. A. R. Thomson, MD—nineteenth to thirty-fourth editions, 1948–84
C. W. H. Havard FCRP—thirty-fifth edition, 1987

Printed in Great Britain by BPCC Wheatons Ltd, Exeter

PREFACE

Black's Medical Dictionary defines and explains a wide range of terms and concepts in use in medicine and in closely related subjects. It includes detailed accounts of many aspects of anatomy, physiology, pathology and therapeutics. It will prove valuable to all those working in fields drawing on medical practice, and to anyone interested in how the body works, and what is happening in medicine today.

This is the thirty-sixth edition of a book first published in 1906. In this edition thirty new sections have been added to topics varying from cluster headaches to cyclical oedema of women. The sections on dentistry, dermatology, diseases of the ear, nose and throat, ophthalmology and psychiatry have been rewritten by specialists in the particular field and I am grateful to Iain Laws, Colin Buckley, Neil Solomons, John Roberts-Harry and Chris Burford for their help in bringing these sections of the dictionary up to date.

Although many completely new subjects have been added to this thirty-sixth edition of *Black's Medical Dictionary* and many more articles have been virtually rewritten, the intention is unchanged: to describe medical theory and practice as clearly and concisely as possible.

A

.BDOMEN is the lower part of the trunk. .bove, and separated from it by the diaphragm r midriff, lies the thorax or chest, and below es the pelvis, or basin, generally described as a eparate cavity though directly continuous ·ith that of the abdomen. Behind lie the spinal olumn and lower ribs which come within a few ıches of the iliac or haunch bones; at the sides he protection afforded to the contained organs ·y the iliac bones and down-sloping ribs is still ıore effective; but in front the whole extent is ·rotected only by soft tissues. The latter consist f the skin, a varying amount of fat, three layers ·f broad, flat muscle, another layer of fat, and ınally the smooth, thin peritoneum which ines the whole cavity. The absence of rigidity llows the necessary distension when food is aken into the stomach, and the various impor-ant movements of the organs associated with ligestion. The shape of the abdomen varies; in hildren it may protrude considerably, though f this is too marked it may indicate disease; in .ealthy young adults it should be either very lightly prominent or slightly indrawn, and hould show the outline of the muscular layer, especially of the pair of muscles running vertically (recti), which are divided into four or five sections by transverse lines; while with advance of age it is quite natural that a certain amount of fat should be deposited on and inside the abdomen.

Contents: The principal contents of the abdominal cavity are the digestive organs, ie. the stomach and intestines, and the associated glands, the liver and pancreas. The position of the stomach is above and to the left when the individual is recumbent, but may be much lower in the erect position. The liver lies above and to the right, lying to a large extent under cover of the ribs, and occupying the hollow of the diaphragm, by which alone both it and the stomach are separated from the lungs and heart. Against the back wall on either side lie the kidneys, protected also to a great extent by the last two ribs; and from the kidneys run the ureters, or urinary ducts, down along the back wall to the bladder in the pelvis. The pancreas lies across the spine between the kidneys, and upon the upper end of each kidney lies a suprarenal gland. High up on the left and partly behind the stomach lies the spleen. The great blood-vessels and nerves, the absorbent vessels and the glands connected with them, lie on the back

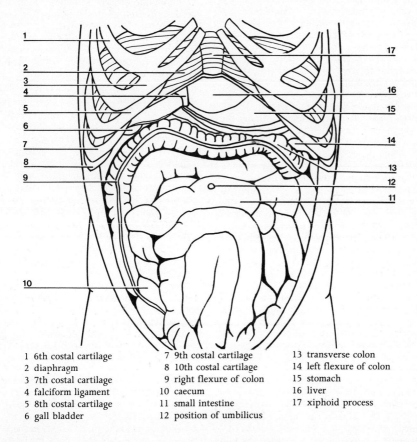

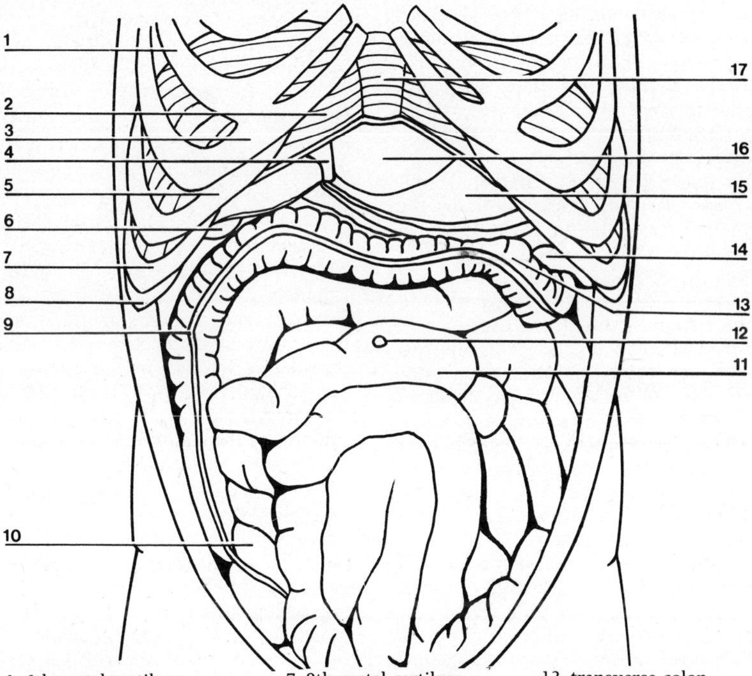

1 6th costal cartilage
2 diaphragm
3 7th costal cartilage
4 falciform ligament
5 8th costal cartilage
6 gall bladder
7 9th costal cartilage
8 10th costal cartilage
9 right flexure of colon
10 caecum
11 small intestine
12 position of umbilicus
13 transverse colon
14 left flexure of colon
15 stomach
16 liver
17 xiphoid process

Contents of the abdomen in position.

wall, and the remainder of the space is taken up by the intestines or bowels (see INTESTINE), the large intestine lying in the flanks on either side in front of the kidneys and crossing below the stomach from right to left, while the small intestine hangs from the back wall in coils which fill up the spaces between the other organs. Hanging down from the stomach in front of the bowels is the omentum, or apron, containing a considerable amount of fat, and helping to protect the bowels from cold and injury. In pregnancy the uterus, or womb, as it increases in size, rises up from the pelvis into the abdomen, lifting the coils of the small intestine above it.

The *pelvis* is that portion of the abdomen which lies within the bony pelvis (see BONE), and contains the rectum or end part of the intestine, the bladder, and, in the male the prostate, in the female the uterus, ovaries, and Fallopian tubes.

ABDOMEN, DISEASES OF: (See under STOMACH, DISEASES OF; INTESTINE, DISEASES OF; DIARRHOEA; LIVER, DISEASES OF; PANCREAS, DISEASES OF; KIDNEY, DISEASES OF; BLADDER, DISEASES OF; HERNIA; PERITONITIS; APPENDICITIS; TUMOURS.)

Symptoms: The symptoms of various diseases will be found under the above headings, and only some general symptoms of abdominal disease, or symptoms, the meaning of which is not plain, but which nevertheless point to trouble in definite organs, will be mentioned here.

PAIN: This is a most important symptom, because the internal organs being devoid of ordinary sensation, pain in them generally means a considerable interference with structure or function. The *site* of the pain may indicate the organ affected. Thus pain under the ribs on the left, or in the pit of the stomach, generally points to the stomach as being at fault. When it is felt on the right high up, and shoots through to the right shoulder, it indicates trouble connected with the liver or gall-bladder. Pain situated on the right, and low down in the iliac region, may arise from a diseased appendix. On the left, and low down, or at the exit of the bowel, it means some rectal trouble. Finally, pain situated vaguely all over the front of the abdomen, especially round the navel, points to inflammation of the peritoneal lining of the abdomen, or to irregularity in movement of the small intestine.

The *character* of the pain is also important. A dull, aching pain is not generally serious, though, if persistent, it may indicate chronic peritonitis or obstruction. (See PERITONITIS; and INTESTINE, DISEASES OF.) A twisting, griping pain is generally, eg. in babies, due to spasmodic movements of the small intestine, often produced by errors in diet, and called colic. A straining pain with frequent calls to stool indicates irritation low down in the large bowel. The pains of stomach trouble are of varied nature. (See DYSPEPSIA.) Sudden, colicky, agonizing pain is often due to the passage of a gall-stone, if situated high up on the right, shooting through towards the back, or to the passage of a renal calculus, if shooting from the back down into the groin. Pain of a dull character slightly to the right of the pit of the stomach, especially when it is relieved by taking food, suggests some trouble in the duodenum.

TENDERNESS on pressure is generally a sign of inflammation either of an organ situated beneath the tender spot or of the peritoneum. (See APPENDICITIS; PERITONITIS.)

VOMITING is an important symptom. (See VOMITING.) When due to irritation of the stomach, it usually ceases as the contents of this organ are brought up. If it persists, it may be due to some obstruction in the bowels, or may be of nervous origin, eg. in sea-sickness, or brain tumour, and have no direct connection with the abdomen.

DIARRHOEA is another important symptom, and may indicate serious trouble. (See DIARRHOEA.)

SWELLING of the abdomen may be so marked as to call the patient's attention to it. This may be due merely to excessive deposit of fat, especially in elderly people – for example, in women at the menopause. (See CORPULENCE; DIET.) Enlargement, of course, occurs in pregnancy. The abdomen in habitual constipation may become more distended, partly by accumulation of gas, or the enlargement may be due to chronic obstruction of the bowels. (See CONSTIPATION; and INTESTINE, DISEASES OF.) Finally, a collection of fluid may produce the swelling (see DROPSY; LIVER, DISEASES OF; HEART, DISEASES OF; PERITONITIS), or it may be due to enlargement of a single organ.

INDRAWING of the abdomen occurs in wasting diseases, and also to a marked extent in meningitis. (See MENINGITIS.)

DISTENSION OF THE VEINS on the surface of the abdomen indicates some interference with the circulation in the portal vein or in the inferior vena cava.

VISIBLE MOVEMENTS are sometimes seen, due to the bowels or stomach being distended and contracting forcibly in the attempt to drive their contents onwards. They indicate (unless they are visible merely on account of extreme thinness of the abdominal wall) some obstruction in the bowel or stomach. (See PERISTALSIS.)

The differentiation of abdominal diseases is often one of the most difficult problems with which even an expert has to deal, and frequently it is only after a period of observation lasting in difficult cases perhaps some weeks that a diagnosis of approximate accuracy can be arrived at. This is partly due to the difficulty or impossibility of feeling the surface and dimensions of the contained organs, eg. the kidneys, especially in stout people; partly to the vagueness of symptoms set up in organs which are very little sensitive to even extreme changes in their structure; and partly to the readiness with which the organs change their relative positions, and to the great changes in shape and position often brought about by previous disease.

'eatment: Details of treatment are given under e headings of the various diseases. On the hole, people are rather too much given to garding abdominal symptoms as trivial and nenable to home treatment. In many cases curable dyspepsia would have been got rid of its early stages if its symptoms had not been eglected, and patients with acute obstruction the bowels may die because a dose of castor l was taken when a doctor should have been nsulted. In this connection one may say that henever the three symptoms of (*a*) abdominal ain, (*b*) vomiting or retching, and (*c*) stoppage the bowels for a day or two, or stoppage llowed by a little diarrhoea, have occurred gether, the case demands skilled medical tention. If severe abdominal pain is directly aceable to some dietetic indiscretion, the fending material should be got rid of speedily y an emetic, if it is still in the stomach (see METICS); or by a purgative if the symptoms are ferable to the bowels (see PURGATIVES). If the ain is griping in character, eg. in babies, relief often given by pressure; thus nurses often lay eir charges stomach downwards across the m, or adults get some relief by lying face ownwards on a pillow. (See COLIC; LEAD-)ISONING.) The application of heat, in the rm of a hot-water bottle, may also give relief. 'hen the pain is agonizing, stronger remedies re necessary. (See COLIC.)

BDOMEN, INJURIES OF: Despite the xposed nature of the abdomen to the front and e thinness of the wall covering the viscera, it surprising how seldom blows and crushes amage the contained organs. This is explained y the fact that the firm muscles, which are erhaps half an inch (12mm) thick, offer the ame type of protection as would be given by a ab of rubber of like thickness tightly tretched, while the fat still further dissipates e effect of violence. When a kick or blow auses rupture of an organ, the violence has enerally been unexpected, and the muscles ave been surprised in a lax condition. It is true at instantaneous death may follow a comparatively trivial blow on the epigastrium or pit of e stomach, and this is due to shock (see HOCK) caused by injury to a nerve-plexus situted in the back of the abdomen in that region. upture of the liver, kidney, or spleen may ccur, with haemorrhage into the surrounding issues, from severe crushes, from falls from a eight, road accidents, etc.; but these are not ecessarily fatal unless some large blood-vessel s torn. Rupture of the bowel occasionally folows a blow or wound and is almost necessarily atal in a few days, unless the abdomen is pened by a surgeon and the torn bowel titched within a few hours of the accident.

People run over by vehicles are liable to have he bladder ruptured. This occurs especially in he case of children, and it happens only when he bladder is full, or nearly so, of urine. In such case the inability to pass water soon after the ccident, provided that it was not passed for some hours previously, or the passage of blood, indicates the necessity of a speedy operation to stitch the torn bladder.

Straining to lift a weight beyond the strength, or excessive straining at stool, may force a loop of the intestine through the muscular part of the abdominal wall, so producing a hernia or rupture. (See HERNIA.)

ABDOMEN, REGIONS OF: For convenience of reference the abdomen is divided into regions by artificial lines. Two are vertical, passing through the middle of the inguinal ligament, a band which crosses the groin obliquely and divides thigh from abdomen; and two are horizontal: the subcostal plane which passes through the lowest part of the costal margin, and the intertubercular plane which passes through the most outwardly projecting points of the iliac or haunch bones. These divide off nine regions named as follows: Epigastrium or pit of the stomach (E), two Hypochondriac regions (H), Umbilical or Navel region (U), two Lumbar or Loin regions (L), Hypogastric region (Hy), and two Iliac regions or Groins (I). The inguinal region on each side is the lower part of the hypogastric region. This contains the inguinal canal which pierces the abdominal wall obliquely.

ABDUCENT NERVE is the sixth nerve rising from the brain and controls the external rectus muscle of the eye, which turns the eye outwards. It is particularly liable to be paralysed in diseases of the nervous system, thus leading to an inward squint.

ABLATION means the removal of any part of the body by a surgical operation.

ABORTIFACIENT is a drug which causes artificial abortion.

ABORTION or MISCARRIAGE, means the separation and expulsion of the contents of the pregnant uterus before the 28th week of pregnancy. The frequency of abortion is not known, but it is estimated that 10 to 15 per cent of pregnancies end in abortion. The common time for abortion to occur is from the 8th to 13th week of pregnancy.

Causes: The cause of the abortion may be found in the mother or in the germ cells, or in some completely extraneous factor.

So far as the mother is concerned, the most common cause is an abnormality of the hormonal balance which controls the course of pregnancy (qv). The main defect is a lack of progesterone (qv). This hormone is secreted by the corpus luteum (qv) in the early weeks of pregnancy and subsequently by the placenta (qv). The function of progesterone is to ensure the safe embedding of the fertilized ovum in the mother's uterus (or womb), and then to ensure that the uterus does not start contracting until the time for labour is due. It is thus obvious why a defective supply of progesterone can result in abortion.

Other maternal causes of abortion include disturbances of other endocrine glands, or hormones, such as hypothyroidism, or myxoedema (qv), and diabetes mellitus (qv); high blood-pressure; glomerulonephritis (qv); any acute illness; congenital abnormalities of the uterus, and any severe emotional disturbance.

Several drugs have achieved a popular reputation as abortifacients, or inducers of abortion, but the reputation is usually fallacious. It is incredibly difficult to induce an abortion by means of drugs in a healthy pregnancy. This even applies to pills containing lead, though there is no doubt that lead can induce an abortion.

Any defect in the germ cells, whether ovum or spermatozoon, may lead to abortion if it is severe enough to cause gross malformation of the embryo.

Finally, reference must be made to criminally induced abortion. This may be attempted in a variety of ways, particularly the introduction of fluids or instruments into the uterus. It is a dangerous practice, as shown by a Ministry of Health investigation into 294 fatal abortions. At least 199 of these were criminal abortions, 105 (53 per cent) of whom died from sepsis. (See also BLIGHTED OVUM.)

Treatment: The treatment depends largely upon whether the abortion is threatened or inevitable. In the case of the former, often a few days rest in bed is all that is necessary, following which the mother takes particular care at the

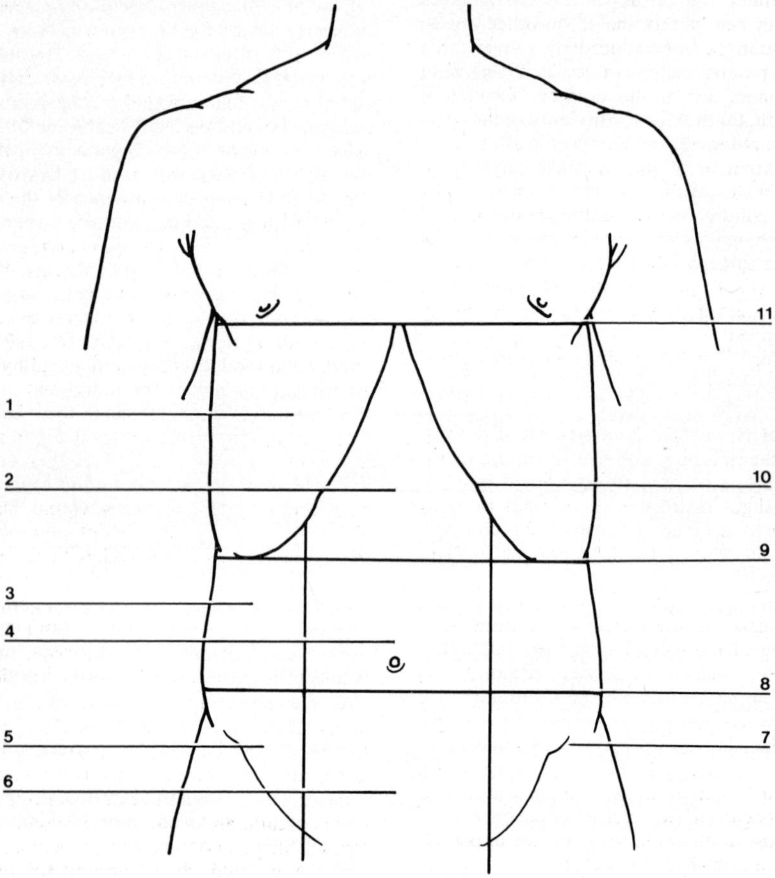

1 hypochondriac region
2 epigastrium
3 lumbar region
4 umbilical region
5 iliac region
6 hypogastric region
7 anterior superior iliac spine
8 intertubercular plane
9 subcostal plane
10 tip of 9th costal cartilage
11 xiphisternal plane

Regions of the abdomen.

xt two period times. If an abortion is inevita-e, the treatment is that of a miniature labour. ore complicated, and requiring skilled super-sion, is the treatment of what is known as an complete abortion (that is, when part of the etus and/or placenta have been retained in e uterus), and – most dangerous of all – the eatment of a septic abortion.

erapeutic abortion: Abortion, or termination pregnancy, is a criminal offence in Britain, t the whole outlook on abortion was changed the Abortion Act, 1967, which came into rce in 1968, and created exceptions to the ffences Against the Persons Act, 1861, which ade it an offence 'unlawfully to administer y poison or other noxious thing or to use any strument or any other means whatsoever ith intent to procure a miscarriage', or to sup-y any such poison or instrument for this pur-se. Under the terms of the 1967 Act, a egnancy can be terminated: in other words, abortion can be induced by a 'registered edical practitioner if two registered medical actitioners are of the opinion, formed in od faith, (*a*) that the continuance of the preg-ncy would involve risk to the life of the preg-nt woman or of injury to the physical or ental health of the pregnant woman or any isting children of her family greater than if e pregnancy were terminated; or (*b*) that ere is a substantial risk that if the child were rn it would suffer from such physical or ental abnormalities as to be seriously andicapped'.

In 1986, 157,000 legal abortions were carried t in England and Wales.

BRASION means the rubbing off of the sur-ce of the skin or of a mucous membrane due some mechanical injury. Such injuries, ough slight in themselves, are apt to allow trance of dirt containing organisms and so to ad to an abscess or some severer form of flammation.

reatment: The most effective form of treat-ent consists in the thorough and immediate eansing of the wound with soap and water. n antiseptic such as 1 per cent cetrimide can en be applied, and a sterile dry dressing.

ENTAL ABRASION is a form of trauma in hich the teeth are worn away. This may be by uxism or excessive use of the toothbrush, articularly if an abrasive toothpaste is used. It sually occurs at the junction of the crown and ot of the tooth and is worst on the upper left eth in a right-handed person.

BSCESS is a localized collection of pus. A inute abscess is known as a pustule (see PUS-ULE), a diffused production of pus is known as ellulitis or erysipelas (see ERYSIPELAS). An bscess may be acute or chronic.

BSCESS, ACUTE: An acute abscess is one hich develops rapidly within the course of a w days or hours. It is characterized by a defi-ite set of symptoms.

Causes: The direct cause is various bacteria. In a few cases the presence of foreign bodies, such as bullets or splinters, or contact with poison-ous plants, such as poison ivy, may produce abscesses, but these foreign bodies may remain for life buried in the tissues without causing any trouble provided they are not contami-nated with bacteria or other micro-organisms.

The micro-organisms most frequently found are *staphylococci*, and next to these *strepto-cocci*, though the latter cause more virulent abscesses, or in general the more serious condi-tion of erysipelas or cellulitis. Other abscess-forming organisms are *Pseudomonas pyocy-anea*, which produces blue or greenish pus; and *Escherichia coli*, which lives always in the bow-els, probably aiding digestion, and under cer-tain conditions wanders into the surrounding tissues and produces abscesses.

The mere presence of micro-organisms is not sufficient to produce suppuration (see IMMU-NITY; and INFECTION); indeed streptococci, which upon occasion produce most disastrous effects, can often be found on the skin and in the skin glands of perfectly healthy individuals. Given the proper micro-organisms in the tis-sues, whether they will produce abscesses or not depends upon the virulence of the organ-ism at the time, and the resisting power of the individual. In the case of bad health, as in dia-betes mellitus, fever, Bright's disease, the tis-sues are less resistant, and cold, injury, or previous disease of a part renders it less able to cope with bacterial invasion. On the other hand, good food, exercise, and a healthy open-air life help to render the individual more or less immune to the ill-effects of these bacteria. They are communicated, principally in a viru-lent form, from one wound to another; but they live also in the air, in dust, and in water. They enter the body generally by a wound, but may also come through the mucous membrane of the intestine when this is rendered less resistant by conditions such as appendicitis; they may also pass through the mucous membranes of the nose, mouth, respiratory and urinary passages, and cause local abscesses, or even through the skin's minute lubricating glands.

When bacteria have gained access, for exam-ple, to a wound, they rapidly multiply, and, by the formation of poisonous substances, irritate the surrounding tissues, and so produce local dilatation of the blood-vessels, slowing of the blood-stream, and exudation of blood corpus-cles and fluid. The leucocytes, or white corpus-cles of the blood, collect around the invaded area, apparently under some attracting influ-ence of the bacteria (chemotaxis), and destroy the latter either by actually devouring and digesting them (see PHAGOCYTOSIS), or by form-ing some substances which cause their death. These white corpuscles undergo a granular fatty degeneration, and in turn die, and form the white constituent of the pus (pus corpus-cles). Meanwhile, the area where these changes have been taking place has been cut off from communication with the rest of the body by plugging of the blood and lymphatic vessels around it. The tissues of the affected area die and are digested by the action of the white corpuscles, and the cavity so produced is distended by fluid and by the white corpuscles which flock to it in increasing numbers till all bacteria have disappeared. The abscess is shut off from healthy tissue by what is known as the abscess wall. The bacteria may find their way along a vessel to some little distance, where the same process takes place, and these secondary abscess cavities may coalesce with the original one.

Symptoms: The classic symptoms of inflammation are *rubor*, *calor*, *tumor* and *dolor*: ie. redness, warmth, swelling and pain; and, besides these, when the abscess is well developed, a considerable amount of fever, perhaps with delirium, sets in, and the temperature rises to 38° to 40°C (100° to 104°F). When the cavity containing fluid has been formed, a sign, known as fluctuation, can be made out. Later, as the abscess is distended almost to bursting, the skin becomes reddish blue, glazed, and thin; and this is known as 'pointing' of the abscess; or if the abscess is very deep-seated the skin over it becomes swollen, and pits on pressure. The lymphatic glands in the neighbourhood may be swollen and tender in an attempt to stop the bacteria spreading to other parts of the body. Immediately the abscess is opened, or bursts, the pain disappears, the temperature falls rapidly to normal, the elasticity of the tissues around the cavity diminishes its bulk, and the healing of the small space left proceeds rapidly. If, however, the abscess discharges into an internal cavity, such as the bowel or bladder, it may heal very slowly, and the reabsorption of its poisonous products may cause general ill-health for long. When an abscess is deep-seated an important sign for diagnosis is provided by examination of the blood. (See LEUCOCYTOSIS.)

Treatment: As soon as there is evidence that pus has formed, we know that the bacteria has been destroyed, and, as the further formation of pus is designed simply to burst a passage to the exterior, we can relieve pain, stop unnecessary destruction of tissue, and shorten the process by opening the abscess. This is done as soon as there is evidence from fluctuation, redness or pitting of the skin that pus has formed. Previous to this, an injection of penicillin, or some other antibiotic to which the causative micro-organism is sensitive, is given.

When the abscess is opened two things are attended to:

(1) That important structures such as arteries in the neighbourhood are not damaged.

(2) That the opening is as far away as possible from a new source of infection like the mouth or anus.

Current practice is to scrape out the abscess after draining its contents and then to close it immediately by sutures. Some surgeons continue to give a dose of the antibiotic daily for five days after operation. Others contend that in the vast majority of cases, only one injecti of antibiotic is necessary – preceding the ope ing of the abscess.

Special varieties of acute abscess: ABSCESS ABDOMEN: When this occurs in the iliac regi it is generally a result of appendicitis (s APPENDICITIS); when in the lumbar region may be the result of this disease 'pointin backwards, or may be the result of inflamm tion in the loose tissue around the kidney (pe inephric abscess). In the upper part of t abdomen it is known as a subphrenic absce and may be the consequence of ulceration fro the stomach or bowels, or of abscess in t liver. All these conditions are very grave.

ABSCESS IN BONE (See BONE, DISEASES OF).

ABSCESS OF BREAST (See BREAST, DISEASES OF).

CEREBRAL AND CEREBELLAR ABSCESS: These a apt to come on suddenly in cases in which t middle ear is diseased, generally after lon standing discharge from the ear. The stoppa of the discharge in such a case is a warning danger. (See EAR, DISEASES OF.)

ABSCESS IN THE FINGER (See WHITLOW).

ILIAC ABSCESS (See APPENDICITIS).

ABSCESS OF THE JAW (See GUMBOIL).

ABSCESS IN THE KIDNEY (See KIDNEYS, DISEAS OF).

ABSCESS OF THE LUNG may follow pneumonia the drawing of some foreign body, such as foo down the windpipe. Being deep-seated, presence may be hard to diagnose. It may bu either into a bronchus, when pus will be sp up, or into the pleural cavity. (See LUN DISEASES.)

ABSCESS IN THE PLEURAL CAVITY is known empyema. (See EMPYEMA.)

ABSCESS, CHRONIC: A chronic abscess one which takes weeks or months for its dev opment. In the majority of cases it tuberculous.

Causes: Some acute abscesses, instead of burs ing, may settle down, become surrounded dense fibrous tissue, and so form chron abscesses, but these are rare. Abscesses m form in the liver as a complication of amoeb dysentery. (See DYSENTERY.) The tubercle bac lus, or *Mycobacterium tuberculosis*, however, generally the cause. How it obtains entrance still in dispute; in the case of abscesses of t neck it is probably through the throat or tons and in the case of abscesses elsewhere, throu the circulation from the lung or intestin canal, owing to infected air or food. A comm source of infection is milk which has not be boiled or pasteurized. Abscesses arise mo commonly from tuberculous deposits in glan or bones, especially in the vertebrae or bones the spine, the epiphyses or large ends of lo bones near a joint, and the ribs. They may sta also in the synovial membranes, ie. membran lining a joint (see JOINT DISEASES), in the loo tissue beneath the skin, quite apart from di ease of any other structure, and, not uncon monly, in the testicle.

ymptoms: There is far less in the way of symp-
oms than in acute abscess. Sometimes the
velling is noticed by accident; it is not hot, red
r in general painful, as is an acute abscess. The
in becomes red only a short time before the
oscess bursts. If the temperature is taken every
our hours it will generally be found that there
a slight rise either in the forenoon or late
fternoon. If the abscess is untreated it gener-
lly enlarges till it bursts, then a ragged wound
left, infection with other organisms takes
lace, and the resulting sinus with 'mixed infec-
on' becomes extremely difficult to heal.

haracter of the pus: The fluid is thin and watery
not thick and white as in an acute abscess) and
ontains little curdy masses. It is not really
ous', as pus corpuscles are almost entirely
bsent, and only fragments of the dead tissues
re found under the microscope.

reatment: For the purpose of discussing treatment it will be assumed that the abscess is
uberculous.

The introduction of the anti-tuberculous
rugs, eg. streptomycin (qv), rifampicin,
thambutol and isoniazid (qv), has revolution-
zed the outlook in tuberculous abscesses and
as removed many of the hazards which were
ttached to them at one time. The general rules
or improving the health of the individual and
esting the affected part still apply, but the
dministration of these drugs shortens the
eriod of treatment and convalescence very
onsiderably. Further details will be found
nder GLANDS; and JOINT DISEASES.

pecial varieties of chronic abscess: ABSCESS OF
HE LIVER: This occurs in persons who have
een the subject of amoebic dysentery (see DYS-
NTERY), frequently after returning in appar-
ntly fair health to a temperate region where
his form of dysentery does not occur. The liver
ecomes enlarged and tender, and there is a
legree of ill-health and slight jaundice.
Amoebiasis, either in the form of amoebic
lysentry or liver abscess, is usually cured by
oral metronidazole (Flagyl). A parentral prepa-
ation is also available. The drug has an
ntabuse effect so that alcohol should not be
aken during treatment with metronidazole. An
lternative method of treatment if
metronidazole is not available or is not effec-
ive is emetine which should be given by subcutaneous injection. Because of possible cardi-
otoxicity the patient should be in bed when
eceiving emetine. Chloroquine is another drug
effective against amoebic abscess; it requires to
e given for 14 days. Sometimes if the liver
bscess is large and painful, aspiration (qv) is
equired to prevent perforation and to hasten
ecovery. The incidence of amoebiasis can be
educed in the tropics by not eating fresh
uncooked vegetable, by not drinking unboiled
water, and by adding iodine-releasing tablets to
drinking water.

SCHIO-RECTAL ABSCESS: This forms at the side of
the rectum. Whether it bursts or is opened, it is
very difficult to keep clean, on account of its
position, and so forms a sinus; or, if it opens
into the bowel, a fistula. (See FISTULA.) It may
occur late in a case of pulmonary tuberculosis,
but may also occur as the first manifestation of
tuberculosis.

RETROPHARYNGEAL ABSCESS: This is due generally to disease of the spinal column in the neck.
It is opened from the side of the neck; otherwise it bursts into the mouth, and the discharges from it lead to rapid falling-off in
health, and to death unless efficient treatment
is instituted.

ILIO-PSOAS ABSCESS: This arises generally from
tuberculous disease of the spinal column in the
lumbar region, and, though this may cure itself,
the abscess bursts into the sheath of the psoas
muscle and passes along the muscle through the
iliac region into the thigh, on the inner side of
which it generally 'points'. Its early symptoms
resemble those of hip-joint disease. (See JOINT
DISEASES.) The opening and scraping of such an
abscess often require large incisions in the
thigh, groin, and lumbar region, and if the
wound becomes the seat of mixed infection the
resulting sinus may last months or years. Fortunately, the introduction of anti-tuberculous
drugs has reduced the risk of this very
considerably.

ACTINOMYCOTIC ABSCESS: This form of chronic
abscess occurs about the jaw or mouth. (See
ACTINOMYCOSIS.)

ABSINTHISM: Absinthe is a greenish liquor prepared by steeping herbs, especially anise and wormwood, in alcohol for several days. It was first introduced into France by soldiers stationed in Algiers between 1830 and 1850, for whom it had been prescribed as a febrifuge (qv), and its employment spread thence into other countries. Its use becomes a habit like that of alcohol, but its effects are more demoralizing. Its habitual use brings on tremors and paralysis, in the arms especially, with delusional insanity.

ABSTRACT: This is a dry powder produced by extracting the active principles from a crude drug with strong alcohol, mixing with sugar of milk, and drying. Abstracts are standardized so as to be twice the strength of the crude drug.

ACACIA GUM, or GUM ACACIA, is a gummy exudation from various species of the acacia tree, which, dissolved in water to form mucilage, is used in coughs and sore throat and in states of irritation of the stomach and bowels.

ACANTHOSIS NIGRICANS, is a darkly pigmented verrucous skin change, usually around the neck and axilla. It may be inherited but is most commonly acquired and is associated with adenocarcinoma, usually of the stomach (see CANCER), and certain hormonal disorders such as the polycystic ovary (qv), Addison's disease (qv) and Cushing's syndrome (qv).

ACAPNIA means a condition of diminished carbon dioxide in the blood.

ACARUS: The group of animal parasites which includes *Sarcoptes scabiei*, the cause of the skin disease known as Itch, or Scabies. This parasite used to be known as *Acarus scabiei*. (See ITCH.)

ACCIDENT PREVENTION IN THE HOME: Over 800,000 accidents in the home requiring emergency treatment are estimated to occur each year in England and Wales. Such accidents in the home are most liable to occur in the young and the old.

In *children* the type of accident varies to a certain extent with age. Choking, and suffocation from food or secretions are the commonest causes of accidents in children under the age of 1 year. This is why there should be no pillow in a baby's cot or pram. When learning to walk there is a tendency to fall, and this may result in a serious accident if the fall is into a fire or a full bath. As inquisitiveness develops, accidents may occur from pulling a saucepan of hot food off the kitchen stove or from sampling medicines. Prevention of burns is of paramount importance. Under the Heating Appliances (Fireguard) Act 1954 all new gas and electric fires must be guarded, but there are still too many old-fashioned gas and electric fires in use without adequate guards. The fireguard mesh must be small enough to exclude little fingers, and the fireguard must be well away from the heated element. Modern paraffin heaters are self-extinguishing if tilted more than 45 degrees. It is now an offence to sell nightdresses made of readily ignited material. Cotton and rayon and the man-made fibres, Acrilan, Courtelle and Orlon, are easily set on fire. Nylon, Terylene and the heavier woollen fabrics are more resistant. The major fire-risk is the wide-skirted dress, apron and nightdress. Girls as well as boys should wear pyjamas. To prevent children poisoning themselves, all medicines, whether tablets or liquid, must be kept in locked medicine cupboards. A point to be remembered here is that the common practice of parents 'bribing' their children to take their medicine as a sweet may have unfortunate, if not fatal, consequences if the child finds the bottle and demolishes the contents on the ground that they are sweets. All paints, polishes, pesticides, petroleum products, turpentine, garden fertilizers, disinfectants and the like must be kept well out of reach. To avoid burning accidents in the kitchen crawling and toddling children should be firmly banned from the kitchen during cooking operations. Falls on stairs are the most dangerous. These should be avoided by having a gate at the top and bottom of the stairs. (See also POISONS.)

In *old age* falls are the major cause of accidents, and they are particularly dangerous at this age because of the ease with which the limbs are broken. Old bones tend to be fragile (see OSTEOPOROSIS), and a fall in old age that would cause no more than bruising in younger life may well result in a broken arm or leg. Prevention consists predominantly of a well-designed home. Stairs should be shallow, carpeted and have a handrail, or preferab two. There should be no polished floors worn-out mats. To prevent slipping, ma should have a rubber-backed underlay. The should be no steps leading down into a roor Lighting must be adequate with easily access ble switches. Central heating is essential f winter warmth. The bath should be shallo with a slip mat inside and outside, and the should be handles on each side for ease of ge ting in and out. To prevent burns, fireguar and fire-resistant clothes are just as essential in childhood, and smoking in bed should discouraged. The risk of poisoning can reduced by ensuring that all medicines a clearly labelled with instructions as to whe and in what dosage they are to be taken. those with failing memory self-administratic should be discouraged as the elderly individu may forget that he has already taken his pr scribed dose.

At all ages accidents may occur from electr shock due to faulty switches and wiring. Tin ering with electric installations is dangerous if not fatal; and many fires are due to faul wiring which has been allowed to age with t house – and the owner. In England in 1984, 2 people died by electric shock in home acc dents. In addition, 45 people died in fir involving electrical equipment. Wounds, to are common, whether caused by knives, ti openers or razors. These are seldom seriou but severe injuries may be caused by mechan cal or powered equipment such as washi machines and mixers in the kitchen or rota lawnmowers and hedgecutters in the garden

All accidents are preventable, it has bee said. This may be true in theory, but not practice. In practice, however, their numb could be radically reduced if first aid was compulsory item in the routine school curric lum. Pending such a move, everyone shou look upon an approved course of first aid essential. Full details of such courses can obtained from the British Red Cross Societ the St. John Ambulance Association, or the S Andrew's Ambulance Association. (See FIRS AID.)

ACCOMMODATION: The process by whic the refractive power of the lens is increased b constriction of the ciliary muscle, producing a increased thickness and curvature of the len Rays of light from an object further than metres away are parallel on reaching the ey These rays are brought to a focus on the retir mainly by the cornea. If the eye is now directe at an object closer than 6 metres away, the ra of light from this near object will be divergir by the time they reach the eye. In order to foc these diverging beams of light, the refractir power of the lens must increase. In other wor the lens must accommodate. This involves t circular part of the ciliary muscle contractin reducing tension in the zonular fibres. The te sion on the lens is thus reduced and, because is normally elastic, the lens assumes a mo rounded shape with more curved surfaces. In so doing, its focusing power (refractive power) is increased and light is focused on the retina once more. The stimulus for accommodation is a clear retinal image. The state of accommodation of the lens is constantly being adjusted to keep the retinal image clear.

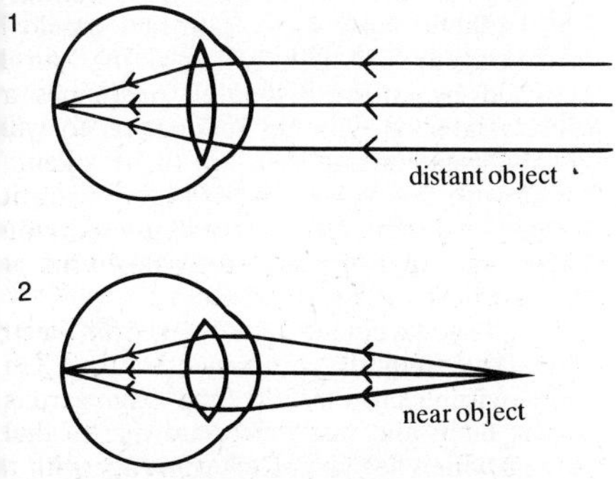

Diagram of eye in relaxed state (1) viewing a distant object and in an accommodated state; (2) with increased convexity of the lens for viewing a near object.

With age the lens loses its elasticity and thus becomes less spherical when tension in the zonule relaxes. This results in an increased long sightedness with age (*presbyopia*) and is manifest by the need for reading glasses in many people by middle age. (See AGE, NATURAL CHANGES IN).

ACCOUCHEUR is a physician who specializes in midwifery.

ACEBUTOLOL (SECTRAL) (see ADRENERGIC RECEPTORS).

ACETABULUM is the cup-shaped socket on the pelvis in which rests the head of the femur or thigh-bone, the two forming the hip joint. (See HIP JOINT.)

ACETAZOLAMIDE is a drug which acts by inhibiting the enzyme carbonic anhydrase. This enzyme is of great importance in the production of acid and alkaline secretions in the body. Acetazolamide has proved of value in the treatment of glaucoma. There is some evidence that it is of value in the prevention of mountain sickness (qv).

ACETIC ACID, also called pyroligneous acid, is prepared by the distillation of wood and subsequent separation from tar. It is also synthesized from acetylene. In the pure form it is solid, being then known as glacial acetic acid. It is the active principle of vinegar, which is prepared from wine by the action of a particular ferment discovered by Pasteur. This grows on the surface of the vine, taking from the air oxygen which it gives up to the alcohol of the wine, so producing acetic acid. Weak acetic acid has all the actions of vinegar, and is less expensive. Strong acetic acid is a caustic and irritant poison.
Uses: In strong solution acetic acid is used to destroy warts or raise blisters. In cases of excessive sweating the weak acid is of value, because, sponged over the skin, it checks perspiration and produces a sense of coolness.

ACETOHEXAMIDE (DIMELOR) is one of the oral hypoglycaemic drugs being used in the treatment of diabetes mellitus. It acts by increasing the output of insulin (see SULPHONYLUREAS).

ACETONE is a chemical substance found in the urine in conditions of starvation, in diabetes mellitus, in prolonged vomiting, and in acute fevers – especially in children. With it occur in the urine beta-hydroxybutyric and acetoacetic acids, particularly in severe cases of diabetes. A large quantity of these acids and of acetone in the urine in diabetes indicates approaching coma. (See also ACIDOSIS.)

ACETYLCHOLINE is one of the substances which mediates the transmission of nerve impulses from one nerve to another, or from a nerve to the organ it acts on such as muscles. Its predominant role is in the parasympathetic nervous system (qv), but it also plays an important part in the transmission of nerve impulses in the brain. Acetylcholine is rapidly destroyed by cholinesterase, an enzyme present in the blood.

ACETYLCYSTEINE is a drug that is used in the treatment of fibrocystic disease of the pancreas (qv) and paracetamol poisoning (qv).

ACETYLSALICYLIC ACID (see ASPIRIN).

ACHALASIA is another term for spasm, but indicates not so much an active spasm of muscle as a failure to relax.

ACHALASIA OF THE CARDIA is a condition in which there is a failure to relax of the muscle fibres round the opening of the gullet, or oesophagus, into the stomach. (See OESOPHAGUS, DISEASES OF.)

ACHEINIA: Absence of the hand.

ACHLORHYDRIA means an absence of hydrochloric acid from the stomach juice; it occurs in about 4 per cent of healthy people and in several conditions, including pernicious anaemia, carcinoma of the stomach and gastritis.

ACHONDROPLASIA is a form of dwarfing in which the arms and legs are abnormally short. It is a hereditary condition, and the commonest form of dwarfism. It affects both sexes and, whilst many are stillborn or die soon after birth, those who survive have a normal expectation of life and good health.

ACHYLIA GASTRICA means the complete absence of ferments and of hydrochloric acid from the gastric juice; in this condition the food is passed from the stomach in a state of incomplete digestion.

ACIDITY is a vague term, more used in popular language than in scientific medicine, and meaning that the reaction of the blood, or of one or more of the secretions, is less alkaline or more strongly acid than normal, while a considerable number of symptoms is rightly or wrongly attributed to the condition.

The blood in health is alkaline, and an elaborate chemical mechanism keeps the degree of alkalinity remarkably constant. This mechanism hinges largely round the relative amounts in the blood of carbonic acid (H_2CO_3) and sodium bicarbonate ($NaHCO_3$): $H_2CO_3/NaHCO_3$. By this and other mechanisms the acids formed in metabolism are neutralized and got rid of through the kidneys and the lungs. These acids are the fixed acids, such as lactic, sulphuric, phosphoric, and carbonic acid which are produced in large amounts daily as a result of tissue activity. The blood in disease never becomes actually acid, except in the terminal stages of life. But the blood may become *less alkaline*: the patient in this state is said to have acidaemia.

ACIDOSIS is a condition in which there is either (i) a production in the body of two abnormal acids – beta-hydroxybutyric and acetoacetic acids, or (ii) a diminution in the alkali reserve of the blood.

Causes: The condition is usually due to faulty metabolism of fat which results in the production of beta-hydroxybutyric and acetoacetic acids. It occurs in diabetes mellitus when this is either untreated or inadequately treated, starvation, persistent vomiting, and delayed anaesthetic vomiting. It also occurs in the terminal stages of Bright's disease when it is due to failure of the kidneys. A milder form of it may occur in severe fevers, particularly in children. (See also ACETONE.)

Symptoms: General lassitude, vomiting, thirst, restlessness, and the presence of acetone in the urine form the earliest manifestations of the condition. In diabetes a state of coma may ensue and the disease end fatally.

Treatment: The underlying condition must always be treated: eg. if the acidosis is due to diabetes mellitus insulin must be given. For the acidosis, alkalis should be given; eg. bicarbonate of soda, either by mouth, or by injection if there is persistent vomiting or if the patient is unconscious. Glucose should also be given, and adequate fluids.

ACIDS are substances which combine with alkalis to form salts. Most are oxygen compounds, have a sour taste, and turn blue litmus red. They are divided into (*a*) mineral or inorganic, and (*b*) vegetable or organic. In strong solution the mineral acids act upon stomach and bowels as irritant poisons, but small quantities in weak solution aid digestion, diminish the alkalinity of the blood, are excreted in the urine, the acidity of which they increase, act as mild astringents and refrigerants, and check excessive sweating. The action of the organic acids varies, but the best known, ie. acetic, citric, lactic, tartaric, while in strong solution acting like mineral acids, in weaker solution after absorption into the blood become decomposed into carbonates, and have precisely the opposite actions: ie. those of alkalis.

Varieties commonly used: (*a*) *Inorganic*: boracic, or boric, chromic, hydrochloric, hydrobromic, nitric, nitro-hydrochloric, phosphoric, sulphuric, sulphurous.

(*b*) *Organic*: acetic, carbolic, carbonic, citric, gallic, hydrocyanic or prussic, lactic, salicylic, tanic or tannin, tartaric.

Uses: The strong mineral acids, especially chromic and nitric, with pure acetic and carbolic from among the organic acids, are used as caustics to remove outgrowths such as corns, warts, piles, and also to destroy diseased tissue in poisoned wounds and spreading sores. In using them, care must be taken not to let the action extend too far and destroy healthy tissue; they are usually applied on a glass rod, and an alkali, oil, or glycerin should be at hand to apply in case a drop falls on the healthy surface.

The astringent action is utilized in excessive sweating. (See also ACETIC ACID.) When the urine is very alkaline there is a tendency to the formation of phosphatic calculi, and catarrh of the bladder is often present; these are relieved by acids among various other substances.

For the use of special acids see under ACETIC ACID; CARBOLIC ACID; SALICYLIC ACID, etc.

ACIDS, POISONING BY: Although most acids have an extremely sour and burning taste, which warns a person drinking one of his error before very much is swallowed, several are so much used in commercial processes, and so easily obtained, that accidental and intentional poisoning by acids is not uncommon.

Symptoms: The symptoms produced are destruction of the skin and mucous membrane about the mouth, great pain in the mouth, throat, and stomach, and sometimes fainting or collapse. There is also later a risk of scarring and contraction of the throat. These are especially the symptoms of poisoning by strong inorganic acids, or by citric, or tartaric in large quantities, while several, such as prussic and

carbolic, have symptoms peculiar to themselves and not due to irritation. For the treatment of poisoning by these last two see PRUSSIC ACID POISONING and CARBOLIC ACID POISONING.
Treatment: Give large quantities of water by mouth, and if possible add alkalis to it – such as cream of magnesia, bicarbonate of soda, or baking soda. If none of these is immediately available, plaster from the ceiling, or soapy water may be used. These neutralize the acid taken and form harmless salts, and also soothe the irritated mucous membrane. On no account must emetics be given. The patient must be treated for shock. Soothing or demulcent substances, such as milk in oil, or barley water, must also be given.

ACINUS is the name applied to each of the minute sacs of which secreting glands are composed, and which usually cluster round the branches of the gland-duct like grapes on their stem. (See GLANDS.)

ACNE, or ACNE VULGARIS, is a chronic skin disease which affects practically all adolescents. Fortunately, in the vast majority of these it is relatively insignificant and only in about 15 per cent of youngsters is it severe enough to require treatment. It usually begins around puberty, achieves its peak in the late teens, and disappears in the early twenties. By the age of 23, some 5 per cent of people have acne severe enough to need treatment, whilst by the age of 40 this figure is down to 1 per cent. There is a rare form of acne which occurs in baby boys, usually in a family with a strong history of acne. This usually disappears around the age of 5 years. Acne may be induced by certain drugs, including the corticosteroids, lithium, phenytoin, rifampicin, and the iodides and bromides. *Industrial acne* occurs in those exposed to vapours of chlorinated naphthalenes used in insulating cable and in those coming in contact with soluble cutting oils of high boiling points.
Causes: Three main factors are necessary for the development of acne: an increased production of sebum (qv); obstruction of the pilosebaceous, or sebaceous, ducts (see SKIN; and SEBACEOUS GLANDS); and the presence of micro-organisms. The activitiy of the sebaceous glands is controlled by testosterone, the male sex hormone, or androgen as it is known. This explains the onset of acne at puberty. In boys the androgen is produced predominantly in the testes as they develop to normal adult activity. In girls it comes predominantly from the adrenal glands. This increased production of sebum, the secretion of the sebaceous glands, is accompanied by blockage of the ducts through which it normally reaches the surface of the skin. It is this accumulation of sebum, which gradually becomes infected with skin micro-organisms, that leads to the formation of the small lumps, or comedones, the characteristic feature of acne. In girls acne tends to flare up in the week preceding menstruation. Sunlight, especially natural sunlight, has a favourable influence on the condition. In some, particularly males who participate in active sports, it tends to be worse on the back after sweating. Mechanical factors may also play a part. Thus acne of the forehead, is seen in tennis players who use head-bands to control their hair, whilst acne on the shoulders and back is not uncommonly seen in young women, due to the pressure of their brassières. The influence of diet is non-proven, though fats and sweets, especially chocolate, have been traditionally associated with it. Stress plays a part, and this has been attributed to acne subjects, especially girls, tending to pick their spots during times of strain and thereby exacerbate the condition.
Symptoms: The eruption occurs predominantly on the face, back and chest, the face usually being the most affected. These are the sites of the eruption because they are the areas most richly supplied with sebaceous glands. The eruption consists of little black spots (blackheads or comedones) which indicate the mouths of blocked sebaceous (or pilosebaceous) ducts, hard pimples generally showing one of these blackheads on the top, and little pustules surrounded by a red area of inflammation which gradually grow, burst and then heal. In more severe cases there may be hard lumps, 12 mm (half an inch) across, which last for weeks or longer, suppurate, and leave a permanent hardness or scar. The amount of scarring of the skin left after the condition has cleared up depends upon the severity of the eruption, but in the majority of cases it clears completely.
Treatment: In milder cases all that is needed is daily washing of the affected parts. Some recommend detergents instead of soap and water, to degrease the skin. Where it is associated with the pressure of a head-band or a brassière, the wearing of these should be given up. The most effective agents for local application are benzoyl peroxide (qv) and retinoic acid (qv) applied once daily. In some cases combining the two, retinoic acid in the morning and benzoyl peroxide in the evening, is more effective. In more severe cases a course of either tetracycline or erythromycin is given. The usual dose is 250 mg twice daily, but this may be increased under medical supervision, for resistant cases and maintained for several months. A course of sunlight therapy is often helpful. Natural sunlight is more efficacious than artificial sunlight, but a three-month course of the latter in hospital during the winter often helps. Those with acne should be discouraged from squeezing out comedones with their fingers or so-called comedone expressors. In those who are left with severe scarring a course of dermabrasion (qv) may remove these blemishes.

ACNE ROSACEA (see ROSACEA).

ACONITE (also known as Wolfsbane, or Blue rocket or Monkshood) is an extremely poisonous plant found in different species all over the

world, and largely grown for its appearance in gardens. All parts of the plant are poisonous. The root has been mistaken for horse-radish, although the resemblance, to those who know horse-radish by sight, is not very great. The root of the horse-radish is long, whitish outside, when scraped remains white, and has the well-known pungent odour. Aconite root is short and stumpy, brown, and when scraped the white cut surface speedily turns pinkish; if it is chewed, the tongue in a few minutes tingles, then becomes numb and swollen, and a burning sensation is felt in the mouth. The action of aconitine, its active principle, is produced by smaller doses than in the case of any other drug; accordingly aconite is a favourite homoeopathic remedy.
Uses: Aconite is seldom used at the present day, although in the form of a liniment it is sometimes used externally to relieve pain, sprains and rheumatism. Tincture of aconite, which is still kept in some households, should never be used without the sanction of a doctor.

ACONITE POISONING: This may occur, as stated above, by mistaking the root for horse-radish, by children eating parts of the plant, or by the administration of too large a dose.
Symptoms: There are characteristic symptoms in the mouth (see ACONITE) after chewing parts of the plant. If a large amount of the poison has been taken into the stomach, vomiting and purging follow after some time. Numbness is felt all over the body. The pulse becomes weak, the breathing laboured, and the face livid. Convulsions may come on, but consciousness is retained.
Treatment: Give plenty of warm water to drink. The poison must be got rid of at once, preferably by washing out the stomach with a solution of tannic acid (6 grams in 4·5 litres [1 gallon]). Alternatively, an emetic may be given, one of the handiest being a tablespoonful of mustard in a cupful of cold water; or, best of all, one or two tablespoonfuls of sal volatile in water, this being also a stimulant. Emetics, however, should not be given if the victim is in a state of collapse. Artificial respiration may be necessary.

ACRIFLAVINE is an aniline derivative. It is an orange-red crystalline powder, readily soluble in water, which gives a rich yellow colour to substances brought into contact with it, and in a solution of 1 in 1000 of water, possesses strong antiseptic powers.

ACROCYANOSIS is a condition, occurring especially in young women, in which there is persistent blueness of hands, feet, nose and ears.

ACRODYNIA (see ERYTHROEDEMA).

ACROMEGALY is a disorder caused by the increased secretion of growth hormone by an adenoma of the anterior pituitary gland. It results in excessive body growth of both the skeletal and the soft tissues. If it occurs in adolescence before the bony epiphyses have fused the result is gigantism. If it occurs in adult life the skeletal overgrowth is confined to the hands, feet, cranial sinuses and jaw. Most of the features are due to overgrowth of the cartilage of the nose and ear and the soft tissues which increase the thickness of the skin and lips. Viscera such as the thyroid and liver are also affected. The overgrowth of the soft tissues occurs so gradually that the patient and spouse are often unaware of the change. It is only relatives who have not seen the patient for many months or years who are aware of the striking change in physical appearance. The local effects of the tumour commonly cause headache and, less frequently, impairment of vision, particularly of the temporal field of vision, as a result of pressure on the nerves to the eye. The tumour may damage the other pituitary cells giving rise to gonadal, thyroid or adrenocortical insufficiency. The diagnosis is confirmed by measuring the level of growth hormone in the serum and by an X-ray of the skull which usually shows enlargement of the pituitary fossa. The treatment consists of removal or irradiation of the pituitary adenoma. This may have to be done via a craniotomy if the tumour is large but can often be done by an approach through the nose and sphenoid sinus. Deep X-ray therapy to the pituitary fossa is also effective treatment but it may take several years for irradiation to achieve its maximum effect. Drugs, such as bromocriptine, which are dopamine agonists, lower growth hormone levels in acromegaly and are particularly useful as an adjunct to radiotherapy.

ACROMION is the part of the scapula, or shoulder blade, forming the tip of the shoulder and giving its squareness to the latter. It projects forward from the scapula, and, with the clavicle or collar-bone in front, forms a protecting arch of bone over the shoulder joint.

ACROPARAESTHESIA is a disorder occurring predominantly in middle-aged women in which there is numbness and tingling of the fingers.

ACTH is the commonly used abbreviation for corticotrophin (qv).

ACTINOMYCIN D (Cosmegen, Lyovac) is an antibiotic isolated from *Streptomyces antibioticus* and *Streptomyces chrysomallus*; it has an inhibitory action on neoplastic cells (see CYTOTOXIC DRUGS).

ACTINOMYCOSIS is an acute or chronic suppurative disease affecting cattle in which it is known as Woody Tongue, and sometimes found in man.
Causes: The direct cause is the ray-fungus or actinomyces known as *Actinomyces israeli*,

which occurs as a commensal (qv) in the mouth. In certain circumstances still rather obscure, but one of which is undoubtedly trauma, such as a fractured jaw or extraction of a tooth, the *A. israeli* becomes active. It then causes hard swellings, abscesses and ulcers, in the pus of which the fungus is found in little yellow balls of a size which can just be made out by the naked eye. These little balls are found to consist of masses of thread-like material matted together, and of club-shaped bodies radiating from a common centre, hence the name of ray-fungus. It used to be thought that the human infection arose from the chewing of straw or grain, or was caught from cattle, but this is now known not to be the case. In over 50 per cent of cases the disease occurs in or about the mouth; in 20 per cent it occurs in the abdomen, and in 15 per cent in the thorax.

Symptoms: These are general bad health, the presence of hard fibrous masses about the mouth or tongue, or in other organs, and the development sooner or later in these masses of abscesses which after bursting form sinuses or ulcers that will not heal.

Treatment: The outlook has been changed completely since the introduction of the antibiotics. The best results are usually obtained with large doses of penicillin, but in some cases chlortetracycline is more effective. Surgical treatment may be required, as in the draining of abscesses.

ACTIVE PRINCIPLES are the portions of a drug which produce its effect, being administered for convenience, or of necessity, with the water, oils, vegetable fibre, etc., which make the bulk of the drug. They are of various chemical nature, but, in general, alkaloids. (See ALKALOIDS.)

ACUPUNCTURE is a traditional Chinese method of treatment by puncture of a part with needles. Its rationale is that disease is a manifestation of a disturbance of Yin and Yang energy in the body, and that acupuncture brings this energy back into balance by what is described as 'the judicious stimulation or depression of the flow of energy in the various meridians'. What is still not clear to the western mind is why needling, which is the essence of acupuncture, should have the effect it is claimed to have. One theory now being mooted is that the technique stimulates the production of pain-relieving endorphins (qv). Of its efficacy in skilled Chinese hands, however, there can be no question.

ACUTE GLOMERULONEPHRITIS (see GLOMERULONEPHRITIS).

ACYCLOVIR is an antiviral drug that is particularly useful in infections by herpes virus.

ADACTYLY: Absence of the digits.

ADDER-BITE (see BITES).

ADDICTS: The Misuse of Drug regulations 1973 require a medical practitioner to notify, in writing, the Chief Medical Officer of any person he considers or has reasonably grounds to suspect is addicted to any of the following substances:

Cocaine Methadone
Dextromoramide Morphine
Diamorphine Opium
Hydrocodone Pethidine
Hydromorphone Phenazocine
Levorphanol Piritramide.

The same regulations also provide that only medical practitioners who hold a special licence issued by the Home Secretary may prescribe diamorphine or cocaine for addicts. Other practitioners must refer any addict who requires these drugs to a treatment centre. All doctors may, however, still prescribe heroin and cocaine for patients, including addicts, for the relief of pain due to organic disease or injury. (See DRUG ADDICTION.)

ADDISONIAN ANAEMIA is another term for pernicious anaemia. (See ANAEMIA.)

ADDISON'S DISEASE: The cause of Addison's disease is a deficiency of the adrenocortical hormones cortisol, aldosterone and androgens due to destruction of the adrenal cortex. It occurs in about 1:25,000 of the population. Although the destruction of the adrenal cortex in Addison's original description was due to tuberculosis, a much more common cause today is auto-immune damage. Rare causes of Addison's disease include metastases from carcinoma, usually of the bronchus, granulomata and haemochromatosis.

Symptoms: The clinical symptoms depend on the severity of the underlying disease process. The patient usually complains of anorexia, nausea and loss of weight. The skin becomes pigmentated due to the increased production of ACTH (qv). Faintness, especially on standing, is due to postural hypotension secondary to aldosterone deficiency. Women lose their axillary hair and both sexes are liable to develop mental symptoms such as depression.

Diagnosis depends on demonstrating impaired serum levels of cortisol and inability of these levels to rise after an injection of ACTH.

Treatment consists in replacement of the deficient hormones and this enable patients to lead a completely normal life and to enjoy a normal life expectancy.

ADENINE ARABINOSIDE is an anti-viral agent that is proving of value in the treatment of certain forms of herpes. (See HERPES SIMPLEX; and EYE, DISEASES OF.)

ADENITIS means inflammation of a gland. (See LYMPHATICS.)

ADENO- is a prefix denoting relation to a gland or glands.

ADENOIDS (see NOSE, DISEASES OF).

ADENOMA means a benign tumour composed of glandular tissue. It may arise in any part of the body in which glandular tissue occurs: eg. the thyroid gland. It must be differentiated from an adenocarcinoma, which is a malignant tumour composed of glandular tissue. (See TUMOURS.)

ADENOVIRUSES are a group of viruses which cause infections of the upper respiratory tract resembling the common cold, and often referred to as febrile catarrh.

ADHESION: This means the uniting together of structures which should normally be separate and freely movable. It is the result of acute or chronic inflammation. The medium by which the attachment takes place may at first be fibrin (qv) as a result of acute inflammation, but later is, in every case, fibrous tissue either in masses or in bands.

Causes: The most important adhesions are those taking place in serous and joint cavities. When one of these structures becomes inflamed there is a great exudation of fluid into the cavity. From this fluid a solid material separates and becomes deposited upon the smooth surface of the cavity. This solid 'fibrin' should, in the course of recovery, be reabsorbed; but, if the inflammation is very severe, or if there is repeated attacks of it, this absorption does not completely take place, the two layers of fibrin on the opposing surfaces of the cavity stick together, and the united mass is 'organized' into the less absorbable fibrous tissue (see FIBROUS TISSUE). As a result there is restricted movement in the parts concerned; thus in the case of a joint there is ankylosis (see JOINT DISEASES); if the inflammation has been pleurisy the lung becomes adherent to the chest wall; if peritonitis, bands are formed between stomach, bowels, and other abdominal organs.

Symptoms: It is generally difficult to tell, except from the history of an inflammatory attack and from the presence of disordered function of internal organs, that adhesions are present (see PLEURISY; PERITONITIS). Sometimes adhesions between loops of bowels may be very serious and cause obstruction, if an old-standing and rigid fibrous band becomes twisted round a loop of bowel (see INTESTINE, DISEASES OF).

Treatment: While the adhesions are still *fibrinous* one expects complete absorption if the inflammation is speedily subdued. If the adhesions are *fibrous*, and show their presence by interference with the function of the organs concerned, one can seldom expect their complete absorption.

Sometimes, eg. when obstruction of the bowels is due to an adhesion, an immediate operation is necessary, and the adhesion is then divided. Adhesions causing limitation of movement in joints can often be broken down by means of manipulation.

ADHESIVE PLASTERS: These are made by spreading upon some supporting material, such as plain or elastic cloth or plastic film, some sticky substance containing drugs of various sorts. The sticky material consists of a mixture of cohesive and adhesive agents, plasticisers and fillers. The cohesive agents include Para rubber, pale crêpe rubber and smoked sheet rubber, polyisobutylene or other synthetic higher polymers with similar properties. The adhesive agents include various resins such as colophony and its derivatives.

Uses: Plasters are generally useful on account of their power of gripping a part and exerting steady pressure on it. They are sometimes used to obtain the absorbent effect of steady pressure combined with warmth and moisture in the treatment of chronic callous ulcers (see ULCERS). In this case the plaster is put on in strips, each of which overlaps the last, and has no holes; it must be changed every few days if it covers an unclean ulcer. Belladonna plaster is used for soothing pain. To support a sprained joint, eg. the ankle, a plaster is often applied in overlapping strips passing round the leg and instep. Plasters of felt are employed to protect corns, bunions, and small sores from abrasion; and 'corn plasters', containing salicylic acid in various strengths, are used to soften and remove corns. (See BLISTERS.)

Mode of application: Most plasters with a rubber basis stick by simply laying the plaster with the adhesive side next to the skin, but some must be warmed. If the plaster is wide, or the surface to be covered is rounded, it is necessary to cut deep notches into the plaster before heating and the edges so formed are allowed to overlap or separate. Plaster strips used to support the ankle or leg should be applied like a bandage (qv).

ADIPOCERE (see PUTREFACTION).

ADIPOSE TISSUE or FAT is a loose variety of fibrous tissue, in the meshes of which lie cells, each of which is distended by several small drops, or one large drop, of fat. This tissue replaces fibrous tissue when the amount of food taken is in excess of the bodily requirements. (See DIET; CORPULENCE.)

ADIPOSIS DOLOROSA, also known as Dercum's disease, is a condition in which painful masses of fat develop under the skin. It is commoner in women than in men.

ADOPTION (see CHILD ADOPTION).

ADRENAL GLANDS (see SUPRARENAL GLANDS).

ADRENALINE is the secretion of the adrenal medulla. (See SUPRARENAL GLANDS.) In the United States Pharmocopoeia it is known as epinephrine. It is also prepared synthetically. When injected it produces the same effect as stimulation of the sympathetic nervous system (qv). Among its important effects are raising of the blood pressure, increasing the amount of glucose in the blood, and constricting the smaller blood-vessels.

It is applied directly to wounds on gauze or lint to check haemorrhage. Injected along with some local anaesthetic it permits painless, bloodless operations to be performed on the eye, nose, etc. It is injected hypodermically to relieve asthma, and to stimulate the heart in collapsed conditions. It is also injected as an antidote in the condition of hypoglycaemia, when too large a dose of insulin has been given.

ADRENERGIC RECEPTORS are the sites in the body on which adrenaline (qv) and comparable stimulants of the sympathetic system (qv) act. Drugs which have an adrenaline-like action are described as being adrenergic. It is now known that there are four different types of adrenergic receptors, known as $alpha_1$, $alpha_2$, $beta_1$, and $beta_2$, respectively. Stimulation of alpha receptors leads to constriction of the bronchi, constriction of the blood vessels with consequent rise in blood-pressure, and dilatation of the pupils of the eyes. Stimulation of $beta_1$ receptors leads to a rise in heart rate and output of the heart, whilst stimulation of $beta_2$ receptors leads to dilatation of the bronchi. The practical implications of this complicated set-up were soon seized upon, particularly from the point of view of discovering useful new drugs.

For long it had been realized that in certain cases of asthma adrenaline had not the usual beneficial effect of dilating the bronchi during an attack; rather it made the asthma worse. This, it was found, was due to its acting on both the alpha and beta adrenergic receptors. A derivative, isoprenaline, was therefore produced which acted only on the beta receptors. This had an excellent effect in dilating the bronchi, but unfortunately also affected the heart, speeding it up and increasing its output –an undesirable effect which meant that isoprenaline, still a valuable drug in the treatment of asthma, has to be used with great care. In due course drugs were produced, such as salbutamol, which act predominantly on the $beta_2$ adrenergic receptors in the bronchi and have relatively little effect on the heart.

The converse of this side of the story was the search for what became known as beta-adrenoceptor-blocking drugs, or beta-adrenergic-blocking drugs. The theoretical argument was that if such drugs could be synthesized, they could be of value in taking the strain off the heart – for example: stress→stimulation of the output of adrenaline→stimulation of the heart→increased work for the heart. A drug that could prevent this train of events would obviously be of value, for example, in the treatment of angina pectoris (qv). And so it proved, and today there is a series of beta-adrenergic-blocking drugs which are subserving a most useful purpose, not only in angina pectoris, but also in various other heart conditions such as disorders of rhythm, as well as high blood-pressure. They are also proving of value in the treatment of anxiety states by preventing disturbing features such as palpitations. An unexpected dividend is that some of them at least appear to be of help in the treatment of migraine.

The first beta-blocker in therapeutic use and probably still the best known is propranolol. Many other beta-blockers are now available and in general they are all equally effective. There are, however, minor differences which may effect the choice in treating an individual patient. Some drugs have intrinsic sympathomimetic activity, which is a manifestation of the ability of these drugs to stimulate as well as to block adrenergic receptors. Oxprenolol, pindolol and acebutolol are members of this group possessing intrinsic sympathomimetic activity and they therefore tend to cause less slowing of the pulse and less coldness of the extremities than the other beta-blockers. Some beta-blockers are lipid soluble and as a result pass the blood brain barrier with ease. They may therefore cause central effects such as sleep disturbances and nightmares. Water-soluble beta-blockers tend not to cross the blood brain barrier and are less likely to have these side effects. Examples of the water soluble beta-blockers are atenolol, nadolol and sotalol. Being water soluble they are excreted by the kidneys and may therefore accumulate in patients with renal impairment.

Some beta-blockers tend to have less effect on the $beta_2$ or bronchial receptors and are therefore called cardio-selective. This is not completely true as if given in larger doses $beta_2$ effects will also occur. Nevertheless metoprolol, atenolol and acebutolol are relatively cardio-selective and have less effect on airways resistance. Despite this, the precaution of avoiding beta-blockers in patients with obstructive airways disease also applies to the so-called selective drugs. Nevertheless the beta-adrenoceptor blocking drugs are most useful in the treatment of hypertension, angina pectoris, secondary prevention of myocardial infarction, migraine, anxiety states, essential tremor, thyrotoxicosis and glaucoma when used topically.

The beta-blockers available at present include:

- acebutolol (Sectral)
- atenolol (Tenormin)
- betaxolol (Kerlone)
- metoprolol (Betaloc, Lopressor)
- nadolol (Corgard)
- oxprenolol (Apsolox, Laracor, Trasicor)
- pindolol (Visken)
- propranolo (Angilol, Apsolol, Bedranol, Berkolol, Inderal, Sloprolol)
- sotalol (Beta-Cardone, Sotacor)
- timolol (Betim, Blocadren)

Labetalol (Trandate) is both an alpha and a beta adreno receptor blocking drug.

ADULTERATION OF FOOD The incidence of adulteration of food has decreased considerably during the last century. The procedure for the inspection of food is laid down in the Food and Drugs Act, 1955, which empowers local authorities to appoint public analysts. A 'sampling officer' is an authorized officer of the local authority, and he may purchase any sample of food (or drug) and submit it for analysis to the local public analyst. In making such a purchase for analysis the following procedure must be followed, otherwise it will not be possible to obtain a conviction of the seller. After the purchase has been completed the purchaser must immediately inform the vendor that he proposes to have the sample analysed. The article must then be divided into three portions and each portion must be separately packed and sealed. One portion is then handed to the vendor, one is sent to the public analyst, and the third is retained by the purchaser.

Examples of adulteration: MILK which contains less than 3 per cent of fat or 8·5 per cent of milk solids other than fat is presumed to be adulterated. The addition of the following to milk is prohibited by law: colouring matter, water, dried or condensed milk or any fluid constituted therefrom, skimmed or separated milk, preservatives of any kind, any thickening substance (except cane or beet sugar to cream). The most common forms of adulteration of milk are the addition of water or the removal of fat. The most satisfactory method of deciding whether or not adulteration with water has taken place is the freezing point method. Milk which freezes above −0·53 °C can be considered to be adulterated. Even more important is the problem of milk-borne disease. (See MILK.)

BUTTER: No preservative may be added to butter and not more than 16 per cent of moisture is permitted by the legal standard. The two most common forms of adulteration of butter are the addition of other fats, eg. cotton-seed oil, and excessive amounts of water.

MARGARINE must not contain more than 16 per cent of moisture or 10 per cent of butter fat. It must be reinforced with 760 to 940 international units of vitamin A and 80 to 100 international units of vitamin D per ounce.

BREAD is usually fairly pure. (See BREAD).

FLOUR: All flour intended for human consumption must contain not less than 1·6 mg of iron, 0·24 mg of vitamin B, and 1·60 mg of nicotinic acid or nicotinamide per 100 grams, and, except in the case of flour containing the whole of the products derived from the milling of wheat, 235 to 390 mg of powdered chalk per 100 grams. If wheat flour should be adulterated with flour of other grains, eg. barley, maize, rye, these can be easily recognized under the microscope.

BAKING POWDERS consist of an acid salt, such as cream of tartar in acid calcium phosphate, and bicarbonate of soda and starch. They act by virtue of the carbon dioxide they evolve in the presence of moisture. They must yield at least 8 per cent of available carbon dioxide and not more than 1·5 per cent of residual carbon dioxide. Neither must they contain more than 15 parts per million fluorine. If carelessly prepared, the acid salt may contain an excess of arsenic. They may also contain alum.

EGG-SUBSTITUTE POWDERS, to give them their correct designation, are virtually baking powders coloured yellow with turmeric or coal-tar dye. Lead chromate has occasionally been found in them.

CUSTARD POWDERS usually consist of coloured and flavoured maize starch, but they have been known to contain sago, rice or potato.

COCOA: There is no standard for cocoa in Great Britain. As sold it usually contains cornflour (or some similar material) and sugar. This is done because pure cocoa is rather indigestible on account of its high fat content.

COFFEE, unless bought as beans, is liable to contain chicory. Chicory can be recognized by the fact that in water it sinks and colours the water brown, whereas coffee floats in the water and scarcely stains it. They can also be differentiated under the microscope.

TEA: Because of the careful examination to which it is submitted by Customs officers, tea is seldom adulterated now as it used to be in the old days with exhausted leaves, leaves from other sources or from green tea 'laced' with indigo or Prussian blue. Cheap tea may still contain a high proportion of tea dust. Unadulterated tea should contain 1·5 to 5 per cent of theine, the alkaloid to which it owes its stimulating action.

SUGAR is usually pure. Sometimes flour may be mixed with it, but this can easily be detected by the presence of sediment when the sugar dissolves. Brown sugar is less highly refined cane sugar containing traces of colouring matter. Demerara sugar, strictly speaking, is a type of cane sugar, which is yellowish-brown in colour, originally obtained from the region of Guyana known as Demerara. Ordinary cane sugar may be adulterated with a synthetic brown dye to simulate brown or demerara sugar.

CHOCOLATES AND SWEETS: Chocolate should contain not less than 10 per cent of ground cocoa nib or 5 per cent of essence of cocoa, to which are added cocoa fat, starch, sugar and milk. Inferior chocolate (usually imported) contains only 2 to 3 per cent of ground cocoa nib; when exposed to a strong light it appears to have a greyish or bluish-grey bloom. Ultra-violet light and X-rays can be used to reveal chemical impurities. Inferior boiled sweets may be contaminated with minute traces of arsenic due to the use of impure glucose instead of sugar.

HONEY may be adulterated with cane sugar or glucose.

JAMS AND MARMALADE are seldom adulterated at the present day. The unofficial standards for jams adopted by the manufacturers are that 'full fruit standard' contains 30 to 45 per cent of fruit, whilst 'lower fruit standard' contains 20 per cent of fruit.

MEAT cannot readily be adulterated except by the sale of unsound or diseased meat. Horseflesh can be distinguished by the fact that it is dark and coarse, has a sickly odour and a soapy feel, and the fat is yellow. As horseflesh contains more glycogen (qv) than oxflesh, the addition of a few drops of a solution of iodine or potassium iodide to a decoction of the flesh will produce a violet coloration.

ARROWROOT may be adulterated with potato starch, rice or wheat flour.

CINNAMON and other similar spices are adulterated with flour and may contain sand.

GROUND GINGER may contain pepper.

PEPPER often contains 1·5 to 3 per cent of sand and grit. This is an example of unavoidable adulteration.

PICKLES, SAUCES AND CHUTNEY often consist principally of vinegar thickened with curry powder, pea-flour and caramel.

MUSTARD is sold mixed with cornflour to keep the mustard grains separate; otherwise it would go solid.

VINEGAR should contain no other acid except acetic acid, no lead or copper and no colouring matter. It has been decided in the courts that non-brewed vinegar containing less than 4 per cent acetic acid is 'not of the nature, substance or quality demanded'. Artificial vinegar is made by diluting acetic acid and it may be coloured with caramel. Sulphuric acid has been used as an adulterant. No preservative may be added to vinegar. It is illegal to describe 'synthetic' or 'artificial' vinegar as 'vinegar'. (See ACETIC ACID.)

ALCOHOLIC BEVERAGES: Whisky may be diluted with water legally; it must not be more than 35 degrees under proof. Some low-grade whiskies may contain potato spirit. Brandy is made from fermented grape juice but inferior brands are made from potato spirit, coloured with burnt sugar and flavoured with various agents, or a little real brandy. Beer may contain arsenic if chemically prepared glucose is used in its manufacture. It may also contain an excessive amount of common salt or excessive preservative: the amount of preservative is limited by Regulations to 70 parts of sulphur dioxide per million. Wines should be made from fermented juice of the grape. Calcium sulphate is sometimes added to wine to increase its dryness and improve its keeping properties: this is known as 'plastering'. If excess is added, this may lead to the formation of sufficient potassium sulphate to produce a purgative effect. To avoid this, not more than 2 grams of calcium sulphate is permitted per litre in France. Artificial colouring matter, especially logwood, may be added to wine. The only preservative allowed in wine is sulphur dioxide, not exceeding 450 parts per million. There is relatively little tampering with foreign wines in Britain, but fraudulent imitations are sometimes sold under the title of 'British wines': eg. water coloured with cochineal, flavoured with essences and thickened with sugar. Cider, because of its acidity, may become contaminated with lead. (See ALCOHOL.)

Preservatives in food: Preservatives such as boric acid, borax, formaldehyde, benzoic acid and sulphur dioxide used to be added often to foodstuffs. Their indiscriminate use led to much trouble and their use is now forbidden by Regulations, with the exception of sulphur dioxide and benzoic acid in specified amounts in specified foods, and sodium or potassium nitrite in ham, bacon and cooked pickled meat. In the case of cooked pickled meat not more than 200 parts per million may be added. Under these Regulations the term 'preservative' does not include salt, saltpetre, sugar, glycerin, alcohol, vinegar, acetic acid or spices. Up to 70 parts of sulphur dioxide or 120 parts of benzoic acid may be added to sweetened mineral waters, but cordials and fruit juices can contain only up to 350 parts of sulphur dioxide or 800 parts of benzoic acid per million parts. Alcoholic wines are not allowed to contain more than 450 parts of sulphur dioxide per million; for beer the upper limit is 70 parts per million, whilst for cider it is 200 parts per million. Sulphur dioxide is also being used in jams and marmalade, the limit being 100 parts per million. Pickles, sauces and chutney may not contain more than 250 parts of benzoic acid per million. Sausages may have sulphur dioxide added as a preservative (450 parts per million).

Food additives: In addition to preservatives other additives to food are used by the manufacturers. These are antioxidants which stop fats and oils from going rancid and destroying vitamins. Two of the most widely used are butylated hydroxyanisole and butylated hydroxytoluene. Emulsifiers and stabilizers are also used to mix foods or prevent them from separating. They are particularly useful in making low-fat table spreads. Examples include locust-bean gum made from carob beans or gum arabic. Emulsifiers are usually natural substances. Flavour enhancers are also used and the best known of these is monosodium glutamate. It is made from sugar-beet or wheat. Additives are also used to make food more colourful. There are 58 permitted colours. The commonest is caramel. Other colouring agents include curcumin which is a yellow extract of turmeric roots. Betacarrotin is also used and this is extracted from carrots. There are also 20 permitted artificial colours, the most commonly used being tartrazine.

The Food Acts make it illegal to put anything into food that will harm health. Government departments have the job of deciding what can safely be put into foods and the manufacturers are required to undertake extensive research before additives are acceptable. Ingredients in food must be listed on labels. Of the permitted additives 280 have been given a number. When an additive has been approved by the European Community it has an E in front of it. From 1 July 1986 it is a legal requirement that additives must be listed in type and chemical name or number in the ingredients' list. The steering group on food surveillance is an advisory committee of the Ministry of Agriculture, Fisheries and Food. It is responsible for monitoring the safety and quality of the national food supply. It does this by reviewing the intakes of individual additives and nutrients and the possibilities of contamination. As a result of the reviews it conducts it recommends to ministers responsible for food quality and safety any measures necessary to ensure that the food intake of the population is both safe and nutritious. The work of the steering group on food surveillance is published in food surveillance papers. These reports are available through HMSO and cost only a few pounds.

ADVERSE REACTIONS TO DRUGS: There are a number of ways in which post-marketing studies permit the detection of adverse drug reactions. In the past techniques such as invididual case reports, the Committee on the Safety of Medicines' yellow card system, monitoring national mortality statistics and case control studies have successfully identified adverse drug reactions. The most useful method, when it is feasible, is the Cohort investigation. This requires that a cohort of patients starting treatment with a particular drug should be identified and the cohort should be sufficiently large to allow rarer adverse reactions to be detected. The system must look at adverse events and not merely suspected adverse reactions suffered by patients from the time of starting treatment to the end of the enquiry.

AEDES AEGYPTI is the scientific name of the mosquito which conveys to man (by biting) the viruses of yellow fever and of dengue or 'breakbone fever'. (See DENGUE; and YELLOW FEVER.)

AEGOPHONY is the bleating or punchinello tone given to the voice as heard by auscultation, when there is a small amount of fluid in the pleural cavity.

AERODONTALGIA is the relatively rare form of dental pain occasionally felt in restored or non-vital teeth by those who fly. It is thought that it is caused by expansion of gas entrapped in the pulp canal of the tooth, resulting from the change in altitude.

AEROPHAGY means air-swallowing, and is the name applied to a habit which some persons, especially when suffering from dyspepsia, contract of swallowing mouthfuls of air. This at first gives relief to the discomfort and pain of indigestion, but later prolongs and aggravates it. The resulting breathlessness can be relieved to some extent by taking peppermint water or chloroform water in doses of a tablespoonful, but the chief necessity is to overcome the habit of swallowing air.

AEROSOL: The pressurised aerosol provides an effective and convenient way of applying drugs directly to the bronchi, thus reducing the risks of unwanted effects accompanying systemic therapy. They are of particular use in asthma. Broncho-dilator aerosols contain either a beta-sympathomimetic agent or ipratropium bromide which is an anticholinergic drug. Of the beta-adrenoceptor agonists isoprenaline was the first compound to be widely used as an aerosol. It did however stimulate beta$_1$ receptors in the heart as well as beta$_2$ receptors in the bronchi and so produced palpitations and even dangerous cardiac arrhythmias. Newer beta-adrenoceptor agonists are specific for the beta$_2$ receptors and thus have a greater safety margin. They include salbutamol (Ventolin) terbutaline (Bricanyl), rimiterol (Pulmadil), fenoterol (Berotec) and reproterol (Bronchodil). Unwanted effects such as palpitations, tremor and restlessness are uncommon with these more specific preparations. In patients who get insufficient relief from the beta-adrenoreceptor agonist the drug ipratropium bromide (Atrovent) is worth adding.

Patients must be taught carefully and observed while using their inhalers. It is important that patients should realise that if the aerosol no longer gives more than slight intransient relief they should not increase the dose but seek medical help. A bronchodilator aerosol can be used regularly three to four times a day for asthma prophylaxis as well as for treatment of an acute attack. Some individuals find it difficult to co-ordinate breathing and activation of the aerosol and this is particularly true of the old, the very young and those with weakness of the hands. Alternative devices such as the Ventolin Rotahaler and the Bricanyl (terbutaline) Spacer are frequently found easier to use.

AESTHESIOMETER is an instrument for measuring the sensation of touch in a person.

AETIOLOGY is the part of medical science dealing with the causes of disease.

AFFUSION is a method of treatment by pouring water upon the body. (See BATHS; DOUCHES.)

AFIBRINOGENAEMIA is a condition in which the blood is incoagulable as a result of absence of fibrin (qv). It is characterized by haemorrhage. There are two forms: (*a*) a congenital form, and (*b*) an acquired form. The latter may be associated with advanced liver disease, or may occur as a complication of labour. Treatment consists of the intravenous injection of fibrinogen and blood transfusion.

AFTERBIRTH, or PLACENTA, is the name given to the thick, spongy disc-like cake of tissue which connects the embryo with the inner surface of the womb, the embryo otherwise lying free in the amniotic fluid. (See AMNION.) The placenta is mainly a new structure growing with the embryo, but, when it separates, a portion of the inner surface of the womb, called the maternal placenta, comes away with it. It is mainly composed of loops of veins belonging to the embryo, lying in blood-sinuses, in which circulates maternal blood. Thus, though no mixing of the blood of embryo and mother takes place, there is ample opportunity for the exchange of fluids, gases, and the nutriment brought by the mother's blood. The width of the full-sized placenta is about 20 cm (eight inches), its thickness 2·5 cm (one inch). One surface is rough and studded with villi, which consist of the loops of foetal veins; the other is smooth, and has implanted in its centre the umbilical cord, or navel string, which is about as thick as a finger and 50 cm (20 inches) long. The longest recorded was 160 cm (63 inches) in length, and the shortest less than 1 cm. It contains two arteries and a vein, enters the foetus at the navel, and forms the sole connection between the bodies of mother and foetus. The name 'afterbirth' is given to the structure because it is expelled from the womb in the third stage of labour (see LABOUR).

AFTERPAINS are pains similar to but feebler than those of labour, occurring in the two or three days following childbirth.
Causes are generally the presence of a blood-clot or retained piece of placenta which the womb is attempting to expel.

AGAMMAGLOBULINAEMIA is a condition found in children, in which there is no gamma-globulin (qv) in the blood. These children are particularly susceptible to infections as they are unable to form antibodies to any infecting micro-organism.

AGAR, or AGAR-AGAR, is a gelatinous substance prepared from seaweed. It is used in preparing culture-media for use in bacteriological laboratories. It is sometimes given for relieving constipation.

AGE, NATURAL CHANGES IN: As age advances, the tissues become more rigid and less elastic. The bones become more brittle. The ligaments are stiffer, so that contortions of the body and limbs become impossible. Fat is deposited beneath the skin in middle life with accompanying increase in weight. It may be absorbed again in old age, leaving the skin wrinkled. Deposition of fat also occurs in internal organs, eg. the heart, weakening their activity. The skin becomes thin, is less well lubricated, and its vessels do not react properly to heat and cold, so that cold is more acutely felt. The chief change is in the blood-vessels, the walls of which become first thicker, then more brittle. This means that obstruction (eg. in the coronary arteries that supply the heart muscle with blood) or haemorrhage (eg. into the brain, with apoplexy) more readily occurs. This change is hastened by alcoholic excesses and some diseases, and the extent to which it has occurred is the measure of the interference with the employments of active life. This thickening of the arteries in the brain and consequent narrowing of their calibre, causing a poorer blood-supply to the brain is one of the chief reasons of mental feebleness in old age. The menopause occurs in women between forty-five and fifty (see MENSTRUATION), and men sometimes about the age of sixty have some months' illness and feebleness, after which strength again returns. Sexual activity tends to diminish but seldom becomes dormant. Loss of elasticity in the lens of the eye brings about the need of spectacles for reading from forty upwards. Another eye change occurs after fifty in the appearance of a whitish ring (arcus senilis) round the cornea, near its edge: this is of no significance. Of more importance is the opacification of the lens known as cataract (qv) which tends to occur after fifty and may so interfere with sight that the lens has to be removed. After sixty the teeth, if still good, may begin to fall out and the hair whitens. (See also CLIMACTERIC; and EXPECTATION OF LIFE.)

AGENE is nitrogen trichloride and was used for many years as a flour improver and bleacher. As a result of experiments that showed that agene produced hysteria in dogs and some other animals, the British and US governments prohibited the use of agene as a flour improver, substituting chlorine dioxide as an alternative.

AGENESIA, or AGENESIS, means incomplete development or the failure of any part or organ of the body to develop normally.

AGGLUTINATION is the adherence together of small bodies in a fluid. Thus, blood corpuscles agglutinate into heaps (rouleaux) when added to the serum of a person belonging to an incompatible blood-group. Bacteria agglutinate into clumps and die when exposed to the presence of antibodies in the blood. This is important in regard to diagnosis of certain diseases due to bacteria. In typhoid fever, for example, the blood of an animal is immunized against typhoid bacilli by repeated injections of these. The blood-serum of the animal, known now as anti-typhoid serum, is issued to laboratories for use when bacilli are found in the excretions of a patient who is possibly suffering from typhoid fever. The bacilli are exposed to the action of a drop of the serum; if the serum shows the power of agglutinating these bacteria, this forms evidence that the bacteria in question are typhoid bacilli. The reaction may also be carried out in the contrary manner: that is to say, the serum from the blood of a patient, who may be suffering from typhoid fever, but in regard to whom the diagnosis is still a matter of doubt, is added to a drop of fluid containing bacteria known to be typhoid bacilli; if these are agglutinated into clumps by the patient's serum, the patient is then known to be suffering from typhoid fever; if they do not agglutinate, his symptoms are due to some other condition.

This reaction for typhoid fever is known as the Widal reaction. Comparable agglutination reactions, using an appropriate serum, are used in the diagnosis of a number of diseases, including glandular fever (when it is known as the Paul-Bunnell reaction), typhus fever (when it is known as the Weil-Felix reaction), undulant fever, and Weil's disease.

AGNOSIA is the condition in which, in certain diseases of the brain, the patient loses the ability to recognize the character of objects through the senses – touch, taste, sight, hearing.

AGORAPHOBIA means a sense of fear experienced in large open spaces and public places, and is a symptom of psychological disorder (see MENTAL ILLNESS). There are said to be 300,000 victims of it in the United Kingdom. Those who suffer from what can be a most distressing condition can obtain help and advice from the Phobics Society, 4 Cheltenham Road, Chorlton cum Hardy, Manchester M21 1QN. (Tel: 061-881 1937.)

AGRANULOCYTOSIS is a condition in which the white corpuscles in the blood of the polynuclear or granular variety become greatly lessened in numbers or disappear altogether. It is usually caused by taking such drugs as amidopyrine, thiourea, sulphonamides, chloramphenicol and the immuno-suppressant drugs.

AGRAPHIA is the loss of power to express ideas by writing. (See APHASIA.)

AGUE (see MALARIA). The term is also sometimes applied to neuralgia (brow ague) and to a state of tremor of the muscles found in various diseases (such as brass founders' ague).

AIDS, or ACQUIRED IMMUNE DEFICIENCY SYNDROME is an incurable disease with a serious prognosis. It is still a rare disease. Only 7981 cases have been reported from the United States of America up to January 1985 and 118 in Britain. The disease is still largely confined to homosexuals, intravenous drug abusers, people from the Caribbean and Central Africa, and haemophiliacs. It is due to an infection with the Human Immunodeficiency virus (HIV). It presents with fatigue, weight loss, fever, diarrhoea and oral candidiasis. However infection results in the full-blown syndrome of AIDS in only a minority of cases. There is no one pathognomonic test for AIDS but the diagnosis can be confirmed by identifying the antibodies to the lymphotrophic virus in the blood. The antibody can be detected in a considerable portion of patients at risk but who do not have any disease. AIDS is transmitted by sexual contact, through parenteral transmission, and by infected blood and plasma products. There are no grounds to suggest that transmission occurs through casual contact and AIDS would seem to be appreciably less infectious than hepatitis B. It is not known how many carriers go on to develop the disease because there seems to be a time lapse of up to five years between documented infection and the onset of symptoms. All the predictions are that the number of cases of AIDS will continue to rise sharply.

The risk of infection as a result of a blood transfusion is extremely low. Infection has occurred in haemophiliacs as a result of treatment with Factor 8 and Factor 9. However, heat-treated Factor 8 is now available and in use and is likely to eliminate the risk of transmission.

Although patients may present with vague symptoms such as lethargy, weight loss and night sweats, the commonest presentation (60 per cent) is a rare type of pneumonia due to pneumocystis carinii; Kaposi's sarcoma accounts for 25 per cent of presentations. Pneumocystis carinii pneumonia is characterised by a persistent non-productive cough, shortness of breath on exercise and fever of several weeks duration. The disease has a slow onset but deterioration is commonly rapid after presentation unless treatment is given. Kaposi's sarcoma manifests itself as a localised red or purple flat or raised lesion anywhere on the skin and may mimic a bruise.

The presence of antibodies to the virus is widespread in certain groups at risk, such as homosexuals with multiple partners and in haemophiliacs.

All blood donors in the United Kingdom are now screened for the presence of the antibody and donors with positive antibodies are removed from the panel. The DHSS has suggested that sexually transmitted disease clinics provide advice and a test where necessary and that facilities for other groups such as organ donors, semen donors and haemophiliacs are provided by District Health Authorities. An important problem now arising is what should be done for and what advice given to the asymptomatic individual who is found to be positive for the virus. There are, after all, for every known case of AIDS fifty to one hundred individuals infected with AIDS virus. Several things are certain: the individual with antibodies is infected by HIV; he or she is almost certainly infectious; over the next two years there is a 10 per cent chance of ill health developing but falling short of the full AIDS syndrome; over five years the figure rises to 25 per cent. The individual continues to be at risk for an unknown period.

When the initial infection with the virus occurs and antibodies to HIV develop, there may be clinical manifestations of a glandular-fever-like illness. There may also be evidence of encephalitis, meningitis or myelitis. It must be remembered that many other conditions cause a glandular-fever-like illness and just a few examples include cytomegalo virus infection, herpes simplex infection and rubella as well as toxoplasmosis.

The profound immune suppression characteristic of AIDS was originally thought to develop soon after the infection. At a recent onference on AIDS in Stockholm (1988) prospective studies showed that the rate of progression from infection to AIDS is slow. In homosexual men it takes an average of 8–10 ears and overall 75–90 per cent of those infected with the virus will develop AIDS. Similar results have been reported in haemophiliacs and subjects infected by transfusion of blood products.

ear	Total
984	77 (73)
985	160 (126)
986	305 (216)
987	653 (283)

JK reports of annual incidence of AIDS cases and umbers known to have died (in brackets)

ransmission category	Male	Female	Total
Iomosexual/bisexual male	1199	—	1199
ntravenous drug abuser (IVDA)	18	6	24
Iomosexual/bisexual male and IVDA	24	—	24
Iaemophiliac	83	1	84
Blood/components recipient: abroad	10	8	18
Ieterosexual:			
presumed infected abroad	27	12	39
presumed infected UK	3	6	9
Child of at-risk/infected parent	5	8	13
Other/undetermined	8	2	10
Totals	1384	45	1429

Cumulative totals of UK reports of AIDS cases, by ransmission category, to 31 March 1988

AIR: The general constituents of air are:

	per cent
Oxygen	20.94
Nitrogen	78.09
Argon	0.94
Carbonic acid	0.03

Besides these there are always ozone, minerals and organic matter in small and variable amounts, and more or less water vapour according to the weather. In the air of towns, sulphurous acid and sulphuretted hydrogen are important impurities derived from combustion. After air has been respired once, the oxygen falls by about 4 per cent and the carbonic acid rises to about 4 per cent, while organic matter and water vapour are greatly increased and the air rises in temperature. The cause of the discomfort felt in badly ventilated rooms and crowded halls is associated with the increase in the temperature and moisture of the air, but a high percentage of carbonic acid may be present without causing any noticeable discomfort or appreciable quickening of the respiration. Microbes are found especially in dusty air, and during coughing, sneezing and loud talking they are expelled from the air passages on droplets of moisture. When epidemic diseases such as influenza are rife, infection is apt to be conveyed through the air by these means, especially in badly ventilated and over-warmed rooms. When the amount of carbonic acid present in the air exceeds 0·1 per cent there is usually a distinct sense of 'stuffiness', which forms the best guide as to the necessity for increased ventilation. The continued breathing day after day of a 'stuffy' atmosphere is apt to produce headache, drowsiness, depression, inability to concentrate on work, dryness of the throat and a tendency to 'catch cold' easily, thus resulting in a gradual deterioration of health. Inadequate ventilation has much to do with the onset of pulmonary tuberculosis as well as with infection by other diseases such as influenza and the common cold. (See VENTILATION.)

Uses (see CLIMATE; INHALATIONS; RESPIRATION; SANITATION; VENTILATION).

AIR-BEDS consist of stout rubber perforated in numerous places by rubber tubes which open on the upper and lower surfaces and add strength to the bed. The bed is pumped up from one end to the desired hardness. Such a bed is both easier for the nurse to manage and more comfortable to the patient than a water-bed. (See RIPPLE BEDS.)

Uses: In general an air-bed is placed under a bedridden person or one suffering from devitalizing disease of the nervous system, in order to prevent the formation of bed sores, by distributing pressure all over the patient's back. Apart from the tendency to bed sores, a patient who is long confined to bed, who is fevered, or who is emaciated, derives a sense of great coolness and comfort from an air-bed.

AIR PASSAGES: These are the nose, pharynx or throat (the large cavity behind the nose and mouth), larynx, trachea or windpipe, and bronchi or bronchial tubes. The air, on entering the nose, passes through a high narrow passage on each side, the outer wall of which has three projections (the nasal conchae) which almost touch the dividing septum between the nostrils, thus making on each side three passages or meatuses, in which the air is warmed, moistened, and relieved of particles of dust. (See NOSE.) Mouth-breathing is, accordingly, a bad habit because the air is not prepared for entrance to the lungs. In the pharynx the food and air passages meet and cross. The larynx lies in front of the lower part of the pharynx and is the organ where the voice is produced (see VOICE) by aid of the vocal cords. The opening between the cords is called the glottis, and shortly after passing this the air reaches the trachea or wind-pipe, a tube 10 to 12·5 cm (4 to 5 inches) long, and 2 cm (¾ inch) wide.

This leads into the chest and divides above the heart into two bronchi, one of which goes to each lung, in which it splits into finer and finer tubes (see LUNGS). The larynx is enclosed in two strong cartilages, the thyroid (of which the most projecting part, the Adam's apple, is a prominent point on the front of the neck) and

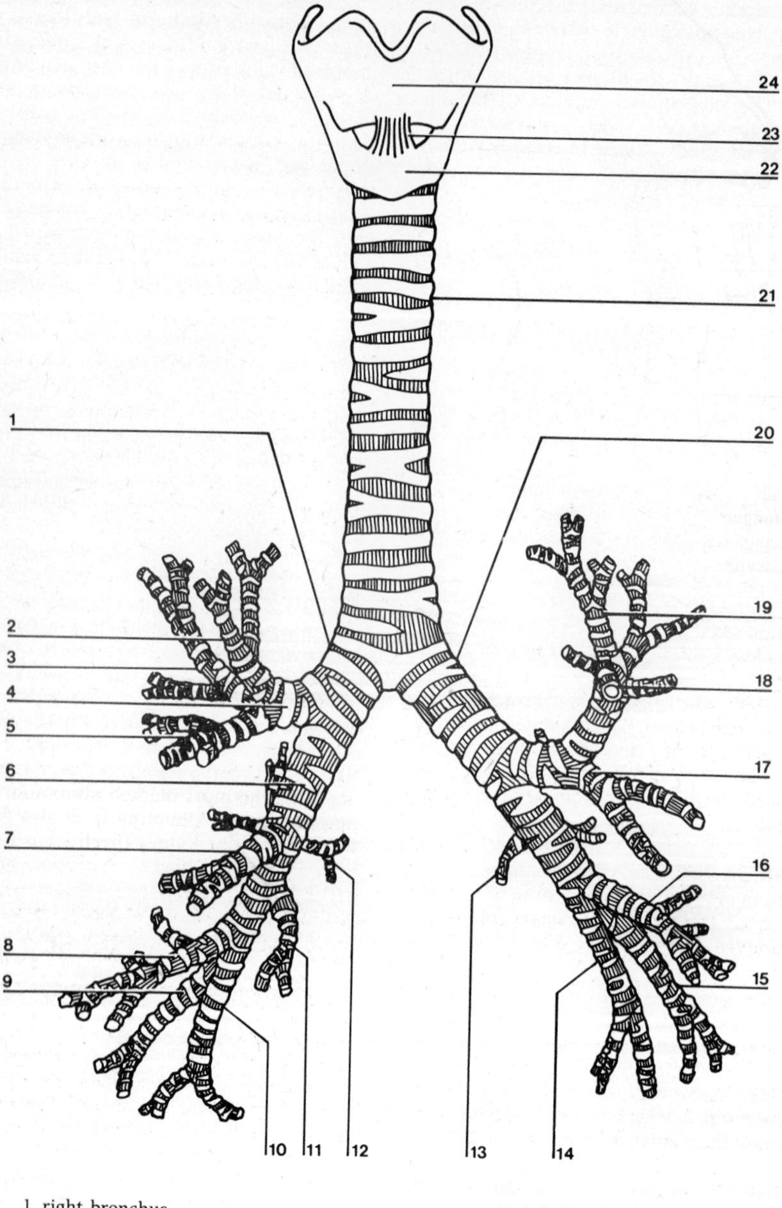

1 right bronchus
2 right apical bronchus
3 right subapical bronchus
4 right eparterial bronchus
5 right pectoral bronchus
6 right hyparterial bronchus
7 right middle lobe bronchus
8 right anterior basal bronchus
9 right axillary basal bronchus
10 right posterior basal bronchus
11 cardiac bronchus
12 right dorsal bronchus
13 left dorsal bronchus
14 left posterior basal bronchus
15 left axillary basal bronchus
16 left anterior basal bronchus
17 left lingular bronchus
18 left pectoral bronchus
19 left apical bronchus
20 left bronchus
21 trachea
22 cricoid cartilage
23 cricothyroid ligament
24 thyroid cartilage

The lower air passages.

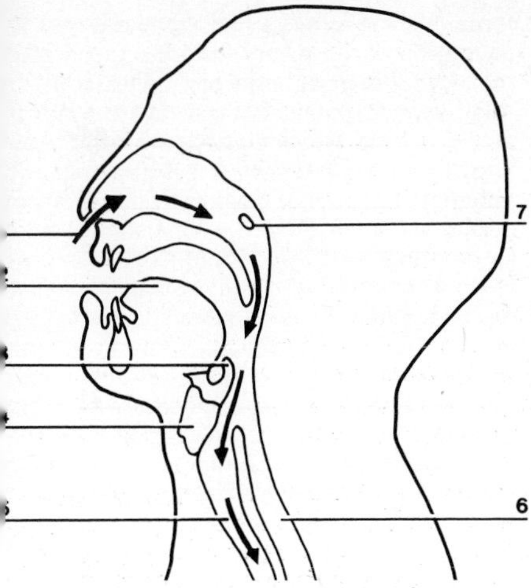

1 air
2 tongue
3 epiglottis
4 larynx
5 windpipe
6 gullet
7 eustachian tube

Vertical section through the middle of the head and neck showing the upper air passages.

.he cricoid (which can be felt as a hard ring ıbout an inch below). Beneath this, the trachea, which is stiffened by rings of cartilage, so that it s never closed in any position of the body, can oe traced down till it disappears behind the oreast-bone.

AIR-SICKNESS: The manifestations of this condition are very similar to those of SEA-SICKNESS (qv). The most satisfactory remedy is hyoscine hydrobromide, (0·3 to 0·5 mg).

AKINESIA means loss, or impairment, of voluntary movement, or immobility. It is characteristically seen in Parkinsonism (qv).

ALASTRIM, or VARIOLA MINOR, is a form of smallpox which differs from ordinary smallpox in being milder and having a low mortality.

ALBINISM: An inherited disorder in which there is an absence or decrease of melanin in the skin, hair and eyes. Those affected tend to have a very fair complexion and blonde or ginger hair. Many have nystagmus, poor visual acuity and a high incidence of squints. There is no treatment. Albinos tend to burn easily in sunlight, so barrier creams and dark glasses may be helpful.

ALBUMINS are proteins. They enter into the composition of all the tissues of the body. Their characters are that they are soluble in pure water; can be dried into a light, flaky, non-crystalline powder; are coagulated by heat, and precipitated by various agents like nitric acid, tannin, alcohol, or perchloride of mercury.

Varieties: Albumins are generally divided according to their source of origin, as muscle-albumin, milk-albumin, blood- or serum-albumin, egg-albumin, vegetable-albumin, etc. These differ both in chemical reactions and also physiologically, for though serum-albumin occurs in the blood, some albumins, eg. egg-albumin, injected direct into the blood are highly poisonous.

Uses: When taken into the stomach they are all converted into a soluble form by the process of digestion (qv), and are then absorbed into the blood, whence they go to build up the tissues gradually worn out in the activity of the body. (See ALBUMINURIA; GLOMERULONEPHRITIS.)

ALBUMINURIA means a condition in which albumin is present in the urine. It is more correctly described as proteinuria, because the other blood proteins are present in the urine as well as albumin, though albumin is far in excess of the others. It is of immense importance because it is often a symptom of serious heart or kidney disease.

Causes: (1) *Kidney disease* is the most important cause of albuminuria, and in some cases the discovery of albuminuria may be the first evidence of such disease. This is why an examination of the urine for the presence of albumin constitutes an essential part of every medical examination. Almost any form of kidney disease will cause albuminuria, but the most frequent form to do this is glomerulonephritis. In the subacute (or nephrotic) stage of glomerulonephritis the most marked albuminuria of all may be found. Albuminuria is also found in infections of the kidney (pyelitis) as well as in infections of the bladder (cystitis) and of the urethra (urethritis). The development of albuminuria in pregnancy is always an indication for the individual to receive careful medical treatment, as it may be the first sign of one of the most dangerous complications of pregnancy: toxaemia of pregnancy, glomerulonephritis, or eclampsia (qv).

(2) *Heart failure* is always accompanied by albuminuria, particularly when the right side of the heart is failing. In severe cases of failure, accompanied by oedema, the albuminuria may be marked. It is due to congestion of the kidneys.

(3) *Fever* is practically always accompanied by albuminuria, even though there is not actual kidney disease. The albuminuria disappears soon after the temperature becomes normal.

(4) *Drugs and poisons*: These include arsenic, lead, mercury, gold, copaiba, salicylic acid and quinine.

(5) *Anaemia*: A trace of albumin may be found in the urine in severe cases of anaemia.

(6) *Functional or orthostatic albuminuria*: Almost any normal person may have a transitory albuminuria after severe muscular exertion or after a cold bath, and it may occasionally appear after eating a large amount of protein: eg. raw eggs. The form commonly known as *orthostatic* or postural albuminuria is

much more common and is of importance because, if the true cause is not recognized, it may be taken as a sign of kidney disease. In the 1914–18 War it was found in 4 per cent of healthy British soldiers, and in an American investigation it was found in 5 per cent of healthy university freshmen. The cause is still doubtful, but it is probably due to temporary congestion of the kidneys caused by adoption of the upright position in individuals with some slight disturbance of the circulation of the blood in the kidneys. At one time it was thought that individuals with this type of albuminuria were more prone to develop glomerulonephritis later in life than individuals in whom it was not present, but this has now been definitely disproved. The features of this type of albuminuria are that it usually occurs in young people, usually between the ages of 8 and 18 years, and that it is not present while the patient is at rest. Thus, the specimen of urine obtained the first thing in the morning, before the individual gets up, contains no albumin, while a specimen obtained later in the day, after the individual has been up and about, will contain albumin.

Albuminuria and Life Assurance: Most companies will not issue a life policy to anyone with permanent albuminuria in case this is due to glomerulonephritis. Even cases in which no serious disease manifests itself have, if the albuminuria persists, a shorter expectation of life than other people, and so require a higher premium. In cases of doubt, tests to measure the function of the kidney may be carried out. If the tests show normal function, then the albuminuria takes on a much less serious aspect.

Treatment: The treatment is that of the underlying disease. (See GLOMERULONEPHRITIS, etc.) In the case of functional albuminuria due to excessive exercise, cold baths, or excessive ingestion of protein, treatment consists of removal of the cause. Individuals who have orthostatic or postural albuminuria are usually adolescents or young adults who are not in good training, and the treatment consists of getting them into good condition.

ALBUMIN WATER is used for administration as a light form of nourishment to patients with weak digestion or suffering from diarrhoea or some condition in which only very small amounts of food can be borne. To prepare albumin water a raw egg is broken in two on the edge of a cup. The white is allowed to escape by passing the yolk from one half of the shell to the other. The white is then whisked for 10 minutes to a stiff froth, 250 ml (½ pint) of cold water is added, and it is allowed to stand for an hour to dissolve. Lemon juice may be added to flavour, and a cupful may be given at one time.

ALCOHOL, more correctly ETHYL ALCOHOL, or ETHANOL, is a liquid obtained by the action of yeast on solutions of sugar, especially of grape sugar or glucose. Carbonic acid gas is also formed in the process and escapes. After fermentation of the sugary fluid has taken place the alcohol is separated from the water by distillation and from the last traces of water by the action of lime, which absorbs the latter. Absolute alcohol contains 99·4 to 100 per cent (by volume) of alcohol. It is a powerful irritant, and even in moderate quantities a poison. Rectified spirit, or spirit of wine, contains 90 per cent of alcohol by volume, and is used to make essences, tinctures and weaker spirits of 80, 70, 60, 50, 45, 25 and 20 per cent strength. Proof spirit contains 57 per cent (by volume) of alcohol. It is called 'proof' spirit, because an old test of its strength was to drench gunpowder with it, set fire to it, and if the gunpowder was ignited the alcohol stood the proof. The legal definition of proof spirit is 'that which at the temperature of 51° by Fahrenheit's thermometer weighs exactly twelve-thirteenth parts of an equal measure of distilled water'. Spirits are described in terms of so many degrees over or under proof (O.P. or U.P.), depending upon the quantity of distilled water which must be added to, or deducted from, 100 volumes of the sample in order to produce spirit of proof strength. Another method of indicating spirit strength, commonly used on the labels of alcoholic drinks, is to give it as a number of degrees, proof spirit being taken as 100 per cent. Thus a spirit said to be 70° would contain 70 per cent of proof spirit: ie. it would be 30° under proof.

	per cent
Rum, Whisky	30
Brandy, Gin	30
Liqueurs	15 to 55
Port, Sherry	15 to 16
Madeira	15 to 16
Champagne	10
Burgundy	about 10
Claret	about 9
Moselle, Hock	about 9
Strong ale	about 8
Cider	2 to 3
Beer	2 to 3

Alcoholic content of alcoholic liquors

Alcohol freezes at a very low temperature and so is used for thermometers for the Arctic regions. It dissolves many things which water does not dissolve, such as fats, oils and resins. Mixed with wood-spirit, it forms methylated spirit, on which no duty is payable but which is, of course, unfit for drinking. It coagulates the tissues, and so has a hardening effect upon skin, wounds, etc.

Effects of alcohol: Alcohol, when drunk, is quickly and completely absorbed. About one fifth of any dose taken is absorbed from the stomach, and almost the whole of the remainder is absorbed in the upper part of the small intestine within two or three hours of having been taken. Very little is excreted by the breath, urine and other channels. This seldom amounts to more than one-twentieth of the quantity swallowed. The remainder is completely used up within twenty-four hours, being oxidized mainly to produce heat. The body can derive one-fifth of the total energy it requires from alcohol, and in this way alcohol spares carbohydrates and fats taken in the food. There is a tendency therefore for both of these to be deposited in the tissues as superfluous fat when alcohol is habitually added to the diet without a decrease of the other food.

The mental effect of alcohol is dependent partly upon its effect on the circulation and partly on its anaesthetic action on the nervous system, dulling small pains and the sense of worry and anxiety. Owing to a similar dulling action upon the higher intellectual faculties, self-criticism and self-control are also to a considerable extent lessened, and this creates the false impression that alcohol is having a stimulating action. Alcohol is not a stimulant, it is a depressant. If a larger dose is taken, the functions of sense perception and skilled movement are to a certain extent dulled and deteriorate, with the result that there is a certain clumsiness of behaviour. The person now begins to make ill-adjusted movements, shows some slurring of speech, and becomes less quick and less capable in performing acts which require decision and promptitude: eg. avoiding a collision when driving a car. In a further stage the intellectual processes of judgment, self-criticism, and self-control are largely suspended and the functions of sense perception and skilled movement become greatly impaired, until ultimately a heavy sleep or stupor supervenes which lasts until the alcohol absorbed by the nervous system has been oxidized and consumed. There is no proof that alcohol in any dose improves the efficiency with which either skilled or unskilled work can be carried out during the few hours while the alcohol acts.

Moderate doses of alcohol increase the secretions of the stomach and thus may aid digestion in persons in whom these secretions are defective. Different wines have very varying effect on different persons in this respect, probably on account of the substances other than alcohol which they contain. When alcoholic beverages are taken habitually over long periods, and especially in the more concentrated form of spirits, they exert a pronounced effect of irritation upon the mucous membrane of the stomach and thus lead to chronic indigestion.

With regard to the action of alcohol on respiration and circulation of the blood, moderate doses have practically no effect upon the breathing, although very large doses have a paralysing effect, and when death occurs from alcohol it is brought about by stoppage of the respiration. As to its 'stimulating' action on the circulation, this is in part brought about by the lessening of mental strain induced by its narcotic and sedative action. It is also due in part to its action in dilating the small blood-vessels, and thus reducing the blood-pressure and possibly relieving strain on the heart.

The popular reputation of alcohol as a means of 'warding off cold' is due largely to its power of dilating the superficial blood-vessels and of dulling the sensory nerves of the skin, so that the skin actually becomes warm, while external impressions are not felt. If at the same time as the alcohol is administered, warmth is applied to the surface of the body by hot blankets, hot bottles, etc., the skin becomes more capable of absorbing the external heat and thus the alcohol acts as a restorative.

The official statistics issued by the Registrar General indicate a heavy mortality among persons occupied in the liquor trade, who are known to consume more than the average amount of alcohol. The experience of insurance companies has made them adverse to admitting on ordinary terms persons who are habitual heavy users of alcoholic beverages.

Uses of Alcohol: *Externally* it is used in the cheap form of methylated spirit to cleanse the skin of oily, fatty, or resinous substances, which water will not remove. Also to harden the skin of the feet before a long walk, or that of the back in persons confined to bed for long periods, and so prevent bed sores (qv).

A *whisky pack* or brandy pack is an old-fashioned remedy to stimulate infants reduced to a state of collapse by diarrhoea or bronchitis.

Internally there are few, if any, absolute indications for the use of alcohol, and during the last fifty years the use of alcohol as a medicine has declined rapidly.

Alcohol may be of value in stimulating the appetite during convalescence. It is also a useful sedative sometimes in old people, particularly in an individual who is used to taking alcohol regularly in moderation. Its value as a stimulant of the heart is doubtful. There is a certain amount of justification for the use of undiluted whisky or brandy in the treatment of fainting, provided this is not due to some serious condition such as haemorrhage. It should never be given to a patient who is suffering from shock. Champagne and brandy-and-soda have a traditional reputation for the relief of vomiting, including sea-sickness.

The popular habit of taking spirits 'to keep the cold out' is a delusion. Alcohol gives a sense of warmth to the skin by bringing the blood there; but, as the blood is rapidly cooled in cold air, the risk of frostbite and even death by freezing is increased, so that experienced hunters and mountaineers will on no account touch spirits on biting cold days or at high altitudes.

In health, there is no necessity for alcohol, and, as so many persons contract the alcohol habit, it would be well for every one to consider the question carefully before embarking on its habitual use. Even far short of drunkenness its constant use in large quantities certainly shortens life. (See ALCOHOLISM, CHRONIC.)

ALCOHOLISM, ACUTE: This is the condition produced by taking excessive quantities of alcohol over a short period. The effects vary greatly according to the hereditary and nervous constitution of the person concerned, his or her age and social surroundings, and to a great extent with the kind of liquor taken, whether it is taken with food, and whether it has been taken for a long time previously.

Varieties: There are many curious effects produced and phases of character brought to light by the disturbance of mental balance, but the three important forms are ordinary drunkenness, alcoholic mania, and delirium tremens.

Symptoms: ORDINARY DRUNKENNESS is too common to need much description. First the person is brightened, his spirits rise, his conversation is witty, the skin becomes flushed, and there is a general sense of well-being. As he becomes really drunk a phase of depression-excitement comes on: the controlling power of reason is lost. A third stage is that in which all feeling of shame is lost, and there is dullness of sense and loss of power, the drunk man or woman reeling or falling and rising with difficulty. The fourth stage is popularly known as 'dead drunk'; the person lies in a state of insensibility, with stertorous breathing and dilated pupils.

ALCOHOLIC MANIA is a state of excitement and fury, leading sometimes to attempts at murder or suicide, comes on after, it may be, only a few glasses of spirits or wine, and lasts some hours or days, without any tendency to dullness or sleep. Some persons who are liable to epileptic attacks have a fit when alcohol is taken even in moderate amount.

DELIRIUM TREMENS is the most serious form, and is popularly known as 'blue-devils', because of the hallucinations accompanying the state. It follows on a long course of drinking which has ended in a bout, or may be brought on by an injury or business worries in a heavy drinker; but it does not follow a single 'spree'. Tremors all over the body, but especially in the hands and tongue, are the first sign of its onset, then complete loss of appetite, sickness, rise of temperature, weak pulse and constant purposeless movements. Finally hallucinations come on: spiders, flies, mice, rats are described on the clothes or floor, or disgusting objects like snakes, toads, and demons; or the bystanders are taken for policemen, hangmen, etc., and the furniture distorts itself into weird shapes. Lastly, delirium of a terrified or raging type comes on, in which there is more or less danger of suicide or homicide. Pneumonia of a serious type is apt to ensue, and if these two be combined the case is usually fatal. When a case of delirium tremens follows upon a very prolonged course of chronic alcoholism the mental state sometimes passes into one of permanent mental feebleness, due to organic changes in the brain. (See also KORSAKOW'S SYNDROME.)

Treatment: Ordinary drunkenness is best treated by letting the person sleep it off, or, if great quantities of alcohol have been rapidly taken, the stomach should be washed out with the stomach-tube. In the second or excited stage, and in alcoholic mania, if the person be uncontrollable, he is to be treated as in *delirium tremens*. In the latter, admission to hospital is necessary, with careful nursing and constant supervision. Chlormethiazole is the best sedative in the acute phase, and promising results are being reported from the use of tranquillizers. If any infection, such as pneumonia is present, full doses of antibiotics are given. A high-calorie, high-vitamin diet should be given, with particular emphasis on a high intake of vitamin B_1 (thiamine).

ALCOHOLISM, CHRONIC: This is the condition of mind and body produced by taking too much alcohol over long periods. Alcoholism accounts for 10 per cent of all admissions to psychiatric hospitals; 20,000 people are admitted to psychiatric hospitals for alcoholism.

Chronic alcoholism is a disease, but it is necessary to differentiate between the chronic alcoholic and the excessive drinker. The latter is able to stop drinking if he is given sufficient good reason for doing so, whereas the victim of chronic alcoholism cannot voluntarily abstain for more than a short while. As one expert has put it: 'The regular heavy drinker lives to drink, but the alcoholic *must* drink to live'. According to the World Health Organization, 'alcoholics are those excessive drinkers whose dependence on alcohol has attained such a degree that they show a noticeable mental disturbance or an interference with their bodily and mental health, their interpersonal relations and their smooth economic and social functioning; or who show the prodromal signs of such development. They therefore need treatment'.

Whatever the reason for drinking, the long-continued consumption of alcohol can result in many medical disorders. The most frequent of these is *gastritis* (qv). Indeed, the most common cause of acute and chronic gastritis is over-indulgence in alcohol. Cirrhosis of the liver (see LIVER, DISEASES) is a frequent complication. Injurious effects on the heart from habitual spirit drinking are not uncommon, and there is an increased tendency for alcoholics to suffer from diseases of the arteries (qv). Peripheral neuritis (qv) is also common. In the early stages this manifests itself by pains in the feet and hands, and tenderness in the calves of the legs, followed later by wrist-drop and foot-drop. In severe cases the cranial nerves may be involved and this may be accompanied by blindness. The fiery visage (see ROSACEA) is a well-known sign of the chronic alcoholic. Finally, there may be severe mental disturbance, such as Korsakow's syndrome (qv) and delirium tremens (see ALCOHOLISM, ACUTE). The full extent of the ravages of alcohol is not known, but in France it is estimated that over 40 per cent of all hospital expenditure is alcohol related.

There are four types of chronic alcoholics: (i) The alcoholic with a good previous personality; about 80 per cent of these make a successful recovery: ie. remain totally abstinent. (ii) The alcoholic whose basic personality is neurotic. About 30 per cent recover, but they are prone to relapse before they finally become abstinent. (iii) The alcoholic whose basic personality is sychotic. The outlook in this group depends entirely upon the psychosis. In a sense they are ot true alcoholics, and treatment is aimed primarily at the psychosis. (iv) The alcoholic whose basic personality is psychopathic. The utlook for this group is extremely bad. The woman psychopath is particularly addicted to lcohol, and she often attempts suicide – and often succeeds. A disturbing feature of recent ears has been the increasing number of women alcoholics. Thus the Alcoholism Community Centre for Education, Prevention and Treatment (ACCEPT) reports that a decade go the ratio of referrals for treatment was one woman to every eight men. In 1978–79 it was two women to every three men, and it is forecast that referrals of women will shortly equal, or exceed, those of men.

The prognosis is good if the patient has a happy home and a good job to return to. Those who are separated or divorced, or the bachelor living on his own, find it more difficult to maintain sobriety. The patient who seeks help has the best chance to recover. Undergoing treatment simply to pacify or please the marital partner, or to avoid being cut out of a will, is a poor prognostic sign. Patients of poor, or limited, intelligence, are unlikely to respond to treatment. Excessive drinking in early adult life s usually found in the neurotic. Violent abnormal behaviour of young people under the influence of alcohol suggests an underlying psychosis, such as schizophrenia, or epilepsy. Alcoholism developing at the menopause suggests a depressive state; if it develops in later life it suggests a senile depressive state and has a poor prognosis. A feature of the chronic alcoholic is that he has few hobbies, few outside nterests, and little interest in other people. His entire life is centred round drinking.

Treatment: To be successful this must practically always be carried out in the first instance n hospital or special clinic. Very few, if any, can be treated at home, and even outpatient treatment is seldom successful without a preliminary period of inpatient treatment.

The essential feature of treatment is the immediate withdrawal of all alcohol over a period not exceeding forty-eight hours. To overcome, or prevent, the inevitable disturbances this causes, the patient is given tranquillizers and intensive vitamin therapy. The disruption of the drinking pattern is then completed either by the so-called vomiting technique, using apomorphine, or by the use of disulfiram. This is a drug which so upsets the patient when he takes alcohol in addition that he develops an aversion to alcohol. An alternative drug, calcium carbimide, is now available which has a similar action.

Once the drinking pattern has been disrupted, the patient then undergoes a course of psychotherapy. Hypnosis is proving particularly useful in this respect. In addition, group therapy is valuable, especially once the patient has recovered and has returned to his normal surroundings. This is the basis of Alcoholics Anonymous, an informal organization of men and women 'for whom alcohol has become a major problem, and who, admitting it, have decided to do something about it'. The address of the General Service Office is PO Box 1, Stonebow House, Stonebow, York YO1 2NJ (0904-644026/7/8/9). Help and advice for relatives of problem drinkers and alcoholics are available from AL-Anon Family Groups, of which there are now 350 in Britain. Details are available from AL-Anon Family Groups, 61 Great Dover Street, London SE1 4YF (Tel: 01-403 0888). Help and advice can also be obtained from ACCEPT (Alcoholism Community Centres for Education, Prevention and Treatment), Clinic, 200 Seagrove Road, London SW6 1RQ (Tel: 01-381 3155); Alcohol Concern, 305 Gray's Inn Road, London WC1X 8QF (Tel: 01-833 3471); and from The Scottish Council for Alcoholism, 137–145 Sauchiehall Street, Glasgow G2 3EU (041-333 9677).

Finally, it must be stressed that there can be no compromise with the alcoholic if he is to be considered cured. Total abstinence is essential for life in every case. There are no exceptions to this rule.

ALCURONIUM is a relaxant drug which is being used by anaesthetists in relatively short operations of around twenty minutes' duration.

ALDOSTERONE is a hormone secreted by the adrenal cortex. It plays an important part in maintaining the electrolyte balance of the body by promoting the reabsorption of sodium and the secretion of potassium by the renal tubules. It is thus of primary importance in controlling the volume of the body fluids.

ALEXIA is another name for word-blindness. (See APHASIA; DYSLEXIA.)

ALFACALCIDOL is a synthetic form (or analogue) of vitamin D. (See VITAMIN.)

ALGESIMETER is an instrument used in measuring the sensitiveness of areas of the skin.

ALGID is that stage of cholera and malaria in which extreme coldness of the body occurs. (See CHOLERA; MALARIA.)

ALIENIST means an expert in the treatment of insanity.

ALIMENTARY CANAL is the passage along which the food passes, in which it is digested (see DIGESTION), and from which it is absorbed by lymphatics and blood-vessels into the circulation. The canal consists of the mouth, pharynx or throat, oesophagus or gullet, stomach, small intestine, and large intestine, in this order. For details see articles under these heads. The total length of the alimentary canal is about 9 metres in man.

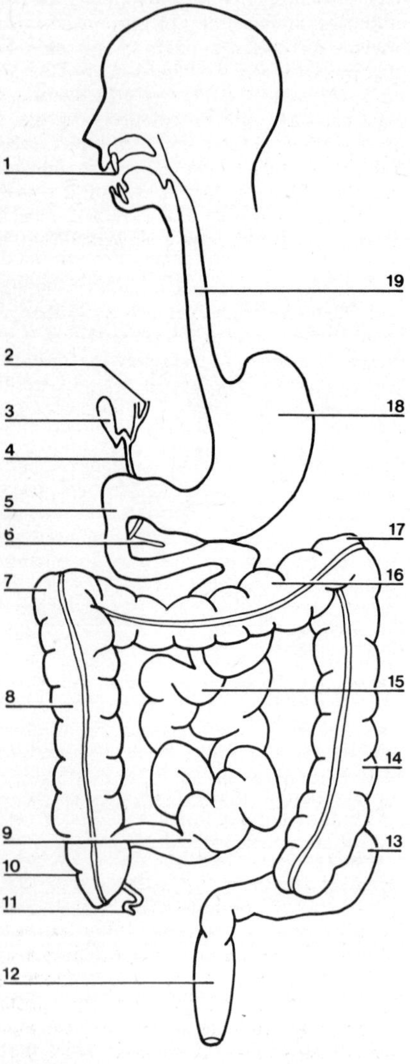

1 mouth
2 hepatic ducts
3 gall-bladder
4 common bile duct
5 duodenum
6 pancreatic duct
7 hepatic flexure
8 ascending colon
9 ileum
10 caecum
11 appendix
12 rectum
13 sigmoid flexure
14 descending colon
15 jejunum
16 transverse colon
17 splenic flexure
18 stomach
19 oesophagus

The alimentary canal.

ALKALI is a substance which neutralizes a acid to form a salt, and turns litmus and oth vegetable dyes blue. Alkalis are general oxides or carbonates of metals.

Varieties: Ammonia, lithia (lithium oxide), po ash (potassium hydroxide) and soda (sodiu carbonate) are the principal ones; the carbo ates of these act as weaker alkalis, and the bicarbonates still weaker. Lime (calciu oxide), magnesia (magnesium oxide), bary (barium oxide) and strontium are called alk line earths, and act as alkalis. Substances whic in the body are converted into alkalis, such acetates, citrates and tartrates, are called 'ind rect' alkalis. In the body protein substanc also act as alkalis, absorbing acids and th preventing the development of gener acidosis.

Uses: In poisoning by acids, one at on administers dilute alkaline solutions (see ACID POISONING BY). Caustic, ie. undiluted, alka are used to destroy warts. Bee-stings and insec bites cause irritation because of an ac injected by the insect, and consequently a relieved by weak alkaline applications. heartburn, bicarbonate of soda (1 · 2G.) is tak after a meal, to sooth irritation and spasm the stomach. The largest use of alkalis is in t treatment of duodenal ulcer and other forms dyspepsia associated with hyperchlorhydr (qv). The most commonly used alkalis for th purpose are magnesium trisilicate, magnesiu carbonate and aluminium hydroxide.

ALKALIS, POISONING BY: People may dri soap-lye, ammonia, caustic soda, caustic po ash, washing soda, pearl ash, spirit of hart horn, by mistake, and when this has been don plenty of water should be given to drink, which should be added, if available, weak aci such as vinegar, orange juice or lemon juic Oily substances, such as olive oil, or white egg, or milk may thereafter be administere On no account must any attempt be made make the patient vomit.

ALKALOIDS are substances found commonl in various plants. They are natural nitrogeno organic bases and combine with acids to for crystalline salts. Among alkaloids, morphi was discovered in 1805, strychnine in 181 quinine and caffeine in 1820, nicotine in 182 atropine in 1833. Only a few alkaloids occur the animal kingdom, the outstanding examp being adrenaline, which is formed in t medulla of the suprarenal, or adrenal, glan Alkaloids are often used for medicinal pu poses. The name of an alkaloid ends in '*ine*' (Latin *ina*).

NEUTRAL PRINCIPLES are crystalline substanc with actions similar to those of alkaloids b having a neutral reaction. The name of a ne tral principle ends in '*in*', eg. digitalin, aloir

The following are the more important alk loids, with their source plants:

Aconite, *from Monkshood.*

Atropine, *from Belladonna (juice of Deadly Nightshade).*
Cocaine, *from Coca leaves.*
Hyoscine, *from Henbane.*
Morphine,
Codeine, *from Opium (juice of Poppy).*
Thebaine,
Nicotine, *from Tobacco.*
Physostigmine, *from Calabar bean.*
Pilocarpine, *from Jaborandi leaves.*
Quinidine, *from Cinchona or Peruvian bark.*
Strychnine, *from Nux Vomica seeds.*

ALKALOSIS means an increase in the alkalinity of the blood, or, more accurately, a decrease in the concentration of hydrogen ions in the blood. It occurs, for example, in patients who have had large doses of alkalis for the treatment of gastric ulcer.

ALKAPTONURIA (see OCHRONOSIS).

ALKYLATING AGENTS are so named because they alkylate or react with certain biochemical entities, particularly those concerned with the synthesis of nucleic acid. Alkylation is the substitution of an organic grouping in place of another grouping in a molecule.

The importance of the alkylating agents in medicine is that by interfering with the growth of cells they have proved of value in the treatment of various forms of malignant disease. Unfortunately they interfere with the growth of normal cells as well as malignant cells, and this restricts their use to a considerable extent.

Nevertheless several of them, including mustine (qv) and thiotepa (qv) have proved of considerable value in the chemotherapy of malignant disease.

ALLANTIASIS is a name for sausage-poisoning. (See FOOD POISONING.)

ALLANTOIN is a crystalline powder which occurs naturally in comfrey root, but is prepared synthetically. It is used in the treatment of skin ulcers to stimulate the formation of the surface epithelial layer of the skin.

ALLANTOIS is a vascular structure which, very early in the life of the embryo, grows out from its hind-gut. The end becomes attached to the wall of the womb. It spreads out at the end, becomes stalked, and develops later into the placenta and umbilical cord (see AFTERBIRTH), which forms the only connection between the mother and embryo.

ALLERGEN is the term applied to any substance, usually a protein, which, taken into the body, makes the body hypersensitive or 'allergic' to it. Thus in hay fever the allergen is pollen.

ALLERGY means special sensitiveness of an individual to certain foods, pollens or other products of plants, animal emanations, insect bites, etc., so that in such an individual conditions like asthma, dyspepsia, nettle-rash, hay fever, eczema and headache are produced. The term anaphylaxis (qv) is given to a similar serious reaction following the injection of serum. The substances that produce allergy, known as allergens, are generally of protein nature and include such ordinary foods as eggs, milk, flour and potatoes; also strawberries, tomatoes, cauliflower, walnuts, pork, shell-fish, salmon, coffee, etc., as well as colouring agents and preservatives in food; it may also be caused by inhalation of dust from feathers (in pillows), of the hair of horses, dogs or cats, of face powder containing orris root, and of pollen, especially from grasses and certain flowers. What happens in allergic individuals is that allergens induce the formation of antibodies. When an allergen comes in contact with its antibody this leads to the release of those substances, such as bradykinin (qv) and histamine (qv), which are responsible for the actual allergic reaction, whether this be asthma, hay fever, eczema or the like.

Symptoms: The reaction in sensitive persons usually appears within a few minutes, but may be delayed for hours. One of the most common effects is nettle-rash or dropsical swellings in various parts; hay fever is another common result; sometimes there is swelling in a joint. Another type of reaction consists in spasmodic contractions of unstriped muscle so that the person affected may become urgently ill with asthma, or may develop spasms in the stomach with painful dyspepsia and vomiting, or in the intestine with symptoms resembling obstruction or severe diarrhoea, or may be troubled by irritability of the bladder. In other cases, neuralgia, headache or attacks of giddiness may come on.

Treatment: It is important to find out the food or other substance to which the individual is sensitive. Sometimes this has been discovered by long personal experience. Skin testing may also be carried out by inoculating into a series of scratches extracts of various foods, etc., likely to cause allergy, and the substance responsible produces a weal (qv) surrounded by redness within a few minutes. When the substance is discovered, it should in future be carefully avoided, or, if it is an ordinary food, the sensitiveness can sometimes be abolished by taking this food constantly in small quantities, very gradually increased. In other cases, particularly of hay fever, it may be possible to desensitize the affected individual by a series of injections of a vaccine made from the substance (eg. pollen) to which he or she is sensitive. Severe symptoms, as in asthma, may be relieved by inhalation or injection of sympathomimotic drugs. There is now available a range of antihistamine drugs (qv) which are of value in treating cases in which the cause of the condition cannot be avoided or is not known.

LABORATORY ANIMAL ALLERGY is an allergic disorder characterized by conjunctivitis, rhinitis (qv), urticaria and asthma, resulting from exposure to allergens derived from animals. It is estimated that there are 4500–8500 cases in the United Kingdom, with asthma occurring in 2500–3500 of them. Whilst the condition may be severe enough in some cases to require the victim to stop working with animals, many can continue working if provided with adequate personal protection, such as masks, airstream helmets, gloves and gowns. In some cases, drugs of the disodium cromoglycate (qv) type may be of value.

ALLOCHEIRIA is the name for a disorder of sensation in which sensations are referred to the wrong part of the body.

ALLOGRAFT is a piece of tissue or an organ, such as the kidney, transplanted from one to another of the same species: eg. from man to man. It is also known as a homograft.

ALLOPATHY is a term applied sometimes by homoeopathists to the methods used by regular practitioners of medicine and surgery. The term literally means curing by inducing a different kind of action in the body, and is an erroneous designation.

ALLOPURINOL is a drug of value in the treatment of gout. It acts by suppressing the formation of uric acid. It is also being used in treatment of uric acid stone in the kidney.

ALOES is the dried juice of a plant which grows in South Africa (*Aloë ferox*) and the West Indies (*A. vera barbadensis*). It acts as a purgative, and, taken in the evening, it acts next morning. Since it tends to cause griping, it is usually combined with other drugs. (See CONSTIPATION.)

ALOIN is an extract from aloes used in pills; the dose is from 15 to 60 mg (¼ to 1 grain).

ALOPECIA is another name for baldness. (See BALDNESS.)

ALOPECIA AREATA is the term given to the disorder in which the hair comes out in patches, resulting in shiny, smooth, bald areas. (See BALDNESS.)

ALUM is either potash alum, potassium aluminium sulphate, or ammonia alum (ammonium aluminium sulphate). It is an astringent, and may be used as a powder to rub into abrasions when bleeding will not stop of itself. As an emetic, a teaspoonful of powdered alum may be given in water. A 1 to 4 per cent solution is used as a mouth-wash in stomatitis and pharyngitis, and a 2 per cent solution is useful when applied to the skin in cases of excessive perspiration.

ALUMINIUM is a light whitish metal which is very malleable and ductile. It is much used for the manufacture of surgical instruments and as a base for artificial dentures. Aluminiur hydroxide is used internally as an antacid an absorbent in dyspepsia. Aluminium powder i used for dusting on the skin around colostom openings (see COLOSTOMY) to protect the ski

ALVEOLITIS means inflammation of the alve oli (see ALVEOLUS) of the lungs caused by a allergic reaction. When the inflammation caused by infection it is called pneumonia an when by a chemical or physical agent it is calle pneumonitis.
EXTRINSIC ALLERGIC ALVEOLITIS is th condition induced by the lungs becoming alle gic (see ALLERGY) to various factors or sub stances. It includes bagassosis (qv), farmer' lung (qv), mushroom-worker's lung (qv budgerigar-fancier's lung (qv) and pigeon breeders' lung (qv). It is characterized by th onset of shortness of breath, tightness of th chest, cough and fever. The onset may be suc den or gradual. Treatment consists of remov of the affected individual from the offendin material to which he has become allergic. Co ticosteroids (qv) give temporary relief. Deser sitization is not a practical proposition.

ALVEOLUS is a term applied to the sockets c the teeth in the jaw-bone. The term is als applied to the minute divisions of glands an the air sacs of the lungs.

ALZHEIMER'S DISEASE is a degenerativ disorder of the cerebral cortex that produces dementia (qv) in middle to late life. The onse is insidious and the first manifestation is usu ally failing memory. Relatives can obtain hel and advice from the Alzheimer's Disease Soc ety, 158/160 Balham High Road, Londo SW12 9BN (01-675 6557).

AMANTADINE is a drug which is being use in the treatment of certain virus infections, an is proving of value in the prevention of certai forms of influenza. It is also used in the trea ment of Parkinsonism (qv).

AMAUROSIS is the term applied to blindnes in which there is no obvious lesion of the eye the blindness being caused by disease of th optic nerve, retina or brain, or being due t hysteria.

AMAUROSIS FUGAX is the term given to sud den transitory impairment, or loss of, vision. I usually affects only one eye, and is commonl due to circulatory failure. In its simplest form i occurs in normal people on rising suddenl from the sitting or recumbent position, when i is due to the effects of gravity. It also occurs i migraine. A not uncommon cause, particularl in elderly people, is transient ocular ischaemi (see ISCHAEMIA), resulting from blockage of th circulation to the retina (qv) by emboli (se EMBOLUS) from the common carotid artery c the heart. Treatment in this last group of case consists of control of the blood pressure if th is raised, as it often is in such cases; the administration of drugs that reduce the stickiness of blood platelets such as aspirin. In some instances removal of the part of the carotid artery from which the emboli are coming may be indicated.

AMBIVALENCE is the term applied to the psychological state in which a person concurrently hates and loves the same object or person.

AMBLYOPIA means defective vision for which no recognizable cause exists in any part of the eye. It may be due to such causes as defective development, hysteria, excessive use of tobacco or alcohol. The most important form is that associated with squinting (qv), or gross difference in refraction between the two eyes. It has been estimated that in Britain 5·7 per cent of young adults have amblyopia due to this cause.

AMBULANCE is a vehicle for conveying sick or injured individuals. Under the National Health Service a comprehensive ambulance service is available for the whole country. There is no charge for this except in the case of patients who are being taken to a nursing home or the pay wards of a hospital. The responsibility for arranging for the ambulance rests with the doctor in charge of the patient. In the case of an emergency, eg. an accident or sudden illness in the street, an emergency ambulance service is available and the quickest way of obtaining an ambulance is through the police. The ambulance service is provided by local health authorities, which not only provide their own ambulances but are allowed to provide them through the agency of other bodies, such as the British Red Cross Society.

There is also a Hospital Car Service run by people who use their own cars to take patients to and from hospital. They are paid an approved mileage allowance by the appropriate local health authority.

AMELIA: This is absence of the limbs, usually a congenital defect.

AMENORRHOEA is the absence of the menstrual flow during the time of life at which it should occur. (See MENSTRUATION.) If menstruation has never occured the amenorrhoea is termed primary. If it ceases after having once become established it is known as secondary amenorrhoea. The only value of these terms is that some patients with either chromosome abnormalities or malformations of the genital tract fall into the primary category. Otherwise the age of onset of symptoms is more important.

The causes of amenorrhoea are numerous and treatment requires dealing with the primary cause. The commonest cause of amenorrhoea is pregnancy. Hypothalamic disorders such as psychological stress or anorexia nervosa also cause amenorrhoea. Poor nutrition or loss of weight by dieting may cause it and any serious underlying disease such as tuberculosis or malaria may also result in the cessation of periods. The excess secretion of prolactin, whether this is the result of a microadenoma (see ADENOMA) of the pituitary gland or whether it is drug induced will cause amenorrhoea and possibly galactorrhoea (qv) as well. Malfunction of the pituitary gland will result in a failure to produce the gonadotrophic hormones with consequent amenorrhea. Excessive production of cortisol, as in Cushing's syndrome, or of androgens, as in the adrenogenital syndrome or the polycystic ovary syndrome, will result in amenorrhoea. Amenorrhoea occasionally follows the use of the oral contraceptive pill and may be associated with both hypothyroidism and obesity. It is thus important to take a careful history with emphasis on psychological factors, weight fluctuations and the use of drugs that may stimulate the release of prolactin, and it is also important to look for evidence of virilisation.

A gynaecological examination is necessary in primary amenorrhoea to exclude malformations of the genital tract. Estimations of the gonadotrophic hormone levels will reveal whether the amenorrhoea is primary ovarian failure or secondary to pituitary disease. In view of the frequent psychosomatic origins of amenorrhoea, reassurance of the patient is of great importance, in particular with reference to marriage and the ability to conceive. When weight loss is the cause of amenorrhoea restoration of body weight alone can result in spontaneous menstruation. Patients with raised concentrations of serum gonadotrophin hormones have primary ovarian failure. It is not amendable to treatment. Cyclical oestrogen/progestogen therapy will usually establish withdrawal bleeding. If the amenorrhoea is due to mild pituitary failure menstruation may return after treatment with clomiphene. Clomiphene is a non-steroidal agent which competes for oestrogen receptors in the hypothalamus. The patients who are most likely to respond to clomiphene are those who have some evidence of endogenous oestrogen and gonadotrophin production.

AMENT is an idiot or mentally deficient person – one having no mind.

AMENTIA is the state of being an ament; mental deficiency from failure of the mind to develop normally.

AMETHOCAINE is a powerful local anaesthetic which is used when a prolonged effect is required. It is also used as a spinal anaesthetic.

AMETROPIA (see REFRACTION).

AMIKACIN is a semi-synthetic derivative of kanamycin (qv) which is proving of value in the treatment of infections caused by micro-organisms resistant to gentamicin (qv) and tobramycin (qv).

AMILORIDE (MIDAMOR) is a diuretic that acts without causing excessive loss of potassium (see DIURETICS).

AMINACRINE HYDROCHLORIDE is a derivative of acridine and is used as a local antiseptic.

AMINES are substances derived from ammonia or amino-acids (qv) which play an important part in the working of the body, including the brain and the circulatory system. They include adrenaline (qv), noradrenaline (qv) and histamine (qv). (See also MONOAMINE OXIDASE INHIBITORS.)

AMINO-ACID is the name given to the ultimate products of digestion of protein foods and from which the protein materials of the body are again built up. They are organic acids in which one or more hydrogen atoms have been replaced by the chemical group NH_2. (See PROTEIN.)

AMINOCAPROIC ACID is one of a group of drugs introduced for the the control of bleeding. These drugs act by inhibiting the fibrinolytic system. This is a complex system which helps to maintain the coagulation mechanism of the blood in such a state that clotting of the blood only occurs when it is necessary. Thus, if fibrinolysis is prevented then the blood will clot more easily and bleeding will stop.

AMINOGLUTETHIMIDE is a drug that inhibits the synthesis of adrenal corticorteroids. It is proving of value in the treatment of cancer of the breast in post-menopausal women.

AMINOPHYLLINE is the name given to a combination of theophylline and ethylenediamine. It is used in the treatment of bronchial asthma.

AMINOPTERIN is an antimetabolite (qv) which is proving of value in the treatment of acute leukaemia (qv).

AMITRIPTYLINE (DOMICAL, ELAVIL LENTIZOL, TRYPTIZOL) (see ANTIDEPRESSANTS).

AMMONIA is a pungent gas formed by heating a mixture of sal ammoniac and quicklime. Dissolved in water it forms spirits of hartshorn, or liquor ammoniae. It is given off slowly from carbonate of ammonia, which is used as smelling salts. Carbonate of ammonia is the chief ingredient in aromatic spirits of ammonia or sal volatile. In chloride of ammonia or sal ammoniac it is fixed. (For ammonia poisoning, see ALKALIS, POISONING BY.)

Uses: Externally, strong ammonia produces blistering. For bee-stings, weak ammonia is applied locally to relieve the pain. (See ALKALI.) Internally it is a powerful stimulant, and therefore a teaspoonful of sal volatile in water is given, or smelling salts are applied to the nose, when fainting threatens. The chloride and the carbonate of ammonia are used as expectorants (qv), whilst the former is also a diuretic (qv).

AMNESIA means loss of memory.

AMNIOCENTESIS is the process whereby a sample of amniotic fluid (see AMNION) is obtained in order to carry out the process of examination known as amnioscopy (qv). It involves inserting a needle through the abdominal wall into the uterus usually between the 12th and 16th week of pregnancy, and withdrawing a sample of the amniotic fluid. The risk of miscarriage following amniocentesis is about 1 to 2 per cent.

Early amniocentesis between the 14th and 16th week of gestation is performed to establish the diagnosis and to terminate the pregnancy of an abnormal foetus. This investigation should only be performed if the mother is prepared to accept termination of pregnancy if the test shows that the foetus is abnormal. A raised concentration of alpha-fetoprotein is found in the amniotic fluid when the foetus has anencephally (qv) or myelomeningocele. The amniotic fluid also contains cells which have been shed from the skin of the foetus and these cells can be cultured. Examination of the cultured cells can reveal the chromosome constitution of the foetus, including the sex, and specific enzyme defects can be sought. Amniocentesis would be undertaken in women who have had a previous infant with Down's syndrome (see MONGOLISM) or in a mother aged over 40 years where the risks of Down's syndrome are considerably greater. It is also indicated in a sex-linked defect in a previous child. It is also possible to predict the risk of infants suffering from the respiraory distress syndrome (see HYALINE MEMBRANE DISEASE) as this is associated with a deficiency of pulmonary surfactant, the correlation of lecithin in the amniotic fluid correlating well with surfactant activity. The main risk of amniocentesis is that of abortion and this is about 1 per cent, or about twice the spontaneous incidence in normal pregnanacies.

AMNION is the tough fibrous membrane which lines the cavity of the womb during pregnancy, and contains from 0·5 to 1 litre (one to two pints) of fluid in which the embryo floats. It is formed from the ovum along with the embryo, and in labour the part of it at the mouth of the womb forms the 'bag of waters'. (See LABOUR.) When a child is 'born with a caul', the caul is a piece of amnion. (See CAUL.)

AMNIOSCOPY is the method whereby the fluid in the amniotic sac (see AMNION) can be assessed without interfering with the course of pregnancy. It is of value in determining hether the foetus is distressed and therefore hether or not labour should be induced, and lso in finding out whether the foetus, or nborn child, is suffering from certain congeni- l diseases, such as mongolism. It is also possi- le to say what is the sex of the child.

MNIOPLASTIN is the membrane prepared om the AMNION (qv) and used in surgery to revent, for example, the brain adhering to the cull after operations on it. The amnioplastin is laced between the skull and the brain. It is also rapped round nerves which have been oper- ted on, to prevent their being bound down by car tissue.

MODIAQUINE is a member of the 4-amino- uinoline series of substances, and is used in he prevention, and treatment, of malaria.

MOEBA is a minute protozoan organism con- isting of a single cell, in which a nucleus is urrounded by protoplasm that changes its hape as the protozoon progresses or absorbes ourishment. Several varieties are found under ifferent conditions within the human body. ne variety, *Entamoeba coli*, is found in the rge intestine of man without any associated isease; another, *Entamoeba gingivalis*, is ound in the sockets of the teeth associated ith pyorrhoea; another, *Entamoeba his- olytica*, is the causative organism of amoebic ysentery (see DYSENTERY). Two, *canthamoeba* and *Naegleria fowleri*, cause the nfection of the brain known as men- ngoencephalitis (qv). *Entamoeba histolytica* ay also cause meningoencephalitis. Other orms are found in the genital organs.

MOEBIASIS (see DYSENTERY).

MOXYCILLIN (see PENICILLIN, ANTIBIOTIC).

MPHETAMINES are a group of drugs closely elated to adrenaline and act by stimulating the ympathetic nervous system. There are now nore than fifty preparations of amphetamine ubstances.

On being inhaled, they constrict the blood- essels in the nose and so ease the congestion or stuffiness' of nasal catarrh. Their indiscrimi- ate use for this purpose is harmful and they hould only be used under medical supervision. Vhen taken by mouth they have a profound timulating effect on the brain, producing a ense of well-being and confidence and increas- ng the capacity for mental work. This effect, owever, is temporary, and its use for this pur- ose, except under medical supervision, is raught with danger.

By virtue of the fact that they inhibit appe- ite, they rapidly achieved a wide-spread repu- ation for slimming purposes. In view of the isks attached to their continued use, they are ow seldom used for this purpose. Indeed there s growing evidence that the dangers of the mphetamines, including the risk of becoming addicted to them, far outweigh their advantages.

AMPHORIC is an adjective denoting the kind of breathing heard over a cavity in the lung. The sound is like that made by blowing over the mouth of a narrow-necked vase.

AMPHOTERICIN is a mixture of antifungal substances derived from *Streptomyces nodosus*, which is proving of value in the treatment of certain of the diseases classified under the heading of mycosis (qv). It is, however, a very toxic substance and is therefore only used in those infections in which the outlook is otherwise hopeless. It is also proving of value in the treatment of certain cases of amoebic meningoencephalitis. (See MENINGOENCEPHALITIS.)

AMPICILLIN (see PENICILLIN, ANTIBIOTIC).

AMPOULE is a small glass container having one end drawn out into a point capable of being sealed so as to preserve its contents sterile. It is used for containing solutions for hypodermic injection.

AMPUTATION means the severing of any limb or part completely from the body. In the case of organs other than limbs the word excision is generally used. An amputation through a joint without sawing of bone is called a disarticulation.

Objects of amputation: In the great majority of cases a limb is amputated because it has been damaged beyond the hope of recovery. It is not always easy to say at once that a limb should, or should not, be removed after an injury, but the three chief points are, as to whether (1) extensive portions of muscle, skin, and bone are so crushed and torn as to make their death and separation inevitable; (2) the great nerves and blood-vessels are divided so as to destroy the viability of the limb; and (3) the laceration is so extensive, or involves joint cavities so as to render cleansing of the wound impossible and endanger the patient from blood-poisoning (qv) due to septic absorption. Often after gunshot wounds, crushes in machinery, or railway accidents, where a decision cannot be made at once, the injured limb is cleaned (blood-vessels tied, sinews stitched, etc.), and a careful watch maintained for some days to see if healing will take place. This is done especially in the case of the hand, where every fragment of tissue is valuable because of the delicate movements the upper limb executes, and where, fortunately, circulation by anastomosis (qv) is good. But in the lower limbs, the chief point is to have a small scar and a sound stump, so that the weight of the body can be borne, and therefore a few cms of length are, if necessary, sacrificed and amputation oftener performed. The more common sites of amputation in the lower limbs are shown in the illustration below. Site 4 is used for injuries in which the whole forefoot is mangled and for severe deformities of the foot.

Site 3, or midleg amputation, is the site of selection for injuries around the ankle, while sites 2 and 1 are reserved for more extensive injuries.

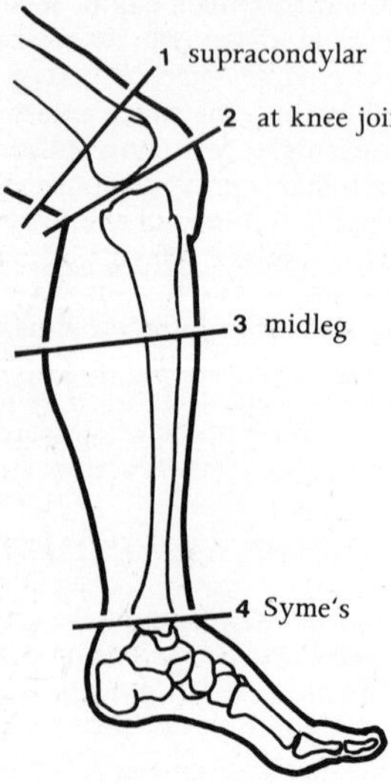

Sites for amputation.

Owing to improvements in surgery which have taken place in recent years, many injured limbs can now be saved which previously would have required to be amputated.

Methods of amputation: The *circular method* is one in which skin, muscles or flesh, and bone are cut or sawn at successively higher levels, so that the skin meets afterwards over the other tissues. It is an old method, and, being rapid, was used before the days of anaesthesia. In the *elliptical method* the tissues are divided in the form of an oblique circle, so that one side of the cut is much lower down the limb than the other. This has the advantage of bringing the resulting scar over to one side of the limb, and thus providing a better covering for the end of the sawn bone.

The *flap method* is one in which a large flap of skin and fibrous tissue is carefully dissected up from the underlying muscles, and, after the limb is removed, laid across the cut surface and stitched at its sides and end. Only one flap may be made, or more often two, which meet end to end and side to side. Sometimes the flap consists of muscle as well as of skin, and occasionally a slice of bone with its covering membrane is included in the flap so as to produce a broad surface of bone when the flap is turned into its final position, and thus to form a better support in the case of lower-limb amputations. The flap method is that most frequently used, partly because with it the scar does not fall opposite the end of the bone, and also because a limb seldom being injured at the same level all round, the formation of a flap enables a larg part to be saved.

Increasing importance is being attached the preservation of the natural knee joint whe ever possible, as this makes such a big diffe ence in allowing the patient to return to a mo or less normal life. Over the last decade t ratio of below-knee amputations to above-kn amputations has risen from 3:10 to over 6:1

Shrinkage of the stump continues for two six months after amputation and obviously permanent artificial limb or prosthesis as it now known, cannot be fitted until su shrinkage is complete. This delay has ma practical disadvantages, and it is now the ge eral practice to initiate physiotherapy immec ately after the operation and to start the patie walking with a temporary prosthesis within week. (See ARTIFICIAL LIMBS; PHANTOM LIMB.)

AMSACRINE (AMSIDINE) (see CYTOTOX DRUGS).

AMYLASE is an enzyme (qv) in pancreat juice which facilitates the conversion of star to maltose. (See PANCREAS.)

AMYL NITRITE is a volatile, oily liquid pr pared by the action of nitric and nitrous aci upon amyl alcohol. It resembles other nitrit in its power of relieving spasms and dilati blood-vessels, and it acts with great rapidi when inhaled, producing its effects in a fe seconds. (See NITROGLYCERIN.)

AMYLOIDOSIS, or WAXY DISEASE, is the co dition in which deposits of complex protei known as amyloid, are found in various par of the body. It is a degenerative conditic resulting from various causes such as chron infection, including tuberculosis and rheum toid arthritis.

AMYLOSE is the name applied to any carb hydrate of the starch group.

AMYLUM is another name for starch.

ANABOLIC STEROIDS: Nitrogen-retaini effect of androgen is responsible for the larg muscle mass of the male. This is called an an bolic effect. Attempts have been made to sep rate the anabolic effects of hormones fro their virilising effects. This is only partially su cessful. Thus anabolic steroids have the pro erty of protein building so that when taken th lead to an increase in muscle bulk and strengt All the anabolic steroids have some androgen activity but they cause less virilisations tha androgens in women. Androgenic side-effec may result from any of these anabolic con pounds, especially if they are given for pr longed periods. Norethandrolone, in additic to its anabolic effect, has a progestation action and so amenorrhoea (qv) or uteri bleeding may result from its withdrawal. A these compounds should therefore be used wi caution in women, and are contra-indicted in men with prostatic carcinoma. Jaundice due to stasis of bile in the intrahepatic canaliculi is a hazard, and the depression of pituitary gonadotrophin production is a possible complication. Norethandrolone and nandrolone phenylpropionate are the most important anabolic steroids.

Anabolic steroids have been used to stimulate protein anabolism in debilitating illness and to promote growth in children with pituitary dwarfism and other disorders associated with interference of growth. Stimulation of protein anabolism may also be of value in acute renal failure, and the retention of nitrogen and calcium is of probable benefit to patients with osteoporosis (qv) and to patients receiving corticosteroid therapy. Anabolic steroids may stimulate bone marrow function in hypoplastic anaemia.

The anabolic steroids in therapeutic use, which can be given by mouth, include: ethyloestrenol (Orabolin), norethandrolone (Nilevar), oxymetholone (Anapolon) and stanozolol (Stromba). Those that require to be given by injection include: nandrolone decanoate (Deca-Durabolin), nandrolone phenylpropionate (Durabolin) and norethandrolone (Nilevar).

ANAEMIA is the condition characterized by inadequate red blood cells and/or haemoglobin in the blood. It is considered to exist if haemoglobin levels are below 13 grams per 100 ml in males and below 12 grams per 100 ml in adult non-pregnant women. No simple classification of anaemia can be wholly accurate, but the most useful method is to divide anaemias into: (*a*) microcytic hypochromic anaemia, (*b*) megaloblastic hyperchromic anaemia, (*c*) aplastic anaemia, (*d*) haemolytic anaemia. In Britain, anaemia is much more common among women than in men. Thus, around 10 per cent of girls have anaemia at the age of 15, whilst in adult life the incidence is over 30 per cent between the ages of 30 and 40, around 20 per cent at 50, and around 30 per cent at 70. Among men the incidence is under 5 per cent until the age of 50, and it then rises to 20 per cent at the age of 70. Ninety per cent of all cases of anaemia in Britain are microcytic, 7 per cent are macrocytic, and 3 per cent are haemolytic or aplastic. (See also SICKLE-CELL ANAEMIA; SPORTS ANAEMIA; and THALASSAEMIA.)

MICROCYTIC HYPOCHROMIC ANAEMIA: This corresponds to a large extent with what used to be known as 'secondary anaemia'. It takes its name from the characteristic changes in the blood.

Causes: (1) *Loss of blood*. (*a*) As a result of trauma. This is perhaps the simplest example of all, when, as a result of an accident involving a large artery, there is severe haemorrhage.

(*b*) Menstruation. The regular monthly loss of blood which women sustain as a result of menstruation always puts a strain on the blood-forming organs. If this loss is excessive, then over a period of time it may lead to quite severe anaemia.

(*c*) Child-birth. A considerable amount of blood is always lost at child-birth, and if this is severe, or if the woman was anaemic during pregnancy, a severe degree of anaemia may develop.

(*d*) Bleeding from the gastro-intestinal tract. The best example here is anaemia due to 'bleeding piles' (see PILES). Such bleeding, even though slight, if maintained over a long period of time, is a common cause of anaemia in both men and women. The haemorrhage may be more acute and occur from a duodenal or gastric ulcer, when it is known as haematemesis (qv).

(*e*) Certain blood diseases, such as purpura (qv) and haemophilia (qv), which are characterized by bleeding.

(2) *Defective blood formation*: (*a*) This is the main cause of anaemia in infections. The micro-organism responsible for the infection has a deleterious effect upon the blood-forming organs, just as it does upon other parts of the body.

(*b*) Toxins. In conditions such as chronic glomerulonephritis and uraemia there is a severe anaemia due to the effect of the disease upon blood formation.

(*c*) Drugs. Certain drugs, such as aspirin and the non-steroidal anti-inflammatory drugs, may cause occult gastro-intestinal bleeding.

(3) *Inadequate intake of iron*: The daily requirement of iron for an adult is 12 mg, and 15 to 20 mg during pregnancy. This is well covered by an ordinary diet, so that by itself it is not a common cause. But if there is a steady loss of blood, as a result of heavy menstrual loss or 'bleeding piles', the intake of iron in the diet may not be sufficient to maintain adequate formation of haemoglobin.

(4) *Inadequate absorption of iron*: This may occur in diseases of intestinal malabsorption.

In many cases the anaemia is found to be due to a combination of two or more of these causes. A severe form of this anaemia in women, known as CHLOROSIS, used to be common, but it is seldom seen nowadays.

Symptoms: These depend upon whether the anaemia is sudden in onset, as in severe haemorrhage, or gradual. In all cases, however, the striking sign is pallor, the depth of which depends upon the severity of the anaemia. The colour of the skin may be misleading, except in cases due to severe haemorrhage, as the skin of many people is normally pale. The best guide is the colour of the internal lining of the eyelid. When the onset of the anaemia is sudden the patient complains of weakness and giddiness, and he loses consciousness if he tries to stand or sit up. The breathing is rapid and distressed, the pulse is rapid, and the blood-pressure is low. In chronic cases the tongue is often sore (glossitis), and the nails of the fingers may be brittle and concave instead of convex (koilonychia). In some cases, particularly in women, the Plummer-Vinson syndrome is present. This consists of difficulty in swallowing and may be accompanied by huskiness; in these cases glossitis is also present. There may be slight enlargement of the spleen, and there is usually some diminution in gastric acidity.

Changes in the blood: The characteristic change is a diminution in both the haemoglobin and the red cell content of the blood. There is a relatively greater fall in the haemoglobin than in the red cell count. If the blood is examined under a microscope the red cells are seen to be paler and smaller than normal. These small red cells are known as microcytes.

Treatment consists primarily of giving sufficient iron by mouth to restore, and then maintain, a normal blood picture. The main iron preparation now used is ferrous sulphate, 200 mg, thrice daily after meals. When the blood picture has become normal, the dosage is gradually reduced. A preparation of iron is now available which can be given intravenously, but this is only used in cases which do not respond to iron given by mouth, or in cases in which it is essential to obtain a quick response.

If, of course, there is haemorrhage, this must be arrested, and if the loss of blood has been severe it may be necessary to give a blood transfusion. Care must be taken to ensure that the patient is having an adequate diet, and a period of rest in hospital, followed by a holiday, is often beneficial. If there is any underlying toxic or infective condition, this, of course, must be adequately treated.

MEGALOBLASTIC HYPERCHROMIC ANAEMIA: There are various forms of anaemia of this type, such as those due to nutritional but the most important is that known as PERNICIOUS ANAEMIA.

PERNICIOUS ANAEMIA: Up until about fifty years ago its cause was unknown and it was an invariably fatal disease. In 1926, two Americans, G. R. Minot and W. P. Murphy, reported that pernicious anaemia responded to treatment with liver. This discovery ranks in importance with that of insulin in the treatment of diabetes mellitus. This form of treatment is based upon the now well-proved fact that pernicious anaemia is due to lack of what is known as the *intrinsic factor*. For the formation of normal red blood corpuscles a substance known as the extrinsic factor is necessary. The efficient absorption of this factor into the body is dependent on the presence of intrinsic factor which is produced normally by the mucosa lining the distal part of the stomach. It is the inability of the patient to produce the intrinsic factor that leads to the onset of pernicious anaemia. In a normal person with adequate amounts of intrinsic factor, approximately 70 per cent of the extrinsic factor (which is vitamin B and is present in meat and other foods) in the daily diet is absorbed into the body. In patients with pernicious anaemia, however, less than 2 per cent is absorbed.

Symptoms: Pernicious anaemia is a disease of middle age, being rare under the age of 40 years. It affects both men and women. The onset is usually insidious, so that the anaemia is usually well developed before medical advice is sought. In addition to the general symptoms and signs already described in the section on microcytic anaemia, the important features of pernicious anaemia are as follows. The patient, who is often prematurely grey-haired, has a characteristic lemon-yellow complexion. The tongue is often sore and appears thinner, smoother, and redder than usual. There is often soreness and excoriation of the corners of the mouth – a condition known as cheilosis. There may be slight enlargement of the spleen. There is a complete absence of free hydrochloric acid in the stomach, even after the injection of histamine.

One of the most serious complications of pernicious anaemia is a disease with the cumbersome title of SUBACUTE COMBINED DEGENERATION OF THE CORD. This, as the name indicates, is a degenerative condition of the spinal cord, and the importance of recognizing its onset is that it can be cured by adequate treatment of the anaemia. Its early manifestations are a sensation of tingling or 'pins and needles' in the legs, accompanied by stiffness. Later, if untreated, the stiffness becomes progressively worse, finally leading to paralysis.

Changes in the blood: The red cells are larger than normal, ie. macrocytes and they appear to be redder than normal. They also vary in shape (*poikilocytosis*) and in size (*anisocytosis*). Occasionally a few primitive red cells (normoblasts) may be found. The total white cell count is diminished: ie. there is leucopenia. The final diagnosis depends upon an examination of the bone marrow, which is found to contain megaloblasts.

Treatment consists of the administration of vitamin B in the form of hydroxocobalamin. It is given by injection. It must always be remembered that a patient with pernicious anaemia requires to take vitamin B for the rest of his or her life.

APLASTIC ANAEMIA is a disease in which the red blood corpuscles are very greatly reduced and in which no attempt appears to be made in the bone marrow towards their regeneration. It is more accurately called hypoplastic anaemia as the degree of impairment of bone marrow function is rarely complete. The cause in many cases is not known, but in rather less than half the cases the condition is due to some toxic substance, such as benzol or certain drugs, or ionizing radiations. The patient becomes very pale, with a tendency to haemorrhages under the skin and mucous membranes, and the temperature may at times be raised. The red blood corpuscles diminish steadily in numbers. Treatment consists primarily of regular blood transfusions. Although the disease is often fatal, the outlook has improved in recent years. About 25 per cent of patients recover when adequately treated, and others survive for several years. In severe cases promising sults are being reported from the use of bone arrow transplantation.

AEMOLYTIC ANAEMIA results from the ccessive destruction, or haemolysis (qv), of e red blood cells. This haemolysis may be due undue fragility of the red blood cells, when e condition is known as congenital aemolytic anaemia, or acholuric jaundice.

NAEROBE is the term applied to bacteria aving the power to live without air. Such orga-isms are found growing freely, deep in the soil, s, for example, the tetanus bacillus.

NAESTHESIA means loss of the power of eling. The word is applied either to loss over a mited area of skin produced by certain ner-ous diseases, by freezing, or by local anaes-etic drugs such as procaine, or to a total loss f feeling and consciousness, in the state pro-uced by a general anaesthetic. When only loss f the sense of pain is meant, without loss of the ense of touch, the correct term is analgesia.

NAESTHETICS are drugs and other mea-ures which produce insensibility to external npressions.

hoice of anaesthetic: At the present day there is large range of anaesthetics to choose from. Many of these require complicated apparatus or their administration, whilst others are otentially dangerous unless used by an exper-enced anaesthetist. The choice of anaesthetic n any one particular case often requires con-iderable judgment, and, except with a highly killed anaesthetist, the sound working rule is hat the doctor should use the anaesthetic of which he has had most experience. In the case f the general practitioner called upon in an mergency to administer an anaesthetic for a urgical operation, this usually means ether or hloroform.

The following is a useful classification of the resent range of anaesthetics.

OLATILE ANAESTHETICS: These include ther, chloroform, nitrous oxide, ethyl chlo-ide, vinyl ether, trichloroethylene, cyclopro-ane and halothane. The last four should only e used by anaesthetists experienced in their se. Mixtures of chloroform and ether are ometimes used. Nitrous oxide has two great dvantages: the patient recovers quickly from he anaesthetic, and there is relatively little ausea and vomiting. Its use for major surgical perations, however, requires considerable kill and special apparatus, and for this purpose herefore it can only be used by an experienced naesthetist. It is now tending to be replaced by yclopropane. Nitrous oxide is an excellent naesthetic for minor surgical operations, for entistry, and in midwifery, but in the first of hese it is tending to be replaced by the basal arcotics. It is often used in endotracheal naesthesia: ie. when the anaesthetic is intro-uced directly into the lungs by means of a tube assed into the trachea. Endotracheal anaes-hesia is employed in operations in the head or neck where a mask or any other anaesthetic apparatus would get in the way of the surgeon. Ethyl chloride is seldom used to maintain anaesthesia; it is more commonly used to induce anaesthesia, especially in children.

BASAL NARCOTICS: These are used to induce anaesthesia, without any distress to the patient, preliminary to the use of some other anaesthetic, under the influence of which the operation in question is to be carried out. In practice they have removed many of the terrors of anaesthesia, so far as the patient is concerned, as they induce loss of consciousness so quickly and painlessly. It is seldom safe to use these basal narcotics to produce a degree of anaesthesia which is sufficient to permit of operations being performed without the addition of some other anaesthetic. They are given either per rectum or intravenously. Thiopentone sodium is the one most commonly used at the present day.

STEROID ANAESTHETICS: Some years ago it was discovered that a state of anaesthesia could be induced by large doses of steroid hormones. Derivatives of these hormones have now been prepared in which the anaesthetic action can be obtained without the hormone action. These include hydroxydione and Althesin.

LOCAL ANAESTHETICS are given by injection to induce loss of sensation in the area to be operated upon, without any general loss of consciousness. For major operations they are more commonly used on the Continent than in this country. Cocaine was the first local anaesthetic to be used, but on account of its toxic properties it has been almost entirely replaced by synthetic preparations. These include procaine hydrochloride, lignocaine and cinchocaine hydrochloride.

SPINAL ANAESTHETICS are used when it is considered inadvisable to induce general anaesthesia and local anaesthesia is contra-indicated. Their two main advantages are that they can be used in patients with diseases of the lung in whom a general anaesthetic may lead to complications, and that they produce excellent relaxation of the muscles. The same anaesthetics are used as for inducing local anaesthesia, with the exception of cocaine, which is never used as a spinal anaesthetic. The solution is injected into the spinal canal by the same technique as in use for lumbar puncture (qv).

EPIDURAL ANAESTHESIA is a form of anaesthesia predominantly used to relieve the severity of labour pains. It is induced by the injection of a local anaesthetic such as lignocaine into the extradural space (see SPINAL CORD).

Stages of anaesthesia: Whatever the anaesthetic employed, the effects are much the same, though some symptoms are more prominent with one anaesthetic, others with another, and in the case of basal narcotics the initial stages are hurried over and the patient plunged almost at once into deep unconsciousness.

STAGE I: There is great rapidity of thought, but disturbance of judgment and power of control. Giddiness, tingling, and other peculiar or pleasant sensations are felt. The patient may be emotional, or may sing, shout or struggle, and then passes off into a dreamy state, with partial loss of sensation. The heart's action becomes stronger and the pupils dilate.
STAGE II: There is a complete loss of consciousness. The speech becomes unintelligible, changing to a mere muttering. There may be muscular spasms of various sorts, also coughing, retching and possibly vomiting. The pupils become small.
STAGE III: There is absolute unconsciousness and complete muscular relaxation, and in this stage surgical operations are performed. The heart's action is weakened, most reflex movements abolished, and the pupil dilates again but is still capable of contracting when the eyelid is raised so that light enters the eye.
STAGE IV: This is the stage of danger; the breathing becomes shallow, the face pallid or livid, the heart weak and irregular, and the pupils widely dilated. If the anaesthetic is not at once removed, breathing and pulse then stop and the person dies.
Uses of anaesthetics: The most evident use of anaesthetics is to relieve the pain of surgical operations and of convulsive diseases. Their use has made possible much more prolonged and delicate operations than could be performed upon the conscious and suffering body. An anaesthetic is also an aid in diagnosis, particularly of abdominal conditions, producing muscular relaxation and allowing the free handling of painful regions. Anaesthetics are also used in medical practice to quiet violent spasmodic states, as in a succession of epileptic fits, in lock-jaw, and in strychnine poisoning. (For the use of local anaesthetics, see ANALGESICS.) (See also CURARE.)

ANALEPTIC means a restorative medicine, or one which acts as a stimulant of the central nervous system: for example caffeine.

ANALGESIA means loss of the power to feel pain without loss of consciousness: eg. in some nervous diseases or due to some drugs. (See also AUDIOANALGESIA; CRYOANALGESIA.)

ANALGESICS are drugs or other measures which cause temporary loss of the sense of pain without unconsciousness and without necessarily loss of the sense of touch. Some act generally on the brain or the nerves to dull pain which is already present (see ANODYNES); others act locally, such as cocaine, benzocaine, procaine and the process of freezing, which are used to prevent pain which would otherwise necessarily be caused by operations. In a position between that of a general anaesthetic and a local analgesic stand drugs such as morphine and scopolamine which are used for the production of a torpid, semi-insensible state like that sometimes used in child-birth (see TWILIGHT SLEEP).

Uses: Local insensibility to pain may be produced in a considerable variety of ways, but most of these fall into one of four classes: (1) infiltration of the region to be operated upon by a solution of the analgesic drug; (2) injection of the solution into or near the nerve trunks which convey the sensations of the part; (3) painting, spraying, or rubbing the surface, especially of mucous membrane, with the drug; and (4) the application of intense cold.

The first drug to be used for local anaesthesia or analgesia in operations was cocaine, which has certain disadvantages in that it is destroyed by boiling, is a dangerous drug of addiction and readily causes symptoms of poisoning, so that it cannot be safely used in doses over 30 mg. Procaine, which is an artificially prepared substance, has largely displaced cocaine because it is many times less poisonous and so can be used in larger doses. Amethocaine is largely used for spinal analgesia. One of the most widely used local anaesthetics at the present moment is lignocaine.

When *infiltration analgesia* is employed, a weak solution of procaine is generally used to which a small amount of adrenaline is added. A long hypodermic needle is used to inject this solution in large quantity into and especially around the part upon which the operation is to be performed. By this means tumours can be removed, the abdomen opened, and similar serious operations, which do not involve great shock to the patient and in which general unconsciousness is not desirable, can be performed.

When general loss of sensation in a region is to be brought about by injecting a nerve trunk or its neighbourhood, stronger solutions (eg procaine 2 per cent) are used in similar quantities. The large nerves of a limb are sometimes treated in this way for the prevention of the shock caused by a severe operation, even when a general anaesthetic is also employed. This method is much used for painless tooth extraction. The two methods of infiltration and regional analgesia are often combined: for example, to perform amputations below the knee or elbow or in removal of a goitre.

Another way of applying the injection method is by *spinal analgesia*, in which sensation is abolished temporarily in the lower limbs by injection of the drug into the spinal canal.

The *surface application* of analgesics is in general only useful in cases in which operations are to be performed upon mucous membranes such as those of the nose or throat, where cocaine and benzamine can readily be applied by painting or spraying.

A transitory analgesia is produced by *freezing* the skin. This is usually effected by spraying a small area with ethyl chloride, which very quickly evaporates, with the production of intense cold.

ANALYSIS means a separation into component parts by determination of the chemical constituents of a substance. The process of analysis is carried out by various means: eg. chromatographic analysis by means of the adsorption column; colorimetric analysis by means of various colour tests; densimetric analysis by estimation of the specific gravity; gasometric analysis by estimating the different gases given off in some process; polariscope analysis by means of the polariscope; volumetric analysis by measuring volumes of liquids. Analysis is also sometimes used as an abbreviation for psycho-analysis (qv).

ANAMNESIS is the term applied to the statement of the past history of some particular case of disease.

ANAPHYLAXIS is a condition of excessive sensitiveness exhibited by certain persons or animals to the injection of foreign material into their tissues. A common example is the pain, swelling, eruption, feverishness and general prostration which occasionally follow the injection of serum containing diphtheria or tetanus antitoxin. An example of a slighter form of anaphylaxis is afforded by people who suffer from nettle-rash, asthma, and similar symptoms when they take some food of which their system is intolerant, or by other people who present similar symptoms when exposed to the emanations of certain animals, eg. horses, cats or fowls. There is an acute form, fortunately rare, known as anaphylactic shock which may occur within minutes of the injection of certain drugs or vaccines to which the injected individual is hypersensitive. It is characterized by severe shortness of breath, marked fall in blood-pressure and acute urticaria (qv). Treatment consists of the immediate intramuscular injection of 1 ml of adrenaline B.P. (See ADRENALINE; ALLERGY.)

ANAPLASIA means the state in which a body cell loses its distinctive characters and takes on a more primitive form; it occurs, for example, in cancer, when cells proliferate rapidly.

ANASARCA is a condition of general dropsy.

ANASTOMOSIS is a term describing the means by which the circulation is carried on when large vessels are narrowed or closed, as by pressure. In the limbs, especially around joints, and in internal organs, small arteries open freely into their neighbours to form a network from which the smallest vessels carry off the blood. By this means pressure from one side, or even the ligature of the main artery to a limb, is prevented from stopping the flow of blood to any part, because so soon as one artery is closed, the other arteries of the limb dilate, through relaxation of their muscle fibres, and the supply of blood passes on as before, but by new channels. Anastomosis is also a term describing the joining together (by operation) of any two parts of the alimentary tract or of blood-vessels.

ANATOMY is the science which deals with the structure of the bodies of men and animals. Brief descriptions of the anatomy of each important organ are given under the headings of the various organs. It is studied by dissection of bodies bequeathed for the purpose or of the bodies of those who die in hospitals and similar institutions, unclaimed by relatives.

ANATOXIN is another name for toxoid (qv).

ANCROD is an enzyme (qv) present in the venom of the Malayan pit viper which destroys the fibrinogen in blood and thereby prevents the blood clotting. In other words it is an anticoagulant (qv).

ANCYLOSTOMIASIS is the parasitic infestation caused by two nematodes, *Ancylostoma duodenale* and *Necator americanus*, perhaps better known as the hookworm. The former is also known as the tunnel-worm on account of the ravages it caused among the men at work on the St Gotthard tunnel. They produce great anaemia, debility, and cardiac weakness, sometimes leading to death. The disease is widespread in the tropics and subtropics, as well as certain mines in Europe. The estimated world prevalence is 700 million cases. *Ancylostoma duodenale* occurs in the Far East, the Mediterranean littoral and the Middle East, whilst *Necator americanus* is found in East, West and Central Africa, Central and South America and the Far East. In recent years these geographical demarcations have been largely broken down. The worms are about 12 mm) (½ inch) long, and inhabit the upper part of the small intestine, often in great numbers; here they embed themselves in the mucous membrane lining the bowel. In certain parts of India it is so common that about 75 per cent of the population are said to be affected; it is also very common in Egypt. The worms embedded in the small intestine produce an enormous number of eggs which pass from the body in the stools; the embryos, finding their way into water, mud, or damp earth, develop rapidly and can maintain their vitality for weeks or months, if moisture is present. In the insanitary conditions so widespread in the areas where the disease occurs, the embryos gain access to the human host through the skin – usually the feet. They may also gain access through the drinking of polluted water. Ultimately, through the bloodstream and the lungs, they gain access to the intestine, where they develop. The disease is a very serious one, partly in consequence of the numbers of people prevented from working by the debility it causes, and partly because death in such debilitated persons is not uncommon.

Treatment: The most effective remedies are tetrachloroethylene, bephenium hydroxynaphthoate, pyrantel embonate, and mebendazole. The anaemia which always accompanies chronic infestation with ancylostoma also needs intensive treatment.

ANDROGEN is the general term for any one of a group of hormones which govern the development of the sexual organs and the secondary sexual characteristics of the male. Testosterone, the androgenic hormone formed in the interstitial cells of the testis, controls the development and maintenance of the male sex organs and secondary sex characteristics. In small doses it increases the number of spermatozoa produced, but in large doses it inhibits the gonadotrophic activity of the anterior pituitary gland and suppresses the formation of the spermatozoa. It is both androgenic and anabolic in action. The anabolic effect includes the ability to stimulate protein synthesis and to diminish the catabolism of amino acids, and this is associated with retention of nitrogen, potassium, phosphorus and calcium. Doses in excess of 10 mg daily to the female may produce virilism.

Unconjugated testosterone is rarely used clinically because its derivatives have a more powerful and prolonged effect, and testosterone itself requires implantation into the subcutaneous fat, using a trocar and cannula for maximum therapeutic benefit. Testosterone propionate is prepared in an oily solution, as it is insoluble in water. It is effective for three days and is therefore administered intramuscularly twice weekly. Testosterone phenylpropionate is a long-acting micro-crystalline preparation, which, when given by intramuscular or subcutaneous injection, is effective for two weeks. Methyl-testosterone is only weakly active by mouth though it is absorbed sublingually. It does however produce a cholestatic jaundice in a significant proportion of patients and is therefore better avoided. Mesterolone is an effective oral androgen and is less hepatoxic. It does not inhibit pituitary gonadotrophic production and hence spermatogenesis is unimpaired. Testosterone undecanoate (Restandol) has recently been introduced and may well prove to be the oral androgen of choice.

The androgens in therapeutic use which can be given by mouth include: mesterolone (Pro-Viron), methyltestosterone (Virormone), testosterone (Testoral), testosterone undecanoate (Restandol). Those that can be given by injection include: testosterone propionate (Virormone), testosterone phenylpropionate, testosterone enanthate (Primoteston Depot), testosterone esters (Sustanon) and drostanolone (Masteril).

ANENCEPHALY is the term given to the condition in which a child is born with a defect of the skull and absence of the brain. Anencephaly is the most common major malformation of the central nervous system. It has an incidence of 0·65 per 1,000 live births. There is complete absence of the cerebral hemispheres and overlying skull and the brain stem and cerebellum are atrophic. If the pregnancy goes to term the infants rapidly die but in 50 per cent of pregnancies associated with anencephaly spontaneous abortion occurs. It is possible to detect the presence of anencephaly in the foetus by measuring the level of alpha foeto protein in the mother's serum or in the amniotic fluid. (See SPINA BIFIDA.)

ANEUPLOIDY is the state in which there is an abnormal number of chromosomes (qv): eg mongolism (qv) and Turner's syndrome (qv).

ANEURINE is an alternative name for vitamin B_1. (See THIAMINE.)

ANEURYSM means a dilatation upon an artery, due to yielding of the vessel-wall and gradual stretching by the pressure of the blood. They are called *dissecting* when the inner coat has given way somewhat suddenly and blood has passed between the coats and torn its way some distance along the vessel wall; *miliary* when the aneurysm is very small and looks like a millet seed on the side of the vessel, which is a form often found on the vessels in the brain. An *arteriovenous aneurysm* is one where there is a communication between an artery and a vein.

Causes: The two main factors responsible for the formation of an aneurysm are (1) strain; (2) weakening of the wall of the artery. The latter is the more important. No amount of strain, whether due to a raised blood-pressure or to muscular effort, will lead to aneurysm formation unless there is some local weakening of the wall of the artery. The two most important causes of weakening of the arterial wall are atheroma (qv) and syphilis (qv). Most aneurysms of the thoracic aorta are due to syphilis. Atheroma is the more common cause of aneurysms in the abdominal aorta. Aneurysms may also be due to loss of the support provided by the surrounding tissues, eg. in the lungs, where an aneurysm may form in one of the branches of the pulmonary artery as a result of destruction of the surrounding tissue by tuberculosis. Occasionally they may be due to congenital defects in the arterial wall: the most common site for such aneurysms is the circle of Willis (qv) at the base of the brain. More rarely they may arise as a result of repeated small trauma and strain in exposed arteries, such as the popliteal artery, which have not much support from the surrounding tissues; popliteal aneurysms were more common in the old coaching days among those who spent most of their working lives on horseback. Small aneurysms, known as *mycotic* aneurysms, may also arise in cases of severe sepsis, as a result of infection of the arterial wall. Aneurysms are more common in men than in women, and particularly among those who perform in hard physical labour.

Symptoms: These vary greatly with the size and position of the aneurysm, but there are some which are characteristic of all forms. If the aneurysm is in a limb, a round *swelling* i noticed, perhaps as large as a walnut or Mandarin orange, which expands and diminishes with each heart-beat. The swelling is generally painless, and the skin over it is unchanged (unlike an abscess). Aneurysms rarely occur farther from the trunk than the elbow or knee. If the aneurysm be internal it is situated upon a great vessel, and is often very large in size before it causes any definite symptoms, which are mainly due to interference with surrounding organs. *Pain* is felt only when the swelling presses upon nerves, upon the air passages, causing great breathlessness, or upon bone, wearing it gradually away. In the latter case pain may be agonizing, although in early cases it is not infrequently taken for mere rheumatic pain. *Breathlessness* or *difficulty in swallowing* may occur where there is a large thoracic aneurysm, from pressure on the windpipe or gullet, also *cough* of a barking, irritating nature, and changes in the voice, from irritation or paralysis of the left recurrent laryngeal nerve. In thoracic and abdominal aneurysm there may be a *bulging* in the upper part of chest or abdomen, as the case may be, which can be felt to throb when one hand is placed on it in front and the other on the back; in a later stage pulsation can also be seen. The *aneurysmal tippet* is the name given to a network of dilated veins which appears upon the chest and shoulders, owing to obstruction of the circulation through the great veins, by a thoracic aneurysm. *Swelling of the skin* or oedema is found with all aneurysms sooner or later from the same cause. Many other signs, such as inequality of the pupils, difference in the pulse on the two sides of the body, and murmurs heard over the swelling, are present in different aneurysms, but can be appreciated only by the trained observer. Congenital aneurysms of the circle of Willis usually cause no symptoms unless they rupture. This results in subarachnoid haemorrhage (qv) or sudden death. By rupturing they are a not uncommon cause of sudden death in apparently healthy young people after exercise.

Treatment: (*a*) MEDICAL: Although the aneurysm tends constantly to increase in size, another tendency is for the blood in contact with the unhealthy wall to clot. If this is encouraged, the aneurysm may become a solid mass, which practically may be looked on as a cure, because there is no more tendency to grow or to burst. If the aneurysm is syphilitic in origin, penicillin is given.

(*b*) SURGICAL: Tremendous advances have been achieved in recent years in the surgical treatment of aneurysms. In many cases, as in aneurysms of arteries in the limbs, all that is required is to ligature the artery above and below the aneurysm, the circulation to the limb being maintained by anastomosis (qv) of the other arteries in the limb. In the case of other major arteries, such as the aorta, the aneurysm is replaced by a graft so that the circulation through the artery can be maintained. This graft may consist of a piece of an artery removed from a cadaver, or of synthetic material such as orlon.

ANGINA means literally choking, and is a term applied to swellings of the throat or other cause of difficulty in breathing, as *tonsillar angina* or quinsy, *laryngeal angina* or laryngitis, *membranous angina* or croup, *anginal scarlatina* or scarlet fever with abscesses round the throat.

ANGINA PECTORIS is a term applied to a painful sensation in the chest, arising for the most part in connection with disease of the coronary arteries.

Causes: Angina pectoris is generally held to be due to an inadequate blood-supply to the myocardium: ie. the heart muscle. The myocardium receives its blood-supply through the coronary arteries. Thus angina pectoris may be due to spasm of the coronary arteries or to narrowing of the lumen of these arteries as a result of arteriosclerosis (qv) or atheroma (qv). It is sometimes due to spasm alone. In the majority of cases it is due either to spasm plus arteriosclerosis (or atheroma) or to arteriosclerosis (or atheroma). Occasionally the defective blood-supply may be the result of disease of the first part of the aorta or of the aortic valve. Because of its association with coronary artery disease, angina pectoris is predominantly a disease of middle age and is more common in men than in women.

Symptoms: The characteristic feature of angina pectoris is the occurrence of pain behind the chest-bone, arising as a result of exertion and relieved by rest. This pain often spreads into the left arm. The amount of exertion necessary to induce the pain varies considerably, and to a certain extent gives some idea of the severity of the condition. Thus, it may only occur on hurrying, whilst in other cases the blood-supply to the myocardium may be so defective that the least exertion, eg. turning over in bed, may be sufficient to induce a severe paroxysm of pain. Aggravating factors are exposure to cold, or exertion immediately following a meal. The paroxysm of pain seldom lasts for more than a few minutes, provided the affected individual remains at complete rest. In most instances the pain is so severe that the affected individual is unable to continue any exertion.

Treatment: The aim of treatment is to prevent the occurrence of pain by persuading the patient to restrict his activities. Thus, he should always rest for at least half an hour after a meal. He should always be warmly clad when he goes out of doors in cold weather. In more severe cases his bedroom should be on the ground floor and should be warmed in the winter. He should always allow himself plenty of time so that he never needs to hurry. If he is overweight he should restrict his diet so as to bring his weight down. Even with all these precautions, attacks of pain may still occur, and for the relief of these glyceryl trinitrate tablets B.P., or trinitrin tablets as they are also known, each containing 500 micrograms, are the most satisfactory. A tablet should be placed in the mouth, as soon as pain is felt, and allowed to melt in the mouth. It should not be swallowed intact, as this delays the onset of relief. Most patients with angina pectoris carry a small supply of these tablets about with them wherever they go, so that they are always available for immediate use. As they tend to lose their potency if not carefully stored, they should be kept in the air-tight container in which they are dispensed, and this should be stored in a cool dry place. A useful guide as to their potency is that a tablet should produce a slight burning sensation when placed under the tongue; if this does not occur a new supply should be obtained. A preparation of glyceryl trinitrate is now available which is applied to the skin once a day and thereby maintains a steady absorption of the drug into the body. It is proving of value in more severe cases in which a steady supply of the drug is necessary to keep the pain under control. An alternative form of treatment is amyl nitrite, which is supplied in the form of small glass 'perles'. One of these, held in a handkerchief, is broken between the fingers and the contents then inhaled. Whilst usually as effective as trinitrin tablets, amyl nitrite is more liable to produce unpleasant side-effects such as headache and giddiness. The precise mode of action of these two preparations is still rather obscure, but all the evidence suggests that they act by reducing the demand of the heart muscle for oxygen. Other drugs used in the treatment of angina pectoris include propranolol (qv), perhexiline, and nifedipine.

Many surgical operations have been recommended for the relief of angina pectoris but few, if any, of them have lived up to the original claims made for them. Recently, however, promising results have been reported with severe cases which were resistant to all forms of medicinal relief, by a grafting operation bypassing the blockage in the coronary arteries.

ANGIOCARDIOGRAPHY means X-raying of the heart after injection into it of a radio-opaque substance.

ANGIOGRAPHY means rendering the blood-vessels visible on an X-ray film by injecting into them a radio-opaque substance. In the case of arteries this is know as *arteriography*; the corresponding term for veins being *venography* or *phlebography*. This procedure demonstrates whether there is any narrowing of the lumen of the vessel.

ANGIOMA is a tumour composed of blood-vessels. (See TUMOUR and NAEVUS.)

ANGIONEUROTIC OEDEMA is a painless swelling in the sub-cutaneous tissues or the sub-mucosa, usually occuring around the face and especially affecting the eyes, lips and tongue. It is similar in many ways to nettle rash (qv). It is caused primarily by food allergy. There is also an hereditary form which is transmitted as an autosomal dominant trait and is due to an enzyme deficiency that inactivates one of the mediators of inflammation called Complement.

ANGIOTENSIN is one of the factors responsible for hypertension, or high blood-pressure. (See ESSENTIAL HYPERTENSION; RENIN.)

ANGIOTENSIN-CONVERTING ENZYME INHIBITORS: The enzyme that converts angiotensin 1 to angiotensin 11 is called angiotensin-converting enzyme. Angiotensin 11 is the most potent endogenous pressor substance produced in the body whilst angiotensin 1 has no such pressor activity. Inhibition of the enzyme that converts angiotensin 1 to angiotensin 11 will thus have marked effects on lowering the blood pressure. Captopril was the first angiotensin inhibitor to be synthesised. It lowers peripheral resistance by causing arteriolar dilatation and thus lowers blood pressure. Enalapril is the most recent angiotensin-converting enzyme inhibitor. It has the advantage of only having to be taken once daily.

ANGITIS, or ANGIITIS, means inflammation of a vessel such as a blood-vessel, lymph-vessel, or bile-duct.

ÅNGSTRÖM UNIT (called after the Swedish physicist) is a measurement of length and equals 1/10000 micrometre, or one-hundred-millionth of a centimetre. It is represented by the symbol Å and is used to give the length of electro-magnetic waves.

ANIDROSIS is the condition in which there is an abnormal diminution in the secretion of sweat.

ANISE, or ANISEED, is the dried fruit of *Pimpinellaanisum*, from which is obtained a volatile oil used as a flavouring agent in some mixtures, as a mild expectorant, and as a remedy for colic in children. (See OILS.)

ANISOCYTOSIS: This refers to a variation in the size of red blood cells.

ANKLE is the joint between the leg bones (tibia and fibula) above, and the talus (the Roman dice-bone) below. It is a very strong joint with powerful ligaments binding the bones together at either side, many sinews running over it, and bony projections from the leg bones, which form large bosses on either side, called the outer and inner malleoli, extending about 12 mm (half an inch) below the actual joint. Two common injuries near the ankle are a sprain, on the inner side, consisting of tearing of the internal ligament; and fracture of the fibula (Pott's fracture) on the outer side. (See also JOINT DISEASES.)

ANKYLOSING SPONDYLITIS (see SPINE, DISEASES AND INJURIES OF).

ANKYLOSIS is a term meaning the condition of a joint in which the movements are restricted by fibrous bands, or by malformation, or by actual union of the bones. (See JOINT DISEASES.)

ANKYLOSTOMA (see ANCYLOSTOMA).

ANODYNES are curative measures which soothe pain. They act by removing the cause of pain, by soothing the irritated nerves of the painful part, or by paralysing the part of the brain by which the painful impression is received. Substances which destroy the power of feeling altogether are called anaesthetics (qv), those which destroy only the power of feeling pain are analgesics (qv).
Varieties: Alkaline applications are anodynes to bee-stings. Prolonged application of either cold or heat is an anodyne in inflammation. Chloroform, camphor and menthol are local anodynes, while internally various synthetic products like aspirin soothe pain in distant parts.
Uses: Opium is the oldest and most powerful anodyne, but can only be used in cases of excessive pain, because of its tendency to habit-formation. Barbiturates dull pain, but with it the mental faculties, so that they also interfere with the performance of everyday duties. Aspirin and paracetamol seem to have the power of dulling only that part of the brain which perceives the pain, and so are most suitable in slighter pains which do not incapacitate though they interfere with ordinary duties. (For further details, see NEURALGIA; HEADACHE; INFLAMMATION; and the various drugs named.)

ANOPHELES is the generic name of a widely distributed group of mosquitoes, certain species of which transmit to man the infecting agent of malaria. *Anopheles maculipennis* and *A. bifurcatus* are both found in England and can both transmit the malaria parasite.

ANOREXIA means loss of appetite. (See APPETITE.)

ANOREXIA NERVOSA is a condition that occurs predominantly in girls in their teens following the onset of puberty. Believing themselves to be overweight, they start dieting but carry this to excess. Even when they have lost a third or more of their weight, they persist in seeking to attain an even lower weight by methods such as inducing vomiting, the abuse of laxatives and excessive exercise. They are consumed with guilt if they eat anything, and are resistant to all appeals, entreaties, bribes or threats. It may occur in older or younger girls or women, and it is rare in males. In a survey of London schools in 1976, the prevalence was found to be 1 in 100 in 16–18 year-old girls in private schools and 1 in 550 in comprehensive schools. The incidence has increased significantly in the last twenty or thirty years.

The precise cause is obscure, but it is predominantly a psychological condition. One view is that the condition represents a 'psychobiological regression' for females who are ill-prepared to meet the responsibilities of adulthood, particularly of adult sexuality. Physically the sufferers revert to a non-menstruating, child-like state, and psychologically many feelings, including sexual ones, are suppressed as a consequence of the starvation'. There is also evidence that some of the victims over-estimate their size, this being more marked the more emaciated they become. Family relationships also play a part. It is a serious condition, with a mortality of around 5 per cent, suicide being the commonest cause of death. Recovery occurs in around 40 per cent of cases. Treatment consists of admission to hospital with close nursing supervision. Recovery is a slow tedious affair, and includes psychotherapy, including family therapy, which is maintained on an outpatient basis once the phobia for food has been overcome.

Those suffering from this condition and their relatives can obtain help and advice from Anorexic Family Aid, Sackville Place, 44 Magdalen Street, Norwich, Norfolk NR3 1JE (0603-621414). (See BULIMIA NERVOSA.)

ANOREXIANT DRUGS reduce appetite. Many of them are synthetic sympathomimetic amines – ie. produce effects simulating those produced by stimulation of the sympathetic nerves. Typical examples are amphetamine (qv), chlorphentermine (qv) and phenmetrazine (qv). In no circumstances should they ever be used except under strict medical supervision.

ANOSMIA means loss of sense of smell. (See NOSE, DISEASES OF.)

ANOXAEMIA means reduction of the oxygen content of the blood below normal limits.

ANOXIA is the term applied to that state in which the body tissues have an inadequate supply of oxygen. This may be because the blood in the lungs does not receive enough oxygen, or because there is not enough blood to receive the oxygen, or because the blood stagnates in the body. (See OXYGEN.)

ANTABUSE (see DISULFIRAM).

ANTACIDS are medicines which correct acidity, either general or stomachic. (See ACIDITY; ALKALI; DYSPEPSIA.)

ANTE- is a prefix meaning before or forwards.

ANTEFLEXION means the abnormal forward curvature of an organ in which the upper part is sharply bent forward. The term is especially applied to forward displacement of the uterus.

ANTENATAL is a term applied to conditions occurring before birth. It is used with reference both to mother and child. (For Antenatal Clinics, see MATERNITY AND CHILD WELFARE.)

ANTERIOR TIBIAL SYNDROME (see MUSCLE).

ANTEVERSION is the term applied to the forward tilting of an organ, especially of the uterus.

ANTHELMINTICS are substances which cause the death or expulsion of parasitic worms.

ANTHRACOSIS is the change which takes place in the lungs and bronchial glands of coal miners, and others, who inhale coal dust constantly. The lungs are amazingly efficient in coping with this problem. During a working lifetime a coalminer may inhale around 5000 grams of dust, but at post-mortem examination it is rare to find more than about 40 grams in his lungs. The affected tissues change in colour from greyish pink to jet black, owing to loading with minute carbon particles. This fine form of dust appears to be almost devoid of any harmful effect.

ANTHRAX is a very serious disease occurring in sheep and cattle, and in those who tend them or handle the bones, skins and fleeces, even long after removal of the latter from the animals. It is sometimes referred to as malignant pustule, wool-sorters' disease, splenic fever of animals or murrain. It is now a rare condition in the United Kingdom. Between 1961 and 1980 there were only 145 cases, 12 of them fatal, in England and Wales. The number of reported cases declined fourfold between 1961–65 and 1976–80, and in 1980 only one case was reported. In 122 cases the disease was a result of occupational exposure. In 23 cases there was no association with occupation: in 15 of these the infection was acquired from handling bone meal as a fertilizer in their gardens or having some other contact with bone meal or bones. One gave a history of handling leather goods while abroad.
Causes: The cause is a bacillus (*B. anthracis*) which grows in long chains and produces spores of great vitality. These spores retain their life for years, in dried skins and fleeces; they are not destroyed by boiling, freezing, 5 per cent carbolic lotion, or, like many bacilli, by the gastric juice. The disease is communicated from a diseased animal to a crack in the skin, eg. of a shepherd or butcher, or from contact with contaminated skins or fleeces. Nowadays skins are handled wet, but if they are allowed to dry so that dust laden with spores is inhaled by the workers an internal form of the disease results. Instances have occurred of the disease being conveyed on shaving brushes made from bristles of diseased animals.
Symptoms: (*a*) EXTERNAL FORM: This is the 'malignant pustule'. After inoculation of some small wound, a few hours or days elapse, and then a red, inflamed swelling appears, which grows larger till it covers half the face or the breadth of the arm, as the case may be. Upon its summit appears a bleb of pus, which bursts and leaves a black scab, perhaps 12 mm (half an inch) wide. At the same time there is great prostration and fever. The inflammation may last ten days or so, when it slowly subsides and the patient recovers, if surviving the fever and prostration.
(*b*) INTERNAL FORM: This takes the form of pneumonia with haemorrhages, when the spores have been drawn into the lungs, or of ulcers of the stomach and intestines, with gangrene of the spleen, when they have been swallowed. It is usually fatal in two or three days.
Treatment: Prevention is most important by disinfecting all hides, wool and hair coming from areas of the world, such as the Middle and Far East, where the disease is commonly found. All hides should be handled wet, so that spores cannot be present in dust; for the internal form is four times as fatal as the external. The hands of workmen must be carefully washed before eating, and working clothes changed. By these means the number of deaths from anthrax in the English woollen manufacturing districts has been reduced to a tenth of the number that occurred fifty years ago, before the disease was understood. An efficient vaccine is now available. Treatment consists of the administration of large doses of penicillin or of one of the tetracyclines. If there is a pustule, this is kept clean, but must not be cauterized or incised.

ANTI- is a prefix meaning against.

ANTIBIOTIC is the term used to describe any antibacterial agent derived from micro-organisms, such as penicillin, streptomycin, chloramphenicol and chlortetracycline.

The discovery and isolation of the penicillin nucleus, 6 amino penicillanic acid (6-APA) in 1958 provided the basis for the synthesis of a large number of new penicillins. These semi-synthetic penicillins now comprise the largest single group of antibiotics in clinical medicine (phenenthicillin, ampicillin, propicillin, azidocillin, carbenicillin, ticarcillin, sulbenicillin, carindicillin, carfecillin, mezlocillin, piperacillin, apacillin, talampicillin, bacampicillin, amoxycillin, pivampicillin, methicillin, nafcillin, oxacillin, cloxacillin, dicloxacillin, flucloxacillin, mecillinam, pivmecillinam). All these compounds are derivatives of 6 amino penicillin acid and at the present time there are sixteen different semi-synthetic penicillins in clinical use.

The cephalosporins are derived from the compound cephalosporin C which is obtained by fermentation of the mould cephalosporium. The cephalosporin nucleus 7 Amino cephalosporanic (7-ICA) acid has been the basis for the production of the semi-synthetic compounds of the cephalosporin nucleus. The first semi-synthetic cephalosporin, cephalothin, appeared in 1962; it was followed by cephaloridine in 1964. The original cephalosporins had to be given by injection but more recent preparations can be given by mouth. The newer preparations are less readily destroyed by beta lactamases and so they have a much broader spectrum of anti-bacterial activity. The newer cephalosporins include cephalexin, cefazolin, cephacetrile, cephapirin, cefamandole, cefuroxine, cephrodine, cefodroxil and cefotaxine. Inactivation of beta lactamase is the basis of bacterial resistance to both the penicillins and the cephalosporins so that attempts to prepare these antibiotics with resistance to beta lactamase is of great importance. A synthetic inhibitor of beta lactamase called clavulanic acid has recently been synthesised. This is used in combination with the penicillins and cephalosporins to prevent resistance. The cephamycins are a new addition to the beta lactam antibiotics. They are similar in structure to the cephalosporins but are produced, not by fungi, but by actinomycetes.

ANTIBODIES are substances in the blood which destroy or neutralize various toxins or 'bodies' (eg. bacteria), known generally as antigens. The antibodies are formed, usually, as a result of the introduction into the body of the antigens to which they are antagonistic, as in all infectious diseases.

ANTICOAGULANTS are drugs which prevent coagulation of the blood. The main ones now in use are heparin (qv), phenindione (qv) and warfarin (qv). Patients who are on anticoagulants require to be under medical supervision, and it is now usual for them to receive from their doctors an Anticoagulant Card with instructions about the use of whatever anticoagulant drug they may be taking.

ANTIDEPRESSANTS are drugs which relieve depression. They are not tranquillisers though some of them have sedative side-effects. There are two main groups of drugs, (i) the tricyclic antidepressants and (ii) the monoamine oxidase inhibitors. The tricyclic antidepressants are generally preferred to the monoamine oxidase inhibitors because they are both more effective antidepressants and they do not share the dangerous drug interactions that characterise the monoamine oxidase inhibitors. Lithium has a mood regulating action but its use is specifically limited to the treatment of manic depressive illnesses.

The antidepressive drugs are most effective in patients with endogenous depressive illness associated with psychomotor and physiological changes such as loss of appetite and sleep disturbances. The antidepressant drugs are oxidised in the liver at very different rates so that different patients on the same oral dose may show a thirty-fold difference in their blood levels. Thus the standard dose may be too much for one patient and not enough for another. The tricyclic antidepressants work by inhibiting the uptake of monoamine into the presynaptic neurone thereby enhancing the availability of the monoamines in the synaptic cleft. The tricyclic antidepressants act predominantly on either serotonin or catecholamine uptake. The tertiary amine such as amitryptyline and clomipramine affects serotonin more than noradrenaline uptake whilst the secondary amines such as nortriptyline and desipramine have more effect on noradrenaline. Unfortunately at the present time the dysfunction of a particular neurotransmitter cannot be correlated with any of the signs or symptoms of depressive illness but a positive response to a particular type of antidepressant in a previous depressive episode or the response of the first degree relative may provide a guideline to the choice of the appropriate drug.

The beneficial effect of the antidepressive takes two to three weeks before it becomes apparent. Patients with anxiety or agitation respond best to a sedative tricyclic such as amitriptyline, doxepin or dothiepin whilst retarded apathetic patients are best treated with a neutral antidepressant such as imipramine or a stimulant tricyclic such as protriptyline, nortriptyline or desipramine. The side-effects of the tricyclics are most commonly anti cholinergic. Dry mouth, blurring of close vision, constipation and occasionally urinary retention are the most common.

The tricyclic antidepressives in common usage are:

AMITRIPTYLINE (Domical, Elavil, Lentizol, Tryptizol)
BUTRIPTYLINE (Evadyne)
CLOMIPRAMINE (Anafranil)
DESIPRAMINE (Pertofran)
DOTHIEPIN (Prothiaden)
DOXEPIN (Sinequan)
IMIPRAMINE (Praminil, Tofranil)
IPRINDOLE (Prondole)
LOFEPRAMINE (Gamanil)
MAPROTILINE (Ludiomil)
MIANSERIN (Bolvidon, Norval)
NOMIFENSINE (Merital)
NORTRIPTYLINE (Allegron, Aventyl)
PROTRIPTYLINE (Concordin)
TRAZODONE (Molipaxin)
TRIMIPRAMINE (Surmontil)
VILOXAZINE (Vivalan).

The monoamine-oxidase inhibitors in common usage are:

PHENELZINE (Nardil)
IPRONIAZID (Marsilid)
ISOCARBOXAZID (Marplan)
TRANYLCYPROMINE (Parnate).

The monamine-oxidase inhibitors are used much less frequently than the tricyclic antidepressants because of their more serious side effects. Tranylcypromine (Parnate) is the most dangerous of the monoamine-oxidase inhibitors because of its stimulant action.

Phenelzine and Isocarboxazid are less stimulant and therefore safer.

ANTIDOTES are remedies which neutralize the effects of poisons. Thus acids have alkalis as antidote and vice versa.

ANTIGEN is the term applied to a substance which causes the formation of antibodies: it is usually a protein that is foreign to the body.

ANTIHISTAMINE DRUGS are drugs which antagonise the action of histamine (qv) and are therefore of value in the treatment of certain allergic conditions. They are also of some value in the treatment of vaso-motor rhinitis. They reduce rhinorrhoea and sneezing but are usually less effective in relieving nasal congestion. All antihistamines are also useful in the treatment of urticaria and certain allergic skin rashes, insect bites and stings. They are also used in the treatment of drug allergies. Chlorpheniramine or promethazine injections are useful in the emergency treatment of angioneurotic oedema and anaphylaxis. Antihistamines are of no value in the treatment of asthma. They have no place in the treatment of patients with chronic bronchitis and emphysema and their sedative actions may actually be harmful.

There is little evidence that any one antihistamine is superior to another and patients vary considerably in their response to them. The antihistamines differ in their duration of action and in the incidence of side-effects such as drowsiness. Most of the antihistamines are short-acting, but some (such as promethazine) work for up to twelve hours. They all cause sedation but promethazine, trimeprazine and dimenhydrinate tend to be more sedating while chlorpheniramine and cyclizine are less so.

Recently three new antihistamines have been introduced with the advantage of being less sedating. These are astemizole, (Hismanal), oxatomide (Tinsed) and terfenadine (Triludan). Astemizole and terfenadine have a peripheral action and cause less sedation; psycho-motor impairment has not been reported. Astemizole does not cause anticholinergic side-effects and is given once daily.

The main disadvantage of antihistamines is that they frequently cause drowsiness. Patients should be warned that their ability to drive or operate machinery may be impaired and that the effects of alcohol may be increased. Other side-effects include headache, dry mouth, blurred vision and gastro-intestinal disturbances and even urinary retention. They should therefore be used with caution in patients who suffer from epilepsy, prostatism, glaucoma and liver disease. The antihistamines available are (in alphabetical order):

ASTEMIZOLE (Hismanal)
AZATADINE MALEATE (Optimine)
BROMPHENIRAMINE MALEATE (Dimotane)
CHLORPHENIRAMINE MALEATE (Piriton)
CLEMASTINE (Tavegil)
CYPROHEPTADINE (Periactin)
DIMETHINDENE MALEATE (Fenostil)
DIMETHOTHIAZINE (Banistyl)
DIPHENHYDRAMINE HYDROCHLORIDE (Benadryl)
DIPHENYLPYRALINE HYDROCHLORIDE (Histryl)
KETOTIFEN
MEBHYDROLIN (Fabahistin)
MEPYRAMINE MALEATE (Anthisan)
MEQUITAZINE (Primalan)
OXATOMIDE (Tinset)
PHENINDAMINE TARTRATE (Thephorin)
PHENIRAMINE MALEATE (Daneral)
PROMETHAZINE HYDROCHLORIDE (Phenergan)
TERFENADINE (Triludan)
TRIMEPRAZINE TARTRATE (Vallergan)
TRIPROLIDINE HYDROCHLORIDE (Actidil).

ANTIMETABOLITES are a group of drugs which have been introduced for the treatment of certain forms of malignant disease. Chemically, they closely resemble substances (or metabolites) which are essential for the life and growth of cells. When introduced into the body they are 'mistaken', so to speak, by the cell for the corresponding metabolite, thereby preventing the cell from making use of the metabolite, or substance, which is essential for its growth. By this means the life of the cell is affected and it ultimately dies.

ANTIMONY is the name applied to a metal and also to its sulphide, a black powder found in nature. The tartrate of potassium and antimony is commonly known as tartar emetic in reference to its chief property. The preparations of antimony are all irritants; hence in large doses they are poisons, producing vomiting, purging, and also paralysis of the heart and nervous system. In moderate amounts they stimulate secretions from the bronchial tubes, intestine and skin, and thus ease cough, move the bowels, and cause free perspiration.
Antidote: Dimercaprol (qv) is the antidote to antimony. Should a poisonous amount be taken by mouth, the stomach should be washed out with strong tea. Failing this, calcium hydroxide or magnesium oxide should be used for this purpose.
Uses: Once a popular constituent, in the form of antimonial wine and James's powder (antimonial powder), of preparations for the treatment of fever and bronchitis, antimony is only used now in the treatment of certain tropical diseases such as kala-azar and schistosomiasis. For this purpose either the trivalent or pentavalent salts are used. These include antimony lithium thiomalate, antimony sodium tartrate, antimony potassium tartrate, sodium antimonylgluconate, stibocaptate and stibophen.

ANTIPERISTALSIS is a movement in the bowels and stomach by which the food and other contents are passed upwards, instead of in the proper direction. (See PERISTALSIS.)

ANTIPHLOGISTICS is an old term meaning remedies used against inflammation, fever, and similar conditions.

ANTI-PSYCHOTIC DRUGS (also known as NEUROLEPTICS). Although many of these drugs have sedative properties they should not be regarded as tranquillisers. They are used to quieten disturbed patients, whether this is the result of brain damage, mania, delirium, agitated depression or an acute behavioural disturbance. They relieve the florid psychotic symptoms such as hallucinations and thought disorder in schizophrenia and prevent relapse of this disorder when it is in remission.

Most of these drugs are dopamine antagonists (see DOPAMINE) and act by blocking dopamine receptors. As a result they can give rise to the extra pyramidal effects of Parkinsonism (qv) and they may also cause hyperprolactinaemia. The extrapyramidal symptoms are the most troublesome side-effects and they can usually be controlled by anticholinergic drugs. The main anti-psychotic drugs are: (i) chlorpromazine (Chloractil, Dozine Largactil), methotrimeprazine (Nozinan, Veractil) and promazine (Sparine, Dolmatil). These drugs are characterised by pronounced sedative effects and a moderate anticholinergic and extrapyramidal effects. (ii) pericyazine (Neulactil), pipothiazine (Piportil) and thioridazine (Melleril). These drugs have moderate sedative effects, marked anticholinergic effects but less extrapyramidal effects than the other groups. (iii) fluphenazine (Doditen), perphenazine (Fentazine) prochlorperazine (Stemetil, Vertigon), sulpiride (Dolmatil) and trifluoperazine (Stelazine), These drugs have fewer sedative effects, fewer anticholinergic effects but more pronounced extrapyamidal effects.

ANTIPYRETICS are measures used to reduce temperature in fever.
Varieties: Cold-sponging, wet-pack, baths and diaphoretic drugs such as quinine, salicylate of soda, and aspirin.
Uses (*see under above headings*).

ANTISEPTICS are substances which have the property of preventing or arresting putrefaction in dead animal or vegetable matter. Air, together with a moderate amount of warmth and of moisture, is necessary for the occurrence of putrefaction, which consists essentially in the breaking up of the complex organic material, and the formation of new and simpler combinations among its constituent elements. During the process, various gases and vapours are evolved, and the lower forms of animal and vegetable life grow and multiply in the putrefying substance. The exciting causes of putrefaction depend upon the growth and activity of micro-organisms (see BACTERIOLOGY). The changes which take place in a wound when organisms gain entrance to it and flourish upon its discharges are collectively known as sepsis or septic processes (see ABSCESS).

Varieties: By exclusion of the air, or even by covering from germ-laden dust, dead matter that does not already contain bacteria may be kept intact for an indefinite time, as shown in the method of preserving meat by hermetically sealing the jars, after destruction of all germs by heat. Again, the preservative influence of a low temperature is well known; extreme cold is a powerful antiseptic. Furthermore, the abstraction of moisture will prevent corruption in dead material. In warm and dry climates, animal food may be preserved by exposure to the sun. In the ancient practice of embalming the dead, which is the earliest illustration of the systematic use of antiseptics, the moister portions of the body were removed before the preservative agents were added. The action of direct sunlight is highly destructive to bacteria, having more effect upon some kinds than upon others.

For practical purposes reliance is chiefly placed on heat and chemical substances which destroy bacteria. Many substances which are strong antiseptics are of little practical use, either because they produce changes in the fluids with which they come in contact of such a nature as to hinder their further action, or because they are too irritating or too destructive when they come in contact with the tissues of the body. Further, some antiseptics act strongly upon certain organisms and less effectively upon others, so that the value of an antiseptic varies in different circumstances.

HEAT is one of the most effective antiseptics and may be applied at a temperature of 100° to 150°C. Dry articles to be disinfected may be brought into contact with steam under pressure, or more simple articles to be preserved from decomposition or sterilized may be boiled for a short period. This method is, however, obviously inapplicable to the living body and to many fragile articles.

BORIC ACID is a weak antiseptic which is used because of its non-irritating qualities. It may be used up to the full strength at which it dissolves in cold water: ie. 1 part in 20 of water.

CARBOLIC ACID, originally introduced by Lord Lister, is a powerful antiseptic: 1 part in 100 of water will in the course of some hours kill most bacteria. Up to a strength of 1 part in 20 of water it may be brought in contact with tissues for a short time, but even this strength is dangerous for prolonged application.

MERCURIC SALTS are among the most powerful antiseptics. Perchloride of mercury (mercuric chloride) may be used for washing the hands in a strength of 1 in 1000 of water. For vaginal douching, it may be used in a strength of 1 in 100,000. Even in the strength of 1 part in 100,000 of water it kills almost all bacteria in a few minutes. The cyanide of mercury is also used, either in lotions of similar strength, or by saturating lint, gauze, or wool for application to wounds. The disadvantage of mercuric salts is that though very powerful they are highly irritating, and secondly, that they are precipitated and rendered useless by the proteins of discharges with which they come in contact.

CRESOL, TRICRESOL, or CRESYLIC ACID, is a mixture of substances obtained from coal-tar, which is less poisonous than carbolic acid. Various preparations sold under propretary names, such as CREOLIN, JEYES' FLUID, and IZAL, are of similar nature and widely used. They are all dark oily liquids which form a white milky emulsion in water. LYSOL and some others contain fluid soap which aids their cleansing and penetrating action. They are all useful general disinfectants for hospital and domestic use. TAR WATER is a popular antiseptic often used because of the cresols and similar substances that it contains.

HYDROGEN PEROXIDE has the double merit of being a strong antiseptic and at the same time non-irritating. It may be freely applied to mucous membranes in the full pharmacopoeial strength, although, even when considerably diluted with water, it is still a powerful germicide. It is essential that it should be fresh, as it rapidly deteriorates by losing oxygen.

IODINE is a strong antiseptic and is specially used in the form of weak solution of iodine (2·5 per cent strength).

IODOFORM has the power of checking septic changes when discharges come in contact with it, probably by its power of giving off iodine. It is sometimes used to impregnate gauze for filling abscesses and other cavities.

CHLORINE GAS is a powerful antiseptic. It is used for the sterilization of water supplies, either as the gas or in the form of chlorinated lime (bleaching powder). CHLORINATED LIME, which gives off chlorine gas, is much used to disinfect drains. Chlorine has the disadvantage of being very irritating and of bleaching and destroying many substances, eg. cloth, leather, with which it comes in contact.

HYPOCHLOROUS ACID, under such names as EUSOL, DAKIN'S SOLUTION, is effective for septic wounds.

SULPHUR DIOXIDE is highly antiseptic. It is used as a food preservative, and also for the disinfection of rooms by fumigation.

FORMALDEHYDE is one of the more powerful antiseptics, and dissolved in water is used as a spray for disinfection of walls and furniture. It is also used in throat lozenges. It is excessively irritating, and therefore cannot be used as an antiseptic for application to the tissues.

POTASSIUM PERMANGANATE is an antiseptic on account of its oxidizing properties. It is used in strengths of 1 part in 4000 of water or weaker as a gargle, douche and as a wash for the hands.

ACRIFLAVINE, PROFLAVINE, and other aniline dyes as well as BRILLIANT GREEN, have a powerful action as antiseptics, and have also a gentle stimulating action on the tissues. They can be used in a strength of 1 part in 1000 of normal saline, and they can be mixed with various other antiseptics without detriment.

ALCOHOL is a powerful antiseptic, and, like ETHER, is used for removing septic matter and grease from the skin.

SILVER NITRATE is a powerful antiseptic used for lotions, eye drops, etc., in the strength of 1 part in 500 or 1000 of water. Other silver salts which are less irritating to the tissues are used in a similar way.

SALTS OF COPPER, SALTS OF IRON, SALTS OF LEAD, CHLORIDE OF ZINC, and compounds of most of the heavy metals act as strong antiseptics, but most of them, on account of their irritating or poisonous action, are not readily applicable for this purpose.

BALSAM OF TOLU, BALSAM OF PERU, and other aromatic substances are mild antiseptics.

CETRIMIDE, a mixture of alkyl ammonium bromides, is most effective for cleaning and disinfecting wounds and as a first-aid dressing in burns. It is also suitable for disinfecting utensils.

CHLORHEXIDINE has proved particularly valuable in obstetric practice, as a skin disinfectant, and in the treatment of burns.

CHLOROXYLENOL is non-irritating and is widely used in obstetric practice.

HEXACHLOROPHANE is a widely used antiseptic. One of its advantages is that it retains its activity in the presence of soap. It is therefore often used in soaps and creams in a concentration of 1 to 2 per cent.

CLIOQUINOL is an iodine-containing preparation used in the form of a cream, lotion or ointment in the treatment of skin infections. The usual strength is 3 per cent. It stains clothing and linen yellow.

POLYNOXYLIN is a condensation product of formaldehyde and urea used as a cream (10 per cent) in the treatment of infections of the skin.

POVIDONE-IODINE slowly liberates iodine on contact with the skin. As an ointment it is used in the treatment of infections of the skin.

Uses: Antiseptics act in various ways. Some of them kill bacteria by drying them: eg. common salt and syrup used as preservatives extract water from bacteria and thus kill them; other antiseptics kill bacteria by oxidation: eg. hydrogen peroxide, potassium permanganate; others coagulate the fluids in and around bacteria: eg. perchloride of mercury; and still others act as bacterial poisons: eg. cresol. The practice of using antiseptics has been in vogue for thousands of years. Thus cedar oil, tar and resins were in use among the Egyptians. Pitch, copper salts, vinegar, etc., were used for wounds by the Romans, while the fumes of sulphur for purification and salt as a preservative of food have been employed from the earliest times. Many of the stronger and more irritating antiseptics are now used as disinfectants (see DISINFECTION).

The methods of applying antisepsis or, as it should more correctly be described, asepsis (qv) in surgery are as follows. The sterilization of the hands of all those participating in an operation varies with the instructions of individual surgeons, but in essence is based upon washing the hands and arms up to the elbows under hot running water, using a sterile nail-brush and some antiseptic such as hexachlorophane soap, for at least five minutes. The hands are then immersed in an alcoholic solution, such as 75 per cent isopropyl alcohol. The skin of the patient is prepared by shaving, followed by a bath using some antiseptic soap. This is often done the day before the operation, and the area to be operated on is then covered by a dressing. On the operating table, and immediately before the operation, a wide stretch of skin in the operation area is cleaned by the antiseptic of the surgeon's choice, usually iodine but always coloured so that the cleansed area is clearly defined. Instruments and dressings are sterilized in autoclaves (qv).

By these means it is ensured that no germs can come in contact with the operation wound. To make doubly sure that such infection should not occur, all modern hospitals are equipped with a Central Sterile Supply Department (CSSD) which supplies all the sterilized material, such as dressings and instruments, required throughout the hospital, whether in operating theatres, wards or casualty departments.

ANTISPASMODICS (see SPASMOLYTICS).

ANTITOXINS, ANTITOXIC SERUM (see SERUM THERAPY).

ANTIVENINE, or ANTIVENOM, is the name given to SNAKE VENOM ANTISERUM, which is produced by the injection of snake venom into animals in small but increasing doses. In course of time the animal becomes immune to the particular venom injected. Native tradition in countries in Africa and Asia where poisonous snakes are common has it that a comparable method provides protection against snake bites in the traditional snake doctors who specialize in the treatment of snake bites. The antiserum prepared from the serum of such immunized animals is effective in neutralizing venom injected by the bite of a snake of the same species. No antiserum effective against all venoms is available. The custom is for each country to prepare antisera able to neutralize the venoms of indigenous snakes. The antivenom active against the venom of the adder is known as Zagreb antivenom. To be of any use, it must be administered as soon as possible after the snake bite. (See BITES AND STINGS.)

ANTROSTOMY is the operation in which an opening is made through the nose into the maxillary antrum. (See ANTRUM.)

ANTRUM means a natural hollow or cavity.

The *maxillary antrum* is now known as the maxillary sinus (see SINUS).

The *mastoid antrum* is situated in the mastoid process, the mass of bone felt behind the ear. It may become the seat of an abscess in cases of suppuration of the middle ear (see EAR, DISEASES OF).

The *pyloric antrum* is the part of the stomach immediately preceding the pylorus (qv).

ANURIA is a condition in which no urine is voided. (See GLOMERULONEPHRITIS; URINE.)

ANUS is the opening at the lower end of the bowel. It is kept closed by two muscles, the external and internal sphincters. The latter is a muscular ring which extends about 25 mm (1 inch) up the bowel, is nearly 6 mm (¼ inch) thick, and is kept constantly contracted by the action of a nerve centre in the spinal cord. In disease of the spinal cord the muscle may be paralysed, and inability to retain the motions results.

ANUS, DISEASES OF (see RECTUM, DISEASES OF).

ANXIETY STATE (see NEUROSIS).

ANXIOLYTICS are drugs for the relief of anxiety. They will induce sleep when given in large doses at night and so are hypnotics as well. Conversely most hypnotics will sedate when given in divided doses during the day. Prescription of these drugs is widespread but it has recently become realised that physical and psychological dependence as well as tolerance to their effects occurs. This is particularly true of the barbiturates but also applies to the benzodiazepines. Withdrawal syndromes may occur if drug treatment is terminated too abruptly. Hypnotic sedatives and anxiolytics should therefore not be prescribed indiscriminately, but reserved for short courses.

AORTA is the large vessel which opens out of the left ventricle of the heart and carries blood to all the body. It is about 45 cm (1½ feet) long and 2·5 cm (1 inch) wide. Like other arteries it possesses three coats, of which the middle one is much the thickest. This consists partly of muscle fibre, but is mainly composed of an elastic substance, called elastin. The aorta passes first to the right, and lies nearest the surface behind the end of the second right rib-cartilage; then it curves backwards and to the left, passes down behind the left lung close to the backbone, and through an opening in the diaphragm into the abdomen, where it divides, at the level of the navel, into the two common iliac arteries, which carry blood to the lower limbs. Its branches, in order, are: two coronary arteries to the heart wall; the brachiocephalic, left common carotid, and left subclavian arteries to the head, neck and upper limbs; several small branches to the oesophagus, bronchi, and other organs of the chest; nine pairs of intercostal arteries which run round the body between the ribs; one pair of subcostal arteries which is in series with the intercostal arteries; four (or five) lumbar arteries to the muscles of the loins; coeliac trunk to the stomach, liver and pancreas; two mesenteric arteries to the bowels; and suprarenal, renal and testicular arteries to the suprarenal body, kidney, and testicle on each side. From the termination of the aorta rises a small branch, the median sacral artery, which runs down into the pelvis. In the female the ovarian arteries replace the testicular.

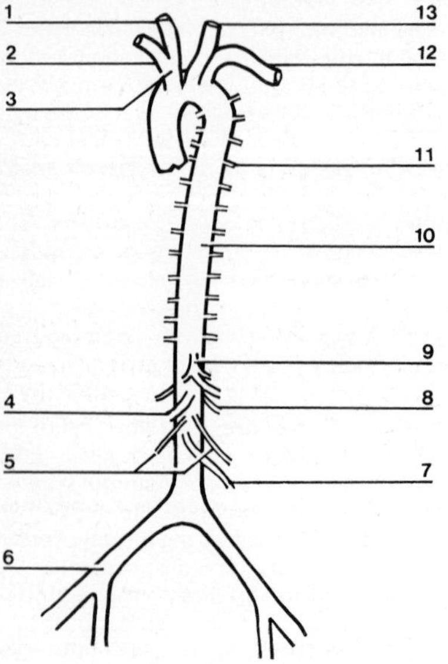

1 right common carotid	8 renal
2 right subclavian	9 common iliac
3 brachiocephalic	10 aorta
4 superior mesenteric	11 intercostal
5 gondal	12 left subclavian
6 right common iliac	13 left common cartoid
7 inferior mesenteric	

Main branches of the aorta.

The chief diseases of the aorta are atheroma and aneurysm. (See ARTERIES, DISEASES OF; ANEURYSM; and COARCTATION OF THE AORTA.)

AORTITIS means a degenerative condition of the lining of the aorta. It is usually produced by syphilis.

AORTOGRAPHY is the technique of rendering the aorta visible in an X-ray film by injecting a radio-opaque substance into it. (See also ANGIOGRAPHY.)

APACILLIN (see ANTIBIOTIC).

APERIENTS are medicines which produce a natural movement of the bowels. (See CONSTIPATION; PURGATIVES.)

APEX is the pointed portion of any organ which has a conical shape. The apex of each lung reaches about 3·5 to 5·0 cm (1½ or 2 inches) above the collar-bone into the neck. In health the apex of the heart can be felt below the fifth rib immediately inside the nipple.

APGAR SCORE is a method of assessing a baby's condition at birth, in which a value of 0, 1 or 2 is given to each of five signs: colour, heart-rate, muscle tone, respiratory (or breathing) effort, and the response to stimulation. A total score of 10 indicates that the newborn child is in excellent condition.

APHAKIA is a term which means absence of the lens of the eye.

APHASIA means a loss of the power of speech, due to injury to the centres which govern this act in the brain. The higher of these centres, which have to do with forming the ideas of speech, putting words together in sentences, and governing the movements of mouth, tongue and larynx, lie on the surface of the cerebral hemispheres, especially of the left; while the lower centres, which directly bring the muscles of the voice organs into action, under superintendence of the higher ones, are in the medulla or hind brain.

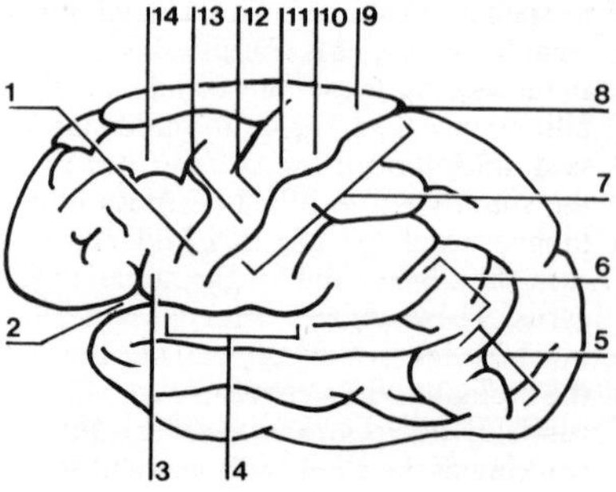

1 movements of tongue	6 memories of written words
2 lateral	7 sensation
3 speech	8 central sulcus
4 hearing	9 movement of leg
5 sight	10 movement of trunk

Areas on the left surface of the cerebrum associated with definite functions.

Causes: The cause is destruction of a portion of the brain, including one of these higher centres, owing to rupture of a blood-vessel, and haemorrhage into the brain tissue; or owing to blocking of a blood-vessel by an embolus (see EMBOLISM), or by clotting of the blood on the diseased wall of a vessel (see THROMBOSIS), any one of which cuts off the supply of blood to the part concerned. The causes are thus the same as in apoplexy (ie. a stroke), and aphasia may be one of the symptoms of an apoplectic seizure, especially when the right side of the body is paralysed, or may occur by itself, according to the extent of brain involved. Other diseases, such as tumours, may also be the cause, the important factor being interference with the functions of certain definite areas of the brain.

Varieties: It was first pointed out by Broca that the inferior frontal gyrus on the left side of the brain in right-handed persons, and vice versa in left-handed persons, is, after death, found to be diseased in those who have, in life, suffered from inability to speak, although the intelligence and powers of silent reading and of writing may have remained. Such a condition is known as *motor aphasia*. But the state is generally more complicated. In addition to Broca's speech area, which governs the movements of the tongue, mouth and larynx that frame words to express ideas, there is a centre in the middle frontal gyrus of the left side, which regulates the power of writing intelligibly, and disease of this region produces loss of power to write rationally, even though the hand remains quite able to hold a pen, this condition being known as *agraphia*. These two forms involve loss of power of *production* of speech and writing, but there are corresponding losses of power of *perception* known as *word blindness* and *word deafness*, the two conditions being grouped together as *sensory aphasia*. In the former of these the afflicted person is unable to read correctly, though his vision is perfect, and he may be able to spell and even to write, though not to read what he writes. This condition is due to disease in the angular gyrus. In word deafness the disability consists in failure to understand what is said, and, though the sufferer hears perfectly, the sounds are to him like those of a foreign tongue which he does not understand; in this case the disease lies in the superior temporal gyrus. There are still more complicated forms in which the disease affects, not the surface of the brain, but the strands of nerve fibres, which run from one centre to another and reduce the working of the whole arrangement to a system.

Symptoms: The disorder generally follows an attack of apoplexy and exists along with some paralysis on the right side of the body. *Aphasia* may come on suddenly and last only a few hours or days, being due then to a passing congestion of the brain, or to a block in the circulation, which is later swept away. Generally it is permanent, and, naturally, a person with aphasia has always some mental impairment. Sometimes he is absolutely without the power of speech, though often a few interjections, like 'Oh dear', 'Yes', or 'No', or meaningless sounds, or even oaths, can be pronounced. When the condition is one of *sensoryaphasia*, names of persons, of places, even of the commonest household articles, are forgotten, a cat is called 'a brush', a bell 'a pen', and so forth, or the person gives meaningless answers to questions, so that conversation becomes very slow or quite impossible.

Treatment: This is as in apoplexy, of which the condition often forms a part (see STROKE). The condition is seldom much improved if it has lasted more than a week without betterment. But in some cases, after the haemorrhage or other cause is long past, improvement is achieved by teaching the afflicted person to read and speak just as one would teach a child, a new part of the brain apparently being educated.

APHONIA means loss of voice. It is caused by some disorder in the throat or in the nerves proceeding to the throat muscles, or by hysteria. (See VOICE.)

APHTHAE (see THRUSH).

APICECTOMY is the minor operation carried out to try to save a tooth which has an abscess on it or which does not respond to root treatment. In this the abscess and the apex of the tooth are removed.

APNOEA means stoppage of breathing, such as occurs when the blood is artificially supplied with too much oxygen; for example, by taking several deep breaths in quick succession. (See ASPHYXIA.)

APO- is a prefix implying separation or derivation from.

APODIA: Absence of the foot.

APOMORPHINE is a crystalline alkaloid closely related to morphine and having a powerful emetic action. Apomorphine hydrochloride is given hypodermically in doses of 2 to 8 mg in cases of poisoning in which the patient is unable to swallow or a very rapid emetic action is desired. It is also used in the treatment of alcoholism.

APONEUROSIS is the term applied to the white fibrous membrane which serves as an investment for the muscles and which covers the skull beneath the scalp.

APOPLEXY (see STROKE).

APOTHECARIES' WEIGHT (see WEIGHTS AND MEASURES).

APPENDICECTOMY, or appendectomy, is the operation for the removal of the appendix vermiformis.

APPENDICITIS is an inflammatory disease starting in the vermiform appendix. (See APPENDIX.)

Varieties: The disease is classified in many ways wth regard to its treatment and its anatomical characters. First of all, one must separate the *acute* from the *chronic* or *relapsing form*. In the latter the person affected is troubled by repeated slight attacks of pain in the right iliac region, perhaps never bad enough to prevent moderate work, but sufficient to be a burden; or there is a sense of constant indefinable weakness and discomfort in this situation. In some cases the slightly inflamed appendix undergoes at times spasmodic, painful contractions: the so-called *appendicular colic*. This may be associated with the presence of concretions in the interior of the appendix or with adhesions between it and neighbouring parts. In other cases the inflammatory process is so mild that no symptoms directly referable to the appendix ever occur, but the patient suffers from constipation, indigestion, or general abdominal discomfort produced in a reflex manner by the disturbance of the appendix. The *acute form* is that which is usually known as an 'attack of appendicitis'. Unless adequately and properly treated, this form may proceed to two very serious forms. *Gangrenous appendicitis* is one in which the inflammation is so intense that the appendix sloughs away, and the bowels communicate, through the opening, with the peritoneal cavity. The other form is *suppurative appendicitis*, in which the inflammation is not quite so severe but the appendix becomes the centre of an abscess. Both of these latter forms are extremely dangerous to life and are often very sudden in their development. It is for this reason that the vast majority of cases of acute appendicitis are operated upon as soon as possible.

Causes: Acute appendicitis is the most common abdominal surgical emergency – certainly in western civilization. It occurs at all ages, but is most common in the first twenty years of life. It tends to be more common in males than in females. The precise cause is not known, but the condition is usually due to a combination of infection and obstruction. What probably happens in most cases is that the appendix becomes obstructed. This may be due to a small mass of faeces accumulating in the appendix or to kinking of the appendix. The contents of the obstructed appendix being infective, the whole appendix rapidly becomes infected, with the dire consequences already described, unless immediate skilled surgical treatment is available.

The widespread popular idea that grapeseeds, apple-pips, and similar small objects have a special faculty for finding out the appendix, lodging there, and setting up appendicitis, is fallacious. Though such objects are found there occasionally, these cases are exceptional, and the small masses of hardened faeces or minute concretions of lime, which are common, are a result of, rather than the cause of, the appendicitis.

Symptoms: An attack of appendicitis comes on as a rule suddenly, without the early feelings of languor and malaise common to most acute diseases. The principal symptoms are: (*a*) sudden pain in the abdomen, often vague in situation at first, but usually settling in the right iliac region. It is generally very severe, and the patient has to lie constantly on his back with the right leg drawn up. (*b*) Disturbance of the digestive functions, consisting in loss of appetite, nausea, often vomiting, and constipation, which has usually been present for a day or two. (*c*) Tenderness to touch in the right iliac region, which in very many cases has its point of greatest intensity defined with curious exactitude at a point called Munro's or M'Burney's point, situated about halfway between the spine of the iliac bone and the navel. (*d*) Fever of a moderate amount, generally about 39°C (102°F). The first three of these occur with varying intensity in other diseases of the abdomen, in which, however, fever is uncommon. Distinct resistance and hardness of the muscles in the right lower quarter of the abdomen can be made out on pressure, and swelling is usually visible in the right iliac region after two or three days. In *gangrenous appendicitis* the symptoms are extreme, the fever high, and death may come on with startling rapidity, if an operation be not performed. In *suppurative appendicitis* an abscess forms with marked swelling, though rarely before the end of the first week, and this also calls for operation in due course.

In some cases an attack is very slight, the bowels around become matted together, an abscess collects in the cavity so formed, and only when it comes near the surface is the condition diagnosed.

Treatment: In no circumstances should a purgative be given. A patient with acute appendicitis seen within thirty-six hours of the onset should be operated on forthwith, the mortality in the hands of good surgeons being very low: around 0·25 per cent. If the case is seen after forty-eight hours of the onset and improvement has set in, some surgeons recommend postponement of the operation until the inflammation has completely subsided; others hold that operation should be done at once. If operation is refused or impossible, the patient should be kept quiet in bed, be given only water by mouth, and perhaps have an injection of morphine. If the case is one of gangrenous appendicitis immediate operation is the only possible course; for the great danger of the disease consists in the production of a general peritonitis through the escape of bacteria and putrescent material in large amount from the interior of the appendix. (See PERITONITIS.)

APPENDIX is a term applied to appendages of several hollow organs. The epiploic appendices are a number of tags of fat hanging from the outer surface of the large intestine. The appendices of the larynx are two pouches, one on either side between the false and true vocal cords. The term appendix is most commonly applied to the vermiform appendix of the large intestine. It is a tubular prolongation of the large intestine with an average length of 9 or 10 cm and a width of 6 mm. It lies in the right lower corner of the abdomen and has peritoneal, muscular and mucous coats similar to those of the rest of the intestine.

APPETITE is the craving for the food necessary to maintain the body and to supply it with sufficient energy to carry on its functions. The ultimate cause of appetite is a question of supply and demand in the muscles and various organs, but the proximate cause is doubtful. Unlike hunger, it is probably an acquired, rather than an inborn, sensation. Thus, a newborn infant experiences hunger, but probably not appetite. Whatever other factors may be concerned, the tone of the stomach is of importance. This is supported by the fact that in conditions associated with poor appetite the tone of the stomach is poor, whilst in conditions such as duodenal ulcer which are characterized by a good, or even excessive appetite, the stomach is often hypertonic. Important factors in stimulating appetite are anticipation and the sight and smell of well-cooked food. Just as, conversely, the sight or smell of badly cooked food may remove all desire for food. Undoubtedly a good appetite is necessary to good digestion, and a perfectly healthy taste and appetite ought to be both a guide to the suitability of foods and a gauge of the amount required. Like every other bodily function, appetite may be out of order. It may be depraved, and may indicate quite unsuitable articles of diet, from toasted cheese in dyspeptics, who know by experience that such an article upsets their digestion, to cinders, hair, pebbles, etc., in the condition known as *pica*, which occurs sometimes during pregnancy, in children, in hysteria, and often in mental disorders. The two chief disorders, however, are excessive increase of appetite and diminution or loss of appetite.

Excessive appetite may be simply a bad habit, due to habitual over-indulgence in good food, and resulting in gout, obesity, etc., according to the other habits and constitution of the person. It may also be a sign of diabetes mellitus or thyrotoxicosis. (See BULIMIA.)

Diminished appetite is a sign common to almost all diseases causing general weakness, because the activity of the stomach and the secretion of gastric juice fail early when vital power is low. It is the most common sign of dyspepsia due to gastritis (see DYSPEPSIA) and of cancer of the stomach. In some cases it is a manifestation of stress or strain such as domestic worry or difficulties at work. Indeed, appetite seems to be particularly susceptible to emotional disturbances.

Diminished appetite in feverish states is a salutary thing, as the digestive functions are reduced in power, and people in these circumstances should restrict themselves to a light diet, consisting mainly of milk and fruit juices, and should rest quietly at the same time. (See also ANOREXIA NERVOSA.)

APPROVED NAMES is the term used for names devised or selected by the *British Pharmacopoeia* Commission for new drugs. The intention is that if any of the drugs to which these Approved Names are applied should eventually be included in the *BritishPharmacopoeia* the Approved Name should be its official title. The issue of an Approved Name, however, does not imply that the substance will necessarily be included in the *BritishPharmacopoeia* or that the Commission is prepared to recommend the use of the substance.

APRAXIA means loss of power to carry out regulated movements. Although there is no muscle weakness or incoordination, there is difficulty in formulating movement patterns.

APYREXIA means absence of fever.

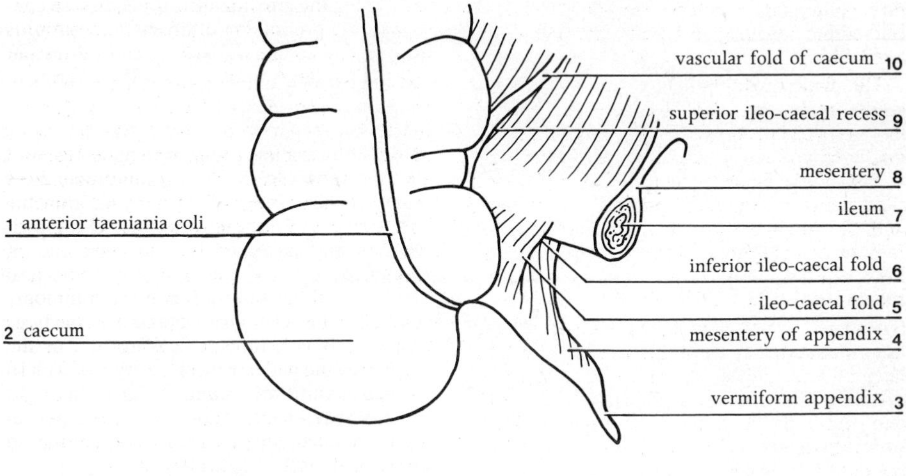

Part of the bowel in the right iliac region showing the relations of the appendix to the ilium and the caecum.

ARACHIS OIL, also known as peanut oil, is the oil expressed from the seeds of *Arachis hypogoea*. It is sometimes used to replace olive oil when the latter is in short supply. It is commonly used as the vehicle for the intramuscular injection of drugs: eg. penicillin.

ARACHNODACTYLY, or MARFAN'S SYNDROME, is a congenital condition characterized by extreme length and slenderness of the fingers and toes and, to a lesser extent, of the limbs and trunk, laxity of the ligaments, and dislocation of the lens of the eye. The antero-posterior diameter of the skull is abnormally long, and the jaw is prominent. There may also be abnormalities of the heart.

ARACHNOID MEMBRANE is one of the membranes covering the brain and spinal cord (see BRAIN). Arachnoiditis is the name applied to inflammation of this membrane.

ARBOVIRUSES are a group of around 200 viruses, which are transmitted to man by arthropods. They include the viruses of dengue (qv) and yellow fever (qv) which are transmitted by mosquitoes.

ARC EYE (see EYE, DISEASE AND INJURIES OF).

ARCUS CORNEALIS (see EYE, DISEASE AND INJURIES OF).

ARENAVIRUSES are a group of viruses, so called because under the electron microscope they have a sand-sprinkled (Latin, *arenosus*) appearance. Among the diseases in man for which they are responsible are lassa fever (qv) in West Africa, Argentinian haemorrhagic fever (mortality rate 3 to 15 per cent), a similar disease in Bolivia (mortality rate 18 per cent), and lymphocytic choriomeningitis, in which deaths are uncommon.

AREOLA literally means a small space, and is the term applied to the red or dusky ring round the nipple, or round an inflamed part. Increase in the duskiness of the areola on the breast is an important early sign of pregnancy.

ARGENTUM is the Latin word for silver.

ARGYLL ROBERTSON PUPIL is a condition (described originally by Dr Argyll Robertson) in which the pupils contract when the eyes converge on a near object, but fail to contract when a bright light falls on the eye. It is found in several diseases, especially in locomotor ataxia and general paralysis of the insane.

ARGYRIA, or ARGYRIOSIS means the effect produced by taking silver salts over a long period, and consists of a deep duskiness of the skin, especially of the exposed parts.

ARGYROL (see SILVER).

ARM is the part of the upper limb between the shoulder and elbow, but is generally taken to include also the forearm and shoulder regions. The upper limb is attached to the body by the strong pectoral muscles in front and by several powerful muscles springing from the spine and ribs behind. The great mobility of the shoulder is largely due to the fact that the only contact with the bones of the trunk takes place between the collar-bone and the upper end of the sternum or breast-bone, the shoulder-blade sliding freely between the muscles of the back as the arm is raised and lowered. The bones of the arm are the clavicle or collar-bone and the scapula or shoulder-blade lying at the upper part of the chest, the humerus, a single bone in the upper arm, and the radius and ulna lying side by side in the forearm. Eight small bones compose the wrist (or carpus) and connect the hand with the lower end of the radius.

The shoulder-joint is of the ball-and-socket variety, the head of the humerus resting against the glenoid cavity of the shoulder-blade. The elbow is a hinged joint formed at the lower end of the humerus above, while the ulna forms the chief part of the joint below, the radius resting lightly against the humerus. When the hand is rotated so as to lie palm up or back up, the radius in the first case lies alongside the ulna and in the latter crosses over it. The chief muscle which bends the elbow is the biceps in front of the upper arm, while the triceps lying behind straightens the limb. A group of muscles attached at the inner side of the elbow act to bend the wrist and fingers; another group of muscles attached to the outer side of the elbow have the general action of straightening and bending backwards the wrist and fingers.

One large artery (brachial artery) runs down the inner side of the upper arm corresponding to the seam of the coat sleeve in position. At the elbow this divides into two branches, the radial and ulnar arteries. The radial artery can be felt pulsating near the wrist and is generally known as the pulse. The ulnar artery lies to the inner side of the forearm, deeply imbedded in muscles. A large group of nerves lies at the inner side of the armpit, and these nerves run downwards to supply the muscles and skin of the arm. The ulnar nerve can readily be felt behind the inner side of the elbow, where it is exposed to bruising and is popularly known as the 'funny bone'. The large radial nerve runs down the back of the upper arm and the outer side of the forearm. At the back of the upper arm it is often damaged, leading then to the condition known as drop-wrist (qv), in which the hand hangs helpless and cannot be raised.

The collar-bone, by reason of its exposed position, is liable to fracture from falls on the shoulder, and the radius is often broken by falls on the palm of the hand. The shoulder-joint, on account of its great mobility, is prone to be dislocated in twists of the upper arm, but the elbow-joint is seldom injured. A small bursa or cavity lies between the skin and the end of the ulna at the point of the elbow, and this is often inflamed as the result of injury, and in the same way as the bursa in front of the knee is affected in the condition known as housemaid's knee. (See BURSITIS.)

ARMPIT, or AXILLA, is the pyramidal hollow between the upper arm and chest, bounded in front by the pectoral or breast muscles, behind by the shoulder-blade and its muscles, and running up to a point beneath the collar-bone. It contains the axillary vessels and nerves which run to the arm, also much fatty tissue, many sweat glands and lymphatic glands. The latter are important, because in poisoned wounds of the arm they may become inflamed, resulting in abscess; and still more, because in cancer of the breast they may become infected with cancer, and have to be removed with the breast. Wounds in the armpit are dangerous on the outer, front, and back walls, because large blood vessels run there.

ARNICA is a medicine derived from *Arnica montana*, a plant of the Western United States and Europe. The tincture of arnica is used as a domestic remedy. Externally the tincture is used as a lotion for application to sprains and bruises, which it relieves by virtue of its weakly irritant action.

ARRHYTHMIA means any variation from the normal regular rhythm of the heart-beat. The condition is produced by some affection interfering with the mechanism which controls the beating of the heart, and includes the following disorders: sinus arrhythmia, atrial fibrillation, atrial flutter, heart block, extrasystole, pulsus alternans, and paroxysmal atrial tachycardia, ventricular tachycardia and ventricular fibrillation. (See HEART DISEASES.)

ARROWROOT is a West Indian plant (*Maranta arundinacea*). As sold, it is a white powder, consisting of almost pure starch, derived from the root of the plant. It is used as an invalid food, because it is easy to digest, but it must, of course, be combined with other forms of nourishment.

ARSENIC is a metal, but is better known by its oxide, white arsenic, by two arsenites of copper, Scheele's green and emerald green, and by two sulphides of arsenic, orpiment or king's yellow, and realgar. It is extensively used in dyeworks, in the manufacture of chemicals, in making enamel, in hardening shot and type, in fly-papers, sheep-dips, yellow and green paints, and is further given to horses to improve their coat. Applied pure, it is a strong germicide and caustic, and in large doses is a powerful irritant to stomach and intestines. When taken over long periods, larger and larger doses can be tolerated, till at last a quantity many times the poisonous dose has no apparent ill-effect. In some parts of the world, as among the mountaineers of Styria, its use has become a habit, and in these people it produces a sense of well-being and greater capacity for sustaining fatigue.

ARSENIC POISONING may be acute or chronic.

Acute: The symptoms are violent purging, vomiting, and great prostration. The treatment is to give an emetic, followed by a purgative such as sodium sulphate.

Chronic poisoning occurs among dyers and paperhangers, or from contamination of food by, or other contact with, green or yellow paint, or wall-paper containing arsenic. It may also occur in those taking so-called tonics containing arsenic. The symptoms are irritability of the eyes and throat, with cough, tendency to sickness, diarrhoea, prostration, and skin eruptions, and often headache, tremors, paralyses, and other nervous signs (see NEURITIS). The treatment is first of all discovery and removal of the source of poisoning, after which one must wait till the arsenic has been gradually expelled from the system by help of fresh air, good food, and tonics. Subjects of arsenic poisoning may be left in a debilitated condition with weak digestion and symptoms of neuritis lasting several years.

In both acute and chronic arsenical poisoning, in addition to the measures outlined, a course of dimercaprol (qv) is now given. This is the most efficient known antidote to arsenic.

ARTERIES are vessels which convey oxygenated blood away from the heart to the tissues of the body, limbs, and internal organs. In the case of most arteries, the blood has been purified by passing through the lungs, and is consequently bright red in colour, but in the pulmonary arteries which convey it to the lungs it is unoxygenated, dark, and like the blood in veins.

The arterial system begins at the left ventricle of the heart with the aorta (see AORTA), which gives off branches that subdivide into smaller and smaller vessels, the final divisions, called arterioles, being microscopic, and ending in a network of capillaries, which perforate the tissues like the pores of a sponge, and bathe them in blood that is collected and brought back to the heart by veins. (See CIRCULATION.)

The chief arteries after the *aorta* and its branches (see AORTA) are: (1) the *common carotid*, running up each side of the neck and dividing into *internal carotid* to the brain, and *external carotid* to the neck and face; (2) the *subclavian* to each arm, continued by the *axillary* in the armpit, and the *brachial* along the inner side of the arm, dividing at the elbow into the *radial* and the *ulnar*, which unite across the palm of the hand in arches that give branches to the fingers; (3) the two *common iliacs*, in which the aorta ends, each of which divides into the *internal iliac* to the organs in the pelvis, and the *external iliac* to the lower limb, continued by the *femoral* in the thigh, and the *popliteal* behind the knee, dividing into the *anterior* and *posterior tibial* arteries to the front and back of the leg. The latter passes behind the inner ankle to the sole of the foot, where it forms arches similar to those in the hand, and supplies the foot and toes by *plantar branches*.

Structure: The arteries are highly elastic, dilating at each heart-beat as blood is driven into them, and forcing it on by their resiliency (see PULSE). Every artery has *three coats*: (*a*) the outer or adventitia, consisting of ordinary strong fibrous tissue; (*b*) the middle or media, consisting of muscular fibres supported by elastic fibres, which in some of the larger arteries form distinct membranes; and (*c*) the inner or intima, consisting of a layer of yellow elastic tissue on whose inner surface rests a layer of smooth plate-like endothelial cells, over which flows the blood. In the larger arteries the muscle of the middle coat is largely replaced by elastic fibres, which render the artery still more expansile and elastic. When an artery is cut across, the muscular coat instantly shrinks, drawing the cut end within the fibrous sheath that surrounds the artery, and bunching it up, so that a very small hole is left to be closed by blood-clot. (See HAEMORRHAGE.)

ARTERIES, DISEASES OF: *Arteriosclerosis*, which is a condition of thickening and rigidity

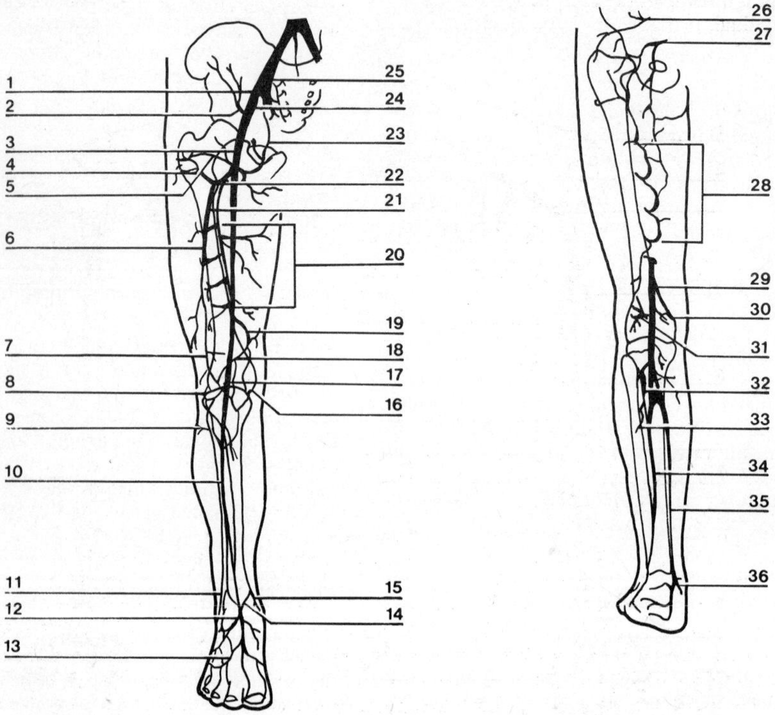

1 external iliac
2 deep circumflex iliac artery
3 femoral artery
4 lateral femoral artery
5 medial femoral circumflex
6 profunda femora
7 superior lateral genicular
8 inferior lateral genicular
9 anterior tibial recurrent
10 anterior tibial
11 lateral malleolar
12 tarsal artery
13 arcuate
14 dorsalis pedis
15 medial malleolar
16 inferior medial genicular
17 popliteal
18 superior medial genicular
19 supreme genu
20 perforating arteries 1-4
21 profunda
22 medial femoral circumflex
23 obturator
24 inferior epigastric artery
25 internal iliac
26 superior gluteal
27 inferior gluteal
28 perforating arteries 1-4
29 popliteal
30 superior medial genicular
31 superior lateral genicular
32 anterior tibial
33 fibular branch
34 peroneal
35 posterior tibial
36 medial malleolus

The arteries of the lower limb, anterior view (left) and posterior view (right).

involving predominantly the inner and middle coat of medium-sized arteries, occurs as a natural change in old age. In some individuals, however, the change occurs earlier. The cause is still obscure, but certain facts are well established, even though they may only be predisposing factors. There is a hereditary tendency, and this is most marked in cases in which it develops at a relatively early age. There is a definite association with high blood-pressure in many cases, but arteriosclerosis can occur without a high blood-pressure. It is much more common in patients with diabetes mellitus than in individuals without this disease. It is also a common finding in gout. The distribution of arteriosclerosis throughout the arterial tree varies considerably. It may give rise to no symptoms, and only does so if it involves certain arteries. Thus, if it involves the arteries to the brain, the individual is liable to have a stroke; if it involves the coronary arteries which nourish the muscle of the heart, it may result in angina pectoris or a coronary thrombosis; if the arteries of the kidney are involved, a form of glomerulonephritis may develop; whilst if the arteries to the legs and feet are involved, gangrene may occur.

Atherosclerosis is a condition characterized by the presence in the inner coat, or intima, of arteries of the degenerative condition known as atheroma. This manifests itself by nodes, or plaques, of yellowish material containing a high proportion of cholesterol (qv) and other lipids (qv). As these plaques enlarge, and the intima increases in thickness, the lumen of the artery becomes smaller and smaller. In due course the lumen of the artery may be so narrowed that it becomes blocked. If this occurs in the coronary arteries, which supply the heart

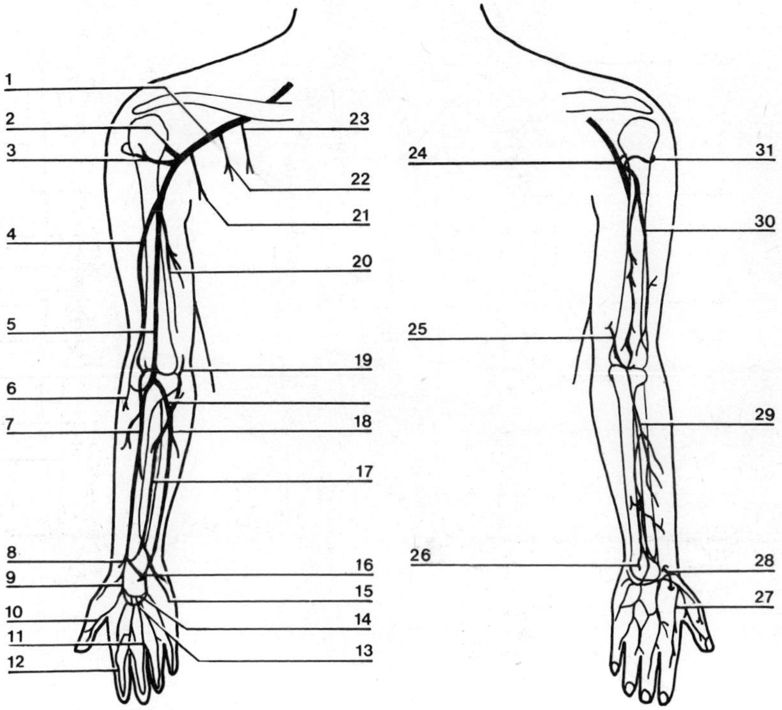

1 axillery
2 posterior humeral circumflex
3 anterior humeral circumflex
4 profunda
5 brachial
6 radial recurrent
7 radial
8 palmar carpal
9 superficial palmar
10 princeps pollicis
11 proper palmer digitals
12 radiallis indicis
13 superficial palmer arch
14 deep palmar arch
15 deep palmar
16 palmar carpal (ulnar)
17 anterior interosseous
18 common interosseous
19 ulnar recurrent
20 superior ulnar collateral
21 subscapular
22 lateral thoracic
23 pectoral branch
24 brachial artery
25 inferior ulnar collateral artery
26 dorsal ulnar carpal artery
27 first dorsal metacarpal artery
28 dorsal carpal radial artery
29 posterior interosseous artery
30 profunda artery
31 posterior humeral circumflex artery

The arteries of the upper limb, anterior view (left) and posterior view (right).

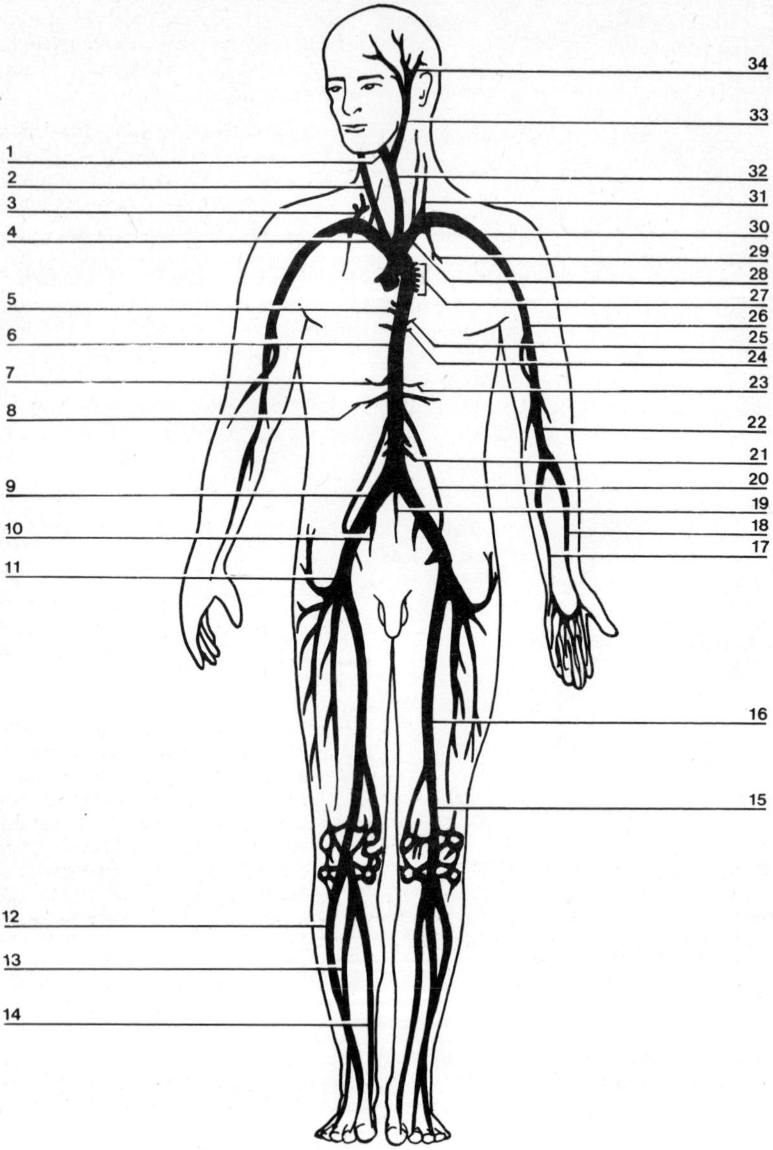

1 internal cartoid
2 vertebral
3 right subclavian
4 brachiocephalic (innominate)
5 oesophageal
6 coeliac
7 middle suprarenal
8 renal
9 common iliac
10 internal iliac
11 external iliac
12 anterior tibial
13 peroneal
14 posterior tibial
15 nophiteal
16 femoral
17 ulnar
18 radial
19 middle sacral
20 spermatic
21 inferior mesenteric
22 brachial
23 superior mesenteric
24 inferior phrenic
25 superior phrenic
26 axillary
27 intercostals
28 left subclavian
29 internal mammery
30 thyrocervical trunk
31 costocervical trunk
32 common carotid
33 external carotid
34 superficial temperal

The chief arteries of the body.

muscle, the result is the all too common coronary thrombosis. If it occurs in the arteries in the brain it causes a stroke. The cause of atherosclerosis is not known, but one factor is the consumption of excessive saturated fats.

Following on atheroma, plates of lime may form in the arteries, or these vessels may, in extreme states, be changed into brittle calcareous tubes, very liable to tearing from slight injuries. When this condition occurs in older people, it is confined to the middle coat and is accompanied by marked calcification; it is known as *Mönckeberg's sclerosis.*

Syphilis and other inflammatory diseases may bring about an *obliterative inflammation*, in which the internal coat becomes greatly thickened (*endarteritis*) and in which the artery is more or less completely blocked. This leads to very serious effects, particularly in the case of arteries supplying the heart and brain. (See also THROMBOANGIITIS OBLITERANS; ANEURYSM.)

ARTERIOGRAPHY (see ANGIOGRAPHY).

ARTERIOLE is a small artery.

ARTERIO-VENOUS ANEURYSM is an abnormal communication between an artery and a vein. It is usually the result of an injury, such as a stab or a gunshot wound, which involves both a neighbouring artery and vein.

ARTERITIS means inflammation of an artery.

ARTHRITIS means inflammation of a joint or joints. The chief forms are osteoarthritis (or osteoarthrosis, as it is now known), rheumatoid, gouty, gonorrhoeal, tuberculous, and traumatic. (See JOINTS, DISEASES OF; GONORRHOEA; GOUT; RHEUMATISM.)

ARTHRODESIS is the operation for fixing a joint in a given position, from which it cannot be moved. It results in a pain-free, stable, strong joint in certain cases of joint disease such as osteoarthrosis of the knee.

ARTHROPATHY is a term applied to any form of joint disease.

ARTHROPLASTY is the term applied to the operation for the making of a new joint as, for example, in advanced cases of osteoarthrosis of the hip, or the loosening of a fixed or stiff joint.

ARTHROPODS are segmented invertebrates with jointed legs. They include a wide range of organisms, such as scorpions, mites, ticks, spiders and centipedes.

ARTICULAR means anything connected with a joint: eg. articular rheumatism.

ARTICULATION is a term employed in two senses in medicine, either meaning the enunciation of words and sentences or meaning a joint.

ARTIFICIAL INSEMINATION is the introduction of semen into the vagina by artificial means. It has long been used in animal breeding, and of recent years has been used to an increasing extent in human beings in an attempt to allow a woman to become pregnant who cannot do so by the normal method. There are two forms of artificial insemination: AIH and AID. In AIH (artificial insemination by the husband) the semen is obtained from the husband. In AID (artificial insemination by a donor) the semen is obtained from a man other than the woman's husband. The former is used when the husband can produce healthy semen but is unable to impregnate his wife; the latter (AID) when the husband is sterile. (See INFERTILITY.)

ARTIFICIAL KIDNEY (see KIDNEY, ARTIFICIAL).

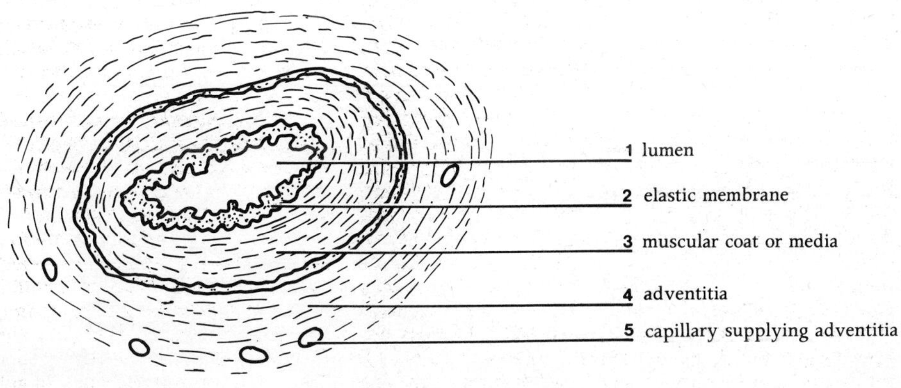

The structure of an artery.

ARTIFICIAL LIMBS AND OTHER PARTS: It is often necessary, for aesthetic or practical reasons, to replace part of the body, lost by injury or disease, with copies of the original, or PROSTHESES as they are now known. From ancient times this has been the case: Herodotus speaks of a man with a wooden foot; the Romans carried the manufacture of limbs to a high degree of efficiency, as witnessed by a leg, the oldest known artificial limb in existence, neatly formed of thin bronze plates, leather and iron, found in a tomb at Capua and dating from around 300 BC; the Etruscans fashioned gold teeth five centuries before the Christian era; Goetz von Berlichingen (1480–1562), to supply his lost right hand, had one made of iron and thus became known as Goetz of the Iron Hand; and Ambroise Paré, who wrote on surgery in the sixteenth century, has a chapter upon artificial limbs. From then there was little advance until 1800 when James Potts, of London, patented an artificial leg made of two hollow wooden cones with a steel knee joint and a wooden ankle joint. It became known as the Anglesey leg after its owner, the Marquis of Anglesey and, with few modifications, remained the basis of British designs until the 1914–1918 War. Since the 1939–1945 War there have been striking advances, particularly in artificial hands, as the result of the introduction of electronics and myoelectric means of control.

Arms: Owing to the very delicate movements which the upper limb has to carry out, it is never amputated if there is any possibility of its being of any use. When amputation is decided upon, as little as possible of the arm is removed. Great strides have been made in the provision of artificial arms and hands, and it is now found that 50 per cent efficiency can be obtained when the amputation has been above the elbow, and 75 per cent efficiency when it is below the elbow. Appliances are now available which allow an individual who has lost an arm to engage, for example, in carpentry, many branches of engineering, and the electrical trades. Such an individual can also write, shoot, play golf and cricket, and even fly-fish.

Legs: An artificial substitute can come much nearer to the usefulness of the original in the lower than in the upper limb. As a result of experience gained in the two World Wars artificial lower limbs are now so efficient that the individual often suffers little disability. This applies particularly to amputations below the knee, but even in the case of amputations high in the thigh many individuals can often resume their old occupations. In addition, they can often ride a bicycle or a horse, or drive a car, whilst tennis and golf are quite normal pastimes. One of the great secrets of success in the fitting of artificial limbs is to restore the patient's morale and to stimulate his sense of independence. As noted in the section on amputation, a considerable time must elapse after amputation, to allow for shrinkage of the stump, before a permanent prosthesis can be fitted. To overcome the practical disadvantages of this delay, a pneumatic post-amputation mobility aid is now available. This fits over the bandaged stump, and is inflated to 40 mm Hg to support a rigid frame. It can be fitted by nurses and paramedical staff without any special training in prosthetics. Using this device patients can now start learning to walk again within a week of their amputation. It is suitable for amputation below, above and through the knee.

Eyes: Artificial eyes are worn both for appearance and to protect the socket from dust, though, of course, vision is impossible. They are made of glass or plastic, and are thin shells of a boat-shape, representing the front half of the eye which has been removed. The stump which is left has still the eye-muscles in it, and so the artificial eye still has the power of moving with the other, though to a less extent, and it is often difficult for this reason to tell at a short distance that a person has a false eye. A glass eye has to be replaced by a new one every year. Plastic eyes have the advantage of being more comfortable to wear, and more durable and of being unbreakable.

Teeth: Where a single tooth is false it is often fitted by a gold peg to the fang of the lost natural one. Where a number are fitted, a plate, either adhering accurately to the gum by suction, or attached to neighbouring teeth by 'crown and bridge work', is employed to carry them. It has been found that in the case of elaborate artificial attachments to roots of teeth suppurative processes of a harmful nature are apt to take place. Less dental work is therefore done at the present day in the form of 'crowning' teeth and attaching artificial teeth by pegs than was formerly carried out.

Nose: The making of a new nose is the oldest known operation in plastic surgery, Hindu records of such operations dating back to 1000 BC. Loss of a nose may be due to eroding disease, war wounds, gun-shot wounds or dog bites. In essence the operation is the same as that practised a thousand years before Christ: namely the use of a skin graft, brought down from the forehead. Alternative sources of the skin graft today are skin from the arm, chest or abdomen. As a means of support the new nose is built round a graft of bone or of cartilage from the ear.

ARTIFICIAL RESPIRATION (see DROWNING, RECOVERY FROM).

ARYTENOID is the name applied to two cartilages in the larynx.

ASBESTOSIS is a form of pneumoconiosis (qv), but its main hazard is the risk of cancer of the lung or pleura, or sometimes of the ovary. It

; caused by the inhalation of asbestos dust, ither in the mining or quarrying of it, or in one f the many industries in which it is used: eg. as n insulating material, in the making of paper, ardboard and brake linings. The number of ases of asbestosis newly diagnosed in England 1 1980 came to 144. Deaths due to asbestos in 984 numbered 2060.

SCARIASIS is the disease produced by infes-ation with the roundworm, *Ascaris lumbri-oides*, also known as the maw-worm. uperficially it resembles a large earthworm. he male measures about 17 cm (7 inches) and e female 23 cm (9 inches) in length. It is a dirt isease, most prevalent where sanitation and leanliness are lacking, particularly in the trop-:s and subtropics. Consumption of food con-aminated by the ova (eggs), especially salad egetables, is the commonest cause of infec-ion. In children, infection is commonly cquired by crawling or playing on contami-ated earth, and then sucking their fingers. fter a complicated life-cycle in the body the dult worms end up in the intestines, whence hey may be passed in the stools. A light infec-ion may cause no symptoms. A heavy infec-ion may lead to colic, or even obstruction of he gut. Occasionally a worm may wander into he stomach and be vomited up.
reatment consists of the administration of evamisole, a piperazine derivative, pyrantel mbonate, or mebendazole.

SCITES means dropsical swelling of the bdomen. (See DROPSY.)

SCORBIC ACID (VITAMIN C) is a substance resent in various natural sources such as fruits nd vegetables, or synthetically prepared. (See ITAMIN.)

SEPSIS is a term, used in distinction from antisepsis', to mean that principle in surgery y which, instead of strong germicides like cor-osive sublimate or carbolic acid being applied o wounds, all the dressings, swabs, and instru-nents used are sterilized by steaming, boiling, r dry heat. Thin, sterilized, india-rubber loves are worn by surgeons and prevent risk of nfection from the hands. Aseptic surgery has he advantage that the germ-destroying activity f the tissues and their healing power after vounds are not lessened by antiseptics which lecrease the vitality of the tissues. Healing is herefore surer and more rapid after an aseptic peration. (See also ANTISEPTICS.)

SH stands for ACTION ON SMOKING AND IEALTH. It is a small charity founded by the Royal College of Physicians in 1971 and sup-orted by the DHSS. Its aim is to alert and nform the public to the dangers of smoking nd to try to prevent the disability and death vhich it causes. It gathers a wide range of infor-nation about smoking and disseminates it to the public to increase knowledge about the dan-gers of smoking and how to give up the habit. It commissions surveys on public attitudes to smoking and brings together working groups on such subjects as giving up smoking and how to prevent children from starting to smoke. It is largely due to the efforts of ASH that the major-ity of adults in the United Kingdom (more than six out of ten) are now non-smokers. ASH works on their behalf by pressing proprietors of public space to provide more smoke-free areas and advising them how to create and operate them. Hundreds of smokers who would like to give up smoking contact ASH for information every month. ASH has a small headquarters staff in London with other national and regional branches in Scotland, Wales, and Northern Ireland. More branches are opening every year. Further information can be obtained from ASH, 5–11 Mortimer Street, London W1N 7RH (Tel: 01-637 9843).

ASPARAGINASE is an enzyme that breaks down the amino-acid, asparagine. This is of no significance to most cells in the body as they can make asparagine from simpler constitu-ents. Certain tumours, however, are unable to do this and therefore, if they cannot receive ready-made supplies of the amino-acid, they die. It is on this basis that asparaginase is prov-ing of promise in the treatment of tumours which, by the administration of asparaginase, are deprived of an essential metabolite – and perish.

ASPARTANE is an artificial sweetener 200 times as sweet as sugar but without the bitter after-taste of saccharine. It has been passed as safe for human use by the Food Additives and Contaminants Committee and at the moment is awaiting parliamentary approval to become available in Britain. It is suitable for diabetics. It is not usable in baking.

ASPERGILLOSIS is a disease caused by inva-sion of the lung by the fungus, *Aspergillus fumi-gatus*. The infection is acquired by inhalation of air-borne spores of the fungus which settle and grow in damaged parts of the lung such as healed tuberculous cavities, abscesses, or the dilated bronchi of bronchiectasis (qv).

ASPERGILLUS is the name applied to a group of fungi including the common moulds. Several of these are capable of infecting the lungs and producing a disease resembling pulmonary tuberculosis.

ASPHYXIA means literally absence of pulse, but is the name given to the whole series of symptoms which follow stoppage of breathing and of the heart's action.
Causes: For practical consideration, by far the most important cause is *drowning*. Human beings are not adapted to extract the oxygen dissolved in water – first, because the amount is only one-third of that required to supply the

needs of the processes of diffusion which take place in the lungs; and, secondly, because the air or fluid taken in through the mouth must return the same way, there being no second opening and rapid constant stream like that by which in fishes a great quantity of water passes over the gills in a short time. *Blockage of the air passages* occurs in some diseases, such as croup, diphtheria, swelling of the throat due to wounds or inflammation, asthma (to a partial extent), tumours in the chest (causing slow asphyxia), and the external conditions of suffocation and strangling. *Poisonous gases* also cause asphyxia. Carbon dioxide in excessive amount in the air, due to the breathing of a number of individuals in a small space, or to the fumes given off in fermentation vats, has often caused death. Carbon monoxide gas is still more deadly, and in the form of 'water gas', or when it is given off, for example, by a stove or charcoal brazier in a badly ventilated room, has killed many people during sleep. (See CARBON MONOXIDE.) Several gases, such as sulphurous acid (from burning sulphur), ammonia, and chlorine (from bleaching-powder), cause involuntary closure of the entrance to the larynx, and thus prevent breathing. Other gases, such as nitrous oxide (or laughing-gas), chloroform, and ether, in poisonous quantity, cause stoppage of breathing by paralysing the respiration centre in the brain.

Symptoms: In the vast majority of cases death from asphyxia is due to insufficiency of oxygen supplied to the blood. The first signs – apart from instinctive efforts to escape from the cause, such as the struggles of a drowning man – are rapid pulse and gasping for breath. Next comes great increase in the pressure of the blood, causing throbbing in the head, with lividity or blueness of the skin, due to failure of aeration of the blood, followed by still greater struggles for breath and by general convulsions. Accordingly, the heart becomes over-distended and gradually weaker, a paralytic stage sets in, and all struggling and breathing slowly cease. When, on the other hand, asphyxia is due to charcoal fumes, coal-gas, and other narcotic influences, there is no convulsive stage, and death ensues gently and may occur in the course of sleep. After death, the right side of the heart, the large veins, and the pulmonary artery are found distended by blood, and this blood is fluid instead of in clots, as it is after a gradual death. These are the chief signs of death by asphyxia, but each cause produces distinguishing signs of its own.

Treatment: So long as the heart continues to beat, recovery may be looked for under prompt treatment. The one essential of treatment is to get the impure blood aerated by artificial respiration. Besides this, the feeble circulation can be helped by various methods. (See under DROWNING, RECOVERY FROM.)

ASPHYXIA NEONATORUM is imperfect breathing in the new-born infant. It has been estimated that it plays a part in about half the deaths which occur during the first month of life. The main causes are serious illness of the mother during the latter months of pregnancy, anaesthetics or analgesics given to the mother during labour, prolonged labour, obstruction to the circulation in the umbilical cord, obstruction of the infant's air passages, intracranial haemorrhage, and congenital heart disease.

ASPIRATION means the withdrawal of fluid or gases from the natural cavities of the body or from cavities produced by disease. It may be performed either for curative purposes, or, very often, a small amount is drawn off for diagnosis of the nature or origin of the fluid. *Pleurisy with effusion* is a condition requiring aspiration, and a litre or more of fluid may be drawn off by an aspirator or a large syringe and needle. *Chronic abscesses* and *tuberculous joints* may call for its use, the operation being done with a small syringe and hollow needle. *Pericarditis with effusion* is another condition in which aspiration is sometimes performed. The spinal canal is aspirated by the operation of lumbar puncture. (See LUMBAR PUNCTURE.) In children the ventricles of the brain are sometimes similarly relieved from excess of fluid by piercing the fontanelle (soft spot) on the infant's head. (See HYDROCEPHALUS.)

ASPIRIN, or ACETYLSALICYLIC ACID, is a white crystalline powder which is used like sodium salicylate as a remedy for rheumatism, chorea, neuralgia, etc., also to reduce fever in infectious diseases. It has some action in relieving pain and producing sleep and is therefore often used for headache and slighter degrees of insomnia. The dose is 300 mg to 1 g.

ASPIRIN POISONING may not be common in relation to the vast amounts that are consumed every year, but nevertheless it is a worrying problem.

In ordinary doses it may induce bleeding from the stomach. This is usually quite mild but it can be severe. In small doses it can produce a severe allergic reaction in individuals who are sensitive to it. This takes the form of asthma and angioneurotic oedema.

When an overdose is taken there is marked over-breathing, sweating and vomiting. Later the individual becomes restless and irritable and there may be convulsions before consciousness is finally lost.

Treatment: The stomach should be washed out preferably with an alkaline solution, and a litre of 5 per cent sodium bicarbonate should be left in the stomach. If there has been much loss of fluid by sweating and vomiting, fluids may need to be given intravenously. In severe cases oxygen may need to be administered.

ASTEREOGNOSIS means the loss of the capacity to recognize the nature of an object by feeling it, and indicates a lesion (eg. tumour) of the brain.

ASTHENIA means want of strength. (See DEBILITY.)

ASTHENOPIA means a sense of weakness in the eyes, coming on when they are used. As a rule it is due to long-sightedness, slight inflammation, or weakness of the muscles that move the eyes. (See VISION.)

ASTHMA is a disorder of respiration characterized by severe paroxysms of difficult breathing, usually followed by a period of complete relief, with recurrence of the attacks at more or less frequent intervals. The term is often incorrectly employed in reference to states of embarrassed respiration, which are plainly due to permanent organic disease within the chest, and which have none of the distinctive characters of true asthma.

Cause: Asthma is an allergic reaction which manifests itself by spasmodic contraction of the smaller bronchial tubes (see ALLERGY). It is this narrowing of the bronchial tubes, often accentuated by swelling of the lining epithelium, that is responsible for the great difficulty in breathing which is the characteristic feature of the condition. There is a large number of substances to which the asthmatic subject may be hypersensitive, contact with which is responsible for an attack. These include pollens; the emanations of certain animals such as cats, dogs, horses; house dust; certain articles of diet; bacteria; the house-dust mite, *Dermatophagoides*; certain industrial agents such as platinum salts (see OCCUPATIONAL DISEASES). Fifty per cent of asthmatics in Japan are said to be allergic to butterflies. The discovery of the substance to which the individual is susceptible may sometimes be difficult. Thus, it may be noted that attacks of asthma occur when the patient goes to bed, and it may be found that these occur because he is susceptible to feathers and the like, with which the pillow is filled. In other instances the difficulty may be due to the fact that the individual is hypersensitive to more than one substance. In many cases the specific susceptibility of the individual may be enhanced by some non-specific conditions, such as emotional disturbance, worry, indigestion or an infection such as a sore throat or a 'cold in the head'. There is another group of asthmatic subjects in whom the asthma is due to sensitization to bacteria responsible for some chronic or repeated infection. For instance, an individual who is subject to repeated attacks of tonsillitis, sinusitis, or nasal catarrh may become sensitized to the causative organism, so that whenever he becomes infected with this organism he is liable to develop attacks of asthma. The reason why asthma does not develop in all such individuals subject to repeated infections, is that such attacks only occur in the individual who has the tendency to develop hypersensitivity or has a family history of such allergic conditions. This tendency is usually hereditary, and it will often be found that the asthmatic subject suffers from other allergic conditions such as hay fever and urticaria (or nettle-rash). Asthma is more common in males than in females, and the first attack usually occurs in childhood. It is estimated that there are 2,000,000 asthmatics in Britain and that around 1 in 20 school children suffer from the disease. Deaths from asthma in Britain in 1984 amounted to 1764.

There is a form of asthma which may not develop until later in life. This occurs in individuals who suffer from chronic bronchitis. A certain proportion of these people ultimately become sensitized to the organisms responsible for their chronic bronchitis, and this sensitization may not develop until middle age.

One other condition to which the term asthma is applied must be carefully differentiated from the condition that has just been described. This is *cardiac asthma*. It consists of sudden attacks of shortness of breath while the patient is resting; it is a grave sign, as it is due to severe heart failure.

Symptoms: The onset of an attack of asthma is usually sudden, although there may exist certain symptoms which warn the sufferer of its approach, such as a feeling of discomfort, drowsiness, irritability, and depression of spirits. The period when the asthmatic paroxysm comes on is generally during the night, or rather in the early hours of morning. The patient then awakes in a state of great anxiety and alarm, with a sense of weight and tightness across the chest, which he feels himself unable to expand with freedom. Respiration is performed with great difficulty, and is accompanied by wheezing noises. His distress rapidly increases, and he can no longer retain the recumbent position, but gets up, and sits or stands with his shoulders raised, his head thrown back, and his whole body heaving with his desperate efforts to breathe. His face is pale or livid, and wet with perspiration, while his extremities are cold; his pulse is rapid, and may be irregular or intermitting. All his clothing must be loose about him; he cannot bear to be touched, and the very presence of others around him seems to aggravate his distress. His one desire is to breathe fresh air; and he will place himself by an open window and sit for hours in the middle of the night, unmindful of the exposure. The paroxysm, after continuing for a variable length of time, often extending over many hours, begins to abate, the breathing becomes easier, and the subsidence of the attack is often marked by the occurrence of coughing with expectoration.

After the cessation of the attack the patient appears to be, and feels, comparatively well. In cases of long standing, however, the subject of asthma comes to bear permanent evidence of its effects. He is easily put out of breath on exertion and he requires to lie with his head elevated, circumstances to be ascribed to organic changes in the chest, which oft-recurring attacks of asthma are liable to induce (see EMPHYSEMA). The asthmatic paroxysms, although occasionally periodic, do not generally observe any regularity in their return. They may recur each successive night for several days, or there may be no return for many weeks or months, this being to a large extent dependent on a renewal of the exciting cause.

Treatment: The treatment of asthma consists in the employment of remedies to allay the paroxysms, and in the adoption of measures likely to prevent their recurrence. During the attack the patient should be placed in as favourable circumstances for breathing as practicable. He usually selects the position easiest for himself. Abundance of air should be admitted to the apartment, and he should be interfered with as little as possible.

In the majority of cases certain drugs are required which should only be taken under medical supervision. These include adrenaline (by injection), ephedrine, aminophylline, isoprenaline, salbutamol, terburaline, and sodium cromoglycate. The latter four are often taken by means of inhalation. In severe cases, corticotrophin, or one of the cortisone group of drugs, is often of value.

To prevent the recurrence of the paroxysms special care must be taken by the sufferer to avoid those influences, whether connected with locality or mode of life, which his experience may have proved to have been the occasion of former attacks. Care must particularly be taken to avoid exposure to those influences apt to bring on bronchitis. Breathing exercises are often of value in reducing the frequency of attacks. In the group of cases found to be due to a particular animal emanation or article of diet, care should be taken to avoid this cause. Thus in those cases due to the house-dust mite preventive measures include daily vacuum-cleaning of the bedroom, the use of synthetic bedding material which should be washed frequently and the enclosure of the mattress in an impervious cover.

The possibility that psychological factors may be responsible, in part at least, should always be borne in mind, and, if present, they should be dealt with if possible. Hypnosis is of value in some cases. (See also OCCUPATIONAL DISEASES.)

ASTIGMATISM is an error of refraction in the eye due to the cornea (the clear membrane in front of the eye) being unequally curved in different directions, so that rays of light in different meridians cannot be brought to a focus together on the retina. The curvature, instead of being globular, is egg-shaped, longer in one axis than the other. The condition causes objects to seem distorted and out of place, a ball for instance looking like an egg, a circle like an ellipse. The condition is remedied by suitable spectacles of which one surface forms part of a cylinder. (See SPECTACLES.)

ASTROVIRUSES are small round viruses wi no distinctive features, which have been is lated from the stools of infants with ga troenteritis (see DIARRHOEA).

ASYNERGIA means the absence of harmon ous and co-ordinated movements betwee muscles having opposite actions – eg. the fle ors and extensors of a joint – and is a sign disease of the nervous system.

ASYSTOLE means arrest of the action of th heart.

ATARACTIC is the term used to describe dru which induce peace of mind. For all practic purposes it is synonymous with tranquilliz (qv). It has never been widely adopted Britain.

ATAVISM means the principle of inheritanc of disease or bodily characters from grandpa ents or remoter ancestors, the parents not ha ing been affected by these.

ATAXIA means loss of coordination, thoug the power necessary to make the movements still present. Thus an ataxic person may have good grip in each hand but be unable to do an fine movements with the fingers, or, if th ataxia be in the legs, he throws these about great deal in walking, though he can lift the le and take steps quite well. This is due to a se sory defect or to disease of the cerebellum. (Se FRIEDRICH'S ATAXIA; LOCOMOTOR ATAXIA.)

ATELECTASIS means collapse of a part of th lung, or failure of the lung to expand at birt

ATENOLOL (TENORMIN) is a drug th antagonises beta adrenergic receptors (qv) an is proving of value in the treatment of hig blood-pressure. One of its practical advantage is that only one dose a day need be taken. (Se ADRENERGIC RECEPTORS.)

ATHEROMA is a degenerative change in th inner and middle coats of arteries. (See ARTE IES, DISEASES OF.)

ATHEROSCLEROSIS is a form of arteriosclе rosis (qv), in which there is fatty degeneratio of the middle coat of the arterial wall.

ATHETOID SPASMS are slow writhing move ments affecting the distal parts of the limb They are due to disease of the extra-pyramid system.

ATHETOSIS is the name for slow, involuntary writhing, and repeated movements of th hands and feet, caused by disease of the brair

ATHLETE'S FOOT is a somewhat loose term applied to a skin eruption on the foot, usuall between the toes. It is commonly due to ringworm (qv), but may be due to other infections, or merely excessive sweating of the feet.

ATLAS is the name applied to the first cervical vertebra. (See SPINAL COLUMN.)

ATONY means want of tone or vigour in muscles and other organs.

ATOPY, meaning out of place, is a form of hypersensitivity characterized, amongst other features, by a familial tendency. It is due to the propensity of the affected individual to produce large amounts of reagin antibodies which stick to mast cells in the mucosa so that when the antigen is inhaled histamine is released from the mast cell. It is the condition responsible for asthma and hay fever. (See also ALLERGY.) It is estimated that 10 per cent of the human race are subject to atopy. (See also ECZEMA.)

ATRESIA means the absence of a natural opening, or closure of it by a membrane. Thus atresia may be found in new-born infants preventing the bowels from moving, and, in young girls after puberty, absence of the menstrual flow may be due to such a malformation.

ATRIAL NATRIURETIC PEPTIDE: The atria of the heart contain peptides with potent diuretic and vaso-dilating properties. It has been known since 1980 that extracts of human atria have potent diurectic and natriuretic effects in animals (see DIURETICS). In 1984 three polypeptide species were isolated from human atria and were called alpha, beta and gamma human atrial natriuretic peptides. Plasma concentration of immuno-reactive atrial natriuretic peptide can now be measured. The levels are low in healthy subjects and are increased in patients with congestive heart failure. Infusion of the peptides into human volunteers causes a natriuresis and diuresis. Atrial natriuretic peptide is thus the most recently isolated hormone.

ATRIUM is the name now given to the two upper cavities of the heart. These used to be known as the auricles of the heart. The term is also applied to the part of the ear immediately internal to the drum of the ear. (Plural: ATRIA.)

ATROPHY is a term used to describe a state of wasting due to some interference with the function of healthy nutrition. It is essential for the maintenance of health that a balance is maintained between the processes of waste and repair. When the appropriation of nutriment exceeds the waste, hypertrophy or increase in bulk of the tissues takes place. (See HYPERTROPHY.) When, on the other hand, the supply of nutritive matter is suspended or diminished, or when the power of assimilation is impaired, atrophy or wasting is the result. Thus the whole body becomes atrophied in many diseases; and in old age every part of the frame, with the exception of the heart, undergoes atrophic change. Atrophy may, however, affect single organs or parts of the body, irrespective of the general state of nutrition, and this may be brought about in a variety of ways. One of the most frequently observed of such instances is atrophy from disuse, or cessation of function.

Thus, when a limb is deprived of the natural power of motion, either by paralysis or by painful joint disease, atrophy of all its tissues sooner or later takes place. This form of atrophy is likewise well exemplified in the case of those organs and structures of the body which subserve important ends during foetal life, but which, ceasing to be necessary after birth, undergo a sort of natural atrophy, such as the thymus gland, and certain vessels specially concerned in the foetal circulation. The ovaries, after the child-bearing period, become shrunken.

Atrophy of a part may also be caused by interruption to its normal blood supply, as in the case of the ligature or obstruction of an artery. Again, long-standing disease, by affecting the nutrition of an organ and by inducing the deposit of morbid products, may result in atrophy, as frequently happens in affections of the liver and kidneys. Parts that are subjected to continuous pressure are liable to become atrophied, as is sometimes seen in internal organs which have been compressed by tumours or other morbid growths.

Atrophy may manifest itself simply by loss of substance; on the other hand, it is often found to co-exist with degenerative changes and the formation of fibrous or fatty growth, so that the part may not be reduced in bulk, although atrophied as regards its proper structure. Thus, in the case of the heart, when affected with fatty degeneration, there is atrophy of the proper muscular texture, but this, being largely replaced by fatty material, the organ may undergo no diminution in volume, but may, on the contrary, be increased in size. Atrophy is usually a gradual and slow process, but sometimes it proceeds rapidly. In the disease known by the name of *acute yellow atrophy of the liver*, that organ undergoes such rapidly destructive change as may result in its shrinking to half, or one-third, of its normal size in the course of a few days.

The term *progressive muscular atrophy* (*wasting* or *creeping palsy*) is applied to an affection of the muscular system, which is characterized by the atrophy and subsequent paralysis of certain muscles, or groups of muscles, and is associated with morbid changes in the anterior part of the grey matter in the spinal cord. This disease begins insidiously, and is often first observed to affect the muscles of one hand, generally the right. Gradually other muscles in the arms and legs become affected in a similar manner, their atrophy being attended with a corresponding diminution in power. (See PROGRESSIVE MUSCULAR ATROPHY *under* PARALYSIS.)

The term *idiopathic muscular atrophy* (also known as *muscular dystrophy*) is applied to a somewhat similar condition affecting young people in whom a progressive degeneration of the muscles occurs. In this condition no change is found in the nervous system after death, the cause apparently acting directly upon the muscles. (See MUSCLES, DISEASES OF.)

ATROPINE is the active principle of belladonna, the juice of the deadly nightshade. Because of its action in dilating the pupils it was at one time used as a cosmetic to give the eyes a full, lustrous appearance. It acts by antagonizing the action of the parasympathetic nervous system (qv). It temporarily impairs vision by paralysing accommodative power. (See ACCOMMODATION.) It has the effect of checking the activity of almost all the glands of the body, including the sweat glands of the skin and the salivary glands in the mouth. It relieves spasm by paralysing nerves in the muscle of the intestine, bile-ducts, bladder, stomach, etc. It has the power, in moderate doses, of markedly increasing the rate of the heart-beats, though by very large doses the heart, along with all other muscles, is paralysed and stopped.

Uses: Externally, liniment of belladonna is used in neuralgia, and other painful conditions. In eye troubles, atropine drops are used to dilate the pupil for more thorough examination of the interior of the eye, or to draw the iris away from wounds and ulcers on the centre of the eye; they also soothe the pain due to light falling on an inflamed eye, and are further used to paralyse the ciliary muscle and so prevent accommodative changes in the eye while the eye is being examined with the ophthalmoscope (qv). Belladonna is employed in cough-mixtures for bronchitis and whooping-cough to dry up the mucus and check spasmodic coughing. In renal colic, gall-stone colic, and other agonizing spasmodic conditions, atropine is given along with morphine by hypodermic injection. It is also used to decrease the amount of gastric secretion in peptic ulcer. It has been used as an antidote in opium poisoning and to muscarine, the poisonous principle of some toadstools.

ATROPINE or BELLADONNA POISONING: This may occur from children eating the berries or leaves of the deadly nightshade (see BERRIES, POISONOUS). The appearance of a patient with atropine poisoning has been described as: 'hot as a hare, red as a beet, blind as a bat, dry as a bone, and mad as a wet hen'. The warning symptoms are: (1) great dryness of the mouth and throat, (2) wide dilatation of the pupils, (3) increased rate of the heart's action. There is sickness later, and the poisoned person has an excited delirium with, at the same time, bodily languor and weakness. If the dose has been very large, paralysis, unconsciousness, and gradual stoppage of heart and breathing ensue.

Treatment: The swallowed material should be got rid of by washing out the stomach followed by a saline purgative such as sodium sulphate, 30 grams in 250 millilitres of water. If breathing becomes feeble, artificial respiration must be performed. The patient should be given plenty to drink and be made to pass water frequently, as the poison is excreted by the kidneys, and may otherwise be reabsorbed. A sedative, such as diazepam or phenobarbitone, is given to control the excitement, as well as neostigmine which is a specific antidote.

AUDIOANALGESIA is a method of relieving the pains of childbirth. It is produced by the patient listening through headphones to a combination of white sound and music. The intensity of the sound is controlled by the woman herself according to the intensity of her pain. Experience suggests that the method is successful in women who are well adapted, like music and have some understanding of labour and delivery.

AUDIOMETRY is the testing of hearing.

AUDITORY NERVE (see VESTIBULOCOCHLEAR NERVE).

AURA is a peculiar feeling which persons, subject to epileptic seizures, have just before the onset of an attack. It may be a sensation of a cold breeze, a peculiar smell, a vision of some animal or person, an undefinable sense of disgust, or the like, but it is very important for persons who experience it, because it gives warning that a fit is coming and may enable a place of safety or seclusion to be reached.

AURICLE is a term applied both to the pinna or flap of the ear and also to the ear-shaped tip of the atrium of the heart.

AURISCOPE is an instrument for examining the ear. The source of illumination may be incorporated in the instrument, as in the electric auriscope, or it may be an independent light which is reflected into the ear by means of a forehead mirror.

AURISTILLAE are ear-drops.

AURUM is the Latin name for gold.

AUSCULTATION is a term in medicine applied to the method employed by physicians for determining, by the sense of hearing, the condition of certain internal organs. The ancient physicians appear to have practised a kind of auscultation, by which they were able to detect the presence of air or fluids in the cavities of the chest and abdomen.

In 1819, the distinguished French physician, Laennec, introduced the method of auscultation by means of the stethoscope with which his name stands permanently associated. For some time previously, physicians, more especially in the hospitals of Paris, had been in the habit of applying the ear over the region of the heart for the purpose of listening to the sounds of that rgan, and it was in the employment of this nethod that Laennec conceived the idea that hese sounds might be better conveyed through he medium of some solid body interposed etween his ear and the patient's chest. He olled up a quire of paper into the form of a ylinder and applied it in the manner just mentioned, when he found that he was able to pereive the action of the heart more distinctly han he had ever been able to do by the immediate application of his ear. He thence inferred hat not merely the heart's sounds, but also hose of other organs of the chest might be rought within reach of the ear by some such nstrument. He therefore had constructed the vooden cylinder, or stethoscope, which bears is name. This instrument was subsequently nodified by Piorry to the form of a thin narrow ylinder, about 18 cm (7 inches) long, with an xpansion at one end for applying to the chest, nd a more or less flattened surface at the other or the ear of the listener.

The binaural stethoscope, consisting of a mall expanded chest-piece and two flexible ubes with ivory or vulcanite ends that fit ightly into the ears of the observer, is the type now generally used. This form is in some ways nore convenient to use, though the sounds are no more clearly heard than with Piorry's instrument, and, in some cases, are less distinct, as he conduction of sound by the flexible tubes is ntirely aerial. Various modifications of the inaural stethoscope have been introduced, uch as the phonendoscope, in which the place of the chest-piece is taken by a small drum. An lectrical stethoscope has been devised, hrough which, by the help of a microphone, elephone, and amplification, the beating of the neart, murmurs, etc., may be heard at a distance from the patient with any desired ntensity.

The numerous conditions affecting the lungs can be recognized and discriminated from each other by means of auscultation and the stethoscope. The same holds good in the case of the heart, whose varied and often complex forms of disease can, by auscultation, be identified with striking accuracy. But in addition to these, its main uses, auscultation is helpful in the investigation of many obscure internal affections, such as aneurysms and certain diseases of the oesophagus and stomach. To the accoucheur the stethoscope yields valuable aid in the detection of some forms of uterine tumours, and especially in the diagnosis of pregnancy – the auscultatory evidence afforded by the sounds of the foetal heart being one of the most reliable of the many signs of pregnancy and giving valuable information concerning the viability of the foetus.

AUTO- is a prefix meaning self.

AUTISM: The term autism was introduced by Kanner in 1943 to describe a disharmony of development in which children are unable to mature socially despite excellent motor skill. Thus, despite their manual dexterity they are unable to form emotional bonds, even with their parents. Because of their disregard of other people they are refractory to discipline. Although they may acquire some language, they communicate little.

Advice and information on autism may be obtained from The National Autistic Society, 276 Willesden Lane, London NW2 5RB (Tel: 01-451 1114).

AUTOCLAVE: This is one of the most effective ways of ensuring that material, eg. surgical dressings, is completely sterilized and that even the most resistant bacteria with which it may be contaminated, are destroyed. Its use is based upon the fact that water boils when its vapour pressure is equal to the pressure of the surrounding atmosphere. This means that if the pressure inside a closed vessel be increased, the temperature at which water inside the vessel boils, will rise above 100°C. By adjusting the pressure, almost any temperature for the boiling of the water will be obtained. This is now one of the most widely used methods of sterilization in hospitals and laboratories.

AUTOGENOUS means self-generated and is the term applied to products which arise within the body. It is applied to bacterial vaccines manufactured from the organisms found in discharges from the body and used for the treatment of the person from whom the bacteria were derived.

AUTO-IMMUNITY is the process whereby an individual develops antibodies to his own tissues. Normally an individual does not develop antibodies to his own tissues, but only to invaders of the body such as micro-organisms. The precise reason why some individuals develop this unfortunate propensity is still obscure but it is proving a fruitful line of investigation into the cause of some diseases of hitherto unknown origin.

AUTO-INTOXICATION means literally self-poisoning, and is any condition of poisoning brought about by substances formed in or by the body.

AUTOLYSIS means the disintegration and softening of dead cells brought about by enzymes in the cells themselves.

AUTOMATISM means the performance of acts without conscious will, as, for example, after an attack of epilepsy or concussion of the brain. In such conditions the person may perform acts of which he is neither conscious at the time nor has any memory afterwards. It is especially liable to occur when persons suffering from epilepsy, mental subnormality, or concussion consume alcoholic liquors. It may also occur following the taking of barbiturates or psychedelic drugs (qv). There are, however, other cases in which there are no such precipitatory factors. Thus it may occur following hypnosis, mental stress or strain, or conditions such as fugues (qv) or somnambulism (see SLEEP). The condition is of considerable importance from a legal point of view, because acts done in this state, and for which the person committing them is not responsible, may be of a criminal nature. According to English law, however, it entails complete loss of consciousness, and only then is it a defence to an action for negligence. A lesser impairment of consciousness is no defence.

AUTONOMIC NERVOUS SYSTEM is part of the nervous system which regulates the functions of some of the internal organs independently of the will power. It consists of two main divisions – the SYMPATHETIC and the PARASYMPATHETIC SYSTEMS (qv).

AUTOPSY means a post-mortem examination, or the examination of the internal organs of a dead body. (See NECROPSY.)

AUTO-SUGGESTION is a peculiar mental state, which sometimes occurs after accidents, in which the will and judgment are partially perverted, so that slight or temporary injuries are greatly exaggerated in the imagination, and the person believes himself to be affected by some serious disability. Examples of this are found in paralysed and insensitive limbs following some minor bruise, for example in a railway accident, and the blindness, deafness, or inability to speak, which sometimes followed concussion in soldiers, especially when the injury was received in the dark. This state is also called 'traumatic suggestion'. The condition often approaches very near to, or is mingled with, the condition of malingering, in which the person consciously suggests to himself or produces some disability from an ulterior motive, as, for example, in some of the prolonged cases of disability following a trifling injury for which a person is in receipt of compensation. The term is also applied to the reverse process, by which, either as a result of suggestion by another person, or suggestion applied by the will-power of the person affected, a cure of such a condition is accomplished.

AVERSION THERAPY is a form of psychological treatment in which such an unpleasant response is induced to his psychological aberration that the patient decides to give it up. Thus the victim of alcoholism is given a drug that makes the subsequent drinking of alcoholic liquors so unpleasant by inducing nausea and vomiting that he decides to give up drinking. (See ALCOHOLISM, CHRONIC; and DISULFIRAM.) Another commonly used method of inducing aversion is an electric shock. Aversion therapy is proving of value in the treatment of alcoholism, drug addiction, sexual deviations, such as transvestism, and compulsive gambling.

AVITAMINOSIS is the condition of a human being or an animal deprived of one or more vitamins.

AVOMINE is the trade name for promethazine theoclate, which is widely, and successfully used as a remedy for travel sickness.

AXILLA is the anatomical name for the armpit (See ARMPIT.)

AXIS is the name applied to the second cervical vertebra. (See SPINAL COLUMN.)

AZAPROPAZONE (RHEUMOX) (see NON-STEROIDAL ANTI-INFLAMMATORY DRUGS).

AZATHIOPRINE (IMURAN) is a cytotoxic and an immunosuppressive drug. In the first of these capacities it is proving of value in the treatment of acute leukaemia. As an immunosuppressive agent, by reducing the antibody response of the body it is proving of value in facilitating the success of transplant operations by reducing the chances of the transplanted organ, eg. the kidney, being rejected by the body. It is also proving of value in the treatment of auto-immune diseases. (See CYTOTOXIC DRUGS.)

AZIDOCILLIN (see ANTIBIOTIC).

AZOOSPERMIA is the condition characterized by lack of spermatozoa in the semen.

AZOTAEMIA means the presence of urea and other nitrogenous bodies in greater concentration than normal in the blood. The condition is generally associated with advanced types of kidney disease.

AZOTE is another name for nitrogen.

B

BABINSKI REFLEX is an abnormal response of the plantar reflex. When a sharp body is drawn along the sole of the foot, instead of the toes bending down towards the sole as usual, the great toe is turned upwards and the other toes tend to spread apart. This response may be obtained in normal infants, but after the age of about two years its presence indicates some severe disturbance in the upper part of the central nervous system.

BACAMPICILLIN (see ANTIBIOTIC).

BACILLI are micro-organisms which are rod-like in form. (See under BACTERIOLOGY.)

BACITRACIN is a polypeptide antibiotic derived from *Bacilluslicheniformis*. It is active against the same range of bacteria as penicillin.

BACK: The back consists mainly of the spinal column and hinder parts of the ribs, and the wide-spreading iliac or haunch bones with the sacrum below. The bones are covered by thick and powerful muscles, which above support and move the head and which below pass round the flanks and downwards into the lower limbs. The skin covering the back is not very sensitive and is not greatly subject to painful conditions. The powerful muscles, of which the chief is the erector spinae, are much subject to minor injuries, the result of twists and strains, and also to rheumatic affections (see LUMBAGO). Diseases and injuries of the spinal column and spinal cord are of a very serious nature (see SPINAL COLUMN; SPINAL CORD).

BACKACHE is a symptom of many diseases. In addition to being the result of local causes, pain may be referred to the back from diseases in deep-seated organs. Medical causes which include inflammatory conditions, neoplasms and metabolic disorders are generally readily recognised but in total they are involved in only 1 or 2 per cent of all cases of chronic persistent backache. Similarly, sensations of pain experienced in the back but originating elsewhere in the body are usually identified by clinical history and laboratory investigations. A large majority of episodes of back pain stem from mechanical or structural disorders. Within this category diagnosis of a prolapsed intervertebral disc as the cause of suffering is relatively straightforward. In many other instances, however, the mechanical abnormalities giving rise to pain remain the subject of speculation. The main causes of back pain are:

(1) Mechanical and traumatic causes.
(*a*) Musculo tenderness and ligament strain.
(*b*) Fractures of the spine.
(*c*) Prolapsed intravertebral disc.
(*d*) Spondylosis.
(*e*) Congenital anomalies.
(2) Inflammatory causes.
(*a*) Osteomyelitis.
(*b*) Tuberculosis.
(*c*) Brucellosis.
(*d*) Paravertebral abcess.
(*e*) Spondyloarthropathy.
(*f*) Ankylosing spondylitis.
(*g*) Reiter's syndrome.
(*h*) Psoriatic arthropathy.
(3) Neoplastic causes.
(*a*) Primary benign tumours.
(*b*) Primary malignant tumours.
(*c*) Metastatic disease.
(4) Metabolic bone disease.
(*a*) Osteoporosis.
(*b*) Osteomalacia.
(*c*) Paget's disease.
(5) Referred pain.
(*a*) Posterior duodenal ulcer.
(*b*) Carcinoma of the pancreas.
(*c*) Pelvic disease–prolapse of the womb. Ovarian inflammation and tumours.
(6) Psychogenic causes.
(*a*) Anxiety.
(*b*) Depression.

People with backache can obtain advice from the National Back Pain Association, Grundy House, 31–33 Park Road, Teddington, Middlesex TW11 0AB (Tel: 01–977 5474).

BACLOFEN is a muscle-relaxing drug that is proving of value in relieving the spasm of muscles in some cases of multiple sclerosis (qv).

BACTERAEMIA is the condition in which bacteria are present in the bloodstream.

BACTERIA is a term which, strictly speaking, means small micro-organisms of a simple primitive form, but the word is now vaguely used to cover a great variety of low microscopic forms of plant life. It is equivalent to terms such as 'germs', 'microbes', 'micro-organisms'.

BACTERICIDE strictly means anything which kills bacteria, but is usually applied to drugs and antiseptics which do this. Hence BACTERICIDAL.

BACTERIOLOGY is the branch of biological science concerned with the study of the lowest forms of plant life, particularly of those which cause disease in men and animals, and putrefaction. It is now tending to be replaced by the more general term, microbiology. (For details on INFECTION; IMMUNITY; ANTISEPTICS; VACCINATION; SERUM THERAPY; and OPSONINS, see these headings.) Although bacteria had been noticed about 1687 by Leeuwenhoek and others after the introduction of the microscope, they were not definitely associated with disease until the nineteenth century. Goodsir, in 1842, described *sarcinae* in the stomach, and Davaine in 1865 noticed the large organisms of anthrax, but Pasteur was the first, about 1865, to make a complete study of the manner in which micro-organisms multiply and produce disease. He was followed by Koch, who in 1876 worked out the complete life-history and spore formation of the bacillus of anthrax. In 1877, Koch published his methods of staining films of bacteria; in 1878 his great memoir on the cause of infectious diseases, describing those kinds of bacteria which produce suppuration in wounds; and in 1881 his method of obtaining pure cultures of different organisms. Koch's methods founded the science of bacteriology.

Classification of micro-organisms: If we include the viruses the micro-organisms which cause disease may be grouped as follows: (1) *Moulds*, of which penicillium, the green cheese-mould, and mucor, a white mould, are examples. These grow on leather, bread, and in fact anything of a nutritious nature which happens to be damp, their spores floating everywhere in the air. One mould is sometimes a cause of pneumonia, another causes disease in salmon, and others produce the various forms of ringworm. (2) *Yeasts*, of which one is of great importance as being the producer of alcohol. (3) *Bacteria* proper. These are again divided, mainly owing to their shape, into *cocci*, which are round; *bacilli*, long, slender rods; *spirilla*, curved or wavy. They have secondary names according to some physical property, such as the power of producing colour, as *Staphylococcus aureus*, which appears under the microscope in grape-like clusters, produces pus in the body, and grows in golden-yellow masses when artificially cultivated. *Streptococci* are cocci arranged in chains; *diplococci* occur in pairs. (4) *Rickettsiae*, named after the bacteriologist, Ricketts, are disease-causing micro-organisms, coccal or rod-shaped, and intermediate in size between bacteria and viruses. Rickettsiae are the infecting agents in typhus and typhus-like fevers, and also of trench fever. *Rickettsiae prowazekii*, the infecting agent of typhus, is conveyed to man by infected lice. Other rickettsial infections – such as Rocky Mountain fever – are conveyed by ticks or fleas. (5) *Viruses* are living agents which cause disease and are so minute that they pass through porcelain filters impassable by ordinary bacteria and cannot be seen with ordinary microscopic methods (ultra-microscopic). They appear to be living crystals of protein, and cause such diseases as poliomyelitis, measles, mumps, chickenpox, the common cold, and influenza.

Properties of bacteria: MOTION: It is doubtful if cocci have this power, but most of the bacilli and spirilla move rapidly and freely, either by quick contortions similar to those of a fish-tail, or by beating the fluid in which they lie by flagella, long whip-like lashes, with which many, such as the bacillus of typhoid fever and the spirillum of cholera, are provided. This power of movement is of immense importance in the spread of disease. The movements become more active if the temperature is raised. Bacteria are attracted to certain substances and repelled by others, this property being known as *positive* and *negative chemotaxis*.

SIZE: It is difficult at first to grasp the extreme smallness of these bodies. Many thousands of them may lie upon the smallest visible speck of dust. The round forms of cocci are between 0·5 and 1·5 micrometres in breadth. The bacillus of anthrax, much the largest disease-producing bacillus, is less than 8 micrometres in length, and most of the bacilli are only 0·25 micrometre or a little more, in breadth.

REPRODUCTION: The moulds have special filaments which produce hundreds of spores, and the yeasts give off little buds from their surface which produce new chains of yeast, but most of the simpler bacteria multiply by growing in size and then splitting into two. As a result of this, long chains are formed in which the individuals lie end to end, or masses, in which they lie side by side. A bacterium may grow and split in about half an hour, with the result that, given favourable circumstances of warmth, food, etc., a single bacterium could, in the course of twenty-four hours, produce nearly 300,000,000,000,000 individuals. Fortunately such favourable circumstances are seldom completely attained in nature. Another important method of reproduction possessed by some bacilli, such as that of anthrax, is by spores. Each bacillus produces only one spore, which, however, is much more tenacious of life than the bacillus and often capable of surviving after being boiled, or after drying for months or years. Each spore again produces a bacillus when it alights in a suitable germinating ground.

Effects of growth: Bacteria produce disease by means of toxins, which are products injurious to the tissues. They are classified into two main groups. Most of them are *endotoxins*. These are toxins that are retained within the bacterial cells, and the bacteria produce their ill-effects wherever they may be in the body. Thus, in pneumonia, due to the pneumococcus which tends to congregate in the lungs, the brunt of the attack from the toxins falls on the lungs, producing the typical signs of consolidation. (See PNEUMONIA.) The other group of toxins is that known as *exotoxins*. These are toxins that pass out from the bacteria into the surrounding medium and then circulate throughout the body, the bacteria themselves tending to 'stay put'. The best example of this type of toxin is that of the bacillus responsible for diphtheria, in which the bacillus tends to congregate on the tonsils while the exotoxin it produces circulates round the body, damaging particularly the cells of the heart.

Some bacilli produce acids by their growth, such as that which turns milk sour. Alcohol, as is well known, is the product of the activity of yeast. Many bacteria also produce brilliant pigments of red, yellow, blue, green, or purple colour, such as the *Pseudomonas pyocyanea*, which produces blue pus in abscesses. Many bacteria produce gases from the substances in which they develop, such as sulphuretted hydrogen, carbon dioxide, marsh gas. Others in the colon play a useful and necessary part in digestion although from time to time when other factors come into play they can produce untoward results such as appendicitis, peritonitis, and other diseases in the neighbourhood of the bowels. Many of the actions of bacteria depend upon ferments which are produced by them and exercise a complicated action. These ferments are sometimes set free in the fluid surrounding the bacteria, and sometimes retained for a time within the bacteria themselves. Most bacteria produce substances which finally stop their growth and activity, checking the excessive growth of, and finally killing their respective bacteria. Some micro-organisms are particularly prone to digest themselves: the process known as autolysis (qv).

Conditions of growth: FOOD: Some bacteria live by taking carbon dioxide and nitrogen from the air and producing complex organic substances in their growth, so that these bacteria are of great importance in some of the operations of farming. Most, however, break down the complex plant and animal bodies into simpler substances. All require some moisture for their growth. Some bacteria are readily killed by drying, thus the vibrio of cholera is killed by two or three hours of drying, but the ordinary bacteria of suppuration may be dried for at least several days, and anthrax spores still survive after drying for several years. A few bacteria live best, or only, in living bodies, being then called parasitic, or, if they produce disease, pathogenic. Others live only in dead matter, and are called saprophytic. The substances on which they grow best are gelatinous or starchy matters containing a little soluble animal substance, like peptone, and a trace of salts, or in fluids like broth, containing much animal or vegetable matter.

WARMTH: The bacteria of putrefaction flourish best at the ordinary temperature found inside a house: ie. about 20°C; the disease-producing bacteria at the temperature of the body: ie. 37°C. Freezing, though it stops growth for the time, does not kill most bacteria, which afterwards take on new activity; but a process of thawing and freezing repeated several times in succession kills all organisms. Boiling, on the other hand, is more deadly to them, and, if continued for a few minutes, kills most bacteria, though not their spores. The latter are killed by super-heated steam at 120°C. Dry heat can be survived at much higher temperatures. A satisfactory method of destruction is intermittent exposure of sterilizing dishes, instruments, and the like at 100°C for twenty to forty-five minutes on each of three successive days. These are exposed to steam rising from boiling water, in a Koch or Arnold's sterilizer, or, equally efficiently, in an ordinary pot with a lid. This kills all bacteria. Next day they are similarly treated, when any spores which have been present have developed into bacteria, and these are likewise killed. A third application of steam, on the day again following, renders certain the freedom from spores and bacteria.

LIGHT: Bacteria develop best in the dark, though some produce their special effects only when exposed to light. Direct sunlight stops their growth, and exposure for several hours to the full light of the sun kills most bacteria, notably those of plague and tuberculosis. The effect of sunlight is increased by dryness, and it has been found, for example, that even anthrax spores, which possess greater vitality than almost any other bacteria, are killed when dried and exposed to sunlight for one and a half hours, although, if moisture is present, a much longer exposure to sunlight is necessary. The effect is still further increased by heat, so that bacteria live for only a very short time in hot, dry, and sunshiny localities. Electric light has a similar, although weaker, action, the violet rays being most powerful in killing bacteria, but the X-rays have very little effect in checking bacterial growth.

AIR: Most bacteria grow with or without fresh air. A certain amount of fresh air is necessary to rapid putrefaction, but a very free supply, and certainly the presence of pure oxygen, tends to destroy bacteria. Bacteria, such as those of tetanus (lock-jaw) and of gas gangrene, can develop only deep in the earth or in deep wounds where oxygen is absent, and these are known as anaerobic bacteria.

Relation to disease: The first bacterium stated to be connected with disease was the anthrax bacillus. Since the introduction of modern bacteriological methods, about 1880, a great number of bacteria responsible for disease have been demonstrated. The proof that a bacterium is the direct cause of any disease depends upon the fulfilment of three conditions laid down by Koch: (1) that the bacterium be always found in the body or its discharges when a certain disease is present; (2) that the bacterium can be isolated and cultivated under laboratory conditions and thus freed from other possible causes of the disease; and (3) that on the inoculation of a healthy man or animal with a culture of the bacterium, which is now free from any possible contamination, symptoms of the original disease appear in the animal inoculated. Thus complete proof has been obtained in the case of a large number of diseases, while in the case of other diseases for some technical reason, such as that the organism cannot be grown in the laboratory or because no animal can be found to suffer typically from the disease, an absolute proof of the connection between the disease and the organism is so far wanting.

Among the diseases which have been definitely shown to be due to particular organisms are the following.

ACUTE INFLAMMATION AND SUPPURATION: Localized inflammation may be due to a great variety of organisms, of which the various *staphylococci* and *streptococci* are the chief. Staphylococci are the most common agents in producing infections of the skin, with pus formation, such as skin pustules, boils, carbuncles, styes and impetigo. They are also liable to infect wounds. Streptococci also cause infections of the skin, including erysipelas. They are also a common cause of cellulitis, tonsillitis, otitis media and puerperal fever, as well as scarlet fever. They are also a causative factor in rheumatic fever and acute glomerulonephritis. One form of streptococcus is the cause of subacute bacterial endocarditis. Streptococci commonly produce more deep-seated, serious, and spreading diseases, such as erysipelas. They also occur in broncho-pneumonia and ulcerative endocarditis. The streptococcus often starts infection of wounds (especially those sustained in war), and indeed may attack any part of the body, resulting in such conditions as peritonitis, meningitis, empyema. Suppuration may also be produced by several bacteria mentioned below as associated with particular diseases.

PNEUMONIA of the acute lobar type is usually due to the pneumococcus or *Diplococcus pneumoniae*. This organism is of several different types, types I and II being much the most common, while type III is found in about 12 per cent of cases of pneumonia. A few cases of pneumonia are due to the *streptococcus*, *Haemophilus influenzae* and *Klebsiella pneumoniae* as it is now known. There is also a form of pneumonia, known as primary atypical pneumonia, which is due to a virus.

CEREBROSPINAL FEVER: This disease is due to the *meningococcus*, which occurs in four types. It appears to gain entrance to the body through the nasal passages, where it is frequently found even in people who do not suffer from the disease.

RHEUMATIC FEVER is commonly associated with a haemolytic streptococcus.

SCARLET FEVER and some allied infections are due to a haemolytic streptococcus.

GONORRHOEA is due to a diplococcus – the gonococcus (or *Neisseria gonorrhoea*, as it is now known).

SYPHILIS is caused by a minute spiral-shaped organism, or spirochaete, known as *Treponema pallidum*. Other diseases due to different varieties of spirochaetes are RELAPSING FEVER, YAWS, SPIROCHAETAL JAUNDICE, and RAT-BITE FEVER.

TUBERCULOSIS is due to one or other of two mycobacteria, known as the human and the bovine types. Tuberculosis in the lung is almost always caused by the human type, while abdominal tuberculosis, as well as tuberculosis of bones and joints, found in children, is due in many cases to the bovine type derived from milk, and tuberculosis of the glands in young children is due to the latter type. Other types of *Mycobacteria tuberculosis* cause similar diseases in birds and fish, while closely allied bacilli are found subsisting in grass.

LEPROSY is caused by the *Mycobacterium leprae* which presents certain close resemblances to the mycobacterium of tuberculosis.

GLANDERS, or FARCY, is caused by *Loefflerella mallei*.

ACTINOMYCOSIS, or WOODY TONGUE, is caused by *Actinomyces israelii*, which is one of a genus of micro-organisms known as actinomyces. The MADURA FOOT OF INDIA is caused by an organism belonging to a closely associated genus.

ANTHRAX, or WOOLSORTERS' DISEASE, is due to a relatively large organism, the *Bacillus anthracis*, which produces spores that may retain their vitality when dried for several years.

TYPHOID FEVER and the group of diseases related to it, such as paratyphoid fever A and B, bacillary dysentery, and forms of food poisoning, are due to *Salmonella typhi*, *Salmonella paratyphi*, and *Shigella sonnei*, and a number of other organisms which resemble one another considerably in their mode of growth, cultural characters, and, broadly speaking, in the effects which they produce on the intestine and the body generally.

DIPHTHERIA is due to the *Corynebacterium diphtheriae*, which is often found in the throat of healthy persons, but which in susceptible persons produces a very severe type of surface inflammation with general toxic effects thoughout the body.

TETANUS, or LOCK-JAW, is produced by the *Clostridium tetani*, which is an anaerobic bacillus growing especially deep in the soil or in dung-heaps. It produces spores which, like those of anthrax, are extremely tenacious of life.

GAS GANGRENE is a disease produced by various anaerobic bacilli, especially the *Clostridium welchii*, which grow deep in highly cultivated soil, and, like the tetanus bacillus, cause infection when such soil is disturbed.

CHOLERA is due to the cholera vibrio, an S-shaped organism which is readily destroyed by drying or by weak antiseptics.

PLAGUE is caused by a rod-shaped bacillus, *Yersiniapestis*, which is transmitted to man through rodents and fleas.

INFLUENZA is due to a virus. Three specific viruses have, so far, been isolated, and others that may take part in the infection are under investigation. At one time it was thought that influenza was due to the *Haemophilus influenzae* (Pfeiffer's bacillus), but it is now known that this is only one of the secondarily infecting organisms that are often found in influenza.

WHOOPING-COUGH is due to a minute oval bacterium, the *Bordetella pertussis*.

MALTA FEVER is due to a minute coccus, the *Brucellamelitensis*.

MALARIA is due to an organism known as the *Plasmodium*. Three different but closely related types cause the three varieties of malaria. The plasmodia belong to a group of micro-organisms known as protozoa. Other diseases which are due to protozoa are: AMOEBIC DYSENTERY, due to the *Entamoeba histolytica*; SLEEPING SICKNESS, due to the *Trypanosoma gambiense*; KALA-AZAR, due to the *Leishmania donovani*, and other closely allied diseases.

TYPHUS FEVER, and the group of diseases associated with it, are caused by a genus of bacteria known as Rickettsiae. These are transmitted to man by lice, ticks or mites. A closely associated genus of bacteria known as Coxiella is responsible for Q fever.

Study of bacteria: It is impossible to go more than very briefly into the highly technical methods employed in a bacteriological laboratory. The material to be examined must be collected in such a way as to prevent contamination by organisms from outside sources, eg. the skin or the air. For example, in collecting matter from the throat to find if the *Corynebacterium diphtheriae* is present, a glass tube plugged with cotton-wool and containing a cotton-wool swab at the end of a piece of wire is used. The throat is rubbed with the swab, which is then carefully withdrawn, reinserted in the tube, and sent to the laboratory. When the urine is to be examined for the presence of bacteria, it is carefully collected into a sterile bottle closed with a sterilized stopper and similarly sent to the laboratory. Similar precautions are taken in the case of material from other sources. The bacteriological methods used fall into four groups.

(1) EXAMINATION BY THE MICROSCOPE: If bacteria are placed in a little fluid upon a glass slide and examined with the aid of a microscope, they appear when magnified some hundreds of times as clear, transparent, often quickly moving particles or lines. For careful observation they must be killed by heat or by some powerful chemical substance, and thereafter stained with appropriate reagents. These are usually aniline dyes of different colours; and the bacteria of different diseases, apart from their size, shape, and general appearance, can often be recognized from the way in which they become stained or fail to stain with certain dyes. Methylene blue is a simple dye generally used for all bacteria. The *Mycobacterium tuberculosis* is distinguished by the peculiar tenacity with which it retains the red fuchsin stain when treated by sulphuric acid and spirit, while from other bacteria this dye can be readily extracted by these reagents. The majority of bacteria are stained a deep purple colour by Gram's stain (successive application of gentian-violet, iodine, and alcohol), but some are readily recognized by being negative to this stain: eg. the gonococcus, meningococcus, and the *Salmonella typhi*. Neisser's stain is much used for the recognition of *Corynebacterium diphtheriae*; it consists of two stains (methylene blue and Bismarck brown) which stain this bacillus in a characteristic variegated manner. Many other bacteria have similar special staining properties by which they can be recognized without further trouble.

(2) CULTIVATION: In general, however, it is not possible to identify an organism with certainty, simply by its appearance, even if suitably stained, and the changes which its growth in large masses produces upon various nutrient substances contained in glass culture tubes must also be observed. In doing this the first necessity is to prepare a nutrient medium and place it in flat covered plates or in glass tubes of which the open end is plugged with a piece of cotton-wool so as to exclude organisms that might enter from the air, while freely admitting the air itself. These tubes and their contents must be carefully sterilized in the manner already indicated; they are then inoculated, by means of a previously sterilized platinum needle or a glass rod, with material containing the organism which it is desired to study; and are finally placed inside an incubator maintained day and night at the temperature of the body. After being incubated for several days the bacteria have multiplied so as to form colonies easily visible to the naked eye, and from these, small fragments are removed by the platinum needle, stained, and microscopically examined.

Among the nutrient substances on which bacteria are grown in the laboratory, the chief are broth, gelatin, agar, potato, and milk. The turbidity produced in broth after some days' growth, the power to liquefy gelatin, the colours produced on the surface of agar or of cut potato, and the curdling of milk form distinctive characters of different bacteria. Again, various sugars may be added to these substances and the bacteria are thus divided into classes according to their power of fermenting the sugar as they grow. The formation of acid by other bacteria is tested by adding to the tubes litmus or some other reagent which changes its colour when acidified, and the development of gas-bubbles is also an important distinguishing mark.

Some bacteria (known as anaerobic bacteria) fail to grow unless the oxygen be extracted from the tubes in which they are placed or an atmosphere of hydrogen gas be provided by means of a special apparatus.

Since many different types of bacteria are as a rule mingled together in the discharge from a diseased part of the body, it becomes necessary to separate these and to obtain for study cultures of each, free from contamination by the others. For this separation, the organisms are either grown upon a medium to which have been added substances that destroy some kinds of bacteria while sparing others; or they are diluted by mixture with a large quantity of sterile fluid, and, drops of this being stroked over the surface of some nutrient material lying on a broad covered glass plate (Petri dish), the individual bacteria produce within a few days widely separated colonies that can be seen by the naked eye and removed for further examination.

(3) AGGLUTINATION or PRECIPITATION is a method much used for the identification of certain bacteria (see AGGLUTINATION). It is usually performed by making a uniform emulsion with water of the bacteria to be identified, and then adding a drop of this emulsion to a drop of immune serum on a microscopic slide. Various stock sera are kept in the laboratory, and one of these is chosen corresponding to the disease to which the bacterium is supposed to belong. If the bacteria on microscopic examination are seen to clump together under the action of the serum, this identifies the bacteria as belonging to the disease from which the serum has been prepared. If the bacteria do not clump, the same process is carried out with another serum until the appropriate serum is found. The same process may be carried out without microscopic examination by placing the bacterial emulsion in small test tubes and adding drops of the sera to these. Precipitation of the bacteria to the bottom of the tube can be seen to take place in a tube containing the corresponding bacteria and serum. This method is much used, for instance, in identifying the meningococcus, and the causative micro-organisms of typhoid and paratyphoid fevers.

(4) INOCULATION OF ANIMALS: For the purpose of making certain which of the many kinds of bacteria derived from a case of disease is its actual cause, or in some instances when the bacteria are so few in number or so difficult to cultivate that they cannot be found, it becomes necessary to inoculate animals like mice,

guinea-pigs, or rabbits with material containing the bacteria, in order, if possible, to reproduce the disease. This inoculation is effected through pricking the skin or puncturing the abdomen by means of a needle and syringe charged with the material in question. Subsequently the animal is humanely killed and its organs examined for signs of the disease.

BACTERIOPHAGE is an agent which affects growing bacteria so as to break them up and destroy them. It is now known to be a virus.

BACTERIOSTATIC: Bringing bacteria to a standstill by preventing their nourishment and growth.

BACTERIURIA means the presence of bacteria in the urine, usually a sign of infection in the kidneys, bladder, or urethra.

BACUP stands for the British Association of Cancer United Patients and their families and friends. It was founded by Dr Vicky Clement-Jones after she was treated for ovarian cancer and it became fully operational on 31st October, 1985. The aim of the association is to provide an information service to cancer patients who want to know more about their illness or who need practical advice on how to cope with it. It does not seek to replace the traditional relationship between the doctor and patient, nor does it recommend specific treatment for particular patients; but its aim is to help patients to understand more about their illness so that they can communicate more effectively and freely with their medical advisors and their families and friends.

The address of the Association is 121–123 Charterhouse Street, London EC1M 6AA and the telephone number of its Cancer Information Service is 01–608 1661.

BAGASSOSIS is an industrial lung disease occurring in those who work with bagasse, which is the name given to the broken sugar cane after sugar has been extracted from it. Bagasse, which contains 6 per cent silica, is used in board-making. The inhalation of dust causes an acute lung affection, and subsequently in some cases a chronic lung disease. (See ALVEOLITIS.)

BAL is the abbreviation for BRITISH ANTI-LEWISITE. (See DIMERCAPROL.)

BALANITIS means inflammation of the parts covered by the prepuce.

BALANTIDIASIS is a form of dysentery caused by a protozoon known as *Balantidium coli*, a common parasite in pigs, which are usually the source of infection. It responds to metronidazole.

BALBUTIES is a medical term for stammering or stuttering.

BALDNESS is generally partial and slowly progressive, and is so universal that it may be looked on as a natural change in age. There is a gradual depletion in hair on the head with age: eg. from an average of 615 per square centimetre at the age of 20 to 30 to 485 at 30 to 50 years of age. It is most common in Caucasoids, less so in Negroes and least common in Mongoloids. It may also occur rapidly in patches, or even every hair on the body may be lost, in the disease called alopecia areata.

Causes: Certain *serious diseases* are associated with partial loss of hair as one of their symptoms; but these diseases are of so much greater importance that the thinness of hair is not taken account of, and as a rule remedies itself as these diseases wear off. Such diseases are acute fevers, myxoedema, syphilis, influenza, anaemia, and great anxiety or nervous shock. Baldness is, to a considerable extent, hereditary, and it is generally preceded for some years by seborrhoeic eczema, a condition of dandruff on the scalp. If it first appears relatively early in life – the twenties or early thirties in men – it is likely to be rapidly progressive and total baldness can be expected within a few years. If it does not set in until later life it tends to progress much less rapidly. In women it seldom tends to be rapidly progressive even though it begins to appear relatively early and actual baldness seldom appears until late middle age, and not always then. Every day, in the healthy scalp, a certain number of hairs reach the end of their existence, and are combed out, being replaced in time by others growing up from below. Each hair-follicle in this way produces many hairs in the course of a person's life, but, if the change is too rapid, the hairs become gradually finer, then downy, until finally the hair-producing power of the follicle wears out. This rapid change is due to the eczematous condition of the scalp. Many skin diseases, like lupus, erysipelas, ringworm, which leave a hardened condition of the scalp behind them, cause baldness, and such cases are made worse by the various stimulating hair washes sold for baldness. Other causes include excessive exposure to ultra-violet light as in prolonged sunbathing, and certain cosmetic procedures such as bleaching, permanent waving, and hair straightening. It can also result from certain hairstyles which impose a mechanical strain on the hair such as the 'ponytail', and by wearing of hair rollers, particularly in bed at night.

Treatment: There is little that can be done to prevent baldness in those predisposed to it.

ALOPECIA AREATA, or patchy baldness, is common on the scalp, but may affect the hair all over the body. It occurs principally in adolescents and young adults. The cause is not known. It is doubtful whether treatment makes any difference. The hair regrows spontaneously in a majority of cases, though sometimes lighter in colour, or even white. Ultra-violet light is beneficial in some cases. The more extensive the areas of baldness, and the more often it recurs, the worse the outlook for regrowth of the hair.

BALNEOLOGY is the department of medical science which deals with the giving of baths. (See BATHS.)

BALSAMS are substances which contain resins and benzoic acid. Balsam of Peru, balsam of tolu, and Friars' balsam (compound tincture of benzoin) are the chief. They are given internally for colds, and aid expectoration, while locally they are used to cover abrasions and stimulate ulcers. Friars' balsam, one teaspoonful, inhaled from a jug of boiling water, is of value in the alleviation of the common cold. Balsam of Peru is given internally in doses of 5 to 15 drops with beaten-up egg; balsam of tolu is similarly administered in doses of 300 mg to 1 g, or is given as the more familiar syrup of tolu in doses of one teaspoonful.

BANDAGES are pieces of material used to support injured parts or to retain dressings in position. The material they are made of includes cotton, calico, gauze, linen, muslin, net, flannel, flannelette, domette crepe, elastic and rubber.

Types: *Triangular bandages* are made by taking a piece of calico 1 metre square and cutting it across cornerwise to form two triangles. The cut side of each is called the 'base', and the opposite right-hand corner is called the 'point'. *Roller bandages* are usually made of open-wove cotton. They are made up in various lengths, and vary in width from 12 mm to 20 cm. *Crepe bandages*, which have a one-way stretch, consist of characteristic fabric of plain weave, in which the warp threads are of cotton and wool and the weft threads are of cotton. They are used in the treatment of mild sprains and strains, as well as a compression bandage over paste bandages in the treatment of varicose ulcers. Much of the elasticity is lost during use, but can be restored by washing the bandage in soapy water. *Domette bandages* consist of union fabric of plain weave, in which the warp threads are of cotton or viscose, or of a combined cotton and viscose yarn, and the weft threads are of wool. It is used mainly for orthopaedic purposes, especially where a high degree of warmth, protection and support is needed. *Elastic bandages* are now available in various forms, their main purpose being to provide firm support as in the treatment of varicose veins. *Plaster of Paris bandages* are bandages impregnated with calcium sulphate, and used as a form of splint. (See PLASTER OF PARIS.) Three more recent forms of bandages are being used to an increasing extent: Netelast, Tubegauz, and Tubifast. *Netelast* is an elasticated net of cellular cotton and elastic in a wide-mesh tubular net. Its great advantage is that it can be applied easily and quickly, can be washed and sterilized, and is available in different sizes. *Tubegauz* consists of seamless, circular cotton tubular material, which can be applied easily and quickly to any part of the body. *Tubifast* is a tubular bandage made from rayon with fine interwoven threads. It has a one way stretch, or elasticity, which provides light pressure and so ensures that it holds itself in position. It is available in three sizes, thus rendering it applicable in a wide range of situations, from babies' arms to adult thighs.

For more detailed instruction in bandaging the reader is referred to "First Aid", the authorized manual of the Saint John's Ambulance Association and Brigade (3rd edition 1972, 10th impression 1978. Hills & Lacey Ltd, London).

BANTI'S DISEASE (see SPLENIC ANAEMIA).

BARAGNOSIS means the inability on the part of a patient to recognize that an object placed in the hand has weight, a condition due to disease of the brain.

BARANY'S TEST is a test for gauging the efficiency of the balancing mechanism (the vestibular apparatus) by applying hot or cold air or water to the external ear.

BARBER'S ITCH (see SYCOSIS).

BARBITURATES: The barbiturate drugs are all derivatives of barbituric acid, so called because it was first prepared on St Barbara's Day (1899). They form a most extensive series of sedative, hypnotic, and anaesthetic drugs, but are being used to a decreasing extent in view of the ease with which they can be abused. They are being replaced largely by the tranquillizers (qv). (See also DRUG ADDICTION.)

BARBOTAGE is the alternate injection and withdrawal of 20 ml of cerebrospinal fluid (qv) into and from the canal of the spinal cord. It is a painless procedure for the relief of otherwise intractable pain due to cancer, and is said to give at least partial relief in around 60 to 70 per cent of cases for periods of up to eight months. Its mode of action is not known.

BARIUM SULPHATE is a heavy white powder used in X-ray diagnosis. The mass of barium forms an opaque shadow and shows the outline of the cavity in which it lies. Thus the physician can see the size and position of the stomach in an X-ray photograph, or can trace a meal in its passage through the bowels.

BARRIER CREAMS are substances applied to the skin before work to prevent damage to the skin by irritants handled at work. They are also used in medicine: eg. for the prevention of bedsores and napkin rashes.

There are three main types of barrier creams:

A **dust barrier** to protect the skin against sensitizing dusts and against substances which, if absorbed, will produce systemic poisoning.

A **water-repellent barrier** for those whose hands are constantly exposed to water, alkalis, and water-soluble oils.

An **oil-repellent or water-miscible barrier,** which is a protective against oils, greases and solvents, and which facilitates their removal without the use of abrasives or oil solvents.

Silicones (qv), which are water repellent, are being used increasingly as barrier creams.

The hands should be clean and dry before applying a barrier cream. The cream should be applied sparingly to the whole of the hands, and not just rubbed into the palms. It is essential to coat the backs of the hands, paying special attention to the sides of the fingers and the webs between. The cream should be well rubbed into the nail folds and under the free edges of the nails. To get the full value from silicone creams, they should be applied twice daily for ten days before exposing the hands to irritants; after this a once-daily application should be sufficient.

A point which is being increasingly emphasized by the experts is that the use of barrier creams must not be allowed to lead to any slackening in the attention paid to other more important protective measures, such as standards of cleanliness in workshops and the wearing of protective clothing.

BARRIER NURSING is the nursing of a patient suffering from an infectious disease in such a way that the risk of his passing on the disease to others is effectively reduced. Thus, precautions are taken to ensure that all infective matter, such as stools, urine, sputum, discharge from wounds, and anything that may be contaminated by such infective matter, such as nurses' uniforms, bedding and towels are so treated that they will not convey the infection. (See NURSING.)

BASAL METABOLISM (see METABOLISM).

BASEDOW'S DISEASE is another name for exophthalmic goitre or Graves' disease. (See GOITRE.)

BASILIC VEIN is the prominent vein which runs from near the bend of the elbow upwards along the inner side of the upper arm. It is generally the vein opened in venesection for blood-letting.

BASILICON OINTMENT is an old name for an ointment of resin, lard, wax, and almond oil.

BASOPHILIA is a term applied to the bluish appearance under the microscope of immature red blood corpuscles when stained by certain dyes. This appearance, with the blue areas collected in points, is seen in lead poisoning and the condition is called punctate basophilia. The term basophilia may also mean an increase in the numbers of basophil cells in the blood.

BAT EARS is the term commonly applied to prominent ears. The condition may be familial, but this is by no means the rule. Strapping the ears firmly back has no effect and is merely a waste of time and an embarrassment to the child. In cases in which the condition is proving a definite embarrassment to the child, it can be rectified by plastic surgery.

BATHER'S ITCH, also called SWIMMER'S ITCH, WATER ITCH, and SCHISTOSOME DERMATITIS, is the term given to a blotchy rash on the skin occurring in those bathing in water which is infested with the larvae of certain trematode worms known as *Schistosomes* (see SCHISTOSOMIASIS). The worm is parasitic in snails. The skin rash is caused by penetration of the skin by the free-swimming larval cercaria. Bather's itch is common in many parts of the world, including USA, Canada, Central and South America, Australasia, Malaysia and Japan. It has also been found in Wales, France, and Germany.

BATHS: The main action of water on the skin is as a vehicle for heat, and baths act largely either by extracting heat from, or adding it to, the body. The sweat glands of the skin excrete around a litre of water daily, containing about one-twentieth part of the nitrogenous waste of the body, and their excretory activity may be greatly increased by baths of high temperature. Baths also exert a mechanical effect by virtue of the fact that water is slightly denser than the human body and therefore causes the body to float on its surface. They also exert an important psychological effect, the heat of a warm bath and the buoyancy of the water allowing a paralysed patient to perform movements of which he thought he was no longer capable. (See also SAUNA.)

VAPOUR BATHS: (1) AROMATIC: The patient sits in a special box, his head protruding through a hole in the lid, while steam from water containing fir-balsam, lavender, etc., circulates round him. Beyond acting as a hot bath this form is of no therapeutic value.

(2) RUSSIAN BATHS have much the same effect as warm-water baths. The bath is generally taken in a room which is filled with vapour, but as good an effect may be obtained from a cabinet, or a tent of blankets, in which the patient sits on a chair some inches over boiling water. In a vapour bath 49°C (120°F) can be borne readily, and the person should remain in the vapour until he breaks into a copious perspiration, usually in about fifteen or twenty minutes. Subsequently a cold douche or bath should be taken, according to the state of his 'reaction'. In Russia it is a common practice immediately after the vapour bath to pour a stream of ice-cold water all over the surface of the body.

DRY BATHS: (1) HOT-AIR BATHS may be taken as the TURKISH or ROMAN bath, in a specially constructed building heated by pipes in the walls, with tepid room, hot room, washing room, and cooling room, through which the bather goes in succession. A hot bath may also be taken in an electric-light cabinet, where the person sits exposed to brilliant light and heat till he sweats copiously, when he takes a cold-water bath.

Such a bath may also be given in bed, the patient lying under a curved wire shield. In hospitals the under-surface of the shield is provided with numerous electric-light bulbs which speedily raise the temperature of the enclosed air to a high degree.

The duration of a Roman bath is about two hours, and it leaves a feeling of great freshness. In either of these baths one may lose 2·7 kg (6 pounds) at one time by sweating. They are useful for reducing weight, and for rheumatism.

The electric-light bath can be given in bed, the lights being underneath a curved shield, 152 cm (5 feet) long, which covers the patient, and there are also smaller shields for single limbs. A dry temperature of 93°C (200°F) can be borne without discomfort for a quarter of an hour, and has excellent results in chronic rheumatism, rheumatoid arthritis and sciatica. When a sick person is being treated by such a high temperature bath, it is necessary that his pulse should be frequently examined, in case the heart's action should become enfeebled.

(2) SAND BATHS are used for rheumatic conditions, the sand being made very hot to purify it, and heaped on the patient when moderately cool.

(3) WAX BATHS are also used for rheumatic aches and pains. Paraffin wax with a melting point of around 46°C (115°F) is placed in a thermostatically controlled tank. The affected hand, or hands, is then dipped in the molten wax about ten times until it is well coated with wax. It is then wrapped in wax-proof paper in a plastic bag and wrapped in a towel for about twenty minutes. The wax is then removed. With care the method can be used at home, the wax being melted in a double saucepan on an electric stove. Because of its inflammability it must not be heated over a naked flame.

MEDICINAL BATHS: (1) ALKALINE BATHS are used to soften the skin in certain skin diseases like general eczema. 170 G of washing soda are added to 135 litres of tepid water.

(2) BRAN BATHS are used to sooth general irritation of the skin. 1·8 kg of bran are boiled and the liquor added to a tepid bath, in which the patient soaks for half an hour.

(3) PEAT and MUD BATHS are used generally for rheumatism at various spas. The patient is covered with a layer of warmed mud, such as fango, lies in it for perhaps twenty minutes, and is then washed clean by a cold douche. Such baths can be taken at a much higher temperature than water baths (39° to 44°C (102° to 112°F)).

(4) MUSTARD BATHS are used for the feet to check colds, and for the whole body as a good general stimulant. For this, a handful of mustard is made into a paste with cold water and stirred into the warm bath.

(5) SEA-WATER BATHS are best taken in the sea. Brine baths are found at various spas. Failing that, about 4 kg of common salt are added to 135 litres of water. The effect is very stimulating. Such baths are used in cases of chronic rheumatism. They are also of value in the treatment of the so-called decubitus ulcers which are liable to occur in patients with spinal cord injuries. The recommended strength for this purpose is 5 per cent crude rock salt and 2·5 per cent magnesium sulphate.

(6) CARBONIC ACID BATHS are used for their stimulating effect upon the skin and upon the body generally. They may be administered by the aid of water which is naturally effervescent, as at Royat, St Moritz, Spa, and Marienbad, where they are specially in vogue for the treatment of heart disorders; or the carbonic acid may be allowed to escape from cylinders in the bath-water; or weak formic acid is mixed with the water in which small cotton bags of washing soda are placed. Such effervescent baths, especially when taken warm, have a marked action in increasing the circulation in the skin and diminishing general arterial blood-pressure.

(7) FOAM BATHS contain some soapy substance such as an extract of quillaia bark, or some detergent preparation, which on stirring produces a copious froth. They usually contain also some substance which adds to the frothy effect by development of carbonic acid gas, and they then have the effects mentioned under carbonic acid baths.

(8) SULPHUR BATHS contain sulphuretted hydrogen, which not only stimulates the skin but is to some extent absorbed. Such baths may be natural as in certain spas, or may be prepared artificially by adding from 112 to 224 G of sulphuret of potassium or of yellow sulphur to 135 litres of hot water. Sulphur baths are specially used in the treatment of skin diseases and in rheumatism.

(9) SITZ BATHS are baths in which only the hips and buttocks are immersed.

(10) SALINE BATHS are baths which are isotonic (qv); ie. contain 9 grams of sodium chloride to 1 litre of water. They are a refreshing, convenient and relatively painfree way of managing large or awkwardly placed wounds on the limbs or trunk, which are septic and contain purulent material which needs to be removed to speed up the healing process.

ELECTRIC BATHS may be given in earthenware, stone or wooden baths. The bath is filled with tepid water, in which the patient lies. An electrode hangs in the water at either end, not touching the patient, and a moderate current is passed through the water. This bath is used in cases of debility and neurasthenia. (See ELECTRICITY IN MEDICINE.)

BCG VACCINE: BCG (*Bacillus Calmette-Guérin*) vaccine, which was introduced in France in 1908, is the only vaccine that has produced significant immunity against the tubercle bacillus and at the same time has proved safe enough for use in human subjects. The original work of Calmette and Guérin has now been amply confirmed by investigators in many parts of the world. BCG vaccination is usually considered for five main groups of people. (1) Schoolchildren: the routine programme in schools usually covers children aged between 10 and 14. (2) Students, including those in teacher training colleges. (3) Children and new-born infants of Asian origin because of the high incidence of tuberculosis in this ethnic group. (4) Health workers, such as nurses, and others likely to be exposed to infection in their work. (5) Household contacts of people known to have active tuberculosis and new-born infants in households where there is a history of tuberculosis. A pre-vaccination tuberculin test is necessary in all age-groups except new-born infants, and only those with negative tuberculin reactions are vaccinated. Complications are few and far between. A local reaction at the site of vaccination usually occurs between two and six weeks after vaccination, beginning as a small papule that slowly increases in size. It may produce a small ulcer. This heals after around two months, leaving a small scar. During 1978, 638,872 school children and students in England were tuberculin tested; 568,321 were found to be negative and of these 563,922 were vaccinated with BCG. In 1986, 518,700 school children, 32,700 babies and 12,600 contacts of tuberculosis cases were vaccinated. (See IMMUNITY; TUBERCULIN.)

BEANS are widely used as a source of food. In the western world they include the kidney bean, or French bean (*Phaseolus vulgaris*) which is the now popular 'baked bean', the scarlet runner bean (*Phaseolus multiflorus*), haricot beans, navy beans and pea beans. In the East, and particularly in China, the most widely eaten bean is the soya bean (*Glycine hispida*) which has twice the protein content of most other beans. Modern methods have now been evolved whereby it can be converted into an acceptable imitation of meat. It is also a constituent of the vegetable milk substitutes being used in the developing countries of Africa, South America and Asia. (See PULSES; SOYA BEANS.)

BEAT ELBOW, BEAT HAND, and BEAT KNEE are terms applied by miners to an inflamed condition with swelling of the elbow, hand or knee. The condition is particularly common in miners, but occurs in other trades also from constant pressure and the ingraining of particles of dirt, caused by the constant use of a tool or pressure in resting on the joints at work. The condition sometimes proceeds to suppuration, but usually subsides under soothing and antiseptic applications.

BECHET'S SYNDROME: This is a syndrome of unknown aetiology. It is characterized by oral and genital ulceration, iridocyclitis and arthropathy. Thrombophlebitis is a common complication and involvement of the central nervous system may occur.

BECLOMETHASONE DIPROPIONATE is a corticosteroid that is proving of value as a cream or ointment in the treatment of certain skin diseases. It is also of value by inhalation in the treatment of asthma and hay fever, and by insertion into the nose in the treatment of perennial rhinitis. (See NOSE, DISEASES OF.)

BED: The bed used in cases of sickness should consist of an iron *frame* of at least 183 cm (6 feet) in length and 99 to 107 cm (3 feet 3 inches to 3 feet 6 inches) in width, and should be provided with a stiff *wire mattress*. A piece of canvas or felt, fixed to the mattress, should form a *mattress cover* to prevent rusting of the wire. Upon this is a mattress of wool, hair, latex, or rubber or plastic foam, or it may have interior springs. The mattress should have a loose cover of cotton, which can be washed from time to time as required, or a plastic or polythene cover. Over the mattress is placed a sheet which is tucked in firmly beneath the mattress all round to form the *under sheet*. The bed is completed by the *upper sheet* and *blankets*, varying in number according to the season of the year, and by a light *bedcover*. Two thin *pillows*, each covered by a linen or cotton pillow-slip, should be supplied, but it is important both in health and in disease that the support for the head should not be too high, and the pillows should simply be sufficient to fill up the distance between the head and shoulder when the patient lies on the side.

The bed should stand with its head towards the wall and the foot towards the centre of the room or ward, and there should be a free passage up either side for access by the attendants. In some diseases and injuries the bed requires special modification. In all cases confined to bed for longer than a few days a *draw sheet* is required. The draw sheet is formed as follows: An ordinary sheet is folded length-wise so that the folded sheet is sufficiently wide to extend from the patient's shoulders to behind the knees. Between the folds of this is placed a mackintosh sheet 0·9 metre (1 yard) square, or it is often more convenient to place the mackintosh sheet beneath the draw sheet, directly upon the under sheet. This folded sheet is pushed at one end under the mattress, carried across the bed, and the superfluous length is folded up and pushed out of the way under the mattress at the other side. From time to time the sheet is pulled through beneath the patient towards the shorter end, thus bringing a fresh piece of sheet beneath the back. In conditions in which the patient perspires profusely, the patient lies directly upon and is covered by a blanket, as the woollen material absorbs the perspiration better than sheets. In cases of *fracture* of a lower limb it is necessary to make the bed more rigid, and for this purpose boards are placed across the wire mattress. In cases of *bronchitis* it is frequently necessary to erect a tent over the bed to retain a moist atmosphere produced by a steam kettle. This can be effected by a light screen placed round the bed and covered with a blanket.

In cases of paralysis, prolonged fever, and other *devitalizing conditions*, the patient may require to be placed upon a mattress which supports his body evenly instead of allowing pressure to come upon its most projecting parts. For this purpose a *water-bed* (qv) may be employed, or, better, an *air-bed* (qv). The water-bed is filled with warm water after it is placed upon the mattress, and care is taken to expel all bubbles of air by stroking it with the hand towards the inlet through which the water is poured. The air-bed is much more easily managed, and is pumped up by an ordinary bicycle pump from time to time without the necessity of removing the patient. The under sheet is laid directly on top of the water-bed, or air-bed.

A *bed rest* must sometimes be provided for patients unable to breathe comfortably in a recumbent position, or in order to change the position from time to time of a patient permanently confined to bed. For this purpose, four or five pillows may be placed behind the patient's back, or, preferably, a rest, consisting of a horizontal part hinged to a cane-backed rest resembling the back of a chair and supported on a strut, is used and furnished with a couple of pillows. In order to give a still further change of position, a *bed table* may be used. This is supported on four legs some 107 cm (3 feet 6 inches) high and is of sufficient width (120 cm (4 feet)) to enable each pair of legs to stand on either side of the bed. Upon this the patient can lean forward.

BED BUG, or *Cimex lectularius*, is a wingless, blood-sucking insect, parasitic on man. It is a flat, rusty brown insect, 5 mm long and 3 mm wide, with an offensive, never forgotten smell, which cannot fly. The average life is 3 to 6 months, but it can live for a year without food. The bed bug remains hidden during the day in cracks in walls and floors, and in beds. It does not transmit any known disease. Eggs hatch out into larvae in 6 to 10 days, which become adult within about 12 weeks. A temperature of 44°C kills the adult in an hour. Various agents have been used to disinfect premises, such as sulphur dioxide, ethylene oxide mixed with carbon dioxide, hydrogen cyanide and heavy naphtha, but a solution of DDT in kerosene is the most effective disinfecting agent.

BED CHANGING: Two methods are adopted for changing the bed-clothes without removing the sick person from the bed. One of these, called medical changing, is generally applicable when the upper part of the body or head is affected. The other, known as surgical changing, is generally used when the lower part of the body is affected or when the lower limbs are the site of fracture or similar disability.

MEDICAL CHANGING: The bed-clothes are first removed until the patient is covered only by a blanket and the upper sheet. The patient is then turned upon one side (right) near the right edge of the bed. The soiled sheet with the draw sheet is then rolled up lengthwise from the right edge of the bed until the roll lies against the patient's back. The fresh sheet is made into a roll lengthwise; one edge is tucked in under the right edge of the mattress and the sheet is unrolled across the bed towards the left until the roll lies alongside the roll of soiled sheet. The patient is next turned on the back and then on the left side near the left-hand side of the bed. He now lies upon the unrolled portion of the fresh sheet. The soiled sheet, which now lies behind his back, is pulled off the bed and the roll of fresh sheet is unrolled and its edge tucked beneath the left-hand edge of the mattress. During this procedure the patient remains covered by the upper sheet and a blanket. A fresh draw sheet is introduced by similar procedure. Finally, the pillows are placed in fresh pillow-slips.

SURGICAL CHANGING: In some cases the under sheet is more conveniently changed from the top or bottom of the bed. To do this the edges of the soiled sheet are pulled out all round from under the edges of the mattress. The sheet is then pulled down under the patient's hips, and, finally, from under the legs. The fresh sheet is now rolled up from top and bottom to the middle, and the double roll is pushed through from the side of the bed beneath the patient's hips while an attendant raises these slightly from the bed. By gently easing up the patient's shoulders the upper half of the sheet is unrolled and tucked in at the top of the mattress, and by similarly elevating his legs slightly the lower half is unrolled and tucked in at the foot of the bed.

CHANGING DRAW SHEET: When it is necessary to insert a fresh draw sheet, the draw sheet is folded up as in the method for changing the under sheet and is introduced either by rolling the patient over or slightly elevating his hips. When the draw sheet requires to be replaced frequently, it is more convenient to place the square of mackintosh on the under sheet and to insert the draw sheet above it separately.

CHANGING NIGHTDRESS: When it is necessary to change the nightdress of a person confined to bed, the fresh nightdress should be warmed; one arm is then slipped out of the soiled nightdress and inserted into the corresponding sleeve of the fresh nightdress. The soiled nightdress is then slipped over the patient's head and removed, and the fresh one is slipped on and arranged. This should be carried out without removing the upper sheet and blankets. In the case of patients too ill to be much disturbed, the nightdress may conveniently be slit down the back.

BED SORES, or PRESSURE SORES, are areas of inflamed skin, tending to ulcerate, which appear upon the body or limbs of those long confined to bed, and especially of those much weakened by disease.

Causes: Sores seldom occur in vigorous people confined to bed by a fractured limb or other minor cause. They appear in those who have not much fat between bones and skin, in the aged, in those suffering from prostrating weakness, and especially in those whose nervous system is at fault and the nutrition of whose skin is consequently impaired: for example in a person with a fractured spine, or with degeneration of the spinal cord. The direct cause may be wrinkles left in the bed-clothes, discharges allowed to soil the invalid's back, and want of daily observation of the places where sores are likely to form.

Symptoms: Very often the invalid feels no pain; sometimes he complains only of a hard place or wrinkle in the bed-clothes. The sites where sores commonly form are where the bones show plainly through the skin in the lower part of the back, on the heels, on the haunch, on one ankle, on the elbows, or on the shoulder blades. At first, for one or two days, there is redness of the skin over a prominence, which quickly turns blue and dusky. Then a black slough forms, and comes away, leaving a raw surface, which widens if not carefully treated.

Treatment: The best treatment is preventive, by keeping the patient's back scrupulously clean and dry, by washing it daily with soap and water, sponging it with spirit in order to dry and harden the skin, and, finally, dusting it with a powder of zinc oxide or boric acid (or instead of using spirit and dusting powder, the skin may be preserved by rubbing in daily a little zinc oxide ointment); by examining night and morning for any sign of redness; and especially by changing the invalid's position, so as to relieve the various prominences from constant pressure. The twice-daily smearing of the skin with barrier creams (qv) containing silicone, such as dimethicone cream, is proving of value. The regular administration of vitamin C (qv) is also of value.

If redness appear over a prominent part, this must be wrapped in dry cotton-wool and the patient at once put on an air ring or air-bed. Superficial sores are treated with 1 per cent gentian violet, or zinc and castor-oil cream. Deeper sores can be treated with cetrimide. When a black, hard slough is forming, and the surface is breaking, infection is almost invariably present and the type of dressing must be changed. Among those that have been recommended are: cod-liver oil; picric acid solutions; tannic acid solutions; eusol; one of the flavine group of antiseptics, eg. proflavine, flavazole. Irradiation of the affected area with ultra-violet light has also been used, in addition to one of these dressings. Whatever dressing is used, sloughs (qv) are removed as they become loosened. When the area has become clean again, a return is made to dry dressings.

BEER (see ALCOHOL).

BEE STINGS (see BITES AND STINGS).

BELCHING (see ERUCTATION).

BELLADONNA (see ATROPINE).

BELL'S PALSY is paralysis of the muscles of the face on one or both sides, causing inability to close the eye, to smile, to show the teeth, and the like, on the affected side. The paralysis is due to damage of the seventh cranial, or facial, nerve. When due to inflammation, it is often temporary, and complete recovery may ensue, but when due to a wound in front of the ear, to fracture of the base of the skull, or to a stroke or apoplexy, it is apt to be permanent, although apoplectic paralysis of the face is more favourable for recovery than that due to injury. (See PARALYSIS.)

BELTS AND BINDERS are commonly worn, not only as articles of dress, but as supports and curative agents.

Uses: Flannel binders give great comfort in cases of lumbago when worn next to the skin. Persons of all ages, with weak and easily tired backs, get great support from wearing a broad belt round the waist. When, however, the upper part of the body is subject to great muscular efforts, as in athletes and navvies, it is a great mistake to encircle the waist tightly with a narrow belt, which ought to run round in the hollow on either side between the summit of the haunch-bone and the hip-joint, and so give full play to the abdominal muscles and those of the loins.

BENDROFLUAZIDE (APRINOX, BERKOZIDE, CENTYL, NEO-NACLEX, URIZIDE) (see BENZOTHIADIAZINES).

BENDS (see CAISSON DISEASE).

BENNETT'S FRACTURE, so-called after an Irish surgeon, Edward Hallaran Bennett (1837–1907), is a longitudinal fracture of the first metacarpal bone, which also involves the carpo-metacarpal joint.

BENZEDRINE is a proprietary name for amphetamine sulphate (see AMPHETAMINE).

BENZENE HEXACHLORIDE is an insecticide which acts more rapidly than DDT but not for such a long time. When first sprayed it is 10 times as toxic to insects as DDT, but its action wears off in 3 to 4 months, whereas that of DDT will persist for up to a year.

BENZHEXOL is a drug that is proving of value in the treatment of Parkinsonism (qv).

BENZOCAINE is a white powder with soothing properties used as a sedative for inflamed and painful surfaces.

BENZODIAZEPINES are the most commonly prescribed anxiolytics. They have a hypnotic action in high dosage and an anxiolytic action in low dosage. They have replaced the barbiturates. The benzodiazepines used as anxiolytics include diazepam (Valium), chlordiazepoxide (Librium), medazepam (Nobrium), chlorazepate (Tranxene), clobazam (Frisium), ketazolam (Anxon), prazepam (Centrax) and bromazepam (Lexotan). Prazepam is long-acting and possibly less sedative.

The benzodiazepines used as hypnotics includes nitrazepam (Mogadon), flunitrazepam (Rohypnol), loprazolam (Dormonoct) and flurazepam (Dalmane), which have a prolonged action. Drugs with a shorter action, and hence less likely to have a hang-over effect, include bromazepam (Lexotan), lormetazepam (Loramet, Noctamid), temazepam (Euhypnos, Normison) and triazolam (Halcion).

The extent of pharmacological dependence with regular, as opposed to intermittent, dosage of benzodiazepines was not fully appreciated until recently. The chief manifestation is a withdrawal syndrome on stopping the drug. The reason for the length of time it has taken to identify the withdrawal syndrome is that it is difficult to distinguish anxiety due to withdrawal from a relapse of the underlying anxiety state. If patients experience a return of their anxiety when they stop taking benzodiazepines it may be the result of a withdrawal syndrome and not a relapse of their disease. Other manifestations of a withdrawal syndrome from benzodiazepines are perceptual disturbances which include an increased sensitivity to all forms of sensory stimuli and a feeling of continuous movement; sometimes symptoms of depersonalisation may occur. Physical symptoms such as weight loss and epilepsy can also occur as a manifestation of withdrawal. The symptoms usually appear within two or three days of stopping a short-acting benzodiazepine and within seven days of stopping a long-acting one. The withdrawal symptoms usually persist for about two weeks but can go on for longer. It has been estimated that 15 per cent of patients who have taken benzodiazepines for a long time will suffer significant withdrawal symptoms when they stop treatment. A recent survey shows that in the U.K. alone one-and-a-quarter-million people have taken a benzodiazepine regularly for a year or more. Thus 200,000 people in the U.K. could be dependent on benzodiazepines. Dependence probably does not occur with intermittent use of short-acting benzodiazepines. Drugs with a short elimination half-life, such as triazolam, temazepam, lorazepam, lormetazepam and oxazepam, are more likely to lead to withdrawal symptoms. It is therefore important for patients who have taken benzodiazepine for a long time to have their medication withdrawn slowly.

BENZOIC ACID is an antiseptic. It, or sodium benzoate, is still given internally in cases of infection along the urinary tract, especially in inflammation of the bladder with decomposition of the urine. Other acids are neutralized in the blood, but benzoic acid is excreted as hippuric acid and acidifies the urine. It is also used as a preservative in certain foodstuffs and beverages: eg. fruit cordials, pickles.

BENZOIN is a balsamic resin, which is an ingredient of inhalations used in the treatment of bronchitis and common colds. The most widely used of these is Friars' balsam. (See BALSAMS.)

BENZOTHIADIAZINES, or THIAZIDES, are a group of diuretics (qv) which are effective when taken by mouth. They act by inhibiting the reabsorption of sodium and chloride in the renal tubules. They also have a blood-pressure-lowering effect. Chlorothiazide was the first member of this group to be introduced. Their main use is to relieve oedema in heart failure.

All thiazides are active by mouth with an onset of action within one to two hours, and a duration of twelve to twenty-four hours. Chlorthalidone (Hygroton) is a thiazide-related compound that has a longer duration of action and only requires to be given on alternate days. The other thiazide drugs available include bendrofluazide (Aprinox, Berkozide, Centyl, Neo-NaClex, Urizide), clopamide (Rinaldix, Viskaldix), cyclopenthiazide (Navidrex), hydrochlorothiazide (Esidrex, Hydrosaluric), hydroflumethiazide (Hydrenox), indapamide (Natrillix), mefruside (Baycaron), methyclothiazide (Enduron), metolazone (Metenix), polythiazide (Nephril) and xipamide (Diurexan).

The loop diuretics are more potent than the thiazides. They are so called because they inhibit re-absorption from the ascending loop of Henle in the renal tubules. Frusemide (Lasix), bumetanide (Burinex) and ethacrynic acid (Edecrin) are the three most important loop diuretics.

BENZOYL PEROXIDE is a bactericide (qv) used in the treatment of acne (qv). It is also used as a bleaching agent in the food industry.

BENZYL BENZOATE is widely used as a lotion in the treatment of scabies (qv).

BENZYLPENICILLIN (see PENICILLIN).

BERBERINE is an alkaloid (qv) derived from the roots and bark of the plant *Berberis aristata*, a deciduous evergreen shrub. It has a broad spectrum antibiotic activity against selective bacteria including vibrio cholera, shigella and pseudomonas, E Coli and proteus. It inhibits the action of the vibrio cholera toxin when administered before or with the enterotoxin in animals and it has been shown to be effective in the treatment of cholera and related diarrhoeas in man. (See CHOLERA.)

BEREAVEMENT There is significantly increased psychiatric and physical morbidity following bereavement. Psychosomatic disorders, common neuroses, affective disorders, alcoholism and suicide may occur. The bereaved who are most at risk are those whose lives are complicated by crises other than bereavement and those who see their families as unsupportive. In the case of those who have been widowed, those whose marriage was ambivalent are particularly at risk and this is sometimes associated with an unrealistic idealisation of the dead partner. Treatment should be directed towards encouragement of the expression of sorrow, anger, guilt, anxiety and helplessness and reassurance about the normality of the physiological accompaniments of grief.

BERGER RHYTHM is the term applied to normal rhythmical changes of electric potential in the brain. The electrical 'waves' can be recorded graphically as in electro-encephalography (qv). A person with epilepsy has abnormal waves.

BERIBERI, called by the Japanese KARKE, is a disease found mainly in Japan, Malaysia, China, Manila, Fiji Islands, India, West Africa, Western Australia and round the Gulf of Mexico, and consists in inflammation of the nerves all over the body. (See NEURITIS.)

Causes: It is found among those living in certain parts of the tropics, whose diet consists mainly of highly milled rice. It also occurs in Newfoundland and Labrador, where the inhabitants' main item of diet is white wheaten flour. In both groups of population the removal of the husk of rice and of the wheat berry leaves the diet very deficient in vitamin B_1 (thiamine). It is the lack of this vitamin that causes the trouble.

Symptoms: The affected person becomes, first of all, for some days feverish and weak; then, though feeling better in general health, he gradually develops symptoms of paralysis, especially of the hands and feet, dropsy, palpitation of the heart and loss of sensation in large areas of the skin, especially about the legs. These pass off, in general, in the course of some weeks, and the sufferer gradually recovers health, or occasionally he gets worse and dies from heart failure.

Treatment: The treatment required is large doses of vitamin B_1 (thiamine) (qv), plenty of nourishing food, and complete rest.

BERKEFELD FILTER is a candle-shaped filter made of diatomaceous earth. It restrains ordinary bacteria but lets through viruses.

BERRIES, POISONOUS: As most berries in Britain are either red or blackish when ripe, their colour is one of the simplest ways of distinguishing them.

Black poisonous berries: One of the most poisonous of these is the *deadly nightshade* (*Atropa belladonna*). Three berries are sufficient to kill a child. Ripening from July onwards, they are dull black in colour, often as large as a small marble, and surrounded by a persistent withered calyx. The plant usually grows in semi-shaded sites and is up to 1 metre (3 feet) in height. Even more poisonous, but fortunately less common, is the *baneberry* (*Actaea spicata*) which grows in woods on limestone in Yorkshire, Lancashire and Westmorland. The berries are nearly 6 mm (¼ inch) in diameter and grow on stems 30 to 60 cm (1 or 2 feet) long. More common is *Herb Paris* (*Paris quadrifolia*), which grows in semi-shaded sites, and has stems up to 60 cm (2 feet) high. The berries are up to 6 mm (¼ inch) in diameter and contain 16 to 20 dark-coloured seeds. The *buckthorn* (*Rhamnus cathartica*) and the *alder buckthorn* (*Rhamnus frangula*) are shrubs up to 6 metres (20 feet) in height which grow in woody thickets on peaty soil. The berries grow in clusters and are about the size of blackcurrants. Each berry contains four seeds. Only on unpruned *privets* (*Ligustrum vulgare* and *Ligustrum ovaliform*) are berries found in quantity. About the size of a pea, the berry has two chambers inside, usually with one or two seeds in each. These berries have caused fatal poisoning in children. The *cherry laurel* (*Prunus laurocerasus*), commonly grown in gardens and parks, produces in late summer small berries very like small black cherries except that the fruit stalk is short and rigid and the berries, up to about twelve in number, are borne along a common stalk 10 cm (4 inches) long. The *spurge laurel* (*Daphne laureola*), which grows sparingly in woodlands in England, produces egg-shaped blue-black berries on stems which grow to about 1·25 metres (4 feet) in height. The *ivy* (*Hedera helix*) produces berries about the size of a pea which ripen in early spring.

Red poisonous berries: These are even more dangerous because their colour is so much more attractive to children. The *woody nightshade* or *bittersweet* (*Solanum dulcamara*), which is common in South and Central England, is a straggling plant which bears clusters of six to eight bright-red translucent berries. These are very like redcurrants except that there is no tuft of old flower parts at the upper end of the fruit and they contain numerous seeds, compared with the six or eight in the redcurrant. The *white bryony* (*Bryonia dioica*) is another scrambling plant of the wayside and wasteland. It is most commonly found in Southern England and is almost entirely absent in the North. The berry is dull scarlet in colour, about a centimetre in diameter and contains three to six large flat, yellow-and-black mottled seeds. Fortunately the taste and odour are unpleasant, which discourages children from eating them. Fifteen berries constitute a fatal dose for children. The *blackbryony* (*Tamus communis*) is another straggling plant. The berries are bright crimson in colour and grow in small bunches. Superficially they are like redcurrants. The *cuckoo-pint* or *lords and ladies* (*Arum maculatum*), which grows in damp woodlands, sometimes in hedgerows, especially on basic soils, produces bright-red berries which ripen from August onwards. The berries, about the size of a pea, grow in clusters of eight to twenty at the upper end of a sturdy, naked, green stem about 15 to 20 cm (6 to 9 inches) long, and bear three small marks at the apex and usually contain three brownish, rough-coated seeds. The *dwarf baytree* (*Daphne mezereum*), which is usually cultivated in gardens because of its heavily scented, pink or purplish flowers from January onwards, bears small clusters of red berries from August onwards. They may be mistaken for redcurrants but can be distinguished by the lack of a tuft of withered flower parts at the upper end of the fruit. The berry of the *yew* (*Taxusbaccata*), which grows naturally in Southern Britain, and is planted widely elsewhere for ornament, ripens from August onwards. The pale, 12 mm (½ inch) long seed is half submerged in a soft, red, juicy cup. This fleshy cup, which has a sickly sweet taste, is not particularly poisonous, but the seed is highly poisonous.

For fuller details see *Bulletin 161, British Poisonous Plants*, published by the Ministry of Agriculture, Fisheries and Food, and obtainable from Her Majesty's Stationery Office.

BERYLLIOSIS is a disease of the lungs caused by the inhalation of particles of beryllium oxide.

BETAMETHASONE is a corticosteroid (qv) which has an action comparable to that of prednisolone, but in much lower dosage. In the form of BETAMETHASONE VALERATE it is used as an application to the skin as an ointment, cream or lotion.

BETATRON (see RADIOTHERAPY).

BETAXOLOL (KERLONE) (see ADRENERGIC DRUGS).

BEZAFIBRATE (BEZALIP) (see HYPERLIPIDAEMIA).

BEZOAR is a concretion found in the stomach and intestines of animals, especially goats, which was formerly used as a remedy against poisoning. It is also occasionally found in man.

BICARBONATE OF SODA, or BAKING SODA (see ALKALI).

BIGUANIDES are a group of chemical substances which act as oral hypoglycaemic agents (that is, reduce the level of the blood sugar when given by mouth), and are proving of value in the treatment of diabetes mellitus. They include metformin (qv). They act by reducing the production of glucose in the liver. (See DIABETES MELLITUS.)

BILE is a thick, bitter, golden-brown or greenish-yellow fluid, secreted by the liver, and stored in the gall-bladder. It consists of water, mucus, pigments (bilirubin and biliverdin), salts of three complex acids (cholic, chenodeoxycholic and deoxycholic acids), cholesterol and some mineral salts, and it is discharged through the bile-ducts into the intestine, a few cms below the opening from the stomach. This discharge is constant, but is much increased shortly after food is taken, and again, some hours later, when the food is digested. Bile is partly an excretion of waste material thrown out by the liver, partly a secretion endowed with some functions in digestion, especially that of fats, and it further aids the absorption of nourishment from the food passing down the bowels, and prevents excessive decomposition by destroying various micro-organisms. About 0·5 to 1 litre (1 to 2 pints) is secreted daily in man, but the greater part of this is reabsorbed with the food, passes into the blood, and ultimately circulates back to the liver, to be again excreted, and so on.

Jaundice is a condition in which the flow of bile becomes obstructed, so that the bile is not poured into the intestine, but circulates in the blood. As a consequence, the bile pigments are deposited in the tissues, and the skin becomes yellow or olive-green, while, at the same time, the stools become grey or white and the urine dark. (See JAUNDICE.)

Bilious headache, or biliousness, is a vague term, applied either to migraine (see HEADACHE) or to the headache and vomiting which occur in acute catarrh of the stomach set up by errors in diet. (See DYSPEPSIA.)

Vomiting of bile occurs in the two last-named conditions, and is also a sign of obstruction of the bowels, but bile may be brought up in any case of persistent vomiting or retching.

BILHARZIASIS is another name for schistosomiasis (qv).

BILIRUBIN is the chief pigment in human bile. It is derived from haemoglobin (qv) which is the red pigment of the red blood corpuscles. The site of manufacture of bilirubin is the reticulo-endothelial system (qv). When bile is passed into the intestine from the gall-bladder, part of the bilirubin is converted into stercobilin and excreted in the faeces. The remainder is reabsorbed into the blood-stream, and of this portion the bulk goes back to the liver to be re-excreted into the bile, whilst a small proportion is excreted in the urine as urobilinogen.

BILIVERDIN is the chief pigment of bile in herbivora and birds. It is a precursor of bilirubin in the production of the latter from haemoglobin, and there is a small amount in human bile.

BINOVULAR TWINS are twins who result from the fertilization of two separate ova. (See MULTIPLE BIRTHS.)

BIO-AVAILABILITY is a term referring to that proportion of a drug which reaches the systemic circulation unchanged after a particular route of administration. The most important factor that determines how much of a drug reaches the circulation is the pre-systemic metabolism in either the intestine or the liver. This is called first pass metabolism. It limits the bio-availability of many lipid-soluble drugs such as the beta blockers, some tricyclic antidepressants and various opiate analgesics (qqv). Food can influence drug bio-availability. The first effect of food is to modify gastric emptying so that the rate of absorption of a drug is reduced. Also calcium in the food may chelate with drugs such as the tetracyclines and reduce their intestinal absorption.

BIOFEEDBACK is a technique whereby an auditory or visual stimulus follows on from a physiological response. Thus, a subject's electrocardiogram (qv) may be monitored, and a signal passed back to the subject indicating his heart rate: eg. a red light if the rate is between fifty and sixty beats a minute; a green light if it is between sixty and seventy a minute. Once the subject has learned to discriminate between these two rates he can then learn to control his heart rate. How this is learned is not clear, but it is claimed that by this biofeedback it is possible to control the heart rate and blood-pressure, relax spastic muscles, and even bring migraine under control.

BIOPSY means the removal and examination of tissue from the living body for diagnostic purposes. For example, a piece of a tumour may be cut out and examined to determine whether it is cancerous.

BIOTIN is one of the dozen or so vitamins included in the vitamin B complex. It is found in liver, eggs, and meat, and it is also synthesized by bacteria in the gut. Absorption from the gut is prevented by avidin, a constituent of egg-white. The daily requirement is small: a fraction of a milligram daily. Gross deficiency results in disturbances of the skin, a smooth tongue and lassitude.

BIRD FANCIER'S LUNG (see PIGEON BREEDER'S LUNG).

BIRTH (see LABOUR): The average length of a child at birth is about 53 cm (21 inches), and the weight 3·2 kg (7 pounds). A *stillborn* child is 'any child which has issued forth from its mother after the twenty-eighth week of pregnancy and which did not at any time after being completely expelled from its mother breathe or show any other sign of life'. *Premature birth* is one which takes place before the natural time (see PREMATURE BIRTH), but in which the child is capable of surviving. A birth which takes place so prematurely that the child must necessarily die is known as an abortion or *miscarriage* (see ABORTION). In only 30 per cent of pregnancies does the child survive to birth. In 15 per cent of cases the pregnancy ends in spontaneous abortion or a stillbirth. In the remaining 55 per cent the foetus, as has been said, 'is presumed to be lost very early in gestation', but the loss cannot be detected.

BIRTH-MARKS are of various kinds. The most common are port-wine marks (see NAEVUS). Pigment spots are found, very often raised above the surface and more or less hairy, being then called moles (see MOLES).

BIRTH RATE: In 1984, the birth rate in England was 12·08 per 1000 population. The mean age at bearing the first child in marriage was 25. During the 1970's there was a fall in all social classes in the numbers of premaritally conceived first births – from 69·4 thousand to 34·7 thousand. In 1980, around half the premaritally conceived births were to teenage mothers. In the birth-rate international stakes, the leader is Nigeria, with a rate of 51·5 births per 1000 population in 1975–80. The lowest rate was in West Germany: 0·5 per thousand in 1980.

BISACODYL is a laxative which acts by stimulation of the nerve endings in the colon by direct contact with the mucous lining.

BISMUTH is a metal, of which the carbonate, subnitrate, salicylate, subgallate and oxychloride are used in medicine.

Uses: In irritative and painful conditions of the stomach or of the bowels, eg. when diarrhoea or vomiting is present, they have a sedative action. The salicylate of bismuth especially is used to check diarrhoea, the usual medicinal dose of it or of the subnitrate being about 1·2 grammes (20 grains). Given internally, bismuth salts turn the stools black. The subgallate is used in the form of suppositories in the treatment of haemorrhoids.

Externally, as dusting powder, they are used, both as a cosmetic and in eczema and other moist conditions of the skin, being commonly mixed, in equal proportions, with starch powder or oxide of zinc, or both.

BITES AND STINGS: Bites of animals are in general to be treated as punctured or lacerated wounds (see WOUNDS), but as animals' teeth are, in general, foul, suppuration is apt to arise if the bite be deep. The bite of some reptiles, scorpions, spiders, etc., causes definite symptoms of poisoning, while, after the bites of several animals, especially the wolf and the dog, there is often a risk of rabies. Wounds which are *septic*, ie. poisoned by bacteria, are dealt with in the section on WOUNDS.

Dog bites are treated by washing (not scrubbing) the bite with soap and water, and then applying hydrogen peroxide or cetrimide. The bite is then covered with a dressing. Penicillin is also given as a rule, and measures taken to prevent tetanus. More active treatment is required if there is possible risk of rabies (qv).

Snake bites are not necessarily poisonous, for not only are many snakes harmless, but people can, like the snake-charmers of India, render themselves immune by the injection under the skin of gradually increasing doses of the poison. It is estimated that the annual death rate from snake bites, throughout the world, is 25,000 to 35,000, of which 20,000 to 25,000 occur in India. In Europe there are probably only 2 or 3 fatal cases every year. The last fatal case reported in England and Wales occurred in 1957, and in the previous fifty years only seven deaths due to snake bite had been reported. There was a fatal case in Scotland in 1975.

The principal poisonous snakes belong to the viper and cobra families, and all inject their poison through a pair of grooved or hollow teeth connected with poison glands. These include in Asia the cobra, the king cobra, the krait, the deboia and the phoorsa; in America the rattlesnake, the copperhead, and the moccasin; in South America the fer-de-lance and the coral snake; in Africa cobras, vipers and the puff-adder; and in Australia the death-adder, tiger snake, copperhead, brown snake and black snake. The sea snakes of the Pacific and Indian Oceans are almost all poisonous. The only poisonous snake in Britain is the adder (*Vipera berus*). It is chiefly found in Scotland, Dartmoor and the New Forest. It is not found in Ireland. In a not inconsiderable number of cases of adder bite the victim is to blame as he has attempted to handle or torment the snake. Adders are not aggressive and usually try to get out of the way of humans.

The symptoms of snake-poisoning are swelling and paralysis of the bitten part, with general depression, palpitation, difficulty of breathing, faintness and later paralysis and convulsions, followed, in severe cases, by death. These symptoms appear within fifteen minutes to an hour after the bite. After the bite of a deboia or of one of the rattlesnakes very severe suppuration may occur in the neighbourhood of the bite in people who recover.

Treatment of an adder bite in Britain consists of immobilizing the limb by splinting, washing the wound with water, and giving an analgesic to relieve the pain. Medical advice should then be sought immediately, no matter how mild may appear to be the immediate effects of the bite. Expert opinion is divided as to whether or not antivenine (qv) should be given. Outside Britain, where the consequences can be much more serious, treatment consists of applying a tourniquet between the bite and the body, to prevent the poison being absorbed into the body. This should be released for a few seconds every fifteen minutes, in order to prevent gangrene. The bite should then be sucked vigorously for five-minute periods at frequent intervals. The serum known as *antivenine* (qv), which is available as an antidote against many snake bites, should be injected intravenously in liberal amounts as soon as possible. Antivenoms are also becoming available which are active against the venoms of individual snakes, such as the carpet viper (*Echis carinatus*) which is widely distributed in Northern Africa, the Middle East, Pakistan, India and Sri Lanka. The individual should also be treated as for shock, ie. resting quietly, kept warm, and given a blood transfusion and oxygen if necessary. As stimulants, sal volatile, strong tea, or coffee may be given, *not* alcohol.

Poisonous fishes exist in most tropical waters, especially round the islands of the Pacific and Indian Oceans, and their venom may be conveyed to man either by poisonous stings or by their bite. The action of the poison is mostly a depressing one upon the heart, and in the case of some of the tropical fishes convulsions and even death may be produced.

Weever fish (known as bishop fish in Cornwall), which are found on Atlantic coasts, as well as on sandy Mediterranean coasts, have poisonous spines which can cause painful wounds –usually in the feet. As the poison is destroyed by heat, the affected foot should be repeatedly bathed in water as hot as the victim can tolerate. A wise precaution is to wear suitable footwear when paddling or bathing.

Jelly-fish around British shores are fairly harmless, with the exception of the so-called Portuguese Man-of-War which occasionally invades our coasts. It has been described as looking 'rather like a pale blue Cornish pastie with a dark line down its back', and has tentacles up to 13 metres (40 feet) in length. The first thing to do in treatment is to withdraw the tentacle if it is still in the skin but this must not be done with the naked hand without the risk of being stung. A glove of wet sand, however, will usually give sufficient protection. The affected part should then be sprayed or gently washed with methylated spirit. Antihistamine preparations may also be helpful, either applied locally as a cream or, in more serious cases, given by mouth or by injection.

The stings of the much more dangerous jellyfish found in North Australian and Pacific and Indian waters may prove fatal unless immediate medical attention is available.

Sea-urchins are a hazard, particularly to skin divers, because of their spines. The main culprit is *Paracentrobus lividus*, a sea urchin found on rocks in the Mediterranean, the Atlantic coasts of France and Spain, and the south coast of England. It has a black body, 2·5 to 5 cm (1 to 2 inches) in diameter, covered with sharp, purple articulated spines 2·5 cm (1 inch) long. The most severe injuries occur from treading on, or diving on to, collections of them on rocks. This produces a severe burning pain. Prevention consists of avoiding rocky shores when swimming or diving. First-aid treatment consists of removal of the spines as soon as possible. This may require the use of a local anaesthetic or anaesthetizing the skin with ethyl chloride (qv). Once removed, an antiseptic dressing should be applied to the affected area until the wound heals. If not removed, the spine may result in a small tender cyst and, if this is burst as a result of pressure on it, there may be a recurrence of severe burning pain.

Toads and salamanders secrete a milky fluid from the skin of the back which is irritating locally, and which, in small animals and weakly children, is said to kill if introduced by a wound.

Centipedes, scorpions and tarantulas (large tropical spiders) kill their prey by poison, and can inflict a very painful, though probably seldom fatal, bite on human beings. The treatment is to apply a ligature as for snake bite at once, and to suck the wound or wash it well with a strong solution of permanganate of potassium. Some other substances have also a reputation as antidotes, such as ammonia, spirit of camphor, tobacco juice, turpentine, and camphor and chloral rubbed up together. An antitoxic serum has been prepared for use against scorpion bite in Egypt. If an abscess forms it is treated like an abscess from any other cause.

Harvest-bugs, fleas, ticks, lice and mosquitoes often cause great irritation of the skin by their bite. Harvest-bugs may bury themselves in the skin and have to be picked out with a needle. Dimethyl phthalate applied to the skin or clothing is an effective repellent. Human beings vary much in their susceptibility to flea bites. The best preventive is dimethyl phthalate. Failing this, smearing the skin with oil of pennyroyal or oil of lavender is helpful, or dusting the underwear and socks with pyrethrum powder, menthol or camphor. Ticks are common parasites of household pets in Britain but seldom attack human beings. In Scotland, however, bites by sheep ticks are accepted as a natural minor hazard of life. The best preventive is dimethyl phthalate or diethyltoluamide. The ticks may be dislodged from the skin by applying the lighted end of a cigarette or the hot end of a match that has just been lit and blown out, or covering it with alcohol, petrol or petroleum jelly. Once bitten, calamine lotion relieves the itching. Lice may be got rid of, if in the hair, by the application of shampoos and lotions containing insecticides. Most preparations contain gamma benzene hexachloride. The lice and nits can then be removed with a fine comb. They may be got rid of from the clothes by baking these in an oven or fumigating with burning sulphur for several hours, or by the use of DDT. (See also under INSECTS IN RELATION TO DISEASE.) Bites by mosquitoes or bugs are soothed by bathing with salt water, by painting with sal volatile or calamine lotion, or by applying an antihistamine cream or ointment. They may be prevented by smearing the skin with dimethyl phthalate (qv), or, if this is not available, camphor water, lime juice or one of the oils of pennyroyal, lavender, cloves or cinnamon.

Trombicula autumnalis is the harvest mite. It is also known as red bug and chigger, and is found in fields, gardens and orchards in the autumn. It is the larva that attacks man by crawling up the legs. The adult, popularly known as the 'money spider', does not attack man. Measuring 1 × 1·5 mm, it can pass through ordinary clothing. It produces itchy red spots, known in Scotland as 'berry bugs' from their occurrence in those who have been picking raspberries and similar soft fruit. Similar trombiculid mites are found in the rest of Europe, America and Asia. In the Far East they are vectors (or carriers) of rickettsial diseases, such as mite-borne typhus (see TYPHUS FEVER.) Relief from the itching is obtained by bathing the affected part with weak ammonia or baking soda, or calamine lotion with or without the addition of 0·5 to 1 per cent phenol. Bites may be prevented by the use of an insect-repellent cream containing demethyl phthalate and diethyltoluamide, which is obtainable from chemists without a prescription. An alternative preventive measure in heavily infested areas is to wear a boiler suit previously soaked in gamma benzene hexachloride in water and then allowed to dry. When put on, the legs of the boiler suit are tucked into the top of Wellington boots.

Ants, bees, wasps and hornets cause great irritation by their stings. Those of ants are allayed by eau-de-Cologne, vinegar or lemon juice. Bees sometimes leave a part of their sting as well as poison in the skin, and this should be looked for first of all and carefully wiped out. The sting of a wasp in the throat, the insect having been taken into the mouth in biting a fruit, has caused death owing to rapid swelling, which blocks the air passage. For bee stings the traditional treatment is the dabbing on of ammonia, bicarbonate of soda or washing blue. For wasp and hornet stings a weak acid, such as vinegar or lemon juice, is said to be better. But the experts claim that in both cases any benefit is psychological. A vaccine (Pharmalgen) is now available for those who are allergic to bee and wasp stings. It is estimated that one in every thousand people in Britain is potentially allergic to bee or wasp stings.

Hairy-caterpillars, by brittle, poisoned hairs, cause an itchy red rash after contact. It is relieved by vinegar or olive oil.

Nettle stings are relieved by bruised dock leaves or raw onion juice.

BITOSCANATE is a drug that is proving of value in the treatment of hookworm infestations.

BITTERS are among the oldest of drugs still prescribed. Wormwood, probably the oldest of them all, though never prescribed as such today, being one of the main constituents of absinthe (qv), is mentioned in the Papyrus Ebers from a tomb in Thebes (1500 BC), and bitters are referred to in the Hippocratic writings (*circa* 400 BC). They are alcoholic extracts of herbs used to stimulate the appetite and to a lesser extent as flavours for tonics and other remedies.

The precise action of bitters is not known, and the modern tendency in medicine is to look upon them as a remnant of the days when medicine was more of an art than a science. It is of course the wise thing to try and find out the cause of any loss of appetite, but often this is not possible. It is in these circumstances that bitters, which are definitely known to increase gastric secretion, often have a beneficial effect in improving the individual's interest in food. Whether or not this is psychological may be open to question but, whatever the reason, if it results in an individual's appetite improving, then something has been achieved.

BLACK CURRANTS, the fruit of *Ribes nigrum*, are a rich source of ascorbic acid (vitamin C). In the form of Black Currant Syrup BPC it is used as a dietary supplement, particularly for children, in a dosage of 5 to 10 millilitres. Ten millilitres contain 7·5 milligrams of ascorbic acid. It is also used as a flavouring agent in cough mixtures.

BLACK DEATH is an old name for plague. (See PLAGUE.)

BLACKFAT TOBACCO DISEASE is a form of pneumonia caused by the smoking of blackfat tobacco, a tobacco flavoured with a mineral oil known as canopus oil. It is a popular tobacco in the West Indies and West Africa, but to date cases of blackfat tobacco disease have only been reported in Guyana.

BLACK DRAUGHT is a powerful purgative preparation, known also as compound senna mixture, and containing Epsom salts, senna and liquorice. The dose is two to three tablespoonfuls.

BLACK DROP is another name for laudanum or tincture of opium. (See OPIUM.)

BLACKHEADS (see ACNE).

BLACK MOTIONS are passed when there is great constipation, and when bismuth or iron is being taken; but the most important cause is blood changed by the digestive processes, and proceeding from ulceration somewhere in the stomach or bowels.

BLACK VOMIT is due to the presence of blood in the stomach. There may be dark masses, as in yellow fever, or a small amount of black sediment like coffee-grounds, as in ulcer of the stomach.

BLACKWATER FEVER is an acute illness characterized by haemoglobinuria ('black water'), jaundice, fever, vomiting, anaemia, and severe haemolysis. It is associated with malignant tertian malaria, and occurs in Central Africa, India and the Far East.

Although the precise cause is still obscure, it is known that the disease may be precipitated in malarial subjects by the taking of quinine or by exposure to cold, by fatigue, and by trauma. Predisposing factors include exposure by non-immune individuals to virulent strains of the malarial parasite and irregular and inadequate treatment of such infections. The mortality rate usually varies between 10 and 20 per cent, but may be as high as 40 per cent.

Symptoms: These are fever, rigor, nausea, bilious vomiting, epigastric discomfort, jaundice and the passage of pinkish, red or port-wine coloured urine – haemoglobinuria. The spleen and liver are enlarged and tender. After a few hours the temperature falls, there is profuse sweating, and the skin becomes jaundiced. Mild cases may recover in a day or two. Severe cases have a succession of attacks.

Treatment: This consists in (1) absolute rest in bed; (2) administration of plenty of alkaline fluids; (3) glucose given intravenously (and sodium bicarbonate if necessary); (4) blood transfusion, and subsequent remedies for anaemia.

BLADDER, DISEASES OF: For diseases of the gall-bladder see GALL-BLADDER, DISEASES OF. (See also URINE.)

The urinary bladder is subject to several diseases, but, partly owing to its inaccessibility, as it lies deep in the pelvis behind the pubic bones, partly owing to general ignorance as to its site and functions, symptoms set up in it are often attributed to the bowels and other organs. Diseased conditions in it are diagnosed in part by the symptoms they set up, in part by chemical and microscopical examination of the urine, and in the more obscure conditions by means of the cystoscope. The *cystoscope* consists of a narrow metal tube fitted up as a telescope, and bearing at its end a small electric lamp by which the cavity is lighted up. The instrument is introduced through the urethra, and shows any tumour or ulcer which may exist, and also whether blood in the urine comes from the bladder wall or runs out of the ureters from the kidneys. (See CYSTOSCOPE.) *Sounding* is another process, consisting in the introduction of a curved solid metal rod, when the presence of a stone is suspected, against which the sound can be felt or heard to strike. *Catheters* are narrow tubes, used to draw off the water when it is not possible to expel this voluntarily, or, when the bladder is to be washed out for some diseased condition. (See CATHETERS.) The following are some of the chief diseased conditions:

CYSTITIS, or INFLAMMATION OF THE BLADDER: **Causes**: Bacteria live readily in the urine but they do not multiply in the healthy bladder. When some cause is present to weaken the bladder wall, or, when bacteria are introduced in large numbers, for example on a dirty catheter, they multiply inside this organ and set up inflammation.

There may be direct infection from neighbouring organs, as the urethra in gonorrhoea. Any cause that prevents the free voiding of the urine, such as stricture or narrowing of the urethra, or enlargement of the prostate gland at the outlet of the bladder, which is a common occurrence in elderly men, may produce a chronic form of cystitis. In women it is commonly associated with prolapse of the womb. A stone, if present, is apt by its irritation to do the same. One of the most frequent organisms found in the urine in cases of cystitis is *Escherichiacoli*. Tuberculous cystitis may be found, due to the *Mycobacterium tuberculosis* which produces a chronic ulcer on the bladder wall. Another very chronic form is caused by the schistosome, a small parasitic worm which may settle in the minute blood-vessels of the bladder wall. This form is very common in Egypt and South Africa. (See SCHISTOSOMIASIS.)

Symptoms: Pain in the region of the bladder or in the small of the back, frequency of making water, and a condition of bad smell, turbidity and whitish sediment in the urine, are the chief facts noticed by the sufferer. In acute cases there may be high temperature and shivering fits. In the chronic form the very frequent desire to pass small quantities of urine is the most marked symptom.

Treatment: Rest in bed and hot applications, like rubber hot water bottles to the lower part of the abdomen, along with simple diet and large quantities of bland fluid, such as barley water, to drink, may be all that is necessary. Large doses of potassium citrate are also helpful, usually combined in a mixture with tincture of hyoscyamus. In the majority of cases, however, it is necessary to give drugs that will destroy the causative organism. In practice this means one of the sulphonamides or antibiotics. The choice is dependent upon which organism is responsible for the infection, and this is determined by submitting a specimen of urine to bacteriological investigation.

STONE, or CALCULUS, in the bladder may be of any size up to that of a hen's or goose's egg, or even larger. The largest one ever seen in England, in 1809, is said to have weighed 1·36 kg (2¾ pounds). An almost equally large one, weighing 1·13 kg 2½ pounds was removed in a London hospital in 1975. There are three varieties of stone: (*a*) URATIC, associated with acidity (see ACIDITY) or with the gouty constitution; (*b*) OXALIC, composed of oxalate of lime, and often associated with a nervous dyspeptic type of temperament; (*c*) PHOSPHATIC, which occur in long-standing cases of inflammation of the bladder, accompanied by constant decomposition of the urine. This is the most common type of stone found in the bladder.

Symptoms: The symptoms of inflammation of the bladder, together with discomfort on movement, and sudden pain immediately after the passing of water, are those generally found.

Treatment: Although control of the diet may reduce the tendency to the formation of stones in the bladder, the only method of treatment once they have formed is surgical removal. In spite of many vaunted claims, there is no drug known which can remove, or dissolve, stones in the bladder. In 1739 a secret remedy sold by Mrs Joanna Stephens was considered so effectual in stones that the secret was bought by the British Government for £5000. It was found to consist of calcined egg shells, soap and aromatic bitters – that is, its essentials were lime, phosphates and alkalis. Surgical removal of the stone (or stones) is carried out by either *litholapaxy* or *lithotomy*. Litholapaxy consists of passing into the bladder through the urethra an instrument known as a lithotrite which crushes the stone, after which the small pieces are removed through the urethra. The advantage of this method is that no incision is required and the patient is only laid up for one or two days. If the stone is larger than 5 cm (2 inches) in diameter, however, or if there are too many stones present, lithotomy has to be performed: ie. the bladder is opened through an incision in the lower abdominal wall and the stone (or stones) are removed in this way.

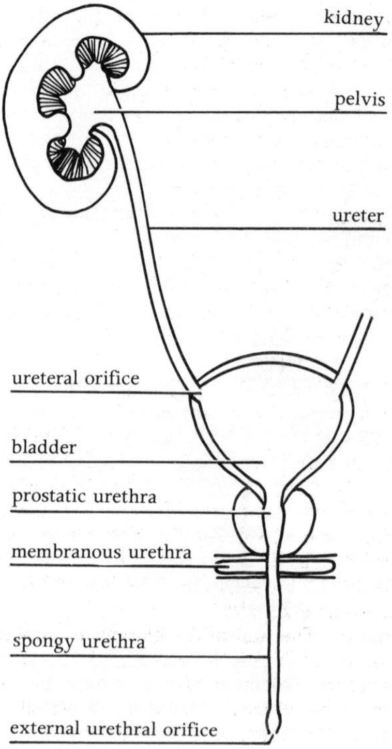

Diagram of the male urinary system.

CANCER: Over 7500 cases of cancer of the bladder are diagnosed every year in Britain, and in 1980 it was responsible for 4013 deaths (2796 men and 1217 women) in England. How many of these cases are occupational in origin is not clear, but it has been stated that contact with benzidine, beta-naphthylamine and alpha-naphthylamine increases the over-all risk of dying from cancer of the bladder 30 times above that of the general population. It is over eighty years now since attention was first drawn to the fact that cancer of the bladder was frequent among workers in the chemical industry. There is new evidence that workers in the rubber and cable-making industries, rodent-control operators, laboratory workers using benzidine, as well as engineering workers using lubricant oils may develop it. Prevention of such industrial cases consists of regular six-monthly screening. In treatment, promising results are being obtained from the use of radio-active isotopes (see ISOTOPE) and doxorubicin (qv).
RUPTURE of the bladder may occur in old men who have long suffered from difficulty in passing water and cystitis, or in healthy people from a blow or crush. (See ABDOMEN, INJURIES OF.)

BLADDERS are sacs formed of muscular and fibrous tissue and lined by a mucous membrane, which is united loosely to the muscular coat, so as freely to allow increase and decrease in the contained cavity. Bladders are designed to contain some secretion or excretion, and communicate with the exterior by a narrow opening through which their contents can be discharged. In man there are two, the *gall-bladder* and the *urinary bladder*.
GALL-BLADDER: This is situated under the liver in the upper part of the abdomen, and its function is to store the bile, which it discharges into the intestine by the bile duct. For further details, see LIVER.
URINARY BLADDER: This is situated in the pelvis, in front of the last part of the bowel. The bladder, in the full state, rises up into the abdomen and holds about 570 ml (a pint) of urine. Two fine tubes, called the ureters, lead into the bladder, one from each kidney; and the urethra, a tube as wide as a lead pencil when distended, leads from it to the exterior, a distance of 4 cm (1½ inches) in the female and 20 cm (8 inches) in the male.
Structure: The wall of the bladder is similar in structure to that of the bowels, and consists of four coats. The inner surface is lined by a soft mucous membrane covered by epithelial cells of irregular shape. This is attached to the muscular coat by a loose, fibrous, sub-mucous coat, in which run numerous blood-vessels. In the muscular coat the muscle fibres are arranged in several layers, and run in various directions, thereby adding greatly to the strength of the wall. On its upper and back part, the bladder possesses a covering of serous membrane, formed by part of the general peritoneal lining of the abdominal cavity, but this outermost coat does not extend down to the base of the bladder, where the latter lies in close contact with the other pelvic organs. The bladder is suspended in position by numerous ligaments, four of which are fibrous bands, while the remaining five are formed by thickened portions of the peritoneum. The base of the bladder is directed downwards and backwards, and in this part are the three openings of the ureters and urethra. The exit from the bladder is kept closed by a muscular ring, which is relaxed every time water is passed.

BLAUD'S PILL is a pill containing carbonate of iron, used in the treatment of anaemia.

BLEEDER is a term applied to persons in whom it is difficult to stop bleeding when some small wound has been sustained. (See HAEMOPHILIA.)

BLEEDING (see HAEMORRHAGE; and BLOOD-LETTING).

BLENORRHOEA means an excessive discharge of mucus or slimy material from a surface, such as that of the eye, nose, bowel, etc. The word catarrh is used with the same meaning, but also includes the idea of inflammation as the cause of such discharge.

BLEOMYCIN is an antibiotic, obtained from *Streptomycesverticillus*, that is being used with a certain amount of success in the treatment of cancer of the upper part of the gut, the genital tract and lymphomas. (See CYTOTOXIC DRUGS.)

BLEPHARITIS means inflammation of the eyelids. (See EYE DISEASES AND INJURIES.)

BLEPHAROSPASM (see EYE, DISEASE AND INJURIES OF.

BLIGHTED OVUM, or BLIGHTED FOETUS, is the term used to describe a condition in which apparently normal development of the embryo and its surrounding membranes continues for a short time and then the embryo dies, leaving the membranes alive for a little longer. The causes are not clear but are assumed to be either defects (possibly hereditary) in the ovum or fertilizing sperm, or some fault in the mother's womb. (See ABORTION; FOETUS.)

BLINDNESS: The statutory definition for the purposes of registration as a blind person under the National Assistance Act, 1948, is that the person is 'so blind as to be unable to perform any work for which eyesight is essential'. Generally this is vision worse than 6/60 in the better eye, or with better acuity than this but where 'the field of vision is markedly contracted in the greater part of its extent'. Partial sight has no statutory definition but there are Department of Health guidelines for registering a person partially sighted. Generally these are vision of 6/24 or worse with some contraction of the peripheral field, or better with gross field defects. The World Health Organization estimated that there were 28–42 million binocularly blind people in the world in 1979. The causes of blindness vary with age and degree of development of the country. In Western society the commonest causes are 'other retinal disease, glaucoma, diabetic retinopathy and senile cataract'. (See also VISION.)

Any blind person, or his or her relatives, can obtain help and advice from the Royal National Institute for the Blind, 224 Great Portland Street, London W1N 6AA (01–388 1266).

NIGHT BLINDNESS (NYCTALOPIA): An inability to see in the dark. It can be associated with retinitis pigmentosa or Vitamin A deficiency.

BLIND SPOT (see VISION, FIELD OF).

BLISTERS AND COUNTER-IRRITANTS: These are employed in cases of both acute and chronic inflammation, on the principle that irritation of the skin causes congestion of the parts immediately below the skin, while it relieves congestion of deep-seated organs through an action upon the nerves that regulate the size of the minute blood-vessels.

Varieties: Substances so employed are spoken of generally as counter-irritants, and divided into *rubefacients*, or substances which merely redden the skin and cause it to peel off; and *vesicants*, or blistering applications, when, in addition, they produce a collection of fluid under the horny layer of the skin; but there is no sharp division between them, most rubefacients producing blisters if left on long enough. The chief *rubefacients* are: mustard, turpentine, cajuput oil, capsicum, tincture of iodine and liniments of ammonia, chloroform, etc., and of *vesicants* we have cantharides or Spanish fly, pure acetic acid, ammonia and chloroform.

The CAUTERY is also used for this purpose. (See CAUTERY.)

Uses: MILDER COUNTER-IRRITANTS are used in cases of bronchitis, congestion of the stomach with vomiting, vague rheumatic pain, sprains and when a prolonged application is desired, so that some swelling or thickening due to chronic inflammation may be absorbed, or some continued pain lessened.

BLISTERS are used (1) to subdue severer forms of pain and inflammation, for example, in pleurisy, pericarditis and sciatica, in which case they are applied a little distance away from the seat of pain; and (2) to promote absorption of thickenings and effusions in joints, etc., in which case the blister is applied to the skin immediately over the affected part.

How to apply a blister or counter-irritant: *Mustard* is made into a paste and spread on muslin or brown paper, and so applied directly to the skin for twenty to thirty minutes, until a warm glow is felt. Mustard leaves can also be purchased and similarly used after moistening. If a more powerful action is desired, mustard may be dusted thickly over the surface of a linseed-meal poultice, and this applied for a similar length of time. After-redness is less if muslin has been placed between the mustard and the skin.

One must be careful not to apply mustard too long in weak persons and children, or a slough may result. For a milder effect the paste may be made with equal quantities of mustard and flour. The skin should be sponged with warm water, dried, and anointed with a little Simple Ointment BP after the mustard is removed.

Turpentine and *cajuput oil* are generally sprinkled, about a teaspoonful at a time, upon flannel cloths, which are then wrung out of hot water, and used for pain in the abdomen or back. (See POULTICES and FOMENTATIONS.)

Tincture of iodine is usually painted on the skin once or twice a day till the epidermis comes off in flakes, but just short of blistering. It is used over joints.

Cantharides blisters are produced by painting on Liquor Epispasticus (blistering fluid), or by applying cantharides plaster, but are never used today in Britain because of their dangers, though they are still in use in some European countries.

Acetic acid, ammonia, and *chloroform* are used by soaking a piece of lint of the required size in one of these fluids, applying it, and covering with a watch-glass till the blister rises.

BLOOD is the fluid which circulates through the arteries, capillaries, and veins, exchanging fluid and gases with the bodily tissues. The latter receive the products absorbed from the food and the oxygen taken up by the blood in its passage through the lungs, while the blood removes from the tissues carbon dioxide to discharge it in the lungs, and various waste products, of which it rids itself in its passage through the kidneys.

Composition: The blood consists, in addition to the fluid, of minute bodies, or corpuscles. These are of three kinds: red corpuscles, white corpuscles and blood platelets. In the *fluid* are dissolved the various salts and proteins which nourish the tissues (see also LYMPH), and also the waste products, such as uric acid, destined for removal from the body. The *red corpuscles* act as the carriers of oxygen; each is a disc, with an average diameter of 7·2 micrometres, hollowed out on either surface, and contains a substance called haemoglobin, which acts as a medium of interchange between the oxygen of the air in the lungs, and the tissues requiring it. Each red blood corpuscle, or erythrocyte as it is technically known, contains about 600 million haemoglobin molecules. There are about 5,000,000 red corpuscles in every cubic millimetre of blood, the blood of women containing slightly fewer than that of men. The *white corpuscles* are of several different kinds, and wander through the walls of the small blood-vessels, upon occasion into the tissues; here they have many functions to perform, of which the chief are the repair of wounds, the absorption of foreign bodies, and the destruction of bacteria; their dead bodies form, when in large numbers, the matter or pus of abscesses. Their number is less than 1 to 500 of the red corpuscles. They are bigger than the red blood cells, ranging in diameter from around 10 to 15 micrometres. The chief varieties of white corpuscles are those with a single large nucleus (monocytes), those with a nucleus consisting of several variously shaped parts (polymorphonuclear), and small corpuscles resembling those formed in the lymphatic glands (lymphocytes). They are also classed according to whether the granules they contain stain with a blue alkaline dye (basophil) or with a red acid dye (eosinophil). The *blood platelets* are extremely minute, and play an important part in clotting. The range of the normal blood count is shown in the table below:

Examination of blood: The corpuscles of the blood may be counted. For this purpose a minute drop is drawn up into a special graduated tube provided with a bulb in which the blood is mixed with a suitable diluting fluid. A drop of this diluted blood is blown out upon a special glass slide on which have been ruled with a diamond a number of lines that divide the surface into areas of a 400th square millimetre in size. A cover glass is then lowered upon the drop and so supported on a raised glass rim that a definite distance (0·1 millimetre) separates it from the ruled surface. The slide is then placed under a microscope, the average number of corpuscles that have settled on each square is counted, and thus the number in one four-thousandth of a cubic millimetre is ascertained. Machines are now replacing man in the execution of this tedious exercise.

Red corpuscles: Men	4·5 to 6·5 million per c.mm
Red corpuscles: Women	4·0 to 5·5 million per c.mm
Haemoglobin: Men	13·5 to 18 G. per 100 ml
Haemoglobin: Women	12·0 to 16 G. per 100 ml
White corpuscles	4000 to 10,000 per c.mm
Neutrophils	2500 to 7000 per c.mm
Eosinophils	50 to 400 per c.mm
Basophils	20 to 200 per c.mm
Lymphocytes	1500 to 3000 per c.mm
Monocytes	200 to 800 per c.mm
Platelets	150,000 to 300,000 per c.mm

Range of normal blood count.

The haemoglobin is estimated by taking a drop in a fine measured tube, diluting it with distilled water in a graduated tube till it assumes the same tint as a known standard, and then, by reading off the amount of water added, the percentage of haemoglobin is obtained.

Dried films are also prepared by smearing the blood on slides and staining these, usually with aniline dyes, methylene blue, and eosin dissolved in methyl alcohol; in these dried films the corpuscles can be examined by a high magnifying power and a differential count can be made of the various forms.

Formation of blood: The average life of a red blood corpuscle is about 120 days. To renew the wear and tear, as well as to make good losses by wounds, constant manufacture is going on in the marrow of the bones, in some glands, and also probably in the spleen, the daily turnover of haemoglobin being about 6·5 grams.

Amount of blood: In health this is around 85 millilitres per kilogram of body weight, or 9 per cent of the weight of the body.

Clotting of blood occurs when blood is shed, and is due to the formation of threads of fibrin which, as it shrinks, squeezes out from its interstices a clear, faintly straw-coloured fluid – serum. (For details of clotting, see COAGULATION.)

Functions of blood: The red corpuscles act as oxygen carriers; the white corpuscles have mainly a defensive action against the onset of infection. The fluid of the blood carries in solution various waste-products such as carbon dioxide to be exhaled by the lungs, urea and salts to be removed by the kidneys; also it distributes foodstuffs, such as sugar and proteins absorbed from the intestine and elaborated by various glands; and it forms a general medium of communication between organs that are chemically inter-dependent; for example, carrying to the stomach the materials for the gastric juice, to the muscles ferments formed in the pancreas, etc., and absorbing secretions needed for the general purposes of the body, like those of the thyroid gland and suprarenal glands.

BLOOD, DISEASES OF (see ANAEMIA; LEUKAEMIA).

BLOOD GROUPS: People are divided into four main groups in respect of a certain reaction of the blood. This depends upon the capacity of the serum of one person's blood to agglutinate the red blood corpuscles of another's in certain circumstances. The reaction depends on antigens, known as agglutinogens, in the red corpuscles and antibodies, known as agglutinins, in the serum. There are two of each, the agglutinogens being known as A and B. Anyone's blood corpuscles may have (1) no agglutinogens, (2) agglutinogen A, (3) agglutinogen B, (4) agglutinogens A and B: these are the four groups.

In blood transfusion, the person giving and the person receiving the blood must belong to the same blood group, or a dangerous reaction will take place from the agglutination that occurs when blood of a different group is present.

Group	*Agglutinogens in the corpuscles*	*Agglutinins in the plasma*	*Frequency in Great Britain*
AB	A and B	None	2 per cent
A	A	Anti-B	46 per cent
B	B	Anti-A	8 per cent
O	Neither A nor B	Anti-A and Anti-B	44 per cent

The four main blood groups.

Rhesus factor: In addition to these A and B agglutinogens (or antigens) there is another one known as the Rhesus (or Rh) factor, so named because there is a similar antigen in the red blood corpuscles of the Rhesus monkey. About 84 per cent of the population have this Rh factor in their blood and are therefore known as 'Rh-positive'. The remaining 16 per cent who do not possess the factor are known as 'Rh-negative'.

The practical importance of the Rh factor is that, unlike the A and B agglutinogens, there are no naturally occurring Rh antibodies, but such antibodies may develop in an Rh-negative person if the Rh antigen is introduced into his or her circulation. This can occur (*a*) if an Rh-negative person is given a transfusion of Rh-positive blood, (*b*) if an Rh-negative mother married to an Rh-positive husband becomes pregnant and the foetus is Rh-positive. If this happens, the mother develops Rh antibodies which can pass into the foetal circulation, where they react with the baby's Rh antigen and cause haemolytic disease of the foetus and newborn. This means that the child may be stillborn or become jaundiced shortly after birth (see HAEMOLYTIC DISEASE OF THE NEWBORN).

As about one in six expectant mothers is Rh-negative a blood-group examination is now considered an essential part of the antenatal examination of a pregnant woman. All such Rh-negative expectant mothers are now given a 'Rhesus card' showing that they belong to the rhesus-negative blood group. This card they should always carry with them. Rh-positive blood should never be transfused to an Rh-negative girl or woman.

BLOODLESSNESS (see ANAEMIA).

BLOOD-LETTING was a practice much in vogue for various ailments a century ago. Indeed, many people had themselves bled regularly for the purpose of avoiding the bad health consequent on over-eating and over-drinking. It came, in time, to be so much abused – many sick people undoubtedly having died, not of the original disease, but of the excessive bleeding practised for its cure – that it fell into almost complete disuse. Certain conditions are, however, benefited by withdrawing blood either from the affected part or from the general circulation. There are three chief methods of blood-letting.

Vein puncture is employed when it is desired to obtain a small quantity of blood for analysis or the performance of various tests. For this purpose a hollow hypodermic needle is pushed into a vein, one of those at the bend of the elbow usually being chosen, while pressure by a band or by the fingers is exerted on the veins in the upper arm. If it is desired to obtain the serum of the blood, the blood is run off into a test tube and allowed to clot. If the blood is required for analysis, clotting may be prevented by adding to the tube, before the blood is drawn off, a few crystals of potassium oxalate or potassium citrate.

Venesection consists in the opening of a vein, usually, owing to its superficial position, one of the veins just above the bend of the elbow. After the desired amount has flowed out, a pad and tight bandage are used to stop the bleeding. This method was used in certain cases of acute heart failure, when life may depend upon quickly and temporarily relieving the strain on the heart. It is also used in the treatment of polycythaemia (qv).

Cupping was at one time used either as dry-cupping to draw blood to the surface, or as wet-cupping to withdraw blood from a congested area. (See CUPPING.)

Leeches were formerly used to draw blood. After they are removed, bleeding is generally free, and may be encouraged, if desired, by warm poultices. They are seldom used for this purpose at the present day.

BLOOD-POISONING is a serious condition, and is known as septicaemia or pyaemia, according as the sufferer is simply poisoned by micro-organisms circulating in the blood, or as he develops, in addition, abscesses at different points over his body, owing to bacteria deposited from the blood. There is a milder form called sapraemia, in which the person becomes fevered and ill owing to the absorption of foul or putrid substances from the bowels or from wounds, but is not dangerously affected, and there is a chronic form called 'hectic fever', in which constant absorption of poisonous material takes place from cavities in the lungs, from diseased bones, etc. (see TUBERCULOSIS).

Causes: Wounds or inflamed areas, especially in bones, joints and veins, may be invaded by specially virulent bacteria, or, owing to great constitutional weakness of the person, for example, in alcoholics or diabetics, the bacteria may find a specially congenial soil for their growth. Women after delivery are specially liable to infection – the condition known as puerperal fever – but this is much less common nowadays as a result of more efficient methods of prevention.

Symptoms: In septicaemia very high temperature, followed speedily by death, may be the only sign. In pyaemia there are, in addition, shivering (rigor), profuse sweating, pains in the joints and muscles and the signs of abscesses at different points, which may last over days or weeks.

Treatment: The introduction of antiseptic surgery by Lord Lister immensely reduced the frequency of blood-poisoning, but the position has been improved out of all recognition by the introduction of the sulphonamides and antibiotics. Which of these should be used in a given case depends upon the causative organism, but in the majority of cases penicillin given intramuscularly is the treatment of choice. Active surgical treatment by amputation, opening of abscesses, antiseptic douches, etc., according to circumstances, may also be necessary.

BLOOD-PRESSURE is the name given to the pressure that must be applied to an artery, say in the arm, in order to stop the pulse in the vessel beyond the point of pressure. It is generally assumed to be equivalent to the pressure to which the blood is subjected by the force of the heart and the elasticity of the vessels, but it is also dependent on the thickness and hardness of the vessel wall, and on the volume of blood thrown out of the heart at each beat.

The blood-pressure is greatest at each heartbeat (systolic pressure) and falls somewhat between the beats (diastolic pressure). The systolic pressure in children is equal to that of a mercury column about 100 mm high, in young adults about 120, and it tends to increase with advancing age as the arteries get thicker and harder, but this is by no means always the case.

The blood-pressure is raised temporarily by exposure to cold, and permanently by kidney disease, by some disorders of the ductless glands, and in the condition known as essential hypertension (qv). A blood-pressure of 180 is not uncommon, and it may be as high as 250 or occasionally even 300 mm. Mental worry combined with lack of sufficient exercise has also an important effect in producing raised blood-pressure. The pressure is below the normal as the result of warmth, eg. after a hot bath, as well as in exhaustion, weakening diseases, fevers and generally in heart failure.

The blood-pressure may be estimated roughly by the pressure with which it is necessary to apply the finger at the wrist in order to obliterate the pulse. It is more exactly measured by means of an instrument known as the *sphygmomanometer*. This consists of a flat rubber bag which is strapped round the arm, and the interior of which communicates by two tubes with either a pressure gauge or a mercury manometer, and with a hand pump. The bag is pumped up so as to constrict the arm, and the systolic pressure is taken as that at which the pulse disappears as felt at the wrist or as heard in the artery at the bend of the elbow.

An abnormally high blood-pressure is often accompanied by disease of the arteries, so that people with greatly raised pressure are specially liable to stroke. In cases associated with advanced disease of the kidneys, the heightened blood-pressure is to some extent a salutary matter, because the circulation of the blood through the diminished vessels of the kidneys is thereby increased. In such a case the general health of the patient is better while the pressure remains moderately high, and if it is reduced too much by drugs and other means the general health deteriorates.

BLOOD-SPITTING (see EXPECTORATION; HAEMOPTYSIS).

BLOOD TRANSFUSION (see TRANSFUSION OF BLOOD).

'BLOWING' OF CANS means the presence of gas in cans of food, the gas resulting from putrefaction or fermentation of the food, or from the action of fruit on the metal of the container, producing hydrogen. The ends of the can or tin bulge and give a tympanitic note on percussion. The food in such cans should not be eaten.

BLUE DISEASE is a popular term for cyanosis. (See CYANOSIS.)

BLUE PILL, or MERCURY PILL, is a purgative. It contains mercury and liquorice. It is also said to stimulate the activity of the liver. The dose is from 250 to 500 mg.

BLUE STONE is copper sulphate.

BOILS, or FURUNCLES, are small areas of inflammation starting in the roots of hairs, and due to the growth of a micro-organism (generally that known as a staphylococcus). When a large number of boils form close together at one time the mass is called a carbuncle.

Causes: The essential cause is bacterial. Diabetics are specially troubled with boils, so that anyone liable to recurrence of boils should be examined in case he may be suffering from diabetes mellitus. People who eat too much food, or who are recovering from an exhausting illness, are also liable to them. Friction, which irritates the hair roots, is an important cause, and therefore boils are commonest on the back of the neck, on the forearm, and on the leg, while those who row or ride have them about the buttocks.

Symptoms: A red swelling forms round a hair, and causes a good deal of irritation and scratching. It gets larger for some days, being, as a rule, not very painful, unless subject to chafing. When, however, the boil begins on the head, in the ear, or in the nose, where the tissues will not stretch readily, the pain may be very great. Even after two or three days the swelling may slowly subside, and the inflammation gradually pass off, the boil being said to 'abort'. In most cases, however, about the sixth or seventh day the top of the boil breaks, and some thin fluid, and perhaps matter, oozes out. The yellowish core, consisting of a small mass of dead tissue, is now seen occupying the interior of the boil, and this comes away about a couple of days later, after which the boil speedily heals. If a boil is not treated, however, the first is apt to be followed by a crop of others in the neighbourhood, owing to the discharge from the first boil infecting other hairs. There is a special danger in boils of the upper lip and nose; for these may lead to inflammation within the head. Generally a boil, though its presence causes great annoyance, does not lead to fever or other general symptoms. But in boils of the ear, or about the face, there may be high temperature and great prostration, which are serious signs. Carbuncles are exhausting, and, in old people, very dangerous.

Treatment: At first the boil should be kept as still as possible, and to this end a piece of antiseptic sticking-plaster with a small hole cut in the centre, through which any discharge can pass, may be applied over the boil and kept in position for several days, when the boil often aborts. Another method to prevent boils coming to a head is to paint the boil and a small area of skin round it night and morning for several days with strong tincture of iodine (10 per cent). If, however, the boil is painful, or if it is proceeding to suppuration, hot fomentations should be applied, or magnesium sulphate paste. Magnesium sulphate paste is very effective, but must be freshly made. Carbuncles, painful boils and boils about the lip and nose may become very dangerous and should on no account be squeezed or fingered. As penicillin is so effective against staphylococcal infection, it has proved of value in the treatment of severe boils and carbuncles. General treatment in the form of good food, and avoidance of alcohol is also necessary. The taking of yeast is said to be of value. New boils are more effectively prevented from forming by rubbing powdered boric acid gently into the skin around the old boil twice a day after washing and drying. In recurrent cases a course of injections of a specially made vaccine or of toxoid may be of value.

BONE forms the framework upon which the rest of the body is built up. The bones are generally called the skeleton, though this term also includes the cartilages which join the ribs to the breast-bone, protect the larynx, etc.

Structure of bone: Bone is composed partly of fibrous tissue, partly of bone earth (phosphate and carbonate of lime), intimately mixed together. As the bones of a child are composed to the extent of about two-thirds of fibrous tissue, whilst those of the aged contain two-thirds of bone earth, one readily understands the toughness of the former and the brittleness of the latter. One speaks of *dense bone*, of which the shafts of the limb bones are composed, the bone being a hard tube surrounded by a membrane, the periosteum, and enclosing a fatty substance, the marrow; and of *cancellous bone*, which forms the short bones and the ends of long bones, in which a fine lace-work of bone fills up the whole interior, enclosing marrow in its meshes. The marrow (qv) of the smaller bones is of great importance. It is red in colour, and in it red blood corpuscles are formed. Even the densest bone is tunnelled by fine canals (Haversian canals) in which run small blood-vessels, nerves and lymphatics, for the maintenance and repair of the bone. Round these Haversian canals the bone is arranged in circular plates called lamellae, the lamellae being separated from one another by clefts, known as lacunae, in which single bone-cells are contained. Even the lamellae are pierced by fine tubes known as canaliculi lodging processes of these cells. Each lamella is composed of very fine interlacing fibres.

Growth of bones: Bones grow in thickness from the fibrous tissue and lime salts laid down by cells in their substance; while the long bones grow in length from a plate of cartilage (epiphyseal cartilage) which runs across the bone about 1·5 cm or more from its ends, and which on one surface is also constantly forming bone till the bone ceases to lengthen about the age of sixteen or eighteen. The existence of this cartilage is important to bear in mind, because in children an injury to it may lead to diminished growth of the limb.

Repair of bone is effected by cells of microscopic size: some called osteoblasts, elaborating the materials brought by the blood, and laying down strands of fibrous tissue, between which bone earth is later deposited; while other cells, known as osteoclasts, dissolve and break up dead or damaged bone. When a fracture has occurred, and the broken ends have been brought into contact, these are surrounded by a mass of blood at first; this is partly absorbed and partly organized by these cells, first into fibrous tissue and later into bone. The mass surrounding the fractured ends is called the callus, and for some months it forms a distinct thickening, which is gradually smoothed away, leaving the bone as before the fracture. If the ends have not been brought accurately in contact a permanent thickening results.

Varieties of bones: Apart from the structural varieties, bones fall into four classes: (*a*) long bones like those of the limbs; (*b*) short bones composed of cancellous tissue like those of the wrist and the ankle; (*c*) flat bones like those of the skull; (*d*) irregular bones like those of the face or the vertebrae of the spinal column (or backbone).

The skeleton consists of over 200 bones. It is divided into an AXIAL part, consisting of the skull, the vertebral column, the ribs with their cartilages, and the breast-bone; and an APPENDICULAR portion consisting of the four limbs. The hyoid bone in the neck, together with the cartilages protecting the larynx and windpipe, may be described as the VISCERAL skeleton.

AXIAL SKELETON: The *skull* consists of the cranium, which has eight bones, viz. occipital, two parietal, two temporal, one frontal, ethmoid, and sphenoid; and of the face, which has fourteen bones, viz. two maxillae or upper jaw-bones, one mandible or lower jaw-bone, two malar or cheek bones, two nasal, two lacrimal, two turbinal, two palate bones, and one vomer bone. (For further details, see SKULL.) The *vertebral column* consists of seven vertebrae in the cervical or neck region, twelve dorsal vertebrae, five vertebrae in the lumbar or loin region, the sacrum or sacral bone (a mass formed of five vertebrae fused together and forming the back part of the *pelvis*, which is closed at the sides by the haunch-bones), and finally the coccyx (four small vertebrae representing the tail of lower animals). The vertebral column has four curves: the first forwards in the neck, the second backwards in the dorsal region, the third forward in the loins, and the

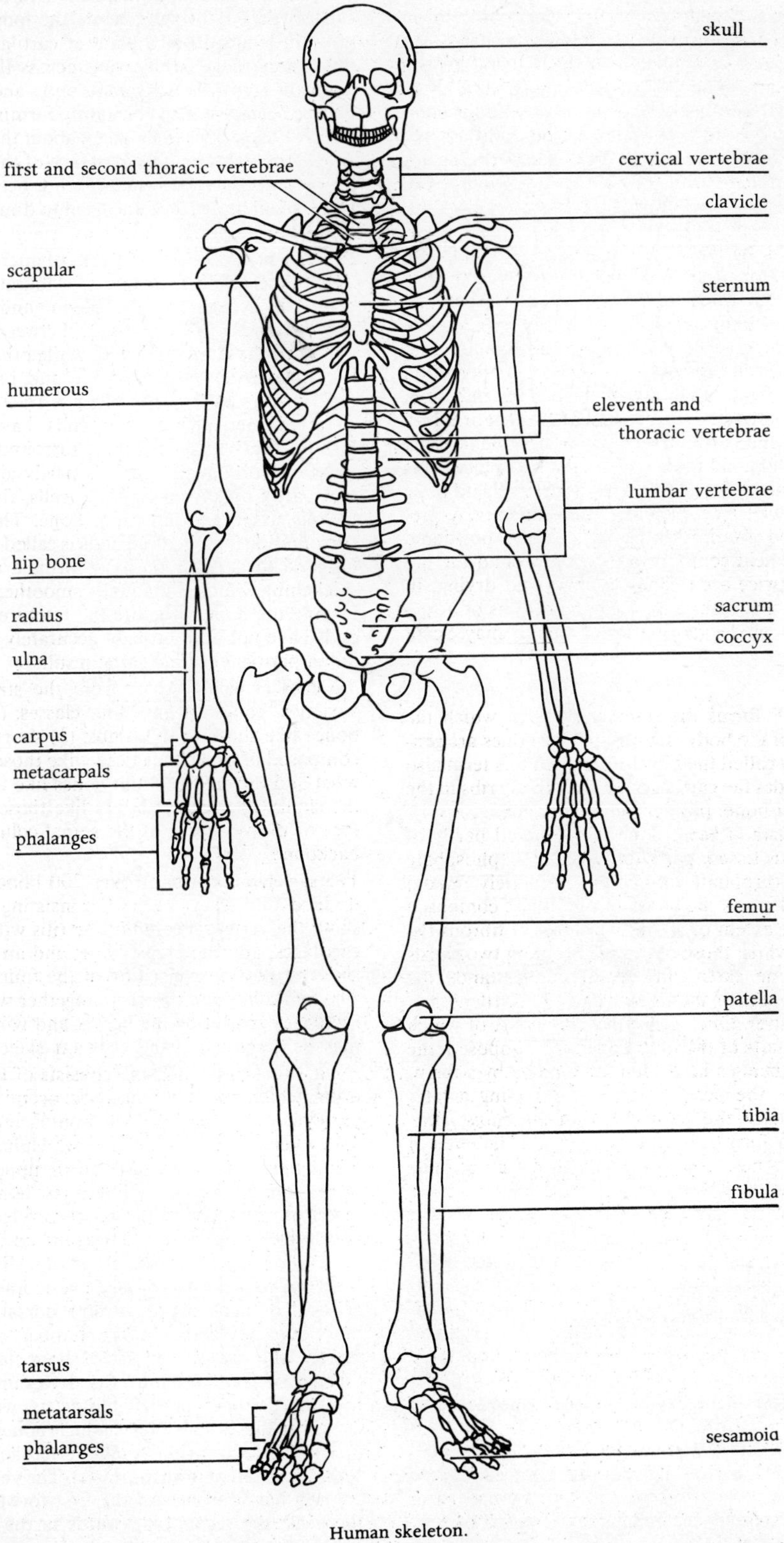
skull
first and second thoracic vertebrae
cervical vertebrae
clavicle
scapular
sternum
humerous
eleventh and
thoracic vertebrae
lumbar vertebrae
hip bone
radius
sacrum
coccyx
ulna
carpus
metacarpals
phalanges
femur
patella
tibia
fibula
tarsus
metatarsals
phalanges
sesamoid

Human skeleton.

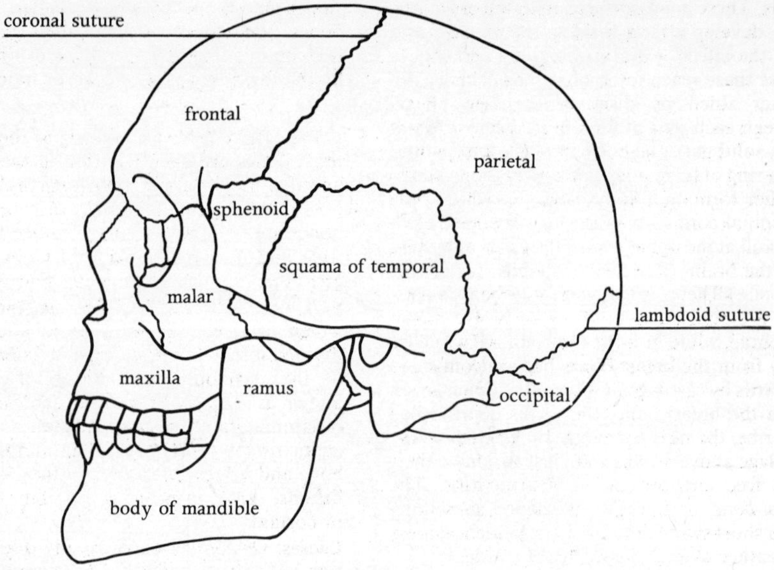

Side view of skull.

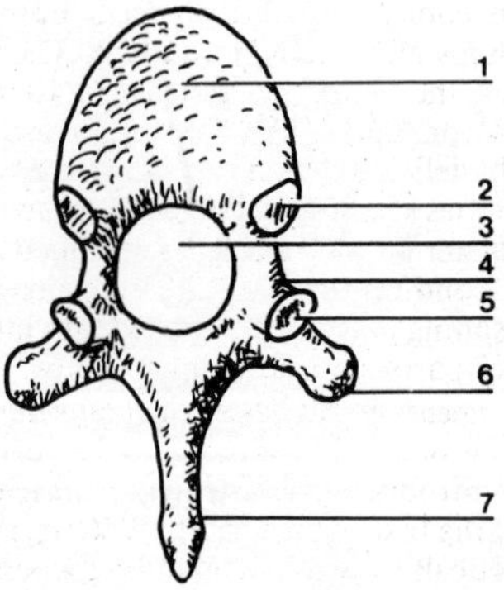

1 body of vertebrae
2 articulas process for the head of corresponding rib
3 neural ring
4 notches by which nerves emege
5 articular process for the vertebrae above
6 transverse process
7 spinous process

Human dorsal vertebra seen from above.

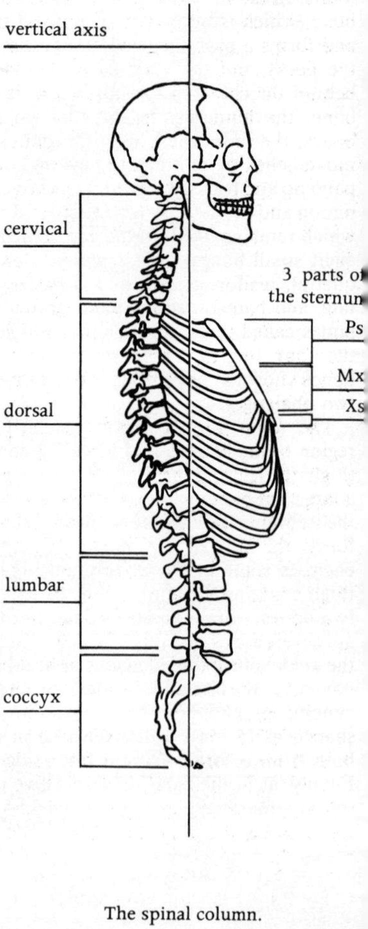

The spinal column.

lowest, involving the sacrum and coccyx, backwards. These are associated with the erect attitude, develop after a child learns to walk, and have the effect of diminishing jars and shocks before these reach internal organs. This is still further aided by discs of cartilage placed between each pair of vertebrae. Each vertebra has a solid part, the body in front, and behind this a ring of bone, the series of rings one above another forming a bony canal, up which runs the spinal cord to pass through an opening in the skull at the upper end of the canal and there join the brain. (For further details, see SPINAL COLUMN.) The *ribs*, twelve in number, on each side, are attached behind to the twelve dorsal vertebrae, while in front they end a few inches away from the breast-bone, but are continued forwards by cartilages. Of these the upper seven reach the breast-bone, these ribs being called true ribs, the next three are joined each to the cartilage above it, while the last two have their ends free and are called floating ribs. The *breast-bone*, or sternum, is shaped something like a short sword, about 15 cm (6 inches) long, and rather over 2·5 cm (1 inch) wide.

APPENDICULAR SKELETON: The *upper limb* consists of the shoulder region and three segments – the upper arm, the forearm, and the wrist with the hand, separated from each other by joints. In the shoulder lie the clavicle or collarbone (which is immediately beneath the skin, and forms a prominent object on the front of the neck), and the scapula or shoulder-blade behind the chest. In the upper arm is a single bone, the humerus. In the forearm are two bones, the radius and ulna; the radius, in the movements of alternately turning the hand palm up and back up (called, respectively, supination and pronation), rotating round the ulna, which remains fixed. In the carpus or wrist are eight small bones – the scaphoid, lunate, triquetral, pisiform, trapezium, trapezoid, capitate, and hamate. In the hand proper are five bones called metacarpals, upon which are set the four fingers, each containing the three bones known as phalanges, and the thumb with two phalanges.

The *lower limb* consists similarly of the region of the haunch and three segments – the thigh, the leg, and the foot. The haunch-bone is a large flat bone made up of three – the ilium, the ischium, and the pubis, fused together, and forms the side of the pelvis or basin which encloses some of the abdominal organs. The thigh contains the femur, and the leg contains two bones – the tibia and fibula. In the tarsus are seven bones: the talus (which forms part of the ankle joint), the calcaneus or heel-bone, the navicular, the lateral, intermediate, and medial cuneiforms, and the cuboid. These bones are so shaped as to form a distinct arch in the foot both from before back and from side to side. Finally, as in the hand, there are five metatarsals and fourteen phalanges, of which the great toe has two, the other toes three each.

Besides these named bones there are others sometimes found in sinews, called sesamoid bones, while the numbers of the regular bones may be increased by extra ribs or diminished by the fusion together of two or more bones.

BONE, DISEASES OF: Owing to the fact that most bones are deeply buried in the muscles, and that they contain in their earthy matter so much indifferent material, diseases in the bones are both apt to escape notice for a long time, and are actually much slower in their progress than similar diseases in other organs.

ACUTE INFLAMMATION is the disease which produces the most rapid effects. It is divided into acute *periostitis*, or inflammation of the enveloping membrane of the bone known as the periosteum (qv); acute *osteitis*, or inflammation of the bony substance itself; and acute *osteomyelitis*, or inflammation in the bone and its central cavity. Of these three conditions, osteomyelitis is by far the most important.

Causes: Osteomyelitis is usually due to infection with the *Staphylococcus aureus*. There is usually a history of a fall or a knock involving the affected limb. The disease is predominantly one of childhood.

Symptoms: In the slighter forms there is pain with tenderness to touch over a bone, which on examination is found swollen, but there are no general symptoms. In more serious cases severe pain comes on suddenly in a limb, one day perhaps after a slight accident. There is much fever, the temperature rising to 40° or 40·5°C (104° or 105°F), often with shivering, and at night delirium. After two or three days the limb becomes swollen, hot, and tender to touch, and still later the skin becomes inflamed and red. If the condition be not treated, general blood poisoning may result, or abscesses may form in other parts, and death may follow.

Treatment: As the *Staphylococcus aureus* is one of the organisms most sensitive to penicillin, the introduction of penicillin has revolutionized the treatment. Instead of being a condition practically always demanding operation and often causing prolonged invalidism, it can now be controlled by penicillin within a short space of time. The earlier treatment with penicillin is instituted, the better the results. Unless penicillin is given at an early stage, it may still be necessary to operate to remove any part of the bone that has been completely destroyed as a result of the infection. Such a dead portion of bone is known as a sequestrum (qv).

CHRONIC INFLAMMATION includes several quite distinct conditions; viz. abscess, necrosis, and exostosis, these conditions usually being due to injury, syphilis, or tuberculosis.

ABSCESS occurs generally in boys about the age of fourteen or fifteen, and the bone usually affected is one of those in the lower limb. The cause is either some local injury or local tuberculous disease.

Symptoms: There is a painful swelling on the bone, usually at the outer or inner side of the knee, and the temperature of the limb may be raised. The pain is generally worse at night and may prevent sleep. This may persist for months or years unless efficiently treated.

Treatment: The treatment is surgical, by having the abscess opened, and the administration of the appropriate antibiotic.

NECROSIS means death of a bone. As already stated, it generally follows acute bone inflammation. It also follows severe fractures, occurs from contact with phosphorus (see OCCUPATIONAL DISEASES), in syphilis, and occasionally at the end of some severe infectious disease like typhoid fever.

Symptoms: Usually in the course of suppuration a passage is burst to the exterior, and remains as a constantly discharging sinus. At the bottom of this lies the dead bone or sequestrum, and an operation must be performed for its removal. Usually about three to six months elapse after the original injury before it is loose and ready for removal. If it be not removed the sinus continues to discharge and amyloidosis (qv) of various internal organs may develop.

EXOSTOSIS is an outgrowth upon a bone, which may be produced by long-continued irritation: eg. the bony growths on the inner side of the knee of those who ride much; or may be a symptom of syphilis; or may be of the nature of a tumour. It may also occur spontaneously.

SYPHILITIC DISEASE of bone in the secondary stage of this disease takes the form of nodes or swellings due to localized inflammation of the periosteal membrane, and in the tertiary stage there are often areas of great hardening with necrosis of pieces of bone.

TUBERCULOUS DISEASE in bone as a rule occurs in young people, but it is also found now and then in a person well up in years (senile tuberculosis). It may occur (*a*) in the bones of the hand or foot, in which case several may be affected; (*b*) in the ends of the long bones, when it is very apt to lead to disease of the neighbouring joint; (*c*) in the vertebrae, where it often results in curvature of the spine, or produces a chronic abscess. (See ABSCESS, CHRONIC.) Caries is the name given to a crumbling condition of the bone produced by this or any other disease.

Symptoms: Generally the health is not first-rate and there may be a history of tuberculosis in other organs. There is generally pain, tenderness, and swelling of the affected part. The whole limb, when a toe or finger is affected, may feel hot. Later the skin may get red and thin and a chronic abscess form and burst, leaving a sinus. Or the condition may heal, leaving the bone only a little thickened. The progress is in any case slow, lasting many weeks or months.

Treatment: The administration of anti-tuberculous drugs is all-important. Rest to the part affected, general exercise of the body in the fresh air, and good food are necessary. When the skin threatens to break, this should be anticipated by an operation, in which the diseased bone, etc., is all scraped away, or even amputation may be advisable in very bad cases. (See further under JOINTS, DISEASES OF.)

TUMOURS: CHONDROMA, a small tumour of cartilage and bone, grows sometimes under the nail of a finger or toe, and causes a good deal of pain and annoyance. It is easily removed, generally by splitting the nail, and does not return. CANCER rarely if ever begins in a bone, though secondary cancers commonly develop inside bones; for example cancer of the breast may be followed by secondary cancer in the bone of the arm or elsewhere. SARCOMA is a tumour sometimes found, especially in the larger bones, causing the bone to break readily, or dilating it to a great size; amputation is necessary for its removal.

RICKETS is a disease of childhood in which the bones do not harden as they ought to do. (See RICKETS.)

ACROMEGALY is a disease in which the bones enlarge in size. (See ACROMEGALY.)

OSTEITIS is a general term applied to inflammatory conditions of bone. It includes *osteitis deformans* (qv), in which the long bones become curved and the skull thickened; also *osteitis fibrosa cystica generalisata* (qv), in which bones become weakened as a result of the presence of cysts.

OSTEOMALACIA is a disease characterized by a gradual loss of lime salts in the bones, so that these become soft and lose their proper form. It is due to lack of vitamin D and of calcium in the diet. (See OSTEOMALACIA.)

OSTEOPOROSIS is a condition characterized by lack of bone quantity, the quality of the remaining bone being normal. (See OSTEOPOROSIS.)

OSTEOGENESIS IMPERFECTA is a hereditary disease of bone, characterized by extreme fragility of the skeleton. (See OSTEOGENESIS IMPERFECTA.)

FIBROUS DYSPLASIA is a rare disease in which areas of bone are replaced by fibrous tissue. (See FIBROUS DYSPLASIA; FIBROUS TISSUE.)

BORAX, or BIBORATE OF SODA, acts in much the same ways as boric acid, but without its acid reaction.

Uses: Its chief use is in the form of a lotion (about 1 part to 30 of water) in all forms of itching and chapping of the skin. In thrush (qv) and other forms of irritation about the mouth in children the honey of borax, smeared on several times a day, is very soothing. To clean the mouth as well as soothe it, borax in honey wiped over the gums and tongue is very efficient. As in the case of boric acid, it should not be used in infants and young children.

BORBORYGMUS means flatulence in the bowels.

BORIC ACID, or BORACIC ACID, is found in volcanic districts, or is prepared from borax. It is a mild antiseptic.
Uses: It is used for dressing wounds, either dusted on as powder or in a lotion (1 part in 30). This lotion, mixed with an equal quantity of warm water, makes a useful eyewash for painful and inflamed eyes. Lint is sold ready soaked in boric lotion, dried, and generally dyed pink; it requires only to be dipped in water and applied. Offensive perspiration of the feet is checked by dipping the stockings in boric lotion and drying them before wearing. Because of the risk of toxic effects it should not be used in the case of infants and young children.

BORNHOLM DISEASE, also known as devil's grip, and epidemic myalgia, is an acute infective disease due to Coxsackie viruses (qv), and characterized by the abrupt onset of pain around the lower margin of the ribs, headache, and fever. It occurs in epidemics, usually during warm weather, and it is more common in young people than the old. The illness usually lasts seven to ten days. It is practically never fatal. The disease is named after the island of Bornholm in the Baltic, where several epidemics have been described.

BOROGLYCERIN is a clear unctuous antiseptic, made by dissolving boric acid crystals in glycerin while hot.

BOTULISM is a rare type of food-poisoning caused by the toxin arising from the presence in improperly preserved foods of the *Clostridium botulinum*. The first symptoms come on a few hours after the food has been taken and consist of vomiting, abdominal pain, and difficulty of vision. Later, nervous symptoms consisting of double vision, drooping of the eyelids, weakness of the facial muscles, dilatation of the pupils, and difficulty in swallowing and breathing appear. The prognosis is extremely grave, the mortality rate being higher than 50 per cent. Fortunately, the condition is rare in Britain. There have only been 21 cases this century in seven different incidents, with 12 deaths. Since the outbreak at Loch Maree in 1922, when eight fishermen died of the disease after eating sandwiches containing duck paste, sixteen cases have occurred in the United Kingdom, with two deaths: one from the 1949 incident, and one from the 1978 incident.

Year	*No. of cases*	*Causes*
1922	8	Duck paste (Loch Maree)
1932	2	Rabbit and pigeon broth
1934	1	Jugged hare
1935	2	Vegetarian nut brawn
	1	Home-made pie
1949	5	Macaroni cheese
1955	1	Pickled fish from Mauritius
1978	4	Tinned Salmon

Recorded incidents of botulism in the United Kingdom since 1922.

During this period several outbreaks of botulism have been reported in Britain, especially in water fowl, broiler chickens, ferrets and mink. Very occasionally it may occur as a result of contamination of a wound by *Clostridium botulinum*. Recently cases have been reported in USA, and one in Britain, of botulism in infants due to the spontaneous formation of botulinum toxin in the infant's gut.
Treatment: An antitoxic serum is available, and this should be given, along with full doses of antibiotics. Because of the nervous signs, such as difficulty in swallowing, skilled nursing is essential.

BOUGIES are solid instruments for introduction into natural passages in the body either in order to apply medicaments which they contain or with which they are coated, or, more usually, in order to dilate a narrow part or stricture of the passage. Thus we have, for example, urethral bougies, oesophageal bougies, rectal bougies, made usually of flexible rubber or, in the case of the urethra, of steel.

BOUILLON is a broth or soup prepared from meat. It is much used in various food preparations and also as a medium for cultivating organisms in bacteriological laboratories.

BOWELS (see INTESTINE).

BOWEN'S DISEASE: This is a form of carcinoma *in situ* in the skin. It presents as an isolated scaling plaque. Round papules appear on the chest and back. It is due to abnormal keratin in the hair follicles and is a genetically determined disease.

BOW LEGS, or GENU VARUM, may be due to an abnormal posture of the limbs in the womb before birth. It often corrects itself, but in more severe or persistent cases, correction may be necessary by means of manipulation, the wearing of a plaster cast, or operation. In the first few years of life, however, a certain amount of bowing of the legs, associated with a tendency to pigeon-toe, may be quite normal and corrects itself as the child grows older. In older children it may be due to bone diseases, such as rickets (qv). Correction of the deformity may be assisted by the wearing of strong shoes with arch support and an outer sole wedge.

BOXING INJURIES rank eighth in frequency among sports injuries. A recent survey of causes of head injuries requiring admission to hospital in Scotland showed golf ranking well ahead of boxing.

According to the 'Report on the Medical Aspects of Boxing' issued by the Committee on Boxing of the Royal College of Physicians of London in October 1969, of 224 ex-professional boxers examined, 37 showed evidence of brain damage which was disabling in thirteen. Commenting on this, the report says: 'This prevalence rate of 17 per cent indicates that one in six of the boxers studied showed evidence of some damage to their nervous systems attributable to boxing but probably only a third of these were affected severely enough to be recognized as "punch drunk"'. The report also notes that 'the Committee has had discussions with members, including medical officers, of the British Boxing Board of Control and appreciate that professional boxing under their auspices is, today, closely and carefully controlled. It is therefore difficult to draw conclusions about the risk of brain damage in professional boxing today'.

In 1984 a report of a working party of the British Medical Association was published. It concludes that there are two main ways in which boxing may lead to structural damage to the brain. The first type of damage occurs as an acute episode in which one or more severe blows leads to loss of consciousness and occasionally to death. Death in the acute phase is usually due to intracranial haemorrhage and this carries a mortality of 45 per cent even with the sophisticated surgical techniques currently available. The second type of damage develops over a much longer period and is cumulative, leading to the atrophy of the cerebral cortex and brain stem. The repair processes of the brain are very limited and even after mild concussion it may suffer a small amount of permanent structural damage. Brain scanning techniques now enable brain damage to be detected during life. Brain damage of the type previously associated with the punch-drunk syndrome is now being detected before obvious clinical signs have developed. Evidence of cerebral atrophy has been found in relatively young boxers including amateurs and those whose careers have been considered successful. The tragedy is that brain damage can only be detected after it has occurred. This report is likely to add momentum to the resolution of the British Medical Association in 1982 "That in view of the proven ocular and brain damage resulting from professional boxing the Association should campaign for its abolition". A leading article in the Journal of the American Medical Association in 1986 argues that professional boxing, already banned in Norway and Sweden, will be illegal in most countries by the end of the century.

BRACHIAL means 'belonging to the upper arm'. There are, for example, a brachial artery, and a brachial plexus of nerves through which run all the nerves to the arm. The brachial plexus lies along the outer side of the armpit, and is liable to be damaged in dislocation at the shoulder.

BRACHYCEPHALIC means short-headed and is a term applied to skulls the breadth of which is at least four-fifths of the length. BRACHYCEPHALY is a characteristic of the Alpine race.

BRACHYDACTYLY is a term applied to the conditions in which the fingers or toes are abnormally short.

BRADYCARDIA means slowness of the beating of the heart with corresponding slowness of the pulse (below 60 per minute). (See HEART DISEASES.)

BRADYKINESIA is a term used to describe the condition in which the movements of the body and limbs are abnormally slow.

BRADYKININ is a substance derived from plasma proteins, which plays an important role in many of the reactions of the body, including inflammation (qv). Its prime action is in producing dilatation of arteries and veins. It has also been described as 'the most powerful pain-producing agent known'.

BRAIDISM, after James Braid, who introduced it into medicine, is another name for hypnotism. (See HYPNOTISM.)

BRAIN: The brain and spinal cord together form the central nervous sytem, the twelve nerves passing on each side from the brain, and the thirty-one from the cord being called the peripheral nervous system, while the complex chains of nerves and ganglia lying within the chest and abdomen, and acting to a large extent independently of the other two systems, though closely connected with them, make up the autonomic system, and govern the activity of the viscera.

Divisions: The brain in its simplest form in lowly vertebrate animals is a thickened part at the front end of the spinal cord, developed in order to govern the organs of special sense, viz. smell, sight, hearing, and taste, lodged near at hand. Higher in the scale, in fishes for example, there are marked bulgings of nervous matter forming the fore-brain, the mid-brain, and the hind-brain, and that part connected with the nerves of the eyes appears to be the highest governing part. In man, however, the part in front of this is specially developed, and not only forms the great bulk of the entire brain, but governs the activities of the rest. This part is called the cerebrum.

The CEREBRUM forms the great bulk of the brain in amount and consists of two cerebral hemispheres which occupy the entire vault of the cranium and are incompletely separated from one another by a deep median cleft, the longitudinal cerebral fissure. At the bottom of this cleft the two hemispheres are united by a thick band of some 200 million transverse nerve fibres: the corpus callosum. Other clefts or fissures, or sulci as they are known, make deep impressions, dividing the cerebrum into lobes. Of these the chief are the lateral sulcus and the central sulcus. The lobes of the cerebrum are the frontal lobe in the forehead region, the parietal lobe on the side and upper part of the brain, the occipital lobe to the back, and the temporal lobe lying just above the region of the ear.

Numbers of shallower infoldings of the surface called furrows or sulci separate raised areas called convolutions or gyri. The outer 3 mm or thereabouts of the cerebral hemispheres consists of grey matter largely made up of ganglion cells, while in the deeper part the white matter consists of medullated nerve fibres connecting different parts of the surface and passing down to the lower parts of the brain. Among the white matter lie several rounded masses of grey matter, the lentiform and caudate nuclei. In the centre of each cerebral hemisphere is an irregular cavity, the lateral ventricle, each of which communicates with that on the other side and behind with the 3rd ventricle through a small opening, the interventricular foramen, or foramen of Monro.

The BASAL NUCLEI consist of two large masses of grey matter imbedded in the base of the cerebral hemispheres in man, but forming the chief part of the brain in many animals. Between these masses lies the 3rd ventricle, from which the infundibulum, a funnel-shaped process, projects downwards into the pituitary body, and above lies the pineal gland. This region includes the important *hypothalamus*.

The MID-BRAIN, or *mesencephalon*, is a stalk about 20 mm long connecting the cerebrum with the hind-brain. Down its centre lies a tube, the cerebral aqueduct, or aqueduct of Sylvius, connecting the 3rd and 4th ventricles. Above this aqueduct lie the corpora quadrigemina, and beneath it are the crura cerebri, strong bands of white matter in which important nerve fibres pass downwards from the cerebrum.

The PONS is a mass of nerve fibres, some of which run crosswise and others are the continuation of the crura cerebri downwards.

The CEREBELLUM lies towards the back, underneath the occipital lobes of the cerebrum.

The MEDULLA OBLONGATA is the lowest part of the brain, in structure resembling the spinal cord, with white matter on the surface and grey matter in its interior. This is continuous through the large opening in the skull, the foramen magnum, with the spinal cord. Between the medulla, pons, and cerebellum lies the 4th ventricle of the brain.

Structure: The brain is made up of grey and white matter. In the cerebrum and cerebellum the grey matter is arranged mainly in a layer on the surface, though both have certain grey masses imbedded in the white matter. In the other parts the grey matter is found in definite masses called nuclei, from which the nerves spring. The grey matter consists mainly of cells in which all the activities of the brain begin. These cells vary considerably in size and shape in different parts of the brain, though all give

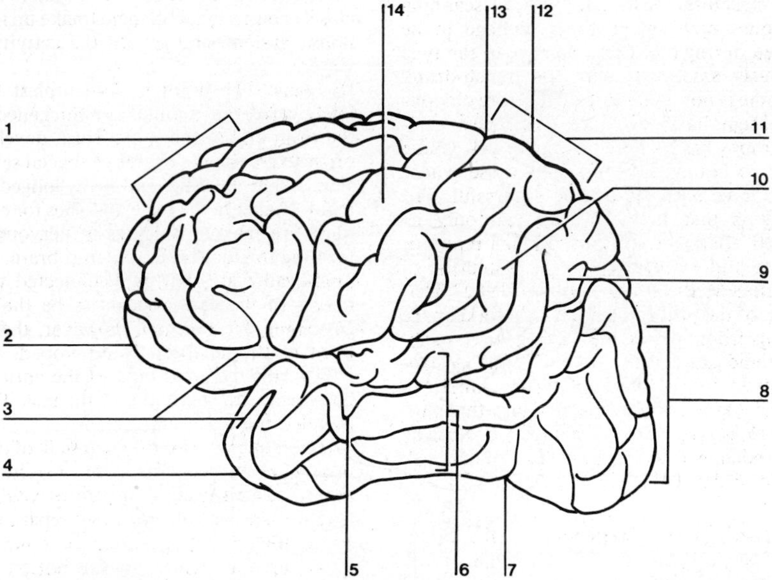

1 frontal lobe
2 frontal pole
3 lateral (sylvian) sulcus
4 temporal pole
5 superior temporal sulcus
6 temporal lobe
7 preoccipital notch
8 occipital lobe
9 angular gyrus
10 supramarginal gyrus
11 parietal lobe
12 postcentral gyrus
13 central sulcus
14 precentral gyrus

Side view of the brain.

off a number of processes, some of which form nerve fibres. The cells on the surface of the cerebral hemispheres, for example, are very numerous, being set in layers five or six deep. In shape these cells are pyramidal, giving off processes from the apex, from the centre of the base, and from various projections elsewhere on the cell. The grey matter is everywhere penetrated by a rich supply of blood-vessels, and the nerve cells and blood-vessels are supported in a fine network of fibres, known as neuroglia. The white matter consists of nerve fibres, each of which is attached, at one end, to a cell in the grey matter, while, at the other end, it splits up into a tree-like structure round another cell in another part of the grey matter in the brain or spinal cord. The fibres have insulating sheaths of a fatty material, which, in the mass, gives the white matter its colour, and they convey messages from one part of the brain to the other (association fibres), or, grouped into bundles, leave the brain as nerves, or pass down into the spinal cord, where they end near, and exert a control upon, cells from which in turn spring the nerves to the body. Both grey and white matter are bound together by a felt-work called neuroglia. The general arrangement of fibres can be best understood by describing the course of a motor nerve fibre. Arising in a cell on the surface in front of the central sulcus, such a fibre passes inwards towards the centre of the cerebral hemisphere, the collected mass of fibres as they lie between the lentiform nucleus and optic thalamus being known as the internal capsule. Hence the fibre passes down through the crus cerebri, giving off various small connecting fibres as it passes downwards. After passing through the pons it reaches the medulla, and at this point crosses to the opposite side (decussation of the pyramids). Entering the spinal cord, it passes downwards to end finally in a series of branches (arborization) which meet and touch (synapse) similar branches from one or more of the cells in the grey matter of the cord (see SPINAL CORD).

Size: The weight of the average male brain is 1·4 kg, ranging from 1·24 to 1·68 kg, of the female brain 1·25 kg, ranging from 1·13 to 1·51 kg, but brains have been found as heavy as 1·8 kg, or, in exceptional cases, even more. The maximum mass of brain tissue is reached at the age of 20, and then decreases steadily.

Functions: The cerebrum is associated with the intellectual faculties in man, and also exerts a guiding influence over the rest of the nervous system. It is not, however, necessary to actual life. If the cerebrum of a frog is destroyed it still breathes and its heart beats, it can hop if pinched, and swim if put in water, but when left alone it sits still till it perishes. If the same happens to a pigeon it can fly when thrown in the air, and can alight, but it does not fly away when threatened, nor will it take food, having lost even the instinct to preserve life. If, on the

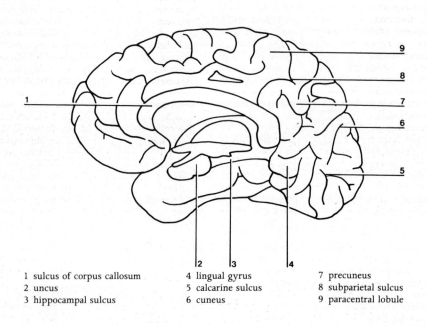

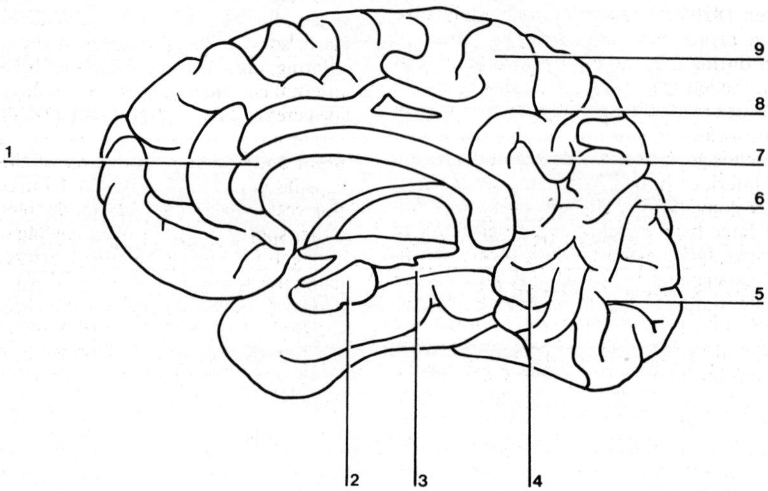

1 sulcus of corpus callosum
2 uncus
3 hippocampal sulcus
4 lingual gyrus
5 calcarine sulcus
6 cuneus
7 precuneus
8 subparietal sulcus
9 paracentral lobule

Vertical section through the middle of the brain.

other hand, the cerebellum of a pigeon is destroyed, the bird cannot maintain its balance, the cerebellum being concerned in the regulation of muscular movements and in preserving the equilibrium of the body.

Plato recognized three mental faculties, which he placed, respectively, in the liver, heart, and brain, these organs being supposed to secrete the 'animal spirits' appropriate to each faculty; and this view was accepted by the medical writers of antiquity. In the Middle Ages the Arabian physicians, however, following Galen's opinion, placed the different mental faculties in the several ventricles of the brain, this theory being adopted by Duns Scotus, Thomas of Aquino, and referred to by Burton in his *Anatomy of Melancholy*.

Descartes (1596–1650) had the fanciful idea that the pineal body was the seat of the mind. After his time it was thought that the whole brain must act together in every process, from the fact that, in cases of severe injury to the head, much substance can be lost from some parts of the brain without impairment of any one definite function or memory.

But it is now known that definite areas of the surface are associated with definite functions. The earliest systematic attempt to localize the functions of the brain to certain areas was made by Gall and Spurzheim, who founded the system of phrenology in the first quarter of the nineteenth century. Although this system was proved to be wrong both as regards the functions of the brain and the philosophic analysis of mental processes, the criticism it called forth gave a great impetus to the attempt to localize the functions of the brain in definite spots. Between 1820 and 1840 it became established that, in people who have lost the power of speech during life, the brain shows some disease in the left frontal lobe after death, and in 1861 Broca made the first definite discovery in cerebral localization by proving that the faculty of speech is governed by a centre in the region of the inferior frontal gyrus, named (after him) Broca's convolution. His discovery was followed later by the important observation of Hughlings Jackson that certain forms of epilepsy, associated with movements beginning in a definite limb, are caused by disease affecting the part of the brain that borders on the central sulcus, and this discovery was confirmed and extended by many experimenters and physicians. Fritsch, Hitzig, Ferrier, Sherrington, Grünbaum and others have shown that definite areas near the central sulcus are associated with the movement of definite parts. Further, the occipital lobes are associated with the sense of sight, the temporal lobe with hearing, and the inner surface of the same lobe with taste and smell. The purely intellectual faculties are probably associated with the frontal lobes, which seem to govern nothing else. The cerebellum has to do with the powers of balancing and of regulating movements. The medulla and pons have important functions, governing many of the processes most essential to life, eg. those of respiration, rate of the heart, swallowing, vomiting, and giving off all the nerves which arise from the brain, except the first four.

Membranes: The brain is separated from the skull by three membranes: the dura mater, a thick fibrous membrane; the arachnoid mater, a more delicate structure; and the pia mater, adhering to the surface of the brain, and containing the blood-vessels which nourish it. Between each pair is a space containing fluid on which the brain floats as on a water-bed. The fluid beneath the arachnoid membrane mixes with that inside the ventricles through a small opening in the 4th ventricle, called the median aperture, or foramen of Magendie.

These fluid arrangements have a great influence in preserving the brain from injury.

Nerves: Twelve nerves come off the brain:

I	Olfactory, to the nose (smell).
II	Optic, to the eye (sight).
III.	Oculomotor
IV.	Trochlear } to eye-muscles.
VI.	Abducent
V.	Trigeminal, to skin of face.
VII.	Facial, to muscles of face.
VIII.	Vestibulocochlear, to hear (hearing and balancing).
IX.	Glossopharyngeal, to tongue (taste).
X.	Vagus, to heart, larynx, lungs, and stomach.
XI.	Spinal accessory, to muscles in neck.
XII.	Hypoglossal, to muscles of tongue.

Blood-vessels: Four vessels carry blood to the brain: two internal carotid arteries in front, and two vertebral arteries behind. These communicate to form a circle (circle of Willis) inside the skull, so that if one is blocked the others, by dilating, take its place. The chief branch of the internal carotid artery on each side is the middle cerebral, and this gives off a small but very important branch which pierces the base of the brain and supplies the region of the internal capsule with blood. The chief importance of this vessel lies in the fact that the blood in it is under specially high pressure, owing to its close connection with the carotid artery, so that haemorrhage from it is liable to occur and thus give rise to apoplexy. Two veins, the internal cerebral veins, bring the blood away from the interior of the brain, but most of the small veins come to the surface and open into large venous sinuses, which run in grooves in the skull, and finally pour their blood into the internal jugular vein that accompanies the carotid artery on each side of the neck.

BRAIN, DISEASES AND INJURIES OF: The signs of brain disease are in general indirect, being manifested by some defect in sensation or in the power of action, or by some peculiarity of conduct. The symptoms are more fully discussed under NERVOUS DISEASES. (See also APHASIA; APOPLEXY; ENCEPHALITIS; EPILEPSY;

HEADACHE; HYDROCEPHALUS; MENINGITIS; MENTAL ILLNESS; PARALYSIS.) The following are some of the conditions more exclusively connected with the brain.

ABSCESS is a very serious condition. It results from wounds of the scalp which suppurate and in which the inflammatory matter does not get free exit, or from suppurating ear disease, in which the discharge from the ear has been stopped. The symptoms are rather vague, but sooner or later there are severe headache and vomiting, with rise of temperature, and often some interference with vision. When the abscess lies in the temporal lobe the temperature is often below normal. The treatment should be prevention, by keeping every scalp wound clean, and by having every case of discharging ear disease under medical supervision (see EAR, DISEASES OF). When it is recognized that an abscess has occurred in the brain, it is customary to trephine the skull and evacuate the abscess, after which recovery often takes place.

ANAEMIA OF THE BRAIN is the cause of fainting when suddenly brought on by weakness of the heart's action. Anaemia of a more chronic type is a cause of sleeplessness in elderly persons, accompanied by weakness of mental power and drowsiness during working hours. It also causes headache, giddiness, and ringing in the ears.

COMPRESSION OF THE BRAIN may be caused by the growth of a tumour in the brain, a collection of blood between the brain and skull from injury of the membranes, or suppuration in the same locality from a neglected scalp wound or fracture of the skull. Unconsciousness coming on some hours after a blow on the side of the head is generally due to a fracture tearing one of the arteries in the membranes and producing a large clot between the skull and brain. The symptoms are vague, but, in addition to unconsciousness, there are generally difficulty of breathing, feeble pulse, and paralysis down one side of the body. The treatment is trephining of the skull (see TREPHINING).

CONCUSSION is a bruising of part of the brain as the result of a blow on the head (generally at the back) or a severe shake of the body. Cases vary in severity from mere giddiness and headache for an hour or two, to complete loss of consciousness lasting for weeks, and include those curious instances of lost memory for facts or even for personal identity which have been much used by novelists. The person lies unconscious and can be roused with difficulty. If he answers questions at all he does so irrelevantly, and shows great irritability of temper, going off to sleep again at once. He lies turned away from the light, with his knees drawn up on the body. Consciousness and convalescence come on very gradually, and for months there may be loss of memory, bad temper, and great susceptibility to the effects of alcohol. Recovery is generally good, but a tendency to epilepsy may remain. The treatment is complete rest in a darkened room, with careful nursing to ensure that no complications develop in the lungs and to prevent the development of bed sores. The urine may need to be drawn off. Once consciousness is regained, there should be a prolonged period of rest in order to prevent persisting or recurring headaches. Even the mildest form of concussion should be followed by a few days' rest. Otherwise there is a tendency to a persisting troublesome headache.

BRAIN FEVER is a popular name for several conditions. One is a state of prostration following some severe mental strain. This is not very serious and passes off in the course of a few weeks of rest. Another condition known under this name is encephalitis lethargica, also known popularly as 'sleepy sickness', in which inflammatory changes accompanied by oedema and haemorrhages take place in parts of the brain, causing a serious and often fatal disorder. (See ENCEPHALITIS LETHARGICA.) Another condition often called by this name is inflammation of the membranes of the brain, or meningitis, which occurs most commonly in children and which may be a dangerous disease (see MENINGITIS).

HAEMORRHAGE into the brain causes apoplexy. (See APOPLEXY.)

LACERATION of the brain may occur in fracture of the skull. When the injury affects the upper part of the cerebrum, it is not of so great importance as the fact of whether the wound is kept clean and free from suppuration, although near the central sulcus damage to the brain may result in paralysis of a limb. When it occurs at the base of the skull serious injury of the brain is apt to result, often ending in death (see FRACTURES).

SOFTENING of the brain is a term used in a strictly scientific sense and in a popular sense. In the former case an actual area of brain tissue softens owing to its blood supply being cut off by plugging of its blood-vessels, or in consequence of some long-standing inflammatory process. The symptoms are then those of apoplexy, though not so sudden as if the cause were haemorrhage. In the popular sense, when people, who have been the subjects of gout, alcoholism, or syphilis, especially elderly people, become gradually dull in intellect, drowsy, absent-minded, emotional, and finally demented, because of their diseased blood-vessels diminishing the blood supply to, and causing deterioration of, the brain, these symptoms are also attributed to 'softening of the brain'.

TUMOURS of the brain produce very insidious and very complex symptoms, depending on the region they affect. Among the general symptoms are headache, giddiness, vomiting independent of food, and tenderness of the head on pressure. Blindness and mental symptoms come on later, owing to rise of pressure inside the skull. Sometimes these tumours are tuberculous or syphilitic in origin, when the general treatment for these diseases is of help. Occasionally a tumour produces definite 'localizing' symptoms indicating its position in the brain. In such cases an operation may be performed for the complete and successful removal of the tumour, or it may be treated with radio-isotopes (see ISOTOPES). As a result of advances in neurosurgery and in nuclear medicine, it is becoming possible to deal successfully with an increasing number of tumours of the brain.

People who have had brain injuries, and their relatives, can obtain help and advice from the National Head Injuries Association, known as Headway, 200 Mansfield Road, Nottingham NG1 3HX (0602-622383).

BRAIN DEATH (see DEATH, SIGNS OF).

BRAN is the meal derived from the outer covering of a cereal grain. It contains little or no carbohydrate, and is mainly used to provide roughage (qv) in the control of bowel function and the prevention of constipation.

BRANDY (see ALCOHOL).

BREAD is one of the cheapest of foods. It is also highly digestible and absorbable, and contains a reasonable amount of protein. In Britain it is made almost exclusively from wheat flour. The wheat germ is made up of bran (13 per cent), inner endosperm (83 per cent), outer endosperm (2 per cent), germ (1 per cent), and scutellum (1 per cent), and each 100 grams contains 9 grams of protein, 2·5 grams of fat, 70 grams of carbohydrate, 36 mg of calcium, 3 mg of iron, and 295 micrograms of thiamine (vitamin B_1). These are approximate figures as the precise amounts vary depending upon the type of wheat used. Unfortunately, the flour made from the wheat grain is too indigestible for most human beings. This 100 per cent wholemeal flour is therefore refined by modern milling processes, in the course of which much of the roughage is removed. In low-extraction flour the bran, germ, scutellum and outer layer of endosperm are all removed. The disadvantage of this from the nutritional point of view is that it involves the loss of much of the bran, iron, calcium and vitamin content of the flour. This loss is relatively slight with 85 per cent extraction, as at this level the germ and scutellum are still retained, and therefore most of the thiamine and iron.

The controversy still rages between the protagonists of high-extraction and those of low-extraction flour. Nutritionally there is no doubt as to the superiority of the former, particularly so far as the vitamin B content is concerned. Some of the other apparent nutritional advantages are counterbalanced by the fact that high-extraction flour is less digestible than 70 per cent extraction flour – which is the normal level of commercial milling. Much of the edge has been taken out of the controversy by the Government regulation, whereby all flour intended for human consumption must be so reinforced that it shall contain not less than 1·65 mg of iron, 0·24 mg of thiamine, and 1·6 mg of nicotinic acid or nicotinamade (one of the vitamin B constituents) per 100 grams, and, except in the case of flour containing the whole of the products derived from the milling of bread, 235 to 390 mg of powdered chalk per 100 grams.

The making of bread, with its spongy texture, from flour is due to the latter containing gluten, the mixture of proteins that constitutes the nitrogenous content of flour. Gluten produces the dough which when blown up by the carbon dioxide released as a result of the fermentation of yeast, remains in the form of a sponge. It is because of this high content of gluten that wheat makes much better bread than other cereals. Rye comes next to wheat as a bread-making grain, but its low content of gluten makes the bread moist and dense, and those not used to it find it rather sour. A typical example of rye bread is the black bread so popular in parts of Europe. Maize contains no gluten and therefore maize meal cannot be used alone to make bread. It can, however, be baked into cakes, and outside Britain is often mixed with wheat flour to make bread. Barley, too, contains little gluten and therefore produces a heavy dough. Mixed with wheat flour, however, it produces a quite acceptable bread. The same applies to oatmeal.

The average nutritional value of the bread made from the current reinforced 70 per cent wheat flour per 100 grams is 8 grams per cent protein, 1·5 grams per cent fat, 53 grams per cent available carbohydrate, 90 mg per cent calcium, 1·8 mg per cent iron, giving a calorie value of 240. When bread is toasted, water is driven off and the calorie value therefore rises – to around 300 Calories per 100 grams. The

	Thiamine	*Nicotinic acid*	*Pantothenic acid*	*Riboflavin*	*Pyridoxine*
	mg	mg	mg	mg	mg
Whole wheat flour	0·40	5·0	1·5	0·16	0·40
Percentage of vitamin remaining					
Extraction rate per cent					
85	89	39	76	52	44
80	63	32	58	47	27
70	20	23	49	33	16

The vitamin content per 100 grams of whole wheat flour and the percentage retained in flour of different extraction rates.

increased digestibility of toast is due to the fact that it is chewed more effectively than bread. Conversely the traditional indigestibility of new bread is due to its moisture making it difficult to chew, and it is therefore swallowed before it has soaked up much saliva.

BREAK-BONE FEVER is another name for dengue (qv).

BREASTS, or MAMMARY GLANDS, are found in the most highly developed class of animals, called the Mammalia, for the purpose of suckling the young. As a rule they are confined to the female sex, though the male has rudimentary nipples, and, even in man, individuals occur in the male sex who have well-developed glands and have been known to produce milk. These glands are developed in the front of the chest, and, in the full-grown female, extend from the second to the sixth or seventh rib, being at the centre about 5 cm (2 inches) thick. There is usually one on each side, but small supplementary breasts are occasionally found in the armpit or low down on the abdomen. In the centre is a dark patch, called the areola, which surrounds the nipple. This areola darkens during pregnancy. This, together with enlargement of the whole breast and dilatation of its veins, forms an important and early sign of this condition. In structure each breast consists of from twelve to twenty compartments, each of which contains a system of branching tubes lined by cells that form the fatty and fluid materials composing the milk. In each section the tubes open on the surface of the nipple by a single small tube, or duct, of which therefore there are twelve to twenty in all. Between these gland tubes lie muscle fibres (which give the breasts their firmness), fibrous tissue, and fat (which is specially plentiful in elderly women).

BREASTS, DISEASES OF: These glands go through great changes during the course of life, becoming considerably enlarged about the age of puberty, afterwards congested at each monthly period, then undergoing great development during pregnancy, so as to be double the usual size during the time of suckling, and finally, with advancing years, undergoing gradual absorption, though, in stout persons, their actual size increases from deposit of fat.

ACUTE INFLAMMATION, or MASTITIS, AND ABSCESS: **Causes**: This is most common during the period of suckling a child, and particularly during the first two months. The infection usually reaches the breast from the nipple, as a result of cracks of the nipple and lack of cleanliness. Another common cause is an indrawn nipple. Passing congestion, producing swelling and tenderness, sometimes appears in boys or girls at the time of puberty, but rarely goes on to abscess formation.

Symptoms: Discomfort in some part of the breast, with increased hardness and fullness, usually towards the lower edge, is first noticed, and, if treatment be then begun, the majority of cases do not go on to an abscess. If the condition remains untreated, definite pain next comes on, especially when the infant sucks, along with redness, swelling, and heat, the general signs of abscess. Finally, the skin over one spot, usually about 6 cms from the nipple, turns purple, and here the abscess bursts.

Treatment: It is essential that every care should be taken to prevent infection of the breast, by scrupulous attention to cleansing of the breast during the later stages of pregnancy and during suckling. This is best done by careful washing with soap and water; scrubbing with a brush is usually unnecessary. If the nipples are retracted during pregnancy, they should be drawn out every day. During suckling, the nipples should be carefully cleaned with sterile (ie. boiled) water each time the baby is put to the breast.

If, in spite of these precautions, the breast becomes hard, tender, or congested, the breast should be firmly bandaged over by a large pad of cotton-wool. The affected breast should be emptied by gentle expression, or this may be done by a breast pump. The common practice today is to start using an antibiotic, usually penicillin, at a very early stage as this reduces the risk of abscess formation. If an abscess forms, it is opened and drained. In severe cases in which it is necessary to wean the baby, the secretion of milk is stopped by taking one of the oestrogenic hormones: eg. stilboestrol (qv). The secretion of milk ceases in about half the women who develop a breast abscess.

CHRONIC INFLAMMATION, or MASTITIS, may take the form of a chronic abscess, but, more commonly, it consists of simple swelling and pain in one part of the breast, often erroneously believed by the affected person to be cancer.

Symptoms: This condition is not due to infection, but to some disturbance of the normal control of the breast exerted by the ovaries and the pituitary gland. It occurs with increasing frequency after the age of 30 years, and is more liable to occur in women who have borne children. Pain is the principal symptom. This is worse just before the monthly period or during the early days of the period. It may be confined to one part of the breast or may involve the whole breast. Both breasts may be involved. One or more swellings may be seen or felt in the breast.

Treatment: The condition is made much worse by the patient allowing her mind to dwell on it and by constant handling of the swelling, so that when the breast is completely covered up and supported by a well-fitting brassiére, complete recovery may speedily take place. The first essential, however, is that medical advice is sought, to decide whether or not the pain and swelling are due to cancer of the breast.

NEURALGIA may be very painful during pregnancy, in pelvic disorders, or in general troubles like anaemia and rheumatism. It is treated like neuralgia elsewhere.

CRACKED NIPPLES are sometimes very troublesome. For their treatment see under Acute Inflammation. When there is a chronic eczematous condition, a nipple-shield should be applied and fixed with plaster or tapes.

TUMOURS: In consequence of the fact that the breast is one of the organs most frequently attacked by cancer, many women render themselves unnecessarily unhappy over some swelling in the breast, taking for cancer what is often simply chronic inflammation, or a cyst or adenoma, the two latter being common non-malignant growths. In every case, immediately a woman discovers a small nodule in her breast she should consult a doctor. If the swelling is not cancer – and usually it is not – her mind will be relieved, and the treatment, whether by operation or not, will not in general necessitate the removal of the breast. If cancer is present, then the earlier an operation is done the more chance there is of a complete cure. A further advantage of early operation for cancer is that it may be possible to remove the growth without removing the whole breast. Such an operation, known colloquially among surgeons as 'lumpectomy', is followed by a course of radiotherapy (qv). (See MASTECTOMY.)

BREATH, DISORDERS OF: The composition of the breath and the changes that air undergoes when it is breathed are described under AIR; the manner in which breathing is affected is described under RESPIRATION. (See also BREATHLESSNESS; CHEST DISEASES; LUNG DISEASES.)

BAD BREATH, or HALITOSIS, is sometimes extremely unpleasant to those around the subject of the trouble, although the smell may be extremely foul without the person himself being conscious of it.

Causes: Frequent causes are bad teeth, infections of the gums (eg. Vincent's angina), chronic tonsillitis, and indigestion. Besides these, an excessively foetid condition is caused by bronchiectasis (qv), by ulceration about the bones of the nose, and by disease of the nose, in which crusts constantly form there (see NOSE, DISEASES OF.) A 'mousey' odour of the breath is often detectable during menstruation or premenstrually. In certain diseases there may be a characteristic odour of the breath: eg. a sweet odour in cases of diabetes mellitus verging on coma; a musty odour (foetor hepaticum) in severe acute liver failure; a urine-like odour in uraemia (qv). Certain drugs, notably paraldehyde and disulfiram, also give a characteristic odour to the breath, as do certain foodstuffs, notably garlic.

Treatment: Careful attention to the hygiene of the mouth is the first essential (see TEETH), or the dental treatment of any defective teeth or infection of the gums. Tonsillectomy may be required if the tonsils are chronically inflamed. In one form of tonsillitis, small cheesy pellets of secretion collect in the hollows of the tonsils and putrefy; the tendency to this is lessened by gargling daily (see GARGLES). Indigestion with furred tongue is also credited with being a frequent cause of bad breath (see DYSPEPSIA). The smell may be temporarily relieved by placing a small drop of some essential oil, such as cloves, occasionally on the tongue, or by various scented sweets, or by means of a mouth wash containing one teaspoonful of concentrated peppermint water BP, and one teaspoonful of salt in 200 millilitres of water.

BREATH-HOLDING: Breath-holding attacks are not uncommon in infants and toddlers. They are characterized by the child suddenly stopping breathing in the midst of a bout of crying evoked by pain, some emotional upset, or loss of temper. The breath may be held so long that the child goes blue in the face. The attack is never fatal and the condition disappears spontaneously after the age of 3 to 5 years, but once a child has acquired the habit it may recur quite often.

The attacks require no treatment as recovery is spontaneous and rapid. In no circumstances should the parents dramatize the situation by slapping, pinching, or drenching the child with water.

BREATHING (see RESPIRATION).

BREATHLESSNESS may be due to any condition which renders the blood impure or deficient in oxygen, and which therefore produces excessive involuntary efforts to gain more air.

Causes: Many diseased *conditions of the lungs* diminish the area available for breathing: eg. pneumonia, tuberculosis, emphysema, bronchitis, collections of fluid in the pleural cavities, and pressure by a tumour or aneurysm.

Pleurisy causes short, rapid breathing to avoid the pain of deep inspiration.

Narrowing of the air passages may produce sudden and alarming attacks of difficult breathing, especially among children: eg. in laryngismus, croup, asthma, and diphtheria (see these headings).

Almost all *affections of the heart* cause breathlessness when the person undergoes any special exertion.

Anaemia is a frequent cause.

Obesity is often associated with shortness of breath.

Among the *general diseases* which may interfere with breathing, uraemia (qv) and the coma which may occur in diabetes mellitus must be noted.

Treatment: In young girls who become breathless on very slight exertion the treatment is generally that for bloodlessness. (See ANAEMIA.) For the treatment of breathlessness in stout people, see CORPULENCE. In all conditions of breathlessness due to disease of a lung, the patient finds most ease in breathing when he lies upon the affected side. In many inflammatory conditions of the air passages much relief is gained from steam inhalations. The subjects of heart disease, if able to go about, should not unduly exert themselves, and are benefited by one of the forms of treatment mentioned under HEART DISEASES. Persons confined to bed by a heart affection are often unable to lie down, and must be provided with a comfortable bed-rest. Their difficulty of breathing is often due to bronchitis (see BRONCHITIS), or to collection of fluid in the chest (see DROPSY), which requires special and energetic treatment. For breathlessness with lividity, oxygen inhalation is often usefully employed.

BRETYLIUM TOSYLATE is one of the drugs introduced for the treatment of resistant cardiac arrhythmias. It acts by inhibiting sympathetic nerve action.

BRIGHT'S DISEASE (see GLOMERULONEPHRITIS).

BRITISH NATIONAL FORMULARY is a pocket book for those concerned with the prescribing, dispensing and administration of medicines. Earlier editions included only those products that had the confidence of the Joint Formulary Committee. However from 1981 onwards the basis of selection has been changed and information is included on most products available to prescribers in the United Kingdom. It is revised twice yearly.

BRITTLE BONE DISEASE is another name for osteogenesis imferfecta (qv).

BROMAZEPAM (LEXOTAN) (see BENZODIAZEPINES).

BROMHEXINE is an expectorant (qv) which is proving of value in the treatment of asthma and chronic bronchitis.

BROMIDES are salts of bromine. The bromides of potassium, sodium, strontium, and ammonium are used in medicine. They act chiefly by depressing activity, and dulling sensibility of the brain.
Uses: Introduced to clinical medicine just over a hundred years ago, the bromides were for long the standard treatment of epilepsy. For this purpose they have now been largely replaced by the barbiturates, or more recent anticonvulsant drugs, but they are still of value in occasional cases of epilepsy which do not respond satisfactorily to the newer drugs. Their other use is as an occasional sedative in mild cases of insomnia: either alone (0·6 to 1·2 G), or in combination with chloral hydrate. They have the disadvantage of tending to produce an eruption, especially about the face. (See BROMISM.) As a result of taking bromides for a long time some people may show symptoms of a disturbed balance of mind, which pass off when the drug is omitted.

BROMIDROSIS means the excretion of evil-smelling perspiration. (See PERSPIRATION.)

BROMISM is the name given to a group of symptoms consisting of acne on the face, mental dullness, sleepiness, weakness, unsteady gait, and bad breath, which shows that too much bromide is being taken.

BROMPHENIRAMINE MALEATE is an antihistamine preparation.

BROMOCRIPTINE is an ergot (qv) alkaloid which is being successfully used in the treatment of acromegaly (qv). It is also proving of value in the treatment of Parkinsonism (qv), the suppression of lactation (qv), and the pain in the breast that sometimes precedes menstruation.

BROMPTON MIXTURE is a prescription of somewhat variable constituents, but consisting basically of morphine, cocaine and whisky (or rum) which for long has had a high reputation as a most effective pain-reliever, particularly in the terminal stages of painful diseases such as cancer.

BRONCHIAL TUBES (see AIR PASSAGES; BRONCHUS; LUNGS).

BRONCHIECTASIS is a condition characterized by dilatation of the bronchi. This is the result as a rule of infection of the bronchial tree leading to obstruction of the bronchi. As a result of the obstruction the affected individual cannot get rid of the secretions in the bronchi beyond the obstruction. This accumulates and becomes infected and gradually weakens the wall of the bronchi which dilate and become an increasingly large deposit of infected material. The initial infection may be due to bacterial or viral pneumonia or the infection of the lungs complicating measles or whooping-cough. Other causes are obstruction of the bronchi by tuberculosis, cancer of the lung or the inhalation into the lungs of a foreign body, such as a tooth during dental extraction. It usually starts in childhood but may not manifest itself until adult life. It manifests itself by the coughing up of large amounts of putrid, foul-tasting, foul-smelling expectoration, which may contain blood. The condition is not immediately dangerous to life, but as a rule it results in a gradual deterioration of health, with night sweats, clubbing of the fingers and toes (see CLUBBING), and an aggravated form of chronic bronchitis.
Treatment consists of getting rid of the accumulated secretion in the dilated bronchi by means of what is known as postural drainage. This consists of the patient lying on the affected side over the edge of the bed with a pillow under him, and the head well down, so as to drain the affected area. This allows the infected secretion to drain to the trachea (or windpipe) whence it is coughed up. This should be carried out for a quarter of an hour night and morning. It helps to increase the amount of secretion got rid of if someone percusses, or firmly taps, on the chest over the affected area. At the same time the patient should take deep breaths and cough firmly to dislodge the secretion and get rid of it.

Should there be a flare-up of the condition, as there often is, this postural drainage should be done four times a day. If the odour is particularly unpleasant, this may be kept in check by inhalations of creosote, or by vaporizing creosote and other aromatic substances in steam near the bed. If there should be a flare-up of the condition due to infection, this is controlled by antibiotics. If the condition is localized to one lobe of the lung, an operation (lobectomy) may be performed to remove the affected lung. Patients with bronchiectasis should be immunized against influenza every autumn, should not smoke, and should ensure that they have a well-balanced diet and as much fresh air as possible.

BRONCHIOLES is the term applied to the finest divisions of the bronchial tubes.

BRONCHIOLITIS is the name sometimes applied to bronchitis affecting the finest bronchial tubes, also known as capillary bronchitis.

BRONCHITIS means inflammation of the mucous membrane of the bronchial tubes. Well known as one of the most common hazards of the climate of Great Britain, bronchitis exists in either an *acute* or a *chronic* form.

(*a*) ACUTE BRONCHITIS, like other inflammatory affections of the chest, often develops following exposure to cold, particularly if accompanied with damp, or sudden change from a heated to a cool atmosphere. It may also arise as the result of inhaling irritating dust or vapours. The exciting cause is infection of the bronchial tree with one or more of the catarrh-producing organisms, and great numbers of these bacteria are commonly found in the expectoration.

Symptoms: The symptoms vary according to the severity of the attack, and more especially according to the extent to which the inflammatory action spreads in the bronchial tubes. The disease usually manifests itself at first in the form of catarrh, or the common cold; but the accompanying feverishness and general constitutional disturbance proclaim the attack to be something more severe, and symptoms denoting the onset of bronchitis soon present themselves. A short, painful, dry cough, accompanied with rapid and wheezing respiration, a feeling of rawness and pain in the throat and behind the breast-bone, and of oppression or tightness throughout the chest, mark the early stages of the disease.

After a few days, expectoration begins to come with the cough, at first scanty and viscid or frothy, but soon becoming copious and of purulent character. In general, after free expectoration has been established the more urgent and distressing symptoms abate; and, while the cough may persist for a length of time, often extending to three or four weeks, in the majority of instances convalescence advances, and the patient is ultimately restored to health, although not infrequently a tendency is left to a recurrence of the disease on exposure to its exciting causes.

When the ear or the stethoscope is applied to the chest of a person suffering from such an attack, there are heard in the earlier stages snoring or cooing sounds, mixed up with others of wheezing or fine whistling quality, accompanying respiration. These are named dry sounds or rhonchi, and they are occasionally so abundant and distinct as to convey their vibrations to the hand applied to the chest, as well as to be audible to a bystander at some distance. As the disease progresses these sounds become to a large extent replaced by others of crackling or bubbling character, which are termed moist sounds or crackles. Both these kinds of abnormal sounds are readily explained by a reference to the pathological condition of the parts. One of the first effects of inflammation upon the bronchial mucous membrane is to cause some degree of swelling, which, together with the presence of a tough secretion closely adhering to it, tends to narrow the tubes. The respired air as it passes through the narrowed tubes gives rise to the dry or sonorous breath sounds, the coarser being generated in the large, and the finer or wheezing sounds in the small divisions of the bronchi. Before long, however, the discharge from the bronchial mucous membrane becomes more abundant and less glutinous, and accumulates in the tubes till dislodged by coughing. The respired air, as it passes through this fluid, causes the moist crackles, above described. In most instances both moist and dry sounds are heard abundantly in the same case, since different portions of the bronchial tubes are affected at different times in the course of the disease.

Such are briefly the main characteristics presented by an ordinary attack of acute bronchitis running a favourable course.

The case, however, is very different when the inflammation spreads into, or when it primarily affects, the minute ramifications of the bronchial tubes which are in immediate relation to the air-cells of the lungs, giving rise to that form of the disease known as *bronchiolitis*. When this takes place all the symptoms already detailed become greatly intensified, and the outlook becomes much more serious in consequence of the interrruption to the entrance of air into the lungs, and thus to the due aeration of the blood. Indeed the condition may become indistinguishable from broncho-pneumonia. The feverishness and restlessness increase, the cough becomes incessant, the breathing extremely rapid and laboured, the nostrils dilating with each effort, and evidence of impending suffocation appears. The surface of the body is pale or dusky, the lips are livid, while breathing becomes increasingly difficult and is attended with suffocative paroxysms which render the recumbent posture impossible. Unless speedy relief is obtained by coughing and expectoration, the patient's strength gives way, somnolence and delirium set in, and death ensues. All this may be brought about in a few days, and such cases, particularly among the very young or the aged, sometimes prove fatal within forty-eight hours.

In addition to the auscultatory signs present in ordinary bronchitis, there generally exist in this form of the disease abundant fine crackles at the bases of both lungs; and the appearance of these organs after death shows the minute bronchi and many of the air-cells to be filled with matter similar to that which had been expectorated, and which has thus acted as a mechanical hindrance to the entrance of the air and caused death by asphyxia.

Acute bronchitis is pre-eminently dangerous at the extremes of life, and mortality statistics show it to be one of the most fatal of the diseases of those periods. This is to be explained not only by the well-recognized fact that all acute diseases tell with great severity on the feeble frames alike of infants and aged people, but more particularly by the tendency which bronchitis undoubtedly has, in them, to become bronchiolitis, and, when it does so, to prove quickly fatal. The importance therefore of early attention to the slightest evidence of bronchitis among the very young or the aged can scarcely be overrated.

Bronchitis is also apt to be very severe when it occurs in alcoholics. Again, in those who suffer from any disease affecting directly or indirectly the respiratory functions, such as tuberculosis or heart disease, the supervention of an attack of acute bronchitis is an alarming complication, increasing, as it necessarily does, the embarrassment of breathing. The same remark is applicable to those numerous instances of its occurrence in children who are, or have been, suffering from such diseases as have always associated with them a certain degree of bronchial irritation, such as measles and whooping-cough.

One other source of danger of a special character in bronchitis remains to be mentioned: collapse of the lung. Occasionally a branch of a bronchial tube becomes plugged up with secretion, so that the area of the lung to which this branch brings air ceases to be inflated on inspiration. The small quantity of air imprisoned in the portion of lung gradually escapes, but no fresh air enters, and the part collapses and becomes of solid consistence. Increased difficulty of breathing is the result, and when a large portion of lung is affected by the plugging up of a large bronchus, a fatal result may rapidly follow, the danger being specially great in the case of children. Fortunately, the obstruction may sometimes be removed by vigorous coughing, and relief is then obtained.

Treatment: In those mild cases which are more of the nature of a simple catarrh little else will be found necessary than confinement in a warm room, or in bed, for a few days, and the use of light diet, together with warm diluent drinks, warm milk being specially beneficial. Additional measures are called for when the disease is more markedly developed. An antibiotic should be given. In the early stages of the disease, when the cough is harsh and unproductive, linctuses give considerable relief. Sedatives are also usually required at night. Opium or morphine must never be given to a patient with bronchitis, because of their depressant effect upon the respiratory centre. In the later stages of the disease, as the cough becomes looser, expectorants (qv) are of value. From the outset of the attack the employment of warm applications to the chest, in the form of an electric pad, medicated wool, or a rubber hot-water bottle, affords great relief. In children, rubbing the chest with some stimulating liniment such as camphorated oil has a similar effect.

In the earlier stages few remedial measures are of greater value than the frequent inhalation of steam. This is accomplished readily enough in the case of adults by the use of an inhaler or simply by breathing over an open-mouthed vessel containing boiling water. In children, in whom this plan cannot be carried out in the same manner, there is in general no difficulty in surrounding them with an atmosphere of steam by erecting over the bed or cot a tent, formed by a screen and blanket, under which can be led the orifice of a tin kettle heated by a spirit lamp or electric heater, and provided with a long spout. Various drugs of soothing or expectorant qualities, such as tincture of benzoin and menthol, can also be added to the water in the kettle, or poured upon a sponge which is placed in the end of the spout, and so inhaled in the steam (see INHALATION).

(*b*) CHRONIC BRONCHITIS **Causes**: This form of the disease may arise as the result of repeated attacks of the acute form, or it may exist altogether independently. It occurs more often among persons advanced in life than among the young, although no age is exempt from it.

It is one of the most common causes of death in this country and is much more common than in any other country. Hence its international reputation as the 'English disease'. Whilst there is probably a constitutional predisposition to the disease, there are in addition six important contributory factors:

(1) Exposure to irritant dust, smoke or fumes either as an occupational hazard or as part of the atmospheric pollution prevalent in industrial areas.

(2) Excessive cigarette smoking

(3) Bad housing

(4) A cold, damp, foggy climate

(5) Obesity

(6) Recurring respiratory infections.

The usual history of this form of bronchitis is that of a cough recurring during the colder seasons of the year, and in its earlier stages, departing entirely in summer, so that it is often called 'winter cough'. In many persons subject to it, however, attacks are apt to be excited at any time by very slight causes, such as changes in the weather; and in advanced cases of the disease the cough is seldom altogether absent.

Chronic bronchitis may arise secondarily to some other ailment. This is especially the case in heart disease, in which it often proves a serious complication.

Symptoms: The symptoms and auscultatory signs of chronic bronchitis are on the whole similar to those pertaining to the acute form, except that the febrile disturbance and pain are much less marked. The cough is usually more troublesome in the morning than during the day. There is usually free and copious expectoration of a thin frothy fluid, and occasionally this is so abundant as to constitute what is termed *bronchorrhoea*.

Chronic bronchitis leads to alterations of structure in the affected bronchial tubes, their mucous membrane becoming thickened or even ulcerated, while occasionally permanent dilatation of the bronchi takes place, often accompanied with profuse foetid expectoration. In long-standing cases of chronic bronchitis, the nutrition of the lungs becomes impaired, and dilatation of the air-sacs (*emphysema*) and other complications result, giving rise to more or less constant breathlessness and leading to deformity of the chest (*barrel-shaped chest*). Chronic bronchitis is liable, in some instances, particularly when accompanied with loss of flesh and strength, to be mistaken for tuberculosis; but, whilst this is a possibility which must always be borne in mind, particularly in the elderly, the physician who carefully regards the history of the case and observes the physical signs and symptoms, will in general be able to distinguish the one disease from the other. In this, too, the examination of the sputum for the presence of the tubercle bacillus is of great importance, the discovery of this organism at once indicating the tuberculous nature of the malady.

Chronic bronchitis does not often prove directly fatal, nor is it necessarily inconsistent with long life. Its chief danger lies in the tendency to intercurrent acute attacks, particularly in the aged; and in this manner it is a disturbingly common cause of death.

Treatment: The treatment to be adopted in chronic bronchitis depends upon the severity of the case, the age of the patient, and the presence or absence of complications. Attention to the general health is a matter of prime importance in all cases, more particularly among persons whose work entails exposure. As severe bronchitis is seldom found in one who has never smoked, smoking – certainly of cigarettes – should be given up. If the victim is overweight, he should take steps to get his weight down. In those aggravated forms of chronic bronchitis in which the slightest exposure to cold air brings on fresh attacks, it may become necessary, where circumstances permit, to enjoin confinement to a warm room, or removal to a more genial climate during the winter months.

When expectoration is difficult, such remedies as squill combined with carbonate of ammonia may prove useful. Alternatively, particularly for the troublesome cough with which the individual with chronic bronchitis tends to awaken in the morning, a hot drink, or an alkaline mixture such as the Compound Sodium Chloride Mixture of the *British Pharmaceutical Codex* 1979, (10 to 20 millilitres in a tumblerful of hot water, sipped slowly) may be effective. The inhalation of vapour containing Friars' balsam or menthol is often followed by marked benefit in this way.

The value of antibiotics in chronic bronchitis is still undecided. Some recommend their routine use every winter, whilst others contend that this is unnecessary and not without its drawbacks. In many cases infection plays a relatively unimportant part, and for such patients antibiotics are obviously of little value, and treatment must consist of the general measures outlined above. In the presence of infection, as exemplified by a purulent sputum and/or the finding of antibiotic-sensitive organisms in the sputum, antibiotics may be of great value. Those who are subject to chronic bronchitis should be vaccinated against influenza every autumn.

Acute attacks of the disease, which are so apt to arise in the chronic form, must be dealt with on the principles already indicated in treating of acute bronchitis.

BRONCHOGRAPHY means rendering the outline of the bronchial tree visible on an X-ray film by means of the injection of a radio-opaque substance through the larynx. This is a simple procedure carried out under general anaesthesia and allows the accurate location of, for example, a lung abscess, bronchiectasis (qv), or a tumour in the lung.

BRONCHOPHONY means the resonance of the voice as heard by auscultation over the site of the large bronchial tubes, and, in diseased conditions, conveyed beyond these by cavities or solidification of parts of the lung.

BRONCHO-PNEUMONIA (see PNEUMONIA).

BRONCHOSCOPE is an instrument constructed on the principle of the telescope, which on introduction into the mouth is passed down through the larynx and windpipe and enables the observer to see the interior of the larger bronchial tubes.

BRONCHUS, or bronchial tube, is the name applied to tubes into which the windpipe divides, one going to either lung. The name is also applied to the divisions of these tubes distributed throughout the lungs, the smallest being called bronchioles.

BROW AGUE is a term used to denote both frontal neuralgia or tic douloureux (see NEURALGIA) and migraine or megrim (see MIGRAINE).

BRUCELLOSIS, also known as UNDULANT FEVER, MALTA FEVER, MEDITERRANEAN FEVER, is a long-continued fever which occurs principally on the shores and islands of the Mediterranean, but is found also in many other countries.

Causes: In Malta and the Mediterranean littoral the causative organism is the *Brucella melitensis* which is conveyed in goat's milk. In Great Britain, the USA, and South Africa, the causative organism is the *Brucella abortus*, which is conveyed in cow's milk. This is the organism which is responsible for contagious abortion in cattle. In Great Britain it is largely an occupational disease. Thus, in 1974, 70 per cent of the cases occurred in farm workers, 10 per cent in veterinary surgeons, and 6 per cent in abattoir workers. Ten per cent probably acquired it from drinking unpasteurized milk. It is now prescribed as an industrial disease (see OCCUPATIONAL DISEASES), and insured persons who contract the disease at work can claim industrial injuries benefit.

The number of recorded cases in England and Wales, and Scotland in recent years is shown in the accompanying table, which demonstrates the relatively high incidence in Scotland. In 1984 there were no deaths from brucellosis in the UK.

Year	England *and Wales*	Scotland
1967	221	188
1968	203	305
1969	198	292
1970	324	325
1971	221	392
1973	217	
1974	162	
1975		113
1976		100
1977	58	
1978	39	
1979	33	76
1980	17	

No of cases of brucellosis in England and Wales, and Scotland 1967—80

Symptoms: The characteristic features of the disease are fever, drenching sweats necessitating a change of night attire and bed linen, pains in the joints and back, and headache. The temperature is usually undulating. There are, however, many atypical cases, and the diagnosis may be difficult. The liver and spleen may be enlarged. The diagnosis is confirmed by the finding of *Br. abortus*, or antibodies to it, in the blood. Recovery and convalescence tend to be slow.

Treatment: Treatment is directed towards relieving the sleeplessness, the pain in the joints, and other symptoms. The condition responds well to one of the tetracycline antibiotics, and also to gentamicin, and co-trimoxazole, but relapse is all too common. In chronic cases a combination of streptomycin and one of the tetracyclines is often more effective.

Prevention: It can be prevented by boiling or pasteurizing all milk used for human consumption. A compulsory eradication programme is now in force, with a view to ensuring that in due course it may be possible to bring the disease under control, as in Scandinavia, the Netherlands, Switzerland and Canada where the disease has disappeared following the eradication of the disease in animals. In January 1980, Scotland was declared a brucellosis attested area, signifying that the disease had been eradicated from all cattle. In Malta it has practically been abolished by ceasing to use goats' milk.

BRUISES, or CONTUSIONS, are more or less extensive injuries of the deeper parts of the skin and underlying tissues, accompanied generally by outpouring of blood from damaged vessels, but unattended by corresponding open wounds.

Varieties: An extensive bruise may be accompanied by a wound, in which case the injury is known as a contused wound. (See WOUNDS.)

The simplest type of bruise is one in which only the deeper layers of the skin are damaged, causing a slight bluish discoloration due to the tearing of minute vessels and the escape of blood into the cellular spaces of the skin. As the result of a severe blow, the muscles may be bruised and torn without any wound in the skin, and the resulting effusion of blood may cause a large swelling which sometimes, though not usually, results in the formation of an abscess. When a bone is bruised, as by a kick on the shin or by a fall upon the knee or elbow, changes similar to those which follow an actual fracture are produced and a permanent thickening of the bone may result. Bruises of this type are of great importance, because an effusion of blood into the cavity of a joint leads to stiffness lasting some weeks, which, if absorption of the blood be not complete, may remain in some degree permanent owing to the formation of adhesions (see ADHESIONS; and JOINTS, DISEASES OF). Further, it is held by many authorities that some slight injury of this nature is sometimes the starting-point of the tuberculous disease which attacks the bones of children. Severe bruises of internal organs, as from a crush or run-over accident, sometimes occur even when the skin has escaped injury and shows no mark (see ABDOMEN, INJURIES OF). Bruising of the brain or spinal cord occasionally occurs in consequence of a severe shaking, as in a railway accident, and is known as concussion (see BRAIN, DISEASES OF).

Appearance of a bruise: The extent of a bruise and the depth of its tint depend upon the amount of blood which has escaped from the vessels, and this again varies according to the violence of the blow and peculiarities of the person injured. In some diseases, like haemophilia and scurvy, extensive bruises are produced by little or no violence. Sometimes a bruise is so sharply limited that it gives a distinct impression of the instrument with which it has been inflicted, whilst in other cases the blood runs downwards and produces a black mark at some distance from the injured part, as seen, for example, in the blackness beneath the eye which may follow an injury of the forehead or temple.

The colour of a bruise is at first black or bluish, later becoming brown, and finally changing to yellow, which fades away as alterations take place in, and absorption occurs of, the blood pigment. (See HAEMATOIDIN AND HAEMIN.) The time occupied in disappearance of a bruise depends largely upon the amount of blood effused, but in moderate bruises ten days or a fortnight must elapse before the injury ceases to be noticeable.

Treatment of slight bruises consists chiefly in preventing the effusion of blood after an injury. This is done by firm pressure over the site for three to five minutes. This may be followed by cold compresses firmly fixed in position by suitable bandages. Ice may also be applied with good results. If it is not convenient to apply cold, various astringent substances may be used in the form of evaporating lotions kept in contact with the part for eight or ten hours; thus a cloth may be wrung out in Goulard's water and applied to the bruise, or the skin may be painted with hazeline or tincture of arnica. In painful bruises one of the best applications is lead and opium lotion. (See GOULARD'S WATER.) The injured part, if a limb, should be elevated in a sling or on a couch.

Mere surface bruises and abrasions are benefited by application of hazeline. If the skin be much ruffled or ingrained with dirt the affected area should be well washed with hot water and soap, and then with some antiseptic such as cetrimide. It may then be advisable to cover the area with an adhesive plastic dressing for a day or so.

BRUIT and MURMUR are words used to describe abnormal sounds heard in connection with the heart, arteries, and veins on auscultation.

BRUXISM or **TOOTH GRINDING** is the habit of grinding the teeth, usually while asleep and without being aware of it. The teeth may feel uncomfortable on wakening. It is very common in children and is of no significance, although more severe forms, even during the waking period, may occur in the mentally retarded. In adults it may be associated with stress or a malpositioned tooth or an overfilled tooth. It is also found in some patients taking drugs, such as fenfluramine and levodopa, which cause minor tremors and reduced muscle control. If the bruxism persists, then excessive wear may result in the loss of enamel and cause pain. Treatment is not very successful unless a cause can be found and removed. A plastic splint fitted over the teeth may help.

BUBO means a swelling of a lymphatic gland in the groin in venereal disease or in plague. (See PLAGUE.)

BUCHU is a remedy derived from the leaves of *Agathosma betulina* and similar plants. It contains volatile oil and mucilage and is administered in inflammatory conditions of the bladder.

BUDGERIGAR-FANCIER'S LUNG is a form of extrinsic allergic alveolitis, resulting from sensitization to budgerigars, or parakeets as they are known in North America. Skin tests have revealed sensitization to the birds' droppings and/or serum. As it is estimated that budgerigars are kept in 5–6 million homes in Britain, current figures suggest that anything up to 900 per 100,000 of the population are exposed to the risk of developing this condition. (See ALVEOLITIS.)

BUERGER'S DISEASE (see THROMBOANGIITIS OBLITERANS).

BULBAR PARALYSIS (see PARALYSIS).

BULIMIA means insatiable appetite of psychological origin.

BULIMIA NERVOSA is a variant of anorexia nervosa (qv). It is characterized by overpowering urges to eat large amounts of food followed by induced vomiting or abuse of laxatives to avoid any gain in weight. Most of the cases are prone to being overweight and all have a morbid fear of obesity. They indulge in bouts of gross overeating, or 'binge rounds' as they describe them, to 'fill the empty space inside'. By their bizarre behaviour, most of them manage to maintain a normal weight. The condition is accompanied by irregular menstruation, often amounting to amenorrhoea. It is most common in women in their 20's. Although there are many similarities to anorexia nervosa, it differs in that there is no attempt at deceit, and it is freely admitted that there is an eating disorder and there is distress about the symptoms it produces. In spite of this, the response to treatment, which is as in anorexia nervosa, is far from satisfactory.

BULLA is another word for blister.

BUMETANIDE (BURINEX) is a diuretic (qv) which is active when taken by mouth. It acts quickly – within half-an-hour – and its action is over in a few hours. (See BENZOTHIADIAZINES, DIURETICS.)

BUNDLE OF HIS, or atrioventricular bundle, is a bundle of special muscle fibres which pass from the atria to the ventricles of the heart and which form the pathway for the impulse which makes the ventricles contract, the impulse originating in the part of the atria known as the sinuatrial node.

BUNIONS (see CORNS AND BUNIONS).

BUPIVACAINE is a local anaesthetic. It is four times as potent as lignocaine (qv).

BURNING FEET is a syndrome (qv) characterized by a burning sensation in the soles of the feet. It is rare in temperate climes but widespread in India and the Far East. The precise cause is not known, but it is undoubtedly associated with malnutrition, and lack of one or more components of the vitamin B complex is the likeliest cause.

BURNING MOUTH is a common complaint. It is most commonly associated with faulty dentures. (See TEETH, DISEASES OF.) Other causes include infections of the mouth. (See MOUTH, DISEASES OF.) It is a not uncommon complaint at the time of the menopause and diabetic subjects are liable to complain of it, especially if their diabetes is not under control. Vitamin deficiency, particularly of certain members of the vitamin B complex, may be responsible. It may be due to a fungal infection following the administration of antibiotics.

BURNS and SCALDS: Burns are injuries caused by dry heat, scalds by moist heat, but the two are similar in symptoms and treatment. Severe burns are also caused by contact with electric wires, and by the action of acids and other chemicals. The burn caused by chemicals differs from a burn by fire only in the fact that the outcome is more favourable, because the chemical destroys the bacteria on the part, so that less suppuration follows.

Severe and extensive burns are most frequently produced by the clothes, for example, of a child, catching fire. This applies especially to cotton garments, which blaze up quickly. It should be remembered that such a flame can immediately be extinguished by making the individual lie on the floor so that the flames are uppermost, and wrapping him in a rug, mat, or blanket. As prevention is always better than cure, particular care should always be exercised with electric fires and kettles or pots of boiling water in houses where there are young children or old people. Equally important is it that children's night-clothes and frocks be made of non-inflammable material. Pyjamas are also much safer than nightdresses. Severe scalds are usually produced by escape of steam in boiler explosions.

Degrees of burns: The French surgeon Dupuytren divided burns into six degrees, according to their depth.

1ST DEGREE: There is simply redness. Such burns may be painful for a day or two. Similar effects are produced by prolonged exposure to sunlight and to X-rays.

2ND DEGREE: There is great redness, and the surface is raised up in blebs. There is much pain, but healing occurs without a scar.

3RD DEGREE: The scarf-skin, or epidermis, or corium, is all peeled off, and the true skin below is in part destroyed, so as to expose the endings of the sensory nerves. This is a very painful form of burn, and a scar follows on healing.

4TH DEGREE: The entire skin of an area is destroyed, with its nerves, so that there is much less pain than in the last form. A scar forms, later contracts, and may produce great deformity.

5TH DEGREE: The muscles also are burned, and still greater deformity follows.

6TH DEGREE: A whole limb is charred. It separates as in gangrene.

In practice, however, today burns are referred to as either *superficial* (or partial thickness) burns when there is sufficient skin tissue left to ensure regrowth of skin over the burned site; and *deep* (or full thickness) when the skin is totally destroyed and grafting will be necessary.

Symptoms: Whilst many domestic burns are minor and insignificant, more severe burns and scalds can prove to be very dangerous to life. The main danger is due to shock (qv). This arises as a result of loss of fluid from the circulating blood at the site of the burn. This loss of fluid leads to a fall in the volume of the circulating blood. As the maintenance of an adequate blood volume is essential to life, the body attempts to compensate for this loss by withdrawing fluid from the uninjured areas of the body into the circulation. This, however, in turn, if carried too far begins to affect the viability of the body cells. As a sequel, essential body cells, such as those of the liver and kidneys, begin to suffer, and the liver and kidneys cease to function properly. This will show itself by the development of jaundice (qv) and the appearance of albumin in the urine. (See ALBUMINURIA.) In addition, the circulation begins to fail with a resultant lack of oxygen (see ANOXIA) in the tissues, and the victim becomes cyanosed (see CYANOSIS), restless and collapsed and, in some cases, death ensues. In addition, there is a strong risk of infection occurring. Particularly is this the case with severe burns which leave a large raw surface exposed and very vulnerable to any micro-organisms. The combination of shock and infection can all too often be life-threatening unless expert treatment is immediately available.

The immediate outcome of a burn is largely determined by its extent. This is of more significance than the depth of the burn. To assess the extent of a burn in relation to the surface of the body, what is known as the Rule of Nine has been evolved. From the figure below it will be seen that the head and each arm cover 9 per cent of the body surface, whilst the front of the body, the back of the body, and each leg each cover 18 per cent, with the perineum (or crutch) accounting for the remaining 1 per cent. The greater the extent of the burn, the more seriously ill will the victim become from loss of fluid from his circulation, and therefore the more prompt should be his removal to hospital for expert treatment. The depth of the burn, unless this is very great and reaches the 5th or 6th degree, is mainly of import when the question arises as to how much surgical treatment, including skin grafting, will be required.

Treatment: This depends upon the severity of the burn. In the case of quite minor burns or scalds, all that may be necessary if they are seen immediately is to hold the part under cold running water until the pain is relieved. Cooling is one of the most effective ways of relieving the pain of a burn. If the burn involves the distal part of a limb, eg. the hand and forearm, one of the most effective ways of relieving pain is to immerse the burned part in lukewarm water and add cold water until the pain disappears. As the water warms and pain returns more cold water is added. After some three to four hours, pain will not reappear on warming, and the burn may be dressed in the usual way. Thereafter a simple dressing – eg. a piece of sterile gauze covered by cotton-wool, and on top of this a bandage or a piece of Elastoplast – should be applied. The part should be kept at rest and the dressing kept quite dry until healing takes place. Blisters should be pierced with a sterile needle, but the skin should not be cut away. No ointment or oil should be applied, and an antiseptic is not usually necessary.

In slightly more severe burns or scalds, it is probably advisable to use some antiseptic dressing. These are the cases which should be taken to a doctor – whether a general practitioner, a factory doctor, or a casualty officer in hospital. There is still no general consensus of expert opinion as to the best 'antiseptic' to use. Among those recommended are chlorhexidine, and antibiotics such as bacitracin, neomycin and polymixin. An alternative is to use a Tulle Gras dressing which has been impregnated with a suitable antibiotic. One of the many methods recommended is to apply a cream containing chlorhexidine and lignocaine (which has the double advantage of being both antiseptic and pain-relieving), covering this with a Tulle Gras dressing, covered in turn by cotton-wool and a crêpe bandage. To ensure that the burn is completely sealed off the ends of the dressing are completely sealed with zinc oxide plaster. The dressing is left on for four or five days before being changed unless the burn becomes painful or there is any evidence of infection (such as redness, swelling and pain), when it is changed immediately.

In the case of severe burns and scalds, the only sound rule is immediate removal to hospital. Unless there is any need for immediate resuscitation, such as artificial respiration, or attention to other injuries there may be, such as fractures or haemorrhage, nothing should be done on the spot to the patient except to make sure that he is as comfortable as possible and to keep him warm, and to cover the burn with a sterile (or clean) cloth such as a sheet, pillowcases, or towels wrung out in cold water. If pain is severe, morphine should be given – usually intravenously. Once the victim is in hospital, the primary decision is as to the extent of the burn, and whether or not a transfusion is necessary. If the burn is more than 9 per cent of the body surface in extent, a transfusion is called for. The precise treatment of the burn varies from hospital to hospital, but the essential is to prevent infection if this has not already occurred, or, if it has, to bring it under control as quickly as possible. A high-protein diet, with ample fluids, is also necessary to compensate for all the protein that has been lost along with the fluid from the circulation. The process of healing is slow and tedious in the case of extensive burns, and involves careful nursing, the

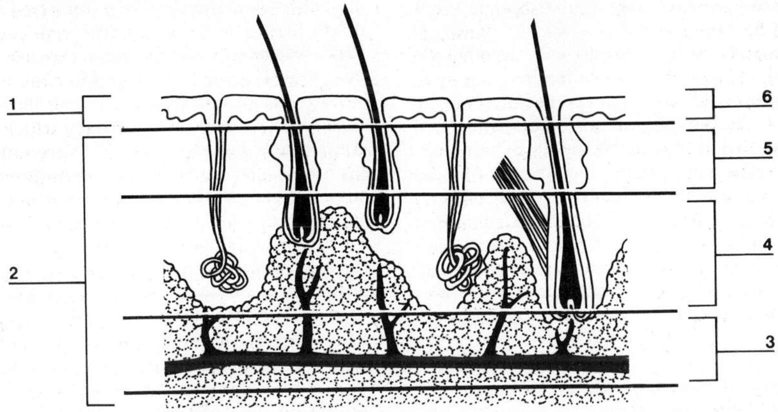

1 Epidermis 2 Dermis
3–4 Full-thickness burn requiring grafting
5 Partial-thickness burn which will usually heal within 3 weeks.
6 Partial-thickness burn which will heal in 7–10 days.

The structure of the skin in relation to the depth of a burn.

maintenance of morale, physiotherapy and occupational therapy. A vital decision is as to whether skin grafting is required, and when this should be initiated.

So far as the ultimate outcome is concerned, the main factor, as has already been noted, is the extent of the burn. The greater this is, the worse the outlook. The outlook is also poor in infants and old people.

Chemical Burns: Phenol or lysol can be washed off promptly before they do much damage. Acid or alkali burns should be neutralized by washing them repeatedly with sodium bicarbonate or 1 per cent acetic acid, respectively. Alternatively, the following buffer solution may be used for either acid or alkali burns: monobasic potassium phosphate (70 grams), dibasic sodium phosphate (70 grams) in 850 millilitres of water. (See also PHOSPHORUS BURNS.)

BURSAE are natural hollows in the fibrous tissues, lined by smooth cells and containing a little fluid. They are situated at points where there is much pressure or friction, and their purpose is to allow free movement without stretching or straining the tissues: for example, on the knee-cap or the point of the elbow, and, generally speaking, where one muscle rubs against another or against a bone. They develop also beneath corns and bunions, or where a bone comes to press in an unwonted manner on the skin.

BURSITIS means inflammation within a bursa. Acute bursitis is of the nature of an abscess, being produced by injury of a bursa, especially on the knee or elbow, when the prominent part of the joint becomes swollen, hot, painful, and red. It is treated as an abscess. (See ABSCESS.)

Chronic bursitis is due to too much movement of, or pressure on, a bursa. For example, the condition of housemaid's knee is a chronic inflammation of the patellar bursa in front of the knee, due to too much kneeling. This condition may consist of either a collection of fluid in the bursa, or, less frequently, in thickening of its walls, producing in either case an elastic swelling over the joint, with pain. In the former case, resting the limb, with counter-irritation (see BLISTERS) over the swelling, or injection of some irritant substance into its interior, forms the treatment; in the latter case, removal by operation.

Chronic bursitis about the sinews round the wrist and ankle is generally called a ganglion. (See GANGLION.)

BUSULPHAN (MYLERAN) is a preparation allied to the nitrogen mustard group of compounds (qv), with an action on dividing cells similar to that of irradiation. It is proving of value in the treatment of chronic myeloid leukaemia. (See CYTOTOXIC DRUGS.)

BUTRIPTYLINE (EVADYNE) (see ANTIDEPRESSANTS).

BUTYROPHENONES are a group of drugs, including haloperidol, which are proving to be effective in the treatment of psychotic illness.

BYSSINOSIS is a pneumoconiosis (qv), or chronic inflammatory thickening of the lung tissue, due to the inhalation of dust in textile factories. It is found chiefly among cotton and flax workers and, to a lesser extent, among workers in soft hemp. It is rare or absent in workers in jute and the hard fibres of hemp and sisal. In 1985 there were 25 deaths from byssinosis in the UK. Six deaths were in males and 19 in females.

C

CACHET means an oval capsule, generally made of rice paper, for enclosing a dose of unpleasant medicine. Cachets are softened by moistening with water prior to swallowing.

CACHEXIA is the feeble state produced by serious disease, such as cancer.

CADAVERIC RIGIDITY is the stiffness which comes on after death. (See DEATH, SIGNS OF.)

CADMIUM POISONING is a recognized hazard in certain industrial processes, such as the manufacture of alloys, cadmium plating and glass blowing (see OCCUPATIONAL DISEASES). It is also now known that sewage sludge, which is used as fertilizer, may be contaminated by cadmium from industrial sources. Such cadmium could be taken up into vegetable crops. Cadmium levels in sewage are carefully monitored; surveys performed of people eating their own vegetables, grown in gardens fertilized with contaminated sludge, have shown no adverse health effects. Cadmium in the form of the sulphide occurs with zinc minerals, and investigations of an old zinc mining area near Shipham in Somerset have revealed a high level of cadmium in the soil and in vegetables grown in it. So far no adverse effect has been detected in those living in the region and eating vegetables grown there. Where an excess of cadmium is consumed it causes gastroenteritis, resulting in diarrhoea and vomiting. The most important source of cadmium is food, particularly some vegetables (cabbage, spinach, lettuce, kale, rhubarb and celery) when grown on soils fertilized with large amounts of contaminated sewage sludge, shellfish and kidneys. Smoking of cigarettes is the second major source of intake. The EEC Directive on the Quality of Water for Human Consumption lays down 5 milligrams per litre as the upper safe level.

CAECUM is the dilated commencement of the large intestine lying in the right lower corner of the abdomen. Into it the small intestine and the appendix vermiformis open, and it is continued upwards through the right flank as the ascending colon.

CAESAREAN SECTION means the delivery of a child by opening the abdomen and womb from in front. It is supposed to get its name from the traditional, but unproven, story that Julius Caesar was so delivered. The more probable explanation is that it was named after Caesarean Law which forbade the burying of a pregnant mother until her baby had first been removed. According to Ovid, Aesculapius, the God of Physic, was born by caesarean section. The first caesarean section in the British Isles is said to have been performed in 1738 by an Irish midwife, Mary Donnally. Her patient, who had been in labour for twelve days, successfully survived the operation. It is performed when delivery by the natural passage is undesirable because of the risk to mother and child: for example, because of bony deformity of the pelvis; also when the mother has died just before labour, so as to save the child.

CAFFEINE is a white crystalline substance obtained from coffee, of which it is the active principle. Its main actions are as a cerebral stimulant, a cardiac stimulant, and as a diuretic. It is also of value in some cases of asthma. It is a constituent of many tablets for the relief of headache, usually combined with aspirin and paracetamol. Granular effervescent citrate of caffeine forms a useful, non-intoxicating stimulant in headache due to tiredness.

CAISSON DISEASE, or COMPRESSED AIR ILLNESS, affects workers in compressed air, such as underwater divers and workers in caissons. Its chief symptoms are pains in the joints and limbs (bends), pain in the stomach, headache and dizziness, and paralysis. Sudden death may occur. The condition is caused by the accumulation of bubbles of nitrogen in different parts of the body.

CAJUPUT OIL is a green oil with a camphor-like smell, used for rubbing over painful joints. Spirit of cajuput in teaspoonful doses is useful for severe colic.

CALABAR BEAN is another name for physostigmine (qv).

CALAMINE, or CARBONATE OF ZINC, is a mild astringent used, as calamine lotion, to soothe and protect the skin in many conditions such as eczema and urticaria.

CALCANEUS is the heelbone or os calcis.

CALCICOSIS is the term applied to disease of the lung caused by the inhalation of marble dust by marble-cutters.

CALCIFEROL, or VITAMIN D_2, is a crystalline substance extracted from irradiated ergosterol, and has the same action as vitamin D. Man attains vitamin D in two ways: from food naturally containing or fortified with vitamin D, or from its production in the skin by the action of ultraviolet light on the precursor 7-dehydrocholesterol. The vitamin D produced in the skin and occurring naturally in food products is cholecalciferol or vitamin D_3 while the product used for food fortification or prescribed as calciferol is the synthetic compound ergocalciferol or vitamin D_2. The biological activity of both ergocalciferol and cholecalciferol is the same and both are metabolised in identical manner. Cholecalciferol itself has little, if any, biological activity and it is metabolised in the liver and subsequently in the kidney to produce the active metabolite one alpha 25-dihydroxy vitamin D and this is known as calcitriol. One alpha cholecalciferol (alfacalcidol) is a synthetic analogue which is rapidly converted to the active metabolite.

The action of vitamin D is to increase the absorption of calcium from the gut and to increase the calcium release from bone. If there is a deficiency of vitamin D from the diet, or if vitamin D is not absorbed adequately, or if renal disease prevents the hydroxylation of cholecalciferol to dihydroxycholecalciferol, the bone disease of osteomalacia (qv) will result. This is a particularly common condition in the Asian immigrant population in Britain who tend to take a diet low in vitamin D and also tend to avoid sunlight on the skin so that the production of ergocalciferol is impaired.

The treatment of osteomalacia is to provide vitamin D. For low-dose treatment the most widely used preparation is Calcium with vitamin D (B.P.C.). Each tablet contains calcium sodium lactate 450 mg, calcium phosphate 150 mg and calciferol 12·5 mcg. For high-dose vitamin D therapy calciferol tablets which contain 1·25 mg of calciferol are usually prescribed. The most common metabolites of vitamin D in therapeutic use are calcitriol (Rocatrol) and alfacalcidol (One-alpha).

CALCIFICATION is the process of deposit of lime salts.

CALCITONIN is a hormone produced by the thyroid gland (qv) which lowers the concentration of calcium in the blood.

CALCIUM is the metallic element present in chalk and other forms of lime. The chief preparations used in medicine are calcium carbonate (chalk), calcium chloride, calcium gluconate, calcium hydroxide (slaked lime), liquor of calcium hydroxide (lime-water), calcium lactate, and calcium phosphate (see LIME). Although still commonly used in the treatment of chilblains, there is little evidence that calcium is of any real value in this condition. Calcium gluconate is freely soluble in water and is used in conditions in which calcium should be given by injection.

Calcium is a most important element in diet; the chief sources of it are milk and cheese. Calcium is especially needed by the growing child and the pregnant and nursing mother.

The recommended daily intakes of calcium are: 500 mg for children, 700 mg for adolescents, 500–900 mg for adults and 1200 mg for pregnant or nursing mothers.

CALCIUM ANTAGONISTS. The influx of calcium is particularly important in the contraction of cardiac and smooth muscle cells. In cardiac muscle it occurs through specialized slow channels during the plateau of the action potential. Analagous channels are important in arterial smooth muscle. The calcium antagonists inhibit the movement of calcium across the cell membrane. Because they relax smooth muscle they have important applications in the treatment of hypertension and angina of effort. Four calcium antagonists are currently available in the United Kingdom. Verapamil (Cordilox) has been available since 1967, nifedipine (Adalat) since 1977, and diltiazem (Tildiem) and lidoflazine (Clinium) were introduced in 1984. All four drugs are rapidly and completely absorbed but undergo extensive first pass metabolism in the liver so that bioavailability is only around 20 per cent. The calcium antagonists are effective in the treatment of angina, both by their action in dilating coronary arteries and also by dilating peripheral arterioles and so reducing cardiac work. They are also effective in the treatment of hypertension by virtue of their effect in dilating arterioles. Their hypotensive effect is additive with that of a Beta-blocker. Only verapamil is effective in cardiac arrhythmias and is the drug of choice in terminating supra ventricular tachycardia. These drugs are particularly useful in patients in whom a Beta-blocker is contra-indicated.

CALCIUM CARBIMIDE is a drug used in the treatment of alcoholism that has the same action as disulfiram (qv) but produces a milder reaction.

CALCULI is the general name given to concretions in, for example, the bladder, kidneys, gall-bladder.

CALIBRE is a talking book service which is available to all blind and handicapped people who can supply a doctor's certificate certifying that they are unable to read printed books in the normal way. Its catalogue contains over 370 books for adults and over 250 for children, and additions are being made at the rate of around three a week. Full details can be obtained from Calibre, Aylesbury, Bucks HP20 1HU (0296 32339 81211).

CALLIPER is a two-pronged instrument with pointed ends, for the measurement of diameters, such as that of the pelvis in obstetrics.

CALLIPER SPLINT is one that is applied to the broken leg in such a way that in walking the weight of the body is taken by the hip bone and not by the foot.

CALLOSITIES are thickenings of the outer skin or epidermis. (See CORNS.)

CALLUS is the new tissue formed round the ends of a broken bone. (See FRACTURES.)

CALOMEL, or SUBCHLORIDE OF MERCURY, is not to be confused with corrosive sublimate or perchloride of mercury, a far more active drug and deadly poison. It is a powerful purgative. (See MERCURY.)

CALORIE is the name applied to a unit of energy. Two units are called by this name. The small calorie, or gram calorie, is the amount of heat required to raise one gram of water one degree centigrade in temperature. The large Calorie or kilocalorie, which is used in the study of dietetics and physiological processes, is the amount of heat required to raise one kilogram of water one degree centigrade in temperature. The number of Calories required to carry on the processes necessary for life and body warmth, such as the beating of the heart, the movements of the chest in breathing, and the chemical activities of the secreting glands, is, for an adult person of ordinary weight, somewhere in the neighbourhood of 1600 Calories. For ordinary sedentary occupations an individual requires about 2500 Calories, for light muscular work slightly over 3000 Calories, and for hard continuous labour about 4000 Calories daily.

Under the International System of Units (SI) (see WEIGHTS AND MEASURES) the kilocalorie has been replaced by the joule, the abbreviation for which is J (1 kilocalorie=4186·8 J). As the term calorie, however, is so well established in medical writing, it has been retained in this edition. Conversion from Calories (or kilocalories) is made by multiplying by 4·186, but a factor of 4·2 is simpler and accurate enough for all practical purposes.

CALUMBA is a bitter. (See BITTERS.)

CALVARIA is another name for the skull cap or vault of the head.

CALX is another name for lime or chalk. It is an old term for the heel.

CALYX means a cup-shaped cavity, the term being especially applied to the recesses of the pelvis of the kidney.

CAMPHINE is another name for oil of turpentine.

CAMPHOR is a solid, crystalline, oily substance distilled from the wood of a species of laurel grown in Japan and Formosa, or made synthetically. It is sold in the form of cubes, or in powder known as flowers of camphor.

Uses: Externally, it is placed among bed-clothes to keep off fleas, lice, and other insect pests, but for this purpose it has now been largely replaced by more efficient insecticides. In gout, and various painful skin conditions, it is rubbed up with menthol, thymol or salol to form an oily liquid which can be smeared over the surface with great relief. Liniment of camphor and camphorated oil (28·5 G of camphor in 228 ml of olive oil) is likewise useful in painful conditions or as a mild counter-irritant to produce a warm glow when rubbed into the chest in bronchitis and similar conditions.

Internally, spirit of camphor in 5 to 30 drop doses and camphor water in tablespoonful doses are used to relieve spasms like hiccup and colic.

Dissolved in oil camphor, is sometimes used by hypodermic injection in the treatment of serious heart failure, but this practice has died out in Britain.

CAMPYLOBACTER is a species of micro-organism found in farm and pet animals, and there is increasing evidence of its transmission from such sources to man. Outbreaks of infection with it have occurred following the drinking of unpasteurized milk from infected cows and eating undercooked meat and poultry. It causes diarrhoea, and it is considered that it may be responsible for 8 per cent of sporadic cases of infective diarrhoea as a result of the inflammation of the small intestine (enteritis) that it produces. During 1981 over 12000 cases were reported in England, but the true prevalence is said to be much greater.

CANALICULUS means a small channel, and is applied to (*a*) the minute passage leading from the lacrimal pore on each eyelid to the lacrimal sac on the side of the nose; (*b*) any one of the minute canals in bone.

CANCELLOUS is a term applied to loose bony tissues as found in the ends of the long bones.

CANCER, CARCINOMA and SARCOMA are general names for forms of tumour to which the term 'malignant' is applied. They are differentiated from benign tumours by four principal criteria: (1) They are not encapsulated, or surrounded by a capsule, and they invade and destroy the tissues in which they arise. (2) They have an unlimited power of disorderly reproduction, quite unlike the orderly way in which the healthy cells of an organ are reproduced. (3) Their cells usually show some loss of differentiation of structure and tend to become more like primitive cells. (4) They are capable of producing metastases, or secondary growths, at a distance from the parent, or primary, tumour. Cancer or carcinoma is composed mainly of epithelial cells, or cells similar to those of skin or of the mucous membrane lining the stomach and bowels, or of secreting glands; but these cells are imperfect in form and arrangement, although they generally retain their characters sufficiently to allow of the organ from which they have come being recognized when a section of the cancer is examined under the microscope. A sarcoma is a tumour developing in the connective tissue of bones, muscles, sinews, etc., and in structure resembling imperfect connective tissue. Sarcoma is less common than cancer in the proportion of about one case of the former to twenty of the latter.

Cancers are classified mainly according to the structure they present on microscopic examination. A cancer growing on skin surface is generally known as an EPITHELIOMA. A cancer arising in the stomach or intestine and presenting an appearance resembling imperfectly formed gland tubules is known as ADENOCARCINOMA. A cancer composed almost entirely of cells without supporting tissue is known as a SOFT CANCER. One in which the cells are much compressed and obliterated by development of fibrous tissue is known as a HARD or SCIRRHUS CANCER; these occur particularly in the breast. Various degenerations also occur in cancers, such as glue-like degeneration (COLLOID CANCER), cystic degeneration, calcareous degeneration. Sarcoma is classified into ROUND-CELLED SARCOMA, SPINDLE-CELLED SARCOMA, etc., according to the microscopic appearances.

Causes: The cause of malignant growths is still undiscovered. Many theories have been advanced, and, considering the fact that cancer is gradually becoming more frequent, it has become of great importance to establish the nature of the cause as a first step towards prevention and treatment. Much has been done in the last few years by various cancer research laboratories to increase our knowledge as to the distribution of cancer in the animal kingdom and among different races, and also to study the mode of spread and conditions of growth in this disease. Cancers occur in animals as well as among human beings, and no race is exempt.

It has been found by experiments on animals that cancer can be transferred directly from one animal to another by inoculating a healthy animal with a small piece of cancerous tissue, and it has further been found that, when transferred in this way through a long succession of animals, the type of cancer produced remains always the same. An important step was taken by Japanese workers who found that cancer could be produced in experimental animals by painting the skin with tar. British workers then isolated the actual chemical substance in tar which produces the cancer, and it was found that this substance is chemically similar to substances present in the healthy body. Does some chemical twist take place and make these normal substances carcinogenic or cancer-producing? Another important factor to be investigated is infection. Many micro-organisms have been incriminated, but the only one that has stood the test of serious investigation is the virus. For example, there is a type of cancer in fowls which is caused by a virus. There is, however, no present evidence that any human cancer is caused by a virus, though viruses are associated with lymphoma (qv). It is also possible that viruses may play a part in the development of some forms of acute leukaemia (qv), of cancer of the breast and of cancer of the cervix uteri, as well as some sarcomas. Another factor in the causation of cancer is the influence of the hormones of the ductless glands. It appears, for example, that the female sex hormone has an effect on the development of breast cancer. Still another factor is heredity. All this, and other work, suggest that cancer is not one disease with one cause, but an abnormal reaction of the tissues to a variety of exciting agents. Some scientists have supposed that no external cause is necessary, but that in early or embryonic life parts of the developing body come to rest, only to start sudden and irregular growth at a later period of life. The structure of some cancers, in which a cancerous growth develops in one part of the body resembling an embryonic structure or some other organ at a distance, lends support to this view.

Several factors are important considerations in the origin of the disease.

OCCUPATION: With the increasing complexity of many industrial processes, evidence is accumulating as to the risk of some of these processes inducing cancer. Thus it is now known that workers with asbestos, vinyl chloride and certain rubber-manufacturing processes, as well as some wool workers, run a higher risk of developing cancer than other members of the community. (See OCCUPATIONAL DISEASES.)

INJURY: Smoking a clay pipe has been observed to bring on cancer of the lip, constant alcoholic indulgence to favour cancer of the throat and stomach, while a scar, eg. of an old ulcer, may be the starting-point. Chimney-sweeps, paraffin workers, and workers in some other special employments have a liability to cancer of the skin, apparently from long-continued irritation. It has also been found by experiments on animals that the prolonged application of tar to an area of skin may result ultimately in development of cancer. There does not seem any reason to suppose that cancer follows mechanical damage caused by a blow or wound, although there is ground for the belief that sarcoma occasionally follows some severe injury, such as fracture of a bone.

LOCALITY: There are undoubtedly wide variations in the incidence of cancer in different parts of the country, apart from the fact that death rates for a given age are higher in urban than in rural areas. The explanation of these geographical differences is still not known.

HEREDITY: Although, strictly speaking, there is no evidence that, in man, cancer is inherited, there is a growing volume of evidence that there may be a familial tendency to develop cancer. Thus, it has been shown that women with carcinoma of the breast or of the uterus have a larger proportion of female relatives with such cancers than would be expected in women in general.

AGE: Cancer is rare before adolescence, the commonest age being between fifty and sixty years. Although cancer is tending to increase in prevalence, there appears from the returns of the Registrar General for England to be no tendency for the number of persons affected below the age of forty-five years to rise, and cancer is now more a disease of old age than formerly. Sarcoma is commoner in younger persons.

SEX: In 1986, in England, the deaths from malignant disease in men were 72,943, compared with 66,146 in women. These figures correspond to a crude death-rate per million living of 2859 males and 2859 females. There is a marked difference in the site of cancer in the two sexes. Thus, in males the most commonly involved site is the lungs, followed by the stomach and the prostate. In women, on the other hand, the breasts and uterus account for one-third of all cancers. The lungs and the larynx are much less commonly involved among women than among men.

CIGARETTE SMOKING: According to the United States Surgeon General (1982) cigarette smoking is the major single cause of cancer mortality in the United States. Tobacco's contribution to all cancer deaths is estimated to be 30 per cent. Reports from the Royal College of Physicians of London have confirmed that smoking is the main cause of lung cancer.

INCIDENCE: Around three out of every ten persons will have contracted cancer at some time in their lives and that two of these three people will die from cancer while the third will die from some other cause.

Symptoms: These vary according to the organs with which the growth interferes. Thus cancer of the stomach tends to cause dyspepsia and, it may be, severe pain; cancer in the bowels is apt to lead to gradually increasing obstruction, which may produce either diarrhoea or constipation; cancer affecting the jaw is apt to set up neuralgia; when the growth originates in the womb, flooding is one of the principal early symptoms; when pressure is exercised upon a vein, dropsy results, and so forth. When the growth takes place on the surface there is a hard swelling, which in time is liable to break down and ulcerate. In all cases, the growth tends to spread by the lymphatic vessels, and the glands in the neighbourhood soon become affected by secondary growths if the original one be not speedily removed. This applies especially to cancer, and is one reason why cancer is so liable to return after apparently complete removal. Sarcoma tends less to spread along the lymphatic vessels, but occasionally minute fragments are carried away to distant organs in the circulating blood. When a cancer begins to ulcerate by invading the skin or an internal mucous membrane, a state of poor health and weakness, called cachexia, results. The duration of symptoms of cancer is extremely variable. When the stomach is affected, these seldom last much longer than six months. When the breast is affected, the duration may be very much longer, especially if the main part of the growth has been removed, and life is then often prolonged for many years. The same applies to cancer of the rectum, when an artificial opening is made so that the growth is not irritated by the passage over it of intestinal contents.

Diagnosis: The earlier cancer is detected, the likelier is it to respond to treatment. Thus all methods available for early diagnosis should be encouraged and practised by both doctors, and patients. In the case of cancer of the breast, the commonest form of cancer in women, the breasts should be palpated regularly and, if a lump is felt, this should be reported at once to the doctor. Other methods for early detection of cancer of the breast are thermography (qv) and mammography (qv). Early detection of cancer of the cervix of the uterus is facilitated by cervical cytology (see UTERUS, DISEASES OF), whilst every woman subject to persistent irregular bleeding from the womb at the menopause should consult her doctor lest this be a sign of cancer. Similarly any middle-aged man or woman with persistent dyspepsia, especially if accompanied by loss of weight, should seek medical advice to exclude cancer of the stomach. More technical devices for this purpose are what are known as 'tumour markers', such as the serum acid phosphatase in cancer of the prostate, calcitonin (qv) in cancer of the thyroid, and chorionic gonadotrophin (see GONADOTROPHIN) in choriocarcinoma (qv).

Mortality: Cancer now stands second in importance as a cause of death, having in England and Wales, in 1984 caused 73,000 deaths as compared with 137,000 due to circulatory heart disease.

About 140,000 new cases of cancer are reported in England and Wales each year, which is equivalent to 29 per 10,000 population. Deaths from cancer accounted for 24 per cent of all deaths in England in 1980. In the same year out of every 1000 cancer deaths in men the site of the cancer was the lung in 391, the stomach in 92 and the intestine in 111. In women the most common site was the breast (201), followed by the lung (141), the stomach (74), the uterus (19), and the cervix of the uterus (34).

The increase in cancer is partly explained by the fact that diagnosis is now more precise and many deaths are registered as due to cancer which formerly would have been attributed to 'old age', 'obstruction of the bowels', etc.; and partly by the fact that more people now reach the ages at which cancer prevails.

Treatment: It should be strongly urged that any person finding a hard swelling under the skin should consult a doctor. In the event of the swelling not being cancer, mental relief will be gained; and if it be cancer, there is at an early stage the chance of the only completely successful remedy at present known: that is thorough removal. The improvement of modern surgical technique and early diagnosis leads now to the possibility of operations which greatly prolong the life of persons affected by cancer, and in some cases permit of permanent recovery. This is admirably demonstrated in the table below, which shows the percentage of patients surviving five years after operation for cancer. Thus it will be seen, for example, that in the case of cancer of the breast, 78 per cent of those diagnosed and treated at an early stage of the disease were alive and well without any signs of cancer five years later, compared with only 6 per cent not diagnosed and treated until a later stage. In the case of certain internal cancers, eg. of the stomach, attempts at complete removal have not, taking all cases together, attained a great measure of success, but much can be done in the way of operations designed for relief of symptoms, which thus prolong life. Much greater success has attended modern operations for complete removal of cancer of the breast and the womb.

	Diagnosed and treated early	*Diagnosed and treated late*
Breast	78	6
Larynx	88	20
Mouth	69	11
Skin	90	14
Cervix uteri	83	3

Percentages of patients with cancer of different parts of the body alive and well with no signs of cancer 5 years after treatment.

Many 'cures' have from time to time been vaunted, such as arsenic paste, turpentine, injections of trypsin, adrenaline and lead salts, but these have all proved useless on trial. In many cases much benefit accrues from combined treatment by surgery, X-rays, and other forms of radiotherapy. (See RADIUM; RADIOTHERAPY; X-RAYS.) Radioactive isotopes are also proving of value in many cases. (See ISOTOPES.)

The most recent development in the treatment of cancer, is chemotherapy. Several chemical substances have been discovered to have an effect on malignant tumours. The major problem here is that, though there are now over thirty anti-cancer drugs, most of them not only damage or kill cancer cells, but also have a harmful effect on the normal cells of the body. They are therefore potentially dangerous and must be used with the greatest of care. Even so there are now at least ten types of cancer which can be cured by chemotherapy in a proportion of patients. These include some of the leukaemias (qv), Hodgkin's disease (qv), choriocarcinoma (qv), and some forms of cancer in childhood.

In the terminal care of patients with inoperable cancer the three essentials are loving care, good nursing and the administration of adequate doses of pain-relieving drugs. It is in providing such care that the modern hospice (qv) is proving so valuable. On the other hand it is a regime that can put considerable strain on the relatives should the patient be nursed at home. Such relatives who are finding the strain too great will obtain valuable help and advice from either The Marie Curie Memorial Foundation, 28 Belgrave Square, London SW1X 8QG (01–235 3325), Cancer Relief Macmillan Fund, Anchor House, 15/19 Britten Street, London SW3 3TY (01–351 7811), or the British Association of Cancer United Patients, 121–123 Charterhouse Street, London EC1M 6AA (01–608 1661 for information).

CANCRUM ORIS, also called WATER CANKER or NOMA, is a gangrenous ulcer about the mouth which affects weakly children, especially after some severe disease, such as measles. It is due to the growth of bacteria in the tissues.

CANDICIDIN is an antibiotic produced by a strain of *Streptomycesgriseus*, which is proving of value in the treatment of certain fungal infections such as candidiasis (qv).

CANDIDA: CANDIDIASIS or MONILIASIS is an infection due to the fungus *Candida albicans*. It is the most common fungal infection. When it infects the mouth it is called thrush and appears as white patches on the throat and tongue. Although it can occur in any debilitated patient, it is particularly common in individuals on prolonged antibiotic treatment. It is cured by the anti-fungal agent Nystatin given as lozenges so that it is retained in the mouth. Candida infections are also common in skin folds and the vulva. Candida is also a common cause of vaginal infection which presents as a vaginal discharge and responds to Nystatin pessaries. Generalized fungal infection may occur in individuals in whom the immune system is compromised, as in patients with AIDS or patients on immunosuppressive drugs. Such more generalized infections require systemic treatment with the anti-fungal drug Ketoconazole given by mouth or Amphotericin by intravenous injection.

CANINE TEETH, or EYE-TEETH, (see TEETH).

CANITIES is the term applied to whitening or greying of the hair (qv).

CANKER is the name applied to small ulcers which form about the mouth and lips as the result of some local irritation, eg. a jagged tooth, or in a condition of dyspepsia and deteriorated general health. (See MOUTH, DISEASES OF.)

CANNABIS INDICA, consists of the flowering tops of *Cannabissativa*.

CANNABIS It is one of the oldest euphoriants. Cannabis does not cause physical dependence but its abuse leads to passivity, apathy and inertia. Acute adverse effects of cannabis include transient panic reactions and toxic psychoses. The panic reactions are characterised by anxiety, helplessness and loss of control and may be accompanied by florid paranoid thoughts and hallucinations. The toxic psychoses are characterised by the sudden onset of confusion and visual hallucinations. Even at lower doses cannabis can precipitate functional psychoses in vulnerable individuals. The acute physical manifestations of short-term cannabis abuse are conjunctival suffusion and tachycardia.

CANNED FOOD, originally popularized in the United States of America, had to overcome considerable prejudice in Great Britain. Such prejudice still persists to a certain extent but, irrespective of the merits of the controversy of fresh versus preserved food, it must be recognized that the advantages of canned food far outweigh the disadvantages. Modern methods of canning are so efficient that not only is the purity of the food preserved but its nutritional value is retained. There is, of course, some loss of vitamin content but this has been much reduced of recent years. Indeed there is probably less loss of vitamins in canning than in average domestic cooking. The further great advantage of canning is that it makes available to many people foodstuffs which otherwise they either would never be able to obtain or could only obtain at certain seasons of the year.

Methods of canning vary according to the foodstuff, but the two essentials of all canning processes are (1) heat treatment of the food and (2) expulsion of all air, after which the can is hermetically sealed. One of the major problems in canning is achieving the optimum temperature that will kill all bacteria but will not affect the nutritive value of the food or spoil its taste. A step to cope with this problem is the introduction of aseptic canning, in which the food is sterilized before it is sealed in sterilized cans. Many canned foods will keep for long periods: eg. canned fish, meat preparations and soups will keep for two years. These, however, are safer figures. Cans of up to 20 years of age have been found to be in good condition, and the contents quite edible.

DANGERS OF CANNED FOOD: Outbreaks of food poisoning caused by canned food are relatively rare unless the food is contaminated after the container is opened, though, as Aberdeen learned to its cost, outbreaks of typhoid fever can occur as a result of the contamination of the contents of cans cooled in contaminated water. And, in 1979, there were several outbreaks of staphylococcal food poisoning in England due to the consumption of faultily canned corned beef from Brazil. In 1960–63 (inclusive), in England and Wales, 63 of the 749 outbreaks of food poisoning, for which information was available, were due to canned food: canned meat on 44 occasions, canned fish on 13 occasions, and canned vegetables on six occasions. The organism most commonly responsible was the staphylococcus. In other cases decomposition of canned fish or meat

may occur due to faulty cans, whilst the acid in fruits or vegetables may lead to erosion of faulty tinplate or soldering, with contamination of the foodstuff with tin or lead.
EXAMINATION OF CANNED FOOD: Most cases of poisoning with canned food could be avoided if cans were examined before use. Canned food is carefully inspected either in the canning factory, if made in this country, or at the port of entry, if imported. About 1·5 per cent of canned meat is rejected in this country. It is a sound rule never to buy a canned food which does not bear a manufacturer's name. Another sound rule is that good cans usually contain good food. Any can which is leaking should be immediately discarded, and much rusting should be regarded with suspicion. 'Blowing', or bulging of the ends of the can, is the most important sign of a faulty can, but this must be differentiated from the bulging of one side of a can due to an indentation in the opposite side. Tapping of a sound can should produce a dull note; if the note is drum-like, this suggests gas-formation in the can due to decomposition. Shaking should produce no sound in a can of meat, but this test, of course, is of no value in the case of canned fruit, which contains syrup. If on opening the can an unpleasant or a stale odour is noted, or if, in the case of meat, there is a loss of firmness of the contents or a fading of the colour, the contents should be discarded.

CANNULA is a tube for insertion into the body, designed to fit tightly round a trocar, a sharp pointed instrument which is withdrawn from the cannula after insertion, so that fluid may run out through the latter.

CANTHARIDES, or SPANISH FLY, is a powder made of the body and wings of a dried beetle, *Cantharis vesicatoria*, which inhabits Spain, Italy, Sicily and Southern Russia.
Action: It is an irritant, first, to the part with which it is brought in contact, and, secondly, to the genital and urinary organs by which it is discharged from the body.
Uses: Its only use is for blistering (see BLISTERS), and it may be applied as a plaster, in a paste, or painted on in ethereal solution called liquor epispasticus but it is seldom used now.

CANTHUS is the name applied to the angle at either end of the aperture between the eyelids.

CAPBENICILLIN (see ANTIBIOTIC).

CAPILLARIES are the minute vessels which join the ends of the arteries to the commencement of the veins. Their walls consist of a single layer of fine, flat transparent cells, bound together at the edges, and the vessels form a mesh-work all through the tissues of the body, bathing the latter in blood with only the thin capillary wall interposed, through which gases and fluids readily pass. These vessels are less than 0·025 mm in width. (See CIRCULATION OF THE BLOOD.)

CAPREOMYCIN is an antibiotic derived from *Streptomycescapreolus*, which is proving of value in the treatment of tuberculosis.

CAPSICUM, or CAYENNE PEPPER, consists of the dried fruits of *Capsicum minimum* and small-fruited varieties of *C.frutescens*. It is irritating when applied either internally or to the skin.
Uses: Externally the powdered pepper is used in an ointment, or in the form of 'Chillie paste', to rub over sprains and bruises, the discoloration of which it helps to remove. Internally, tincture of capsicum is given for some forms of dyspepsia, and is said to be useful (in 15-drop doses before meals) to allay the craving for alcohol.

CAPSULE is a term used in several senses in medicine. The term is applied to a soluble case, usually of gelatine, for enclosing small doses of unpleasant medicine. *Enteric-coated capsules*, which have been largely superseded by enteric-coated tablets, are capsules treated in such a manner that the ingredients do not come in contact with the acid stomach contents but are only released when the capsule disintegrates in the alkaline contents of the intestine.

The term is also applied to the fibrous or membranous envelope of various organs, as of the spleen, liver or kidney. It is also applied to the ligamentous bag surrounding various joints and attached by its edge to the bones on either side.

CAPTOPRIL is a drug that has been introduced for the treatment of patients with severe hypertension (qv) resistant to other hypertensive agents. It acts by lowering the concentration in the blood of angiotensin II which is one of the factors responsible for high blood-pressure. (See ANGIOTENSIN; RENIN.)

CAPUT MEDUSAE is the term describing the abnormally dilated veins that form round the umbilicus in cirrhosis of the liver.

CAPUT SUCCEDANEUM is the temporary swelling which is sometimes found on the head of the new-born infant. It is due to oedema in and around the scalp, caused by pressure on the head as the child is born. It is of no significance and quickly disappears spontaneously.

CARAWAY FRUIT, generally called caraway seed, is used to prepare caraway water and caraway oil. A tablespoonful of the former or 2 drops of the latter on sugar is useful for checking colic, griping pains in children, and flatulence.

CARBACHOL is a drug which stimulates the parasympathetic nervous system. It is given, for example, for paralysis of the gut and for retention of urine due to atony.

CARBAMAZEPINE is a drug which is proving of value in the treatment of trigeminal neuralgia (see TRIGEMINAL NEURALGIA). It is also of value in the treatment of certain cases of epilepsy. Because of its occasional action in causing aplastic anaemia and jaundice it must only be used under careful medical supervision.

CARBARYL is a broad-spectrum insecticide effective against lice. It was introduced because lice began to show resistance to DDT and gamma benzene hexachloride. It is particularly effective against head lice. (See INSECTS IN RELATION TO DISEASE.)

CARBENICILLIN (see PENICILLIN).

CARBENOXOLONE is a derivative of glycyrrhetinic acid, the active principle of liquorice, which is proving of value in the treatment of gastric ulcer.

CARBIMAZOLE is at present one of the most widely used drugs in the treatment of hyperthyroidism. It acts by interferring with the synthesis of thyroid hormone in the thyroid gland.

CARBOHYDRATE is the term applied to an organic substance in which the hydrogen and oxygen are usually in the proportion to form water. Carbohydrates are all, chemically considered, derivatives of simple forms of sugar and are classified as monosaccharides (eg. glucose), disaccharides (eg. cane sugar), polysaccharides (eg. starch). Many of the cheaper and most important foods are included in this group, which comprises sugars, starches, celluloses and gums. When one of these foods is digested, it is converted into a simple kind of sugar and absorbed in this form. In the disease known as diabetes mellitus (qv), the most marked feature consists of an inability on the part of the tissues to assimilate and utilize the carbohydrate material. Each gram of carbohydrate is capable of furnishing slightly over 4 Calories of energy. (See DIET.)

CARBOLIC ACID, or PHENOL, is a coal-tar preparation, first introduced into medicine by Lord Lister.

Action: Carbolic acid first paralyses and then destroys all forms of life, having a specially destructive action upon lowly organisms like bacteria. It has a softening action upon tissues, pus, etc., and it also vaporizes readily, so that it has much greater penetrating power than alcohol, perchloride of mercury, and other powerful antiseptics, which have a hardening action that retards their germicidal power. It dulls pain when applied to an inflamed part, by benumbing the nerves around.

It must never be forgotten that pure carbolic acid, or even a weak lotion too long applied, may painlessly kill the skin and cause it to slough. This effect is lessened by smearing the damaged part with glycerin or with oil.

Internally it has similar actions, and even in moderate doses it is a poison, being first of all an irritant and on absorption a narcotic.

Carbolic acid is used as a standard antiseptic for comparison of the power of other substances to kill germs.

Uses: Because of the risk of producing gangrene or ulceration, carbolic acid must never be used in a compress or dressing on the skin. In the pure form it is sometimes used as a cauterizing agent to sterilize septic areas. In the pure form it is also used in minute amounts in the treatment of ulcers of the cornea. In very weak solution it is used as a throat gargle. As a 2½per cent solution in glycerin it is useful in treatment of infections of the ear. A further use is in the treatment of haemorrhoids and varicose veins. As a 1 per cent lotion it is of value in the treatment of itching conditions of the skin.

As a disinfectant 1 in 20 of water (or 5 per cent) is the convenient strength, and is used to put in the bottom of the sputum-dish of consumptives, to steep the sheets soiled by typhoid-fever cases, to swab the floors and walls of sickrooms. Lysol is now more commonly used for this purpose.

CARBOLIC ACID POISONING may be due to accident or suicide. No bottle containing carbolic lotion should ever be kept near other medicine bottles, as a few teaspoonfuls may cause death.

Carbolic acid poisoning may also come on slowly through gradual absorption from dressings by a wound. The urine generally is black for a day or two before the case gets serious.

Symptoms: If the acid has been swallowed there is a sense of burning about the mouth and throat, followed by numbness, and the skin and mucous membrane of the mouth show white where the acid has touched them. Unconsciousness and stupor soon come on, and death follows usually in a few hours.

Treatment: Olive oil, or any fatty substance like milk or cream, should be administered at once, and the stomach washed out or emptied by an emetic in several tumblerfuls of tepid water. Large doses are also given internally of Epsom salts or sulphate of magnesium, which combines with the carbolic acid and renders it harmless.

CARBON DIOXIDE, or CARBONIC ACID, is the gas formed by the tissues and exhaled by the lungs (see AIR and VENTILATION). It effervesces from aerated waters and sparkling wines, and is used in baths for stimulation to the skin (see BATHS). Carbon dioxide in cylinders, combined with oxygen, is used to control breathing in anaesthesia and in cases of carbon monoxide poisoning.

CARBON DIOXIDE SNOW is formed when carbon dioxide (CO_2), stored under pressure in a cylinder, is allowed to escape through a small nozzle. This sudden expansion lowers its temperature to about −70°C and the CO_2 is obtained as a white powder or 'snow', which is then compressed into a cake or tube for application to the skin. It is a most effective method of freezing a localized area, and is commonly used in the treatment of warts (qv).

CARBON MONOXIDE is a colourless and odourless gas, the presence of which in a room is undetectable by the occupants. Hence its danger because it has 300 times the affinity for oxygen that haemoglobin (qv) has. It converts haemoglobin into carboxyhaemoglobin, and thereby deprives the tissues of the body of oxygen, as there is no haemoglobin left to pick up oxygen in the lungs and carry it throughout the body. Being odourless the unfortunate occupants of the room – or garage – have no idea that they are breathing it, and therefore they cannot take avoiding action by turning off the source of the carbon monoxide or getting out into fresh air. The result is that they become unconscious in the contaminated atmosphere and, all too often, by the time they are found, they are dead. Carbon monoxide has a special action on the ganglia at the base of the brain, and, if sufficient amounts are inhaled, permanent destructive changes occur in this vital part of the nervous system. What makes carbon monoxide poisoning all the more dangerous is its insidious onset, which so impairs the mental faculties at an early stage that, in the words of one expert, 'the person affected may be brought to the very verge of unconsciousness without appreciating in the least degree that anything is wrong'. Hitherto one of the commonest causes of carbon monoxide has been coal gas, particularly if inadequately combusted in a badly ventilated room, as in a water heater in a bathroom, but this risk has been brought under control in Britain as a result of the introduction of so-called natural gas, which contains no carbon monoxide. This, however, does not mean that natural gas is absolutely safe in this respect. It still suffers from the defect of all carbon-containing fuel, whether coal, oil, coke, wood, or manufactured (or town) gas or natural gas. This is that when burned in the absence of sufficient oxygen, or, whenever, for any reason, combustion is incomplete, carbon monoxide is formed. In the case of gas the risk is particularly high with water heaters in inadequately ventilated bathrooms, and with portable gas fires. The gas industry no longer permits the use or sale of the latter, but unfortunately there are still an unknown number in use. Anyone who owns such a portable gas fire should get rid of it at once. So far as gas water heaters in bathrooms are concerned, it is essential to ensure that it has a flue and that this is adequate and is neither blocked nor faulty. Three golden rules recommended by one of the British Gas Boards for the use of gas water heaters are:

1. Do not block any permanent means of ventilation, eg. an air-vent.
2. Leave the window or door open while the water heater is in use.
3. Turn off the gas before entering the bath.

The same care about maintaining adequate ventilation must be observed with all forms of heating derived from carbon-containing fuel, as listed above. Perhaps the greatest risk in this respect today is from the use of oil heaters in rooms in which all sources of ventilation, such as windows and ventilators, have, for all practical purposes, been hermetically sealed. This is one of the major reasons why deaths in the home from carbon monoxide poisoning, other than piped gas, have increased fivefold in the last two decades. Coke braziers are yet another recurring cause of carbon monoxide poisoning. Not the least important, however, is the exhaust gas of petrol vehicles. This is why the engine of a car must *never* be switched on in a garage unless the garage doors are open, and the car must be run out into the open air the moment the engine has been started. A further useful precaution is always to run the car into a garage front first, so that the exhaust pipe is jutting out towards the open air. The main manifestations of carbon monoxide poisoning are shown in the table below. One of the most striking signs of carbon monoxide poisoning is the cherry-red appearance of the victim's face. This is due to the large amount of carboxyhaemoglobin in the blood.

Carbon monoxide, which has a deleterious effect on arteries, aggravating the arterial disease which occurs in high blood-pressure (see

Degree of saturation of haemoglobin with carbon monoxide per cent	*Signs and symptoms*
0 to 10	No symptoms
10 to 20	Tightness across the forehead Possibly headache Flushed skin Yawning
20 to 30	Headache Dizziness Palpitations on exercise
30 to 40	Severe headache Weakness Dizziness Nausea Collapse (possibly)
40 to 50	As above, with increased respiratory rate and pulse rate, and more possibility of collapse
50 to 60	Syncope Coma Cheyne-Stokes' respiration
60 to 70	Coma Weakened action of the heart and breathing Death imminent or actually takes place
70 to 80	Respiratory failure Death
90	Immediate arrest of the heart

The manifestations of carbon monoxide poisoning, according to the amount of carbon monoxide in the blood. The limit of safety is 18 to 20 per cent

ESSENTIAL HYPERTENSION) and coronary thrombosis (qv), is present in cigarette smoke. The concentration is lowest in low tar cigarettes and highest in middle tar cigarettes which should therefore be avoided.

Treatment of carbon monoxide poisoning consists of the immediate removal of the victim into the open air, followed by artificial respiration (qv) and, if available, the inhalation of oxygen and carbon dioxide. In this context 'immediate' means 'instant'. Speed is the essence of success, and may literally make all the difference between life and death. Artificial respiration should be given by the Schafer method, and the mixture of oxygen and carbon dioxide should contain 5 per cent of carbon dioxide. If the victim has been unconscious, he must rest in bed for the next twenty-four hours; otherwise there is a liability for him to collapse. Such collapse is particularly likely to occur on exertion.

CARBOXYHAEMOGLOBINAEMIA is the term applied to the state of the blood in carbon monoxide poisoning, in which this gas combines with the haemoglobin, displacing oxygen from it. (See CARBON MONOXIDE.)

CARBROMAL is a white powder with soporific action, given in doses of 300 mg to 1 G.

CARBUNCLE like a boil, is an infection of a hair follicle and sebaceous gland or of a sweat gland, but unlike a boil it does not remain localized but spreads more deeply. The infecting organism is usually a staphylococcus. (See BOILS; KIDNEYS, DISEASES OF.)

CARCINOGENESIS is the means or method whereby the changes responsible for the induction of cancer are brought about.

CARCINOMA is another name for cancer (qv).

CARDAMOM, AROMATIC TINCTURE OF, is a bright red fluid, prepared from the seeds of *Elettaria cardamomum*, useful to relieve spasm and flatulence, and much used to colour medicines. (See CARMINATIVES.)

CARDIA is a term applied to the upper opening of the stomach which lies immediately behind the heart.

CARDIAC DISEASE (see HEART DISEASES).

CARDIAC MASSAGE is the procedure used to restart the action of the heart if it is suddenly arrested. For long the only recognized method of doing this was by opening the chest wall and massaging the heart directly by hand. This is perfectly feasible if the heart stops beating during an operation. Elsewhere, however, it is seldom a practicable proposition.

Recently it has been shown that in many cases the arrested heart can be made to start beating again by rhythmic compression of the chest wall.

This is done by placing the patient on a hard surface – a table or the floor – and then placing the heel of the hand over the lower part of the sternum and compressing the chest wall firmly, but not too forcibly, at the rate of 60 to 80 times a minute. At the same time artificial respiration must be started by the mouth-to-mouth method. (See DROWNING, RECOVERY FROM.)

CARDIAC PACEMAKER: The rate and rhythm of the heart are controlled by a small collection of specialized nervous tissue known as the sinuatrial node, situated at the base of the heart (see HEART). This is the natural pacemaker of the heart – or cardiac pacemaker. When the impulse sent out by this pacemaker cannot reach all parts of the heart (a condition known as heart-block), the heart either stops or contracts in an irregular manner. (See HEART DISEASES.)

In these cases the natural pacemaker can be replaced by an artificial pacemaker which, for all practical purposes, is a battery which stimulates the heart and allows it to beat at normal speeds. Most pacemakers are powered by mercury cells. Batteries powered by lithium-iodide batteries are also available, as well as an isotope-powered one, the potential longevity of which is 20 to 30 years, compared with two years for mercury batteries and 10 years for lithium batteries. The majority of cardiac pacemaker units are normally adjusted to deliver 65 to 75 impulses a minute. The pacemaker is either fixed to the outside of the chest or implanted in the armpit, and connnected to an electrode catheter which is passed through the main vein in the neck, into the heart. Approximately one person in every 2000 of the population in the United Kingdom has a pacemaker.

Under the Motor Vehicles (Driving Licences) Amendment Regulations 1973, which came into force on January 1, 1974, patients with heart disease whose condition has been brought under control by the fitting of a pacemaker can be given a licence to drive provided they satisfy the following conditions: (a) that their driving vehicle is not likely to be a source of danger to the public; (b) that the applicant has made adequate arrangements to receive regular medical supervision by a cardiologist throughout the currency of the licence and is complying with these arrangements.

There are many possible sources of electrical interference with pacemakers. These include the anti-theft devices in shops and libraries, and airport weapon detectors. Surgical diathermy is a common source of interference. Short-wave heat treatment of the type used in physiotherapy departments should not be applied to pacemaker patients. Inhibition of what is known as a demand pacemaker by low frequency acupuncture has been reported, and some dental apparatus, including the ultrasonic cleaner, is a potential danger. Overall, however, the risks from interference are very slight. Their efficacy is demonstrated by the report from Guy's Hospital of pacemaker patients who have achieved county standard at athletics, competitive swimmers and scuba divers as well as many golfers.

CARDIOANGIOGRAPHY means rendering the outline of the heart visible on an X-ray film by injecting a radio-opaque substance into it.

CARDIOLOGY is the term applied to that branch of medical science devoted to the study of the diseases of the heart.

CARDIOMYOPATHIES are diseases of heart muscle of unknown cause. There are three distinct varieties: (1) *Hypertrophic cardiomyopathy* is characterised by massive ventricular hypertrophy. This hypertrophied muscle is not efficient and cannot relax adequately so that the ventricles do not fill properly during diastole. (2) *Congestive cardiomyopathy* is characterised by dilatation of both ventricles causing severe impairment of contraction. (3) *Restrictive cardiomyopathy* –organic material collects around the endocardium and myocardium which restricts the inflow of blood to the ventricles.

The disorder usually presents with congestive cardiac failure for which there does not appear to be a known cause.

CARDIOSPASM means the spasmodic contraction of the muscle surrounding the opening of the oesophagus into the stomach: also termed ACHALASIA OF THE CARDIA. (See OESOPHAGUS, DISEASES OF.)

CARFECILLIN (see PENICILLIN, ANTIBIOTIC).

CARIES, dental decay, is the material remaining after the calcified structure of the tooth has been removed in dental disease. This is probably initiated by bacteria. As the decay is removed a hole develops and the tooth may collapse.

CARINDICILLIN (see ANTIBIOTIC).

CARMINATIVES are preparations to relieve flatulence, and any resulting griping, by the bringing up of wind, or eructation (qv). Their essential constituent is an aromatic volatile oil, usually of vegetable extraction. As in the case of bitters, their precise mode of action is not known, but in practice, when swallowed, they induce a pleasant taste which may be accompanied by an increased flow of saliva. This is followed by a sensation of warmth as they are swallowed, and sooner or later there ensues the bringing up of wind. There is a large variety of carminatives, many of which are referred to elsewhere, such as caraway, cardamon, chamomile, cinnamon, cloves, dill, ginger, nutmeg and peppermint. Most of them are now used more for their flavouring effects either in medicine or in the kitchen, but, again as in the case of bitters, if used in moderation in correct dosage, they can undoubtedly help the individual to renew his or her interest in food, and thereby increase, or at least restore, his interest in life. Whether this is accompanied by the bringing up of wind is incidental.

CARNEOUS MOLE is an ovum which has died in the early months of pregnancy. It usually requires no treatment and evacuates itself.

CAROTENE is a colouring matter of carrots, other plants, butter and yolk of egg, and is the precursor of vitamin A, which is formed from carotene in the liver. (See VITAMIN.)

CAROTID BODY is a small reddish-brown structure measuring 5 to 7 × 2·5 to 4 millimetres, situated one on each side of the neck, where the carotid artery divides into the internal and external carotid arteries. Its main function is in controlling breathing so that an adequate supply of oxygen is maintained to the tissues of the body.

CARPAL TUNNEL SYNDROME is a condition characterized by attacks of pain and tingling in the first three or four fingers of one or both hands, which usually occur at night. It is caused by pressure on the median nerve as it passes under the strong ligament that lies across the front of the wrist. It often responds to rest induced by fixing the wrist in a plaster splint. If it does not respond to this treatment, the pressure is relieved by surgical division of the compressing ligament.

CARPUS is the Latin term for the wrist, composed of eight small bones firmly joined together with ligaments, but capable of a certain amount of sliding movement over one another. (See WRIST.)

CARRAGEEN, or IRISH MOSS, is derived from the sea-weed, *Chondrus crispus*. It is pleasantly soothing and in the form of a jelly is sometimes added to an invalid diet. Its main dietetic value is on account of the iron, calcium, and iodine which it contains.

CARRIERS OF DISEASE (see INFECTION).

CARTILAGE is a hard but pliant substance forming parts of the skeleton, eg. the cartilages of the ribs, of the larynx and of the ears. Microscopically, cartilage is found to consist of cells arranged in twos or in rows, and embedded in a ground-glass-like material devoid of blood-vessels and nerves. The end of every long bone has a smooth layer of cartilage on it where it forms a joint with other bones (articular cartilage), and in young persons up to about the age of sixteen there is a plate of cartilage (epiphyseal cartilage) running right across the bone about 12 mm (half an inch) from each end. The latter, by constantly thickening and changing into bone, causes the increase in length of the bone.

(See BONE.) In some situations there is found a combination of cartilage and fibrous tissue, as in the discs between the vertebrae of the spine. This fibro-cartilage, as it is known, combines the pliability of fibrous tissue with the elasticity of cartilage. (For cartilages of the knee, see KNEE.)

CARUNCLE is the name applied to any small fleshy eminence, whether normal or abnormal.

CASCARA SAGRADA is the bark derived from *Rhamnus purshiana*, or *Rhamnus frangula*, from which a liquid and a solid extract of powerful purgative action are prepared. The full dose for one administration is ½ to 1 teaspoonful of the liquid extract or 100 to 250 mg of the solid. But it is best taken in small doses of 5 or 10 drops of the fluid extract after each meal, or night and morning; gradually this may be decreased and finally left off, the bowels continuing regular in action. The elixir of cascara is a pleasanter preparation, of which the dose is ½to 1 teaspoonful.

CASCARILLA is an aromatic bitter tonic derived from the bark of *Croton eluteria* (see BITTERS). The dry bark has been used as a substitute for tobacco during attempts to break off the habit of smoking.

CASEATION is a process which takes place in the tissues in tuberculosis and some other chronic diseases. The central part of a diseased area, instead of changing into pus and so forming an abscess, changes to a firm cheese-like mass which may next be absorbed or may be converted into a calcareous deposit and fibrous tissue, and so healing results with the formation of a scar.

CASEIN is that part of milk which forms cheese or curds. It is produced by the union of a substance, caseinogen, dissolved in the milk, with lime salts also dissolved in the milk, the union being produced by the action of rennin, a ferment from the stomach of the calf. The same change occurs in the human stomach as the first step in the digestion of milk, and therefore when milk is vomited curdled it merely shows that digestion has begun.

CASTOR OIL is a thick colourless oil pressed from the seeds of *Ricinis communis*, the castor-oil plant. Owing to its general action over the whole intestine it is perhaps the best purgative for a single administration, though, in consequence of the fact that its action is often followed by slight constipation, it is unsuitable for frequently repeated use.

The dose for an adult is from one teaspoonful to two tablespoonfuls. To a child one year old a teaspoonful may be given. To help to disguise its nauseous flavour, the cup in which it is given should be scalded out with hot water, of which a little remains in the bottom; the oil is next poured in, and upon it a little brandy or whisky in the case of an adult. The oil may be then swallowed without leaving too much taste behind. In the case of a child, lemon juice may be substituted for the brandy or whisky.

CASTRATION is the operation for removal of the testicles or ovaries.

CASTS of hollow organs are found in various diseases. Membranous casts of the air passages are found in diphtheria and in one form of bronchitis, and are sometimes coughed up entire. Casts of the interior of the bowels are passed in cases of mucous colitis associated with constipation, and casts of the microscopic tubules in the kidneys passed in the urine form one of the surest signs of glomerulonephritis.

CATALEPSY is a term applied to a nervous affection characterized by the sudden suspension of sensation and volition, accompanied by a peculiar rigidity of the whole, or of certain muscles, of the body. The subjects of catalepsy are in most instances females of highly nervous or hysterical temperament. The exciting cause of an attack is usually mental emotion operating either suddenly, as in the case of a fright, or more gradually in the way of prolonged depression. Sometimes the typical features of the disease are exhibited in a state of complete insensibility, together with a statue-like appearance of the body, which will retain any attitude it may be made to assume during the continuance of the attack. In this condition the whole organic and vital functions appear to be reduced to the lowest possible limit consistent with life, and to such a degree as to simulate actual death. The attack may be of short duration, passing off within a few minutes. It may, however, last for many hours, and in rare instances persist for several days; and it is conceivable that in such cases the appearances presented might be mistaken for real death, as is alleged to have happened occasionally. Catalepsy is sometimes associated with epilepsy and with grave forms of mental disease. From what has been stated it follows that the successful treatment of such a disease as catalepsy must depend upon the due recognition of both its corporeal and mental relations. (See ECSTASY; HYSTERIA; SLEEP.)

CATAMENIA is another term for menstruation.

CATAPHORESIS is a method of treatment by introduction of medicine through the unbroken skin by means of an electric current. (See IONIZATION.)

CATAPLASM is another name for poultice.

CATAPLEXY is a condition in which the patient has a sudden attack of muscular weakness affecting the whole body. (See also NARCOLEPSY.)

CATARACT: An opacity of the lens.

Classification: One method is by the cause of cataract formation:

Age related (senile) With age, changes occur within the lens which render it gradually opaque. These changes begin at about the age of fifty years and are progressive at a variable rate during later life. Changes include lens protein aggregation, increased amounts of insoluble lens protein and increased pigmentation of the lens nucleus. These changes occur in eyes that are otherwise perfectly healthy (see AGE, NATURAL CHANGES IN).

Trauma (see EYE INJURIES): This is the commonest cause of monocular cataract in the young. Cataract may be the result of penetrating or blunt injury, infra-red energy, electric shock or ionizing radiation (the commonest cause is following irradiation of an ocular tumour).

Metabolic disorders: *Diabetes* can produce two types of cataract. The commoner is the 'age related' cataract which develops at an earlier age and is more rapidly progressive in diabetics than in non-diabetics. True diabetic cataracts can occur at any age. Other metabolic conditions associated with cataracts include *galactosaemia*, *Fabry's Disease*, *Wilson's Disease* and *hypoparathyroidism*.

Drugs can cause cataracts, in particular steroids.

Associated with other eye conditions, eg. *uveitis*, *acute glaucoma*, *retinitis pigmentosa*.

Congenital cataracts: These may be *hereditary*, ie. passed on genetically from one generation to the next. They may be present due to infection of the patient's mother during pregnancy. Typically *rubella* can cause cataracts in this way. Certain congenital syndromes are associated with cataracts, eg. *Down's syndrome*.

The acquired form of cataracts results in a progressive deterioration in vision. In senile cataracts this occurs fairly slowly over months or years. Traumatic cataracts can develop over a few hours with subsequent rapid loss of vision. Congenital cataracts are usually detected in routine examination of a child, or because there is a family history. Treatment of a cataract is undertaken for a variety of reasons: *(a)* in order to improve vision; *(b)* where the cataract is causing or is likely to cause complications that may damage the eye with consequent permanent loss of vision; *(c)* where the presence of a cataract may hinder treatment of other eye disorders because the doctor cannot see well enough through the cataract. Cataracts do not need to be removed just because they are there.

Types of cataract surgery: The two common forms of cataract extraction are (i) INTRACAPSULAR EXTRACTION: the zonule is first dissolved with chymotripsin (an enzyme) and the whole lens (capsule, cortex and nucleus) is removed in its entirety by means of a cryoprobe (a device whose tip can be frozen so that it sticks to the lens). This method was the more common until a few years ago. (ii) EXTRACAPSULAR EXTRACTION: a small hole is made in the anterior lens capsule; the cortex and the nucleus are then removed through this small hole, leaving the posterior part of the lens capsule in place. This is now the commoner method of surgery. Modern surgery requires the use of an operating microscope. Surgery can be performed under local or general anaesthetic and the length of stay in hospital varies from 24 hours to a few days in uncomplicated cases. An estimated 500,000 cataract operations are performed in the USA each year. Having had a cataract removed the eye is made long sighted. An alternative means of focusing light on the retina must be found. The three usual alternatives are cataract glasses, contact lenses or a perspex intra-ocular lens (or implant). Implants by and large give the best results, but are not suitable for all patients.

CATARRH is a state of irritation of the mucous membranes, particularly those of the air passages, associated with a copious secretion of mucus. This complaint, so prevalent in damp and cold weather, usually begins as a nasal catarrh or coryza, with a feeling of weight about the forehead and some difficulty in breathing through the nose, increased on lying down. Fits of sneezing, accompanied with a profuse watery discharge from the nostrils and eyes, soon follow, while the sense of smell and to some extent that of taste become considerably impaired. There is usually present some amount of sore throat and of bronchial irritation, causing hoarseness and cough. Sometimes the vocal apparatus becomes so much inflamed (laryngeal catarrh) that temporary loss of voice results. There is always more or less feverishness and discomfort, and often an extreme sensitiveness to cold. After two or three days the symptoms begin to abate, the discharge from the nostrils and chest becoming thicker and of purulent character, and producing when dislodged considerable relief to the breathing. On the other hand, the catarrh may assume a more severe aspect and pass into some form of pulmonary inflammation. (See BRONCHITIS; CHILLS AND COLDS.)

The term catarrh is also applied to describe a state of irritation, accompanied by abnormal secretion of mucus, in the stomach (see DYSPEPSIA), in the bowels (see DIARRHOEA; and INTESTINE, DISEASES OF), in the bladder (see Cystitis under BLADDER, DISEASES OF), and in other mucous surfaces.

CATATONIA is a symptom of mental disease in which the patient remains rigidly in the same position, behaving very much like a statue. Catatonia minor is a term applied to the group of symptoms occurring in the mental disease, schizophrenia, in which the patient shows peculiar mannerisms, continuing to repeat the same words or actions. (See MENTAL ILLNESS.)

CATECHOLAMINES are substances produced in the body from the dietary amino-acids (qv), phenylalanine and tyrosine. They include adrenaline (qv) and noradrenaline (qv).

CATECHU is a reddish extract from the leaves of the *Uncariagambier*, containing much tannin and acting as an astringent. Compound catechu powder, containing catechu, kino, rhatany, cinnamon and nutmeg, and tincture of catechu is given in diarrhoea, and catechu lozenges are useful in relaxed sore throat.

CATGUT is used in surgery for tying cut arteries and stitching wounds. It is made from the fibrous coat of the intestines of animals, especially of the sheep, requires very careful purification, and in the tissues is gradually absorbed – in about five to ten days – as it is itself an animal substance. Hardened catgut is catgut which has been treated with a suitable hardening agent to prolong the time taken for it to be absorbed; catgut hardened by treatment with chromium compounds is known as chromicized catgut.

CATHARTICS are substances which produce an evacuation of the bowels. (See PURGATIVES.)

CATHETERS are hollow tubes used for passing into various organs of the body, either for investigational purposes or to give some form of treatment.

Varieties: *Cardiac catheters* are introduced through a vein in the arm and passed into the heart in order to diagnose some of the more obscure forms of congenital heart disease, and often as a preliminary to operating on the heart. *Endotracheal catheters* are used to pass down the trachea into the lungs, usually in the course of administering anaesthetics (qv). *Eustachian catheters* are small catheters that are passed along the floor of the nose into the Eustachian tube (qv) in order to inflate the ear. *Nasalcatheters* are tubes passed through the nose into the stomach to feed a patient who cannot swallow: so-called nasal feeding. *Rectal catheters* are catheters passed into the rectum in order to give injections. *Suprapubic catheters* are catheters passed into the bladder through an incision in the lower abdominal wall just above the pubis, either to allow urine to drain away from the bladder, or to wash out an infected bladder. *Ureteric catheters* are small catheters that are passed up the ureter into the pelvis of the kidney, usually to determine the state of the kidney, either by obtaining a sample of urine direct from the kidney or to inject a radio-opaque substance preliminary to X-raying the kidney. (See PYELOGRAPHY.) *Urethral catheters* are catheters that are passed along the urethra into the bladder, either to draw off urine or to wash out the bladder. It is these last three types of catheters that are most extensively used, and will now be described in detail.

Urethral catheters may be made of plastic, rubber, gum elastic (or silkweb), silver or glass. Plastic and rubber catheters are now those most widely used. They may be straight or bent. The straight catheters have the eye near the tip, which is solid in order to make introduction of the catheter easier. The bent catheters have one or two bends, which makes it easier to pass them in a patient with an enlarged prostate. There is also an olive-headed catheter, which has a moulded tip to make it easier to pass the catheter through a urethra which has a stricture. A whistle-tipped catheter has an open tip, and is used when there is a risk of the catheter becoming obstructed as may happen, for instance, if there is much bleeding with large clots of blood. Indwelling, self-retaining catheters are used when a catheter needs to be left in for some time. They have a small balloon at the tip which, when inflated, keeps the catheter in position and prevents its coming out.

Suprapubic catheters, which are not now used as much as at one time, are larger than urethral catheters and are usually made of rubber. *Ureteric catheters* are long, thin and graduated. They are made of terylene base, nylon web, gum elastic, or plastic on nylon web.

Sterilization: The cleaning and sterilization of catheters is of paramount importance. After use, catheters must be carefully cleaned at once. This is done by rinsing them through with running water, and then syringing through with cetrimide. The outside is then well washed with soap and water. Rubber, silver and glass catheters are sterilized by being placed in boiling water. Once the water has again come to the boil, the catheter is boiled for ten minutes. Plastic (vinyl) catheters can be sterilized by boiling, or by autoclaving at 120°C at 15 pounds pressure for fifteen minutes, after which they must be removed at once from the autoclave. Gum elastic catheters are difficult to sterilize, which is one reason why they are being given up. The introduction of disposable catheters, which are only used once and then discarded, has led to their being used to an increasing extent. They are sterilized by gamma radiation.

Uses: The use of any form of catheterization of the bladder, whether urethral, ureteric or suprapubic, must be made under the strictest possible sterile conditions. Not only must the catheter be sterilized, but the hands of those passing the catheter must be prepared with the same care as for a surgical operation, and the opening of the urethra must be sterilized with the utmost care so as to avoid passing any infection into the bladder. The greatest gentleness must be exercised in introducing the catheter. This applies particularly in passing a urethral catheter in men, in whom the urethra is so much longer than in women.

CAT-SCRATCH FEVER is a disease, probably due to a virus, which is characterized by enlargement of the glands. In spite of the name, there is a history of a cat scratch in only about half the cases; in others the infection is acquired through a puncture of the skin by a splinter or thorn. The glandular swelling is usually slight and of short duration, but in some cases may go on to abscess formation which requires aspiration. The infection is not controlled by penicillin.

CAUL is the piece of amnion which sometimes covers a child when he or she is born.

CAULIFLOWER EAR is the term applied to the distortion of the external ear produced by repeated injury in sport. Initially it is due to a haematoma (qv) in the auricle (see EAR). To prevent deformity the blood should be drawn off from this haematoma as soon as possible, and a firm pressure bandage then applied. Subsequent protection can be given to the ear by covering it with a few layers of two-way stretch strapping wound round the head.

CAUSTICS and CAUTERIES are used to burn diseased tissues, the former by chemical action, the latter by their high temperature.

Varieties: The chief chemical caustics in use are acetic, lactic, chromic, carbolic and nitric acids, caustic soda and caustic potash, arsenic in paste, and silver nitrate or lunar caustic. Of cauteries there are Corrigan's button cautery, the electro cautery, consisting of a platinum point heated by an electric current, the galvanocautery, in which a wire is heated with a galvanic current, and Paquelin's cautery, which has a hollow metal point kept hot by benzine constantly blown into it, and diathermy (see DIATHERMY).

Uses: Caustics are used to destroy warts, small tumours, etc. The cautery is used, mildly heated, as a counter-irritant instead of a blister in sciatica, neuralgia, rheumatic pains, etc. (see BLISTERS). The galvanocautery is used to reduce inflamed tissues about the nose and throat. Paquelin's cautery was at one time much in vogue for removal of small growths, conversion of foul ulcers and poisoned wounds into healthy burns, and operations upon very vascular organs like haemorrhoids.

CAVERNOUS BREATHING indicates a peculiar quality of the respiratory sounds heard on auscultation over a cavity in the lung.

CEFAMANDOLE (see ANTIBIOTIC).

CEFAZOLIN (see ANTIBIOTIC).

CEFODROXIL (see ANTIBIOTIC).

CEFOTAXINE (see ANTIBIOTIC).

CEFOXITIN is a semi-synthetic antibiotic, given by injection, which is proving of value in the treatment of infections due to Gram-negative micro-organisms such as *Proteus* which are resistant to many other antibiotics.

CEFUROXINE (see ANTIBIOTIC).

CELLS are the microscopic particles which build up the tissues, of which they are the smallest structural divisions. There are around 10 billion in the human body.

Every cell consists essentially of a cell-body of soft albuminous material called cytoplasm, in which lies a kernel or nucleus which seems to direct all the activities of the cell. Within the nucleus may be seen a minute body, the nucleolus; and there may or may not be a cell-envelope around all. (See also MITOCHONDRIA.)

Cells vary much in size, ranging in the human body from 0·0025 mm to about 0·025 mm.

All animals and plants consist at first of a single cell (the egg-cell, or *ovum*), which begins to develop when fertilized by the sperm-cell derived from the opposite sex. Development begins by a division into two new cells, then into four, and so on till a large mass is formed. These cells then arrange themselves into layers, and form various tubes, rods, and masses which represent in the embryo the organs of the fully developed animal. (See FOETUS.)

When the individual organs have been laid down on a scaffolding of cells, these gradually change in shape and in chemical composition. The cells in the nervous system send out long processes to form the nerves, those in the muscles become long and striped in appearance,

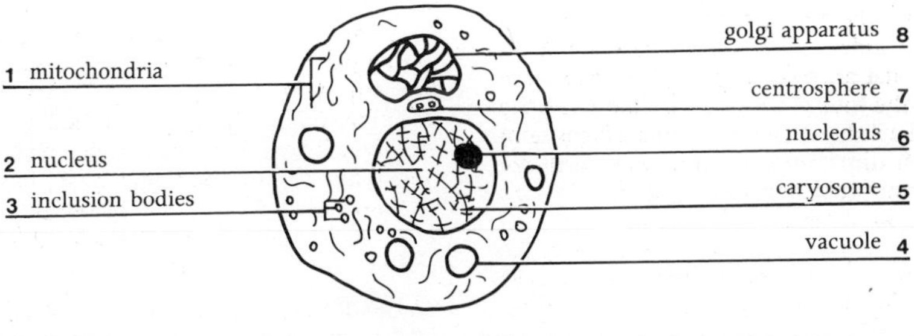

A semi-diagrammatic representation of a cell.

and those which form fat become filled with fat droplets which distend the cells. Further, they begin to produce, between one another, the substances which give the various tissues their special character. Thus, in the future bones, some cells deposit lime salts, and others form cartilage; while, in tendons, they produce long white fibres of a gelatinous substance. In some organs the cells change little: thus the liver consists of columns of large cells packed together, while many cells, like the white blood corpuscles, retain their primitive characters almost entire.

Thus cells are the active agents in forming the body, and they have a similar function in repairing its wear and tear. Tumours (qv), and especially malignant tumours, have a highly cellular structure, the cells being of an embryonic type, or, at best, forming poor imitations of the tissues in which they grow.

CELLULITIS means an inflammation taking place in cellular tissue and usually refers to infection in the subcutaneous tissue. (See ABSCESS; ERYSIPELAS.)

CELLULOSE is a carbohydrate substance forming the skeleton of most plant structures. It is colourless, transparent, insoluble in water and is practically unaffected by digestion. In vegetable foods it therefore adds to the bulk, but it is of no value as a food-stuff. It is found in practically a pure state in cotton-wool.

CELLULOSE PHOSPHATE is a drug which prevents the absorption of calcium from the gut. For this reason it is used in patients with a high level of calcium in the urine (hypercalciuria) to prevent the formation of stones in the kidneys, and also for the treatment of stones in the kidneys in such patients.

CEMENT (see TEETH).

CEMENT BURNS arise as a result of prolonged contact of the skin with builders' cement. They are due to quicklime which constitutes 65 per cent of cement. As they are chemical, and not thermal, burns, the victim feels no immediate pain and therefore allows the contact to persist. The precautions that should be taken include adequate protection of the hands and feet, and avoidance of prolonged contact of the skin with cement.

CENSOR is a term applied to the mental influence which prevents certain subconscious thoughts and wishes from coming into consciousness unless they are disguised so as to be unrecognizable.

CENTENARIANS (see EXPECTATION OF LIFE).

CENTRE is a term applied to a collection of nerve cells which give off nerve fibres and control some particular function: eg. the speech centre and the vision centre in the brain.

CEPHACETRILE (see ANTIBIOTIC).

CEPHALEXIN (see ANTIBIOTIC).

CEPHALOSPORINS have been described as 'a valuable and versatile group of broad-spectrum, non-toxic antibiotics'. Most of them available at the moment are semi-synthetic derivatives of cephalosporin C, an antibiotic originally derived from a sewage out-fall in Sardinia. They include cephaloridine, cephalothin, cephalexin, cephradine, and cephalozin. The term is sometimes used to include a group of semi-synthetic antibiotics with a comparable range of antibacterial action, but derived from a species of streptomyces. Strictly speaking this group, which includes cefoxitin (qv), should be described as cephamycins. The indications for the use of individual members of the group vary. Some are active when given by mouth. Some have to be given by injection. One of their valuable features is that they are sometimes active against micro-organisms that have become resistant to penicillin, such as the gonococcus.

CEPHAPIRIN (see ANTIBIOTIC).

CEPHRODINE (see ANTIBIOTIC).

CERATE is a medicinal preparation, intended for external application, made with a basis consisting of wax in whole or in part which can be spread on the skin without melting: eg. camphor cerate, compound menthol cerate.

CEREAL is the term applied to any plant of the nature of grass bearing an edible seed. The important cereals are wheat, oats, barley, maize, rice and millet. Along with these are usually included tapioca (derived from the cassava plant), sago (derived from the pith of the sago palm) and arrowroot (derived from the root of a West Indian plant), all of which consist almost entirely of starch. Semolina, farola and macaroni are preparations of wheat.

	per cent
Water	10 to 12
Protein	10 to 12
Carbohydrate	65 to 75
Fat	0·5 to 8
Mineral matter	2

Composition of cereals

	Water	Protein	Fat	Carbo-hydrate	Cellu-lose	Ash
Wheat	12·0	11·0	1·7	71·2	2·2	1·9
Oatmeal	7·2	14·2	7·3	65·9	3·5	1·9
Barley	12·3	10·1	1·9	69·5	3·8	2·4
Rye	11·0	10·2	2·3	72·3	2·1	2·1
Maize	12·5	9·7	5·4	68·9	2·0	1·5
Rice (polished)	12·4	6·9	0·4	79·4	0·4	0·5
Millet	12·3	10·4	3·9	68·3	2·9	2·2
Buck-wheat	13·0	10·2	2·2	61·3	11·1	2·2

Composition of certain cereals.

Cereals consist predominantly of carbohydrate. They are therefore an excellent source of energy. On the other hand, their deficiency in protein and fat means that to provide a balanced diet, they must be supplemented by other foods rich in protein and fat, such as meat, milk and eggs.

CEREBELLUM AND CEREBRUM (see BRAIN).

CEREBRAL PALSY is the term used to describe a group of conditions characterized by varying degrees of paralysis and occurring in infancy or early childhood. In some 80 per cent of cases this takes the form of spastic paralysis: hence the lay description of them as 'spastics'. The incidence is believed to be around 2 or 2·5 per 1000 of the childhood community. In the majority of cases the abnormality dates from before birth or occurs during birth. Among the pre-natal factors are some genetic malformation of the brain, a congenital defect of the brain, or some adverse effect on the foetal brain as by infection during pregnancy. Among the factors during birth that may be responsible are trauma to the child or prolonged lack of oxygen such as can occur during a difficult labour. This last factor is considered by some to be the most important single factor. In some 10 to 15 per cent of cases the condition is acquired after birth, when it may be due to kernicterus (qv), infection of the brain, cerebral thrombosis or embolism, or trauma. The congenital form is commoner in boys than girls, and a high proportion of the cases are first-born children.

The disease manifests itself in many ways. The victim may be spastic or flaccid, or the slow, writhing involuntary movements, known as athetosis, may be the predominant feature. These involuntary movements often disappear during sleep and may be controlled, or even abolished, in some cases by training the child to relax. The paralysis varies tremendously. It may involve the limbs on one side of the body (hemiplegia), both lower limbs (paraplegia), or all four limbs (tetraplegia). Mental subnormality is not uncommon.

The outlook for life is good, only the more severely affected cases dying in infancy. Although there is no cure, much can be done to help these unfortunate children, particularly if the condition is detected at an early stage. Little can be done to help those who have severe mental subnormality, but much can be done for those with normal intelligence by team work, giving attention to education, physiotherapy, occupational therapy and speech training. In this way many of these handicapped children are now reaching adult life as useful members of the community. Much help in dealing with these children can be obtained from the Spastics Society, 12 Park Crescent, London W1N 4EQ (01–636 5020); and the Scottish Council for Spastics, 22 Corstorphine Road, Edinburgh EH12 6HP (031–337 9876).

CEREBROSPINAL FEVER is another name for cerebrospinal meningitis. (See under MENINGITIS.)

CEREBROSPINAL FLUID is the fluid within the ventricles of the brain and bathing its surface and that of the spinal cord. It is normally under a pressure of 60 to 150 mm of water and contains 0 to 5 lymphocytes per c.mm. In each 100 millilitres of cerebrospinal fluid there are normally between 10 to 20 mg of protein (mostly albumin), 50 to 80 mg of glucose, and 725 to 750 mg of chlorides.

CEREBROVASCULAR ACCIDENT (see under STROKE.)

CERECLOTH means linen or cotton cloth impregnated with wax and made antiseptic for use in dressing wounds.

CEREVISIA is the Latin name for yeast.

CERUMEN is the name for the wax-like secretion found in the external ear.

CERVICAL means anything pertaining to the neck, or to the neck of the womb.

CERVICITIS means inflammation of the cervix uteri or neck of the womb.

CERVIX UTERI is the neck of the womb or uterus and is placed partly above and partly within the vagina. (See UTERUS.)

CETRARIA, or ICELAND MOSS, is a substance used in the form of decoctions, jellies or lozenges in irritable states of the mouth and throat.

CETRIMIDE (also known as CETAVLON) is the official name for a mixture of alkyl ammonium bromides. It is a potent antiseptic, and as a 1 per cent solution is used for cleaning and disinfecting wounds, and in the first-aid treatment of burns. As it is also a detergent, it is particularly useful for cleaning the skin, and also for cleansing and disinfecting greasy and infected bowls and baths.

CHAFING OF THE SKIN occurs in infants at the natural folds, eg. groins, armpits, elbows, where two moist surfaces constantly rub one another; in stout elderly people at similar positions; and generally where the clothes cause friction or pressure, as in the armpits or on the feet of those who walk great distances.

To prevent chafing the folds of the skin should be kept specially clean by washing with warm water and super-fatted soap, carefully dried, and then dusted with fuller's earth or any dusting-powder, such as a mixture of starch, zinc oxide and subnitrate of bismuth in equal parts.

CHAGAS' DISEASE, or American trypanosomiasis, is a disease widespread in Central and South America, and caused by the *Trypanosoma cruzi*. The disease is transmitted by the biting bugs, *Panstrongylus megistus* and *Triatoma infestans*. It occurs in an acute and a chronic form. The former, which is most common in children, practically always affects the heart, and the prognosis is poor. The chronic form is commonest in adolescents and young adults and the outcome depends upon the extent to which the heart is involved. There is no effective drug treatment. It has been suggested that Charles Darwin acquired the disease during his historic voyage on *The Beagle* and that it was the chronic form that turned him into an invalid for 40 years of his life after his return home and ultimately was responsible for his death in 1882. (See also SLEEPING SICKNESS.)

CHALAZION (see EYE, DISEASES AND INJURY OF).

CHALICOSIS is a disorder of the lungs found among stonecutters, and due to the inhalation of fine particles of stone.

CHALK is calcium carbonate.

CHALK-STONES (see GOUT).

CHALYBEATE tonics or waters are those containing salts of iron. (See IRON.)

CHAMOMILE TEA is a bitter made by infusing chamomile flowers in boiling water for fifteen minutes and then straining. It is used cold in wineglassful doses.

CHANCRE means the primary lesion of syphilis.

CHANCROID means a soft or non-syphilitic venereal sore. It is caused by a micro-organism known as *Haemophilus ducreyi*. It is usually acquired by sexual contact, and responds well to treatment with sulphadimidine (qv). There were 80 cases in England in the year ended June 30, 1983.

CHANGE OF LIFE (see CLIMACTERIC; MENSTRUATION).

CHAPPED HANDS occur in cold weather, when the activity of the sweat and sebaceous glands is reduced and there is therefore less natural protection of the skin. If the hands are then degreased by prolonged immersion in soapy water, and afterwards exposed to cold air, the skin becomes inelastic and cracks.

Prevention: A mop should be used for washing up, and household rubber gloves worn when using strong bleaching solutions, ammonia or degreasing compounds for cleaning ovens. A barrier cream (qv), such as petroleum jelly or lanolin, may be used, but most housewives find these too greasy. A more effective, and less greasy barrier cream is the *British Pharmacopoeia* Oily Cream. Adequate drying of the hands is essential, and the hands should be protected from cold weather so far as possible.

Treatment: Once chapping has occurred, a cream, such as the Oily Cream just mentioned or another *British Pharmacopoeia* preparation, Aqueous Cream, should be applied every night at bedtime. After it has been applied, the hands should be covered with thin cotton gloves. The painful cracks which are so liable to form at the fingertips are best treated with a paint consisting of equal parts of tincture of benzoin and collodion.

CHAPPED LIPS (see LIPS).

CHAPPED NIPPLES (see BREASTS).

CHARCOAL as used in medicine is a black powder prepared from vegetable matter such as sawdust, peat, cellulose residues and coconut shells by carbonization and activation. Its medicinal value is a result of its ability to absorb both gases and chemicals. It is available in the form of a powder, granules, tablets or biscuits.

Uses: Its traditional use is in the treatment of flatulence in a dose of 4 grams, on the principle that it absorbs the intestinal gases, but its value in this role is doubtful. It is also used in the treatment of poisoning with many drugs such as aspirin, paracetamol, barbiturates and morphine, all of which it absorbs. Here the dosage is much higher – up to 50 grams in water. A strawberry-flavoured preparation is now available which makes it more palatable and easier to administer to children. This is supplied as a powder containing 20 grams in a 200-millilitre bottle. The powder is stable for several years. When needed, the bottle is filled with water and the suspension swallowed. Another traditional use is as a deodorizing application to foul ulcers.

CHARCOT-LEYDEN CRYSTALS are sharp crystals found in the sputum of those suffering from asthma, and of those affected by some blood diseases.

CHARCOT'S JOINTS is the name applied to a painless swelling and disorganization of the joints which is the result of damage to the pain fibres that occurs in diabetic neuropathy and tabes dorsalis. (See TABES.)

CHARPIE is linen waste, formerly used to absorb discharges, but now replaced by absorbent cotton-wool.

CHAULMOOGRA OIL, or HYDNOCARPUS OIL, is a volatile oil obtained from the seeds of an Asiatic shrub, *Hydnocarpus wightiana*, which was at one time widely used in the treatment of leprosy. It has now been largely replaced by sulphones and other drugs. (See LEPROSY.)

CHEILOSIS is an eczematous condition of the lips, especially at the angles of the mouth, and believed to be due to deficiency in the diet of one of the vitamins in the vitamin B complex – riboflavin. ANGULAR STOMATITIS and PERLECHE are other terms used to describe the condition, which may be associated with a red, sore tongue; fine desquamation at the junction of nose and lip, just inside the nose, and in the ears; eczema of the scrotum and perineum.

CHEIROPOMPHOLYX is the term applied to a disease of the skin in which little blisters filled with clear fluid suddenly appear on the hands and fingers. (See also POMPHOLYX.)

CHELATING AGENTS are compounds that will render an ion (usually a metal) biologically inactive by incorporating it into an inner ring structure in the molecule. (Hence the name from the Greek *chele*=claw.) When the complex formed in this way is harmless to the body and is excreted in the urine, such an agent is an effective way of ridding the body of toxic metals such as mercury. The main chelating agents are dimercaprol (qv), penicillamine (qv) and sodium calciumedetate (qv).

CHEMOSIS: Swelling of the conjunctiva. (See EYE, DISEASES AND INJURIES OF.)

CHEMOTAXIS means the property possessed by certain cells of attracting or repelling other cells.

CHEMOTHERAPY is the treatment of disease by chemical substances. In the modern sense it dates from the discovery by Paul Ehrlich, in 1910, of the action of Salvarsan ('606') in destroying the spirochaete of syphilis. This organic arsenical preparation revolutionized the treatment of syphilis. The next great advance in chemotherapy was the introduction of the sulphonamides in 1935. Just as Salvarsan had revolutionized the treatment of syphilis so did the sulphonamides revolutionize the treatment of infections with the streptococcus, pneumococcus, gonococcus and similar organisms. They remained supreme in the treatment of such infections as septicaemia, pneumonia, and certain forms of meningitis, until the introduction of penicillin during the 1939–45 War. Subsequently a series of new antibiotics (qv) have been discovered, including streptomycin, chloramphenicol and the tetracyclines.

Chemotherapy has also played an important rôle in tropical medicine: eg. mepacrine and proguanil for the treatment of malaria; the amidines in the treatment of sleeping sickness in man, and the sulphones in the treatment of leprosy.

In the last two decades it has played an increasing part in the treatment of cancer (qv).

CHENODEOXYCHOLIC ACID is one of the bile acids (see BILE), which is used in the treatment of cholesterol gall-stones (see GALL-BLADDER, DISEASES OF).

CHENOPODIUM OIL, distilled from American wormseed, is used in the treatment of roundworms and hookworms in doses of 0·2 to 1 ml.

CHEST, or THORAX, is the upper part of the trunk. It is enclosed by the breast-bone and rib-cartilages in front, by the twelve ribs at each side, and by the hinder parts of these along with the spinal column behind. Above, it is continued by an opening a few inches wide, through which pass the windpipe, gullet and large blood-vessels, into the root of the neck; while, below, its cavity is separated from that of the abdomen by a thin dome-shaped plate of muscle, the diaphragm or midriff. Between each pair of ribs lie two thin muscular layers, the intercostal muscles, which fill up the spaces between the ribs, and move the chest wall in respiration. Its outlines are further covered and moulded behind by four layers of muscles, sometimes several inches thick, and by the shoulder-blade with its muscles, and in front by the two pectoral muscles which pass from the ribs to the upper arm. Further, there is a more or less plentiful layer of fat beneath the skin, and in this fat lie the breasts, extending in the female from the second rib down to the seventh.

Contents: The chest contains the lungs, one on each side, with the end of the windpipe, which divides into right and left bronchial tubes, to the two lungs; the heart in the middle and projecting on the left almost to the nipple, with the great vessels which carry blood from and to it; the gullet, which passes down on the left side of the spinal column to enter the abdomen through an opening in the diaphragm; the thoracic duct of the absorbent system, which runs up to enter a vein in the neck; and various important nerves which control the contained organs. Each lung is enclosed in a smooth, double membrane, the pleura (see LUNGS), and the heart in a similar membrane, the pericardium.

CHEST, DEFORMITIES OF: The healthy chest is gently rounded all over, its contour being still more rounded in women by the breasts, and in transverse outline it should present an oval shape slightly flattened behind and having a proportion of about 10 to 7·5 between its side-to-side and front-to-back measurements. The angle at the lower end of the breast-bone formed between the edges of the rib cartilages of the two sides should be about four-fifths of a right angle. An interval of about two inches should exist between the twelfth rib and the haunch-bone. The circumference varies from 84 cm (33 inches) for a man of 152 cm (5 feet) in height to about 102 cm (40 inches) for a man of 183 cm (6 feet).

Long chest is one in which the shoulders slope downwards, the ribs incline downwards as they come forwards more than they should do, the lower ribs touch or almost touch the haunch-bones, and the circumference is small. Further, the neck is long, the throat prominent, and the shoulder-blades stand out behind, the chest for this reason being also called the winged or alar chest. Traditionally, this form is said to predispose to tuberculosis and other lung diseases, probably because the lungs are never properly expanded, but this long chest can be much improved and the circumference rapidly increased by proper exercises.

Flat chest is often a consequence of lung diseases, and flatness is sometimes found along with too great length. In this form, the ribs and their cartilages grow too straight in front, so that the chest loses in fullness. This form is partly curable in youth by exercises.

Barrel chest is one in which the ribs are too horizontal, the shoulders raised, and the chest short. It is the opposite in every respect of the long chest. The curves of the chest resemble those of a barrel and the ribs the hoops. This form is due to too great expansion of the lungs, especially in the disease called emphysema (qv). The chest being blown out almost to its full capacity at expiration, inspiration is made very laborious.

Rickety chest is due to rickets in early life, and usually the head and other bones are also affected. (See RICKETS.) There is a hollow down each side owing to the yielding of the soft growing ribs in early life under the pressure of the atmosphere. There is, however, a protrusion of the front of the chest, so that the lungs are not pressed on, or specially liable to disease. Frequently the chest shows, down each side, a row of nodules placed at the junction of the ribs with their cartilages, and known as the 'rickety rosary'. Sometimes the lower part of the chest is much bulged out from moulding over the liver and other abdominal organs.

Pigeon breast is one in which the cross-section of the chest becomes triangular, the breast-bone forming a sort of keel in front, like that in the pigeon's breast. It is due to the ribs becoming straightened so as to push the breast-bone straight forwards, and is caused by some obstacle to the entrance of air in early life.

Bulging of the chest may be due to curvature of the spine, which makes a projection behind, and consequently, the chest being shortened, causes the breast-bone to bend on itself and project in front. When the spine twists to one side, that side becomes flattened, the other side bulging and the contained organs being pushed into it.

Hollowing of the chest is found in many conditions. In tuberculosis, when the lung becomes chronically solidified in its upper part, and later probably develops a cavity, it shrinks, and the chest wall to some extent falls in beneath the collar-bone. In pleurisy of long standing the lung is apt to collapse, i.e undergo a shrinking process and lose its air spaces, so that the whole chest wall of that side sinks inwards under atmospheric pressure.

CHEST DEVELOPMENT is of great practical importance in view of the fact that persons with long and flat chests suffer more often from serious lung disease than those who have good chest capacity. The muscles which come into action in taking a breath fall into two classes: (1) the muscles of ordinary inspiration, including the diaphragm, and the intercostal muscles, which suspend one rib from that next above it; and (2) the muscles of forced inspiration, including most of the muscles of the neck, the shoulder and the abdomen, which come into play in taking an extra deep breath.

The lungs rise a distance of 12 to 36 mm (half to one and a half inches) above the collar-bone into the root of the neck, and this portion is little expanded except in forced breathing. It is here that tuberculosis is liable to make its first appearance, and, though cause and effect are not quite clear, there can be little doubt that the deficient expansion, and consequently sluggish circulation, play an important part in this location of the disease.

Although violent exercise like football has an indirect influence in expanding the chest by necessitating deep breathing, other forms of athletics add mainly to the size and strength of the muscles on the chest without increasing its capacity. Probably the only exercise which attains the latter thoroughly is forced breathing.

CHEST DISEASES (see LUNGS, DISEASES OF; HEART DISEASE; ANEURYSM; ANGINA PECTORIS; PLEURISY; PNEUMONIA; BRONCHITIS; TUBERCULOSIS): Chest diseases are of special importance, because the lungs and heart are perhaps the most important organs in the body, and are especially difficult to treat, as these are the only organs which cannot rest for a few minutes without death becoming imminent. Further, they are so closely placed and so intimately associated by the circulation of the blood, that when one suffers from disease, either acute or chronic, the other is rarely unaffected.

Symptoms: Owing to the rigid nature of the chest wall, changes in the enclosed organs rarely become visible to the eye. *Pain* is a very important symptom. Very severe pain may, it is true, be caused by muscular rheumatism in the chest wall (the condition called pleurodynia) or by neuralgia, but when of a stabbing character and felt at the end of every breath it suggests pleurisy as a cause. Pain about the heart may be caused by indigestion, but if severe, and especially if brought on by exertion, is seldom found without some slight or serious heart disease. Pain in the precordium brought on usually by physical effort is known as angina pectoris (see ANGINA PECTORIS). Severe persistent pain of a boring character is suggestive of an aneurysm (see ANEURYSM). *Expectoration* of blood may occur both in heart and in lung disease, and various other characters are noteworthy in the sputum (see EXPECTORATION). *Breathlessness* is an important sign of lung and heart diseases (see BREATHLESSNESS). *Other organs* are prone to be affected by disease of either heart or lungs; thus in tuberculosis the digestive system sometimes gives the first sign of ill-health, and in heart disease congestion of the liver, or swelling of the feet, may be for long the main trouble. *Cough* is one of the best-known symptoms of respiratory disease, either of tuberculosis or of bronchitis, but it may be due to irritation of other parts of the respiratory system, or even of the stomach.

Treatment: Rest is the most important factor in the treatment of all chest conditions, because, when the body is quiet, the circulation of the blood becomes slower, the rate of pulse and respiration slackens, and so the heart and lungs have a partial rest. Pain is soothed by the application of hot-water bottles, or counter-irritants to the chest. Fresh air is specially necessary in lung disease (see TUBERCULOSIS). Infections are controlled by the sulphonamides or antibiotics. Various drugs called expectorants are given to act upon the lungs, or similar drugs are inhaled (see EXPECTORANTS; INHALATIONS). Oxygen is much used both in affections of the heart and of the lungs. In the case of the heart, there are several drugs by which the action of this organ can be slowed, or quickened, or made more regular: for example, digitalis.

CHEST INJURIES: Injuries due to moderate violence are not usually serious, resulting generally in muscular bruises or in fractured rib (see FRACTURES). If the ribs do not penetrate the lung, union and recovery are rapid, but, if the lung is injured, various complications, such as emphysema, effusion of blood and entrance of air into the pleural cavity, abscess in the lung, traumatic pneumonia, may ensue. Penetrating wounds of the lungs, as by a bullet or stab, are apt to lead to similar complications, but do not necessarily produce serious effects unless a large vessel is severed. Simple fractures of ribs may be serious in old people, and bronchitis often follows their occurrence. Wounds of the heart are generally at once fatal from haemorrhage, but this organ has been so seriously injured as to require stitching, and yet recovery has ensued.

CHEYNE-STOKES BREATHING is a type of breathing seen in some serious nervous affections, such as brain tumours and stroke, and also in the case of persons with advanced disease of the heart or kidneys. When well marked it is a sign that death is impending, though milder degrees of it do not carry such a serious implication in elderly patients. The breathing gets very faint for a short time, then gradually deepens till full expirations are taken for a few seconds, and then gradually dies away to another quiet period, again increasing in depth after a few seconds and so on in cycles.

CHICKENPOX, or VARICELLA, is an acute contagious disease predominantly of children, though it may occur at any age, characterized by feverishness and an eruption on the skin. The name, chickenpox, is said to be derived from the resemblance of the eruption to boiled chick-peas.

Causes: The disease occurs in epidemics affecting especially children under the age of ten years. It has no connection with smallpox, to which it bears a superficial resemblance. It is due to a virus, and the condition is an extremely infectious one from child to child.

Symptoms: There is an incubation period of fourteen to twenty-one days after infection, and then the child becomes feverish or has a slight shivering, or may feel more severely ill with vomiting and pains in the back and legs. Almost at the same time, and at all events within twenty-four hours, an eruption consisting of red pimples which quickly change into vesicles filled with clear fluid appears on the back and chest, sometimes about the forehead, and less frequently on the limbs. These vesicles during the second day may show a change of their contents to turbid, purulent fluid and within a day or two they burst, or, at all events, shrivel up and become covered with brownish crusts. An important point of difference between this eruption and that of smallpox is that these vesicles keep on appearing for several days, so that vesicles are seen at all stages of development, whilst in those of smallpox all parts of the rash are at the same stage at one time. In a slight case there may be only eight or ten of these vesicles, or there may be several hundreds. The small crusts have all dried up and fallen off in little more than a week and recovery is almost always complete.

Treatment: The child must be isolated from susceptible children for a week from the appearance of the rash or until all the vesicles are dry, but there is no need to wait until the scabs have separated. A patient need not be confined to bed unless the temperature is raised, but he should be kept in one room. If the rash appears on the face, care must be taken to prevent scratching or pock marks may remain. Calamine lotion or a simple dusting powder relieves the itchiness. No other treatment beyond isolation is required.

CHIGGER is another name for *Trombicula autumnalis*, popularly known as the harvest mite (see BITES AND STINGS).

CHILBLAIN, or ERYTHEMA PERNIO, is an inflamed condition of the skin of the hands or feet, or even of the ears, occurring in persons of defective circulation and in those of poor health.

Causes: Chilblains are found especially in childhood and adolescence. Under-feeding, poor clothing and a defective circulation favour their appearance. People who suffer from them have habitually cold and numb hands and feet, and are subject to chills and colds in the head.

In these people tight footwear is often sufficient to bring on chilblains of the feet, and warming the hands at the fire when they are cold produces chilblains on the fingers, the skin becoming engorged with blood in consequence of the irritation or warmth, and later losing its vitality.
Symptoms: There are three stages in the development of a chilblain:

(1) The skin, usually of the little toe, the outer side of the foot, or the inner side of the hand, becomes purple and very itchy.

(2) Blebs, containing a thin yellow fluid, form on this discoloured area, which becomes very painful.

(3) These blebs break and leave behind an ulcerated surface very difficult to heal.

True chilblains should not be confused with a cracked or chapped condition of the hands, feet, lips, or ears brought on by cold wind, or washing with hot water during cold weather in people of robust constitution but delicate skin.
Treatment: Preventive treatment is the best. Good food and warm clothing improve the general condition upon which chilblains depend. Regular exercise improves the circulation. The person liable to chilblains should wear wide footwear and thick woollen socks in winter, and, before going into the open air, should always put on gloves. Garters and constrictions round the wrist or ankle, which interfere with the circulation, should be avoided and india-rubber shoes should not be worn. If the hands and feet are cold they should be rubbed for warmth, not held before the fire. In the first stage the chilblain may be rubbed with hazeline snow or cream, or painted with tincture of iodine. Carefully controlled irradiation with ultra-violet light is often beneficial. Voyagers to the Arctic regions rub the part with a mixture of whisky and soap. In the second and third stages some simple ointment, like boracic, and a dressing of wool are best, or the part may be painted with compound tincture of benzoin.

CHILD ADOPTION: In Great Britain around 2·5 per cent of all liveborn infants, or 25,000 per annum, are legally adopted. Adoption and illegitimacy are closely interrelated. In England and Wales 80 per cent, and in Scotland 90 per cent, of adopted children are illegitimate. Conversely in England and Wales 30 per cent, and in Scotland nearly 40 per cent, of illegitimate children are adopted. The majority of parents who adopt children are between 25 and 35 years of age, and only some 10 per cent are 40 or over. A mother cannot give formal consent to the placement of her infant until the baby is 6 weeks old, although informal placement may take place earlier. Thereafter there must be a probation period of three months before court proceedings can take place. Thus, few adoptions can be formally legalized before the age of 6 months. The number of children under the age of six months adopted in 1986 was 243 males and 229 females. Between the age of six and eight months the figures were 427 males and 402 females. Between 9 and 11 months the figures were 155 males and 116 females and at a year old 200 males and 213 females were adopted. In the year 1986, 4,244 children were adopted at the age of one or over.

Adoption can be carried out in three ways. (i) Through an adoption agency; this accounts for approximately 70 per cent of adoptions. (ii) By the mother directly placing the infant with adoptive parents; this accounts for nearly 30 per cent of adoptions. A high proportion of such adoptions are adoptions by the mother (now married) of her own baby or adoption by her relatives. (iii) Through a third party acting as an intermediary between mother and adoptive parents; this accounts for only 1 to 3 per cent of all adoptions. Of infants who are legally adopted, some 72 per cent are adopted by non-relatives, and 28 per cent by relatives.

There are two types of registered adoption agency: the voluntary adoption society, and the local authority acting as an adoption agency. In England and Wales approximately two-thirds of agency placements are carried out by voluntary societies and one-third by local authorities. In Scotland the proportions are approximately equal. For many years voluntary societies have had a national organization: the Standing Conference of Societies Registered for Adoption. This has now been replaced by a national organization: the Association of British Adoption and Fostering Agencies, which includes both voluntary adoption societies and local authorities acting as adoption agencies. Its address is: 40 Brunswick Square, London WC1 (tel. no. 01–407 8800).

CHILD-CROWING is another name for laryngismus. (See LARYNGISMUS.)

CHILD DEVELOPMENT: A child normally smiles at six weeks of age. It is vocalising by the age of three months. By the age of four months a grasp reflex is established whereby an object placed in a baby's hand is grasped by the fingers though it is not till the age of nine months that the child will actually grasp an object. A child is usually sitting without support between the ages of five to twelve months. It can follow a rolling ball or falling object at the age of six months. This is an important sign of development; visual attention is related to intelligent quotient so it provides information about intellect as well as about actual vision. A normal child walks between the ages of nine months to two years.

Learning takes place relatively slowly until the age of nine months, after which it proceeds at a fast rate. Children who mature earlier do better at school than those who mature late. By the age of three a child should be able: (1) to point correctly to his nose, eyes or mouth when asked to do so; (2) to name familiar objects like cup, pencil, or key when shown to him; (3) to name three simple objects in a picture shown to him; (4) to say whether he is a boy or girl; (5) to give his last name; (6) to repeat three numbers when named to him.

At the age of six a normal child should be able: (1) to point to right hand, left, ear, etc. as named; (2) when shown a picture of a figure from which parts have been left out, to name the missing parts; (3) to give an explicit reply to simple questions such as 'what should you do if you find that the house is on fire?'; (4) to count objects up to thirteen; (5) to name correctly coins shown to him; (6) to repeat correctly a simple sentence of twelve or fifteen words. An intelligent six-year old child should know the meaning of around 13,000 words. Two years later this figure should double. At the age of nine a normal child should be able: (1) to give the correct day, month and year; (2) to arrange a series of weights in proper order; (3) to repeat backwards four stated figures; (4) to make a simple sentence containing three stated words.

CHILDREN, FEEDING OF (see INFANT FEEDING).

CHILDREN, PECULIARITIES OF: The fact that children cannot put into words, or cannot correctly estimate, the nature of troubles and pains from which they suffer, coupled with the great importance of remedying as early in life as possible any physical or mental defect, or any bad habit, makes the observation of their peculiarities of great importance.

Activity: For some weeks after an infant is born the only signs of intelligence, apart from the performance of the merely animal functions, consist in *constant movements* of the lips, head, and limbs. The fingers are constantly opened and shut, the legs drawn up and down, and the lips pouted, while the child is awake; and the vigour of these movements gives a good idea of the vitality of the child. At about the third or fourth month the child should begin to develop the power of attention, as shown by his staring fixedly at any bright or moving object presented to him and ceasing other movements while his attention is so engaged. During the sixth month teething begins. A delay in teething is one of the signs of rickets (see TEETH). About the end of the first year of life the child should be gaining the power to stand and walk (see GAIT).

Crying in early childhood is a manifestation of either pain, or hunger, or discomfort. The most common pain is that known as 'gripes' and associated with indigestion, in which the cry is of a wailing character, with a note of ill-temper (see COLIC). In head pain the cry is of a sharp, piercing nature. In older children frowning is a common symptom of headache, especially when it is due to eye-strain (see VISION, DISORDERS OF).

Temperature is not much of a guide to disease in children, because the temperature-regulating mechanism is easily thrown out of gear.

Fullness under the eyes may be a symptom of glomerulonephritis.

An open mouth in breathing, especially when deafness and shortness of breath accompany it, is usually due to enlargement of the tonsils and adenoids in the throat. A child so affected is generally found to snore when asleep (See NOSE, DISEASES OF.) Accompanying these symptoms in older children we find broadening of the bridge of the nose, narrow nostrils, and often narrowing of the roof of the mouth with projecting front teeth.

The expression of the face is often of great importance. Brain disease causes contractions of the facial muscles producing the appearance of emotions quite foreign to childhood, and causing the deep lines which, in middle-aged persons, are supposed to denote character. The head, too, is often drawn back in such a case, and the back arched. Deep hollowing of the eyes during an attack of gastroenteritis (qv) and vomiting is a grave sign, indicating dehydration. The size of the cranium is large in children compared with that of the face. At birth the proportion is about eight to one, though the face rapidly grows in size. On the top of the head is the fontanelle or soft spot, which at birth is about a square inch in size, and gradually closes as the bones grow till, at the end of the second year, it should have disappeared. Premature closure, with narrowing of the forehead, is often, though not necessarily, associated with mental deficiency. Late closure, with the development of a lofty, 'intellectual'-looking forehead, is one of the signs of rickets.

Limping may be due to many causes. These include injury resulting in a fracture, dislocation of a joint or bruised muscles, disease of a joint such as congenital dislocation of the hip (see DISLOCATIONS), or tuberculosis (see JOINTS, DISEASES OF), a mild degree of cerebral palsy (qv), and inequality of the length of the legs (qv). At the age of 1 to 2, the likeliest causes are injury, congenital dislocation of the hip or cerebral palsy. At the age of 2 to 5, trauma, cerebral palsy and transient synovitis of the hip (see JOINTS, DISEASES OF) are likely causes. To these at the age of 5 to 10 should be added Perthe's disease (qv) and Köhler's disease (qv). In older children the possibility of its being feigned or hysterical should always be considered, and at all ages the first thing to do is to exclude its being due to a nail in the sole of a shoe, crinkling of the sole of the shoe or ill-fitting shoes.

Nervousness may show itself by twitching movements of hands and feet, and a shy, nervous child is apt to be unintentionally clumsy. Twitchings and grimaces may show the beginning of St. Vitus's dance, and children are apt to be punished for these quite involuntary peculiarities, such punishment only aggravating the condition. Convulsions in young children are due to many causes (see CONVULSIONS), and when some nervous disease is the cause they form a serious symptom. Although much more common in children, they are not by any means as grave as fits of similar severity in adults. The involuntary or unconscious passing of urine, or enuresis (see

NOCTURNAL ENURESIS), showing itself generally by wetting of the bed, is usually a bad habit in a nervous child and capable of correction by careful psychological treatment, but is occasionally due to physical conditions needing correction.

Bad habits in children include such actions as persistent sucking of the thumb or tongue, biting the nails, rolling or nodding the head in a rhythmic manner, knocking the head violently on the pillow, rhythmic swaying of the body, eating of dirt. These habits all consist in a morbid exaggeration of some normal action which has an extraordinary fascination for the children who practise it. They should be corrected at an early stage, firmly yet tactfully and without any fuss, by checking the child and making him carry out some other activity on each occasion when the habit is noticed. Advice should be sought at a child-guidance clinic or from the family doctor if the habit persists.

Left-handedness is often taken for a sign of stupidity, and children are punished when they do not use the right. This is a great mistake, because the condition is due to the fact that the side of the brain governing the left hand has developed in advance of the other. The child may, however, be taught to do certain things with the right hand, and so attain a condition of ambidexterity.

Delay in talking is much commoner in boys than in girls. It may be due to several causes, such as deafness, mental retardation, abnormalities of the lips, tongue or palate, or merely under-stimulation of the child. Fifty per cent of all children are using words with meaning by the age of 12 months, and 97 per cent by the age of 21 months. Half of all children join words into simple sentences by 23 months and 97 per cent by the age of 3 years. In the development of speech, girls are usually more advanced than boys. In addition there are some children whose speech is still difficult to understand at the age of 4 years as a result of poor articulation or omission or substitutions of consonants.

Sleep should be longer the younger the child. Some children can do with relatively little sleep and will lie quite happily in bed for an hour or more before falling asleep, whilst they may waken relatively early in the morning. Rigid rules therefore cannot be laid down.

	Hours a Day
During first year	20
During second year	14–16
From second to fourth year	12–14
From fourth to sixth year	10–12
From sixth to twelfth year	10
From twelfth to sixteenth year	9

Approximate requirements of sleep at different ages.

CHILLS and COLDS form a subject of some importance because, although in general trivial ailments, on occasion they can be the prelude to serious diseases.

Causes: The so-called 'common cold' may follow some chill to the surface, such as exposure to a draught of cold air, breathing in a foggy atmosphere, wetting of the feet on a cold day, sudden immersion in water, some persons being specially liable after one of these to develop a catarrh of the respiratory passages and feverish state. These, however, are only predisposing factors, and the primary cause is a virus. Often a 'cold in the head' runs through all the members of a family or school or a group of persons employed together, and such an 'infectious cold' is due to the causative virus passed from one person to another by sneezing or coughing.

Varieties and symptoms: A cold in the head with catarrh of the nose is known to every one; the catarrh sometimes extending up into the frontal sinuses and causing a severe browache, or involving the maxillary sinuses (see SINUS) and causing face-ache, or even spreading up the Eustachian tubes and causing inflammation of the middle ear with painful earache. Generally, these secondary affections disappear as the cold gets well, but suppuration may result in these various cavities, most commonly in the middle ear, though seldom in the frontal sinus. When the throat is the part affected, inflammation of the tonsils may result. (See TONSILLITIS.) In persons who use the voice much, or in those who take too much in alcohol, the larynx is a weak point, and laryngitis, with huskiness or even temporary loss of voice, is the common result of a chill. The cold may affect the respiratory passages farther down and bronchitis then results, or if the surfaces of the air spaces in the lungs be inflamed, pneumonia is the condition produced. When the air passages from the larynx downwards contain mucus, coughing results, this being a series of involuntary explosive expirations designed to force the irritating substance up into the mouth, from which it is spat out. Some persons have a liability, as the result of a chill, to catarrh not of the respiratory, but of the alimentary system, as shown by ensuing dyspepsia or diarrhoea. It should be remembered that a so-called 'cold' is the commencement of several infectious and serious diseases, such as measles, whooping-cough, influenza, and tuberculosis. Medical advice should therefore be sought whenever this apparently trivial malady lasts more than a few weeks. Finally a chilly sensation is a frequent accompaniment of some nervous shock either of a severe nature or even of some minor type.

Treatment: There is little one can do in the treatment of a cold. Most people have their pet remedies, and most of these are harmless. On 'catching a cold', with a temperature above normal, the best thing to do is to go to bed and stay there at least 24 hours, if not two days. In this way the course of the cold will be cut short, and at the same time the sufferer will not be exposing other people to his infection. The best way to prevent colds is to isolate the infected by keeping them in bed. Equally important is it that those suffering from a cold should not cough or sneeze indiscriminantly as their secretions are loaded with the causative organism, which is why health, and not merely politeness, demands coughing or sneezing into a handkerchief. On the other hand, this means that the handkerchief becomes loaded with micro-organisms. It has been reported that 15,000 organisms can be removed from a used handkerchief during thirty seconds of gentle manipulation, which is why disposable paper handkerchiefs should be used when one has a cold, sore throat or the like. Vaccines seem to be ineffectual in the prevention of colds.

CHIMERA is an organism, whether plant, animal or human being, in which there are at least two kinds of tissue differing in their genetic constitution. In recent years it has become possible to combine together two embryos (qv) at a very early stage of development so that they develop as a single individual. Such an animal, which thus can have four parents, instead of two, is an example of a chimera.

CHINCOUGH is another name for whooping-cough. (See WHOOPING-COUGH.)

CHIRETTA, or CHIRATA, is a favourite bitter, resembling gentian. (See BITTERS.)

CHIROPODY is that part of medical science which is concerned with the health of the feet. The modern chiropodist is a specialist capable of providing a fully comprehensive foot health service. This includes the palliation of established deformities and dysfunction both as short term treatment for immediate relief of painful symptoms and long term management to secure optimum results. This requires the backing of effective appliances and footwear services. It also involves curative footcare, including the use of various therapeutic techniques, including minor surgery and the prescription and provision of specialized and individual appliances. Chiropody also has a preventative role which includes inspection of children's feet and the detection of foot conditions requiring treatment and advice and also foot health education. The chiropodist is trained to recognise medical conditions which manifest themselves in the feet, such as circulatory disorders, diabetes mellitus and diseases causing ulceration.

The scope of practice of chiropodists is defined by the Society of Chiropodists as comprising the maintenance of the feet in healthy condition and the treatment of their disabilities by methods covered by the syllabus of training hitherto approved by the Department of Health. A chiropodist should confine his practice to this field of work and to such forms of advice and treatment as his training and experience qualify him to give. The only course of training in the United Kingdom recognised for the purpose of state registration by the Chiropodists Board of the Council for Professions Supplementary to Medicine is the Society of Chiropodists 3-year full-time course. The course includes instruction and examination in the relevant aspects of anatomy and physiology, local analgesia, medicine and surgery, as well as in podology and therapeutics. The registered address of the Society of Chiropodists is 53 Welbeck Street, London W1N 7HE (01–486 3381).

CHIROPRACTOR is a term applied to a person who practises chiropractic. This is a system of adjustment by hand of supposed minor displacements of the spinal column. These minor displacements, or subluxations (qv) of the spine, chiropractors contend, affect the associated or neighbouring nerves. The claim of chiropractic is that by manipulating the affected part of the spinal column the patient's complaint, whatever it may be – for example, backache – is relieved.

CHIRURGEON is an obsolete method of spelling surgeon.

CHLAMYDIA is a genus of micro-organisms which include those responsible for non-specific urethritis (qv), ornithosis (qv), psittacosis (qv), and trachoma (qv). They are also widespread in birds and animals.

CHLOASMA: This is an increase in the melanin pigment of the skin as a result of hormonal stimulation. It is commonly seen in pregnancy and sometimes in women on the contraceptive pill. It mainly affects the face.

CHLOPRPROMAZINE (CHLORACTIL, DOZINE, LARGACTIL) (see ANTI-PSYCHOTIC DRUGS).

CHLORAL HYDRATE is a substance which when taken internally in moderate doses, produces sound, dreamless, refreshing sleep, like natural sleep. It acts rapidly, within about half-an-hour, and its effect lasts for about eight hours. It is, however, dangerous in large doses, and people taking it frequently may contract a habit for it. It should not be taken in conjunction with alcohol. In safe doses it does not lessen pain appreciably, as opium does, and so will not cure sleeplessness due to this cause. In dangerous doses it paralyses and slows the heart, slows respiration, and reduces body temperature.

Uses: It is given in doses of 300 mg to 1·2g, or in the form of syrup of chloral, a teaspoonful, but should only be taken under medical observation. It is particularly useful in children (as the syrup) and in old people. *Externally* chloral is an antiseptic, and a lotion of strength 500 mg of chloral to each 28·5 ml of water is used for cleansing unhealthy ulcers, and some forms of eczema. Chloral and camphor, rubbed together in equal parts, form a clear fluid, as do chloral and menthol, and either of these is useful for painting on to the skin in cases of neuralgia or of gouty pain.

CHLORAL POISONING is by no means infrequent, because, the sleep-producing effect of the drug passing off after repeated administrations, the sleepless person is apt to increase the dose too far.
Symptoms: Occasionally, though seldom, there is gastric pain and sickness after a large dose. Usually the result is a speedy and deep sleep, passing gradually into coma, the pulse growing feebler, and the respirations embarrassed till death peacefully ensues.
Treatment: The patient must be persistently irritated and roused as in opium poisoning. The stomach should be at once emptied by stomach tube or emetic. The extremities of the body must be kept warm, and stimulants given. Leptazol and ephedrine are said to be useful. Artificial respiration may be needed.

CHLORAMBUCIL (LEUKERAN) is a derivative of nitrogen mustard (qv), which is proving of value in the treatment of chronic lymphatic leukaemia (qv) and Hodgkin's disease (qv). It is given by mouth. (See CYTOTOXIC DRUGS.)

CHLORAMINE is a white powder with powerful antiseptic action, which is non-irritant and non-poisonous.

CHLORAMPHENICOL, or CHLOROMYCETIN, is an antibiotic derived from a soil organism, *Streptomyces venezuelae*. It is also prepared synthetically. It is active against a wide range of organisms, but its most striking feature is its activity against certain rickettsias (qv). It has proved effective in the treatment of typhus, scrub typhus, Rocky Mountain spotted fever, typhoid and paratyphoid fevers. Its activity against certain organisms not susceptible to the sulphonamides and penicillin is proving of value. Particularly is this true of its use in the treatment of meningitis due to *H. influenzae*. It is given by mouth.

It is an antibiotic, however, that must be administered with discrimination because in certain individuals it may cause aplastic anaemia (qv), particularly if given for too long a period or in repeated courses.

CHLORAZEPATE (TRANXENE) (see BENZODIAZEPINES).

CHLORDANE is an insecticide which has been used sucessfully against flies and mosquitoes resistant to DDT, and for the control of ticks and mites. It requires special handling as it is toxic to man when applied to the skin.

CHLORDIAZEPOXIDE, the proprietary name of which is LIBRIUM, is a widely used anti-anxiety drug. (See TRANQUILLISERS, BENZODIAZEPINES.)

CHLORETONE, or CHLORBUTOL, is a white powder with an odour like camphor. Applied to the surface of the skin or mucous membrane it has a soothing and antiseptic effect, and internally it acts as a hypnotic.

CHLORHEXIDINE, also known as HIBITANE, is an antiseptic which has a bacteriostatic action against many bacteria.

CHLORINATED LIME, also known as CHLORIDE OF LIME, is a white powder made by passing chlorine gas over slaked lime. Chlorine is a greenish gas, heavier than air, with a pungent, choking smell, and highly poisonous to all forms of bacterial life. By virtue of its power to give off chlorine, chlorinated lime is a powerful bleaching agent and disinfectant, especially when mixed with an acid. To disinfect rooms, chlorinated lime may be mixed with an equal bulk of water acidulated with sulphuric acid, and exposed on flat dishes for some hours. To disinfect water-closets and drains, 450 g (1 pound) of the chlorinated lime may be mixed with 4·5 litres (1 gallon) of water and poured down the drain.

To disinfect swimming baths it should be added in such an amount that the free chlorine, after combining with any organic matter in the water, is left in a concentration of 0·25 to 1 part per million parts of water. It is an efficient disinfectant for drinking water when added in the proportion of 28·3 grammes to 9000 litres (1 ounce to 2000 gallons). The residual taste of chlorine can be removed by adding a small crystal of sodium thiosulphate, about the size of a grain of rice, to a quart jug of water.

CHLORINE (see CHLORINATED LIME, and SODIUM HYPOCHLORITE).

CHLORMETHIAZOLE (HEMINEVRIN) is a useful hypnotic particularly for elderly patients because of its freedom from hang-over effect. It is particularly useful in the acute withdrawal symptoms of alcoholism. Dependance may occur occasionally and therefore the length of period for which the drug is used should be limited. Side-effects include sneezing, conjunctival irritation and occasional headache.

CHLORODYNE is another name for the *British Pharmaceutical Codex* preparation known as Chloroform and Morphine Tincture, which contains morphine hydrochloride. The dose is 0·3 to 0·6 millilitre. It is a useful soothing remedy in diarrhoea.

CHLOROFORM is a colourless, volatile liquid, half as heavy again as water, and, unlike ether, non-inflammable. It was discovered by Liebig in 1831, and is a compound of carbon, hydrogen, and chlorine ($CHCl_3$). It does not dissolve to a large amount in water, but mixes readily with alcohol or ether. It dissolves sulphur, phosphorus, fats, resins, and most substances which contain a large proportion of carbon; it is therefore very useful as a cleansing agent. It was introduced into medicine in 1847 by Sir J.

Y. Simpson, who was then in search of a substance which could produce unconsciousness for operative purposes more conveniently than ether, introduced a short time previously by Morton in America. (See ANAESTHETICS.)

Uses: Chloroform is used as a solvent of fats, resins, etc., in many chemical processes.

Externally as the liniment of chloroform it is a useful application for rheumatic and similar pains, having both a soothing and a mildly counter-irritant action.

Internally its chief use is by inhalation to produce insensibility to pain during surgical operations, in painful and convulsive diseases such as gall-stone colic, and during child-birth. By mouth, small doses have also the effect of relieving vomiting, especially in seasickness. For this purpose 1 to 5 drops may be taken on a lump of sugar.

CHLOROMA, or GREEN CANCER, is the name of a disease in which greenish growths appear under the skin, and in which a change takes place in the blood resembling that in leukaemia.

CHLOROPHYLL is the name of the green colouring matter of plants. Its main use is as a colouring agent, principally for soaps, oils and fats. It is also being found of value as a deodorant dressing to remove, or diminish, the unpleasant odour of heavily infected sores and wounds.

CHLOROQUINE, which is a 4-aminoquinoline, was introduced during the 1939–45 War for the treatment of malaria. It has also been found of value in the treatment of the skin condition known as chronic discoid lupus erythematosus, and of rheumatoid arthritis.

CHLOROSIS is a form of anaemia which receives its name from the yellow or faintly greenish-grey complexion of those suffering from it. Very common before the 1914–18 War, it is scarcely ever seen now. (See ANAEMIA.)

CHLOROTHIAZIDE is a potent benzothiadiazine (qv) diuretic which is active when taken by mouth. It has also a blood-pressure-lowering effect when used in conjunction with other hypotensive drugs.

CHLOROTRIANISENE (TACE) is a synthetic oestrogen (qv) which is active when taken by mouth. (See OESTROGENS.)

CHLOROXYLENOL, or DETTOL, is an antiseptic which is used for treating cuts, abrasions and wounds. It is also widely used in obstetric practice. It is only slightly soluble in water (1 in 3000).

CHLORPROMAZINE is chemically related to the antihistamine drug, promethazine. It is one of the antipsychotic drugs, and is being used extensively in psychiatry on account of its action in calming psychotic activity without producing undue general depression or clouding of consciousness.

CHLORPROPAMIDE (DIABENESE, MELITASE) is one of the oral hypoglycaemic agents. It is a sulphonamide derivative and acts by stimulating the release of insulin from the pancreas. As it has a prolonged action, it need only be given once a day. Those taking chlorpropamide should bear in mind that in around 10 per cent of people it causes undue sensitivity to alcohol, resulting in severe flushing of the face, headache and a feeling of intoxication. (See also DIABETES MELLITUS, SULPHONYLUREAS.)

CHLORTETRACYCLINE. (See TETRACYCLINES.)

CHLORTHALIDONE (HYGROTON) (see BENZOTHIADIAZINES).

CHOKE-DAMP (see DAMP).

CHOKING is the process which results from an obstruction to breathing situated in the larynx (see AIR PASSAGES). It may occur as the result of disease causing swelling round the glottis (the entrance to the larynx), or of some nervous disorders that interfere with the regulation of the muscles which open and shut the larynx, but generally it is due to the irritation of a piece of food or other substance introduced by the mouth, which provokes coughing but only partly interferes with breathing. In the act of swallowing, all food passes over the top of the larynx, and, as a preliminary to swallowing, the glottis is automatically closed by approximation of the sides of the larynx at their upper edge, over which the bolus of food is shot into the gullet. When, as the result of some nervous disease, such as a form of paralysis of the mouth and throat muscles, or simply of an attempt to speak or laugh during eating, this preliminary closure is not complete, a piece of food is apt to lodge in, or some fluid to trickle down into, the larynx. The mucous membrane lining the upper part of the latter being specially sensitive, coughing results in order to expel the cause of irritation. At the same time, if the foreign body is of any size, lividity of the face appears, due to partial suffocation (see ASPHYXIA).

Treatment: If coughing is vigorous the choking person should be let alone, a glass of water being put within reach, because a gulp of cold water often dislodges the particle, and, at all events, stimulates more vigorous coughing. The choking person should take slow, deep inspirations, which do not force the particle farther in (as sudden catchings of the breath between the coughs do), and which produce more powerful coughs. If the coughing is weak, one or two strong blows with the palm of the hand over either shoulder blade, timed to coincide with coughs aid the effect of the coughing. In the case of a child the patient may be held up by the legs, when the substance causing the obstruction is more readily dislodged. If this is not effective, firmly held by the ankles, the child is swirled around for half a minute or so.

If this fails to dislodge the foreign body, what is known as the Heimlich manœuvre should be tried. If the victim is standing or sitting, stand behind him and wrap your arms round his waist. Grasp the closed fist of the bottom hand with the other hand, and place the thumb side of the first against the abdomen slightly above the navel and below the ribs. Then press your fist against the abdomen with a quick upward thrust. Repeat several times if necessary. If the victim is lying down, whether semi-conscious or unconscious, kneel astride his hips facing him. With one hand on top of the other, place the heel of the bottom hand on the abdomen slightly above the navel and below the ribs. Press into the abdomen with a quick upward thrust. Repeat several times if necessary. Should the victim vomit, turn him quickly on his side and wipe out his mouth to prevent him inhaling the vomited material. The essence of the manœuvre is the quick upward thrust, which quite often causes the foreign body to shoot out of the mouth. Another method in adults is to draw the thighs up towards the body with the knees bent. The thighs are then pressed suddenly and violently into the abdomen.

If this fails, an attempt should be made to remove the foreign body as follows. The bystander should pass his right forefinger along the side of the patient's tongue, forcing the teeth apart first, if necessary, with a knife handle, and keeping them apart by the fingers of the other hand with a napkin rolled round them. The forefinger should be passed as far down the throat as possible, its point then turned towards the middle line and hooked forwards towards the root of the tongue. After a few attempts the foreign body will very likely be dislodged and pulled up into the mouth.

Sometimes, however, the foreign body may be too small to catch; for example, death has been recorded in consequence of a fragment of cabbage leaf which lay over the opening of the larynx like a valve, completely preventing the entrance of air. As the opening is only a slit about 6 mm (a quarter of an inch) from side to side and less than 25 mm (one inch) from before backwards, such an accident may well happen. In this case, if the sufferer is livid and unconscious, and if no medical man is obtained within five minutes, someone at hand may undertake to open the larynx below the obstruction, and admit air to the lungs, but, on account of its dangers, this is suitable only in extremest cases. For this purpose a sharp-pointed knife, such as a penknife, should be taken, the prominent Adam's apple in front of the neck felt for, and the knife pushed boldly into the throat at a point 12 mm (half an inch) below the prominence (in a full-grown person). The knife must be pushed in exactly in the middle line, straight backwards to the depth of 12 mm (half an inch), and the cut extended 12 mm (half an inch) downwards. After this, artificial respiration (see DROWNING) may be necessary, and, if there be any bleeding from the wound in the neck, a bystander should press gently with his fingers on the edge from which it comes, at the same time pressing the edges of the wound apart so as to allow the air to enter. By this procedure, lives have been saved when the obstruction could not be dislodged through the mouth.

CHOLAEMIA is a vague term applied to conditions in which the bile is not excreted from the body to its usual extent, but circulates in the blood. (See JAUNDICE.)

CHOLAGOGUES are substances which increase the flow of bile by stimulating evacuation of the gall-bladder. The great majority of these act only by increasing the activity of the digestive organs, and so producing a flow of bile already stored up in the gall-bladder. Substances which stimulate the liver to secrete more bile are known as CHOLERETICS.

CHOLANGIOGRAPHY is the process whereby the bile ducts and the gall-bladder are rendered radio-opaque and therefore visible on an X-ray film. (See IOPANOIC ACID; SODIUM DIATRIZOATE.)

CHOLANGITIS is the term applied to inflammation of the bile ducts.

CHOLECYSTECTOMY means the removal of the gall-bladder by operation.

CHOLECYSTITIS means inflammation of the gall-bladder (qv).

CHOLECYSTOGRAPHY is the term applied to the process whereby the gall-bladder is rendered radio-opaque and therefore visisble on an X-ray film. (See IOPANOIC ACID; SODIUM DIATRIZOATE.)

CHOLECYSTOKIN is the hormone (qv) released from the lining membrane of the duodenum (qv) when food is taken, and which initiates emptying of the gall-bladder (qv).

CHOLELITHIASIS means the presence of gall-stones in the bile-ducts and/or in the gall-bladder. (See GALL-STONES.)

CHOLERA belongs originally to Asia, more particularly to India and Bangladesh, where epidemics are known to have occurred at various times for several centuries. It was not, however, till 1817 that the attention of European physicians was specially directed to the disease by the outbreak of a violent epidemic of cholera at Jessore in Bengal. This was followed by its rapid spread over a large portion of British

India, where it caused immense destruction of life among both natives and Europeans. By 1823 it had extended into Asia Minor and Russia in Asia, and it continued to advance steadily though slowly westwards, and spread onwards to England, appearing in Sunderland in October 1831, and in London in January 1832. The disease subsequently spread through North and Central America, reaching even to the military posts on the upper Mississippi. In 1835 it was general throughout North Africa, after which this epidemic disappeared.

About the year 1841 another great epidemic of cholera appeared in India and China, and soon began to extend in the direction traversed by the former, but involving a still wider area. This epidemic appears to have been even more deadly than the former, especially in Great Britain and France.

A third great outbreak of cholera took place in the East in 1850, entering Europe in 1853. It was specially severe throughout both North and South America.

A fourth epidemic visited Europe again in 1865-66, but was on the whole less extensive and destructive than its predecessors. In 1884, and again in 1892 and 1893, there were outbreaks in the middle of Europe, the last one being specially severe in Hamburg and some other cities, but, apart from occasional cases brought by ship, there has been no epidemic in Britain or in the United States for many years.

In 1977, a world total of 60,000 cases of cholera was notified, affecting thirty-four countries, including several around the Eastern Mediterranean. In 1980, four imported cases were notified in England.

In 1971 what is known as the el tor bio-type of *Vibriocholerae* entered Europe from the Far East. Between 1970 and 1978 twenty imported cases of this type of cholera were reported in England and Wales, but there was no spread of infection. Neither were there any deaths. In view of the high standard of sanitation in Britain, the possibility of such imported cases leading to an epidemic is most remote. There were only nine cases of cholera notified in 1986 in the UK.

Causes: The cause of the disease is the *Vibrio cholerae*, or comma-bacillus, discovered by Koch. This organism is constantly found in the discharges from the bowels of those suffering from the disease. The most important mode of transmission is by means of contaminated water, but the infection is also conveyed by flies, which contaminate food with infected faeces. The crowding which occurs under conditions of war and famine also favours epidemics.

Symptoms: The incubation period is a few hours to five days. The disease varies in severity from mild cases which do not feel ill enough to take to bed, to cases which are fatal within twenty-four hours. Over 90 per cent of cases, however, are of the so-called *Cholera gravis* type, in which three stages are recognized.

The *first stage*, which lasts for three to twelve hours, is of sudden onset with painless diarrhoea and vomiting. The stools rapidly become frequent and copious, resembling rice-water and containing flakes of fibrin. This is soon followed by agonizing cramps, first in the limbs and then in the abdomen. The patient complains bitterly of thirst and becomes restless and exhausted, with cold bluish skin, sunken eyeballs, and husky voice. The pulse is weak and the temperature taken in the rectum is 38·3° to 40°C) (101° to 104°F).

The *second stage* is termed the stage of collapse, or algid stage. The symptoms now advance with rapidity. The signs of collapse increase. The surface of the body becomes colder and assumes a dusky blue or purple hue, the skin is dry and wrinkled, indicating the intense draining away, in the evacuations, of the fluids of the body. The features are pinched and the eyes more deeply sunken, the pulse at the wrist is imperceptible, and the voice is reduced to a hoarse whisper (the 'vox cholerica'). There may be complete suppression of the urine.

In this condition, death often takes place in less than one day, but, in epidemics, cases are sometimes observed in which the collapse is so sudden and complete as to prove fatal in one or two hours without any great amount of previous purging or vomiting. In most instances the mental faculties are comparatively unaffected, although in the later stages there is generally more or less apathy.

Reaction may, however, take place, and this constitutes the *third stage*. It consists in the arrest of the alarming symptoms of the second stage, and the gradual but evident improvement in the patient's condition. The pulse returns, the surface assumes a natural hue, and the bodily heat is restored. Before long, the vomiting ceases, and, though diarrhoea may continue for a time, it is not of a severe character and soon subsides, as do also the cramps. The urine may remain suppressed for some time, and on returning is often found to be albuminous.

Even in this stage, however, the danger is not past, for relapses sometimes occur which speedily prove fatal; while, again, the reaction may be of imperfect character, and there may succeed an exhausting fever (the so-called *typhoid stage* of cholera), which may greatly retard recovery, and under which the patient may sink at a period even as late as two or three weeks from the start of the illness.

The death-rate varies tremendously: from over 50 per cent in epidemics to around 5 per cent among patients who have received adequate treatment. The outcome is worst in children and old people. Many mild cases are probably never detected in countries where the disease is epidemic.

The bodies of persons dying of cholera are found to remain long warm, and the temperature may even rise after death. Muscular contractions have been observed to take place after death, so that the position of the limbs may become altered.

Treatment: PREVENTIVE TREATMENT: When cholera threatens to invade any place, however favourably circumstanced as to its hygienic condition, increased vigilance will be requisite on the part of those entrusted with the care of the public health. Cholera may be introduced into a community by one or more individuals who have themselves only suffered from the first or milder stage of the disease (cholera diarrhoea), since the discharges from the bowels abound in the infective organisms, and, where sanitary arrangements are deficient, may readily contaminate the water of a locality.

Where suspicion attaches to the water, it should be boiled or chlorinated before being used; milk should also be boiled. Water and food should be protected against pollution with flies, and houses should be fly-proofed. Instructions should be issued by the authorities warning all persons against the use of unwholesome food, unripe fruit, and excesses of every kind, and recommending early application for medical advice where there is any tendency to diarrhoea. The discharges from cholera patients should be treated, as soon as passed, with strong disinfectants (see DISINFECTION), and special care should be taken that they are not disposed of in places where they can contaminate drinking-water. In 1893 Haffkine introduced a vaccine for preventive inoculation against cholera, and this seems to afford a certain amount of protection over a period of some six months. It is recommended for all those going to subtropical or tropical Africa or Asia and wherever there is an outbreak.

CURATIVE TREATMENT: Strict rest in bed is essential. All but a small percentage of cases can now be treated successfully by the administration by mouth of electrolyte solutions. This can be accomplished effectively and economically by the distribution of packets containing pre-weighed amounts of glucose, sodium chloride, potassium chloride and sodium bicarbonate to be added to measured volumes of boiled water in hospital, local treatment centres and, most importantly, in the home, even in the most rural and underdeveloped areas. In severe cases an intravenous infusion is necessary. The infusion fluid consists of two volumes of isotonic sodium chloride (0·9 per cent) plus one volume of sodium lactate (1·75 per cent) or sodium bicarbonate (1·4 per cent). An alternative is the so-called Dacca solution:

Sodium chloride	5 grams
Sodium bicarbonate	4 grams
Potassium chloride	1 gram
Water	to 1 litre

A blood-pressure below 70 mm of mercury, especially if there is associated cyanosis, restlessness, cramps, and cold extremities, is an indication for immediate transfusion with isotonic saline solution.

Chemotherapy is useful only in reducing the period during which the vibrio remains in the stool. For this purpose, chlortetracycline, or one of the insoluble sulphonamides (eg. sulphaguanidine) should be used.

CHOLERETIC is the term applied to a drug that stimulates the flow of bile (qv).

CHOLESTEROL is a sterol, which is one of a class of solid alcohols; these are waxy materials derived from animal and vegetable tissues. It is widely distributed throughout the body, being especially abundant in the brain, nervous tissue, adrenal glands and skin. It is also found in egg yolk and gall-stones. It plays an important role in the body, being essential for the production of the sex hormones, as well as the repair of membranes. It is also the source from which bile acids are manufactured. The total amount in the body of a man weighing 70 kilograms (10 stones) is around 140 grams, and the amount present in the blood is 3·6 to 7·8 m.mol per litre or 150 to 250 milligrams per 100 millilitres.

A high blood-cholesterol level – that is, one over 6 m.mol per litre or 238 mg per 100 ml – is undesirable as there appears to be a correlation between a high blood cholesterol and atheroma (qv), the form of arterial degenerative disease associated with coronary thrombosis and high blood-pressure. This is well exemplified in diabetes mellitus (qv) and myxoedema (qv), two diseases in which there is a high blood cholesterol, sometimes going as high as 20 m.mol per litre; patients with these diseases are known to be particularly prone to arterial disease. There is also a familial disease known as hypercholesterolaemia, in which members of affected families have a blood cholesterol of around 18 m.mol per litre, or more, and are particularly liable to premature degenerative disease of the arteries.

The rising incidence of arterial disease in western countries in recent years has drawn attention to this relationship between high levels of cholesterol in the blood and arterial disease. The available evidence indicates that there is a relationship between blood-cholesterol levels and the amount of fat consumed. Thus, in Cape Town it has been shown that in men aged 45 the mean blood-cholesterol level was 234 mg per 100 ml in the European community and 166 mg per 100 ml in the Bantu community, and this was correlated with the basic difference between the diets of the two communities: 40 per cent of the calories in the European's diet was fat, compared with 20 per cent or less in the Bantu's diet. The suggestion was therefore made that the rising incidence of coronary heart disease, and other manifestations of arterial disease, such as high blood-pressure and strokes, might be arrested by persuading those living in western communities, such as Western Europe and USA, to eat less fat. One of the troubles is that the blood-cholesterol level bears little relationship with the amount of cholesterol consumed, most of the cholesterol in the body being produced by the body itself. Thus, it has been reported that even eating ten eggs, and eggs are the only rich source of cholesterol in the diet, does not usually raise the level of cholesterol in the blood.

On the other hand, it has been shown that diets containing fats with a high proportion of what are known as saturated fatty acids raise the blood-cholesterol level, whereas those with fats containing a high proportion of unsaturated fatty acids lower it. Fats with a high proportion of fatty acids include animal fats such as butter, dripping and the like, whereas the fatty acids with a high proportion of unsaturated fatty acids are predominantly vegetable oils such as olive oil, corn oil, and sunflower oil. The recommendation therefore is that people should reduce their consumption of 'saturated' fats and concentrate on 'unsaturated' fats. Unfortunately, what should have been kept as a straight scientific investigation has become bedevilled with emotional overtones, and it is difficult to give an objective scientific opinion on the present status of the controversy. There is little doubt that there is a tendency to eat too much animal fat today. It is also generally admitted that, if an individual's blood cholesterol is on the high side, even if he is not suffering from diseases such as diabetes mellitus, then it is wise for him to curtail his intake of saturated fats, just as he should aim at avoiding obesity. The same probably applies to a man who has had a coronary thrombosis. Whether there is any need to go further than this is problematical, and much more scientific investigation will be necessary before the medical profession is justified in recommending any striking alteration in our eating habits –except to advise moderation in all things.

CHOLESTYRAMINE (QUESTRAN) is a drug that is proving of value in the treatment of the pruritus, or itching (qv), which occurs in association with jaundice. This it does by 'binding' the bile salts in the gut and so preventing their being reabsorbed into the bloodstream, where their excess in jaundice is responsible for the itching. It is also proving useful in reducing the level of cholesterol and triglycerides in the blood and thereby, like clofibrate (qv), helping to reduce the incidence of coronary artery heart disease. (See CORONARY THROMBOSIS, HYPERLIPIDAEMIA.)

CHOLINE is one of the many constituents of the vitamin B complex. Lack of it in the experimental animal produces a fatty liver. It is found in egg-yolk, liver, and meat. The probable daily human requirement is 500 mg, an amount amply covered by the ordinary diet.

CHONDROMA is a tumour composed in part of cartilage. (See TUMOURS.)

CHOREA, or ST VITUS'S DANCE, is a disorder of the nervous system occurring for the most part in children, and characterized mainly by involuntary jerking movements of the muscles. The name, St. Vitus's dance, was originally applied to those remarkable epidemic outbursts of combined mental and physical excitement which for a time prevailed among the inhabitants of some parts of Germany in the Middle Ages. It is stated that sufferers from this dancing mania were wont to resort to the chapels of St Vitus, the saint believed to possess the power of curing them. The name was transferred to the disease at present under consideration, with which it has evidently nothing to do, and the original application has been to a great extent lost sight of. The term, SYDENHAM'S CHOREA, is also applied to this disorder to distinguish it from Huntington's chorea, a disease of hereditary nature which appears late in life and is accompanied by mental defects.

Causes: Chorea is a condition resulting from involvement of the central nervous system by the same factor (or factors) as are responsible for acute rheumatism (qv). It is more common in girls than in boys, in the proportion of 3:1. Like acute rheumatism it is rare under the age of 3 years and uncommon under the age of 5 years. There is no definite evidence that it is hereditary, but it is more likely to occur in excitable, intelligent, ambitious children than in the phlegmatic child. There may be a history of some precipitating factor such as a fright or worry over an impending examination. It forms an occasional but rare complication of pregnancy.

Although chorea is the manifestation of acute rheumatism which is most likely to occur without manifestations of rheumatism elsewhere, the main importance of chorea is that about one-third of children who develop it show evidence of rheumatism elsewhere in the body, and usually in the heart. Recurrences occur in about one-third of the cases, usually within a year of the first attack. Such recurrences are more common in girls than in boys. If the heart is not involved in the first attack, it is unlikely to be affected in recurrent attacks.

Symptoms: The characteristic features are: (1) involuntary, purposeless, incoordinated movements; (2) weakness of voluntary movements; (3) loss of precision of movement; (4) psychological disturbances. The symptoms are usually preceded by changes in the temper and disposition, the child becoming sad, irritable and emotional, while at the same time the general health is impaired. The first thing indicative of the disease is a certain awkwardness or fidgetiness of manner, together with restlessness, the child being evidently unable to continue quiet, but frequently moving the limbs into different positions. In walking, too, slight dragging of one limb may be noticed. The convulsive muscular movements usually show themselves first in one part, such as an arm or a leg, and in most instances they may remain localized to that limited extent, whilst in all cases there is a tendency for the disorderly symptoms to be more marked on one side than on the other. The child when standing or sitting is never still, but is constantly changing the position of the body or limbs in consequence of the sudden and incoordinate action of muscles or groups of them. These symptoms are aggravated when purposive movements are attempted, or when the child is watched. Sometimes the disorder is first noticed owing to the frequency with which the child drops cups, plates and similar articles. Speech is affected, and the taking of food becomes a matter of difficulty. When the tongue is protruded, it comes out in a jerky manner, and is immediately withdrawn, the jaws at the same time closing suddenly and sometimes with considerable force. The heart may be affected as in acute rheumatism, and this may lay the foundation of permanent heart disease (see HEART DISEASES). Usually, there is a remission of the symptoms during sleep.

This disease occasionally assumes a very acute and aggravated form, in which the disorderly movements are so violent as to render the patient liable to be injured and to necessitate forcible control of the limbs or the employment of anaesthetics to produce unconsciousness. Such cases are rare but of very grave character, if, as is common, they are accompanied with sleeplessness, and they may prove fatal by exhaustion. In the great majority of cases, however, complete recovery is to be anticipated sooner or later, the symptoms usually continuing for from one to two months, or even sometimes longer.

Treatment: The first step in treatment is to provide the patient with complete physical and mental rest. Under suitable conditions the disease tends to recover of itself. These conditions, however, are all-important, and embrace the proper feeding of the child with a full nutritious diet, the absence of all sources of excitement and annoyance, such as being laughed at or mocked by other children, and the removal of any causes of irritation and of irregularities in the general health. Confinement to bed is necessary – usually for four to six weeks. Of medicinal remedies the most serviceable are sodium salicylate and aspirin, especially the latter. After recovery the general health of the child should for a long time receive attention, and care should be taken to guard against excitement, excessive study or any exhausting condition, physical or mental.

In the rare instances of the acute form of this malady, where the convulsive movements are unceasing and violent, the only measures available are the use of full doses of chloral, or injections of hyoscine or morphine. It is these cases which tend to end fatally. (See also HUNTINGTON'S CHOREA.)

CHORIOCARCINOMA is a form of cancer affecting the chorion (qv), in the treatment of which particularly impressive results are being obtained from the use of methotrexate.

CHORION is the more external of the two foetal membranes. (See AFTERBIRTH.)

CHOROID (see EYE).

CHOROIDITIS (see UVEITIS).

CHRISTMAS DISEASE is a hereditary disorder of blood coagulation which can only be distinguished from haemophilia (qv) by laboratory tests. It is so called after the surname of the first case reported in this country. About one out of every ten patients clinically diagnosed as haemophiliac has in fact Christmas disease. It is due to lack in the blood of Factor IX.

CHROMAFFIN is a term applied to certain cells and organs in the body, such as part of the adrenal glands, which have a peculiar affinity for chrome salts. These cells and tissues generally are supposed to secrete substances which have an important action in maintaining the tone and elasticity of the blood-vessels and muscles.

CHROMIC ACID is used in several industries, particularly in chromium plating. Unless precautions are taken it may lead to dermatitis of the hands, arms, chest and face. It may also cause deep ulcers, especially of the nasal septum and knuckles.

Uses: The chief medicinal use of chromic acid is as a caustic for the treatment of warts and indolent ulcers. It is also sometimes used in a 2 or 3 per cent solution for the treatment of sweating feet.

CHROMOSOMES are the rod-shaped bodies to be found in the nucleus of every cell in the body. They contain the genes, or hereditary elements, which establish the characteristics of an individual. They occur in pairs, and human beings possess forty-six, made up of twenty-three pairs. The number of chromosomes is specific for each species of animal. (See HEREDITY; SEX CHROMOSOMES.)

CHRYSAROBIN, or GOA POWDER, is a substance derived from a concretion which forms on the stems of the *Araroba* plant, powdered and purified. It is used in various skin diseases, especially psoriasis. It stains the clothes a deep violet colour. These stains may be removed with benzol or weak chlorinated lime in water.

CHYLE is the milky fluid which is absorbed by the lymphatic vessels of the intestine. The absorbed portion consists of fats in very fine emulsion, like milk, so that these vessels receive the name of lacteals (L. *lac*, milk). This absorbed chyle mixes with the lymph and is discharged into the thoracic duct, a vessel as large as a quill, which passes up through the chest to open into the jugular vein on the left side of the neck, where the chyle mixes with the blood.

CHYLURIA means the passage of chyle (qv) in the urine. This results in the passing of a milky-looking urine. It is one of the manifestations of filariasis (qv), where it is due to obstruction of the lymphatics (qv) by the causative parasite.

CHYME is the name given to the partly digested food as it issues from the stomach into the intestine. It is very acid and grey in colour, containing salts and sugars in solution, and the animal food softened into a semi-liquid mass. It is next converted into chyle.

CHYMOPAPAIN is an enzyme (qv) obtained from the paw-paw, which is being used in the treatment of prolapsed intervertebral discs (qv). When injected into the disc it dissolves it.

CHYMOTRYPSIN is an enzyme (qv) produced by the pancreas (qv) which digests protein. It is used as an aid in operations for removal of a cataract (see ZONULOLYSIS), and also by inhalation to loosen and liquefy secretions in the windpipe and bronchi.

CICATRIX is another word for scar.

CILIA is a term applied to minute, lash-like processes which are seen with the aid of the microscope upon the cells covering certain mucous membranes: eg. the trachea (or windpipe) and nose and which maintain movement in the fluid passing over these membranes. They are also found on certain bacteria which have the power of rapid movement.

CIMETIDINE is a drug that is proving of value in the treatment of peptic ulcer (qv). It acts by reducing the hyperacidity of the gastric juice by antagonising histamine receptors in the stomach.

CIMEX LECTULARIUS (see BED BUG).

CINCHONA is the general name for several trees in the bark of which quinine is found. This bark is also known as Jesuit's bark, having been brought first to notice by Spanish priests in South America and brought to Europe first by the Countess of Cinchon, wife of the Viceroy of Peru, in 1640. The red cinchona bark is that which contains most quinine, and from which it is usually prepared. (See QUININE.) Various extracts and tinctures are made direct from cinchona bark, and used in place of quinine.

CINNAMON is the bark of *Cinnamomum zeylanicum*, a species of laurel grown in Sri Lanka (Ceylon). It has a stimulating action upon the stomach, and assists digestion; hence its use as a condiment. It is also an antispasmodic.

Uses: In flatulent dyspepsia and in sea-sickness, cinnamon powder (600 mg) is very useful. For the same purposes, or for relieving griping, four drops of oil of cinnamon may be taken on sugar, or one tablespoonful of cinnamon water (distilled) may be similarly used.

CIRCLE OF WILLIS, or CIRCULUS ARTERIOSUS, is a circle of arteries at the base of the brain, which is formed by the junction of the basilar, posterior cerebral, internal carotid and anterior cerebral arteries. Congenital defects may occur in these arteries and lead to the formation of aneurysms (qv).

CIRCULATION OF THE BLOOD: This principle was demonstrated for the first time by William Harvey in 1628. Harvey proved, first of all, mainly by the examination of living animals, that the arteries contain only blood. Secondly, he showed by three main propositions that this blood must go round from arteries to veins in a continuous circuit. (1) The quantity of blood passing from the veins into the heart in the course of a whole day is so great that it is quite impossible it could all be manufactured from the food. (2) The blood in the arteries passes in a constant stream to all the members of the body, and does not return by the same route. (3) The blood in the veins flows incessantly to the heart, and does not ebb and flow, as is shown by the valves in veins and in the heart, and by the fact that veins when pressed on do not fill from above. Having proved these points, he assumed there must be 'pores in the flesh' through which the blood 'percolated' from the ends of the arteries to the commencements of the veins. The last link in the evidence was supplied some thirty years later by Malpighi, an Italian scientist, who with the help of the microscope showed these 'pores' to be the minute vessels now called capillaries.

The course of the circulation is as follows: The veins pour their blood, coming from the head, trunk, limbs and abdominal organs, into the right atrium of the heart. This contracts and drives the blood into the right ventricle, which then forces the blood into the lungs by way of the pulmonary artery. Here it is contained in thin-walled capillaries, over which the air plays freely, and through which gases pass readily out and in. The blood gives off carbon dioxide (CO_2) and takes up oxygen (see RESPIRATION), and passes on by the pulmonary veins to the left atrium of the heart. The left atrium expels it into the left ventricle, which forces it on into the aorta, by which it is distributed all over the body. Passing through capillaries in the various tissues, it enters the veins, which ultimately unite into two great veins, the superior and the inferior vena cava, these emptying into the right atrium. This complete circle is accomplished by any particular drop of blood in about half a minute.

In one part of the body there is a further complication. The veins coming from the bowels, charged with food material and other products, split up, and their blood undergoes a second capillary circulation through the liver. Here it is relieved of some food material and purified, and then passes into the inferior vena cava, and so to the right atrium. This is known as the portal circulation.

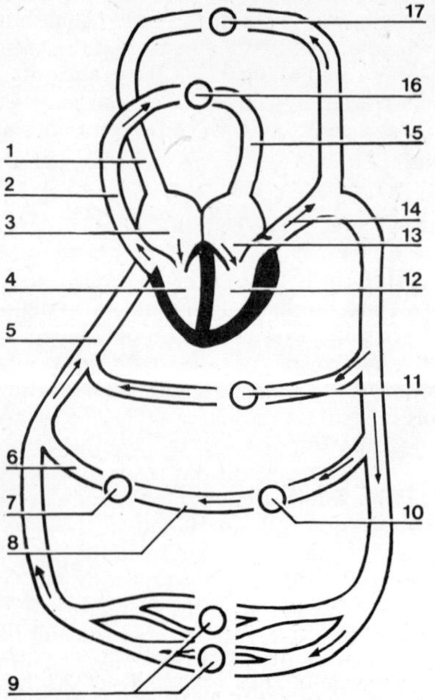

1 superior vena cava
2 pulmonary
3 right atrium
4 right ventricle
5 inferior vena cava
6 hepatic vein
7 liver
8 portal vein
9 limbs
10 intestines
11 kidney
12 left ventricle
13 left atrium
14 aorta
15 pulmonary vein
16 lungs
17 head

General plan of the circulation.

The circle is maintained always in one direction by four valves, situated one at the outlet from each cavity of the heart. (See HEART.)

The blood in the arteries going to the body generally is bright red, that in the veins dull red in colour, owing to the former being charged with oxygen, the latter with carbon dioxide (see RESPIRATION). For the same reason the blood in the pulmonary artery is dark, that in the pulmonary veins bright. There is no direct communication between the right and left sides of the heart, the blood passing from the right ventricle to the left atrium through the lungs.

In the embryo, before birth, the course of circulation is somewhat different, owing to the fact that no nourishment comes from the bowels nor air into the lungs. Accordingly, two large arteries pass out of the navel, and convey blood to be changed by contact with maternal blood (see AFTER-BIRTH), while a large vein brings this blood back again. There are also communications between the right and left atria, and between pulmonary artery and aorta. The latter is known as the ductus arteriosus. At birth all these extra vessels and connections close and rapidly shrivel up.

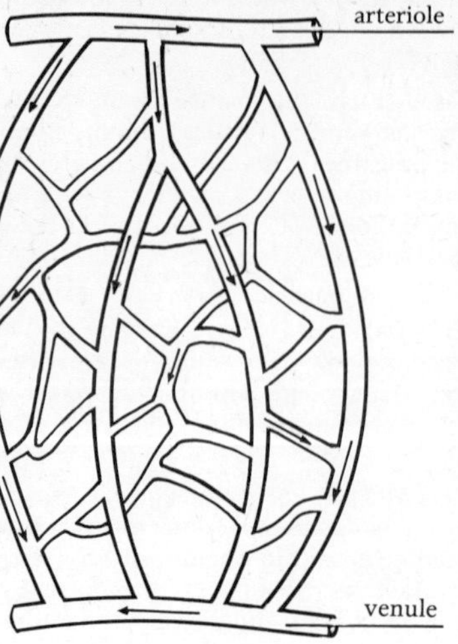

Diagram of the capillary bed. The direction of the blood flow is shown by the arrows.

CIRCULATION, DISORDERS OF: The steady maintenance of the circulation depends upon two factors: (1) the power and regularity of the heart; and (2) the condition of the walls of the vessels, especially of the small arteries. The arteries are not rigid tubes, nor are they merely elastic tubes of a definite size, for each vessel has the power of dilating and contracting within wide limits, so as to let a larger or smaller stream of blood pass through. These motions are controlled by constricting and dilating nerves governed by the nervous system, and upon the action of these, more than upon the heart, depends the state of circulation in various parts. For example, when cold strikes the skin the constrictor nerves are stimulated, the vessels contract, and the blood is driven from the skin, which becomes pallid. On the other hand, blushing is due to loss of control by these nerves over the vessels, or, when the redness is extreme, to stimulation of the dilating nerves by some emotion powerfully affecting the nervous system. Similar changes occur, under other conditions, in all the organs.

Causes and symptoms: *Inflammation* in its early stages is associated with great redness and swelling, due to excessive inflow of blood to the inflamed part through widely dilated arteries. *Congestion* is a condition sometimes due to inflammation, sometimes to an obstruction to the veins which should carry off the blood, or very often to the feebleness of the heart, which cannot drive the blood upwards from dependent parts like the feet, or like the back portions

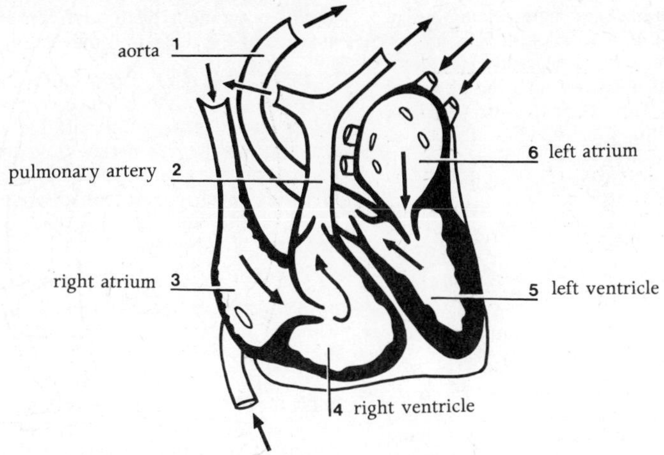

Diagram of the heart opened from in front to show the action of the valves.

of the lungs in bed-ridden persons. In old persons with diseased vessels, in which blood-clots are liable to form, congestion of the brain readily takes place from such obstructions. In weak persons, or those exhausted by illness, lying constantly on the back, congestion of the lungs is very apt to come on. Congestion of the lungs with bronchitis, and congestion of the liver and stomach with various disorders of digestion, are common results of valvular disease of the heart (see HEART DISEASES). *Oedema* and *varicose veins* are similar disorders often due to obstruction to veins. Oedema is also a usual result of heart disease and of kidney disease (see OEDEMA; VEINS, DISEASES OF). *Bloodlessness* of parts is a disorder in the opposite direction, due to spasm and extreme narrowing of arteries (see RAYNAUD'S DISEASE). A local blanching often precedes *chilblains*, which occur in people of sluggish circulation. *Coldfeet and hands*, especially at night, form a milder variety of the same condition. *Insomnia* in elderly people is sometimes due to disordered circulation in the brain, because the vessels are extremely narrowed by disease.

Treatment: Where any failure of the heart is present, the case is treated by various cardiac drugs, by rest, and by graduated exercises. Some cases of disordered circulation depending on the vessels are benefited by cold baths and daily vigorous exercises, while good diet, warm clothing and tonics are of importance for their cure. (See also CHILBLAIN.)

CIRCUMCISION: There is virtually no medical or surgical reason for circumcision in the new-born infant. The prepuce is not normally retractable in infancy so this is not an indication for circumcision. By the age of one the prepuce is retractable in most boys. The Americans are more enthusiastic about circumcision. And the reason offered is that cancer of the penis occurs only when a foreskin is present. This is however a rare disease and is unlikely to occur if cleansing is adequate. In the uncircumsized adult there is an increased transmission of herpes and cytomegalo viruses during the reproductive years but this can be reduced by adequate cleansing. Phimosis is an indication for circumcision. Haemorrhage infection and meatal stenosis are rare complications of circumcision.

CIRRHOSIS, or FIBROSIS, is a diseased condition, in which the proper tissue is replaced by fibrous tissue similar to scar tissue. The name cirrhosis was originally given by Laennec to the disease as occurring in the liver, because of its yellow colour. (See LIVER DISEASES.)

CIRSOID ANEURYSM is the term applied to the condition in which a group of arteries become abnormally dilated and tortuous.

CISPLATIN (NEOPLATIN, PLATINEX, PLATOSIN) (see CYTOTOXIC DRUGS).

CITRIC ACID is the acid which gives their sharp taste to lemons, limes, unripe oranges, currants and raspberries. It is practically identical in action and appearance with tartaric acid, which is obtained from grapes and other fruits, although the two differ in chemical composition. It is similar also to malic acid, found

in apples, pears and the berries of the mountain ash.
Uses: These vegetable acids and their salts (citrates and tartrates) are changed, on absorption into the blood, into alkaline substances, and act therefore to correct acidity (see ACIDITY). The acids themselves have the power of allaying thirst by stimulating the flow of saliva, and also of creating a feeling of coolness. For both these reasons they are much used for cooling drinks in fever. When, in addition, the stomach is irritable, they are best taken in the form of effervescing drinks, which soothe this organ.

CITRINE OINTMENT, or NITRATE OF MERCURY OINTMENT, is used for stimulating sluggish ulcers, and also, diluted with olive oil, in cases of eczema.

CLAUSTROPHOBIA means the fear of being in a confined space, or the fear experienced while in it.

CLAVICLE is another name for the collar-bone (qv).

CLAVUS is a form of neuralgia about the head, often found in hysterical people and others, compared by them to the pain of driving in a nail (see NEURALGIA). The term is also applied to a corn, or thickening of the horny epithelium upon the foot (see CORNS).

CLAW-FOOT, or PES CAVUS, is a familial deformity of the foot characterized by an abnormally high arch of the foot accompanied by shortening of the foot, clawing of the toes and inversion, or turning inwards, of the foot and heel. Its main effect is to impair the resilience of the foot resulting in a stiff gait and aching pain. Milder cases are treated with special shoes fitted with a sponge rubber insole. More severe cases may require surgical treatment.

CLAW-HAND is a condition of bending and wasting of the hand and fingers, especially of the ring and little fingers. The condition is generally due to paralysis of the ulnar nerve. A somewhat similar condition is produced by contraction of the fibrous tissues in the palm of the hand, partly due to rheumatic changes and partly to injury caused by the constant pressure of a tool against the palm of the hand. (See DUPUYTREN'S CONTRACTURE.)

CLAW-TOES (see CLAW-FOOT).

CLEANLINESS (see ANTISEPTICS; ASEPSIS; BATHS; DISINFECTION).

CLEFT FOOT is a rare congenital abnormality characterized by the absence of one or more toes and a deep central cleft that divides the foot into two. It is sometimes known as lobster foot or lobster claw. It may be accompanied by other congenital defects, such as cleft hand, absent permanent teeth, cleft lip and palate, absence of the nails, and defects of the eye.

CLEFT HAND is a rare congenital abnormality characterized by the absence of one or more fingers and a deep central cleft that divides the hand into two. It is sometimes known as lobster hand. It may be accompanied by other congenital defects, such as cleft foot, absent permanent teeth, cleft lip and palate, absence of the nails and defects of the eye.

CLEFT PALATE is the term applied to a fissure in the roof of the mouth (palate) and/or the lip which is present at birth. It is found in varying degrees of severity in about 1 in 700 children. Modern plastic surgery can greatly improve the appearance of the baby and often further cosmetic surgery later will not be necessary. The parent of the child who has cleft lip and/or palate will be given detailed advice specific to his case. In general the team of specialists involved are the paediatrician, plastic surgeon, dentist or orthodontic specialist, and speech therapist. (See PALATE, MALFORMATIONS OF.)

CLICKING FINGER is a condition in middle-aged people in which the victim finds on wakening in the morning that he or she cannot straighten the ring or middle finger spontaneously, but only by a special effort, when it suddenly straightens with a painful click. Hence the name. In due course the finger remains bent at all times unless a special effort is made to straighten it with the other hand. The condition is due to a swelling developing in one of the tendons of the affected finger. If the tendon sheath is slit open surgically, the condition is relieved. Many cases recover spontaneously if the patient is prepared to wait.

CLICKING THUMB is a comparable condition sometimes found in the new-born baby, and occasionally in adults. In the baby, surgery should not be resorted to, as the condition practically always clears up spontaneously. In the adult it can be such a nuisance that it should probably be operated on at a fairly early stage.

CLIMACTERIC was a word originally applied to the end of certain epochs or stages in the life of an individual, at which some great change was supposed to take place. (See also MENOPAUSE.)

CLIMATE IN RELATION TO DISEASE: Climate is of great medical importance, both because various diseases are found in one part of the world and not in others, so that it becomes necessary to know the reasons for this difference, and because removal of a diseased person to new conditions of air, warmth, moisture and the like, is often a valuable means of cure.

The broad division of climates is into hot, temperate and cold climates.

(*a*) **Hot climates** are generally considered as extending to about 35° from the equator, and possessing an average temperature throughout the year of about 29°C (84°F). In the Southern Hemisphere, Montevideo, Cape Town and Sydney lie just at the edge of this band, while north of the equator the limit divides the northern from the southern states of North America, skirts the south of Algeria, the north of India, and excludes Japan from the hot region. Generally speaking, there are, in this region, a wet and a dry season, but near the equator, two wet and two dry seasons.

(*b*) **Temperate climates** are those from about 35° to 55° of latitude, and have a mean temperature of about 3·3°C (38°F) in winter and 31°C (68°F) in summer. These regions include the northern states of USA, the south of Canada, Central and Southern Europe, and, in the East, Japan.

(*c*) **Cold climates** are those from 55° latitude to the poles. The cold is much modified, however, in some localities by ocean currents, so that Scotland, at the same latitude as Labrador, enjoys a temperate though moist climate, the surrounding seas and air being warmed by the Gulf Stream.

But, in estimating the effect of climate, far more than mere distance from the equator has to be considered. The degree of moisture in the air and presence of the sea near at hand, the rarefaction of the air in consequence of altitude, the difference between night and day temperatures, and the presence or absence of dust and bacteria are all of vital importance. For these reasons climates are classed into four sub-varieties: (1) seaboard and ocean climates; (2) inland low climates; (3) mountain climates; (4) dry climates.

(1) SEABOARD AND OCEAN CLIMATES: The important features of these climates are the large amount of moisture in the air, the relatively high content of oxygen compared with mountain air, and the presence of salt and iodine. The air of the high seas is also free from dust and bacteria. Further, large expanses of water warm and cool more slowly than the earth, so that a seaboard climate tends to be more uniform than inland climates. The cases for which seaside air is most suitable are those convalescent from acute diseases, and those worn out by business or social worries.

(2) INLAND LOW CLIMATES include most of the health resorts to which people go in order to drink mineral waters. The general character of inland climates is the great variation between the summer and winter temperature, but, as most of these places are resorted to only in the open part of the year, the climate goes often by the vague name of 'relaxing', in contradistinction to the 'bracing' climate of mountains. Diseases of the heart and other parts of the circulatory system are treated at some of the less relaxing of these resorts, such as Nauheim, where graduated exercises aid the restful action of the climate.

(3) MOUNTAIN CLIMATES have, as their chief character, the rarity of the air, by reason of which the breathing and heart-beats are increased in rate, and a feeling of buoyancy and increased strength given to the whole system. Further, the air is drier and less laden with dust and bacteria, and there is greater difference between the day and night and between the sun and shade temperatures than at lower levels.

(4) DRY CLIMATES or DESERT CLIMATES combine warmth and dryness. In addition, the air is relatively clear of bacteria, though apt to be dusty, and the nights are cold. Such climates are found in Egypt, Australia, some of the Western States of the USA, and, in a milder degree, on the Pampas of South America and the tablelands of Cape Province in South Africa. These are suited especially for chronic rheumatism and chest diseases.

CLINDAMYCIN is an antibiotic which is used in the treatment of serious infections. This restriction is imposed because it is liable to cause severe colitis. It is active against a wide range of micro-organisms.

CLINICAL means literally 'belonging to a bed', but the word is used to denote anything associated with the practical study or observation of sick people as clinical medicine, clinical thermometers.

CLINICAL PSYCHOLOGY: Psychology is the scientific study of behaviour. It may be applied in various settings including education, industry and health care. Clinical psychology is concerned with the practical application of research findings in the fields of physical and mental health. Training in clinical psychology involves a degree in Psychology followed by post graduate training. Clinical Psychologists are specifically skilled in applying theoretical models and objective methods of observation and measurement and in therapeutic interventions aimed at changing patient's dysfunctional behaviour, including thoughts and feelings as well as actions. Dysfunctional behaviour is explained in terms of normal processes and modified by applying principles of normal learning, adaption and social interaction.

Clinical Psychologists are involved in health care in the following ways: (1) Assessment of thoughts, emotions and behaviour using standardised methods. (2) Treatment based on theoretical models and scientific evidence about behaviour change. Behaviour change is considered when it contributes to physical, psychological or social functioning. (3) Consultation with other health-care professionals about problems concerning emotions, thinking and behaviour. (4) Research on a wide variety of topics including the relationship between stress, psychological functioning and disease, the aetiology of problem behaviours, methods and theories of behaviour change. (5) Teaching other professionals about normal and dysfunctional behaviour, emotions and functioning.

Clinical Psychologists may specialise in work in particular branches of patient care, including surgery, psychiatry, geriatrics, paediatrics, mental handicap, obstetrics and gynaecology, cardiology, neurology, general practice and physical rehabilition. Whilst the focus of their work is frequently the patient, at times it may encompass the behaviour of the health-care professionals.

CLINICAL TRIALS: Voltaire defined medical treatment as the act of pouring drugs, of which one knew nothing, into a patient, of whom one knew less. This derisive appraisal of the therapeutics of his time was nearly true as there were virtually no drugs of significant therapeutic value and any benefit the patient received was usally a placebo effect.

The development of effective medical treatment only dates back 50 years or so. When useful drugs did become available in the 1940s and the 1950s doctors realised the importance of evaluating their effectiveness. This lead to the introduction of the so-called clinical trials. Systematic measures were introduced to assess the efficacy initially of new medicines and, later, of surgical operations. This is now done by controlled, randomised clinical trials which compare the new treatment under evaluation either with a placebo or the previous standard treatment. If possible this is done on a double blind basis when neither the patient nor the doctor knows at the time whether the test treatment or the control is being administered: this enables bias to be removed.

CLINICS (see MATERNITY AND CHILD WELFARE).

CLINIFEED (see ENTERAL FEEDING).

CLOBAZAM (FRISIUM) (see BENZODIAZEPINES).

CLOFAZIMINE is a drug used in the treatment of leprosy.

CLOFIBRATE (ATROMIDS) (see HYPERLIPIDAEMIA).

CLOMIPHENE is a drug that stimulates ovulation, or the production of ova, through the medium of the pituitary gland. It is thus being used in the treatment of female infertility. One of its hazards is that, if given in too big doses, it may produce multiple births.

CLOMIPRAMINE (ANAFRANIL) is an antidepressant drug. (See ANTIDEPRESSANTS.)

CLOMOCYCLINE is one of the tetracyclines (qv).

CLONAZEPAM is a drug that is proving of value in some cases of epilepsy, and in the restless legs syndrome (qv). (See TRANQUILLISERS.)

CLONIC is a word applied to short spasmodic movements.

CLONIDINE is a drug originally introduced for the treatment of high blood-pressure. It is an alpha$_2$ adrenoreceptor agonist. It is also proving of value in the prevention of attacks of migraine. If it is used in the treatment of high blood-pressure, its use must not be stopped abruptly as this may result in a sudden rise of blood-pressure within a matter of hours to a dangerously high level. This is not likely to arise with the smaller doses used in the treatment of migraine.

CLONING, from the Greek *klon* meaning a cutting such as is used to propagate plants, is essentially a form of asexual reproduction. The initial stages have been successfully achieved in rabbits. In essence the technique consists of destroying the nucleus of the egg and replacing it with the nucleus from a body cell of the same species – either a male or a female. This provides the egg with a full complement of chromosomes (qv) and it starts to divide and grow just at it would if it had retained its nucleus and been fertilized with a spermatozoon. The vital difference is that the embryo resulting from this cloning process owes nothing genetically to the female egg. It is identical in every respect with the animal from which the introduced nucleus was obtained.

CLOPAMIDE (RINALDIX, VISKALDIX) is a diuretic which is proving of value in the treatment of oedema due to heart disease, cirrhosis of the liver and nephrosis. (See BENZOTHIADIAZINES.)

CLOSTRIDIUM is the genus, or variety, of micro-organisms that produce spores which enable them to survive under adverse conditions. They normally grow in soil, water and decomposing plant and animal matter, where they play an important part in the process of putrefaction (qv). Among the important members of the group, or genus, are *Clostridium welchii*, *Cl. septicum* and *Cl. oedematiens*, the causes of gas gangrene (qv); *Cl. tetani*, the cause of tetanus (qv); and *Cl. botulinum*, the cause of botulism (qv).

CLOT is the term applied to any semi-solid mass of blood, lymph or other body fluid. Clotting in the blood is due to the formation of strings of fibrin produced by the action of a ferment. Milk clots in a similar manner in the stomach when exposed to the action of the ferment rennin. Clotting occurs naturally when blood is shed and comes in contact with tissues outside the blood-vessels. It occurs also at times in diseased vessels (*thrombosis*), producing serious effects upon the organs supplied by these vessels. Clots also form sometimes in the heart when the circulation is feeble and irregular. (See COAGULATION; EMBOLISM; THROMBOSIS.)

CLOTRIMAZOLE is a drug that is proving of value in the treatment of certain fungal or yeast infections, such as aspergillosis (qv) and cryptococcosis (qv).

CLOVES are the unexpanded flower-buds of a species of myrtle, *Eugenia caryophyllus*, from the Indian Archipelago. Oil of cloves is an antiseptic, checks griping, and masks bad breath. It may be taken in doses of 2 or 3 drops on a lump of sugar, or one tablespoonful of infusion of cloves may be similarly used. Cotton-wool dipped in clove oil and put in a hollow tooth relieves toothache temporarily.

CLOXACILLIN (see PENICILLIN, ANTIBIOTIC).

CLUBBING is the term applied to the thickening and broadening of the finger tips and, less commonly, the tips of the toes, that occurs in certain chronic diseases of the lungs and heart. It is due to interstial oedema especially at the nail bed leading to a loss of the acute angle between the nail and the skin of the finger. It is associated with lung cancer, empyema, bronchietasis and congenital cyanotic heart disease.

CLUB-FOOT, or TALIPES, is a deformity in which the foot is permanently twisted at the ankle-joint, so that the sole no longer rests on the ground in standing.

Varieties: The foot can be twisted in four directions. The heel may be pulled up so that the person walks on his toes (*talipes equinus*), or the toes may be bent up so that he walks on his heel only (*talipes calcaneus*), or the sole may look inwards so that he walks on the outer edge of the foot (*talipes varus*), or outwards so that he walks on the inside of the foot (*talipes valgus*). These are usually combined, the heel being drawn up and the sole turned inwards (*equino-varus*) or the heel resting on the ground and the sole looking outwards (*talipes calcaneo-valgus*). A more important division is into those cases in which the deformity exists at birth, which are generally at first fairly easily rectified; and into those cases which are acquired later in life as the result of some disease, which do not yield to such simple treatment.

Causes: The cases found at birth are due to some arrest of development resulting in a congenital deformity (talipes equino-varus), or some faulty position of the foetus in the womb (talipes calcaneo-valgus). *Talipes equino-varus* occurs in about 1 per 1000 live births, is twice as common in boys as in girls, and in half the cases involves both feet. Children of affected parents are more likely to have club-foot than those of non-affected parents. Those which are acquired later may be caused by some spasm in the muscles of the one side of the leg (cerebral palsy), or by paralysis of the muscles on the side of the leg away from the deformity (poliomyelitis), or by rigidity due to the scar following a burn or inflammation.

Treatment: *Talipes calcaneo-valgus*, which is almost always due to a faulty position of the foot in the womb, and often involves both feet, responds well as a rule to manipulation. All that is required in most cases is that the affected part should be moulded into the *equino-varus* position each time mother attends to the babe. It is only in the more severe cases that the foot may need to be strapped into the correct position, or fixed in this position in plaster of Paris for a few weeks. The ultimate result is excellent, but there may be a tendency for the condition to relapse when the child starts walking. This is controlled by a wedge on the heel of the shoe. *Talipes equino-varus* is the most important of all forms of club-foot, and treatment depends upon the cause. If it is due to a congenital deformity, the baby must be referred to a specialist as soon as possible. The sooner treatment is begun the better. This consists of stretching and strapping under medical supervision, the baby being seen regularly by the doctor who does the re-strapping as the foot comes into the normal situation, and the mother being taught to stretch the foot regularly between visits to the clinic. In the more severe cases an operation may be needed if the condition has not responded to non-surgical treatment by the age of 2 or 3 months. In the cases which develop as a result of disease or injury after birth, treatment consists of splinting, strengthening the weakened muscles by massage and electrical stimulation. In the more severe cases operation for transplanting tendons may be necessary.

CLUSTER HEADACHES: This is a distinct entity separate from migraine, although it is sometimes referred to as migrainous neuralgia. The name derives from the fact that the headaches cluster in periods of six to twelve weeks at certain times of the year. The headache is usually on one side and often around the eye. Lacrimation and running of the nose are frequently associated. A chronic form in which attacks persist for more than six months exists. Prophylactic treatment with Lithium carbonate is usually effective.

CLYSTER is another name for enema.

COAGULATION of the blood is the process whereby bleeding (or haemorrhage) is normally arrested in the body. The process is summarized in the following diagram:

prothrombin + calcium + thromboplastin
|
thrombin + fibrinogen
|
fibrin

Prothrombin and calcium are normally present in the blood. Thromboplastin is an enzyme which is normally found in the blood platelets and in tissue cells. When bleeding occurs from a blood-vessel there is always some damage to tissue cells and to the blood platelets. As a result of this damage, thromboplastin is released and comes in contact with the prothrombin and calcium in the blood. In the presence of thromboplastin and calcium prothrombin is converted into thrombin, which in turn interacts with fibrinogen, a protein always present in the blood, to form fibrin. Fibrin consists of needle-shaped crystals, which, with the assistance of the blood platelets, form a fine network in which the blood corpuscles become enmeshed. This meshwork, or clot as it is known, gradually retracts until it forms a tight mass which prevents any further bleeding. It will thus be seen that clotting, or coagulation, does not occur in the healthy blood-vessel because there is no thromboplastin present. There is now evidence suggesting that there is an anti-thrombin substance present in the blood in small amounts, and that this substance antagonizes any small amounts of thrombin that may be formed as a result of small amounts of thromboplastin being released.

COAGULUM is the Latin term for a clot.

COAL-MINER'S LUNG (see ANTHRACOSIS).

COARCTATION OF THE AORTA is a narrowing of the aorta in the vicinity of the insertion of the ductus arteriosus. It is a congenital abnormality. Satisfactory results are now obtained from surgical treatment.

COBALAMINS are a group of substances which have an enzyme action (see ENZYME) and are essential for normal growth and nutrition. (See also CYANOCOBALAMIN; HYDROXOCOBALAMIN.)

COBALT-60 is a radioactive isotope which is being used as a substitute for radium and high-voltage X-rays in the treatment of malignant disease. (See RADIOTHERAPY.)

COBALT EDETATE is an antidote for prussic acid poisoning (qv).

COCAINE: Coca leaves are obtained from two South American plants, *Erythroxylum coca* and *Erythroxylum truxillense*, and contain an alkaloid, cocaine, which has marked effects as a stimulant, and, locally applied, as an anaesthetic by paralysing nerves of sensation. The dried leaves have been used from time immemorial by the South American Indians, who chew them mixed with a little lime. Their effect is to dull the mucous surfaces of mouth and stomach, with which the saliva, produced by chewing them, comes into contact, thus blunting, for long periods, all feeling of hunger. The cocaine, being absorbed, produces on the central nervous system a stimulating effect, so that all sense of fatigue and breathlessness vanishes for the time. It was by the use of coca that the Indian post-runners of South America were able to achieve their extraordinary feats of endurance. The continued use of the drug, however, results in emaciation, loss of memory, sleeplessness and general breakdown. (See DRUG ADDICTION.)

Uses: Before the serious effects that result from its habitual use were realized the drug was sometimes used by hunters, travellers and others to relieve exhaustion and breathlessness in climbing mountains, to steady the nerves, and to dull hunger. The chief use in medicine is by local application to dull pain. Internally it is prescribed along with morphine or heroin for the relief of pain in advanced cancer. (See BROMPTON MIXTURE.) Here the risk of addiction is a secondary consideration. Otherwise it is practically only used in the treatment of diseases of the eye, and diseases of the ear, nose and throat. In the eye it is used as an anaesthetic in the form of eye-drops. It is also used in the form of lamellae to induce anaesthesia of the eye. A 5 per cent spray solution is used to anaesthetize the throat and nose, whilst pastilles and lozenges containing 1·5 to 10 mg are used to reduce irritation of the throat and hoarseness. Artificial chemical compounds closely allied to cocaine are injected hypodermically in order to render painless small operations, such as amputation of the fingers, and by injection into the spinal canal to enable major operations to be done on the lower limbs without pain. (See PROCAINE HYDROCHLORIDE.)

COCCUS is the name applied to a rounded form of bacterium. (See BACTERIOLOGY.)

COCCYDYNIA, or COCCYGODYNIA, means the sensation of severe pain in the coccyx.

COCCYX is the lower end of the spinal column, resembling a bird's beak and consisting of four nodules of bone, which represent vertebrae, and correspond to the tail in lower animals. They are deeply buried in the muscles in man, but in occasional cases they project backwards, and are surrounded by a fold of skin, so as to form an actual tail.

COCHLEA is the part of the inner ear concerned with hearing. (See EAR.)

COCILLANA is the bark of *Guarea rusbyi*, a South American plant with properties similar to those of ipecacuanha. It is used as a remedy in coughs.

CODEINE is one of the active principles of opium (qv). In the form of codeine phosphate it is widely prescribed for the relief of a useless, irritative cough, and also along with aspirin for the relief of headaches and rheumatic pains. It tends to be somewhat constipating.

COD-LIVER OIL is made by purification of the oil pressed from the fresh liver of the cod (*Gadus callarius*). Its principal value in medicine arises out of its high content of vitamin D, the vitamin used in the prevention and treatment of rickets. The official cod-liver oil of the *British Pharmacopoeia* contains not less than 85 international units of vitamin D per gram. Cod-liver oil is also a rich source of vitamin A, the official cod-liver oil of the *British Pharmacopoeia* containing not less than 600 units of vitamin-A activity per gram. The protective dose of vitamin D for infants and children is around 400 international units daily.

Human milk contains enough vitamins for the breast-fed baby provided the mother has enough vitamins in her diet and enough vitamin D from the action of sunlight on her skin, or by taking vitamin tablets during pregnancy and lactation when prescribed by her medical adviser. Cow's milk contains less vitamin D than human milk, but in Britain all baby foods contain added vitamin D (as well as vitamins A and C). There is therefore no need to give the bottle-fed baby vitamins as long as he or she is receiving vitamin-supplemented baby milks. Neither is there any need to give the breast-fed baby vitamin supplements as long as the mother has had sufficient of a mixed diet during pregnancy, has been out in the sunshine, and taken any prescribed vitamin tablets. When, however, the weaning process is begun, and the baby starts taking cow's milk, vitamin supplements are necessary.

COELIAC DISEASE is a wasting disease of childhood in which there is inability to absorb fat from the intestines; there is therefore an excess of fat in the stools. It is the result of a constitutional intolerance of gluten (a constituent of wheat flour) which damages the lining membrane of the small intestine. This in turn interferes with the absorption of fat. Treatment is by means of a gluten-free diet. People with coeliac disease, or parents or guardians of coeliac children can obtain help and guidance from the Coeliac Society of the United Kingdom, PO Box 220, High Wycombe, Bucks HP11 3HY. (See also GLUTEN; MALABSORPTION SYNDROME; SPRUE.)

COELIOSCOPY is a method of viewing the interior of the abdomen in patients in whom a tumour or some other condition requiring operation may be present but cannot with certainty be diagnosed. The examination is carried out by making a minute opening under local anaesthesia, and inserting an instrument bearing an electric lamp and telescopic lenses like that for examining the bladder (cystoscope) into the abdominal cavity. Certain of the abdominal organs can then be directly inspected in turn.

COITUS is sexual intercourse. *Coitus interruptus* (see CONTRACEPTION).

COLCHICUM, the bulb of *Colchicum autumnale*, or meadow-saffron, has long been used as a remedy for gout. How it acts is not quite certain.

Uses: Its main use is in gout, for which colchicine, the active principle of colchicum, in doses of 0·5 mg every one or two hours until the pain is relieved, followed by 0·5 mg thrice daily for about a week, is the form generally employed. Demecolcine, a derivative of colchicine, is sometimes of value in the treatment of chronic myelogenous leukaemia.

COLD, INJURIES FROM (see CHILBLAIN; FROST-BITE; HYPOTHERMIA; also CHILLS AND COLDS).

COLD SORES (see HERPES SIMPLEX).

COLD, USES OF: The application of cold to the surface of the body is capable of influencing the progress of disease in deep-seated parts to a considerable extent by acting on the blood at the surface, or through the nerves which end in the skin. Cold is applied for five chief purposes:

(a) **To subdue pain**: In headache, a wet cloth to the forehead, or sponging with an evaporating mixture of vinegar and water, or eau-de-Cologne and water, is a well-known remedy. Sprains, if treated by holding the injured joint at once under running water, are much relieved. Later on, however, cold applications do harm, rather than good, by preventing the absorption of the effused blood. The pain of pleurisy may also be relieved by the application of an ice-bag to the side. Small operations may be done painlessly after freezing the skin of the part by spraying ethyl chloride over it.

(b) **To lessen inflammation**: Ice-bags are used in inflammatory conditions to prevent the formation of an abscess. In meningitis, or inflammation of the membranes of the brain, they often give some relief when applied to the head.

(c) **To reduce high temperature**: In any fever, sponging the arms and legs, one by one, with tepid water, is harmless and often very soothing. When the temperature runs very high, eg. to 40·5 to 41·8°C (105° or 107°F), wrapping the patient in a wet sheet and rubbing it with ice, or by putting him in a cold bath may be life-saving. (See also under TYPHOID FEVER; WET PACK.)

(d) **To stop haemorrhage**: In cases of increasing haemorrhage under the skin, for example, a bruised and blackening eye or a sprain, the amount of bleeding, and consequent discoloration, are lessened by applying compresses containing ice or some cooling lotion.

(e) **As a general stimulant**: Some diseases are systematically treated in certain countries by cold bathing: for example, typhoid fever. Others are benefited by an alternation of hot and cold bathing: for example, chronic rheumatism. (See also HYPOTHERMIA; CRYOANALGESIA; CRYOSURGERY.)

COLD WEATHER ITCH is a common form of itchiness that occurs in cold weather. It is characterized by slight dryness of the skin, and is particularly troublesome in the legs of old folk. The dryness may be accompanied by some mild inflammation of the skin. It may be exacerbated by excessive central heating. Over-washing with soap should be avoided. A non-alkaline substitute for soap such as Aqueous Cream BP is often beneficial. Relief is obtained from the use of emollients such as E45, applied regularly and always after a bath. Rough winter clothing should not be worn next to the skin.

COLDS (see CHILLS AND COLDS).

COLECTOMY is the operation for removing the colon.

COLESTIPOL (COLESTID) (see HYPERLIPIDAEMIA).

COLIC: By this term is generally understood an attack of spasmodic pain in the abdomen.
SIMPLE COLIC commonly arises from the presence in the alimentary canal of some indigestible matter, which excites spasmodic contraction of the muscular coats of the intestines. The pain of colic is relieved by pressure over the abdomen, and there is no attendant fever – points which are of importance in distinguishing it from inflammation.

Attacks of this form of colic may occur in connection with a variety of causes other than that above mentioned: eg. from accumulations of faeculent matter in the intestines in the case of those who suffer from habitual constipation; as an accompaniment of nervous ailments and not infrequently as the result of exposure to cold and damp, particularly where the feet become chilled, as in walking through snow. Similar attacks of colic are apt to occur in infants, especially those who are fed artificially; and in such cases it will generally be found that a temporary change of diet will be necessary. The duration of an attack of simple colic is seldom long, and in general no ill consequences follow from it. It is, however, not free from risk, especially that of sudden obstruction of the bowel from twisting, or invagination of one part within another (intussusception) during the spasmodic seizure, giving rise to a very grave condition. Colic is also a serious symptom when due to obstruction of the bowel by a tumour or similar condition. (See INTESTINE, DISEASES OF; INTUSSUSCEPTION.)
LEAD COLIC (*Syn.* painters' colic, *colica Pictonum*, Devonshire colic, dry belly-ache) is due to the absorption of lead into the system. This disease had been observed and described long before its cause was discovered. Its occurrence in an epidemic form among the inhabitants of Poitou was recorded by Francis Citois, in 1617, and the disease was thereafter termed *colica Pictonum*. It was supposed to be due to the acidity of the native wines, but it was afterwards found to depend on lead contained in them. About the middle of the eighteenth century this disease, which had long been known to prevail in Devonshire, was carefully investigated by Sir George Baker, who traced it to the contamination of the native beverage, cider, with lead, either accidentally from the lead-work of the vats and other apparatus for preparing the liquor, or from its being sweetened with litharge. (See LEAD POISONING.)
BILIARY COLIC and RENAL COLIC are the terms applied to that violent pain which is produced, in the one case where a biliary calculus or gall-stone passes down from the gall-bladder into the intestine, and in the other where a renal calculus descends from the kidney along the ureter into the bladder. (See GALL-STONES; and KIDNEY, DISEASES OF.)
Treatment: The treatment of colic consists in means to relieve the spasmodic pain, and in the removal, where possible, of the cause upon which it depends. When the attack appears to depend on accumulations of irritating matter in the alimentary canal, a brisk purgative, such as castor oil, will, in addition, be called for. It must be borne in mind that abdominal pain may indicate the onset of acute appendicitis or be a sign of, say, perforation of a peptic ulcer: in such cases purgatives must on no account be given.

Pressure upon the abdomen may relieve the pain partially if not completely. This may be effected, in the case of a baby, by laying him face downwards across the nurse's arm, and in the case of older people by laying a hot-water bottle upon the abdomen, or by lying face downward upon a folded-up pillow. The various substances known as carminatives (qv) or anti-spasmodics (see SPASMOLYTICS) also aid in giving relief.

COLISTIN is an antibiotic isolated from the soil organism, *Bacillus polymyxa* var. *colistinus*. It is active against many Gram-negative organisms, and is proving of value in the treatment of gastro-intestinal and genito-urinary infections.

COLITIS means inflammation of the colon, the first part of the large intestine. *Mucous colitis*, once a fashionable disease, is now recognized not to be a form of colitis and has been named *mucomembranous colic*, or *spastic* or *irritable colon*. It is caused by painful spasms of the colon and occurs in nervous types of individuals. Treatment consists of dealing with the underlying nervous condition, the avoidance of all aperients, and a full diet without an excess of roughage. *Acute catarrhalcolitis* occurs as part of an acute gastro-enteritis, usually due to food poisoning. The treatment is as for acute diarrhoea (qv). *Chronic catarrhal colitis* is usually due to the abuse of aperients and purgatives.
ULCERATIVE COLITIS is the most important form of colitis. It is an acute condition, the cause of which is not known. Although apparently precipitated at times by exposure to cold

or damp or by dietetic indiscretions, these are not the primary cause. It is predominantly a disease of young adults. Once an individual has had the disease, it is very liable to relapses.

Symptoms: The onset may be sudden or insidious. In the acute form there is severe diarrhoea and the patient may pass up to twenty stools a day. The stools, which may be small in quantity, are fluid and contain blood, pus and mucus. There is always fever, which runs an irregular course. In other cases the patient first notices some irregularity of the movement of the bowels, with the passage of blood. This becomes gradually more marked. There is seldom actual pain except immediately prior to the passage of a stool, but there is always a varying amount of abdominal discomfort. The constant diarrhoea leads to emaciation and weakness, and there is always a well-marked anaemia. The acute form may be rapidly fatal, but as a rule the acute phase passes into a chronic stage. The chronic form is liable to run a prolonged course, and the majority of cases are subject to relapses for many years.

Treatment: Rest in bed is essential during the acute stage and as long as there is fever. The diarrhoea is controlled by Corticosteroids which may be given either by mouth or by enema. The diet should be bland and nourishing and should contain a minimum of roughage: ie. a low-residue diet (see DIETS). The anaemia which is always present is treated by means of iron preparations. In some cases it may be necessary to use surgical measures to control the condition: eg. by removing more or less of the affected colon. Corticosteroids, along with sulphasalazine (qv), have become the basic treatment. Another drug proving useful in this condition is azathioprine (qv). Once a patient has recovered and is back to work again, it is essential for him to remain on a low-residue diet, and to be particularly careful in avoiding unnecessary exposure to cold and damp; otherwise the condition is liable to recur. In the prevention of recurrences, sulphasalazine is proving most effective.

Patients and their relatives can obtain help and advice from the National Association for Colitis and Crohn's Disease, 98A London Road, St. Albans, Herts AL1 1NX (0727–44296).

COLLAGEN is the most abundant protein in the body. It is the major structural component of many parts of the body and occurs in many different forms. Thus it exists as thick fibres in skin and tendons. It is also an important constituent of the heart and blood vessels. With calcium salts it provides the rigid structure of bone. It also occurs as a delicate structure in the cornea of the eye, and in what is known as the basement membrane of many tissues including the glomeruli of the kidneys and the capsule of the lens of the eye. It plays a part in many diseases, hereditary and otherwise. Among the inherited abnormalities of collagen are those responsible for aneurysms of the circle of Willis (qv) and for osteogenesis imperfecta (qv). On boiling it is converted into gelatin.

COLLAGEN DISEASES is a term used to describe a group of diseases, including acute rheumatism and rheumatoid arthritis, which are characterized by changes in the collagen of the tissues. The precise cause of these changes is not known, but they are probably a sensitization reaction to an unknown toxin, and they respond to cortisone and corticotrophin.

COLLAPSE is a condition of extreme weakness of all the bodily powers, and especially of the nervous system. It forms the termination of many severe diseases, such as cholera, typhoid fever, irritant poisoning. It is closely allied to the condition of surgical shock, but, whilst in collapse from the conditions mentioned the chief feature is feebleness of the heart's action, in shock there are numerous other prominent symptoms. (See SHOCK.)

Symptoms: The face is pale and drawn, the forehead sometimes covered with cold sweat, the eyes sunken and glassy. The voice is weak, the breathing shallow, and the pulse rapid and feeble or imperceptible. The temperature is usually reduced to 35·6° or 36·1°C (96° or 97°F). Generally the patient lies on his back, paying no attention to what is proceeding around him.

Treatment: The patient should be allowed to lie quietly on his back in a darkened room, well covered, and surrounded by hot bottles to maintain the body heat. Stimulants are also necessary.

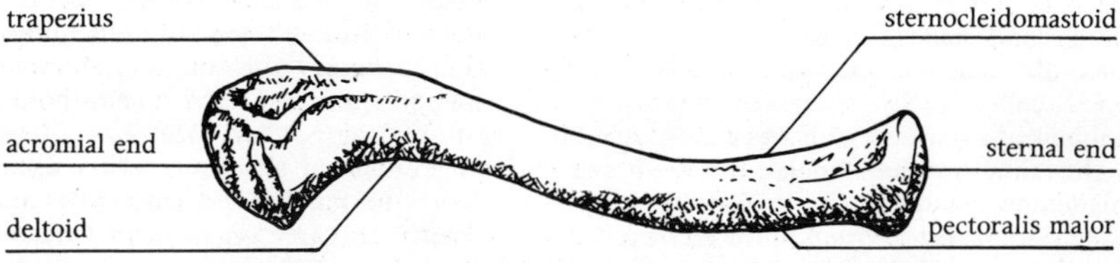

The right clavicle; superior aspect (*see text on following page*).

COLLAPSE THERAPY is the term applied to the method of treating diseases of the lung by bringing about collapse of the diseased part through removing the supporting ribs (thoracoplasty), or introducing air into the pleural cavity (artificial pneumothorax).

COLLAR-BONE, or CLAVICLE, is the bone which runs from the upper end of the breast-bone towards the tip of the shoulder across the root of the neck. It supports the upper limb, keeps it out from the side, and gives breadth to the shoulders. The bone is shaped like an '*f*' with two curves, which give it increased strength. It is, however, liable to be broken by falls on the hand or on the shoulder, and is the most frequently fractured bone in the body. (See FRACTURES.)

COLLARGOL is a form of colloidal silver which mixes readily with water and any albuminous fluids, and has an antiseptic action. It is used especially for application to the eyes in inflammatory conditions.

COLLES'S FRACTURE is a fracture of the lower end of the radius close to the wrist, caused usually by a fall forwards on the palm of the hand, in which the lower fragment is displaced backwards. (See FRACTURES.)

COLLODIONS consist basically of a thick, colourless, syrupy liquid, made by dissolving guncotton (pyroxylin) in a mixture of ether and alcohol or with acetone. When painted on the skin the solvent evaporates, leaving a tough film behind. *Flexiblecollodion*, or collodion as it is often referred to, contains 1·6 per cent of pyroxylin, with colophony, castor oil and alcohol (90 per cent) in solvent ether. It should be kept in a well-sealed container. Being relatively elastic, it does not crack through the movements of the skin. *Salicylic acidcollodion* contains 12 per cent of salicylic acid.
Uses: Collodion is mainly used as a covering for wounds after these have been cleaned. The objection to its use is that, if a wound, or the surface round it, be not absolutely clean, the discharges from the wound are retained by the collodion, and may carry infection deeply into the tissues. *Salicylic acidcollodion* is sometimes used in the treatment of corns and warts.
Mode of application: The wound having been cleaned thoroughly, dried, and all bleeding stopped, collodion is painted over it with a camel-hair brush. Before this has time to dry, a very thin film of cotton-wool is laid on it and painted down with more collodion. Then another film of cotton-wool, followed by collodion, and so on till five or six layers of each have been applied, successful application depending on the films of wool being as thin as possible, and upon each layer being applied before that beneath it has had time to dry completely.

COLLOID is the name given to a type of cancer of internal organs, in which a glue-like substance collects in the interior of the tumour. The term is also applied to substances existing in a colloidal solution, and to the viscid iodine-containing material in the spaces of the thyroid gland.

COLLOIDAL SOLUTIONS are solutions in which a substance very finely divided into particles is suspended in another substance, as, for example, metals like silver and iron suspended in the form of minute particles in water or glycerin. The two constituents of the colloidal solution are called phases – the particles being known as the internal phase, and the medium in which they are suspended, the continuous or external phase. The term, suspensoid, is applied to colloids in which the particles consist of pure solid, and the term, emulsoid, is applied to those in which the particles absorb some of the liquid in which they are suspended.

COLLYRIUM means an eye-lotion.

COLOBOMA simply means a defect, but its use is usually restricted to congenital defects of the eye. These may involve, the lens, the iris, the retina or the eyelid.

COLOCYNTH, or BITTER APPLE, is the fruit of a species of cucumber, *Citrullus colocynthis*, growing on the Mediterranean shores. The dried white pulp is a powerful purgative. It is administered usually as colocynth and hyoscyamus pill, the hyoscyamus being incorporated to counteract the severe griping of the colocynth. It has largely been superseded by less drastic purgatives.

COLON is the first part of the large intestine. (See INTESTINE.)

COLONOSCOPE is an instrument for viewing the interior of the colon. It is made of fibre glass which ensures flexibility, and incorporates a system of lenses for magnification and a lighting system.

COLOSTOMY is the operation for the establishment of an artificial opening into the colon. This acts as an artificial anus. The operation is carried out when there is an obstruction in the colon or rectum that cannot be overcome, or in cases, such as cancer of the rectum in which the rectum and part of the colon have to be removed. Such a colostomy opening can be trained to function in such a way that the patient can carry on a normal life, eating a more or less normal diet. Anyone wishing help or advice in the practical management of a colostomy should get in touch with the British Colostomy Association, 38/39 Eccleston Square, London, SW1V 1PB (01-828 5175). (See STOMA.)

COLOSTRUM is the first fluid secreted by the mammary glands for two or three days after childbirth. It contains less casein and more albumin than ordinary milk.

COLOUR BLINDNESS (see VISION, DEFECTIVE COLOUR VISION).

COLPITIS is a term applied to inflammation of the vagina. (See WHITES.)

COLPOMICROSCOPY is a refinement of colposcopy (qv), whereby it is possible to examine the cervix uteri under a magnification of 270 by the insertion of a microscope tube into the vagina.

COLPORRHAPHY is an operation designed to strengthen the pelvic floor in cases of prolapse of the uterus.

COLPOSCOPY is the method of examining the vagina and cervix by means of the binocular instrument known as the colposcope. It is proving of particular value in the early detection of cancer of the cervix.

COLTSFOOT is the name given to the leaves of *Tussilago farfara* or *Tussilago petasites*, the butter burr, used in the form of a decoction for the treatment of coughs.

COMA is a state of profound unconsciousness, in which not only can the sufferer not be roused, but there are not even reflex movements when the skin is pinched, the eyeball touched, etc. The breathing is generally stertorous, but deep, and the heart's action is strong. The cause of coma is usually apoplexy, but it may also be due to high fever, diabetes mellitus, glomerulonephritis, alcohol, epilepsy, cerebral tumour, meningitis, injury to the head, overdose of insulin, carbon monoxide poisoning, poisoning from opium and other narcotic drugs. Though usually of relatively short duration, and terminating in death, unless yielding to treatment, it may occasionally be long-lasting. The longest recorded case is that of the woman who died in the USA in 1978 at the age of 43, after having been in a coma for thirty-seven years following an operation for removal of her appendix. (See UNCONSCIOUSNESS.)

COMEDONES (see ACNE).

COMMENSAL is the term applied to micro-organisms which live in or on the body (eg. in the gut or respiratory tract, or on the skin) without doing any harm to the individual.

COMMISSURE means a joining, and is a term applied to strands of nerve fibres which join one side of the brain to the other, to the band joining one optic nerve to the other, to the junctions of the lips at the corners of the mouth, etc.

COMMITTEE ON SAFETY OF MEDICINES (CSM): The Committee for Safety of Drugs was set up in 1963 in response to the thalidomide disaster. When the Medicines Act became law in 1971 this Committee was replaced by the Committee on Safety of Medicines. The CSM is an advisory committee which scrutinises drugs at three stages: before clinical trials (clinical trial certificate stage), before a drug is advertised or marketed (product licence stage), or after marketing, the stage at which most doctors first have a direct interest in its work. Until 1981 the first stage in the assessment of new products required the granting to the company concerned of a clinical trial certificate, without which the product could not be tested in man. The issue of a trial certificate requires detailed animal evidence of toxicology and of teratogenic effects. A product licence is normally valid for five years, after which it has to be renewed. Before such a licence is granted efficacy must be shown for each of the proposed indications and appropriate warnings about side effects, contra-indications and interactions given.

COMMON COLD (see CHILLS AND COLDS).

COMMOTIO CEREBRI is another term for concussion of the brain.

COMMUNITY HEALTH COUNCIL (see NATIONAL HEALTH SERVICE).

COMPENSATION is a term applied to the counterbalancing of some defect of structure or function by some other special bodily development. The body possesses a remarkable power of adapting itself to even serious defects, so that disability due to these passes off after a time. The term is most often applied to the ability possessed by the heart to increase in size, and therefore in power, when the need for greater pumping action arises in consequence of a defective valve or some other abnormality in the circulation. A heart in this condition is, however, more liable to be prejudicially affected by strains and diseased processes, and the term 'failure of compensation' is applied to the symptoms that result when this power becomes temporarily insufficient.

COMPLEMENT is a normal constituent of blood serum which plays an important part in the antibody-antigen reaction which is the basis of many immunity processes. (See IMMUNITY.)

COMPLEX is the term applied to a combination of various actions or symptoms. The term is particularly applied to a set of symptoms occurring together in mental disease with such regularity as to receive a special name.

COMPLEXION (see ACNE; SKIN DISEASES; SUNBURN).

COMPOSITOR'S DISEASE is a form of lead poisoning which occasionally attacks those who handle metal type. (See LEAD POISONING.)

COMPRESS is the name given to a pad of linen or flannel wrung out of water and bound to the body. It is generally wrung out of cold water, and may be covered with a piece of waterproof material. It is used to subdue pain or inflammation. (See COLD.) A hot compress is generally called a fomentation. (See FOMENTATIONS.)

COMPRESSED AIR ILLNESS (see CAISSON DISEASE).

COMPRESSION SYNDROME (see MUSCLE).

COMPUTED TOMOGRAPHY: Tomography is an X-ray examination technique in which only structures in a particular plane produce clearly focussed images. Whole-body computed tomography was introduced in 1977 and has already made a major impact in the investigation and management of medical and surgical disease. The technique is particularly valuable where a mass distorts the contour of an organ, eg. a pancreatic tumour, or a lesion which has a density different from that of surrounding tissue, eg. a metastasis in the liver. Computed tomography can distinguish soft tissues from cysts or fat, but in general soft tissue masses have similar appearances, so that distinguishing an inflammatory mass from a malignant process may be impossible. Computed tomography is particularly useful in patients with suspected malignancy. It can also define the extent of the cancer by detecting enlarged lymph nodes, indicating lymphatic spread. The main indications for computed tomography of the body are: mediastinal masses, suspected pulmonary metastases, adrenal disease, pancreatic masses, retroperitoneal lymph nodes, intra-abdominal abscesses, orbital tumours and the staging of cancer.

CONCEPTION signifies the complex set of changes which occur in the ovum and in the body of the mother at the beginning of pregnancy. The precise moment of conception is that at which the male element, or spermatozoon, and the female element, or ovum, fuse together. Only one-third of these conceptions survive to birth, whilst 15 per cent are cut short by spontaneous abortion or stillbirth. The remainder – over one half – are lost very early during pregnancy without trace. (See FOETUS.)

CONCRETIONS are masses of various sizes and substances which form in many of the tissues and smaller cavities of the body in certain circumstances.

Varieties and causes: There is a special liability to the deposit of lime salts in damaged or degenerating tissues. The reason for this is probably much the same as that for the similar deposit from hard water inside kettles and boilers. The tissues in question being inactive do not produce sufficient carbon dioxide to keep dissolved the lime salts in the fluids circulating past and through them. Accordingly, healed-up areas in the lungs, which have been the seat of tuberculosis, the remains of dead parasites and other foreign bodies, degenerated blood-vessels, tumours and scars generally, are apt to have lime deposited in and around them till masses of considerable size are formed. The tartar on the teeth, some stones in the bladder, and the calculi sometimes found in the ducts of salivary glands in the cheek or beneath the tongue, are examples of a similar deposit of lime and phosphates, due to the action of bacteria.

Hair-balls, which are common in the stomachs of lower animals that lick themselves, occur sometimes in mentally deranged patients who have a habit of chewing their hair, and may reach the size of walnuts or larger. (See also BEZOAR.)

Various glands produce secretions, which, by a gradual process of sedimentation build up solid masses in the ducts of these glands. Examples of this are found in the gall-stones, formed of cholesterin separated from the bile, in the uratic stones found in the kidney or bladder of persons suffering from acidity, in the plugs of hardened wax which often give trouble in the ear, and in the cheese-like masses which accumulate in the tonsils and give rise to foetor of the breath.

Gout is a disease in which the pain is due to sharp uratic crystals which are deposited on the surfaces of joints, the same crystals being deposited in other tissues also, at a later stage of the disease, so that large solid masses called 'chalk-stones' are ultimately formed. (See GOUT.)

CONCUSSION OF THE BRAIN (see BRAIN).

CONDIMENTS (see DIET).

CONDURANGO is the dried stem bark of *Marsdenia condurango*, a South American plant which is used as a bitter tonic.

CONDYLE is the name given to a rounded prominence at the end of a bone: for example, the prominences at the outer and inner sides of the knee on the thigh-bone (or femur). The projecting part of a condyle is sometimes known as an *epicondyle*, as in the case of the condyle at the lower end of the humerus (qv) where the epicondyles form the prominences on the outer and inner side of the elbow.

CONDYLOMA means a localized, rounded swelling of mucous membrane about the opening of the bowel, and the genital organs, sometimes known as 'genital warts' or 'ano-genital warts'. There are two main forms of them: *Condyloma latum*, which is syphilitic in origin, and *Condyloma acuminatum*, which often occurs in association with venereal disease, but is only indirectly due to it, being primarily a virus infection.

CONDY'S FLUID is a powerful disinfectant containing permanganates. (For its action and uses, see PERMANGANATE OF POTASSIUM.)

CONFECTIONS, also known as conserves and electuaries, form a method of prescribing certain bulky drugs mixed into a paste with sugar or honey. The best known confections are those of senna and sulphur, both of which are aperient in action. Compound confection of guaiacum, better known as 'Chelsea Pensioner', is an old remedy for constipation and rheumatic pains in elderly people, having received its name from the success of its use among the men of that hospital. It contains guaiacum resin, rhubarb, potassium acid tartrate, nutmeg, sublimed sulphur and honey. The dose of all these confections is about a teaspoonful or more.

CONGENITAL deformities, diseases, etc., are those which are either present at birth, or which, being transmitted direct from the parents, show themselves some time after birth.

CONGESTION means the accumulation of blood in a part due to over-filling of its blood-vessels. The condition may be due to some weakness of the circulation (see CIRCULATION, DISORDERS OF), but as a rule is one of the early signs of inflammation (see ABSCESS; INFLAMMATION).

CONGESTION TREATMENT is a method sometimes used to stimulate the process of repair in both acute and chronic states of inflammation. It depends upon the principle that when the blood-vessels of an inflamed part are artificially dilated the number, and consequently the activity, of phagocytes (see PHAGOCYTOSIS) are increased. The congestion is brought about either by obstructing the return of blood (eg. in a limb) by means of an elastic bandage, or by diminishing the atmospheric pressure in the case of flat or outlying parts (eg. the back or the finger) by means of a suction cup or cylinder from which a rubber tube leads to a suction pump.

CONIUM (see HEMLOCK).

CONJUGATE DEVIATION is the term for describing the persistent and involuntary turning of both eyes in any one direction, and is a sign of a lesion in the brain.

CONJUNCTIVA (see EYE).

CONJUNCTIVITIS (see EYE, DISEASES AND INJURIES OF).

CONOVID (see NORETHYNODREL).

CONSOLIDATION is a term applied to solidification of an organ, especially of a lung. The consolidation may be of a permanent nature due to formation of fibrous tissue, or may be temporary, as in acute pneumonia.

CONSTIPATION, or COSTIVENESS, means a condition in which the bowels are opened too seldom or incompletely, the motions as a consequence being dry and hard. It should, however, be borne in mind that, though most persons have in health one daily movement of the bowels, some perform this act twice, while in others a motion once in two or more days is perfectly natural. Constipation is a chronic condition, and must be carefully distinguished from acute obstruction of the bowels, a much more serious condition. (See INTESTINE, DISEASES OF.) Great variations, however, take place in colour (see STOOLS), in amount, and in consistency, according to the nature and quantity of the food and drink taken.

Causes: The uncommon causes of constipation are mechanical –that is, obstruction by stricture of the bowel, by tumour, by adhesive bands. The common causes are (1) habit, (2) 'a greedy colon', which absorbs water too quickly, (3) a spastic colon, the muscle of which remains in a state of spasm, (4) lack of tone of the colon muscle, sometimes because of too little vitamin B_1 in the diet, (5) a diet which has not enough 'roughage' in it to stimulate the intestine to activity. Of these, habit is probably most important. Constant neglect to respond to the sensation in the rectum which indicates that it is full and needs emptying leads to retention of faeces, which become dry and hard. The condition is aggravated by the use of purgatives.

Symptoms and effects: The stools are dark, hard, and passed with difficulty, and in small amount. In severe, persistent cases there may be swelling of the abdomen, from the retention of large masses of the remnants from digestion. Colic may occur in long-standing cases, in which the accumulation in the lower part of the bowel is beginning to affect the rest of the gut. Piles, which are a cause of increasing constipation, are often brought on by inattention to the bowels to begin with. Headache and lassitude may be present, but this is largely due to the pressure of the accumulated faeces in the rectum, not to any so-called toxic effect.

Treatment: Assuming that there is no organic cause, such as tumour or other source of mechanical obstruction, the most important matter is the regulation of the daily habits. The person concerned should take a certain amount of exercise daily. Above all things, a habit of opening the bowels, at the same time every day, should be cultivated; a definite hour should be fixed, preferably after a meal, and best after breakfast, and, no matter whether there be a sensation that the bowels will move or not, the attempt should unfailingly be made. The diet is of importance. On the whole, in cases of constipation this errs in being too concentrated and too unirritating. As a rule, the diet should be changed to include brown bread, green vegetables, and fruit, especially fruit like prunes, which have a large indigestible residue, while a considerable amount of fluid should be taken. The juice of an orange or grapefruit, or a glass of water, first thing in the morning may help. There is much to be said for adding a dessertspoonful of wheat bran (in the form known as miller's bran) to the breakfast cereal, or lunch or dinner sweet.

The use of aperients and purgatives has usually exaggerated the condition, and as a general rule should be given up.

CONSTITUTION, or DIATHESIS, means the general condition of the body, especially with reference to its liability to certain diseases.

CONSUMPTION (see TUBERCULOSIS).

CONTACT LENSES are lenses worn in contact with the eye, behind the eyelids and in front of the cornea. They may be worn for cosmetic, optical or therapeutic reasons. The commonest reason for wear is cosmetic, many short-sighted people preferring to wear contact lenses instead of glasses. Optical reasons for contact-lens wear include cataract surgery (usually unilateral extraction) and the considerable improvement in overall standard of vision experienced by very short-sighted people by wearing contact lenses instead of glasses. Therapeutic lenses are those used in the treatment of eye disease, 'bandage lenses' are used in certain corneal diseases: contact lenses can be soaked in a particular drug and then put on the eye so that the drug slowly leaks out on to the eye. Contact lenses may be hard, soft or gas permeable. Hard lenses are more optically accurate (because they are rigid), cheaper and more durable than soft. The main advantage of soft lenses is that they are more comfortable to wear. Gas permeable lenses are so called because they are more permeable to oxygen than other lenses, thus allowing more oxygen to reach the cornea.

	Hard lens	*Soft lens*
Cost	Cheap	Expensive
Fitting	Straightforward	Simpler
Adaptation time	Can be considerable	Much shorter
Wearing time	Limited	Longer
Comfort	May cause discomfort	Very comfortable
Visual acuity	Good	Poorer; may be unstable
Stability	May be displaced, or ejected from eye	Rarely displaced or ejected
Durability	Resistant to mishandling	More easily damaged
Length of service	Usually long	Limited
Care	Simple	More difficult

Relative advantages and disadvantages of hard and soft contact lenses.

CONTAGION means the principle of spread of disease by direct contact with the body of an affected person.

CONTINUED FEVERS are typhus, typhoid and relapsing fevers, so called because of their continuing over a more or less definite space of time.

CONTRACEPTION is the prevention, by artificial means, of fertilization of the ovum following sexual intercourse. The most favoured method of contraception is the 'Pill'. Oral contraceptives are synthetic steroids consisting of an oestrogen in addition to a progestogen. Because of the risk of thrombosis the oestrogen content of most oral contraceptives was reduced in 1970 to 50μg. These compounds inhibit ovulation, render the cervical mucus impenetrable to the sperm and diminish the receptivity of the endometrium to implatation. Although ovulation may be inhibited by progestogen alone, the addition of oestrogen maintains the endometrium and gives better control of the menstrual cycle. Twenty-two oral contraceptive tablets have been approved by the Family Planning Association and there is little doubt that these tablets provide the most efficient method of birth control available.

Low Oestrogen Dose Preparation
Oestrogen Progestogen
1 Microgynon 30 0·03mg ethinyloestradiol 0·15mg levonorgestrel
2 Ovranette 0·03mg ethinyloestradiol 0·15mg levonorgestrel
3 Eugynon 30 0·03mg ethinyloestradiol 0·25mg levonorgestrel
4 Ovran 30 0·03mg ethinyloestradiol 0·25mg levonorgestrel
5 Conova 30 0·03mg ethinyloestradiol 2·00mg ethynodioldiacetate
6 Brevinor 0·035mg ethinyloestradiol 0·50mg norethisterone
7 Ovysmen 0·035mg ethinyloestradiol 0·50mg norethisterone
8 Norimin 0·035mg ethinyloestradiol 1·00mg norethisterone

Medium Oestrogen Dose Preparations
Oestrogen Progestogen
9 Demulen 50 0·05mg ethinyloestradiol 0·50mg ethynodiol diacetate
10 Ovulen 50 0·05mg ethinyloestradiol 1·00mg ethynodiol diacetate
11 Eugynon 50 0·05mg ethinyloestradiol 0·50mg DL-norgestrel
12 Ovran 0·05mg ethinyloestradiol 0·50mg DL-norgestrel
13 Minilyn 0·05mg ethinyloestradiol 2·50mg lynestrenol
14 Orlest 21 0·05mg ethinyloestradiol 1·00mg norethisterone acetate
15 Minovlar 0·05mg ethinyloestradiol 1·00mg norethisterone acetate
16 Minovlar ED ethinyloestradiol 1·00mg norethisterone acetate
17 Norlestrin 0·05mg ethinyloestradiol 2·50mg norethisterone acetate
18 Gynovlar 21 ethinyloestradiol 3·00mg norethisterone acetate
19 Anovlar 21 0·05mg ethinyloestradiol 4·00mg norethisterone acetate
20 Ortho-Novin 1/50 0·05mg mestranol 1·00mg norethisterone
21 Norinyl 1 0·05mg mestranol 1·00mg norethisterone
22 Norinyl 1/28 0·05mg mestranol 1·00mg norethisterone

Side-effects are infrequent. Premenstrual tension, menorrhagia, irregular cycles and a mucoid vaginal discharge are suggestive of oestrogen excess and they may be relieved by a change to an oral contraceptive with a more dominant progestogen action. Breast discomfort, acne, abdominal cramps and a dry vagina are suggestive of a progestogen excess and a change to a tablet with less progestogenic action is indicated if such symptoms prove troublesome.

Triphasic Low Oestrogen, Low Progestogen Combination: The hormone content of these pills varies throughout the cycle. There are three different strengths of pill and they must be taken in the right order for 21 days, as marked on the packet, followed by 7 pill-free days. The progestogen is given throughout the cycle, the dose being increased at mid-cycle and again in the last 10 days to prevent breakthrough bleeding. It may help those women in whom the standard oral contraceptive has been associated with breakthrough bleeding or the absence of withdrawal bleeding. Triphasic contraception is claimed to provide reliable contraception, with few unwanted effects.

Logynon 0·03/0·04/0·03mg 0·05/0·075/0·125mg
Trinordiol 0·03/0·04/0·03mg 0·05/0·075/0·125mg
Logynon ED 0·03/0·04/0·03mg 0·05/0·075/0·125mg

Progestogen-only Oral Contraceptives: Preparations that contain only progestogen exert their contraceptive effect by making the cervical mucus thick and scanty during the cycle. This prevents the passage of the sperm and also to some extent the implantation of the ovum. These preparations are less efficient that the oestrogen-progestogen mixtures and they often cause irregular bleeding at frequent intervals. Their main advantage is that they do not have the side-effects of oestrogen on venous thrombosis and carbohydrate tolerance.

Norgeston 0·03mg levonorgestrel
Microval 0·03mg levonorgestrel
Neogest 0·075mg DL-norgestrel
Micronor 0·35mg norethisterone
Noriday 0·35mg norethisterone
Femulen 0·5mg ethynodiol acetate

Mode of Administration: One tablet of oestrogen-progestogen combination is taken daily from the fifth day after the onset of menstruation for 20 days. Withdrawal bleeding occurs within 3 or 4 days of completion of the course and the first day of the withdrawal bleed is taken as the first day of the subsequent menstrual cycle. The progestogen-only pill is begun on the first day of the period and is taken every day even during menstruation.

Harmful Effects: There is an increased risk of thrombo-embolic disease in women receiving the oestrogen-progestogen mixtures. One in every 2000 women on the pill is admitted to hospital each year with venous thrombosis, compared with 1 in 20,000 women not on oral contraceptives. There is also an increased risk of developing cerebral arterial thrombosis; this is of the same order as that for venous thrombo-embolism. The risk of thrombo-embolism is related to the oestrogen content of the pill. In 1970 the oestrogen content of most oral contraceptives was reduced to 50μ and, although it is too early to assess the effect, it seems probable that the incidence of thrombo-embolism will be reduced.

Contra-indications to the oral contraceptive include thrombo-embolic disorders, markedly impaired liver function, known or suspected carcinoma of the breast or uterus, and undiagnosed genital bleeding. Amenorrhoea may follow the stopping of the contraceptive pill. This is sometimes associated with galactorrhoea. It is not a common event and a return to ovulation can be expected within the first three cycles after stopping oral contraceptives in 98 per cent of women. The amneorrhoea is due to failure of the hypothalamus to recover from supression induced by prolonged exposure to pregesterone and oestrogens.

It is important to keep the risk of oral contraception in perspective and to appreciate that abortion is now the most common cause of maternal mortality.

Starting an Oral Contraceptive: The combined oestrogen-progestogen pill should be started on the first day of menstruation. The cycle of the first month is often shortened so bleeding starts on approximately the 22nd day. The next course should then be started after a seven day break. The progestogen-only pill should be started on the first day of menstruation. An additional contraceptive will be needed for the first 14 days. This type of pill is taken every day without a break. The contraceptive effect is maximal at about four hours after the pill is taken. After childbirth a woman who is bottle feeding should start the combined pill during the fourth week. Starting the combined pill earlier increases the risk of thrombosis.

If a woman forgets to take a combined pill and the interval is less than 12 hours it should be taken as soon as it is remembered; the next pill should be taken at its normal time. No additional precautions are then necessary. If however a pill has been forgotten for more than 12 hours it should be taken together with the next pill and additional contraception used for the next 14 days. If a woman is on the progestogen-only pill the contraceptive affect is dependant on the cervical mucus being made impenetrable to the sperm. This effect increases for four hours after ingestion but then wanes towards the end of the 24 hours. If taking the pill has been delayed for 4 to 24 hours an additional contraceptive will be needed for the first 48 hours after taking the forgotten pill. If the pill has not been taken for 48 hours barrier contraception should be used for the next 14 days.

If a woman changes from one combined oral contraceptive to another, the new pill should be started the day after the last of the previous pills have been taken, there being no break. Breakthrough bleeding is unlikely during this six-week changeover period. If a woman is changing from a combined pill to a progestogen-only pill the progestogen-only pill should be started the day after the last combined pill in the packet. If a woman is changing from a progestogen-only pill to a combined pill, the new pill should be started on the first day of bleeding.

Post-coital hormone contraception: this is sometimes called the 'morning after pill'. It is little use if the earliest episode of unprotected intercourse has occurred more than 72 hours previously. The regime consists of 100μg of Ethinyloestradiol and 50μg of Levonorgestrel followed by the same dose 12 hours later. There is a failure rate of about 2 per cent and ectopic pregnancy is a rare complication.

NON-HORMONAL METHODS OF CONTRACEPTION: Other methods of contraception include the *occlusive* (or Dutch Cap) which covers the entrance to the womb and thereby prevents entrance of spermatozoa, and the *sheath* or *condom*, which prevents spermatozoa entering the vagina. Other methods include *coitus interruptus* or withdrawal of the penis from the vagina before ejaculation. With the *rhythm method* intercourse is restricted to the so-called safe period; that is the period during each monthly menstrual cycle when conception cannot take place because there is no ovum available for the spermatozoa to impregnate.

Spermicides are available as jellies, creams, pessaries and foams. They work both by forming a physical barrier to the sperm and by immobilizing the sperm. They are not effective if inserted more than an hour before intercourse. There is some variation in the reported effectiveness of spermicides.

Over recent years vasectomy or sterilization of the husband has become more popular. (See SAFE PERIOD; STERILIZATION; VASECTOMY.)

A survey carried out by the Office of Population Surveys in 1983 showed that 50 per cent of women between the ages of 18 and 19 were on the oral contraceptives. Four-fifths of women between the ages of 25 and 39 are taking the Pill. Of the various methods of contraception used 28 per cent of women take the Pill regularly, 22 per cent were sterilised or their partners were sterilised. 13 per cent used the sheath or condom and 10 per cent used other methods of contraception. The oral contraceptive is the most popular method of contraception in those under the age of 30 whereas sterilisation is the most popular in the older age groups.

CONTRACTURE means the permanent shortening of a muscle or of fibrous tissue. Contraction is the name given to the temporary shortening of a muscle.

CONTRE-COUP means an injury in which a bone, generally the skull, is fractured, not at the spot where the violence is applied, but at the exactly opposite point.

CONTROLLED DRUGS: Preparations which are subject to the prescriptions requirements of the Misuse of Drugs Regulations 1973 are distinguished throughout the British National Formulary by the symbol CD (controlled drugs). Prescriptions for these drugs must be signed and dated by the prescriber who must give his address. The prescription must always be in the presriber's own handwriting and provide the name and address of the patient and the total quantity of the drug or preparation or the number of dose units in both words and figures. The pharmacist is not allowed to dispense a controlled drug unless all the information required by law is given on the prescription.

CONTUSION (see BRUISES).

CONVALESCENCE means the condition through which a person passes after having suffered from some acute disease, and before complete health and strength are regained. Many diseases have special dangers during convalescence: for example, after typhoid fever the effects of overeating may be disastrous; after measles, pneumonia, and other diseases of the respiratory tract, there is a greater risk than usual of the onset of tuberculosis in susceptible individuals; and, while convalescence from scarlet fever is proceeding, there is a special risk of kidney inflammation. These are guarded against by working the body at low pressure for a time, exposing it to no strain, partaking of a moderate diet, and taking an ample allowance of rest and sleep, till all the functions have regained their usual activity and vigour. For further details see under each disease.

CONVOLUTIONS (see BRAIN).

CONVULSIONS are rapidly alternating contractions and relaxations of the muscles, causing irregular movements of the limbs or body generally, and usually accompanied by unconsciousness. They form really only a symptom of some other trouble, often, in children, of a trifling nature, but, on account of the alarm they cause and their occasional seriousness, they are treated often as a disease by themselves.

Causes: The most common cause of convulsions in adults is epilepsy (qv). As the vast majority of convulsive seizures occur in children, however, only these will be dealt with here. The relative frequency of convulsions in infants and young children is probably due to an instability of the immature nervous system. An American investigation showed that in a group of 8823 otherwise normal children, some 6 per cent had had one or more convulsions. Some children are more liable to develop convulsions than others, and this is probably due to a neurotic inheritance.

In young infants convulsions may be due to *birth injuries*, usually the result of a difficult labour. The convulsions in these cases are due to damage of the brain, either by bleeding from torn blood-vessels or concussion of the brain

	I	II	III
Acts	Dangerous Drugs Acts 1965 and 1967; Dangerous Drugs (No. 2) Regulations 1964; Dangerous Drugs (Notification of Addicts) Regulations 1968; Dangerous Drugs (Supply to Addicts) Regulations 1968	Drugs (Prevention of Misuse) Act 1965	Pharmacy and Poisons Act 1933; Poisons List (No. 2) Order 1968; Poisons (No. 2) Rules 1968
Drugs controlled	Opiates including Morphine Heroin* Synthetic analgesics, eg.: Pethidine Methadone Cocaine* Cannabis*	Amphetamines* and some similar substances Lysergic acid diethylamide (LSD 25)* and some similar substances, including mescaline	All those named in the Poisons List including barbiturates and the drugs named in columns I and II *Note:* Barbiturates and the drugs mentioned in columns I and II are included in Part I of the Poisons List and Schedule IV of the Rules
Main provisions	(a) Offence to possess without authority (b) Offence to import and export except under licence (c) Persons authorized to possess have to keep records of drug movements (d) Drugs to be kept under lock and key by persons authorized to possess (e) Medical practitioners must notify all cases of persons addicted† to drugs controlled under the Act of 1965 (f) Heroin and cocaine may be prescribed only for an addict, by a specially licensed medical practitioner	(a) Offence to possess without authority (b) Offence to import except under licence	(a) Offence for a poison in Part I of the Poisons List to be sold retail otherwise than by an authorized seller of poisons from registered premises (b) Offence for substances named in Schedule IV to the Poisons Rules to be sold except on a prescription given by a duly qualified practitioner (c) Records of sales of Schedule IV substances are not required, but private prescriptions must be retained for two years
Penalties	Summary—£250 fine and/or 12 months' imprisonment Indictment—£1000 fine and/or 10 years' imprisonment	Summary—£200 fine and/or 6 months' imprisonment Indictment—unlimited fine and/or two years' imprisonment	£50 fine

* Drugs commonly obtained illegally
† As defined in the Regulations

Summary of statutory provisions for the control of drugs in England and Wales.

In older infants convulsions may be due to the irritability of the brain often associated with *rickets*. This is the condition known as tetany, and before the introduction of the routine administration of vitamin D to infants and children, it was one of the most common causes of convulsions in older infants and young children. Other metabolic causes include hypoglycaemia and hypokalaemia.

A sudden *rise of temperature*, such as may occur in any infection, may induce convulsions in an infant and young child. This is most likely in pneumonia, and it would appear as if in the child a convulsion was the equivalent of the chill or rigor which occurs in adults. *Irritation* elsewhere in the body may cause convulsions in the predisposed child. This is most likely to occur with irritation in the bowels, eg. the eating of unripe or indigestible food, colic, worms or even constipation. Infection of the kidneys or bladder may also be responsible, as may be earache, particularly if of sudden onset. The role of teething as a cause of convulsions has been exaggerated, but there is no doubt that, if painful, the teething process may occasionally produce convulsions.

Diseases of the brain, such as meningitis, encephalitis and tumours, or any disturbance of the brain due to bleeding, blockage of a blood-vessel, or irritation of the brain by a fracture of the skull, may also be responsible for convulsions.

Asphyxia, such as may occur in a young child during a paroxysm of whooping-cough, may also bring on convulsions. Breath-holding (qv), a not uncommon condition in infants and young children, may also persist long enough to bring on convulsions. These breath-holding attacks follow a severe bout of crying, at the end of which the infant holds his breath. As a rule, the worst that happens is that the infant holds his breath until he is blue in the face, and then starts breathing again. Occasionally, however, the breath-holding persists until there is a convulsion. An occasional breath-holding attack need not be taken too seriously but, if it is repeated, medical advice should be sought.

Finally, it must never be forgotten that *epilepsy* can occur in infants and young children.

Treatment: Convulsions are rarely dangerous to life unless they occur as part of a dangerous condition which is already threatening the child's life. The time-honoured custom is to put the child in a hot bath, but this is seldom necessary. On the other hand, tepid sponging may help if there is fever. If there is any possibility of the child biting his tongue, a spoon or a spatula should be put between the teeth. There is seldom any need to restrain the movements unless they are severe enough to throw the child off the bed or couch. If the convulsions persist, it may be necessary to give parenteral benzodiazepines. As a rule a sedative, or an injection of one of the barbiturates, controls the convulsions. Once these are under control, the cause of the convulsions must be sought and the necessary treatment given.

COOLEY'S ANAEMIA, or THALASSAEMIA, is a condition in which there is an inherited defect in the production of normal haemoglobin, resulting in a severe degree of anaemia.

CO-ORDINATION means the governing power exercised by the brain as a whole, or by certain centres in the nervous system, to make various muscles contract in harmony, and so produce definite actions, instead of meaningless movements. It is bound up intimately with the complex sense of localization, which enables a person with his eyes shut to tell, by sensations received from the bones, joints and muscles, the position of the various parts of his body. The power is impaired in various diseases, such as locomotor ataxia. It is tested by making the patient shut his eyes, moving his hand in various directions, and then telling him to bring the point of the forefinger steadily to the tip of the nose, or by other simple movements.

COPAIBA is a mixture of oil and resin in a thick yellow fluid, obtained by cutting into the bark of *Copaifera lansdorfii*, a South American tree. It is excreted by the mucous membranes, especially of the urinary and respiratory organs, which it stimulates.
Uses: It is used in various chronic inflammations of the urinary organs, and as an expectorant in chronic bronchitis.

COPPER is an essential nutrient for man, and all tissues in the human body contain traces of it. The total amount in the adult body is 100 to 150 mg. Many essential enzyme systems are dependent on traces of copper. On the other hand, there is no evidence that dietary deficiency of copper ever occurs in man. Infants are born with an ample store, and the normal diet for an adult contains around 2 mg of copper a day. It is used in medicine as the two salts, sulphate of copper (blue stone) and nitrate of copper. The former is, in small doses, a powerful astringent, and in larger doses an irritant. Both are caustics when applied externally.
Uses: Externally, either is used to rub on unhealthy ulcers and growths, with the view of stimulating the granulation tissue to more rapid healing. In very small amounts copper is necessary for the formation of red blood corpuscles. It is therefore sometimes necessary to give copper as well as iron to cases of anaemia, especially in children. In a concentration of 0·5 to 1 part per million, copper sulphate is used to prevent the growth of algae in, for example, swimming pools.

COPPER POISONING is rare. Copper itself is harmless, but sulphate of copper (blue vitriol) and acetate of copper (verdigris) are now and then taken as poisons. The use of copper salts in very small quantities to colour canned peas is said to lead to occasional unpleasant symptoms, while adverse effects have also, though rarely, been reported from stewing fruit in copper-lined vessels. (See also WILSON'S DISEASE.)
Treatment: If one of the salts above named has been taken by mistake, the treatment is that for any irritant poison: milk or white of egg as an antidote, followed by washing out the stomach. Penicillamine or sodium calciumedetate should also be given.

COPROLALIA is the condition in which insane people give utterance to filthy and obscene words.

CORDOTOMY, or CHORDOTOMY, is the surgical operation of cutting the antero-lateral tracts of the spinal cord to relieve otherwise intractable pain. It is also sometimes known as TRACTOTOMY.

CORNEA (see EYE).

CORNEAL GRAFT (KERATOPLASTY): If the cornea becomes damaged or diseased and vision is impaired, it can be removed and replaced by a corneal graft. The graft is taken from the cornea of a human donor. Some of the indication for corneal grafting include keratoconus, corneal dystrophies, severe corneal scarring following herpes simplex, alkali burns or injury. Because the graft is a foreign protein, there is a danger that the recipient's immune system may set up a reaction causing rejection of the graft. Rejection results in oedema of the graft with subsequent poor vision. Once a corneal graft has been taken from a donor, it should be used as quickly as possible. Corneas can be stored for a short while in tissue-culture medium at low temperature.

The Department of Health and Social Security has drawn up a list of suitable eye-banks to which people can apply to bequeath their eyes, and an official form is now available for the bequest of eyes. (See also DONORS; TRANSPLANTATION.)

CORNS and BUNIONS: A corn is a localized thickening of the cuticle or epidermis, of a conical shape, the point of the cone being directed inwards and being known as the 'eye' of the corn. A general thickening over a wider area is called a callosity. Bunion is a condition found over the joint at the base of the great toe, in which not only is there thickening of the skin, but the head of the metatarsal bone, in consequence of bending outwards of the toe by pointed or too short boots, becomes unduly prominent beneath thickened skin. Hammer-toe is a condition of the second toe, often caused by short boots, in which the toe becomes bent at its two joints in such a way as to resemble a hammer.

Causes: The cause of bunions is ill-fitting footwear. Corns are due similarly to the pressure of tight or badly fitting footwear, or, when on the under-surface of the foot, to unevenness in the sole. The skin grows more rapidly in consequence of the irritation, and becomes changed by the pressure into a species of horn. Where the corns are between the toes, they become moist and sodden, and are called soft corns.

Treatment: The first requisite is to wear sufficiently large and properly shaped shoes. The inner side of the sole should be straight, not cut away to a point, and the width of the sole at the level of the little toe should be as great as that of the bare foot when the weight of the body is thrown on it. Relief from the pain of a corn may be obtained by wearing a ring of felt (corn plaster) round the corn, so as to free it from pressure and distribute the pressure of the boot over the surrounding skin. To remove the corn, the foot should be soaked in hot soapy water, and the corn then cut or scraped away with a knife or pair of scissors. After drying, the site of the corn should be covered with a small piece of soap plaster, or painted inside the felt ring with salicylic acid collodion. This consists of 12 grams of salicylic acid in 100 ml of flexible collodion. This preparation softens and breaks up the corn, which may be picked away gradually or rubbed down with pumice-stone. After the corn is removed, the skin of the foot should be hardened by daily bathing for some time in salt water or in spirit. A tendency to bunions, flat foot, and corns can sometimes be checked by wearing shoes of which the sole is slightly thicker along the inner side than on the outer side.

Soft corns and the deformities of bunion and hammer-toe should be treated by wearing socks made like gloves with a compartment for each toe, or in slighter cases by inserting a piece of boracic lint each morning in the spaces between the toes. In bad cases of bunion the opening of the boot should run forwards to between the first and second toes, where the lace, or a peg known as a 'toe-post', is fixed to the sole in order to keep the great toe in its proper place; or a rubber pad may be worn between the toes. In old-standing cases of bunion and hammer-toe, an operation in which the protruding toe joint is excised may be necessary for cure.

Individuals who are liable to corns and bunions would be well advised to place themselves in the hands of a well-qualified and experienced chiropodist.

CORONARY is a term applied to several structures in the body encircling an organ in the manner of a crown. The coronary arteries are the arteries of supply to the heart which arise from the aorta, just beyond the aortic valve, and through which the blood is delivered to the muscle of the heart. Disease of the coronary arteries is a very serious condition producing various abnormal forms of heart action and the disease, angina pectoris.

CORONARY ARTERIES: The right coronary artery arises from the right sinus of the valsalva and passes into the right atrio-ventricular groove to supply the right ventricle, part of the intraventricular septum and the inferior part of the left ventricle. The left coronary artery arises from the left sinus and divides into an anterior descending branch which supplies the septum and the anterior and apical parts of the heart, and the circumflex branch which passes into the left antrio-ventricular groove and supplies the lateral posterior surfaces of the heart. Small anastomoses exist between the coronary arteries and they have the potential of enlarging if the blood flow through a neighbouring coronary artery is compromised.

CORONARY THROMBOSIS is the acute, dramatic manifestation of ischaemic heart disease, one of the major killing diseases of western civilization. In 1985, ischaemic heart disease was responsible for 163,104 deaths in England, compared with an annual average of 109,064 in England and Wales in the period 1958 to 1960. The alternative name for ischaemic heart disease is coronary artery disease. The underlying cause is disease of the coronary arteries, which carry the blood supply to the heart muscle (or myocardium). This results in narrowing of the arteries until finally they are unable to transport sufficient blood for the myocardium to function efficiently. One of three things may happen. If the narrowing of the coronary arteries occurs gradually, then either the individual concerned will develop angina pectoris (qv) or he will develop signs of a failing heart. (See HEART DISEASES.)

If the narrowing occurs suddenly or leads to complete blockage, or occlusion, of a major branch of one of the coronary arteries, then the victim collapses with acute pain and distress. This is the condition commonly referred to as a coronary thrombosis because it is usually due to the affected artery suddenly becoming completely blocked by thrombosis (qv). More correctly, it should be described as coronary occlusion, because the final occluding factor need not necessarily be thrombosis. Alternatively, it is sometimes referred to as myocardial infarction, this describing the destructive changes produced in the myocardium by lack of its blood supply. (See INFARCTION.)

Causes: The precise cause is not known, but there is a wide range of factors which play a part in inducing coronary artery disease. In the first place it is commoner in men than in women. It is more common in those in sedentary occupations than in those who lead a more physically active life. There is a strong familial element, and it is more likely to occur in those with high blood-pressure than in those with normal blood-pressure. It is more common among smokers than non-smokers. The Royal College of Physicians in its report 'Smoking and Health' (1983) stated that 30 per cent of heart disease deaths are attributable to smoking. It is often associated with a high level of cholesterol (qv) in the blood. This in turn has been linked with an excessive consumption of animal, as opposed to vegetable, fats. In this connection the important factors seem to be the saturated fatty acids of animal fats which would appear to be more likely to lead to a high level of cholesterol in the blood than the unsaturated fatty acids of vegetable fats.

Symptoms: The presenting symptom is the sudden onset, often at rest, of acute, agonizing pain in the front of the chest. This rapidly radiates all over the front of the chest and often down over the abdomen. It is often accompanied by nausea and vomiting, so that suspicion may be aroused of some acute abdominal condition such as gall-stone colic or a perforated peptic ulcer. The victim soon becomes collapsed, with a pale, cold sweating skin, rapid pulse and difficulty in breathing. There is usually some rise in temperature.

Treatment is immediate relief of the pain by injections of morphine. Whether or not admission to hospital is necessary is an open question to be decided in each case by the medical attendant. The essentials of subsequent treatment are absolute rest, the continued administration of drugs to relieve the pain, the administration of drugs that may be necessary to deal with the heart failure that commonly develops and the irregular action of the heart that quite often develops, and the administration of oxygen. A recent development has been the establishment in major hospitals of what are known as coronary care units, to which patients with coronary thrombosis can be admitted for constant supervision. Such units maintain an emergency, skilled, round-the-clock staff of doctors and nurses, as well as all the necessary instruments, drugs and resuscitation apparatus that may be required. A controversial form of treatment at the moment is the administration of anticoagulant drugs. Theoretically, these should be of value to patients with thrombosis, to prevent the thrombus spreading. Carefully controlled clinical trials, however, have given no clear picture of whether or not these drugs are indicated.

The outcome varies considerably. The first few days are the critical ones from the point of view of recovery. If these are survived, then with a first coronary thrombosis the outlook is quite good provided the patient does not have a high blood-pressure and is not overweight. Following recovery, there should be a gradual return to work, care being taken to avoid any increase in weight, unnecessary stress and strain, and to observe the golden rule about moderation in all things. Cigarette smoking should be given up. At one time, patients who had had a coronary thrombosis were kept in bed for prolonged periods. Today, however, in uncomplicated cases the aim is to get them up and about as soon as possible. Most patients are in hospital for about ten days and back at work in three months.

CORONAVIRUSES, so called because in electron micrographs the spikes projecting from the virus resemble a crown, are a group of viruses which have been isolated from people with common colds, and have also been shown to produce common colds under experimental conditions. Their precise significance in the causation of the common cold is still undetermined.

CORPORA QUADRIGEMINA form part of the mid-brain. (See BRAIN.)

CORPULENCE (see OBESITY).

COR PULMONALE is another name for pulmonary heart disease, which is characterized by hypertrophy and failure of the right ventricle of the heart as a result of disease of the lungs or disorder of the pulmonary circulation.

CORPUSCLE means a small body. (See BLOOD.)

CORPUS LUTEUM is the mass of cells formed in the ruptured Graafian follicle in the ovary from which the ovum is discharged about fifteen days before the onset of the next menstrual period. When the ovum escapes the follicle fills up with blood. This is soon replaced by cells which contain a yellow fatty material. The follicle and its luteal cells constitute the corpus luteum. The corpus luteum begins to disappear after ten days, unless the discharged ovum is fertilized and pregnancy ensues. In pregnancy the corpus luteum persists and grows and secretes the hormone, progesterone (qv).

CORRIGAN'S PULSE is the name applied to the collapsing pulse found with incompetence of the aortic valve. It is so called after Sir Dominic John Corrigan (1802–80), the famous Dublin physician, who first described it.

CORROSIVES are poisonous substances which corrode or eat away the mucous surfaces of mouth, gullet and stomach with which they come in contact. Examples are strong mineral acids like sulphuric, nitric and hydrochloric acids, caustic alkalis, and some salts like chlorides of mercury and zinc. (See POISONS.)

CORROSIVE SUBLIMATE, or PERCHLORIDE OF MERCURY, is a powerful antiseptic and an irritant poison. It is not to be confounded with subchloride of mercury or calomel. (See ANTISEPTICS; DISINFECTION; MERCURY.)

CORTICOSTEROIDS is the generic term for the group of hormones with a cortisone-like action. Many chemical modifications of the cortisone molecule have been prepared in an attempt to dissociate therapeutic action from side effects. Analogues are already available with no mineralo-corticoid effects and steroids with a gluco-corticoid activity and no inflammatory action have been synthesised. The main corticosteroid hormones currently available are cortisone, hydrocortisone, prednisone, prednisolone, methyl prednisolone, triamcinolone, dexamethasone, beta-methasone and paramethasone. They are used clinically in three quite distinct circumstances. First they constitute replacement therapy in states of adrenocortical insufficiency or hypopituitarism. In this situation the dose is physiological, namely the equivalent of the normal adrenal output under similar circumstances, and it is not associated with any side effects. Secondly, steroids are used to depress secretory activity of the adrenal cortex in conditions where this is abnormally high or where the adrenal cortex is producing abnormal hormones, as occurs in some hirsute women. The third application for corticosteroids is in suppressing the manifestations of disease in a wide variety of inflammatory and allergic conditions and in reducing antibody production in a number of auto-immune diseases. The inflammatory reaction is normally part of the body's defence mechanism and is to be encouraged rather than inhibited. However, in the case of those diseases in which the body's reaction is disproportionate to the offending agent, the steroid hormones can inhibit this undesirable response and although the underlying condition is not cured as a result it may resolve spontaneously. When such compounds are used for anti-inflammatory properties, the dose must be pharmacological; that is it must exceed the normal physiological requirement. Indeed, the necessary dose may exceed the normal maximum output of the healthy adrenal gland, which is about 250 to 300 mg cortisol per day. When doses of this order are used there are inevitable risks and side effects. A drug induced Cushing' syndrome will result.

Corticosteroid treatment of short duration, as in angioneurotic oedema of the larynx or other allergic crises, may at the same time be life-saving and without significant risk. Prolonged therapy of such connective tissue disorders, such as polyarteritis with its attendant hazards, is generally accepted because there are no other agents of therapeutic value. Similarly the absence of alternative medical treatment for such conditions as auto-immune haemolytic anaemia and auto-immune thrombocytopenia purpura establishes steroid therapy as the treatment of choice, which few would dispute. The place of steroids in such chronic conditions as rheumatoid athritis, asthma and eczema, is more debatable.

Although one must be aware of the side-effects, it is possible to become so obsessed with the risks of therapy as to underestimate the misery and danger of unrelieved chronic asthma or the incapacity, frustration and psychological trauma of rheumatoid arthritis. On the other hand, a form of treatment with the hazards of steroid therapy should never be undertaken lightly or until other established remedies have failed.

The incidence and severity of side effects is related to the dose and duration of treatment. Prolonged daily treatment with 15 mg of prednisolone, or more, will cause hypercortisonism. Less than 10 mg prednisolone a day may be tolerated by most patients indefinitely. When used in pharmacological doses, steroid therapy is associated with certain side effects which are so common as to be almost invariable but are not usually of serious consequence. These include gain in weight, fat distribution of the cushingoid type, acne and hirsutism, amenorrhoea, striae and increased bruising tendency. The more serious complications which fortunately occur much less frequently include infection, dyspepsia and peptic ulceration, gastrointestinal haemorrhage, adrenal suppression, osteoporosis, psychosis, diabetes mellitus, myopathy and potassium depletion.

CORTICOTROPHIN is the *British Pharmacopoeia* name for the adrenocorticotrophic hormone of the pituitary gland, also known as ACTH. It is so called because it stimulates the functions of the cortex of the suprarenal glands. This results, among other things, in an increased output of cortisone, Although first isolated from the pituitary gland in 1933, it was not until the discovery, in 1949, of the effect of cortisone and corticotrophin in rheumatoid arthritis that it came into general use. No means of synthesis has yet been discovered, and the only available sources are the pituitary glands of animals. It is only active when given by intravenous or intramuscular injection, but there are preparations available, which give a more prolonged action and which are given subcutaneously. As its action is predominantly the same as that of cortisone, the action of the two is discussed together in the section on cortisone (qv).

CORTISOL is another name for hydrocortisone (qv).

CORTISONE, originally known as Compound E, was isolated from beef adrenal glands in 1936 by workers at the Mayo Clinic. Its chemical name is 11-dehydro-17-hydroxycorticosterone. Mainly because of difficulties in obtaining adequate amounts, little interest was taken in it until, in 1949, Hench and Kendall and their colleagues demonstrated its dramatic, if transitory, effect in rheumatoid arthritis. The precise mode of action of cortisone is still not known. Among other things, it prevents (or delays) the proliferative changes in the tissues which are the normal response to infection and in allergic conditions. Among the conditions which have been shown to benefit from cortisone are rheumatoid arthritis, rheumatic fever, gout, certain eye conditions, certain skin conditions and Addison's disease.

Cortisone has two disadvantages which will always tend to restrict its use. One is that in chronic conditions such as rheumatoid arthritis the effect of cortisone is merely temporary, and tends to stop when administration is stopped. The other is that cortisone has certain toxic effects, and therefore it must only be used under medical supervision.

For all practical purposes corticotrophin (qv) and cortisone have the same action. (See also BETAMETHASONE; DEXAMETHASONE; HYDROCORTISONE; PREDNISOLONE; PREDNISONE; and TRIAMCINOLONE.)

CORYZA is the technical name of a 'cold in the head'.

COSTAL means anything pertaining to the ribs.

COSTALGIA means pain in the ribs.

COSTIVENESS (see CONSTIPATION).

COT DEATH is the term applied to the unexpected death of an apparently healthy baby, usually during sleep. It is also known as the Sudden Infant Death Syndrome, and it is estimated that probably at least 1800 such deaths occur every year in Britain. Most babies who die in this way have been healthy, or only slightly unwell, the day before death. Death occurs silently and suddenly, the baby being found dead in his cot in the morning. Over half these deaths occur between the ages of 2 and 6 months, and boys are more affected than girls. They are more common in social classes III, IV and V (see SOCIAL CLASSES), and the incidence is highest in the winter. Most of the infants have been bottle fed.

The cause is still not really known. Smothering by a soft pillow may account for a few of the deaths, and a certain number are due to an infection of the lungs, such as broncho-pneumonia or bronchitis, usually due to a virus. There is some evidence that these infants have an innate tendency to poor control of their breathing and are therefore likely to stop breathing should they have even a mild infection such as a cold. One possibility is that they may be associated with allergy to milk. Another is that they may be due to a sudden upset of the fluid balance of the baby as a result of bottle feeding. Yet another is that they may be associated with a deficiency of vitamin E. Another possible cause is the spontaneous production of botulinum toxin in the gut of young babies. All that can really be said at the moment, however, is that the baby most likely to die in this way is one who was underweight when born, comes from a poor family, whose mother is young and already has several children, who has been bottle fed, has been unwell during the preceding fortnight and has signs of a cold in the head when put to bed. Bereaved parents can obtain help and advice from the Foundation for the Study of Infant Deaths, 15 Belgrave Square, London SW1X 8PS (Tel: 01-235 1721/0965).

CO-TRIMOXAZOLE is an antibacterial agent which is proving of value in a wide range of infections. It is a combination of two antibacterial agents: trimethoprim and sulphamethoxazole.

COTTON WOOL, or ABSORBENT COTTON as it is now technically named by the *British Pharmacopoeia*, is a downy material made from the hairs on cotton plant seeds (*Gossypium herbaceum*). It is used in medicine for a great variety of purposes, including protection to injured parts, by reason of its combined warmth and cheapness. It is highly inflammable. It may be medicated with various substances, such as capsicum, capsicum cottonwool being used as a counter-irritant (qv) for use in dressings in the treatment of painful rheumatic conditions.

COUGH is a sudden indrawing of air with the glottis (qv) wide open. This is followed by a blowing out of air against a closed glottis. The glottis then suddenly opens and the air in the lungs is expelled under high pressure – up to 300 millimetres of mercury and at a speed of 960 kilometres (600 miles) an hour. Its purpose is to rid the air passages and windpipe of what are colloquially known as foreign bodies, including the excessive mucus and other secretions produced in infections of the lungs and upper air passages, such as bronchitis and sore throat. As such secretions contain many microorganisms, it is clear what an important part coughing plays in spreading the common cold and other infections of the nose, throat and lungs. It is a reflex action (qv) produced by stimulation of nerve endings in the air passages and may therefore be induced by irritation of these nerve endings by inflammation without any secretion. This results in the dry irritable cough which can be such a troublesome feature of the early and late stages of acute bronchitis, tracheitis (qv) and laryngitis (qv). Conversely the inability to cough in inflammatory conditions of the lungs, such as bronchitis and broncho-pneumonia, especially in old folk, is an ominous sign, and every effort must be made to stimulate coughing so far as this is possible.

COUGH SYNCOPE is the loss of consciousness that may be induced by a severe spasm of coughing. This is the result of the high pressure that may be induced in the chest – over 200 millimetres of mercury – by such a spasm. This prevents the return of blood to the heart, the veins in the neck begin to bulge and the blood-pressure falls. This may so reduce the blood flow to the brain that the individual feels giddy and may then lose consciousness. (See FAINTING.)

COUNTER-IRRITANTS (see BLISTERS AND COUNTER-IRRITANTS).

COWPOX is a disease affecting the udders of cows, on which it produces vesicles. It is communicable to man, and there has for centuries been a tradition that persons who have caught this cowpox from cows do not suffer afterwards from smallpox. This formed the basis for Jenner's experiments on vaccination. (See VACCINATION.)

COXA VARA is a condition in which the neck of the thigh-bone is bent so that the lower limbs are turned very much outwards and lameness results.

COXSACKIE VIRUSES are a group of viruses so-called because they were first isolated from two patients with a disease resembling paralytic poliomyelitis, in the village of Coxsackie in New York State. Thirty distinct types have now been identified. They constitute one of the three groups of viruses included in the family of enteroviruses (qv). They are divided into two groups: A and B. Despite the large number of types of group A virus (24) in existence, evidence of their role in causing human disease is limited. Some, however, cause aseptic meningitis, and others cause a condition known as herpangina (qv). Hand, foot and mouth disease (qv) is another disease caused by the A group. All 6 types of group B virus have been associated with outbreaks of aseptic meningitis, and they are also the cause of Bornholm disease (qv). Epidemics of type B_2 infections tend to occur in alternate years. In 1981, 427 cases were reported in England and Wales, over 60 per cent of which were in children under the age of 5. Of the 12 fatal cases, 5 occurred in infants under the age of 1 month. The most common features of these cases were respiratory tract infection, gastroenteritis, meningitis, Bornholm disease, or non-specific fever.

CRAB-LOUSE is another name for *Pediculus pubis*, a louse that infests the pubic region. (See PEDICULOSIS.)

CRACKED-POT SOUND is a peculiar resonance heard sometimes on percussion of the chest over a cavity in the lung, resembling the jarring sound heard on striking a cracked pot or bell. It is also heard on percussion over the skull in patients with diseases of the brain such as haemorrhages and tumours, and in certain cases of fracture of the skull.

CRADLE is the name applied to the cage which is placed over the legs of a patient in bed, in order to take the weight of the bed-clothes off the legs.

CRADLE CAP, or CRUSTA LACTEA as it is technically known, is the form of seborrhoea of the scalp which is not uncommon in nursing infants. It usually responds to an ointment containing equal parts of Salicylic Acid Ointment of the *British National Formulary*, Sulphur Ointment BP, and White Soft Paraffin BP.

CRAMP is a painful spasmodic contraction of muscles, most commonly occurring in the limbs, but also apt to affect certain internal organs. This disorder belongs to the class of diseases known as local spasms, of which other varieties exist in such affections as tetany and colic. The cause of these painful seizures resides in the nervous system, and operates either directly from the great nerve centres, or, as is generally the case, indirectly by reflex action, as, for example, when attacks are brought on by some derangement of the digestive organs.

NIGHT CRAMP is most common in the elderly, during pregnancy, in diabetics and in those with peripheral vascular disease. It comes on suddenly, often during sleep, the patient being aroused by an agonizing feeling of pain in the calf of the leg or back of the thigh. During the paroxysm the muscular fibres affected can often be felt gathered up into a hard knot. The attack in general lasts but a few seconds and then suddenly departs, the spasmodic contraction of the muscles ceasing entirely; or, on the other hand, relief may come more gradually during a period of minutes or even hours. Even after the sharp pain has gone there is often a persisting ache. The cause is not known. It is more common in older people, but has been reported in soldiers during their preliminary period of training. It is also common in pregnancy.

Treatment: This painful disorder can be greatly relieved and often entirely removed by firmly grasping or briskly rubbing the affected part with the hand, or by anything which makes an impression on the nerves, such as the application of some cold substance to the part, or occasionally by warmth. Even a sudden and vigorous movement of the limb, in such a direction as to stretch the affected muscle, will often succeed in terminating the attack, though this may also exacerbate the condition. If troublesome during pregnancy, the mother should restrict her milk intake to 0·5 litre (1 pint) a day and take calcium gluconate tablets with or without vitamin D. In men and non-pregnant women, in whom the condition is irritatingly recurrent, 60 to 300 mg of quinine bisulphate, or 600 mg of calcium lactate the last thing before going to bed, have a high reputation as a preventive.

Causal relationship	Treatment or prevention
Effort:	
Footballer's	Oral slow sodium may have some benefit
Stitch	Adequate training with muscle relaxation
Swimmer's	Avoid unusually cold water; relaxation training
Miner's	Sodium replacement; slow sodium orally
Writer's	Learn to write with opposite hand.
At rest:	
Nocturnal	Quinine 60 mg at night; diazepam 5 mg; diphenhydramine; phenytoin 100 mg; procainamide 250 mg; dantrolene 25 mg; methoxyphenamine HCL 100 mg; avoid caffeine
Pregnancy	No satisfactory treatment; preferably no drug treatment
Local irritation	Treat infection; in arthritic conditions anti-inflammatory drugs; maintain muscle movements and mobility
Secondary to disease:	
Profuse diarrhoea	Replace sodium and potassium loss
Renal salt wasting	Replace sodium
Vascular occlusive disease	Vasodilators doubtful; surgery
Motor neurone disease	No effective treatment known
Neoplastic peripheral nerve involvement	Dantrolene 25 mg daily; must be delayed effect
Strychnine poisoning	Diazepam
Tetanus	Diazepam
Black-widow spider bite	*d*-tubocuranine

Treatment for various types of cramp. After *Journal of the Royal Society of Medicine*.

SWIMMER'S CRAMP includes usually spasm of the arteries as well as of the muscles, due to cold and exertion, so that death is apt to occur from stoppage of the heart. If treatment can be applied, friction of the limbs, warmth, and hot drinks are essential.

CRAMP OF THE STOMACH, or GASTRALGIA, is usually a symptom in connection with some form of gastric disorder (see STOMACH, DISEASES OF). For cramp affecting the muscular wall of the bowels, see COLIC.

HABIT SPASMS, or FUNCTIONAL SPASMS, are liable to occur in individuals of almost any handicraft, and are often extremely troublesome.

Spasmodic Wry-neck is one of the most frequent forms which the disease takes. This comes on in shoemakers, tailors, and people generally whose employment necessitates their following, with the head, movements which the hands are making. The result is that the muscles of the neck assume the unpleasant habit of drawing the head to one side whenever the slightest attempt is made to turn and look at anything. Indeed, although actually a rare disease, no muscle or group of muscles which is specially called into action in any particular occupation is exempt from liability to this functional spasm, which is therefore ascribed to over-use of the parts concerned.

Treatment: In the treatment of habit spasms, the only effectual remedy is absolute cessation for a time (it may be a month or longer) from the work with which the attack is associated. It is sometimes recommended that the opposite hand or limb be used, so as to afford the affected part entire rest, but this may be followed by the extension of the disorder to that locality also. Special forms of penholder and other mechanical contrivances have been suggested so as to enable the occupation to be carried on, but they do not afford any relief to the disease, for the cure of which entire rest is important. There is often a strong psychological element in such cases, and psychotherapy is indicated. Where the spasmodically acting muscles are not of great importance to the bodily economy, their action can be controlled by division of their nerves of supply. For example, spasmodic wry-neck can be checked by division of the spinal accessory nerve on one side of

the neck. Such a procedure is out of the question in the case of the hand.
HEAT CRAMPS are painful contractions of muscles occurring in men (eg. stokers) working in high temperatures. The cramps are due to excessive loss of salt in the sweat, and can be cured, and prevented, by giving salt water to drink. (See also HEAT STROKE.)

CRANIAL NERVES are those arising from the brain. (See BRAIN.)

CRANIUM is the part of the skull enclosing the brain as distinguished from the face.

CRASIS is the term applied to the individual temperament or constitution. (See CONSTITUTION.)

CREAM is the oily or fatty part of milk from which butter is prepared. Various medicinal preparations are known also as cream, eg. *cold cream*, which is a simple ointment containing rose-water, beeswax, borax, and almond oil scented with oil of rose.

CREAM OF TARTAR is another name for bitartrate of potassium.

CREATINE is a nitrogenous substance, methylguanidine-acetic acid. In the adult human body there are about 120 grams of it, and 98 per cent of this is present in the muscles. Much of the creatine in muscle is combined with phosphoric acid as phosphocreatine, which plays an important part in the chemistry of muscular contraction.

CREATINE KINASE is an enzyme (qv) which is proving of value in the investigation and diagnosis of muscular dystrophy (qv), in which it is found in the blood in greatly increased amounts.

CREATININE is the anhydride of creatine and is derived from it. It is purely a waste product.

CREEPING ERUPTION is a skin condition caused by the invasion of the skin by the larvae of various species of nematode worms. It owes its name to the fact that as the larva moves through and along the skin it leaves behind it a long creeping thin red line. (See STRONGYLOIDIASIS.)

CREMATION (see DEAD, DISPOSAL OF THE).

CREOSOTE is a clear, yellow liquid, of aromatic smell and burning taste, prepared by distillation from pine-wood or from beech-wood, the product of the latter being of better quality. It mixes readily with alcohol, ether, chloroform, glycerin, and oils.

It is a powerful antiseptic and disinfectant. It has also a soothing action upon parts with which it is brought into contact. It is unchanged after absorption into the blood, and, being excreted by the lungs and exhaled on the breath, it exercises an effect upon these organs.
Uses: Creosote is an ingredient of some disinfectant fluids. It is also used in the form of a vapour, containing creosote 5 ml, and light carbonate of magnesia 2 G, in water 28·5 ml, of which a teaspoonful is added to a pint (570 ml) of hot water and inhaled in cases of suppurating throat, foetid breath, etc. In cases of seasickness, it is sometimes given in doses of 2 to 10 drops to check the vomiting. It has also been used for the temporary alleviation of toothache, the aching cavity being filled with cotton wool soaked in creosote.

CREPITATIONS is the name applied to certain sounds which occur along with the breath sounds, as heard by auscultation, in various diseases of the lungs. They are signs of the presence of moist exudations in the lungs or in the bronchial tubes, are classified as fine, medium, and coarse crepitations, and resemble the sound made by bursting bubbles of various sizes.

CREPITUS means a grating sound. It is found in cases of fractured bones when the ends rub together; also in cases of severe chronic arthritis by the rubbing together of the dried internal surfaces of the joints.

CRESOL is an oily liquid obtained from coal tar. It is a powerful antiseptic and disinfectant.
Uses: It is used combined with soap to form a clear saponaceous fluid known as lysol, which can be mixed with water in any proportions. For the disinfection of drains it is used at a dilution of 1 in 20; for heavily infected linen 1 in 40; for floors and walls 1 in 100.

CRETA is a Latin name for chalk.

CRETINISM is a disease which is due to defective thyroid function in foetal life or early in infancy. The clinical recognition of hypothyroidism (qv) during the first week or months of life is difficult. However if the infant has feeding problems, is constipated and fails to thrive, and is excessively sleepy, hypothyroidism should be considered. The physical signs include a typical facies, a hoarse voice, coarse or thin hair and a large tongue, umbilical hernia and large anterior fontanelle. If the diagnosis is delayed numerous neurological abnormalities occur with abnormal gait, speech difficulties and poor co-ordination. If the disorder is not treated early mental retardation will be permanent. In a population in North London screened for congenital hypothyroidism in 1980 only 40 per cent of the cases were clinically recognized before the age of three months. Experience in Switzerland and North America is similar. An early diagnosis, therefore, necessitates biochemical screening if the benefits of early treatment are to be utilised. A recent review showed that 55 per cent of infants treated in the first six weeks of life had an I.Q. of 90 or more but only 36 per cent of those starting treatment from 7 to 12 weeks of age achieved this level. Without early diagnosis one third of patients with cretinism will require special schooling and one quarter will have an I.Q. of less than 70.

Screening programmes for congenital hypothyroidism have thus been established in North America, some European countries and the United Kingdom. The incidence of primary hypothyroidism detected by such programmes is about 1:4400 live births. The screening programmes utilise cord blood serum, or capillary serum taken by a heel prick on day 5; the blood is used to assay the level of Serum Thyroxine and Serum TSH.

Treatment consists in giving thyroxine (qv) regularly.

CREUTZFELDT-JAKOB DISEASE is a rapidly progressive dementia occurring between the ages of forty and sixty-five. It is an uncommon disease in which dementia develops rapidly so that a normal healthy individual can be totally helpless within a year. The disease can be transmitted to animals by the innoculation of brain tissue from patients with the disease, after an incubation period of 11 to 71 months. The transmissible agent is thought to be a slow virus.

CRISIS is a word used with several distinct meanings.

1. The usual meaning is that of a rapid loss of fever and return to comparative health in certain acute diseases. For example, pneumonia, if allowed to run its natural course, ends by a crisis, usually on the eighth day, the temperature falling in twenty-four hours to normal, the pulse and breathing becoming slow and regular, and the patient passing from a partly delirious state into natural sleep. The opposite mode of ending to crisis is by lysis: for example, in typhoid fever, where the patient slowly improves during a period of a week or more, without any sudden change.

2. A popular use of the word crisis, and still more frequently of critical, is to signify a dangerous state of illness in which it is uncertain whether the sufferer will recover or not.

3. The word crisis is also used to signify a paroxysm of pain in the larynx, stomach, or bowels occurring during the course of locomotor ataxia (qv).

CROHN'S DISEASE (see ILEITIS).

CROTON OIL is a powerful purgative, seldom used now, producing copious watery evacuations.

Externally, croton liniment is used as a counter-irritant.

CROUP is a household term for a group of diseases characterized by swelling and partial blockage of the entrance to the larynx, occurring in children and characterized by crowing inspiration. There are various causes including diphtheritic laryngitis (see DIPHTHERIA), acute laryngitis, and the condition known as spasmodic croup or laryngismus stridulosus. It is an account of this last condition which will be given here. (See also LARYNGO-TRACHEO-BRONCHITIS.)

The important thing to remember about any form of croup is that it is always potentially dangerous – particularly in the case of an infant – because of the narrowness of the entrance to the larynx and therefore the comparative ease with which it may be blocked, thereby leading to suffocation of the infant.

Symptoms: The attack usually comes on at night, when the child is in bed, and follows a chill caught during the day, or an ordinary cold that has lasted perhaps for some days. The breathing is hoarse and croaking (hence the name of the disease), the voice thin, the cough paroxysmal and metallic in tone, and the air passes in with a harsh, loud noise. The child is frightened and excited at first, but later becomes feeble and livid. Still later, pallor, sweating, and great struggling for breath come on, and may last half-an-hour or several hours. After this the symptoms begin to abate, gradually pass away, and the child falls asleep, but there is always a danger that the larynx may become completely blocked, in which case death ensues in a few minutes. A fatal termination is rare if the child receives proper treatment, and the alarming symptoms usually abate on the day following the attack, to return, it may be, on the succeeding night. A child who has once had croup is liable to have future attacks, and so should be specially guarded against cold and damp till he has outgrown the tendency.

Treatment: The child should be put into a hot bath to which a tablespoonful of mustard has been added, and a tent should be made with a blanket over the bath, so that he may inhale the steam. When he is put back into bed the tent should be put over the bed and the nozzle of a steam kettle brought within it. To the water in the kettle may be added a teaspoonful of compound tincture of benzoin, of creosote inhalation (see CREOSOTE), or of other soothing substance (see INHALATION). At the beginning, an attack may be checked by the administration of a teaspoonful of ipecacuanha wine every ten minutes till vomiting takes place. Sometimes, when the spasm of the laryngeal muscles seems very great, inhalation of chloroform is resorted to.

CRUCIATE LIGAMENTS are two strong ligaments in the interior of the knee-joint, which cross one another like the limbs of the letter X. They are so attached as to become taut when the lower limb is straightened, and they prevent over-extension or bending forwards at the knee.

CRURAL means something connected with the leg.

CRUSH SYNDROME is the term given to a condition in which kidney failure occurs in patients who have been the victims of severe crushing accidents. The fundamental injury is damage to muscle. The limb swells. The blood volume falls. Blood urea rises; there is also a rise in the potassium content of the blood. The patient may survive; or he dies with renal failure. Post-mortem examination shows degeneration of the tubules of the kidney, and the presence in them of pigment casts.

CRUTCH-PALSY (see DROP-WRIST).

CRYMOTHERAPY is the term applied to the treatment of disease by refrigeration. The two main forms in which it is now used are HYPOTHERMIA (qv) and REFRIGERATION ANAESTHESIA. Perhaps the best example of the latter is when a gangrenous leg in chronic diabetes mellitus or arteriosclerosis is kept by means of ice bags at a temperature of 5°C for from 1 to 5 hours. This form of anaesthesia much reduces the risks of shock and infection.

CRYOANALGESIA is the induction of analgesia (qv) by the use of cold produced by means of a special probe. The use of cold for the relief of pain dates back to the early days of man. Two millennia ago, Hippocrates was recommending snow and ice packs as a preoperative analgesic. The modern probe allows a precise temperature to be induced in a prescribed area. Among its uses is in the relief of chronic pain which will not respond to any other form of treatment. This applies particularly to chronic facial pain.

CRYOPRECIPITATE: When frozen plasma is allowed to thaw slowly at 4°C, a proportion of the plasma protein remains undissolved in the cold thawed plasma and stays in this state until the plasma is warmed. It is this cold insoluble precipitate that is known as cryoprecipitate. It can be recovered quite easily by centrifuging. Its value is that it is a rich source of Factor VIII, which is used in the treatment of haemophilia (qv).

CRYOSCOPY means the method of finding the concentration of blood, urine, etc., by observing their freezing-point.

CRYOSURGERY is the use of cold in surgery. Its advantages include little associated pain, little or no bleeding, and excellent healing with little or no scar formation. Hence its relatively wide use in eye surgery. The coolants used include liquid nitrogen with which temperatures as low as −196°C can be obtained, carbon dioxide (−78°C) and nitrous oxide (−88°C).

CRYPTOCOCCOSIS is a rare disease due to infection with a yeast known as *Cryptococcus neoformans*. Around 5 to 10 cases are diagnosed annually in the United Kingdom. It usually involves the lungs in the first instance, but may spread to the meninges and other parts of the body; including the skin. It responds well as a rule to treatment with amphotericin B, clotrimazole, and flucytosine.

CRYPTOCOCCUS is a genus of yeasts. *Cryptococcus neoformans* is widespread in nature and present in particularly large numbers in the faeces of pigeons. It occasionally infects man, as a result of the inhalation of dust contaminated by the faeces of pigeons, causing the disease known as cryptococcosis.

CRYPTORCHIDISM means an undescended testis. The testes normally descend into the scrotum during the seventh month of gestation. Until then the testis is an abdominal organ. If the testes do not descend before the first year of life they usually remain undescended until puberty and even then descent is not achieved in some instances. Fertility is impaired when one testis is affected and is usually absent in the bilateral cases. The incidence of undescended testis in full term children at birth is three and a half per cent falling to less than two per cent at one month and 0·7 per cent at one year. Because of the high risk of infertility undescended testes should be brought down as early as possible and at the latest by the age of two. Sometimes medical treatment with human chorionic gonadotrophin is helpful but frequently surgical interference is necessary. This is the operation of orchidopexy.

CRYSTAL VIOLET (see GENTIAN VIOLET).

CUBEB is the fruit of *Piper cubeba*, used similarly to copaiba (qv).

CULDOSCOPY is a method of examining the pelvic organs in women by means of an instrument comparable to a cystoscope (qv) inserted into the pelvic cavity through the vagina. The instrument used for this purpose is known as a culdoscope.

CUPPING is used in cases of deep-seated congestion to draw blood to the surface. It causes sudden dilatation of the superficial blood-vessels, and so probably contracts those of underlying organs. But whatever the explanation, it gives relief in difficulty of breathing due to asthma, bronchitis and pleurisy and brings relief in lumbago and various forms of rheumatic pain, though its current popularity in Britain is low. Cupping is of two kinds: *dry-cupping* and *wet-cupping*. To dry-cup, one takes a cupping-glass (or an ordinary thick glass tumbler), puts a few drops of methylated spirit upon a fragment of blotting-paper into it, ignites this, and, while it is still burning, claps the mouth of the glass tightly on the back of the patient. A vacuum is produced, and the skin swells up into the glass as blood rushes into its small blood-vessels. This is repeated four, six, or eight times in different places. Wet-cupping is rarely used these days. The skin is first dry-cupped, the swollen skin is next scarified with a lancet or a special instrument for the purpose, and then the cupping-glass is again applied, and blood drawn off into it. The vacuum for dry- or wet-cupping may also be produced by a suction bulb.

CUPRUM is the Latin word for copper.

CURARE, known also as CURARA, WOORALI, WOURARI, URARI, and TICUNAS, is a dark-coloured extract from some trees of the *Strychnos* family. It is used by the South American Indians as an arrow poison, and is extremely potent, its action depending upon a crystalline alkaloid: *d*-tubocurarine chloride. This alkaloid paralyses the nerve endings in muscle. For many years it was considered to be much too dangerous for use in man, but research has shown that the pure alkaloid can be used with safety. Its main use is in anaesthesia, where the muscular relaxation it produces is of invaluable assistance to the surgeon. With the aid of tubocurarine adequate muscular relaxation can be obtained with a lesser degree of anaesthesia than would be required were the drug not being used. It is a drug, however, that should only be used by a skilled anaesthetist. Its action is antagonized by neostigmine. It has also been used in the treatment of spastic conditions.

CURDLED MILK (see CASEIN).

CURETTE is a spoon-shaped instrument used in surgery for scooping out the contents of any cavity of the body: eg. the uterine cavity.

CUSHING'S SYNDROME was described in 1932 by Harvey Cushing, the American neurosurgeon. It is due to the excess production of cortisol. It can thus result from an adrenal tumour secreting cortisol of from a pituitary tumour secreting ACTH and stimulating both adrenal cortexes to hypertrophy and secrete excess cortisol. It is sometimes the result of ectopic production of ACTH from non-endocrine tumours in the lung and pancreas. The patient gains weight and the obesity tends to have a characteristic distribution over the face, neck and shoulder and pelvic girdles. Purple striae develop over the abdomen and there is often increased hairiness or hirsutism. The blood pressure is commonly raised and the bone softens as a result of osteoporosis. The best test to establish the diagnosis is to measure the amount of cortisol in a 24-hourly specimen of urine. Once the diagnosis has been established it is then necessary to undertake further tests to determine the cause.

CUSPARIA, or ANGOSTURA, is the dried bark of *Galipea officinalis*, a tree of tropical America. An infusion is used as a bitter, in doses of one, two, or more tablespoonfuls.

CUTANEOUS means belonging to the skin. (See SKIN; SKIN DISEASES.)

CUTICLE (see SKIN).

CUTS (see WOUNDS).

CUT-THROAT is an injury which may be due to suicide or murder, an expert being able to tell at a glance the one from the other. Death, when it occurs at once, is usually due to bleeding from the large vessels of the neck, and later may be caused by inflammation of the air passages. Another danger is that air will enter the large veins in such amount as to bring the circulation of the blood to a standstill. In a case of cut-throat, if any vessel is seen to bleed, the haemorrhage should be checked by pressure with the finger till surgical assistance can be obtained.

CYANIDES are salts of hydrocyanic or prussic acid. They are highly poisonous, and are also powerful antiseptics. (See PRUSSIC ACID; WOUNDS.) Double cyanide of mercury and zinc is specially powerful as an antiseptic used to impregnate gauze and cotton wool for dressing wounds.

CYANOCOBALAMIN is the name given by the British Pharmacopoeia Commission to vitamin B_{12}. It is a red cobalt-containing substance, and it owes its name to the fact that it contains cyanide and cobalt. Vitamin B_{12} was first isolated in 1948 and was found to be an effective substitute for liver in the treatment of pernicious anaemia. (See ANAEMIA.) It has now been replaced by hydroxocobalamin (qv) as the standard treatment for this condition. (See COBALAMINS.)

CYANOSIS is a condition of blueness seen particularly about the face and extremities, accompanying states in which the blood is not properly oxygenated in the lungs. It appears earliest through the nails, on the lips, and the tips of the ears, and over the cheeks. It may be due to blockage of the air passages, or to disease in the lungs, or to a feeble circulation, as in heart disease. (See METHAEMOGLOBINAEMIA.)

CYBERNETICS is the science of communication and control in the animal and in the machine.

CYCLAMATES are artificial sweetening agents which are about 30 times as sweet as cane sugar. After being in use since 1965, they were banned by Government decree in 1969 because of adverse reports received from the USA.

CYCLICAL OEDEMA: This is a syndrome in women characterized by irregular intermittent bouts of generalized swelling. Sometimes the fluid retention is more pronounced before the menstrual period. The eye lids are puffy and the face and fingers feel stiff and bloated. The breasts may feel swollen and the abdomen distended and ankles may swell. The diurnal weight gain may exceed 4 kg. The underlying disturbance is due to increased loss of fluid from the vascular compartment, probably from leakage of protein from the capillaries increasing the tissue oncotic pressure. Recent evidence suggests a decrease in the urinary excretion of dopamine may contribute as this catecholamine has a natriuretic action. This may explain why drugs that are dopamine antagonists, such as chlorpromazine, may precipitate or aggravate cyclical oedema. Conversely bromocriptine, a dopamine agonist, may improve the oedema.

CYCLIZINE HYDROCHLORIDE, or MARZINE, is an antihistamine drug (qv) which is mainly used for the prevention of sickness, including sea-sickness.

CYCLOFENIL (ONDONID) (see OESTROGENS).

CYCLOPHOSPAMIDE (ENDOXANA) (see CYTOTOXIC DRUGS).

CYCLOPHOSPHAMIDE (NAVIDREX) is a nitrogen mustard derivative (qv) which is proving of value in the treatment of various forms of malignant disease, including Hodgkin's disease and chronic lymphatic leukaemia. (See BENZOTHIADIAZINES.)

CYCLOPLEGIA denotes paralysis of the ciliary muscle of the eye, which results in the loss of the power of accommodation in the eye. (See ACCOMMODATION.)

CYCLOPROPANE is one of the most potent of the anaesthetics given by inhalation. Its advantages are that it acts quickly, causes little irritation to the lungs, and its effects pass off quickly.

CYCLOSERINE is an antibiotic derived from an actinomycete, which is of value in the treatment of certain infections of the genito-urinary tract, and of limited value in the treatment of tuberculosis.

CYCLOSPORIN A is a drug that is proving of value in preventing the rejection of transplanted organs such as the heart and kidneys. (See TRANSPLANTATION.)

CYCLOTHYMIA is the state characterized by extreme swings of mood from elation to depression, and vice versa.

CYCLOTRON is a machine in which positively charged particles are so accelerated that they acquire energies equivalent to those produced by millions of volts. From the medical point of view its interest is that it is a source of neutrons. (See RADIOTHERAPY.)

CYESIS is another term for pregnancy.

CYPROHEPTADINE is a drug originally introduced as an antihistamine drug (qv), but is now known to be effective in stimulating appetite and allowing underweight children and adults to gain weight.

CYPROTERONE ACETATE (ANDROCUR) is an anti-androgen. It inhibits the effects of androgens at receptor level. It is therefore useful in the treatment of hirsutism in women and in the treatment of severe hypersexuality and sexual deviation in men. (See OESTROGENS.)

CYSTEAMINE is a drug used in the prevention and treatment of radiation sickness (qv), and the treatment of paracetamol poisoning (qv).

CYSTIC FIBROSIS (see FIBROCYSTIC DISEASE OF THE PANCREAS).

CYSTITIS means inflammation of the bladder. The presenting symptom is usually dysuria; that is, a feeling of discomfort when urine is passed and frequently a stinging or burning pain in the urethra. There is also a feeling of wanting to pass water much more often than usual and yet there is very little urine present when the act is performed. Cystitis may be associated with a dragging ache in the lower abdomen. The urine usually looks dark or stronger than normal. It is frequently associated with haematuria, which means blood in the urine and is the result of the inflammation. It is a common problem; over half the women in Britain suffer from it at some time in their life. The cause of the disease is a bacterial infection of the bladder, the germs having entered the urethra and ascended into the bladder. The most common organism responsible is called E. coli. This organism normally lives in the bowel where it causes no harm. It is therefore likely to be present on the skin around the anus so that there is always a potential for infection. The disease is much more common in women because the urethra, vagina and anus are very close together and the urethra is much shorter in the female than it is in the male. It also explains why women commonly suffer cystitis after sexual intercourse and honeymoon cystitis is a very common presentation of bladder inflammation. In most cases the inflammation is more of a nuisance than a danger but the infection can spread up to the kidneys and cause pyelitis (qv) or pyelonephritis (qv) which are much more serious disorders.

In cases of cystitis the urine should be cultured to grow the responsible organism. The relevant antibiotic can then be prescribed. Fluids should be taken freely not only for an acute attack of cystitis but also to prevent further attacks, because if the urine is dilute the organism is less likely to grow. Bicarbonate of soda is also helpful as this reduces the acidity of the urine and helps to relieve the burning pain, and inhibits the growth of the bacteria. Careful hygiene, in order to keep clean down below, is also important. (See BLADDER, DISEASES OF.)

CYSTOGRAM is an X-ray picture of the urinary bladder.

CYSTOMETER is an instrument for measuring the pressure in the urinary bladder.

CYSTOSCOPE is an instrument for viewing the interior of the bladder. It consists of a narrow tube carrying a small electric lamp at its end, a small mirror set obliquely opposite an opening near the end of the tube, and a telescope which is passed down the tube and by which the reflection of the brightly illuminated bladder wall in the mirror is examined. It is of great value in the diagnosis of conditions like ulcers and small tumours of the bladder.

Fine catheters can be passed along the cystoscope, and by the aid of vision can be inserted into each ureter and pushed up to the kidney, so that the urine from each kidney may be obtained and examined separately in order to diagnose which of these organs is diseased.

CYSTS are hollow tumours, containing fluid or soft material. They are almost always simple in nature.

Varieties: (*a*) RETENTION CYSTS: In these, in consequence of irritation or other cause, some cavity which ought naturally to contain a little fluid becomes distended or the natural outlet from the cavity becomes blocked. Wens (qv) are caused by the blockage of the outlet from sebaceous glands in the skin, so that an accumulation of fatty matter takes place. Ranula (qv) is a clear swelling under the tongue, due to a collection of saliva in consequence of an obstruction to a salivary duct. Cysts in the breasts are, in many cases, the result of blockage in milk ducts, due to inflammation. Cysts also form in the kidney as a result of obstruction to the free outflow of the urine.

(*b*) DEVELOPMENTAL CYSTS: Of these, the most important are the huge cysts that originate in the ovaries. The cause is doubtful, but the cyst probably begins at a very early period of life, gradually enlarges, and buds off smaller cysts from its wall. The contents are usually a clear gelatinous fluid. Very often both ovaries are affected, and the cysts may slowly reach a great size, often, however, taking a lifetime to do so.

A similar condition sometimes occurs in the kidney, and the tumour may have reached a great size in an infant even before birth (congenital cystic kidney).

Dermoid cysts are small cavities, which also originate probably early in life, but do not reach any great size till fairly late in life. They appear about parts of the body where clefts occur in the embryo and close up before birth, such as the corner of the eyes, the side of the neck, the middle line of the body. They contain hair, fatty matter, fragments of bone, scraps of skin, even numerous teeth.

(*c*) HYDATID CYSTS are produced in many organs, particularly in the liver, by a parasite which is the larval stage of a tapeworm found in dogs. They occur in people who keep dogs and allow them to contaminate their food. (See TAENIASIS.)

CYTARABABINE (CYTOSAR) (see CYTOTOXIC DRUGS).

CYTO- is a prefix meaning something connected with a cell or cells.

CYTOGENETICS is the study of the structure and functions of the cells of the body, with particular reference to the chromosomes (qv).

CYTOLOGY is the study of cells.

CYTOMEGALOVIRUSES are a group of viruses belonging to the herpesvirus group. They are so-called from the swollen appearance of infected cells (*cytomegalo* = large cell). Their importance is that they are responsible for the condition of cytomegalic disease of the newborn. The virus is transmitted from the mother either to her unborn baby while still in the uterus or to the baby during birth. In some cases the baby may show no evidence of infection, but in others it may cause a fatal disease characterized by jaundice and an enlarged liver and spleen. In those who recover from this severe form of the disease, there may be permanent mental retardation. In England and Wales, around 400 babies a year are born mentally retarded because the mother was infected with the virus in pregnancy.

CYTOMETER is an instrument for counting and measuring cells.

CYTOPLASM is the name given to the protoplasm (qv) of the cell body. (See CELL.)

CYTOSTATIC means the slowing, or stopping, of the growth of cells.

CYTOTOXIC means being destructive to cells. Many cytotoxic drugs are now available for the treatment of cancer and to suppress the immune system to prevent rejection of organ transplants. In some patients with cancer the treatment with cytotoxic drugs, or chemotherapy (qv), is given with the aim of curing the disease. Under these circumstances some degree of drug-related toxicity is acceptable. Patients with acute leukaemia and lymphomas as well as some carcinomas can be be cured with cytotoxic drugs. They are frequently used in combination because of the enhanced response achieved when given in this way.

The cytotoxic drugs include: (1) the alkylating agents which act by damaging DNA, thus interfering with cell reproduction. Cyclophosphamide (Endoxana), ifosfamide (Mitoxana), chlorambucil (Leukeran), kelphalan (Alkeran), busulphan (Myleran), thiotepa and mustine are examples of alkylating agents.

(2) There are a number of cytotoxic antibiotics used in the treatment of cancer–doxorubicin (Adriamycin), bleomycin, actinomycin D (Cosmegen, Lyovac), mithramycin (Mithracin), amsacrine (Amsidine) are examples. They are used primarily in the treatment of acute leukaemia and lymphomas.

(3) Antimetabolites–these drugs combine irreversibly with vital enzymes systems of the cell and hence prevent normal cell division. Methotrexate (Emtexate), cytarabine (Cytosar), fluorouracil (Efudix), mercaptopurine (Puri-Nethol) and azathioprine (Imuran) are examples.

(4) Another group of cytotoxic drugs are the vinca alkaloids such as vincristine (Oncovin) and vinblastine (Velbe).

(5) Some newer cytotoxic drugs have been introduced, such as cisplatin (Neoplatin, Platinex and Platosin). This cytotoxic agent is particularly useful in the treatment of carcinoma of the ovary and teratomas of the testis.

D

DACRYOCYSTITIS (see EYE, DISEASES AND INJURIES OF).

DACTYLITIS means inflammation of a finger or toe.

DANAZOL (DANOL) inhibits pituitary gonadotrophin secretion and is used in the treatment of endometriosis, menorrhagia and gynaecomastia. The dose is usually of the order of 100 mg twice daily and side-effects may include nausea, dizziness, flushing and skeletal muscle pain. It is mildly androgenic.

DANDELION (see TARAXACUM).

DANDRUFF, or SCURF, is the white scales cast off from the scalp. (See SEBORRHOEA.)

DANGEROUS DRUGS: This term is applied to certain drugs which are scheduled under the Dangerous Drugs Act, and which must be dispensed only under certain stringent regulations. These include morphine, cocaine, ecgonine, diamorphine (commonly known as heroin), extracts and tinctures of Indian hemp and opium, as well as any preparation containing one part in 500 or more of morphine or one part in 1000 or more of cocaine, ecgonine, or diamorphine. Prescriptions containing any of these drugs must be written, dated, and signed by a practitioner, and must give the name and address of the person for whom the prescription is intended, as well as the total amount of the drug to be applied.

All other poisonous substances are scheduled in twelve classes, the important ones from the medical point of view being those included in the first and fourth schedules. The substances included in the First Schedule are those containing the more deadly poisons, which may not be sold by chemists except to persons known to the seller, and the name and address of the purchaser must be entered in a book. The Fourth Schedule includes drugs such as barbituric acid and its derivatives. A prescription for any substance in Schedule Four must contain the prescriber's name, the name and address of the seller, and the date on which the prescription was dispensed. It must not be dispensed more than once unless the prescriber directs that it be dispensed a stated number of times or at stated intervals.

In 1968, further regulations were introduced. Under the Dangerous Drugs (Notification of Addicts) Regulations, 1968, a doctor is required to pass to the chief medical officer at the Home Office full details of any person he is attending whom 'he considers or has reasonable grounds to suspect' to be addicted to any of the drugs listed in the Schedule to the 1965 Dangerous Drugs Act. These drugs include morphine, heroin, pethidine, dextromoramide. Under the Dangerous Drugs (Supply to Addicts) Regulations, 1968, it is an offence to provide cocaine or heroin or any of their derivatives to patients other than on licence issued by the Secretary of State and in accordance with the Regulations. Such licences are not issued for use in general practice, but only to individual doctors for use in a clinic, hospital or institution approved for the purpose.

On July 1, 1973, the Misuse of Drugs Act, 1971, and the regulations under it (Misuse of Drugs Regulations, 1973) came into force. The Act, which combines and extends the Dangerous Drugs Acts, 1965, and 1967, and the Drugs (Prevention of Misuse) Act, 1964, applies to the whole of the United Kingdom. The main practical changes introduced by this new legislation are: (*a*) Dangerous Drugs are now referred to as Controlled Drugs. (*b*) Nine drugs are added to the list of such Controlled Drugs, including amphetamine, codeine, dexamphetamine, methaqualone, and pholcodine. (*c*) Notification of addiction is required in respect of the following drugs: cocaine, dextromoramide, diamorphine (heroin), dipipanone, hydrocodone, hydromorphone (Dilaudid), levorphanol, methadone, morphine, omnopon, papaveretum, opium, oxycodone, pethidine, phenazocine, piritramide. (*d*) A new category of drugs has been introduced, including the hallucinogens (eg. lysergic acid diethylamide) and cannabis, which can only be prescribed under special licence. (*e*) Some tightening up of prescribing rules for doctors of Controlled Drugs.

DANTROLENE is a muscle-relaxing drug that is proving of value in relieving the muscular spasm in some cases of multiple sclerosis (qv).

DAPSONE is one of the most effective drugs in the treatment of leprosy.

DARTOS is the thin muscle just under the skin of the scrotum which enables the scrotum to alter its shape.

DAY BLINDNESS is a condition in which the patient sees better in a dim light or by night than in daylight. It is only found in conditions in which the light is very glaring, as in the desert and on snow, and is relieved by resting the retina, for example by wearing coloured glasses for a time.

DDT is the generally used abbreviation for the compound which has been given the official name of dicophane. It was first synthesized in 1874, but it was not until 1940 that, as a result of research work in Switzerland, its remarkable toxic action on insects was discovered. This work was taken up and rapidly expanded in Great Britain and the USA, and one of its first practical applications was in controlling the spread of typhus. This disease is transmitted by the louse, one of the insects for which DDT is most toxic. Its toxic action against the mosquito has also been amply proved, and it thus rapidly became one of the most effective measures in controlling malaria. DDT is toxic to a large range of insects in addition to the louse and the mosquito; these include house-flies, bed-bugs, clothes-moths, fleas, cockroaches, and ants. It is also active against many agricultural and horticultural pests, including weevils, flour beetles, pine sawfly, and most varieties of scale insect.

DDT has thus had a wide use in medicine, public health, veterinary medicine, horticulture, and agriculture, both in temperate and tropical zones. Like all potent preparations, however, its indiscriminate use is not without danger. Thus, it is toxic to bees and a number of parasites of fruit pests, and may therefore do as much harm as good if used indiscriminately as a horticultural spray. Again, if used to kill fleas in animals such as cats, which lick themselves, care must be taken in using it, as it may be toxic when swallowed. It is quite safe when applied to the skin, either in man or animals, in a watery solution, but if applied in an oily solution it may be rapidly absorbed and produce toxic effects. When used for domestic purposes or on animals, it is usually applied as a 5 per cent dust. Full details concerning its use may be obtained from the many leaflets and booklets issued by the manufacturers, by government departments, and by agricultural and horticultural institutes.

Finally, there is the most worrying factor of all: the increasing number of species of insects which are becoming resistant to DDT. Fortunately, to date newer insecticides have been introduced which are toxic to DDT-resistant insects, but there is a certain amount of anxiety as to whether this supply of new insecticides can be maintained.

DEAD, DISPOSAL OF THE: Practically, only three methods have been used from the earliest times: (*a*) burial; (*b*) embalming; (*c*) cremation.
(*a*) **Burial** is perhaps the earliest and most primitive method. It was customary to bury the bodies of the dead in consecrated ground around the churches till the earlier half of the nineteenth century, when the utterly insanitary state of churchyards led to legislation for their better control, and now that cemeteries are supposed to be situated outside towns and in proper sites, the interment of the dead should seldom be a menace to the health of the living. Burials in Britain take place usually upon production of a certificate from a registrar of deaths, to whom notice of the death, accompanied by a medical certificate, must be given without delay by the nearest relatives.
(*b*) **Embalming** is still used to a certain extent, particularly in the USA. The process consists in removing the internal organs by small openings and filling the body cavities with various aromatics of antiseptic power, the skin being swathed in bandages or otherwise protected from the action of the air. Bodies are also preserved by injecting the blood-vessels with strong antiseptics like perchloride of mercury. In certain circumstances bodies become naturally changed to a non-putrefying substance known as adipocere. (See PUTREFACTION.)
(*c*) **Cremation** provides a much speedier reduction of the body to its simple components than does burial, and one devoid of any harmful tendencies to the living. Not the least of its advantages is the amount of space that is saved. It is being used to an increasing extent.

In order to prevent any abuse, special certificates are required, and the necessary forms for these are obtained from the cremating authority. The law does not distinguish in England or the USA between cremation and burial, but special formalities are insisted upon by the crematorium authorities. The process of incineration takes between one and two hours. About 2·3 to 3·2 kg (5 to 7 pounds) of ash result from the combustion of the body, and there is no admixture with that from the fuel.

DEAD FINGERS (see RAYNAUD'S DISEASE).

DEADLY NIGHTSHADE is the popular name of *Atropa belladonna*, from which atropine is procured. Its poisonous black berries are sometimes eaten by children. (See ATROPINE; BERRIES, POISONOUS.)

DEAFNESS is divided into three classes, according to the section of the ear at fault.
EXTERNAL EAR, or EXTERNAL ACOUSTIC MEATUS, is the passage, about 33 mm (1½ inches) in length, leading inward from the surface to the drum, or tympanic membrane. When the deafness has its cause in this part, it is due simply to obstruction of the passage by a tumour, by a foreign body, such as a pea, or a polypus, or, most commonly of all, by a plug of hardened wax.

MIDDLE EAR is the tympanic cavity separated by the tympanic membrane from the outer ear, and communicating with the mastoid antrum, a hollow in the skull, behind, and with the Eustachian (or auditory) tube, which leads to the throat, beneath. These communications are important: the connection with the throat explains the deafness that accompanies a cold in the head and other forms of inflammation which spread from the nose and throat up into the middle ear; while the connection with the antrum shows why suppuration in the antrum can cause great destruction of the delicate mechanism in the middle ear. Acute inflammation in the throat, for example in measles, or chronic conditions like adenoids in children, are liable to produce middle-ear disease, perforation of the drum, and deafness. Tearing of the drum in consequence of, for example, an explosion, as a rule heals and leaves no deafness; but a perforation following inflammation in the antrum or middle ear is accompanied by suppuration, discharge from the ear, and other changes, and generally attended by impairment of hearing unless effective treatment is instituted at an early stage. It is a peculiarity of deafness in middle-ear disease that the hearing is often better during a loud noise: for example, a conversation is more clearly heard while church bells are ringing, or in the noise of a railway train.

INTERNAL EAR AND BRAIN constitute the receptive and perceptive apparatus for sound, the outer and middle ear forming parts of the conducting and collecting apparatus. Certain fevers like typhus and typhoid, tumours of the brain, meningitis, Menière's disease, mumps, and fractures of the base of the skull may all bring on a greater or less degree of deafness by interference with the perceptive apparatus. Some drugs produce a temporary deafness, notably quinine and certain antibiotics, particularly dihydrostreptomycin and streptomycin.

The human ear, it has been said, is such a remarkable instrument that the largest sound that can be tolerated without pain and almost instantaneous permanent damage is five million times the smallest that can be heard at all. It is poor, however, compared with the whale and dolphin which have an acoustic frequency register of 150 to 150,000 Hz (the human range is only 20 to 18,000 Hz).

In spite of its versatility there is a limit to what the human ear will tolerate, and the amount of noise in our midst is causing increasing anxiety.

Boiler-maker's disease is a condition of deafness long recognized to be due to a gradual wearing out of the nervous mechanism by the constant noise of hammering, and comes on in a few years, especially in boiler-makers, but also in others similarly subject to constant noise. The term, boiler-maker's disease, is now a misnomer as there are so many working conditions under which noise is a major hazard to hearing. The amount of deafness due to excessive noise at work is turning out to be much higher than was suspected, and at long last steps are being taken to reduce to a minimum the amount of unnecessary noise in industry. The current view is that for an eight-hour working day an acceptable upper limit of noise is around 90 decibels. Where the amount of noise cannot be reduced to a safe level, then workers must be supplied with effective ear-protection. No ear-protector, however, is an effective substitute for a safe level of sound. In medicolegal terms, 'impairment' of hearing means hearing loss, 'handicap' implies that the loss of hearing has social consequences, whilst 'disability' is reserved for those in whom the damage leads to difficulties in employment.

Attempts are also being made to reduce the amount of noise in the community at large. Thus under the Road Traffic Acts the present noise limits, measured at a distance of not less than 5·2 metres (17 feet), are: 80–89 decibels for motor-cycles depending on size of engine, 87 decibels for cars, 88 decibels for light commercial vehicles and 92 decibels for heavy commercial vehicles.

The hereditary form of deafness known as otosclerosis (qv) comes on in several members of some families shortly after puberty, owing to hardening changes in the inner ear.

It is estimated that 1·75 million people, that is 3·5 per cent of the population of England and Wales, are affected by deafness. In those over the age of 75, more than half have impaired hearing.

Treatment: Deafness due to causes in the external ear is readily dealt with, and, considering the frequency of hardened wax, it is a good and safe procedure to syringe out the ear with a tumblerful of warm water containing a teaspoonful of sodium bicarbonate. The stream of water is directed along the upper wall of the passage and flows out below. In cases where deafness accompanies nasal catarrh, adenoids, enlarged tonsils, etc., these conditions must be remedied. (See NOSE, DISEASES OF.) In a case of perforation of the drum, accompanied by a chronic discharge, particular care must be taken to keep the ear clean; otherwise there is a danger not only of increased deafness but of retained matter infecting some neighbouring part, and causing a dangerous abscess in the brain, meningitis, or suppuration in the mastoid antrum. (See EAR, DISEASES OF.) Boiler-maker's deafness generally improves if the occupation be changed; otherwise it grows steadily worse. Deaf-mutism is a condition where deafness has been complete from early life, usually from birth, and the child has never learned to speak, though the voice-producing organs are perfect. Such children can with patience be taught to carry on a fluent conversation by means of lip-reading, or by the finger language and signs. Where adults are concerned there are wide variations in the ability to lip-read. Some are born lip-readers, the majority have a reasonable ability, some find it most difficult. What is important in the care of both adults and children is that full advantage be taken of whatever capacity they may have for hearing. Even a minimum of hearing ability makes lip-reading much more effective. (See also DUMBNESS; HEARING AIDS; PRESBYACUSIS.)

A large range of effective hearing aids is now available, including the Medresco hearing aid supplied under the aegis of the National Health Service. These instruments are highly successful in the case of many deaf people,though not of great use in others. Each instrument requires to be carefully tuned for the deaf person using it. Before deciding to use a hearing aid the advice of an ear specialist should be obtained. The Royal National Institute for the Deaf, 105 Gower Street, London, WC1E 6AH (01-387 8033, Fax 01-388 2346), provides a list of clinics where such a specialist can be consulted. It also gives reliable advice concerning the purchase and use of hearing aids. (See also HEARING AIDS.)

DEAMINATION is the process of removal of the amino group, NH_2, from amino-acids not required for building up body protein. This is carried out mainly in the liver by means of an enzyme, deaminase. The fatty acid residue is either burnt up to yield energy, or is converted into glucose.

DEATH, CAUSES OF: Although the final cause of death is usually failure of the vital centres which govern the beating of the heart and the act of breathing, the practical question is the disease or injury which leads to this failure. A general idea of the extent to which different causes operate in terminating life can be obtained from the table below.

Ischaemic heart disease	157,506
Malignant disease	138,326
Respiratory disease (excluding tuberculosis)	36,895
Cerebrovascular disease	71,470
Motor vehicle accidents	5,481
Accidental falls	3,841
All other accidents	3,649
Suicide and self-inflicted injury	4,315
Congenital anomalies	3,119
Diabetes mellitus	4,457
Tuberculosis	753

Some of the principal causes of death in England in 1984.

The principal causes of death in England in 1984 were ischaemic heart disease, which accounted for 31 per cent of all male deaths and 24 per cent of all female deaths, cerebral vascular disease, which accounted for 10 per cent of all male deaths and 10 per cent of all female deaths. Cancer of the respiratory organs accounted for 10 per cent of all male deaths and cancer of the digestive organs for 8 per cent of all male deaths, whereas cancer of the digestive organs accounted for 7 per cent of all female deaths.

DEATH RATE: In 1984, the death rate in England was 11·3 per thousand. In Scotland, in 1979, it was 12·72 per thousand. In the international death stakes, based on what is known as the Standardized Mortality Ratio (SMR), which is a more satisfactory method of comparison, England occupies an intermediate position with an SMR of 87 in 1980. The range of SMRs is 71 (Iceland) to 121 (Portugal) for males, and 75 (Iceland) to 127 (Hungary) for females.

DEATH, SIGNS OF: There are some minor signs, such as relaxation of the facial muscles, which produces the staring eye and gaping mouth of the *Hippocratic countenance*, as well as a loss of the curves of the back, which becomes flat by contact with the bed or table; *discoloration of the skin*, which becomes of a wax-yellow hue, and loses its pink transparency at the finger-webs; *absence of blistering and redness* if the skin is burned (Christison's sign); and *failure of a ligature* tied round the finger to produce, after its removal, the usual change of a white ring, which, after a few seconds, becomes redder than the surrounding skin in a living person.

The only certain sign of death, however, is *stoppage of the heart*, and to ensure that this is permanent it is necessary to listen over the heart, that is, over the chest at the inner side of the nipple, for five minutes. This can be done by means of a stethoscope or by listening directly with the ear on the chest. *Stoppage of breathing* should also be noted, and this can be confirmed by observing that a mirror held before the mouth shows no haze, that a feather placed on the upper lip does not flutter, or that the reflection on the ceiling from a cup of water placed on the chest of the dead person shows no movement. An important sign is that if a cut is made in the skin or a vessel is opened no bleeding takes place after death.

In the vast majority of cases there is no difficulty in ensuring that death has occurred. The introduction of organ transplantation, however, and of more effective mechanical means of resuscitation, such as respirators, whereby an individual's heart can be kept beating almost indefinitely, has raised difficulties in a minority of cases. To solve the problem in these cases the concept of '*brain death*' has been introduced. In this context it has to be borne in mind that there is no legal definition of death. Death has traditionally been diagnosed by the irreversible cessation of respiration and heart-beat. In the Code of Practice drawn up in 1983 by a Working Party of the Health Departments of Great Britain and Northern Ireland, however, it is stated that 'death can also be diagnosed by the irreversible cessation of brain-stem function'. This is described as 'brain death'. The brain-stem consists of the mid-brain, pons and medulla oblongata which contain the centres controlling the vital processes of the body such as consciousness, breathing and the beating of the heart (see BRAIN). This new concept of death, which has been widely accepted in medical and legal circles throughout the world, means that it is now legitimate to equate brain death with death, that the essential component of brain death is death of the brain-stem, and that a dead brain-stem can be reliably diagnosed at the bedside.

Four points are important in determining the time that has elapsed since death. *Hypostasis*, or congestion, begins to appear as livid spots on the back, often mistaken for bruises, three hours or more after death. It is due to the blood running into the vessels in the lowest parts. *Loss of heat* begins at once after death, and the body has become as cold as the surrounding air after 12 hours, though this is delayed by hot weather, death from asphyxia, and some other causes. *Rigidity*, or rigor mortis, begins in six hours, takes another six to become fully established, remains for twelve hours and passes off during the succeeding twelve hours. It comes on quickly when extreme exertion has been indulged in immediately before death. Conversely it is slow in onset and slight in death from wasting diseases. It is slight or absent in children. It begins in the small muscles of the eyelid and jaw and then spreads over the body. *Putrefaction* is variable in time of onset, but usually begins in 2 or 3 days, as a greenish tint over the abdomen. (See PUTREFACTION.)

DEBILITY means a state of weakness.

DECIBEL is the unit of hearing. One decibel is the least intensity of sound at which a given note can be heard. The usual abbreviation for decibel is dB.

DECIDUA is the name of the soft coat which lines the interior of the womb during pregnancy and which is cast off at birth.

DECOCTION is a preparation made by boiling various plants in water and straining the fluid.

DECOMPENSATION means a failing condition of the heart in a case of valvular disease.

DECUBITUS is the name applied to the peculiar positions taken up in bed by patients suffering from various conditions. For example, patients with pleurisy or pneumonia prefer to lie upon the affected side; patients suffering from peritonitis, on the back; much exhausted people, far down in the bed.

The bed sores (qv) which such patients are liable to develop are known as decubitus ulcers.

DECUSSATION is a term applied to any point in the nervous system at which nerve fibres cross from one side to the other: eg. the decussation of the pyramidal tracts in the medulla, where the motor fibres from one side of the brain cross to the other side of the spinal cord.

DEFAECATION means the act of opening the bowels. (See CONSTIPATION; DIARRHOEA.)

DEFICIENCY DISEASE is the term applied to any disease resulting from the absence from the diet of any substance essential to good health: eg. one of the vitamins.

DEFORMITIES may be present at birth, or they may be the result of injuries, or disease, or simply produced by bad habits, like the curved spine occasionally found in children. (See BURNS; CHEST, DEFORMITIES OF; CLUB-FOOT; FINGERS; FLAT-FOOT; KNOCK-KNEE; LEPROSY; PALATE, DEFECTS OF; PARALYSIS; RICKETS; SCAR; SKULL; SPINE, DISEASES OF; JOINTS, DISEASES OF.)

DEGENERATION means a change in structure or in chemical composition of a tissue or organ by which its vitality is lowered or its function interfered with. Degeneration is of various kinds, the chief being fatty, fibroid (see CIRRHOSIS), calcareous (see CONCRETIONS), waxy, colloid, and mucoid.

Causes of degeneration are, in many cases, very obscure. In some cases heredity plays a part, particular organs, for example the kidneys, tending to show fibroid changes in successive generations. Fatty, fibroid, and calcareous degenerations are part of the natural change in old age. Defective nutrition may bring them on prematurely, as may excessive and long-continued strain upon an organ like the heart. Various poisons, like alcohol, play a special part in producing the changes, and so do the poisons produced by various diseases, particularly syphilis and tuberculosis.

DEGLUTITION means the act of swallowing. (See CHOKING.)

DELHI BOIL is a form of chronic sore occurring in Eastern countries, caused by a protozoan parasite, *Leishmania tropica*. (See LEISHMANIASIS.)

DELIRIUM is a condition of altered consciousness in which there is disorientation (as in a confusional state), incoherent talk and restlessness but with hallucination, illusions or delusions also present.

DELIRIUM (CONFUSION) The *milieu interieur* of some old people is so fragile that acute confusion or acute brain syndrome is a common effect of physical illness. Elderly people are often referred to as being 'confused'; unfortunately this term is often inappropriately applied to a wide range of eccentricities of speech and behaviour as if it were a diagnosis. It can be applied to a patient with the early memory loss of dementia (qv), forgetful, disorientated and wandering; to the dejected old person with depression, often termed Pseudo-Dementia (Arie); to the patient whose consciousness is clouded in the delirium of acute illness; to the apranoid deluded sufferer of late-onset schizophrenia or even to the patient presenting with the acute dysphasia and incoherence of a stroke.

DELIRIUM TREMENS is the form of delirium most commonly due to withdrawal from alcohol, if dependent on it. There is restlessness, fear or even terror accompanied by vivid, usually visual, hallucinations or illusions. The level of consciousness is impaired and the patient may be disorientated for time, place and person.

Treament is, as a rule, the treatment of causes. (See also ALCOHOLISM, ACUTE.) As the delirium in fevers is due partly to high temperature this should be lowered by tepid sponging (see COLD, USES OF). Careful nursing is one of the keystones of successful treatment, which includes ensuring that ample fluids are taken and nutrition is maintained. As for any withdrawal from alcohol dependence, sedation will be needed for delirium tremens, as an in-patient with medication such as benzodiazepines or chlormethiazole, on a gradually reducing basis. Care must be taken to exclude gross medical problems such as Wernicke's encephalopathy and it may be wise to give vitamin supplements by mouth or intramuscularly.

DELIVERY means the final expulsion of the child in the act of birth. (See LABOUR.)

DELTA WAVES is the term given to abnormal electrical waves observed in the electro-encephalogram. (See ELECTRO-ENCEPHALOGRAPHY.) The frequency of the normal alpha waves is ten per second. That of the delta waves is seven or less per second. They occur in the region of tumours of the brain, and in the brains of epileptics.

DELTOID is the powerful triangular muscle attached above to the collar-bone and shoulder-blade, and below, by its point, to the humerus, nearly half-way down the outer side of the upper arm. Its action is to raise the arm from the side, and it covers and gives roundness to the shoulder.

DELUSIONS are errors in judgment, regarding simple facts, which interfere with the ordinary conduct of life. Thus a man may have the delusion that he has no stomach and refuse to take food. No amount of argument or demonstration will convince the subject of a delusion as to the error of his belief. The existence of a delusion, of such a nature as to influence conduct seriously is one of the most important signs in reaching a decision to arrange for the compulsory admission of the patient to hospital for observation. (See MENTAL ILLNESS.)

DEMENTIA: Severe dementia occurs in 5 per cent of individuals aged over 65; mild intellectual impairment is present in an additional 10–15 per cent (benign senile forgetfulness); the incidence of significant dementia rises to 20 per cent in those aged over 80. The predominant causes of dementia are Senile Dementia of the Alzheimer Type (SDAT) and Multi-Infarct Dementia (MID), occurring in a ratio of 70:30, and both types must be distinguished from the reversible Dementia Syndrome which develops over a few months. SDAT is characterized by defects in orientation, memory, intellectual function, judgement and activity; it is an acquired persistent loss of intellectual function with impairments in at least three of the following spheres of mental activity; language, memory, visio-spatial skills, personality and cognition (eg. abstraction, judgement, mathematics). These defects in function tend to be preceded by memory loss, specifically, short term, occurring in the two to three years prior to presentation.

DEMETHYLCHLORTETRACYCLINE, or LEDERMYCIN, is a tetracycline (qv) preparation which is effective in relatively low dosage and is said to be more stable than other tetracycline preparations.

DE MORGAN SPOTS, so called after the English physician who first described them, are small haemangiomas (qv) which occur in the skin of middle-aged people. They seldom exceed 3 millimetres in diameter. There are usually only one or two in any one individual, though occasionally they may be more widespread. They are of no significance.

DEMULCENTS are substances which sooth or protect the surface of the alimentary canal.

Varieties: Mucilaginous substances like gum, isinglass, Iceland moss; oils like olive, linseed, and almond oils; starchy substances like arrowroot; also glycerin, borax, honey, and mild alkalis, and fine powders like subnitrate of bismuth.

Uses: They are used in cases of inflammation, particularly of the throat and stomach, in gargles or draughts, to protect these parts from the irritation of their own secretions; and after injury, such as that due to swallowing a corrosive poison, in order to soothe the pain and encourage healing in the injured part.

DENGUE, also called BREAK-BONE FEVER, DANDY-FEVER, and THREE-DAY FEVER, is a disease of tropical and sub-tropical regions caused by an arbovirus (qv) transmitted to man by the mosquito, *Aëdes aegypti*. It is a sudden and short infectious fever, with an incubation period (see INCUBATION) of a few days, characterized mainly by swelling and pains in the joints, and by skin eruptions.

Symptoms: It usually begins suddenly with pain in a joint and fever. Next appears redness of the face, spreading later over the body, very much like the rash of measles. This itches intensely. There are also sore throat and running of the eyes, and the muscles and joints generally become very painful. These symptoms endure for about three days, and then gradually pass off, leaving the person very weak. After two or three days a relapse generally takes place, very similar to the first attack. There may be a third or even a fourth relapse, and recovery from the weakness and pains in the joints is often slow, sometimes lasting over months. Death hardly ever occurs.

Treatment: Aspirin, with or without codeine, usually relieves the pains and reduces the temperature though in more severe cases pethidine may be needed to bring relief. Calamine lotion eases the itching of the rash.

DENGUE HAEMORRHAGIC FEVER is a more acute form of the disease which occurs predominantly in young children and seems to be confined largely to the indigenous population of South-east Asia.

DENTINE (see TEETH).

DENTIST is a person who diagnoses disease in the mouth, treats it and prevents its recurrence. There are a number of different groups. There is the *general dental practitioner* who is concerned with primary dental care. The *community dental practitioner* is part of the public-health team and is largely concerned with monitoring dental health and treating the young and the handicapped. In the *hospitals and dental schools* are those who are involved in only one of the specialities. The *restorative dentist* is concerned with the repair of teeth damaged by trauma and caries, and the replacement of missing teeth. The *orthodontist* is involved in the correction of jaws and teeth which are misaligned or irregular. This is done with appliances which may be removable or fixed to the teeth which are then moved with springs or elastics. *Oral and maxillo-facial surgeons* are those who carry out surgery to the mouth and face. This not only includes removal of buried teeth but also treatment for fractured facial bones, removal of cancers and the repair of missing tissue and the cosmetic restoration of facial anomalies such as cleft palate or large or small jaws.

DENTITION (see TEETH).

DEODORANTS are substances which remove or lessen objectionable odours. Some, which have a powerful odour, simply cover other smells, but the most effective act by giving off oxygen, so as to convert the objectionable substances into simple and harmless ones.

Varieties: Volatile oils of plants, such as eucalyptus and turpentine, chlorine water and chlorinated lime, peroxide of hydrogen, charcoal, dry earth, sawdust, and potassium permanganate are among the most powerful.

Uses: The main use is to purify sewage, bilge-water, and water-closets. Many powerful deodorants act, at the same time, as disinfectants. They are also used in sick-rooms to cover the smell of discharges, and the like. For the manner of use see under the individual deodorants. (See also PERSPIRATION.)

DEOXYCORTONE ACETATE is a synthetic corticosteroid (qv).

DEPILATION is the process of destroying hair; substances and processes used for this purpose being known as depilatories. The purpose may be effected in three ways: (1) by removing the hairs at the level of the skin surface; (2) by pulling the hairs out (epilation); (3) by destroying the roots and so preventing the growth of new hairs.

Shaving is the most effective way of removing superfluous hairs. Rubbing morning and night with a smooth pumice-stone is said to be helpful. The alkaline sulphides used as depilatories tend to erode the skin as well as the hairs. Electrolysis and diathermy have a limited use.

DEPRESSION (see MENTAL ILLNESS).

DEPRESSOR is the name given to a nerve by whose stimulation motion, secretion, or some other function is restrained or prevented: eg. the depressor nerve of the heart slows the beating of this organ.

DEQUALINIUM CHLORIDE is an antibacterial and antifungal compound which is of value in the treatment of infections of the mouth, gums, and throat, and in certain skin conditions.

DERBYSHIRE NECK is a name for goitre, which was fairly common in Derbyshire. (See GOITRE.)

DERMABRASION, or 'surgical planing', is a method of removing the superficial layers of the skin, which is sometimes useful in the removal of tattoos and superficial blemishes of the skin.

DERMATITIS means inflammation of the skin, though its differentiation from eczema is by no means clear. Indeed, different dermatologists (or skin specialists) use the two terms in quite different ways. For the present purpose only three forms of dermatitis will be considered here: contact dermatitis, light dermatitis, and exfoliative dermatitis. (See also DERMATITIS under OCCUPATIONAL DISEASES.)

Atopic Dermatitis (see NEURODERMATOSES).

Contact Dermatitis is dermatitis caused by contact between the skin and some substance to which the skin is sensitive. The skin eruption may vary from mere redness to severe inflammation of the skin. The onset may be gradual or sudden, depending upon how sensitive the individual is to the incriminating substance. A large range of substances can produce contact dermatitis, including cosmetics such as lipstick, hair dyes, shampoos, perfumes, nail varnish, face powder and rouge; nylon hair nets; rubber sponges; dyes used in clothing; nickel, chromium and rubber, as used in suspenders; contraceptives; paints and varnishes; and plants. So far as plants are concerned, the most important in Britain is the indoor primula, *Primula abconica*; next comes chrysanthemum, anthemis (the stinking mayweed) and the giant hogweed. Medicaments applied to the skin as ointments, lotions and the like are an increasing cause of contact dermatitis. For this reason antibiotics, such as penicillin, are seldom used in the form of such local applications in case they should render the patient sensitive. Not only does this expose patients to the unnecessary discomfort of a contact dermatitis, it may also mean that they can no longer be given the antibiotic in question, when it may be a life-saving measure. The diagnosis of the condition is usually fairly simple, one of the important factors being the localization of the dermatitis. Thus, if it occurs on the thigh in a woman it may well be due to her suspenders, whereas if it occurs in the armpit it may be due to some dye in clothing or to some deodorant spray. In doubtful cases the diagnosis can usually be settled by what is known as a patch test. This consists of applying a small amount of the suspected sensitizing substance to an area of normal skin. If the individual is sensitive to the substance in question, an area of dermatitis appears beneath the patch in twenty-four to forty-eight hours, and the test is said to be positive.

Prevention consists in the first instance of finding the cause and then making sure the afflicted individual has no further contact with it.

Treatment varies with the severity of the condition. In relatively mild cases the application of calamine lotion is often all that is necessary. In more severe cases this is supplemented by the application of a corticosteroid (qv). The area involved should not be washed with soap, but cleaned with olive oil, or an emulsion of water and Emulsifying Ointment, BP. When the condition has become chronic, with thickening and scaliness of the skin, there is often quite intense itching, and the resultant scratching makes the condition worse. In such a case the application of Compound Zinc Paste, BP, to which coal tar has been added, brings relief and aids healing.

Dermatitis herpetiformis is a bullous, or blob-like, eruption often mistaken for eczema or scabies. It is associated with a sensitivity to gluten (qv). It responds to a gluten-free diet or to the administration of dapsone (qv).

Light Dermatitis, or LIGHT ERUPTION, is a dermatitis, with reddening and blistering of the skin, which occurs on exposure to sunlight. It is recognized by the fact that it occurs on the parts of the body normally exposed to sunlight –the face, neck and hands – and that its incidence is between April and September. It takes two main forms. One is an exaggerated form of sunburn, and this soon passes off. The other occurs in individuals who are photo-allergic. In other words, they have been rendered allergic, or sensitive, to sunlight by some substance. This may be a drug, and the drugs most likely to be responsible are the phenothiazines which include some of the antihistamine drugs and some of the tranquillizers, and the sulphonamides. Eosin in lipstick and perfume in cosmetics may also be the responsible sensitizing agent. In some individuals no sensitizing agent can be implicated, and it is assumed that this form of the condition, sometimes referred to as *polymorphic light eruption*, is due to some innate sensitivity in the individual's skin. It is this form of the condition which is most likely to be seen in children.

Treatment consists of treating the dermatitis as already outlined. To protect the skin a sun-screen, oil or cream should be applied which contains some substance such as titanium dioxide that absorbs the ultra-violet rays in sunlight which cause the trouble. For the unfortunate minority for whom no remedy can be found, the only remedy is the wearing of shady hats, long sleeves and gloves.

Exfoliative Dermatitis, or ERYTHRODERMA as it is also known, is a condition which begins with patches of erythema, or reddening of the skin, followed by gradual thickening of the skin which then begins to desquamate, or peel off. It gradually spreads until practically the whole of the body is involved. It is rare before the age of 50, and is three times more common in men than in women. In over half the cases it occurs in people with some other skin condition, usually chronic eczema or psoriasis. In about a third no cause can be found, and in the remainder it develops in patients with Hodgkin's disease (qv), mycosis fungoides (qv) or chronic leukaemia (see LEUKAEMIA).

Treatment: No matter what the underlying cause, treatment consists of large doses of corticosteroids. (See also SKIN DISEASES.)

DERMATOGLYPHICS is the study of the patterns made by the ridges and crevices of the hands and the soles of the feet. It has become an important study in medicine because of the help it provides in the diagnosis of certain diseases, such as mongolism. It is also proving of value in certain other congenital diseases. Thus, a recent study showed abnormal palmar findings in 64 per cent of patients with congenital heart disease (qv) compared with only 17 per cent of patients with acquired heart disease.

DERMATOMYOSITIS is an auto-immune disease, characterized by erythema of the skin and wasting of the muscles.

DERMATOPHYTES: These are fungal infections. They are commonly seen as athlete's foot, scalp ringworm, tinea corporis and nail infection. They are due to fungi that normally inhabit the keratin tissue of the skin, hair and nails.

DERMOGRAPHIA, also known as DERMOGRAPHISM and URTICARIA FACTITIA, is a condition in which tracings made on the skin leave a distinct swollen, reddish mark. It occurs in allergic individuals, in whom the stimulus of scratching the skin produces an excessive amount of histamine. (See ALLERGY.)

DERMOID CYST (see CYSTS).

DERRIS is the dried root of several species of Derris, the active constituent of which is rotenone. It is used as an insecticide and larvicide, and also for the control of warble fly in cattle. A form known as Prepared Derris used to be widely used in the treatment of scabies.

DESFERRIOXAMINE is a chelating agent which is proving of value in the treatment of iron poisoning and thalassaemia.

DESIPRAMINE (PERTOFRAN) (see ANTIDEPRESSANTS).

DESQUAMATION means the scaling off of the superficial layer of the epidermis.

DETERGENTS are substances which clean the skin surface. This means that, strictly speaking, any soap, or soap-like substance used in washing, is a detergent. At the present day, however, the term is largely used for the synthetic detergents which are now used on such a large scale. These are prepared by the cracking and oxidation of high petroleum waxes with sulphuric acid. The commoner ones in commercial preparations are aryl alkyl sulphate or sulphonate and secondary alkyl sulphate.

Considering their widespread use they appear to cause relatively little trouble with the skin, but more trouble has been reported with the so-called 'biological' detergents that were introduced some years ago. They are so named because they contain an enzyme (qv) which destroys protein. As a result they are claimed to remove proteins – stains such as blood, chocolate, milk or gravy, which are relatively difficult for ordinary detergents to remove. Unfortunately these 'biological' detergents may cause dermatitis of the hands. In addition, they have been reported to cause asthma in those using them, and even more so in workers manufacturing them.

DETOXICATION means reduction or removal of the toxic properties of poisons or remedies. (See VACCINES.)

DEVONSHIRE COLIC is caused by drinking cider which has been stored in contact with lead, so that colic comes on as a result of lead poisoning. (See COLIC; LEAD POISONING).

DEXAMETHASONE is a corticosteroid derivative. As an anti-inflammatory agent it is approximately 30 times as effective as cortisone and eight times as effective as prednisolone. On the other hand, it has practically none of the salt-retaining properties of cortisone.

DEXTRAN is the name given to a group of polysaccharides which was first discovered in sugar-beet preparations which had become infected with certain bacteria. Of recent years, a homogeneous preparation of it, with a consistent molecular weight and free from protein, has been introduced as a substitute for plasma for transfusion purposes.

DEXTRIN is a soluble carbohydrate substance into which starch is converted by diastatic ferment or by heat. It is thus contained in toast, the crust of bread, biscuits, and breakfast foods. It is a white or yellowish powder which, dissolved in water, forms mucilage. Animal dextrin, also known as glycogen (qv), is a carbohydrate stored in the liver after meals, often in considerable amounts.

DEXTROMORAMIDE is a potent, habit-forming analgesic, or pain-reliever, which is active whether taken by mouth or given by injection.

DEXTROSE is another name for purified grape sugar or glucose.

DIA- is a prefix meaning through or thoroughly.

DIABETES INSIPIDUS is a disease characterized by excessive thirst and the passing of large volumes of urine which have a low specific gravity and contain no abnormal constituents. It is either due to a lack of the antidiuretic hormone normally produced by the hypothalamus and stored in the posterior pituitary gland, or to a defect in the renal tubules which prevents them responding to the antidiuretic hormone vasopressin. When the disorder is due to a vasopressin insufficiency, a primary or secondary tumour in the area of the pituitary stalk is responsible for one third of cases. In another one third of cases there is no apparent cause and such idiopathic cases are sometimes familial. A further one third of cases result from a variety of lesions including trauma, basal meningitis and granulomatous lesions in the pituitary stalk area. When the renal tubules fail to respond to vasopressin this is usually because of a genetic defect transmitted as a sex-linked recessive characteristic and the disease is called nephrogenic diabetes insipidus. Metabolic abnormalities such as hypercalcaemia and potassium depletion render the renal tubule less sensitive to vasopressin and certain drugs such as lithium and tetracycline may have a similar effect.

If the disease is due to a deficiency of vasopressin, treatment should be with the analogue of vasopressin called desmopressin which is more potent than the natural hormone and has less pressor activity. It also has the advantage in that it is absorbed from the nasal mucosa and so does not require to be injected.

Nephrogenic diabetes insipidus cannot be treated with desmopressin. The urine volume can, however, usually be reduced by half by a thiazide diuretic. Diabetes insipidus is a relatively rare condition and must be differentiated from diabetes mellitus (qv) which is an entirely different disease.

DIABETES MELLITUS is a syndrome, the most characteristic feature of which is an elevation in the concentration of glucose in the blood with consequent glycosuria (qv). This abnormal elevation of blood glucose level may only occur after the intake of food and may be asymptomatic. When, however, the disease is more florid and more severe, large quantties of glucose are lost in the urine and as a result of the osmotic diuresis polyuria (qv) results, with consequent thirst. As a result of the loss of calories in the urine, body weight is lost, and physical energy is reduced. In 1889 Mering and Minkowski found that diabetes frequently followed removal of the pancreas from animals. This defect was established in 1909 to be due to the failure of the pancreas to produce a hormone which was given the name insulin. Insulin was however not isolated until 1921 when it was successfully obtained for the first time by Banting and Best.

Symptoms: The main symptoms of diabetes are thirst, polyuria and tiredness. Weight loss results and is usually associated with a good appetite. As a result of the sugar in the urine, which provides an excellent growth medium for bacteria and fungi, infection is common in the region of the groin so that balanitis (qv) and pruritis vulvae (see PRURITUS) are common presenting symptoms. Eczema of various parts of the body may result from the presence of sugar in the sweat and as a result of the reduced vitality of tissues, boils and carbuncles may occur anywhere over the skin. Cataracts are common complications of diabetes and the disease damages retinal vessels, leading to haemorrhages and exudates at the back of the eye and proliferation of new blood vessels which may result in blindness. Diabetes is associated with the development of peripheral vascular disease and with peripheral neuropathy and damage to the kidneys.

Diabetes mellitus is a syndrome and thus has many causes:

(1) It may be primary. Type 1 diabetes mellitus is insulin dependent and tends to occur in young people with a peak age of onset of between 12 and 14 years. The onset of the disease is usually rapid and the patient is commonly underweight. Ketosis results if insulin is not given, and this may lead to coma. The disease is due to low or absent endogenous insulin.

Type 2 diabetes mellitus is not insulin dependent and it is sometimes further sub-divided into obese and non-obese groups. This variety of diabetes tends to affect the older age groups, the peak age of onset being more than 50 years. The onset is insidious and ketosis does not develop. Insulin secretion is normal or even increased in the early stages and the diabetes frequently responds to diet alone, although oral hypoglycaemic agents are needed in some instances. There is a tendency to insulin resistance and there is no particular HLA association.

(2) Another variety of diabetes occurs during pregnancy and remits afterwards. This is called gestational diabetes mellitus.

(3) Finally, diabetes mellitus may occur secondary to certain other diseases. For example, disorders of the pancreas such as chronic pancreatitis or haemochromatosis may result in destruction of the islet cells and resultant insulin deficiency. It may also be hormonal or drug induced. For example, diabetes is common in Cushing's syndrome as a result of the enhanced gluconeogenesis produced by the raised blood levels of cortisol. It is also frequently a feature of acromegaly because growth hormone is an insulin antagonist. It may result from a phaeochromocytoma due to the excess mobilisation of glycogen induced by the raised levels of adrenalin. It may also be secondary to primary aldosteronism as a result of hypokalaemia impairing carbohydrate tolerance. Similarly, hypokalaemia produced by diuretics may also predispose to diabetes mellitus and exogenous steroids used in the treatment of a variety of auto-immune and hypersensitivity diseases may provoke diabetes mellitus.

Diabetes mellitus is a common disease with a prevalence of 1 to 1·5 per cent. It has been known for centuries that diabetes tends to occur in families, although the precise mode of genetic transmission is uncertain. Less than 20 per cent of patients with type 1 diabetes mellitus have first degree relatives with the disease and only about 25 per cent of the offspring of two diabetic patients are likely to develop the disorder. In type 2 diabetes, however, 60 per cent of the children of two type 2 diabetic patients will themselves develop the disease by the age of 60. Immunological factors may also be important for there is a well recognised association between type 1 diabetes and many organ-specific auto-immune diseases. The role of viral infection is also possibly important. There is an increased prevalence of diabetes in the winter and it is known that viruses such as Coxsackie virus can damage pancreatic islet cells in animals. Type 2 diabetes is certainly multifactorial for although there is a genetic background environmental factors play an important part in the development of diabetes.

Treatment: The aim of treatment is to restore carbohydrate metabolism to as near normal as possible, and the two main guides as to how successfully this is being attained are the blood-sugar concentration and the amount of sugar and ketone bodies (eg. acetone) in the urine. The patient's general health is also of importance here, but it will usually be found that there is a direct correlation between the first two and the patient's sense of well-being. The one important exception to this occurs in the case of middle-aged and elderly diabetics, many of whom feel better with a rather high blood-sugar level than they do when the blood-sugar level is brought down to within normal limits. In other words, the diabetic must not become too introspective about the amount of sugar he finds on testing his urine, nor must the doctor attach all his interest to the concentration of sugar in the blood of his diabetic patients. Generally speaking, once a diabetic patient has been stabilized in his treatment, there is no need for him to test his own urine provided he is feeling well and is attending his doctor or his diabetic clinic at regular intervals. Conversely, it is equally important that the moment he begins to feel unwell, eg. develops dyspepsia, a cough, or 'a cold', he should report at once to his doctor.

The treatment of uncomplicated diabetes mellitus can be divided into two sections: (1) diet; (2) insulin. These can, again, be divided into two stages: (*a*) stabilization; (*b*) maintenance.

DIET: Of recent years the tendency has been to give the diabetic patient as liberal a diet as possible, except in the case of the obese patient in whom it is essential to obtain a reduction of weight. It has also been recognized that, as diabetes mellitus practically always persists for the rest of the patient's life, dietetic restrictions should be reduced to a minimum so that he should be able to lead as normal a life as possible. The simplest and most satisfactory way of attaining this is to control the amount of carbohydrate in the diet. This may amount to as much as half the energy content of the diet provided this is in the form of what are known as polysaccharides: eg. bread, potatoes, cereals, beans. This increase in carbohydrate is accompanied by a reduction in the amount of fat, which should not exceed 35 per cent of the energy content of the diet. The diet should also contain ample fibre, taken, for example, in the form of wholemeal bread, cereals and bran. There is no need to buy diabetic speciality foods; not only are they relatively expensive, but they have no advantage over ordinary food and are often unpalatable. Unless medically contraindicated, diabetics may take most alcoholic drinks except sweet wines and liqueurs, provided allowance is made for their energy contribution to the diet. A point to bear in mind is that beers and lagers specially brewed for diabetics have a relatively high alcohol content and are expensive. It should be remembered, however, that diabetics may be susceptible to alcohol-induced hypoglycaemia. They should therefore guard against excessive alcohol intake and avoid drinking on an empty stomach. Practically all soft drinks, such as Lucozade, Ribena, Coca-Cola, Pepsi-Cola, lemonade and other fizzy drinks are banned. Artificial sweeteners such as saccharin may be used, but many diabetics prefer to get used to taking their tea and coffee unsweetened.

When diabetes mellitus is first diagnosed, it is usual to initiate treatment by diet alone unless the condition is very severe, when the immediate use of insulin may be called for. The usual initial diet is one containing 100 grams of carbohydrate daily. If the diabetes improves on this diet, then it is gradually increased by 50-gram stages every two or three weeks, so long as the blood-sugar level remains satisfactory. In milder cases such dietetic control may be all that is necessary, but if it is impossible to control the diabetes in this way, then insulin is necessary.

INSULIN: The *British National Formulary* lists 27 insulin preparations, which now include the first of the new human insulins. All these have to be given by injection – usually subcutaneously, but they can also be given intravenously in an emergency. Insulin pumps are now available which maintain a supply of insulin more comparable to the way in which insulin is supplied from the pancreas in a non-diabetic individual. They incorporate means for increasing the dose of insulin when it is most needed: ie. before a meal. This is done either manually or electronically. The pump is usually worn in a pouch, attached to a belt round the waist or a shoulder harness. The essential difference between these nine forms is their duration of action. Thus, the action of insulin injection begins in 20 to 30 minutes and reaches its maximum in 4 to 5 hours. With protamine zinc insulin the blood sugar begins to fall in 5 to 11 hours, and the maximum effect is obtained in 15 to 20 hours. With globin insulin the effect begins in 1 to 2 hours, and reaches a maximum in 8 to 16 hours. Isophane insulin begins to act in 2 hours and its action persists for 24 hours. Insulin zinc suspension has a fairly rapid onset of action which persists for 24 hours. Insulin zinc supension (amorphous) has also a fairly rapid onset of action, but this lasts for only 12 to 16 hours. Insulin zinc suspension (crystalline) has a somewhat delayed onset of action which persists for 24 hours (see INSULIN).

In stabilizing a new case of diabetes which requires insulin, it is advisable to use insulin injection. The amount of insulin is gradually increased every four or five days until a satisfactory blood-sugar level is attained. The subsequent course of treatment depends upon the individual response of each patient. The aim in an active patient, who is not overweight, is to allow him to take a diet containing 200 to 300 grams of carbohydrate daily. In the case of children, 300 grams of carbohydrate daily should be considered the minimum if full health and adequate growth are to be maintained. In the case of the obese patient, a diet of 1100 Calories, containing 60 grams of carbodydrate daily, is the optimum one to obtain a reduction in weight without undue discomfort to the patient. Once on insulin it is essential that the carbohydrate intake be steady from day to day and that it is taken at regular intervals throughout the day. This means that most of it is taken at the three main meals – breakfast, lunch and supper, leaving a little over to be taken as snacks in mid-morning and mid-afternoon.

Once the patient is stabilized on a given diet and insulin injection, a decision is then taken as to whether the maintenance insulin is to be insulin injection or one of the others. The theoretical advantage of the delayed-action insulins is that they maintain a steadier blood-sugar level throughout the 24 hours; their practical advantage is that they involve only one injection every day instead of two. The final decision in each case as to which form of insulin to use is one to be decided by the medical attendant in charge of the case.

Oral hypoglycaemic agents: Certain sulphonamide and biguanide derivatives have been introduced which, when taken by mouth, lower the level of the blood sugar. The available evidence indicates that, as a substitute for insulin, they are used by 30 per cent of all diabetics. Their use is restricted to those mild, or relatively mild, diabetics in whom: (i) Diet alone fails to bring the blood sugar within or near normal limits. (ii) The dietary restriction required to control the diabetes causes progressive loss of weight or severe hunger. (iii) The withdrawal of insulin is not followed by relapse into significant acidosis. They should not be used during pregnancy. A point to remember is that alcohol may dangerously potentiate their hypoglycaemic effect. The sulphonamide derivatives, or sulphonylureas as they are technically known, act chiefly by stimulating the release of insulin from the pancreas. The biguanides act chiefly by reducing the amount of glucose produced in the liver. (See BIGUANIDES; CHLORPROPAMIDE; GLIBENCLAMIDE; GLYMIDINE; METFORMIN; SULPHONYLUREAS; and TOLBUTAMIDE.)

Dangers: The danger which is always present in cases of diabetes is the occurrence of *acidosis*, which, in severe cases, proceeds to *diabetic coma*. An indication of the presence of this condition is given when a large amount of acetone along with sugar is found in the urine. This is a dangerous condition unless it is immediately treated with full doses of insulin.

This type of coma must be carefully differentiated from *hypoglycaemic coma*, which is due to an overdose of insulin resulting in an extreme fall in the blood-sugar concentration. Milder forms of hypoglycaemia are relatively common, manifesting themselves by a sinking feeling, a sensation of hunger, a feeling of sickness, giddiness, or breaking out in a sweat. The treatment consists of the administration of sugar in some form – by mouth if the patient is conscious, by intravenous injection if the patient is unconscious. Every diabetic subject on insulin should carry sugar about with him, in the form of lumps of sugar or barley sugar, so that he can easily avert an attack should he feel it coming on.

This is a particularly important point for the 150,000 diabetics in Great Britain who are potential motorists. Diabetes is not a disqualifying disability for a driving licence, though it is recommended that those taking insulin should not drive heavy goods vehicles or public service vehicles. Insulin, however, is legally a drug, and a driver with symptoms of hypoglycaemia may be charged with driving while under the influence of drugs. Every diabetic driver therefore should keep an emergency supply of lumps of sugar permanently in his or her car.

Another serious danger incurred by the subject of diabetes is the occurrence of *gangrene* in the skin, especially about the toes. In order to avoid this, special care must be taken to keep the feet in a healthy condition by frequent washing, treatment of corns and abrasions, and avoidance of tight shoes. A regular visit to a chiropodist is a wise precaution. All forms of infection, such as boils, must be treated with special care on ordinary principles. *Necrobiosis lipoidica diabeticorum* is an unsightly, though, fortunately, uncommon blemish of the skin which occasionally occurs. It is usually on the shin and practically always in women. It sometimes goes on to ulceration. There is no effective treatment. The frequency with which *chest complications* supervene in diabetes has been mentioned, and special precautions must be taken to avoid these. It is also essential that diabetics should have their eyes examined and tested at least once a year. This is essential to detect at as early a stage as possible the onset of retinopathy (qv) as it is now amenable to laser therapy. After 20 years of diabetes around 80 per cent of patients have retinopathy. Fortunately in many instances this remains of a mild form. Occasionally, however, it flares up, and leads on to blindness. After 30 years of diabetes around 7 per cent of patients are blind. In England and Wales there are some 8000 registered blind diabetics, most of whom are over the age of 60.

Although diabetes is now the third most frequent cause of death in industrialized countries, after heart disease and cancer, many diabetics live to a ripe old age provided the condition is diagnosed at an early stage and the rules of healthy living as outlined in this section are adhered to.

People with diabetes mellitus, or their relatives, can obtain advice from the British Diabetic Association, 10 Queen Anne Street, London W1M 0BD (01-323 1531, Fax 01-637 3644).

DIACHYLON (see LEAD).

DIAGNOSIS is the art of distinguishing one disease from another, and is essential to scientific and successful treatment. The name is also given to the opinion arrived at as to the nature of a disease. It is in diagnosis more than in treatment that the highest medical skill is required, and, for a diagnosis, the past and hereditary history of a case, the symptoms complained of, and the signs of disease found upon examination are all weighed. Many methods of laboratory examination are also used at the present day in aiding diagnosis.

DIALYSIS is the process whereby crystalloid and colloid substances are separated from a solution by interposing a semipermeable membrane, such as cellophane, between the solution and pure water. The crystalloid substances pass through the membrane into the water until a state of equilibrium, so far as the crystalloid substances are concerned, is established between the two sides of the membrane. The colloid substances do not pass through the membrane.

This is the principle upon which the artificial kidney works. (See KIDNEY, ARTIFICIAL.) When, as in the artificial kidney, the patient's blood is used, the process is known as *haemodialysis* (qv). An alternative technique is to circulate the dialysing fluid through the abdominal cavity, thus using the peritoneum (qv) as the semi-permeable membrane. This is the process known as *peritoneal dialysis*.

DIAMORPHINE and DIACETYLMORPHINE are other names for heroin (qv).

DIAPEDESIS (see INFLAMMATION).

DIAPHORESIS is another name for sweating. (See PERSPIRATION.)

DIAPHORETICS are remedies which promote perspiration. By imperceptible perspiration, or insenble perspiration as it is technically known, the body loses around 500 ml (1 pint) of moisture daily. Under exertion or in a heated atmosphere, this natural function of the skin is increased, sweating more or less profuse follows, and, evaporation going on rapidly over the whole surface, little or no rise in the temperature of the body takes place. In some forms of disease, such as fevers and inflammatory affections, the action of the skin is arrested, and the surface of the body feels harsh and dry, while the temperature is greatly elevated. The occurrence of perspiration often marks a crisis in such diseases, and is in general regarded as a favourable event. (See PERSPIRATION.)

Varieties and uses: Many means can be used to induce perspiration, among the best known being baths, either in the form of hot-vapour or hot-water baths, or the exposure of the body to a dry and hot atmosphere or to beams of electric light in a special apparatus. (See BATHS.) Such measures, particularly if followed by the drinking of hot liquids and the wrapping of the body in warm clothing, seldom fail to cause copious perspiration. Numerous medicinal substances have a similar effect, one of the oldest of these being Mindererus spirit (acetate of ammonia). Opium acts as a diaphoretic, when in combination with ipecacuanha, as in Dover's powder, and alcohol, as well as aspirin, and similar drugs, also produces perspiration. (See under these headings.) When employed at the start of a common cold, diaphoretics sometimes check it or at least ameliorate it. In certain circumstances, diaphoretics, particularly in the form of baths, may be unsafe, especially where there is any affection of the heart or lungs attended with embarrassed respiration.

DIAPHRAGM, or MIDRIFF, is the muscular partition which separates the cavity of the abdomen from that of the chest. It is very thin and is of a dome shape, extending up on the right side to the space beneath the fourth rib, on the left to that beneath the fifth. In contact with its lower surface are, on the right side, the liver, right kidney, and suprarenal body, and to the left the stomach, pancreas, left kidney, suprarenal body, and spleen; while upon its upper surface lies the heart, with a lung on either side. The diaphragm is attached by its edge to the lower margin of the chest all round, and consists of muscular fibres meeting round a trefoil-shaped piece of fibrous tissue in the centre. It completely shuts off the above-named cavities from one another, being pierced only by openings for the gullet, the aorta, and the inferior vena cava, with a few minute openings for nerves and small vessels. The diaphragm is of great importance in respiration, playing the chief part in filling the lungs. During deep respiration its movements are responsible for 60 per cent of the total amount of air breathed and in the horizontal posture, or in sleep, an even greater percentage.

DIAPHYSECTOMY is the operation whereby a part of the shaft of a long bone (eg. humerus, femur) is excised.

DIAPULSE is a form of pulsed high-frequency electrical energy, consisting of pulsed short-wave bursts of energy of 1000 watts maximum, with an average input of 36 watts. It is used as a form of physiotherapy, particularly in the treatment of severe sprains.

DIARRHOEA or looseness of the bowels, is really a symptom of some disease situated in the bowels, but deserves special mention because of its potentially serious import.

Varieties and causes: Diarrhoea forms the chief symptom of several serious diseases, but it would be a great mistake to imagine that, by checking the diarrhoea, the disease is of necessity successfully treated. For example, the severity of an attack of cholera or dysentery is gauged mainly by the extent to which diarrhoea is present; in typhoid fever, people fed upon ordinary diet have much diarrhoea, so that this is a usual feature in early stages of this disease; in tuberculous ulceration of the intestine diarrhoea occurs which may be the first evidence of the disease. In some diseases of the liver, kidneys, lungs, or heart, diarrhoea ensues as a result of congestion of the bowels, or through the bowels taking up in part the eliminating functions of the damaged organs. In such cases the diarrhoea may actually be a salutary thing. These special forms are considered under the headings of the respective diseases which produce them. Recurring attacks of diarrhoea occur in some cases of habitual constipation, owing to irritation caused by the presence of hard faecal masses.

Catarrhal diarrhoea is the ordinary form, and in it the intestinal mucous membrane is in much the same condition of congestion and swelling as the nasal mucous membrane during a 'cold in the head', and secretes, in great amount, clear, viscid mucus of a similar nature. This catarrhal diarrhoea may be produced in a slight degree by indigestible food, by nervous excitement, or as the result of a chill. In a severer form, it may be due to infection by micro-organisms of the food-poisoning group (see FOOD POISONING), or to drugs such as mercury and arsenic. Atmospheric conditions may also play a part, some people developing an attack of diarrhoea upon a change of weather, just as others develop a catarrhal condition in the air-passages.

Diarrhoea in infants is such a serious condition that it requires separate consideration. One of its features is that it is usually accompanied by vomiting. Some ten per cent of the cases in this country are due to the dysentery organisms (qv) and will not be considered here. The remainder constitute the group of cases now usually referred to as infantile gastroenteritis. The condition is rare after the age of fifteen months, and the majority of cases occur between the ages of two and four months. The younger the infant, the higher the mortality rate. This is the type of diarrhoea which used to be known as 'summer diarrhoea' because of its high incidence in the late summer, but during recent years this seasonal incidence has tended to disappear. The precise cause is still obscure, but certain strains of the organism known as *Escherichia coli* (*E. coli*) are responsible for some cases, whilst in others a virus, often the rotavirus (qv), is the cause. One predisposing factor is artificial feeding. The condition is rare in breast-fed babies, and when it does occur in these it is usually less severe. The environment of the infant is also important. The condition is highly infectious and, if a case occurs in a maternity home or a children's hospital, it tends to spread like wildfire. This is why such an institution is closed to all further admissions if a case of infantile gastroenteritis occurs; and is not opened until the infection has been completely eradicated. A third factor is infection elsewhere in the body, particularly in the ear or the mastoid.

Lienteric diarrhoea is a chronic form, in which a movement of the bowels occurs shortly after every meal. The condition may become so aggravated that food passes rapidly and undigested through the body, and the sufferer becomes very thin.

Pancreatic diarrhoea is a form occasionally met in children of imperfect development, in consequence of failure by the pancreas to secrete its proper digestive fluid.

Ulcerative colitis is a serious condition characterized by the passage of frequent stools containing blood. (See COLITIS.)

Diarrhoea may also be a symptom of ulceration or gangrene of the bowels, and is then associated with the passage of *blood and mucus*, or even of shreds of membrane produced by the destruction of the inner surface of the bowels.

Treatment: The treatment of diarrhoea which is an incident of special diseases like cholera, typhoid fever, dysentery, is considered under these heads.

ACUTE DIARRHOEA, it must be remembered, is often merely a symptom either of one of the above diseases or of some local disease like intussusception, so that if the symptom be treated as if it were the real disease, the consequence may be disastrous to the sick person. Assuming that we are dealing simply with cases of uncomplicated *catarrhal diarrhoea*, we may consider the treatment of an adult and child separately. In the case of both, rest in bed is essential until the diarrhoea has subsided.

In adults, if the attack has followed the eating of some indigestible substance, a dose of a purgative may be given. To control the diarrhoea the two most effective drugs are kaolin and opium. Kaolin may be given in doses of one tablespoonful thrice daily; alternatively, in doses of 2 g it may be combined in a mixture with 0·6 ml of chlorodyne. If the diarrhoea lasts more than a couple of days, an enema consisting of starch cream (115 g) with laudanum (20 drops) is useful, given every six hours. If there is much discomfort with distension of the abdomen, a turpentine stupe (qv) may be of value. During the first twenty-four hours of an acute attack, no food should be given, but the individual must be given ample water. In less acute cases barley water may be given. This, as in the case of water, should be given in small amounts at frequent intervals. After the severer symptoms of diarrhoea have passed off, the affected person must exercise great caution for several days in respect to diet. A gradual return should be made to ordinary food, consisting at first of eggs, milk, and milk puddings, followed later by fish, and only after the lapse of several days by meat and vegetables.

In infants treatment is highly specialized, and much depends upon efficient nursing. The child or infant must be completely isolated from all other children. Drugs play little part in the treatment. Opium and its derivatives are badly tolerated by these infants and should not be used. The evidence concerning the value of the sulphonamide drugs and antibiotics is contradictory, but recent reports suggest that when the infant is not responding to dietetic treatment and the temperature is raised, one of the sulphonamides or one of the antibiotics should be given. Severe cases should receive such therapy from the outset. If there is any evidence of infection elsewhere in the body, eg. the ear, this must be treated at once. When there is no evidence of dehydration, ie. the infant has not lost much fluid in the stools or the vomit, the infant should be starved for twelve to twenty-four hours, but during this period should be given plenty of fluid to drink in small amounts at frequent intervals. In early cases in which there is not much loss of fluid in the stools, or dehydration as it is technically known, a suitable drink is one level 5-ml teaspoonful of salt and eight level teaspoonfuls of sugar in 1 litre of water. In more severe cases, a suitable drink is Oral Rehydration Salts solution as recommended by the World Health Organization: 3·5 grams sodium chloride; 2·5 grams sodium bicarbonate; 1·5 grams potassium chloride; 20 grams glucose dissolved in 1 litre of water. An alternative is the Sodium Chloride and Dextrose Oral Powder of the *British National Formulary*, which can be obtained from any chemist. One of these powders should be dissolved in 500 millilitres. When feeding is reinstituted, this should consist of half-strength, half-cream National Dried Milk, alternating with the glucose-saline mixture, in frequent small feeds. After 24 hours, if progress is maintained the infant is given half-strength, half-cream milk. The strength of the milk is gradually increased until, usually within a matter of five to seven days, the infant is able to take all feeds of full-strength National Dried Milk. Should the baby be breast-fed, there is no need to stop this unless it appears to aggravate the diarrhoea.

When dehydration is severe, the outlook is much more serious, and adequate fluid must be given either subcutaneously or intravenously. The fluid is usually glucose in saline, but some prefer to use Hartman's solution (isotonic sodium lactate) instead of the saline. During the first twelve or twenty-four hours of intravenous administration, nothing is given by mouth. By the end of this time vomiting has usually stopped, and then feeding by mouth can be started very gradually.

TODDLER DIARRHOEA is a form of diarrhoea in otherwise healthy-looking infants who are growing normally, in which frequent loose stools are passed containing undigested food. The cause is not known and no treatment is needed. It usually clears up after the age of about 2 years.

CHRONIC DIARRHOEA requires, above all things, full investigation to try and determine the cause. Kaolin in doses of 1 teaspoonful or more in water after meals has sometimes a beneficial effect. Drugs such as codeine phosphate or diphenoxylate (lomotil) are useful.

DIASTASE is a mixture of enzymes obtained from malt. These enzymes have the property of converting starch into sugar. It is used in the preparation of predigested starchy foods, and in the treatment of dyspepsia, particularly that due to inability to digest starch adequately. It is also used for the conversion of starch to fermentable sugars in the brewing and fermentation industries.

DIASTASIS is a term applied to separation of the end of a growing bone from the shaft. The condition resembles a fracture, but is more serious because of the damage done to the growing cartilage through which the separation takes place, so that the future growth of the bone is considerably diminished.

DIASTOLE means the relaxation of a hollow organ. The term is applied in particular to the heart, to indicate the resting period between the beats (systole), while blood is flowing into the organ.

DIATHERMY is a process by which electric currents can be passed into the deeper parts of the body so as to produce internal warmth and relieve pain; or, by using powerful currents, to destroy tumours and diseased parts bloodlessly. The form of electricity used consists of high-frequency oscillations, the frequency of oscillation ranging from 10 million to 25,000 million oscillations per second.

The so-called ultra-short-wave diathermy (or short-wave diathermy, as it is usually referred to) has replaced the original long-wave diathermy, as it is produced consistently at a stable wave-length (11 metres) and is easier to apply. In recent years microwave diathermy has been developed, which has a still higher oscillating current (25,000 million cycles per second, compared with 500 million for short-wave diathermy).

When the current passes, a distinct sensation of increasing warmth is experienced and the temperature of the body gradually rises; the heart's action becomes quicker; there is sweating with increased excretion of waste products. The general blood-pressure is also distinctly lowered. The method is used in painful rheumatic conditions, both of muscles and joints, and in severe cases of neuritis, such as sciatica.

By concentrating the current in a small electrode, the heating effects immediately below this are very much increased, and the method may be used to produce the effects of a cautery in surgical conditions. It differs from ordinary forms of cautery because it is cold when brought into contact with the patient, and gradually becomes heated by the current. Its surgical application has been used in treating malignant ulcers, particularly of the mouth, throat, and bladder, where ordinary surgical means are not readily available. (See MICROWAVES.)

DIATHESIS is another name for constitution (qv).

DIAZEPAM (VALIUM) (see TRANQUILLIZERS, BENZODIAZEPINES).

DIBUTYL PHTHALATE is an insect repellent. It is less effective than dimethyl phthalate (qv), but has the advantage of being harmless to clothing and resists washing better. When rubbed into clothing it may give protection for up to a fortnight.

DICEPHALUS is the term applied to a foetal 'monster' having two heads.

DICHLORALPHENAZONE is a non-barbiturate sedative, consisting of a complex of chloral hydrate (qv) and phenazone (qv).

DICHLOROPHEN is a drug for the treatment of tapeworm infestations. The dose is 70 mg per kg body weight, given as a single dose or in three divided doses eight-hourly.

DICLOFENAC (VOLTAROL) (see NON-STEROIDAL ANTI-INFLAMMATORY DRUGS).

DICLOXACILLIN (see ANTIBIOTIC).

DICOPHANE is the official name for DDT (qv).

DICROTIC pulse is one in which at each heartbeat two impulses are felt by the finger. A dicrotic wave is naturally present in a tracing of any pulse as recorded by an instrument for the purpose, but in health it is imperceptible to the finger. In fevers, a dicrotic pulse indicates considerable prostration, in which the heart continues to beat violently while the small blood-vessels have lost their tone. (See PULSE.)

DIELDRIN is one of the most effective insecticides available as it combines a prolonged action with a highly lethal action on insects. In addition, it is toxic to a wide range of insects. On the other hand, it is more toxic to man than DDT, and must therefore be handled with care.

DIENOESTROL is a synthetic oestrogen closely related to stilboestrol (qv). It is not as potent as stilboestrol, but as it would appear to be less toxic, it may, for this reason, have certain advantages over stilboestrol.

DIET is a subject of the greatest importance. Information as to the change in diet necessary in special diseases will be found in the sections on these diseases, and what will be said here refers to general principles of feeding. Details regarding the diet of young children are given under INFANT FEEDING.

Dietetic principles: The body is, in many respects, comparable to an engine. Like a piece of machinery it requires fuel to supply the muscles, etc., with energizing power for the various bodily activities, and it likewise needs building materials to repair loss from wear and tear. For the latter purpose, food containing nitrogen is necessary, the protein of which the muscles and other tissues are composed being replaceable only by fresh nitrogen-containing protein. For the necessary supply of energy protein would suffice but, as its use for this purpose would throw upon the kidneys and other excretory organs the necessity of getting rid of a large residue, fats and carbohydrates (including starch and sugars), which contain only carbon, hydrogen, and oxygen, are more convenient for the purpose. In addition to these three varieties of food, water must be taken in sufficient quantity to make up for the loss by the urine, sweat, etc., and also various salts, of which, however, there is always a surplus in the food. Certain substances known as vitamins, which are present in small quantities in a variety of foods, are also essential, as are certain minerals.

The protein requirement of the average man lies between 70 and 100 grams a day, or a bit more than 1 gram of protein for every kilogram of body weight a day. Growing children require, in proportion to their weight, a greater allowance of protein than adults.

The scientific mode of expressing the food requirements is stated in terms of energy-producing power. Kilocalorie, or large Calorie, is the name applied to the amount of heat necessary to raise the temperature of a kilogram of water from 15° to 16°C, and of these Calories of energy 4·1 are obtainable by burning a gram of protein or of carbohydrate, and 9·3 by combustion of the same amount of fat. In estimating the energy expended by an individual in climbing a mountain, doing his daily work, and the like, one expresses it as so many Calories, while the amount of food which is burned up in the body by the process may be similarly stated.

Occupation	*Energy expenditure (kCal./day)* *Mean*	*Min.*	*Max.*
		Men	
Elderly retired	2330	1750	2810
Office workers	2520	1820	3270
Colliery clerks	2800	2330	3290
Laboratory technicians	2840	2240	3820
Elderly industrial workers	2840	2180	3710
Building workers	3000	2440	3730
University students	2930	2270	4410
Steel workers	3280	2600	3960
Farmers	3420	2900	4000
Army cadets	3490	2990	4100
Coal miners	3660	2970	4560
Forestry workers	3670	2860	4600
		Women	
Elderly housewives	1990	1490	2410
Middle-aged housewives	2090	1760	2320
Laboratory technicians	2130	1340	2540
Assistants in department store	2250	1820	2850
University students	2290	1380	2500
Factory workers	2320	1970	2980
Bakery workers	2510	1980	3390

Daily rates of energy expenditure by individuals in Scotland with various occupations. *Davidson and Passmore.*

Quantity of food: The total daily amount of food necessary for a fair-sized man, doing average hard work, should provide over 3000 Calories of energy, and since about 110 grams of the daily food must be protein, to supply wear and tear, this leaves 2500 Calories to be supplied by carbohydrate and fat together. For a diet giving about 3000 Calories a day these may be suitably provided thus: carbohydrate, 400 grams; fat, 110 grams; protein, 90 grams; – providing respectively 1640, 1020 and 370 Calories.

The degree of physical activity plays a large part in deciding how many calories an individual requires. The table below shows the recommendation of the Department of Health and Social Security for individuals undertaking varying degrees of activity. In western communities, such as the United Kingdom and the USA, the emphasis today must be on the number of Calories consumed by those in sedentary occupations, as they are tending to consume far more calories than are good for them, and are thereby putting on weight.

Age	*Occupation*	*Calories*
Men		
18–35	Sedentary	2700
	Moderately active	3000
	Very active	3600
35–65	Sedentary	2600
	Moderately active	2900
	Very active	3600
65–75	Sedentary	2350
75 and over	Sedentary	2100
Women		
18–55	Most occupations	2200
	Very active	2500
55–75	Sedentary	2050
75 and over	Sedentary	1900
Pregnancy		2400
Lactation		2700

Recommended average daily intake of Calories for adults in the United Kingdom. The ages are from one birthday to another. Thus 18 to 55 means from the 18th birthday up to, but not including, the 55th birthday.

Quality of food: After the energizing power of a substance has been ascertained, there remain several other factors which determine its suitability as a food. *Digestibility* is one of the most important, for, while petroleum, sawdust, and the like have a high energy-producing power, they are absolutely useless as foods. *Absorbability* is also of importance, for few substances are completely absorbed into the system, and some, like vegetable proteins, are even rejected if taken as food in large amounts, and passed by the bowels unchanged. Thus a considerable amount of all food eaten, and especially of the coarser kinds, remains unused. *Satisfying power* is of great importance, and depends partly upon the bulk of the food and partly upon its preparation. Except in certain special circumstances, such as food for invalids, food should not be capable of too rapid digestion. Hence also the value of cooking certain foods with fat, which, when it penetrates the other food, retards digestion. To a certain extent, the more satisfying a food is the less digestible it proves; and this is one of the chief reasons why different foods and different methods of cooking suit persons of diverse physique and digestive powers. *Preparation* by cooking is also important. The effect of cooking is partly to develop flavours in the food, and so make it more palatable and digestible; partly to kill organisms and animal parasites which may be present in it; and, mainly, in the case of meats, to soften the connective tissues which bind the meat proper, and, in the case of vegetables, to burst or tear the fibres and capsules of cellulose which surround the starchy and sugary material. *Cheapness* may also be very important. Animal protein, as beef, forms the dearest food, and bread is by far the cheapest. Among the cheapest and most efficient forms of protein food are skimmed milk, cheese and fish. Fat has double the energy-producing power of carbohydrates, but butter is more than four times as expensive as its equivalent in bread. Hence fatty foods are called 'rich foods'. Nevertheless margarine falls into the list of cheap foods and is quite as nutritious as butter, and, since September 1939, all margarine has had the vitamins A and D added up to the level of some butter. *Freshness* is important, since preserved foods tend to lose their vitamins, and the daily diet should include vegetables, fruit, milk, butter, cheese.

The main objection to *vegetarianism* – at least in its extreme form – lies in the enormous bulk of vegetable food necessary, mainly in consequence of the relatively large amount of water it contains. Thus, if one were to subsist on nothing but lentil porridge, about 2·25 kg (5 pounds) of it would be necessary daily; or if one lived solely on green vegetables and succulent fruits, the impossible weight of about 13·5 kg (30 pounds) every day would be necessary to a fairly hard-working healthy man. Those vegetarians who add milk, eggs, and cheese to their food reach at once a healthy and rational diet.

Age (years)	*Calories*
Boys and Girls	
0 to 1	800
1 to 2	1200
2 to 3	1400
3 to 5	1600
5 to 7	1800
7 to 9	2100
Boys	
9 to 12	2500
12 to 15	2800
15 to 18	3000
Girls	
9 to 18	2300

Recommended average daily intake of Calories for children and adolescents in the United Kingdom. The ages are from one birthday to another. Thus, 0 to 1 means from birth up to, but not including, the first birthday.

External conditions produce great differences in the need for food. In cold climates, or in people unusually exposed to the weather, a special addition of fats or carbohydrates must be made to the diet in order to maintain the body heat. For the same reason a tall, spare man requires a much greater supply of these foods than a short, fat man of the same weight. Such a difference in configuration may mean the necessity for adding one-quarter or more of the amount of food.

Age and sex are important considerations. A woman requires around four-fifths of the diet of a man about the same size and build, the reduction affecting chiefly the starchy and sugary elements of her food. Children require much more protein – ie. building material – in proportion to their size than adults; whilst old people, on the other hand, if they wish to keep healthy, should be sparing eaters, particularly of animal foods.

Articles of diet: Further details, regarding the various articles in common use as foods, are given under BREAD; CANNED FOODS; CEREAL; MILK; PROTEIN; INFANT FEEDING. Some of the substances added to foods are mentioned under ADULTERATION OF FOODS. The articles of food which may most suitably be taken in various diseased conditions are mentioned under the headings of the various diseases.

Diet for athletes and manual workers: For long it has been traditional for athletes in training to eat large amounts of meat. There is, however, no evidence to suggest that this is necessary. Carbohydrate, and not protein, is the best source of energy. Although there is still considerable difference between theory and practice, the views of dietitians and athletes are now converging, and it is now generally accepted that a simple and sufficient diet is what is required. The same holds true for manual workers. In the case of an athlete, it is probably advisable for him to go on a lighter diet for a day or two before the contest for which he is training, making certain that this contains ample carbohydrate. There is probably also much to be said in favour of taking glucose shortly before the event. There is also some evidence that the requirements of certain components of the vitamin B complex increase with exercise, so that care should be taken to ensure that there is ample vitamin B in the diet. Ample fluids should also be taken, but there is no evidence that alcohol is of any advantage.

The total daily Calories should be about 4500, and the following list gives some indication of the foods to be taken:

Foods for Calories – Dripping, suet, butter, margarine, bacon, cheese, bread, flour, sugar, jam, syrup, dried fruits, potatoes, cereals.
Foods for first-class proteins – Milk, cheese, eggs, meat, fish.
Foods for vitamins – Vitamin A: dairy foods, liver, tomatoes, green and yellow vegetables. Vitamin B: yeast, liver, kidney, whole-meal bread, bacon, ham, wheat germ. Vitamin C: citrus fruits, swedes, potatoes, green vegetables, liver. Vitamin D: fat fish, summer milk, and butter.

Invalid diet: One of the advances of recent years has been the recognition of the importance of diet in the treatment of disease. Whilst this is best exemplified in the case of diabetes mellitus, there are many other conditions in which special diets are ordered. Thus, in chronic constipation a high-roughage diet is indicated, containing whole-meal bread, bran, vegetables (particularly salads and coarse green vegetables), fruit, nuts and the drinking of plenty of water. In chronic cholecystitis a low-fat diet is necessary, whilst in jaundice a diet rich in first-class protein and carbohydrate is prescribed. Low-Calorie diets are the most effective for obesity, whilst a low-sodium diet is an essential part of the treatment of oedema.

In febrile conditions the diet depends upon the expected duration of the fever. Thus, in a long-continued fever, such as typhoid fever, the essentials are that the diet should have a high Calorie value (3000 Calories), a large proportion of carbohydrate (380 grams), adequate protein (70-80 grams), and be given in easily digestible form in small amounts every two hours.

On the other hand, in fevers of short duration, eg. pneumonia, the amount of nourishment taken is not of such importance. If the individual is receiving ample fluid, including at least two pints (1 litre) of milk daily, there is little to worry about for several days. Again, small feeds should be given every two hours. To increase the nutritional value of the diet, and yet still impose no strain upon the digestive organs, glucose may be added to the water the patient drinks, and this can be flavoured with fruit juice, the addition of which ensures an adequate intake of vitamin C. If the patient desires more food, this may be given in the form of eggs (lightly boiled or poached), milk puddings (eg. junket, arrowroot), or jellies.

During convalescence it is necessary to give as nourishing a diet as possible. On the other hand, digestion is sometimes not satisfactory, and the appetite is fickle.

DIETETICS: Dietitians apply dietetics, the science of nutrition, to the feeding of groups and individuals in health and disease. They are primarily advisors and teachers. Their training requires a four-year degree course in the nutritional and biological sciences. The role of the dietitian can be divided into four main areas.
(1) Preventive – by liaising with Health Education Departments, schools and various groups in the community. They plan and provide nutrition education programs including in-service training and the production of educational material in nutrition. They are encouraged to plan and participate in food surveys and research projects which involve the assessment of nutritional status.
(2) Therapeutic – they provide advisory services to physicians and surgeons and their patients who require specific dietary therapy as all or part of their treatment. They teach patients in hospitals to manage their own dietary treatment and ensure a supportive follow-up so that they and their families can be seen to be coping with the diet. They advise catering departments on the adaptation of menus for individual diets and on the nutritional value of the food supplied to patients and staff. They advise Social Services departments so that meals on wheels have adequate nutritional value.
(3) Industry – the advice of dietitians is sought by industry in the production of product information literature, data sheets and professional leaflets for manufacturers of ordinary foods and specialist dietetic food. They give advice to the manufacturers on nutritional and dietetic requirements of their products.
(4) Education – dietitians are required to teach nutrition and dietetics to student dietitians and students of many other disciplines at universities and colleges.

DIETHYLCARBAMAZINE CITRATE is a derivative of piperazine, which is proving of value in the treatment of filariasis and other parasitic diseases.

DIETL'S CRISES (see KIDNEY, DISEASES OF under MOVABLE KIDNEY).

DIFLUNISAL (DOLOBID) (see NON-STEROIDAL ANTI-INFLAMMATORY DRUGS).

DIGESTION, ABSORPTION, and ASSIMILATION are the three processes by which food is incorporated in the living body. In digestion, the food is softened and converted into a form which is soluble in the watery fluids of the body, or, in the case of fat, into very minute globules. In absorption, the substances formed are taken up from the bowels and carried throughout the body by the blood. In assimilation, these substances, deposited from the blood, are united with the various tissues for their growth and repair. For the maintenance of health each of these must proceed in a regular manner. Transit time through the digestive tract in young and middle-aged people in Britain averages two to four days, all but twelve hours of this being in the colon. Transit time is probably longer in the elderly.

SALIVARY DIGESTION begins as soon as the food enters the mouth. Saliva runs from the minute orifices of the salivary gland ducts, and contains a ferment named ptyalin, which actively changes the starch of bread, potatoes, and the like, into sugar. The object of chewing is not only to bruise the food, and make it more permeable for the gastric juice, but also to mix the starchy parts thoroughly with saliva. This process goes on, after swallowing, for the first twenty minutes or half-hour that the food remains in the stomach, after which the action of the saliva is checked by the acid of the gastric juice.

GASTRIC DIGESTION begins a little time after the food enters the stomach, the gastric juice exuding rapidly from the openings of the minute glands with which the interior surface of this organ is covered. The gastric juice begins to be secreted even before the food enters the stomach, at the sight and smell of food (psychic secretion). This juice contains ferments or enzymes, named pepsins, which have the power to break down the proteins of food into smaller molecules containing fewer amino-acids and to clot milk. There are also present free hydrochloric acid, which aids the action of the pepsin and prevents putrefaction of the food, and acid salts, such as phosphate of soda, which have a similar action. The slow, churning movements which take place in the walls of the stomach have the effect of thoroughly mixing the food and gastric juice, and, to a slight extent, of breaking up the former. The main function of the stomach is to render the ingested food soluble, and mix it thoroughly with the gastric juice until it assumes a gruel-like consistency. This material, known as *chyme*, is then passed through the pylorus into the intestine. Very soon after soft food has been taken, waves of movement may be seen on X-ray examination, the orifice at the lower end of the stomach (pylorus) opens, and the food is squeezed quickly in small quantities into the bowel; but if any hard food comes in contact with the stomach wall near the exit the orifice at once closes. Gastric digestion of a simple meal of tea, bread, butter and jam should be complete in about an hour, a meal containing milk, eggs or light meat requires three or four hours, while a heavy dinner with soup, meat, fruit, and wine or beer is not entirely treated by the stomach till six or seven hours have elapsed. Hence the English plan of taking the heavy meal of the day (dinner) in the evening is a sound one, giving time during the night for the later stages of digestion.

INTESTINAL DIGESTION: The softened food, or chyme, which leaves the stomach is exposed in the bowels to the action of four factors: (*a*) bile, (*b*) pancreatic juice, (*c*) intestinal juice, (*d*) bacteria. Bile is collected from the liver and gall-bladder into the common bile-duct, which, together with the duct from the pancreas, opens into the duodenum a short distance from the exit of the stomach. The bile consists mainly of complex salts and pigments, which assist in digesting the fats of the food, and partly of waste products removed from the blood. The pancreatic juice contains four powerful ferments, which have the following effects: lipase breaks down fats into glycerol and fatty acids; amylase completes the digestion of starch; and trypsin and chymotrypsin carry on the breaking down of proteins begun in the stomach. Intestinal juice contains small amounts of enzymes which (1) complete the breakdown of proteins into the constituent amino-acids; (2) act upon the disaccharides, maltose, sucrose and lactose, converting them into the monosaccharide glucose; (3) split fats into fatty acids and glycerin. Bacteria are normal inhabitants of both small and large intestine. In the former they have a fermentive, in the latter a putrefactive, action. In the former they act upon carbohydrate to produce acetic, butyric, and lactic acids. In the latter, bacteria decompose protein into such products as histamine, phenol, cresol, indole, skatole. These are no longer believed to be responsible for the ill-effects of constipation. The intestinal bacteria also play an important and valuable role in the manufacture of certain components of the vitamin B complex.

ABSORPTION: The only substance absorbed from the stomach to any extent is alcohol. Water is quickly passed from the stomach into the intestine, and considerable quantities are there absorbed in a few minutes. But it is only after subjection to digestion in the intestine for several hours that the bulk of the food is taken up into the system. The semi-solid chyme which leaves the stomach is converted into a yellowish fluid of creamy consistence called chyle by the action of bile and pancreatic fluid. From this the fats, in the form of a fine emulsion, are taken up by lymph vessels called lacteals, and ultimately reach the blood, while sugars, salts, and amino-acids formed from proteins pass directly into the small blood-vessels of the intestine. The process is facilitated by the extreme unevenness of the intestinal wall, which is folded into many ridges and pockets, while, in microscopic structure, the surface is covered by fine finger-like processes named villi, which are bathed in the fluids passing down the intestine. Further, absorption is probably assisted by the leucocytes, or white cells of the blood, wich are increased in numbers after a meal, and which have the power of wandering out of the blood-stream and taking up particles into their substance. Food materials are absorbed almost exclusively by the small intestine. The large intestine, or colon, absorbs water and salts. The food is passed down the intestine by the contractions of its muscular coat, and, finally, the indigestible residue, together with various waste substances excreted from the liver and intestinal walls, is cast out of the body in the stools.

ASSIMILATION takes place more slowly, the blood circulating through every organ, and each taking from it what is necessary for its own growth and repair. Thus the cells in the bones extract lime salts, muscles extract sugar and protein, and so forth. When the supply of food is much in excess of the immediate bodily requirements it is stored up for future use, fat being deposited in various sites, sugar being converted into glycogen in the liver. The greater bulk of nutriment is assimilated by the muscles for heat production and work, the sugar and amino-acids being built up into a substance which forms the permanent part of the muscle. The substance so formed undergoes chemical changes, and is broken down to form carbonic acid, lactic acid and other waste products as the muscle does work. Various hormones, such as insulin, which is an internal secretion of the pancreas, circulate in the blood and are concerned in these processes. For all these processes to function satisfactorily an adequate daily intake of water is necessary; about 1·5 litres (3 pints) are drunk or taken with the food and absorbed daily, a similar amount being discharged from the body in the urine, perspiration, and other excretions.

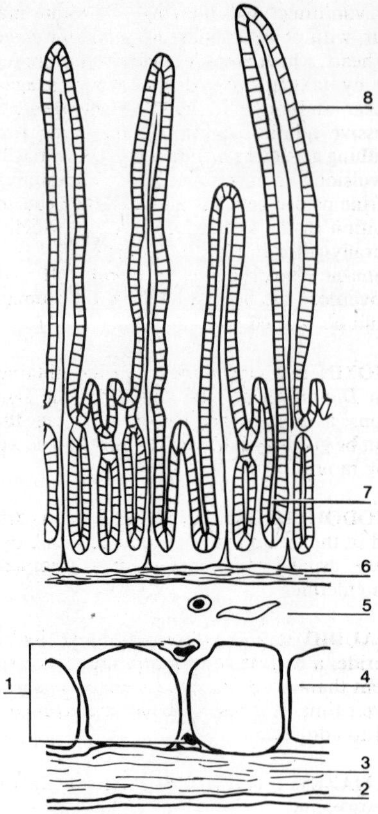

1 nerve plexuses
2 serous coat
3 longitudinal muscular coat
4 circular muscular coat
5 submucosa
6 muscularis mucosae
7 crypt of Lieberkühn
8 villus

Section of small intestine (jejunum), showing four of the villi with which the inner surface is covered. Magnified 110 times.

DIGITALIS is the leaf of the wild fox-glove, *Digitalis purpurea*, gathered when the flowers are at a certain stage, dried, and powdered. The leaf contains several active principles, which can be extracted in various ways. Its action is to strengthen involuntary muscular contraction, particularly that of the muscle fibres in the heart and blood-vessels. It is one of the most valuable remedies we have in cases of disease of the heart, associated with atrial fibrillation. Upon the heart it has the double action of increasing the strength of each beat and of lengthening each intervening pause (diastole), so that the muscle of the damaged organ obtains longer periods for rest and repair. It promotes the excretion of sodium by the kidney and so has a diuretic effect.

Uses: Digitalis may be given as a powder, as tincture, as infusion and also in the form of sugar-coated 'granules' which contain the active principle of the drug. The most common form of administration is the powder given in the form of a tablet. Its action is particularly useful when the heart failure is due to atrial fibrillation, the condition in which the heart rate is wholly irregular. In such cases the digitalis slows the heart rate by abolishing many of the weak heart-beats. (See also DIGOXIN.)

DIGITALIS POISONING may occur from taking medicinal doses over too long a period, or from taking a single overdose. There are nausea and vomiting, and blurring of vision may occur, with objects appearing yellow or green. The heart, which is made slower and more regular by taking small doses, becomes again quicker and more irregular as the result of excessive administration. At the same time breathing gets more difficult, and there may be convulsions or unconsciousness. The amount of urine passed gets less and less, thus causing retention in the system of the drug, which is naturally got rid of by the kidneys.

Treatment: The drug must be stopped. If a single overdose has been swallowed, the stomach should be washed out.

DIGOXIN is a crystalline glycoside obtained from *Digitalislanata*. It is used for the same purpose as digitalis, and has the advantage that it can be given by intravenous injection as well as by mouth.

DI-IODOHYDROXYQUINOLINE is a drug used in the treatment of chronic amoebic dysentery, usually as a supplement to treatment with emetine.

DILAUDID is a dihydromorphinone hydrochloride, a derivative of morphine. It is more potent than morphine, but its effect lasts for a shorter time. It is just as liable as morphine to lead to addiction.

DILTIAZEM (TILDIEM) (see CALCIUM ANTAGONISTS).

DILUENTS are watery fluids of a non-irritating nature, which are given to increase the amount of perspiration or of urine, and carry solids with them from the system. Examples are water, milk, barley-water, and solutions of alkaline salts.

DIMENHYDRINATE, or DRAMAMINE, is a drug which is widely used, with considerable success, in the treatment of travel sickness.

DIMERCAPROL is the official name for BAL (British Anti-Lewisite), the antidote to lewisite poisoning which was discovered during the 1939–45 War. It was subsequently found to be an excellent antidote to poisoning with certain heavy metals, including arsenic, mercury and gold, and it is now widely used for this purpose.

DIMETHYL PHTHALATE is an organic compound which was found, during the 1939–45 War, to be a most effective repellent for mosquitoes. It is also effective against flies, midges, blackflies, mites, fleas and ticks. Under the proprietary names of MYLOL and SKEETOFAX, it is available as a cream and as a liquid. This is smeared on the face, arms, hands, legs or other exposed parts of the body. It has to be re-applied every three or four hours. Care must be taken not to allow it to get into the eyes or to come into contact with plastic spectacle-frames. It does not kill, but merely prevents the insect from alighting on the skin.

DINOESTROL (ARMO-NOESTROL) (see OESTROGENS).

DIOCTYL SODIUM SULPHOSUCCINATE is a faecal-softening agent that is proving useful in the treatment of constipation in old people.

DIODONE is a complex, organic, iodine-containing preparation. It is used primarily for contrast radiography of the kidney passages, but can also be used for contrast radiography of the biliary tract.

DIOPTRE is a term used in the measurement of the refractive or focusing power of lenses; one dioptre is the power of a lens with a focal distance of one metre and is the unit of refractive power. As a stronger lens has a greater refractive power, this means that the focal distance will be shorter. The strength in dioptres therefore is the reciprocal of the focal length expressed in metres.

DIPHENHDYRAMINE is a widely used antihistamine drug (qv).

DIPHENOXYLATE is a drug chemically related to pethidine that is proving of value in the treatment of travellers' diarrhoea by quietening down the gut. It has no anti-infective action.

DIPHTHERIA is an acute infectious disease, which is accompanied by a membranous exudation on a mucous surface, generally on the tonsils and back of the throat or pharynx.

Causes: The infection is essentially a local one in the throat due to the development there of the *Corynebacterium diphtheriae*, and the general symptoms are referable to the absorption of toxins (qv) which damage the heart muscle and the nerves. Among the first signs of the disease is inflammation of the throat, where a membrane develops, composed partly of the dead surface of mucous membrane and partly of products effused from the blood and lymph. In this membrane the causative organisms swarm, along with many other varieties of organisms, particularly streptococci.

The disease is generally conveyed by direct contagion, as by kissing an affected person, using his cup or spoon, or receiving a drop of saliva or fragment of membrane upon the lips or face through incautiously approaching him when he is coughing. The organism grows freely in milk, and infection may be conveyed in this way.

Three strains of *Corynebacterium diphtheriae* are now recognized as causing clinical diphtheria: *gravis*, *intermedius*, *mitis*. *Gravis* and *intermedius* strains are almost always virulent; about 10 per cent of *mitis* strains are non-virulent.

It is predominantly a disease of the autumn and winter and, although it occurs at all ages, it is commonest in childhood. It is rare under six months of age as the young infant has a transmitted immunity from the mother.

A method known as the *Schick test* has been devised for detecting the susceptibility of individuals to diphtheria. A minute quantity of toxin filtered off from growing diphtheria bacilli is injected with a very fine needle into the skin of the arm. Individuals possessing naturally a considerable amount of antitoxic power show no reaction, but if the individual has very little resisting power to diphtheria, an area of inflammation is produced on the skin at the site of the injection.

In 1984 only two cases of diphtheria, with no deaths, were notified in England and Wales, compared with over 45,000 cases and 2400 deaths in 1940, the year in which a national immunization campaign was launched. The substance injected is diphtheria toxoid, which is diptheria toxin so treated that it is harmless but will produce antibodies to the diphtheria bacillus and thereby give the injected individual an immunity to the disease. Since 1971 there have only been three deaths from the disease: one in 1971, one in 1975, and one in 1982. The disease, however, is still common in many lands, and we in Britain are therefore vulnerable to renewed outbreaks, particularly from cases imported from overseas unless a high level of immunity is maintained in our children by vaccination.

Very few children are immunized solely against diphtheria at the present day. They are more usually given a combined vaccine against diphtheria, tetanus and whooping-cough. (See VACCINES.)

Symptoms: The severity of diphtheritic inflammation in general, and the fact that it is accompanied by serious constitutional symptoms, suffice usually to distinguish this disease from croup, which, although resembling diphtheria, differs from it in being a merely local inflammation of the larynx. There are several other diseases of the throat, such as acute suppurative quinsy, which are even more liable to be mistaken for diphtheria. The diagnosis may be difficult, even for a skilled physician.

In doubtful cases, the deciding point is the taking of a throat swab. A swab of cotton-wool mounted on a wire is rubbed against the throat, and then sent to a bacteriologist for examination. A culture of the organisms from the swab is made upon dried serum, for 16 to 24 hours at body temperature, and if the organisms found in the resulting culture be pronounced to be *Corynebacterium diphtheriae*, the case can be safely diagnosed as one in which this disease is present.

Cases of diphtheria differ as to their intensity from the mildest forms, which resemble an ordinary sore throat, to those of the most severe character (such as the gangrenous form), in which the disease is hopelessly intractable from the first.

Following an incubation period of two to six days after infection, symptoms set in like those commonly accompanying a cold: chilliness and depression. Sometimes very severe disturbances usher in an attack, such as vomiting and diarrhoea. A slight feeling of uneasiness in the throat is experienced along with some stiffness of the back of the neck. When looked at, the throat appears reddened and somewhat swollen, particularly in the neighbourhood of the tonsils, the soft palate, and upper part of pharynx, while along with this there are tenderness and swelling of the glands at the angles of the jaw. The affection of the throat spreads rapidly, and soon the characteristic exudation appears on the inflamed surface in the form of greyish-white specks or patches, increasing in extent and thickness until a yellowish-looking membrane is formed. This deposit is firmly adherent to the mucous membrane beneath, or is incorporated with it, and, if forcibly removed, it leaves a raw, bleeding, ulcerated surface, upon which it is reproduced in a short period. The appearance of the exudation has been compared to wet parchment or washed leather, and it is dense in texture. It may cover the whole of the back of the throat, the cavity of the mouth, and the posterior nares, and may spread downwards into the air passages and into the alimentary canal, while any wound on the surface of the body is liable to become covered with it. As it loosens, it becomes decomposed, giving a most offensive and characteristic odour to the breath. There are pain and difficulty in swallowing, but, unless the disease has affected the larynx, no affection of the breathing. The voice acquires a snuffling character. When the disease invades the posterior nares, an acrid, foetid discharge, and sometimes also copious bleeding, take place from the nostrils.

Along with these local phenomena there is evidence of severe constitutional disturbance. There may not be great fever, and the temperature seldom rises above 39° to 39·5°C (102° or 103°F), but there are marked depression and loss of strength. The pulse becomes small and rapid, the countenance pale, the swelling of the glands in the neck increases, which, along with the presence of albumin in the urine, testifies to a condition of blood-poisoning. Unless favourable symptoms emerge, death takes place within three or four days or sooner, either from the rapid extension of the membrane into the air passages, giving rise to asphyxia, or from a condition of general collapse, which is sometimes remarkably sudden owing to sudden failure of the heart, for which the diphtheria toxin has a special predilection. For the same reason death occasionally takes place suddenly during convalescence, from acute dilatation of the weakened heart, if a considerable effort be made at too early a period. Death may also ensue if the temperature rises excessively.

In cases of recovery, the change for the better is marked by an arrest in the extension of the membrane, the detachment and expectoration of that already formed, and the healing of the ulcerated mucous membrane beneath. Along with this, there is a general improvement in the symptoms, the power of swallowing returns, and the strength gradually increases, while the glandular enlargement of the neck diminishes, and the albumin disappears from the urine. These favourable symptoms should appear within three or four days, but it may be many weeks before full convalescence is established. During this period it is particularly necessary in the case of diphtheria to guard against premature over-exertion, and for this reason patients are kept in bed for several weeks even though feeling quite well.

Even when diphtheria ends quite favourably, certain sequels may follow, generally in a period of two or three weeks after all the local evidence of the disease has disappeared. These effects, which are due to neuritis caused by the effect of the diphtheria toxin upon various nerves, may occur after mild as well as after severe attacks, and they are principally in the form of paralysis affecting the soft palate and throat, causing difficulty in swallowing, with regurgitation of fluid through the nose, and giving a peculiar nasal character to the voice. Another form of paralysis is one affecting the muscles of the eye, and producing loss of the power of accommodation and consequent difficulty in reading which often lasts for a period of several months; another form may be paralysis of a limb, or of both legs, or even of the respiratory muscles. These symptoms, however, after continuing for a variable length of time, almost always ultimately disappear.

Treatment: The first essential of treatment is the immediate injection of *antitoxin*. (See SERUM THERAPY.) Every moment of delay increases the danger to the patient. As diphtheria antitoxin contains horse serum, the possibility of an anaphylactic reaction (see ANAPHYLAXIS) must be borne in mind. In addition to antitoxin, the patient is given penicillin daily for five days, as this antibiotic has a bactericidal action on *C. diphtheriae*. Erythromycin is also effective.

The second essential is *complete rest in bed* for at least three weeks. Adequate nourishment should be freely administered in the form of milk, soup, etc., as long as there exists the power of swallowing, and when this fails, fluids, in the form of Hartmann's solution (qv), glucose and plasma, should be given by infusion or by nasal catheter. The strict maintenance of the recumbent position is of great importance in preserving the strength of the heart. If the infection spreads to the larynx (laryngeal diphtheria), additional antitoxin is given and the patient is kept in a steam tent. If obstruction to breathing is not relieved by this, it may be necessary to perform the operation of tracheotomy (qv).

Most cases of diphtheritic paralysis recover without special treatment. In cases in which the respiratory muscles are paralysed, it may be necessary for a time to resort to artificial respiration till the paralysis passes off, by means of some form of apparatus which rhythmically inflates and deflates the chest.

As the disease is notifiable a case of diphtheria should be notified immediately to the community physician, and arrangements made for urgent admission to a hospital for infectious diseases. Cases are isolated until cultures from three successive nose and throat swabs, taken at intervals of not less than two days, are negative.

If a case of diphtheria occurs in a closed community, such as a school, a daily examination of the throats of all contacts should be made during the incubation period, and throat swabs should be taken. Those with positive throat swabs should be given an intramuscular injection of antitoxin and also penicillin. They must also be isolated until three successive throat swabs free of virulent *C. diphtheriae* are obtained. The Schick test should be carried out on all contacts, and those who give a positive reaction should be given a course of toxoid immunization.

DIPHYLLOBOTHRIUM LATUM is a fish tapeworm which infests man and may cause a form of megaloblastic anaemia. (See ANAEMIA.)

DIPLEGIA is extensive paralysis on both sides of the body. (See PARALYSIS.)

DIPLO- is a prefix meaning twofold.

DIPLOCOCCUS is a group of bacterial organisms which have a tendency to occur in pairs: eg. pneumococci.

DIPLOE is the layer of spongy bone which intervenes between the compact outer and inner tables of the skull.

DIPLOPIA means double vision. It is due to some irregularity in action of the muscles which move the eyeballs, in consequence of which the eyes are placed so that rays of light from one object do not fall upon corresponding parts of the two retinae, and two images are produced. It is a symptom of several nervous diseases, and often a temporary attack follows an injury to the eye, intoxication, or some febrile disease like diphtheria.

DIPROSOPUS is the term applied to a foetus which has two faces instead of one.

DIPSOMANIA is a morbid and insatiable craving for alcohol. (See ALCOHOLISM, CHRONIC.)

DIPYGUS is the term applied to a foetus which has a double pelvis.

DISABLED PERSONS now have a wide range of services available to help them to lead as normal and active a life as possible. Officially, the disabled include those with significant impairment of any kind, including impairment of sight and hearing, mental subnormality, and chronic illness as well as disablement due to accidents and the like.

Financial help is available for the disabled as follows: *Invalidity benefit* for those who have paid national insurance contributions. *Non-contributory invalidity pension* for those who have not been able to work and pay national insurance contributions. *Attendance allowance* for disabled persons who are dependent on others: for example, need frequent attention to bodily needs. *Invalid care allowance* for people who have stopped working to look after an invalid. Normally, housewives cannot draw this benefit. *Mobility allowance* is intended for people aged 5 to 65 (60 for women) who are unable or virtually unable to walk. At present it is only payable up to the age of 58, but this is being gradually extended. Full details of all these can be had from a local Department of Health and Social Security Office. If asked, someone from the local office will call to see the disabled person in his own home.

Social services are provided by Local Authority Social Services Departments. Those laid down under the Chronically Sick and Disabled Persons' Act 1970 include: (1) Practical help in the home (usually through home helps or aids to daily living). (2) Provision of, or help in obtaining, a radio, television, library or similar facilities. (3) Provision of lectures, games, outings or other recreational facilities outside the home, and assistance in taking advantage of available educational facilities. (4) Assistance in carrying out adaptations in the disabled person's house. (5) Assistance in taking holidays. (6) Provision of meals whether in the disabled person's home ('Meals on Wheels') or elsewhere (Luncheon Centres). (7) Help in obtaining a telephone. Many of these facilities will involve the disabled person in some expense, but full details can be obtained from the local Social Services Department, which will, if necessary, send a social worker to discuss the matter in the disabled person's home. A warning is necessary here to the effect that, owing to lack of funds and staff, many Local Authority Social Service Departments are unable to provide the full range of services.

Aids to daily living: There is now a wide range of aids for the disabled. Full details of these can be obtained from:

Aids North, Mea House, Ellison Place, Newcastle-upon-Tyne NE1 8XS (091-232 2855).

Birmingham Disabled Living Centre, 260 Broad Street, Birmingham B1 2HF (021-643 0980).

Disabled Living Centres Council, c/o TRAIDS, 76 Clarendon Park Road, Leicester LE2 3AD (0533-700747).

Disabled Living Foundation, 380–384 Harrow Road, London W9 2HU (01-289 6111) – national information service and equipment centre on aids and equipment for people with disabilities.

Medical Aid Department, British Red Cross Society, 76 Clarendon Park Road, Leicester LE2 3AD.

Merseyside Centre for Independent Living, Youens Way, East Prescot Road, Liverpool 14.

National Demonstration Centre, Pinderfields General Hospital, Wakefield, West Yorkshire WF1 4DG (0924-375217, ex. 2510/2263).

Scottish Council on Disability, Information Department, Princes House, 5 Shandwick Place, Edinburgh EH2 4RG (031-229 8632).

Aids cannot be bought at these centres.

Aids to mobility and transport: The Department of Health and Social Security invalid vehicles are no longer provided, having been replaced by the mobility allowance. The major car manufacturers make specially equipped or adapted cars, and some have official systems for discounts. Details can be obtained from local dealers. Help can also be obtained from Motability, Gate House, West Gate, Harlow, Essex CM20 1HR (0279-635666) which provides advice to enable the disabled to make the most of the mobility allowance, and financial assistance for buying, adapting or running a car. The disabled travelling in a car, either as a passenger or driver, may be eligible for an orange badge if they have considerable difficulty in walking or if they are blind. It allows the holder some parking concessions, and is obtainable on a doctor's certificate. A wide variety of wheelchairs is available from the Department of Health and Social Security Appliance Centres which issue them on permanent loan and maintain them.

For help in making full use of these facilities the disabled should consult their general practitioner. Citizens' Advice Bureaux are another useful source of information.

(See also REMPLOY.)

DISARTICULATION is the amputation of a bone by cutting through the joint of which the bone forms a part.

DISCHARGE is the term applied to abnormal emissions from any part of the body. It usually applies to purulent material: eg. the septic material which comes away from an infected ear, or nose.

DISCISSION is the term applied to an operation for destroying a structure by tearing it without removal: eg. the operation of needling the lens of the eye for cataract.

DISINFECTION is the process of rendering harmless any persons, articles, rooms, and the like, which are liable to communicate disease. *Disinfectants* are potent, but toxic, preparations or procedures which are able to destroy micro-organisms but not necessarily resistant spores. (See BACTERIOLOGY.) *Antiseptics* are substances which kill or prevent the growth of micro-organisms, and which can safely be applied to living tissue without harming it. *Germicides* are measures or preparations which kill germs or micro-organisms. *Deodorants* are substances which suppress foul smells, and, although many deodorants are disinfectants, they are so only on much more effective application than is necessary to subdue smell. Thus charcoal exposed in a sick-room clears away smell but does not disinfect the room, and eucalyptus sprinkled on the floor renders the air of a room sweet, but does not destroy the germs of disease in the room.

FORMS OF DISINFECTANT: **Light and fresh air** are too apt to be neglected. There can hardly be found a more powerful disinfectant than direct sunlight, for few bacteria can survive exposure to it in the open for an hour. This applies, for example, with special force to the tubercle bacillus.

Heat is of great importance. Exposure to moist heat at 100°C or 212°F (ie. boiling in water) kills bacteria in five to ten minutes but longer exposures to higher temperatures (eg. 15 minutes at 121°C) are necessary to kill off resistant spores. (See BACTERIOLOGY). Steam under pressure, as in the autoclave (qv), is the most effective means of sterilization for materials that will withstand damp and moisture, such as clothes and dressings. For instruments, such as knives and scalpels, however, dry heat is necessary, as in a hot-air oven. A higher temperature and a longer exposure (eg. 160°C for an hour) are necessary than with moist heat.

CRUDE CARBOLIC in a dilution of 1 in 20 is used for disinfecting clothing and bedding. Although it does not harm fabrics or affect colours or metals, it is liable to stain, due to the presence of impurities.

PURE PHENOL is a satisfactory disinfectant in a dilution of 1 in 100. Although not as efficient as crude carbolic, it has the advantage of not staining.

CRESOL, in the form of a 1 per cent emulsion of saponified cresol, is an excellent disinfectant.

IZAL, CYLLIN AND LYSOL are other satisfactory coal-tar disinfectants. Izal and cyllin, which have a carbolic coefficient of 20, are used in a dilution of 0·5 per cent, whilst lysol, with a carbolic coefficient of 5 to 10, is used in a 1 per cent solution.

PERCHLORIDE OF MERCURY in a 1 in 1000 solution is a potent disinfectant, killing organisms in thirty minutes. Its use is restricted by the fact that it corrodes metals, and is not suitable for disinfecting faeces and sputum, as it forms insoluble compounds with albuminous material. Because of its extreme toxicity and the fact that it forms a colourless solution like water, it is coloured blue to prevent accidents. The following formula gives a 1 in 960 solution: mercury perchloride 14 grams, hydrochloric acid 28·5 ml, aniline blue 300 mg, water 13·5 litres.

FORMALDEHYDE may be used either as a gaseous disinfectant or in solution as formaldehyde solution (formalin).

POTASSIUM PERMANGANATE, which is a disinfectant by virtue of being a powerful oxidizing agent, is a useful and safe disinfectant. Its use is restricted by the fact that it is rendered inert by organic matter. Five minutes in a 1 in 1000 solution of permanganate is an effective way of sterilizing drinking and eating utensils. Although it stains textiles, the stain can be removed by oxalic acid or lemon juice. Condy's fluid contains potassium permanganate.

SODIUM HYPOCHLORITE is unstable in solution and corrodes metal, but in 1 in 3000 solution it is a useful disinfectant for floors and latrines.

LIME, one of the cheapest of disinfectants, kills organisms in a few hours in a 1 per cent solution.

CHLORINATED LIME (bleaching powder) is less stable than lime. It has the further disadvantage of being destructive to fabrics. In a 0·5 to 1 per cent solution it kills most organisms in one to five minutes.

HYDROGEN CYANIDE, which, because of its intense toxicity, must only be used by experienced personnel, is used for destroying bed bugs and for fumigating ships.

SULPHUR DIOXIDE is also used for fumigating ships.

METHODS OF DISINFECTION: **The person**: The hands must always be carefully disinfected after being in contact with an individual suffering from an infectious disease, or before dressing a wound. The best method is to wash the hands thoroughly in plenty of warm water, using an antiseptic soap such as hexachlorophane soap and a sterilized nail-brush. The hands should then be carefully rinsed in one of the following: pink potassium permanganate solution; perchloride of mercury solution (1 in 2000); biniodide of mercury solution (1 in 1000 solution in water); 75 per cent isopropyl alcohol; or 1 in 500 parts of 90 per cent alcohol. An alternative measure is to apply chlorhexidine cream to the hands after drying them.

Dressings and instruments: The former are now sterilized by high-pressure steam sterilization. Surgical instruments can be sterilized by boiling in water for ten to twenty minutes, but more usually nowadays instruments are sterilized by autoclaving.

Rooms: Provided reasonable precautions are taken during the illness, disinfection of the sick-room is not now considered necessary in the case of ordinary infectious diseases such as measles and diphtheria. Thorough washing with soap and water and plenty of fresh air are all that are required. At the beginning all unnecessary ornaments and hangings should be removed and the room should be kept well ventilated. During the illness dusting and sweeping must be reduced to a minimum and carried out only with damp dusters and mops. Recent work has shown that certain organisms remain alive in dust and in fluff from blankets for considerable periods. To overcome spread of infection by this means blankets and floors are now

being treated by oil in hospitals. If it is considered necessary to disinfect a room after an infectious illness, the first preliminary is to burn articles of little value and to send bedding and mattresses for steam disinfection. The only satisfactory way of disinfecting a room is by a spray, and for this purpose the best is formalin: 230 ml to 4·5 litres, and 4·5 litres for every 111 square metres of surface. A room sprayed in this way in the morning can be occupied again the same evening, provided all windows and doors are kept open during the spraying.
Clothes and bedding: Bed linen, blankets and similar articles should be soaked in cresol or a 5 per cent solution of carbolic acid for twelve hours before being washed. It should be remembered that if soiled linen is boiled without preliminary soaking it will be permanently stained, and that blankets do not stand repeated boiling or steam disinfection. Putting them out in the sunshine and fresh air has been described as 'one of the cheapest and most effective ways of disinfecting them'. Other articles, such as boots and leather materials, which cannot be soaked in disinfectant or destroyed, should be left in the room during disinfection, and afterwards exposed to the open air for an entire day. Where a central disinfecting station exists, arrangements should be made with the local health authority to have the disinfecting done there.
Sputum, stools and other discharges: Sputum and discharges from the nose should be collected in gauze and burnt. If there is sufficient sputum to justify a sputum flask, this should contain a 5 per cent solution of carbolic acid. The bed-pan should also contain 5 per cent solution of carbolic acid, or cresol. After use, more disinfectant should be added, well mixed with the contents and allowed to stand for two hours before being emptied down the water-closet.

DISINFESTATION means the destruction of insect pests, especially lice, whether on the person or in dwelling-places.

DISLOCATIONS are injuries to joints of such a nature that the ends of the opposed bones are forced more or less out of connection with one another. Besides displacement of the bones, there is more or less bruising of the tissues around them, and tearing of the ligaments which bind the bones together.
Varieties: Dislocations, like fractures, are divided into simple and compound, the bone in the latter case being forced through the skin. This seldom occurs, since the round head of the bone has not the same power to wound as the sharp end of a broken bone. Dislocations are also divided according as they are (1) congenital, ie. present at birth in consequence of some malformation, or (2) acquired at a later period in consequence of injury, the great majority falling into the latter class.
Causes: The causes of dislocation are similar to those of fracture, the fact as to whether a bone or a joint gives way depending upon the manner in which force is applied, and still more upon the relative strength of bones and joints. Thus in very young and very old persons dislocations are rare, because the bones are relatively easily broken, and thereby the joints are saved from damage. Congenital dislocations are mainly due to some defect in development of the bones.

Signs and symptoms: The injured limb is useless, but, as a rule, there is little pain, unless the dislocated bone presses upon some nerve trunk. When the limb is compared with that of the opposite side, the joint is found to be unduly prominent in one place, and shows an abnormal hollow in another. Further, there is loss of movement at the joint in question, but no grating (crepitus) as in a case of fracture. Each joint shows further special signs dependent upon its conformation.

Treatment: So far as temporary treatment is concerned, nothing is necessary but a splint, bandage, sling or the like, to keep the injured part moderately quiet, becase there is not the same danger of damage to nerves, vessels, and the like, by the rounded head of the bone as by the sharp fragments of a fracture. The greatest care is necessary in reduction, ie. putting the dislocated bone back in place, for great damage may be done by an unskilled person in the way of breaking the bone, tearing nerves and blood-vessels, or even leaving the bone dislocated in a new direction. After reduction to the natural position, the limb must be fixed for a time so as to prevent a recurrence, which will take place if it be used at once. The length of time depends upon the severity of the injury; as a rule, after about ten days, gentle movements are made to prevent the joint becoming stiff, and the bandages, and the like, left off after about three weeks. But care in using the limb is necessary for much longer.

SHOULDER: This may be reduced in one of two methods. (*a*) By *manipulation*, in which the bone is gently worked back into place by a method too complicated for description here. (*b*) By *extension*. The injured person lies on his back upon a couch or upon the floor. The operator then, sitting down by the injured side opposite the patient's hip and facing towards his shoulder, grasps the limb with one hand by the wrist, with the other above the elbow, while at the same time he places his foot, from which the shoe has been removed, in the armpit, on the edge of the shoulder-blade, to steady it, and give him something against which to pull. He then pulls on the injured arm gently, steadily, and strongly, first in a direction parallel with the injured person's body, and, if this is unsuccessful, at right angles to it, pressing all the while with his foot against the edge of the shoulder-blade. The injured person must at the same time relax all his shoulder muscles. The bone goes into place generally with a snap, and the appearance of the joint is then like that of its fellow.

ELBOW: This joint may be dislocated backwards by a fall on the hand, or forwards by a fall on the point of the elbow. In both cases it is reduced by bending steadily across the knee of the operator, who at the same time pulls on the forearm.

WRIST: This joint is seldom dislocated, and the dislocation is readily replaced by pressure, and is then kept in position by a well-padded splint on the palm and front of forearm. A fracture of the lower end of the radius (Colles's fracture) is sometimes mistaken for a dislocated wrist.

FINGERS AND TOES may be dislocated and are difficult to reduce, because the tight ligaments close round the displaced bone, and because of the difficulty in grasping the finger to pull on it. This may be overcome by winding strips of sticking-plaster round the finger, or by a device of interlacing tapes known as the 'Indian puzzle'. Dislocation of the thumb at its base is particularly hard to reduce, and may even require an operation to enlarge the opening through which the bone has passed.

HIP: This joint, being extremely strong, is seldom dislocated, and, when dislocated, is very difficult to reduce. The head of the thigh bone usually passes backwards and upwards, so that the limb appears much shortened and the toes turned inward. Reduction is effected by a special form of manipulation, or, failing this, by extension. For the latter, the injured person lying on his back, the limb is pulled straight downwards, one assistant steadying the pelvis by pressing one of his hands upon each iliac spine, and another pulling the whole thigh outwards by means of a towel passed round it as high up as possible. A very steady, powerful pull is necessary if reduction is to be effected.

CONGENITAL DISLOCATION OF THE HIP is commoner in girls than in boys. Its incidence is between 2 and 3 per 1000 births. If detected at, or soon after, birth, the results of treatment are excellent. This is why the routine examination of the newborn baby always includes a careful examination of the hips. Any undue instability of the hip, particularly if accompanied by a clicking sound on movement of the hip, indicates the probable presence of dislocation. When diagnosed within the first few days of life, treatment merely consists of the application for a few months of a simple splint maintaining the hips in abduction and flexion, and the results are excellent. If the condition is not detected at this stage it is often missed until the child starts walking, when she is seen to have a characteristic waddling gait. Treatment at this stage is more complicated and less satisfactory.

KNEE: This joint is very seldom dislocated, and such an injury to it is specially severe, being accompanied by the tearing of strong ligaments.

ANKLE: This joint is hardly ever dislocated, most severe injuries near it being fractures of the leg bones.

SPINE: Dislocation of the spine is only produced by great violence, and is usually combined with fracture. Very often pressure on, or tearing of, the spinal cord takes place, which may produce paralysis of the lower limbs, or even death from shock.

JAW: This joint is sometimes dislocated forwards when the mouth is very widely opened, as in yawning or singing. It can usually be replaced by a person pressing downwards with his thumbs upon the farthest back teeth and at the same time pressing up the chin. He should take care that his thumbs do not get bitten.

DISODIUM CROMOGLYCATE is a drug that is proving of value in the treatment of asthma when given as an inhalation.

DISOPYRAMIDE is a drug that is proving of value in the prevention, and treatment of disturbances of the rhythm of the heart, particularly in those which occur following a coronary thrombosis (qv).

DISORIENTATION: Orientation in a clinical sense includes a person's awareness of time and place in relation to himself and others, the recognition of personal friends and familiar places and the ability to remember at least some past experience and to register new data. It is therefore dependent on the ability to recall all learned memories and make effective use of memory. Disorientation can be the presenting feature of both delirium (qv) (confusion) and dementia (qv); delirium is reversible, developing dramatically, and accompanied by evidence of systemic disease, dementia is a gradually evolving, irreversible condition.

DISPLACEMENT is a term used in psychological medicine to describe the mental process of attaching to one object painful emotions associated with another object.

DISSEMINATED SCLEROSIS (see MULTIPLE SCLEROSIS).

DISTICHIASIS is the term applied to the condition in which there are two complete rows of eyelashes in one eyelid (or in both).

DISTOMA is a general term including various forms of trematodes, or fluke-worms, parasitic in the intestine, lung and other organs.

DISTRICT HEALTH AUTHORITY (see NATIONAL HEALTH SERVICE).

DISULFIRAM, or ANTABUSE, the full chemical name of which is tetraethylthiuram disulphide, is used in the treatment of alcoholism. It is relatively non-toxic by itself, but when taken in conjunction with alcohol it produces most unpleasant effects: eg. flushing of the face, palpitations, a sense of oppression and distress, and ultimately sickness and vomiting. The rationale of treatment therefore is to give the alcoholic subject a course of disulfiram and then demonstrate, by letting him take some alcoholic liquor, how unpleasant are the effects. If the patient is co-operative, the results of treatment are often very satisfactory. It is a form of treatment, however, that is not without risk, and it must therefore be given under skilled medical supervision.

DIURETICS are substances which produce diuresis, that is, a copious excretion of urine by the kidneys.

Varieties: There is a host of substances which can produce diuresis, although only a small proportion of these are now used. Water, for instance, is an excellent diuretic, and if the diminished output of urine is due to inadequate intake of fluid or excessive loss of fluid through other channels, eg. sweating, diarrhoea, water is often the best diuretic to rectify matters. Salts of potassium, calcium chloride and ammonium chloride produce diuresis by temporarily altering the chemistry of the blood. Urea acts as a diuretic by stimulating the glomeruli of the kidneys. Vasodilators (qv) act as diuretics by increasing the blood supply to the kidneys. Among the vasodilators used for this purpose are caffeine, theophylline, aminophylline and theobromine. Spirit of nitrous ether, a popular constituent of fever mixtures, falls into this group, but is a much weaker diuretic than the others mentioned. Gin used to be a commonly used diuretic; here there was a twofold action – the alcohol acted as a vasodilator and the oil of juniper acted as a mild irritant of the kidney, thereby acting as a stimulant to the excretion of urine. Needless to say, gin is never used now for this purpose. The digitalis group of drugs act as diuretics in cases of oedema due to heart failure; this they do mainly by improving the action of the heart: in this way they increase the circulation through the kidneys and thereby increase the output of urine.

The most widely used diuretics are benzothiadiazine (qv) derivatives. However over the last decade many new diuretics have been introduced. The so-called loop diuretics (because they act on the ascending loop of Henle in the renal tubules) are more powerful than the benzothiadiazines. In fact the loop diuretics are the most potent of all diuretics. They include frusemide (Aluzine, Diuresal, Dryptal, Frusetic, Frusid, Lasix), bumetanide (Burinex), ethacrynic acid (Edecrin) and piretanide (Arelix).

There are potassium-sparing diuretics. Spironolactone itself is an aldosterone antagonist and therefore preserves potassium. Amiloride (Midamor) and triamterene (Dytac) are also potassium-sparing diuretics, acting directly on the renal tubule. There are also osmotic diuretics. Mannitol is the main drug in this group. It is not metabolised by the body and it is not absorbed by the renal tubule and hence retains water within the tubular lumen by osmosis. Mannitol, however, requires intravenous administration. The other diuretics may be given by mouth but intravenous preparations for most of them are available.

The main indication for diuretics is in the oedema that results from heart failure. They are also indicated in ascites secondary to liver disease and in oedema secondary to the nephrotic syndrome.

DIVERTICULITIS is inflammation of diverticula (see DIVERTICULUM) in the large intestine. It is characterized by pain in the left lower side of the abdomen, which has been aptly described as 'left-sided appendicitis' as it resembles the pain of appendicitis but occurs in the opposite side of the abdomen. The onset is often sudden, with fever and constipation. It may, or may not, be preceded by diverticulosis (qv). Treatment consists of rest in bed, no solid food but ample fluid, and the administration of tetracycline. Complications are unusual but include abscess formation, perforation of the colon, and severe bleeding.

DIVERTICULOSIS means the presence of diverticula (see DIVERTICULUM) in the large intestine. Such diverticula are not uncommon over the age of 40, increasing with age until over the age of 70 they may be present in one-third to one-half of the population. They mostly occur in the lower part of the colon, and are predominantly due to muscular hyperactivity of the bowel forcing the lining of the bowel through weak points in the bowel wall, just as the inner tube of a pneumatic tyre bulges through a defective tyre. There is increasing evidence that the low-residue diet of western civilization is a contributory cause. The condition may or may not produce symptoms. If it does, these consist of disturbance of the normal bowel function and pain in the left side in the lower abdomen. If it is causing symptoms, treatment consists of a high-residue diet (see DIET) and an agar (qv) or methylcellulose (qv) preparation.

DIVERTICULUM means a pouch or pocket leading off a main cavity or tube. The term is especially applied to protrusions from the intestine, which may be present either at the time of birth as a developmental peculiarity, or which develop in numbers upon the large intestine during the course of life. The process of formation of these intestinal pockets is known as diverticulosis, and inflammation of them as diverticulitis.

DIZZINESS is a vague symptom and it is important to establish what the individual means by dizziness. It may encompass a feeling of disequilibrium, it may be light-headedness, faintness, a sensation of swimming or floating, an inbalance or unsteadiness or episodes of mental confusion. It may be true vertigo which is an hallucination of movement (see VERTIGO). These symptoms may be due to diseases of the ear, eye, central nervous system, cardiovascular system, endocrine system or they may be a manifestation of psychiatric disease. It is a common symptom in the elderly and by the age of eighty two thirds of women and one third of men have suffered from the condition.

DNA is the abbreviation for deoxy-ribonucleic acid, one of the two types of nucleic acid (qv) that occur in nature. It is the fundamental genetic material of all cells, and is present in the nucleus of the cell (qv) where it forms part of the chromosome (qv) and acts as the carrier of genetic information. The molecule is very large, with a molecular weight of several millions, and consists of two single chains of nucleotides (see NUCLEIC ACID) which are twisted round each other to form a double helix (or spiral). The genetic information carried by DNA is encoded along one of these strands. A gene (qv), which represents the genetic information needed to form protein, is a stretch of DNA containing, on average, around 1000 nucleotides paired in these two strands.

To allow it to fulfil its vitally important function as the carrier of genetic information in living cells, DNA has the following properties. It is stable so that successive generations of species maintain their individual characteristics, but not so stable that evolutionary changes cannot take place. It must be able to store a vast amount of information. For example, an animal cell contains genetic information for the synthesis of over a million proteins. It must be duplicated exactly before each cell division to ensure that both daughter cells contain an accurate copy of the genetic information of the parent cells (see CELLS).

DOBUTAMINE is a drug which acts on sympathetic receptors in cardiac muscle and increases the contractility and hence improves the cardiac output but has little effect on the cardiac rate. It is particularly useful in cardiogenic shock. It must be given by intravenous infusion.

DOG BITES (see BITES AND STINGS; RABIES).

DOLICHOCEPHALIC means long-headed and is a term applied to skulls the breadth of which is less than four-fifths of the length.

DOMETTE BANDAGE is a bandage of union fabric of plain weave, in which the warp threads are of cotton and the weft threads of wool. It is used especially when a high degree of warmth, protection and support is needed. (See also BANDAGES.)

DONORS: The inception, and increasing amount, of transplantation (qv) have created an ever-growing demand for donors of eyes, kidneys and other organs of the body. This is in addition to the already existing demand for blood donors. There is still also a demand for bodies for dissecting purposes in the anatomy department of our medical schools.

Those who wish to bequeath their bodies for dissection purposes should get in touch with: H.M. Inspector of Anatomy, Department of Health, 158–160 Great Portland Street, London, W1N 5TB (01–872 9302, ext. 48301), who will give full advice as to the correct procedure to be followed.

There is a steadily increasing demand for blood for transfusion (see TRANSFUSION OF BLOOD), as the present supply scarcely meets the demand. More donors are therefore required. There are fifteeen blood transfusion centres in England, four in Scotland and one in Wales. Details of how to become a donor can be obtained through general practitioners, the local community physician at the local town hall, from any hospital, or, in the case of those in employment in large organizations, from the organization's medical officer. Alternatively, in Wales full details can be obtained from the Director of the Welsh Regional Blood Transfusion Centre, Rhyd-Lafar, St Fagans, Cardiff CF5 6XF (0222–890302). In Scotland such details can be obtained from the Secretary of the Scottish National Blood Transfusion Service, Royal Infirmary, Edinburgh EH3 9HB.

In the case of organs of the body, such as the eyes, kidneys, the liver and the heart, the problem is that, to be capable of transplantation, they must be removed from the body within a matter of a few hours of the death of the donor. In practice this means that it is highly desirable that the permission of the donor for such removal is obtained in advance in writing. If the matter is left until after the death of the donor, there is inevitable delay in getting permission from the relatives to remove the organ in question. Not only, as in the case of a sudden death due to road accident, may this be difficult, but it may cause unnecessary distress to the relatives at a time when they are already emotionally upset.

So far as corneal grafting (qv) is concerned, the Department of Health and Social Security has drawn up a list of suitable eye-banks to which people can bequeath their eyes, and an official form is available for the bequest of eyes. Copies of this can be obtained on application to the Department at: Alexander Fleming House, Elephant and Castle, London, SE1.

In the case of kidney transplantations the Department of Health and Social Security has prepared a kidney donor card to be signed by the donor and countersigned by the donor's next of kin. Copies of this card can be obtained in any pharmacy, or from general practitioners. The card, when duly signed, should aways be carried about by the donor, so that it is readily available, even though his (or her) death should occur unexpectedly – as in a road accident. Although the number of kidneys becoming available for transplantation has been increasing, there is still an urgent need for more.

No special arrangements have been made to date for obtaining permission for the transplantation of hearts, livers or lungs, and other organs, but anyone who is willing to become a donor of one or more of these should sign, and have countersigned, a form comparable to the kidney donor card.

DOPAMINE is a catecholamine (qv) and a precursor of noradrenaline (qv). Its highest concentration is in that portion of the brain known as the basal nuclei (see BRAIN) where its function is to convey inhibitory influences to the extrapyramidal system. There is good evidence that dopamine deficiency is one of the causative factors in Parkinsonism (qv).

DOSAGE: Many factors influence the activity with which drugs operate. Among the factors which affect the necessary quantity are age, weight, sex, idiosyncrasy, genetic disorders, habitual use, disease, fasting, combination with other drugs, the form in which the drug is given, and the route by which it is given.

Age is but one factor. Normally, a young child requires a smaller dose than an adult. There are, however, other factors to be taken into consideration. Thus, children are more susceptible than adults to some drugs such as morphine, whilst they are less sensitive to others such as atropine. Various methods have been introduced for calculating roughly and quickly the dose generally suitable for a child of any given age. One, for instance, is:

$$\text{adult dose} \times \frac{\text{age next birthday}}{20}$$

Another formula is:

$$\text{adult dose} \times \frac{\text{weight in pounds}}{150}$$

Yet another is:

$$\frac{\text{age} \times \text{adults dose}}{\text{age in years} + 12}$$

Another formula based on the surface area of the child is:

$$\text{adult dose} \times \frac{\text{surface area in square metres}}{1{\cdot}82}$$

There is, however, no simple way of calculating the dose of a drug for an infant child. The body weight is probably the best and simplest, but it must be used with discrimination, bearing in mind the other factors that have to be taken into consideration. An approximate rule of thumb, based on children of average height and weight, and assuming an adult dose of 100 mg is:

Age years	*Average weight* kg	*Dose* mg
1	10	25
7	25	50
12	40	75
Adult	70	100

Old people, too, often show an increased susceptibility to drugs. This is probably due to a variety of factors, such as decreased weight in many old people; diminished activity of the tissues and therefore diminished rate at which a drug is utilized; and diminished activity of the kidneys resulting in decreased rate of excretion of the drug.

Weight and sex have both to be taken into consideration. Women require slightly smaller doses than men, probably because they tend to be lighter in weight. The effect of weight on dosage is partly dependent on the fact that much of the extra weight of a heavy individual is made up of fatty tissue which is not as active as other tissue of the body. In practice, the question of weight seldom makes much difference unless the individual is grossly overweight or underweight.

Idiosyncrasy occasionally causes drugs administered in the ordinary dose to produce unexpected effects. Thus, some people are but little affected by some drugs, whilst in others certain drugs, such as potassium iodide, or atropine, produce excessive symptoms in minute doses. In some cases this may be due to hypersensitiveness, or an allergic reaction, to the drug. This is a possibility that must always be borne in mind, particularly with penicillin. As a rule the individual has had the drug in question previously. Penicillin comes into this category; so much so that an individual who is known to be allergic to penicillin is strongly recommended to carry about with him wherever he goes a card to this effect. The carrying of such a card may well prevent his being given in some emergency a dose of penicillin that could possibly prove fatal.

Habitual use of a drug is perhaps the influence that causes the greatest increase in the dose necessary to produce the requisite effect. The classical example of this is opium and its derivatives. Arsenic is another example that was often encountered in the days when arsenical drugs were one of the great stand-bys in the Pharmacoepia.

Disease may modify the dose of medicines. This can occur in several ways. Thus, in serious illnesses the patient may be more susceptible to drugs, such as narcotics, that depress tissue activity, and therefore smaller doses must be given. Again, absorption of the drug from the gut may be slowed up by disease of the gut, or its effect may be enhanced if there is disease of the kidneys, interfering with the excretion of the drug.

Fasting aids the rapidity of absorption of, and also makes the body more susceptible to the action of, drugs. Partly for this reason, as well as to avoid irritation of the stomach, it is usual to prescribe drugs to be taken after meals, and diluted with water.

Combination of drugs is now frowned upon as it is often difficult to assess what their combined effect may be. In some cases they may have a mutually antagonistic effect, which means that the patient will not obtain full benefit from the prescription. In other cases the combination may have a deleterious effect, whilst in others again the combination may so enhance the effect on the patient as to produce harmful effects.

Form of administration is important in two respects. In the first instance, there is a tendency today to give a drug in the form of the active principle rather than, say, the leaf from which it is obtained as was the case at one time. This means, of course, that a smaller dose of the active principle is required than of the leaf or the tincture. In the second place, it involves the question of whether the drug is given as a tablet, a mixture or a powder. Various factors have to be taken into consideration; but today the common practice is to give a drug in tablet form, mainly because of the convenience of both patient and prescriber.

Route of administration naturally affects dosage. In Britain, medicines are given *by mouth* whenever possible, unless there is some degree of urgency, or because the drug is either destroyed in, or is not absorbed from, the gut. In these circumstances, it is given *intravenously*, *intramuscularly* or *subcutaneously*. In some cases, as in cases of asthma or bronchitis, the drug may be given in the form of an *inhalant* or *aerosol* (qv), in order to get the maximum concentration at the point where it is wanted: that is, in the lungs. If a local effect is wanted, as in cases of diseases of the skin, the drug is applied *topically* to the skin. On the Continent there is a tendency to give medicines in the form of a *suppository* which is inserted in the rectum.

Recent years have seen developments whereby the assimilation of drugs into the body can be more carefully controlled. These include, for example, what are known as transdermals, in which drugs are built into a plaster that is stuck on the skin, and the drug is then absorbed into the body at a controlled rate. This method is now being used for the administration of glyceryl trinitrate (qv) in the treatment of angina pectoris (qv), and of hyoscine hydrobromide in the treatment of travel sickness (qv). Another is a new class of implantable devices. These are tiny polymers infused with a drug and implanted just under the skin by injection. They can be tailored so as to deliver drugs at virtually any rate – from minutes to years. A modification of these polymers now being investigated is the incorporation of magnetic particles which allow an extra burst of the incorporated drug to be released in response to an oscillating magnetic field which is induced by a magnetic 'watch' worn by the patient. In this way the patient can switch on an extra dose of drug when this is needed: insulin, for instance, in the case of diabetics. In yet another new development, a core of drug is enclosed in a semi-permeable membrane and is released in the stomach at a given rate. (See also LIPOSOMES.)

Genetic disorders are now coming to assume an increasing importance. Perhaps the classical example is the individual who suffers from a congenital deficiency of the enzyme known as glucose-6-phosphate dehydrogenase. Such individuals develop an acute haemolytic anaemia (see ANAEMIA) if they are given certain drugs, including phenacetin or a sulphonamide.

DOTHIEPIN (PROTHIADEN) is a drug that is being used in the treatment of depression. (See ANTIDEPRESSANTS.)

DOUBLE VISION (see SQUINT).

DOUCHE is an application of water to the body, directly, through a pipe.

Action: Douches fall into two divisions: (*a*) those which act by virtue of some substance which they contain, such as astringent douches, cleansing douches; (*b*) those which act by virtue of their temperature, producing the effects which have been described under BATHS, and COLD, USES OF, with the distinction that douches act locally and so produce an action, upon one part only, greater than if the application were made to the whole body at one time.

Uses: (*a*) MEDICATED AND CLEANSING DOUCHES are used as a rule to wash out infected cavities. Thus, *bladder douches* are used in inflammation of this cavity, containing, for example, either half-saturated boric lotion; or oxycyanide of mercury, 1 in 10,000; or chlorhexidine, 1 in 5000 given at a temperature of 43°C (110°F). Such a douche is administered by means of a douche-can holding 1 litre (2 pints) or more, connected by rubber piping with a three-way or T-shaped tube of glass, which, on its other two ends, has an outflow tube and a tube leading to a catheter introduced into the bladder. The douche-can, being suspended at a height of 1 metre (3 feet) or so above the bed on which the patient lies, is filled with fluid, which runs into the bladder as soon as the outflow tube is pinched. When sufficient has entered, it can be at once drawn off by pinching the inflow tube and releasing the outflow. This is repeated several times. *Vaginal douches* of chloroxylenol solution ('dettol'), 4 ml in 0·5 litre; potassium permanganate, 1 in 500; boric acid, 1 in 50; or normal saline (ie. 4 G in 1 litre), at a temperature of 40°C (104°F) are used in some cases of leucorrhoea or 'whites'. A 1 litre (2 pints) or larger douche-can is used at a height of 1·5 or 2 metres (5 or 6 feet). It leads by an rubber tube to a large nozzle, which should be made of glass for ready disinfection. Such a douche is sometimes used at a temperature of 46°C (115°F), or as hot as the hand can bear, in order to obtain also the soothing and constricting action of a hot douche on the blood-vessels of the surrounding parts.

(*b*) TEMPERATURE DOUCHES may be hot or cold, or in general the two alternated. The action upon the circulation has been explained under the heading of BATHS, with the exception that the douche acts strongly upon a single part. Douching, combined with massage, is a useful procedure for rheumatism, neuralgia, and other pains. The Scotch douche consists of an alternate hot water or steam douche and a cold douche. It is used for similar purposes, and it is important that the hot stream should be given first, and that it should last four or five times as long as the cold stream. Such a douche acts powerfully upon the skin and nerves, and can be continued for a few minutes only.

DOVER'S POWDER, also known as IPECACUANHA AND OPIUM POWDER, is made from 10 per cent each of powdered opium and ipecacuanha, with 80 per cent of lactose. (See OPIUM.) Still one of the most popular remedies in medicine, it was introduced by Captain Thomas Dover (1660–1742), one of the most romantic figures in the history of medicine. Perhaps his greatest claim to fame is that he was a member of the privateering expedition which rescued Alexander Selkirk from Juan Fernandez, an island off the coast of Chile. It was upon the story of Alexander Selkirk that Daniel Defoe based *Robinson Crusoe*.

Uses: It is widely used as a diaphoretic, analgesic and sedative in the treatment of feverish colds and influenza. It is also an excellent remedy for dry, hacking coughs. The dose is 300 to 600 mg.

DOWN'S SYNDROME (or MONGOLISM) is a variety of mental subnormality, in which the patient has Mongolian-like eyes, a snub nose, high cheek-bones, a large tongue, a small round skull, and short, thick hands and feet. Another characteristic feature is the palm print, which reveals distinctive markings; the most distinctive of these is the so-called four-finger line. The condition is being increasingly referred to as Down's syndrome (or disease) after Dr. J. L. H. Down, the London doctor who first described it in 1866.

The incidence is approximately 1 per 600 births, but the incidence in the community is lower than this, as many Down's syndrome victims die in infancy. This high death-rate is due partly to the fact that these children have a much higher incidence of other congenital deformities, such as malformations of the heart, than other children, and partly to their lower resistance to infection.

It is much commoner in children born to older women. Thus, the risk of having a Down's child in women over 45 is more than 1 in 60, compared with less than 1 in 1000 in women under 30. Forty per cent of children with Down's syndrome are born to mothers over 40, 30 per cent to those aged 35 to 40. For mothers who give birth to a Down's child when they are younger the chances of a subsequent child being affected is relatively high. Precise figures in this respect can be misleading, and the best advice for a young mother who has had a Down's child, and who wishes to know the risk of her having another, is to go and discuss the matter with her family doctor.

In 95 per cent of cases the cause is the presence of an extra chromosome (qv) in the ovum. The cause of this extra chromosome is not known. In the remaining cases the cause is a fault in the division of the germ cells known as translocation.

The degree of mental backwardness varies considerably. Up to a third of all severely mentally handicapped children of school age have Down's syndrome. It has been estimated that 6 per cent of Down's children are probably capable of profiting appreciably from attendance at schools for the educationally subnormal. Practically all who survive to school age gain some benefit. Most eventually acquire some degree of speech, and about 5 per cent learn to read. They practically never learn to write. Most learn to wash, dress and feed themselves, and many are able to run simple errands.

There is no known cure for the condition, but much can be done for them, especially if they can be kept at home rather than sent to an institution. Parents of such children seeking advice and help are recommended to get in touch with the Down's Syndrome Association, 12–13 Clapham Common Southside, London SW4 7AA (01–720 0008).

DOXEPIN (SINEQUAN) (see ANTIDEPRESSANTS).

DOXORUBICIN (ADRIAMYCIN) is a drug that is proving of value in the treatment of acute leukaemia, lymphoma, and various forms of sarcoma and cancer, including cancer of the bladder. (See CYTOTOXIC DRUGS.)

DOXYCYCLINE is a wide-spectrum, long-acting antibiotic of the tetracycline group (qv), which is active against a wide range of microorganisms, including the causative organism of scrub typhus.

DRACUNCULIASIS, or DRACONTIASIS, is the disease caused by the guinea-worm, *Dracunculus medinensis*. It has been described as the oldest known human parasite, and is believed to be the Mosaic fiery serpent that harassed the Israelites on the shores of the Red Sea. It is found in India, Arabia, Iran, the Nile valley, East and West Africa, where it afflicts 20–40 million people. The female may attain a length of 120 cm (4 feet). It is transmitted by *Cyclops*, a fresh-water crustacean, and man is infected by drinking contaminated water. The worm causes no trouble for about a year, when it approaches the surface of the body and causes a local painful swelling which is usually accompanied by fever. The essential treatment, ie. removal of the worm, has changed little since Biblical days. Mebendazole, metronidazole and thiabendazole are proving of value in controlling the disease.

DRAINS (see SEWAGE AND SEWAGE DISPOSAL).

DRAMAMINE is the trade name for dimenhydrinate, a drug widely used in the treatment of travel sickness.

DRASTICS are substances which have a violent purgative action, such as croton oil, jalap, scammony. (See PURGATIVES.)

DRAUGHT, or DRAFT, is a small mixture intended to be taken at one dose. It consists generally of two or four tablespoonfuls of fluid.

DRAW SHEET (see BED).

DREAMS (see SLEEP).

DRENCH is an old term still used in parts of England for a draught of medicine.

DREPANOCYTOSIS is another term for sickle-cell anaemia (qv), which is characterized by the presence in the blood of red blood corpuscles sickle-like in shape. The anaemia is a severe one and afflicts black people.

DRESSINGS (see WOUNDS).

DROP ATTACKS are attacks, usually in a middle-aged woman, whose legs suddenly 'give way', so that she falls to the ground without any warning. There is no loss of consciousness. In some cases the loss of tone in the muscles, responsible for the fall, may persist for several hours. In such cases moving the patient or applying pressure to the soles of the feet may restore the tone to the muscles. In most cases, however, recovery is immediate. The cause is probably a temporary interference with the blood supply to the brain. In others there may be some disturbance of the vestibular apparatus which controls the balance of the body. (See EAR.)

DROP-FOOT is a condition in which there is difficulty in raising the front part of the foot from the ground, or in which, when the condition is severe, the foot hangs limp.
Causes: The commonest form is that due to neuritis of the nerve (anterior tibial) supplying the muscles on the front of the leg. It may be caused by alcohol, lead poisoning or trauma to the leg, or it may follow some infection such as typhoid fever or diphtheria. In drop-foot from these causes, there are apt to be disturbances of sensation on the leg also. Drop-foot may occur in children who have had poliomyelitis, but in this condition there is no sensory disturbance. It is also liable to occur in patients who are confined to bed for any length of time. In order to prevent this occurring the weight of the bedclothes should be taken off the patient's feet by means of a cradle (qv). If the condition is not so severe as to prevent the patient from going about, he walks by lifting the foot high so as to prevent the toes from catching on objects on the ground.
Treatment: If the condition is due to neuritis, it tends gradually to become better as the neuritis passes off. (See NEURITIS.) While the condition lasts, it is usual for the patient to wear a shoe the front part of which is supported by an elastic band attached to the front of the leg, in order to prevent the weak muscles from being over-stretched and the toes from dropping. Massage and electrical treatment are also required to maintain the tone of the affected muscles.

DROPPED BEAT means the missing out of a regular beat of the heart. It can be detected either by listening to the heart or by feeling the pulse. It may be due to *heart block* (qv) or to an *extrasystole* (qv). Dropped beat due to extrasystole is of no great significance.

DROPSY, or HYDROPS (see OEDEMA).

DROP-WRIST, or wrist-drop, is a condition in which, owing to partial or complete paralysis of the muscles which extend the hand, the latter droops at the wrist.
Causes: Perhaps the commonest form is that known as crutch-palsy, in which, owing to the constant pressure of a crutch in the armpit, the large nerve (radial) that controls the extensor muscles of the forearm becomes damaged, and hence the muscles in question are paralysed. The same effect may be produced when a person sleeps with his head resting on the upper arm, or with the arm over the back of a chair. A blow on the back of the arm may produce a similar condition. Poisoning by alcohol or by lead may cause the condition, which may also be brought about by a chill.
Treatment: The forms due to pressure on the nerve or to chill require only rest and application of massage and electricity to the muscles to prevent their wasting, for recovery usually takes place gradually but surely. In the cases due to lead, the appropriate treatment for lead poisoning is necessary.

DROSTANOLONE PROPIONATE (MASTERIL) is an anti-cancer drug which is proving of value in the treatment of some advanced cases of cancer of the breast. (See ANDROGENS.)

DROWNING, RECOVERY FROM: In Britain, deaths from drowning numbered 971 in 1984. Two-thirds of these are accidental and one-third suicidal. An analysis by the Royal Life Saving Society of 715 fatal drowning accidents in Great Britain in 1973 shows that 21 per cent of these occurred while swimming, bathing or paddling, 16 per cent from boats, 4·4 per cent while fishing, and 21 per cent among children playing near water. This last group included five children drowned in private swimming pools. Thirty per cent of these drowning fatalities occurred in children under 16 years of age; 14 per cent of them in the 0 to 5 years age-group. In drowning, death as a rule ensues from asphyxia (see ASPHYXIA), although, in falls from a height upon water, or in cases where the body in falling has encountered blows upon the head or abdomen, death may be due to shock. In the latter case, instead of the signs of asphyxia, the skin is pale, the face placid, and the lungs are empty of water because no attempts at breathing have taken place. In slight cases of shock the chances of resuscitation are rather more hopeful than in cases of asphyxia, because little water has been drawn into the lungs, and because there has been no struggling. Artificial respiration must be persisted in until the signs of death are unmistakable. External cardiac compression will be necessary in addition if the heart has stopped. Speed and immediate treatment on withdrawal from the water are of paramount importance. Recovery is more likely in the case of sea-water drowning than fresh-water drowning.

The specific gravity of the body being slightly greater than that of water, it sinks at first; then if the person is able to struggle, his efforts bring him to the surface, only to sink again as he becomes exhausted. This may be repeated several times. In these struggles, water mixed with air is drawn into the air-passages, and the two are churned up with mucus into a froth which forms a great obstacle to the entrance of air into the lungs during subsequent attempts at resuscitation. The first step in this process should be taken *on the instant the body is drawn from the water*, without delay for any examination, removal of clothing, or the like, and consists in the attempt to restore breathing by *artificial respiration*. Before beginning the actual movements of artificial respiration a few seconds should be spent in getting rid of as much water as possible from the lungs and air-passages: for example, a child may be held up by its heels, and the water will run out of his mouth; when an adult is lying prone on the ground, the operator's arms can be linked round the patient's middle, which is then raised, and water will flow out of the mouth. Any seaweed or other matter in the mouth should be quickly removed by the finger. According to the St John Ambulance Association, the St Andrew's Ambulance Association and the British Red Cross Society, expired air resuscitation, or the mouth-to-mouth (or -nose) method, is the method of choice.

1. **Expired-air resuscitation** consists of the old Biblical method of breathing direct into the victim's mouth. Careful investigations have indicated that it is a more efficient method of artificial respiration than any of the more indirect methods.

As in all methods of artificial respiration, speed is the essence of success. Briefly, the technique is as follows:

(1) Lay the victim on his back and kneel opposite his ear. (2) Turn his head towards you and extend it to the sniffing position. (3) Open his mouth, and sweep a finger round the mouth and throat to remove any obvious debris. (4) Place the thumb of the right hand between the teeth and grip the lower jaw in the centre and hold it forwards so that the lower front teeth protrude. (5) Close the victim's nose by pinching the nostrils with the thumb and index finger of the left hand. (6) Take a deep breath and, placing your mouth over the victim's mouth, sealing it, blow forcefully in adults, gently in children, and with puffs of the cheeks in infants, so that the chest is seen to rise. (7) Remove your mouth and allow passive expiration. (8) Repeat about 20 times a minute at first; later slow down to 15.

Three important points to remember are: (i) The victim's head must be extended: ie., bent backwards. (ii) The lower jaw must be kept thrust forwards. (iii) You must take a deep breath each time.

2. **Schafer's prone-posture method**: Immediately on removal from the water, place the patient face downwards on the ground, with a folded coat under the lower part of the chest, and lose no time by removing clothing. Turn the victim's face a little to one side, so that the mouth and nose are not obstructed. Let the operator *kneel astride* of, or to one side of, the victim, facing his head, and let him place his hands over the lower part of the patient's back, one on each side (on the lowest ribs). Let him throw the weight of his body forward upon his hands, so as to press the air (and water if there is any) out of the patient's lungs. Then let him immediately raise his body to take the pressure off and allow the patient's chest to expand. Repeat these movements twelve or fifteen times per minute.

This method has the advantages of extreme simplicity and great effectiveness. Further, no time is lost in freeing the air passages of water and mucus, which may drain from the mouth during the whole procedure; there is no trouble caused by the tongue falling backwards into the throat, as in the face-up methods. The introducer of the method also claimed that, while the amount of air taken into the lungs of an average-sized healthy person is about 5850 millilitres per minute, the amount that can be drawn in by this method is about 6760 millilitres.

3. **Rocking method,** originally recommended by Dr F. C. Eve, is carried out by securing the patient face-down on a stretcher. The stretcher is then rocked at the rate of 12 to 15 double rocks per minute. It is an excellent form of artificial respiration provided the stretcher and suitable appliances for rocking it are available.

After-treatment for drowning: As soon as the patient makes efforts at breathing, these measures are stopped. But no such effort may be made for twenty minutes, an hour, or even, in some recorded cases, for more than an hour, and still the person may recover, so that artificial respiration should be persevered with so long as there is the slightest sign of life. Efforts must next be made to restore the feeble circulation, and, in cases in which the body has been long in water or much exposed during artificial respiration, to regain the body warmth. To this end the patient should be wrapped in hot blankets, with hot bottles to the sides and feet, and the arms and legs should be rubbed upwards towards the body. So soon as the power of swallowing returns, sips of hot water, and teaspoonfuls of hot brandy and water, or hot coffee, may be administered. Ammonia, nitrite of amyl, or smelling salts may for the same purpose be now and then held to the nose. Finally, if the patient shows a tendency to sleep, this should be encouraged. All patients require admission to hospital for assessment of their respiratory function and to exclude the complications of hypoxia.

Immersion hypothermia: This is responsible for a large number of unnecessary deaths every year, particularly in young people who have been involved in sailing or boating accidents. The summer sea temperature around southern Britain is about 15°C. An unprotected adult of average weight in such water will cool to dangerous levels within two hours. A thin person will reach this critical stage in an hour; a fat one, with his layers of protective insulating fat, may survive indefinitely. Children, particularly boys, who are on average thinner than girls, may be at risk within half-an-hour. Survival times are greatly increased if thick conventional clothing, as well as a lifejacket, is worn, and are shortened for those who swim about rather than float still in a lifejacket, thus retaining their heat. In practice this means that the way to prevent this potentially fatal lowering of body temperature is on abandoning ships or small craft to put on thick clothing, or special insulated clothing such as thermofloat jackets if available, as well as an efficient lifejacket, and to float still while awaiting rescue. A further precautionary measure for yachtsmen is never to take even small amounts of alcohol in exposed conditions unless a large meal is eaten at the same time.

A point to be borne in mind by rescuers, if several people are involved, is that the quietest people are most likely to be reaching a dangerously low temperature, that small boys are most at risk, and that older girls and women are the most likely to remain in good condition if all cannot be rescued on the first rescue trip. Equally important is it to remember that a small child drifting away from shore, holding a float, needs immediate rescue if he or she is not to risk cooling to a dangerous degree.

Treatment consists of getting the victim into warm surroundings as quickly as possible, preferably a bath of water as hot as the attendant can stand with his own hand – about 45°C. The temperature should be a little lower for conscious patients. The hot bath should be tried even though the victim is apparently dead. Cardiac massage (qv) should be given at half the normal rate if the heart is stopped. In most cases the hot bath will cause rapid recovery, and it is best to discontinue the bath as soon as the victim is clearly improving. Excessive rewarming may do harm, especially in older people. Once a healthy victim of acute immersion is recovering, and has been taken from the bath and allowed to rewarm slowly, lying flat under blankets in a warm place, all is likely to be well. In the case of older people, or those in whom there has been evidence of the heart being affected, removal to hospital for further treatment and investigation is indicated. First and foremost, however, is the necessity for taking prompt action to raise the body temperature to normal limits. (See also HYPOTHERMIA.)

DRUG ADDICTION: A wide range of drugs comes into this category of drugs of addiction or dependence. Some, such as aspirin, are comparatively harmless in this respect. Others, such as the morphine-like drugs, are among the greatest social evils of the day. The characteristics of some of these drugs are shown in the table below. *Physical dependence* is the result of an adaptation of the body to a drug so that if the concentration of the drug falls below a certain level the body is unable to function properly. This produces what is known as the *abstinence syndrome*, characterized by the individual becoming ill and remaining ill until he receives a further dose of the drug. *Tolerance* means that a larger and larger dose of the drug is needed in order to produce the same effect. Drug dependence can develop without tolerance; conversely, tolerance may occur without any concurrent dependence. *Psychic dependence* is a complex factor not yet fully understood. Basically it is the state of mind induced in an individual by a certain drug. It may include what is shown in the table as '*overpowering need*', but not necessarily so. As is shown in the table, psychic dependence may occur in individuals who do not have an overpowering need to take the drug in question, as in the case of cannabis and LSD. On the other hand, overpowering need is always accompanied by psychic dependence. *Acquired desire* is perhaps best illustrated in the case of cannabis. Devotees of cannabis have to learn to enjoy the drug. If they fail, they may give it up. If, however, they are unfortunate and acquire a desire for the drug, then psychic dependence develops and pleasure is associated with this dependence. *Psychotoxic effects* appear as disturbances in the normal behaviour pattern of the individual. They may vary with the drug being used and are influenced by the psychological make-up of the individual. *Psychotic on withdrawal* is part and parcel of the abstinence syndrome, which develops when the individual stops taking the drug.

The number of addicts in England known to be receiving narcotic drugs from medical practitioners in treatment of their addiction at the end of 1984 was 5869, but this is not a guide to the total number of people who abuse drugs of various kinds; the number of these cannot be reliably estimated. The official view is that the total number of addicts may be of the order of 10,000 with a further 10,000 habitual users of barbiturates. Unofficial, but reliable, medical sources put the figure at nearer 40,000.

Morphine and heroin: Opium and all its derivatives (heroin (qv) is a derivative of morphine) are the classical example of drugs of addiction, with a history stretching back into very early times. Dangerous though they are in western civilization, it has to be borne in mind that by some Oriental peoples opium is widely used, not in an excessive and pernicious manner, but almost in the same sense as tobacco or alcohol is used in the West. Indeed, in the East opium smoking is used as an aid to contemplative serenity, and there can be no doubt that the habit in such a culture by someone brought up in its traditions can be a relatively harmless procedure. Equally, however, it should be noted that opium smoking can be grossly abused in the East as well as in the West. The two great dangers of opium in this sphere, apart from addiction – and whatever expert discussion there may be as to what is meant by addiction, opium is unquestionably accepted as a drug of addiction – are the tolerance the individual develops to it, and the appalling effects of sudden stoppage of its use. The first means that the individual has to take larger and larger doses, whilst the second means that he (or she) is unable to stop the habit alone as the moment dosage is reduced to any appreciable extent he becomes violently ill with what are known as 'withdrawal symptoms'. There is some quite impressive evidence that these withdrawal symptoms can be controlled, if not actually suppressed, by electro-acupuncture (see ACUPUNCTURE). The rationale of this may be that (a) the level of certain enkephalins (qv) are low in morphine and heroin addicts; (b) electro-acupuncture increases the output of these enkephalins.

Until comparatively recent years the vast majority of opium addicts were what were known as 'therapeutic' addicts or professional addicts. Therapeutic addicts were individuals who had acquired the habit as a result of having been prescribed some form of the drug for quite legitimate medical reasons. Professional addicts were doctors, nurses or pharmacists who had acquired the habit through being in constant contact with it and therefore open to the temptation offered by easy access to the drug in times of depression, overwork or emotional stress and strain. Today, however, the picture is completely changed. Not only have the majority of addicts of morphine-like drugs started the habit on their own initiative, but many are taking the much more dangerous heroin.

The addict to this group of drugs degenerates steadily, physically and mentally. His face becomes sallow, his appearance prematurely aged, and his muscles wasted. His memory becomes bad, he suffers from insomnia, and he complains of generalized aches and pains. The appetite fails and the liver functions inefficiently. He loses interest in his work and his surroundings. His character changes, and a person who previously was honest and truthful becomes utterly untrustworthy and an inveterate liar. Delusions of various sorts develop, and under their influence criminal acts may be performed. The death-rate is high, particularly among heroin addicts. In one series it was found to be 28 times the average death-rate. In another series the mean age of death was 24·8 years. In most of the cases the causes of death are either related to use of the drug or what has been described as 'non-natural'. Thus, an analysis of the causes of death among non-therapeutic heroin addicts in the United Kingdom between 1955 and 1966 showed that 22 per cent were due to suicide or violent death, and 61 per cent were due to suicidal overdose, narcotic overdose (accidental), sudden death (related to addiction) and septic conditions. The high incidence of sepsis is due to the septic conditions under which the addict injects the drug.

Cannabis: Cannabis, or Indian hemp, is a plant which subserves the eminently practical purpose of providing fibre for the making of cord and textiles; it also provides one of the oldest euphoriants. Its terminology has become increasingly involved in recent years. The resin (hashish) or the dried flowers (marijuana) may be smoked in cigarettes or through a water pipe. The elixir may be drunk, marijuana may be eaten, and the drug is also taken as snuff. Currently used slang terms are 'grass' and 'pot', and a marijuana cigarette is known as a 'stick' or a 'joint'.

The propensities of the drug have been known for thousands of years. The Chinese were using it as an anaesthetic in surgery 2000 years ago, and it has been claimed that 'soma', a potent hallucinogenic potion referred to in Indian writings around 800 BC, contained cannabis. Herodotus, writing around 400 BC, refers to the Scythians as throwing some mysterious seeds on to red hot stones, and then inhaling the vapour, and it has been said that the seeds were probably those of cannabis. It was probably not until around the 10th century AD that the use of cannabis became widespread in Africa and Asia. How it became introduced to Britain is not quite clear, but the probability is that the habit came from the United States of America, to which it was introduced from Mexico, where marijuana smoking is a long-established practice, around the 1930s. Its widespread use throughout Asia is almost part and parcel of the cultural life, the Brahmin in India using it, for example, to help him say his prayers.

When marijuana is smoked, the effects appear quickly, reach a peak in two hours and then pass off. The physical effects are quickening of the pulse, a rise in blood-pressure, congestion of the eyes, frequency of passing of urine, and often nausea and vomiting or diarrhoea. The psychological effects vary according to the individual, but by and large are dependent upon the mood of the individual when he

Drugs	*Physical Dependence*	*Tolerance*	*Over-powering Need*	*Acquired Desire*	*Psychic Dependence*	*Psycho-toxic*	*Psychotic on With-drawal*
Morphine-like	+	+	+		+	+	+
Barbiturates and other hypnotics	+	+	+		+	+	+
Cocaine			+		+	+	
Amphetamine	+	+	+	+	+	+	
Cannabis				+	+	+	
LSD and other Hallucinogens		+		+	+	+	
Inhalation Drugs		?	+*	+	+		
Aspirin		?	+*	+	+	+	
Caffeine		+		+	+		
Nicotine		+		+	+		
Alcohol	+	+	+	+	+	+	

* Only some of the users display this.

Comparison of the characteristics of drugs of dependence. *The Practitioner.*

takes the drug. If he is in an optimistc mood he will become exhilarated; if he is depressed he will become even more depressed. The ideal that the users of marijuana aim at has been described as a 'mood of pleasant euphoria, which is accompanied by a feeling that his thoughts are coming more quickly, that the world is more intensely interesting, and by a general loosening of inhibition'. This is what is meant by being 'high'. The expert regular smoker may achieve this without intoxicating or incapacitating himself, but all too often the individual becomes increasingly restless and lethargic, or dreamy and withdrawn, and there may be transient disorientation. Tremors and unsteadiness of gait may develop, and in the initiate the feeling of loss of control may evoke unpleasant anxiety. Whether or not it can produce a psychotic state is open to question. According to one expert in this field, 'marijuana releases what is latent in the individual's thoughts and emotions, but does not evoke responses which would be totally alien to him in his undrugged state'.

Although marijuana is not as vicious an addiction-forming drug as heroin, its potentialities for evil, and the risk of the user becoming dependent on it, are such as to justify steps to bring its use strictly under control or to render its use illegal in Britain. As has been pointed out over and over again, the argument that the stable personality might be able to continue using the drug without any deleterious effect, does not justify anyone, and particularly the adolescent and young adult, embarking on its use. Equally, whilst there is no logical reason why the use of marijuana need necessarily lead on to the use of heroin, all the evidence indicates that the individual – and again particularly the adolescent and young adult – who embarks on the use of marijuana sooner or later is liable to find himself (or herself) in the company where the temptation to try heroin may be so overwhelming and tempting as to brook no refusal – with dire effects.

Hallucinogens: The hallucinogenic drugs include lysergic acid diethylamide (LSD as it is popularly known), dimethyltryptamine, mescaline, psilocybin and psilocin. They are a group of compounds that since ancient days American Indians have used as intoxicants to produce ecstatic states for religious occasions. LSD is the one most widely used today in western civilization. It produces distortion of perception, visual and emotional changes, emotionally charged fantasies that may induce extreme states of panic, feelings of omnipotence or bodily and mental dissolution, panic reactions or transcendental calm and psychotic or near-psychotic reactions.

The value of LSD in the field of treatment is still a matter of debate, but there seems little doubt that under skilled supervision, and used with the utmost caution and care, it can prove of value in the treatment of certain neuroses and phobic states. One experienced worker in this field has summed up the position as follows: 'One cannot emphasize too strongly the need for all LSD therapy to be carried out in a carefully controlled environment by trained staff working as a therapeutic team with their patients. If this is done, much can be achieved with a group of patients who often otherwise defy our therapeutic efforts: the phobic states, the sexual neuroses and some inadequate and neurotic psycopaths'.

Otherwise, *pace* Aldous Huxley, the propensities for evil in this group of drugs are such that there can be no questioning the ban on its use except by specified medical practitioners and psychiatrists. There is more than a suspicion that they can produce genetic damage.

Phencyclidine: Next to cannabis, phencyclidine is the most widely abused street drug in the USA. It is also known as PCP, angel dust, crystal, elephant and horse tranquillizer, killer weed, super weed, monkey dust, peace pill, goon, surfer and scuffle. It was originally introduced as an anaesthetic but withdrawn from use for this purpose because of the vivid dreams and hallucinations experienced by patients on coming round from anaesthesia. It is still used, however, as an animal anaesthetic. It is widely sold in combination with other drugs of abuse such as barbiturates, amphetamines, heroin and cocaine. It produces a state closely resembling schizophrenia (qv) which may persist for up to two weeks. In this state there is a feeling of sensory isolation and of depersonalization which can be terrifying to the individual in question, accompanied by hallucinations, predominantly of hearing. This is accompanied by aggressive behaviour, users feeling that they have superhuman strength and invulnerability. More cases of homicide and suicide are associated with PCP than with any other drug of abuse.

Amphetamines: These drugs were originally introduced as stimulants of the nervous system. It was then found that they inhibited appetite, and as a result they were used widely in the treatment of obesity. The first warning of the dangers of amphetamines was given by the finding that a disturbingly high number of housewives, who had originally been prescribed these drugs for obesity, were becoming dependent upon them as a means of keeping up their spirits and counteracting household blues. The next warning was the finding that a number of patients on amphtetamines were developing a psychosis, with ideas of persecution and hallucinations. Then, somewhere in the early 1960s, youngsters started taking them for the 'kicks' they obtained. Initially this reaction takes the form of euphoria (feeling pleased with oneself and the world), a tendency to talkativeness, and diminution of inhibitions. In due course, with larger doses, and especially if the drug is taken by injection rather than by mouth, restlessness develops, rapid, often slurred speech, irritability and anxiety, unsteadiness, dilatation of the pupils and dryness of the mouth. If this last item is relieved by alcohol the results can be catastrophic. The effects are heightened if, as tends to happen, the amphetamines are taken with other drugs, such as the barbiturates.

Barbiturates and tranquillizers: For the anxiety-ridden, immature, unstable, highly wrought individual the barbiturates and tranquillizers can prove such a boon and anchor amid the emotional storms of life that it is scarcely surprising that, having once sampled their efficiency, he or she is reluctant to dispense with their aid. Whether this is a true state of addiction, in the strict sense of the term, may be arguable, but certainly these members of the community become reliant, if not dependent, on them. This may be at least a partial explanation of the fact that between 1962 and 1968, in England and Wales, the number of National Health Service prescriptions for tranquillizers rose from 6·6 million to 16 million. By 1984 the number of prescriptions for hypnotics and tranquillisers had risen to 32,843,000. The number of prescriptions for barbiturates had fallen to 1,837,000. The fall in the number of prescriptions for barbiturates reflects the recognition by doctors of the dangerous potentialities of these compounds. It is now becoming increasingly recognised that dependance develops to the benzodiazepine tranquillisers and hopefully the number of prescriptions for these drugs will fall over the next few years. The disturbing development in recent years has been the increasing use of barbiturate-like drugs by the younger generation. These are often taken by injection, and usually in conjunction with other drugs such as the amphetamines, as in the notorious 'purple hearts'. A recent survey showed that 62 of 65 heroin addicts interviewed had taken barbiturates and 52 of these had injected the drug.

The main dangers of this group of drugs are threefold. In the first place, the individual may become so dependent on them that he, or she, refuses to go to bed at night without taking one or more tablets, even though the original cause of sleeplessness has been removed. Unless the dose has been carefully worked out, the individual may well waken up in the morning with the equivalent of a 'hangover' and find it difficult to 'come to' sufficiently to do an efficient day's work. The next stage is that the individual may start taking the prescribed tablet to cope with any problem that may crop up during the day. This, in turn, may lead to experimenting with other more dangerous drugs, such as the amphetamines, or even heroin.

Cocaine: The action of this drug is described under COCAINE. It is generally taken nasally or hypodermically by its addicts. A hypodermic dose of around 60 mg may produce after a few minutes a feeling of suffocation, anxiety and faintness, but this rapidly passes off and is followed by mental exhilaration, rapidity of thought, and a feeling of buoyancy. After a short time, however, this passes off, and as dose after dose is taken, a reaction of deeper and deeper depression ensues upon each. At the same time, dyspepsia, loss of appetite, restlessness, sleeplessness, forgetfulness and failure of the power to apply the mind to any task appear. Finally, the person may pass into a state of melancholia or mania. Marked physical deterioration, in the form of emaciation and digestive disorders, is also found. In the United Kingdom the number of known cocaine addicts has risen rapidly in recent years. Many of these use the drug in combination with heroin. This combination was introduced in London as a result of a mistaken belief on the part of some doctors that the combination was safer than either drug alone. In fact, the combination is much more dangerous and almost impossible to treat with any degree of success.

Inhalation drugs: These include benzenes, paint thinners, glue, amphetamines and ether. In some instances, as in the case of benzedrine inhalers, once widely prescribed for relieving the congestion in nasal catarrh, and of certain inhalers used by asthmatic subjects, the habit was acquired as a result of the inhaler being prescribed by a doctor for a perfectly legitimate purpose. The patient, however, derived so much pleasure and comfort from the inhaler that he found it increasingly difficult to dispense with it, even though there was no longer any physical need for it. Ether addiction is predominantly an occupational hazard of anaesthetists. Other anaesthetics, notably nitrous oxide, may have the same propensity, but ether seems to be the most dangerous in this respect. There is, however, some evidence that abuse of nitrous oxide may induce a condition comparable to subacute combined degeneration of the cord (qv).

Other drugs: These include caffeine, nicotine and aspirin. They also include many hypnotics, such as chloral hydrate and bromides, which are less of a problem today in view of their diminishing use. By and large this form of dependence seldom causes much trouble and can usually be controlled, with the possible exception of nicotine. (See also GLUE SNIFFING.)

Treatment: Psychic dependence occurs in all types of drug-dependency and is characterised by a psychological need to continue to take the drug, either to produce a feeling of pleasure or well-being or to avoid discomfort. Physical dependency is characterised by the development of specific physiological disturbances when the drug is withdrawn and by the relief of these withdrawal symptoms by the drug itself. Tolerance develops when, after repeated administration of certain drugs, the effect of the drug gradually diminishes and increasingly large doses are required to produce the same pharmacological effect. Drugs of abuse are classified according to whether they are mainly cerebral depressants, cerebral stimulants or hallucinogens. The cerebral depressants are mainly either narcotic analgesics or barbiturates.

The long-term treatment of opiate addicts in the UK is based on a drug dependency clinic. Oral methadone dispensed at these clinics is more effective than injected heroin in reducing doses for the majority of addicts but a significant minority illegally obtain a supply of heroin elsewhere. Therapeutic communities which rely on peer group confrontation to foster development of a sense of personal responsibility provide the ideal psychotherapeutic approach but obviously require an initial degree of commitment and motivation from the addict. With the stimulant drugs, such as cocaine, amphetamines, phenmetrazine, which produce marked psychological but not physical dependency, withdrawal can lead to rebound depression, irritability and profound fatigue. By withdrawing the stimulant drugs cautiously, these may be avoided but sometimes they require treatment in their own right. With the hallucinogens, of which LSD, psilocybin and mescaline are the main drugs, there is no physical dependency but they produce marked emotional change with ecstasy, anxiety and hallucinations.

The treatment of the 'bad trip' requires that the patient should be calmed down and told that he is experiencing a temporary adverse reaction to a drug and that the disturbing thoughts and sensations will gradually disappear. Tranquillisers will reduce agitation.

DRUG INTERACTIONS: Drugs in combination may cause serious adverse effects from which each individual drug in similar dosage is free when given separately. There may be a direct chemical or physical interaction such as the inactivation of heparin by protamine. One drug may alter the intestinal absorption of another. Calcium lactate reacts with phytic acid from vegetables. Tetracyclines chelate calcium, magnesium and iron salts with the formation of non-absorbed, pharmacologically inactive complexes. Calcium, aluminium, magnesium and iron salts also interfere with the absorption of tetracycline. Drugs may interact with each other by one drug displacing another from the plasma protein to which it is bound. Drugs such as warfarin are 99 per cent bound to plasma albumin, leaving only 1 per cent free to exert a pharmacological effect. The number of such binding sites is limited. If another drug that binds to the same site is given the warfarin will be displaced and an increased anti-coagulant effect will result.

One drug may accelerate the metabolism of another drug. This process is known as enzyme induction and hypnotics such as barbiturates and glutethimide, anticonvulsants such as phenytoin and carbamazepine, analgesics such as phenylbutazone, antibiotics such as rifampicin and griseofulvin, and diuretics such as spironolactone will induce the enzymes in the liver concerned with drug oxidation so that all drugs excreted in this way will be metabolised more quickly with a fall in the serum concentration. Drugs that metabolise by oxidation in the liver include tricyclic antidepressants, oral anticoagulants, phenothiazines and corticosteroids. An opposite effect may occur on occasions when one drug may inhibit the metabolism of another drug. The metabolism of the oral hypoglycaemic drugs tolbutamide and chlorpropamide is inhibited by phenylbutazone and dicoumarol. The metabolism of phenytoin is inhibited by the antituberculous drug isoniazide. The metabolism of the antidepressive nortriptyline is inhibited by perphenazine and haloperidol. The metabolism of the anticoagulant warfarin is inhibited by allopurinol and cimetidine.

Multiple prescribing should therefore be avoided whenever possible, especially in certain areas of prescribing in which drug interactions are known to be more likely to be dangerous. These areas are: (1) anticoagulant therapy; (2) cytotoxic therapy; (3) monoamine oxidase inhibitors; (4) antidiabetic drugs, and (5) digoxin.

DRUGS: The sale and supply of medicines are controlled by part III of the Medicines Act 1968, the underlying principle of which is that medicines should normally be sold under the supervision of a pharmacist, but it also enables the Health Ministers to modify the application of this principle. Thus, the Medicines (General Sale List) Order lists the medicines which can with reasonable safety be sold or supplied at non-pharmacy premises. These are the medicines where the hazard to health, the risk of misuse, or the need to take special precautions in handling is small, and where wider sale than in pharmacies would be a convenience to the purchaser. At the other end of the scale the Medicines (Prescription Only) Order specifies the medicines which may only be supplied in accordance with the prescription of a doctor, dentist or veterinarian. These are the medicines whose use in treatment needs to be supervised by a practitioner because their use involves a known or potential toxic hazard. In between these two categories are the medicines (unlisted) which can be sold only at pharmacies under the supervision of a pharmacist. Exemptions from the pharmacy sale restrictions are contained in the Medicines (Pharmacy and General Sale – Exemption) Order and the Medicines (Exemption from Restriction in the Retail Sale or Supply of Veterinary Drugs) Order. These include exemptions for particular products such as homoeopathic products; for professional groups, such as state registered chiropodists; and for agricultural merchants selling or supplying medicines to farmers. There is also an Order, the Medicines (Retail Sale or Supply of Herbal Remedies) Order, specifically relating to herbal remedies. (See also DOSAGE; PRESCRIPTION; SAFETY OF DRUGS.)

DRUGS IN PREGNANCY: Unnecessary drugs during pregnancy should be avoided because of the adverse effect of some drugs on the foetus which have no harmful effect on the mother. Drugs may pass through the placenta and damage the foetus because their pharmacological effects are enhanced as the enzyme systems responsible for their degradation are undeveloped in the foetus. Thus if the drug can pass through the placenta the pharmacological effect on the foetus may be great whilst that on the mother is minimal. Warfarin may thus induce foetal and placental haemorrhage and thiazide administration may produce thrombocytopenia in the new born. Many progestogens have androgenic side effects and their administration to a mother for the purpose of preventing recurrent abortion may produce virilisation of the female foetus. Tetracycline administered during the last trimester commonly stains the deciduous teeth of the child yellow.

The other dangers of administering drugs in pregnancy are the teratogenic effects. It is understandable that a drug may interfere with a mechanism essential for growth and result in arrested or distorted development of the foetus and yet cause no disturbance in the adult in whom these differentiation and organisation processes have ceased to be relevant. Thus the effect of a drug upon a foetus may differ qualitatively as well as quantitatively from its effect on the mother. The susceptibility of the embryo will depend on the stage of development it has reached when the drug is given. The stage of early differentiation, that is from the beginning of the third week to the end of the tenth week of pregnancy, is the time of greatest susceptibility. After this time the risk of congenital malformation from drug treatment is less although the death of the foetus can occur at any time.

DRUNKENNESS (see ALCOHOLISM, ACUTE and CHRONIC).

DUCT is the name applied to a passage leading from a gland into some hollow organ, or on to the surface of the body, by which the secretion of the gland is discharged: eg. the pancreatic duct and the bile duct opening into the duodenum, and the sweat ducts opening on the skin surface.

DUCTLESS GLAND is the term applied to any one of certain glands in the body the secretion of which goes directly into the blood stream and so is carried to different parts of the body. These glands – the pituitary, thyroid, parathyroid, adrenal and reproductive – are also known as the ENDOCRINE GLANDS (qv). Some glands may be both duct glands and ductless glands. For example, the pancreas manufactures a digestive juice which passes by a duct into the small intestine. It also manufactures, by means of special cells, a substance called insulin which passes straight into the blood.

DUCTUS ARTERIOSUS is the blood-vessel in the foetus through which blood passes from the pulmonary artery to the aorta, thereby by-passing the lungs, which do not function during intra-uterine life. (See CIRCULATION OF THE BLOOD.) The ductus normally ceases to function soon after birth and within a few weeks is converted into a fibrous cord. Occasionally this obliteration does not occur: a condition known as patent ductus arteriosus. This is one of the more common congenital defects of the heart, and one which responds particularly well to surgical treatment. Closure of the duct can also be achieved in some cases by the administration of indomethacin. (See HEART DISEASES.)

DUCTUS DEFERENS, or VAS DEFERENS, is the tube which carries spermatozoa from the epidydimis to the seminal vesicles. (See TESTICLE.)

DUMBNESS means an inability to pronounce the elementary sounds which make up words.

Varieties: The important classification of cases of deficient power of speech is into (*a*) those associated with deafness and (*b*) those in which hearing is good. In a case associated with deafness, the person may be dumb merely because he has been born deaf, and, having no knowledge of sound, cannot understand or make intelligible sounds, although provided with good voice mechanism; or a person who has lost his hearing by some disease in childhood may be unable to speak otherwise than as a child for the same reason. It is estimated that 1 per 1000 deaf children are so deaf that natural speech is impossible. When hearing is good, on the other hand, dumbness is due generally to some mental defect or sometimes to some failure in the organs of voice production.

Causes: Deafness is the most important cause, because the one most capable of treatment. Of those due to some congenital brain-deficiency, some arise in children of parents who were themselves deaf-mutes. Another class of cases, in which there is also mental deficiency, arises from brain disease, such as that due to syphilis. Those children who are mentally bright and whose hearing is good have occasionally some structural defect, such as tongue-tie or enlarged tonsils and adenoids in the throat, which allow of attempts at speaking but prevent proper formation of words. Dumbness is sometimes a hysterical manifestation. Lisping and lalling speech are slight forms of dumbness due to inefficient control of the voice mechanism, but can generally be cured by careful training. (See STAMMERING; VOICE.)

Treatment: A dumb child is cut off from other people and so cannot develop normally, unless adequately treated; a careful examination should be made of any child who does not speak by two years of age. Deafness is easily discovered by finding that the child pays no attention to noises made behind its back. Mental ability can be measured by special tests. Physical obstructions, like tongue-tie or large tonsils, should be removed if present.

Deaf-mutes may be trained to read the lips and throat movements of others by sight, and to use their powers of voice through a complicated process, which should begin about the age of six or seven. It is hard for adults to pick this up, and people who are to be instructed in this method should not learn the finger language first.

The training required for this 'oral' method is long, and, if the deaf person is to gain a modulated voice and a fair command of language, the constant attention of an expert tutor is necessary all through childhood and youth. In England and Wales a local education authority can compel a parent of any child of two years of age or over to submit the child for medical examination. If this shows that special educational treatment is required, the authority must provide such treatment. In the case of deaf-mutes, attendance is compulsory between the ages of 5 and 16.

Training in lip-reading should be started as soon as possible, and special educational methods should be begun as soon as possible after the age of two years.

DUODENAL ILEUS is the term applied to dilatation of the duodenum due to chronic obstruction of the duodenum, caused by an abnormal position of arteries in the region of the duodenum pressing on it.

DUODENAL ULCER has much in common with gastric ulcer. (See STOMACH, DISEASES OF.) The two together are known as peptic ulcers, and in recent years there has been a tendency for the two forms of ulceration to be regarded as modifications of one entity known as peptic ulcer, rather than as separate disease entities. Part of the reason for this is that, as increasingly detailed statistics have become available, it has become clear that the incidence of the disease (or diseases) has been changing over the last century. Be all that as it may, it is abundantly clear that, as one authority has expressed it, 'peptic ulcer in general is still a large health problem' in Britain, probably as many 'as one in ten of the population suffering at some time or other during his or her lifetime from ulcer-type dyspepsia'.

Duodenal ulcer is ten to fifteen times more common than gastric ulcer. The age incidence of the two forms of ulcer differs. Thus, duodenal ulcer occurs at any age from 20 years onwards, whereas gastric ulcer usually occurs after the age of 40. Duodenal ulcer is three times as common in men as in women; indeed, in some series the ratio between men and women is as high as ten. In gastric ulcer, on the other hand, the sex ratio is less than two men to one woman. Gastric ulcer is rare in women until after the menopause. Here it should be noted that these figures, and the whole of this section, are concerned with chronic peptic ulcer. It is such ulcers that are practically always referred to when mention is made of duodenal or gastric ulcer. Acute peptic ulcers are quite uncommon. Indeed, there is some evidence that they may be an entirely different disease from chronic peptic ulcers. This does not mean, however, that chronic peptic ulcers, whether duodenal or gastric, do not pass through stages when their manifestations can be justifiably described as acute. There is also a different social incidence between the two forms of ulcer. Duodenal ulcer is more common in the upper social classes, although it is to be found in all classes, but gastric ulcer is more common among the lower social classes. There is also a higher incidence of duodenal ulcer in individuals who belong to blood group O. (See BLOOD GROUPS.) Not the least interesting observation in the field of peptic ulcer is that the large increase in incidence since the turn of the century has been due to the increase in duodenal ulcers. There is some statistical evidence that this 'epidemic' is now on the wane, and that the incidence of duodenal ulcer in Britain is beginning to fall.

There is no general consensus of expert opinion as to the precise cause of peptic ulcers. What probably happens is that there is some abrasion, or break, in the lining membrane (or mucosa) of the stomach and/or duodenum, and that it is gradually eroded and deepened by the gastric juice. What is not known, however, is why this only occurs in some people. After all, the probability is that such abrasions occur in everyone of us at some time or other, but it is only in a minority that these develop into peptic ulcers. Equally puzzling is why the acid and pepsin in the gastric juice erode the stomach (or duodenum) lining downwards into the depth of the wall of the stomach (or duodenum), but does not erode, or digest, it all along the surface of the lining. Needless to say, all sorts of theories have been advanced to explain these discrepancies. None is proven, but some are probable, whilst others have practical implications. Thus, mental stress and strain are probably provocative factors, thus explaining the increased incidence of duodenal ulcer in managers and executives. Smoking seems to accentuate, if not cause, duodenal ulcer, and the drinking of alcohol is probably harmful. The apparent association with a given blood group, and the fact that relatives of a patient with a peptic ulcer are unduly likely to develop such an ulcer suggest that there is some constitutional factor.

Symptoms and signs: These are similar in some ways to those of gastric ulcer, but there are certain differences. The presenting symptom is pain in the middle of the upper part of the abdomen, or somewhat to the right. This tends to come on two or three hours after a meal, and to be relieved by taking food (eg. a glass of milk). It also tends to occur during the night. The pain varies in intensity, and, if not treated, may persist for up to an hour. The appetite is not usually affected, and, though the individual tends to remain thin, there is not usually much loss of weight. Vomiting is not common. When it does occur, it usually means that the ulcer is causing obstruction of the exit of the food from the stomach into the duodenum. The main finding on examination is tenderness over the area of pain, accompanied by stiffening, or guarding, of the overlying muscles. The diagnosis is clinched by the radiological demonstration of what is known as a 'niche' in the duodenum. This niche is the actual ulcer, and it is made visible by giving the individual some radio-opaque substance, such as barium sulphate, to swallow. This fills up the ulcer crater, which is then visible when an X-ray is taken, or when the duodenum is studied by fluoroscopy (qv). Direct visualisation of the ulcer by fibroscopy has become more popular over recent years. (See FIBEROPTIC ENDOSCOPY.) Another method of examination is gastric analysis. (See TEST MEAL.) In patients with duodenal ulcer this usually reveals a high gastric acidity.

As in the case of a gastric ulcer, the patient with a duodenal ulcer is liable to two complications: perforation of the ulcer, and haemorrhage (see HAEMATEMESIS). If the bleeding from the ulcer is slight, there may be no vomiting of blood (or haematemesis), the blood being passed down the gut. In the course of its passage through the gut it is chemically altered and becomes black in colour. Then, when it is finally passed in the stools, the stools are dark and shiny, or tarry, in appearance. (See MELAENA.)

Treatment consists basically of rest, a diet, and the administration of alkalis. In severe cases a period of rest in bed may be advisable. This in itself has a most beneficial effect. No complicated dietetic regime is called for nowadays. The basis of the diet is the avoidance of all condiments, a minimum of fried food, and something to eat every two hours. The rationale of this is to counteract the increased acidity of the gastric juice. In practice, two-hourly feeding means breakfast, lunch and dinner (or supper), with a glass of milk mid-morning, a snack in mid-afternoon and a snack the last thing at night on going to bed. The basis of the snacks should be milk or something milky. Strong tea and coffee should be avoided, as should smoking. Alcohol is better avoided, but a glass of wine with food will do no harm. There is a large range of alkalis to be chosen from, and the individual choice should be made in conjunction with the family doctor. The management of duodenal ulcers has ben revolutionised by the advent of the histamine receptor antagonists which inhibit gastric acid secretion and allow the ulcer to heal. Both cimetidine and rantidine reduce the hyperacidity of the gastric juice. If the ulcer does not respond to adequate medical treatment along these lines, or if it leads to obstruction of the pylorus (qv), then operation is called for. Operation is also indicated should perforation occur. A perforated duodenal (or gastric) ulcer is an emergency, and must be dealt with immediately. The majority of surgeons still favour immediate operation. Should a haemorrhage occur, the treatment depends upon its severity. As a rule, a blood transfusion is called for.

DUODENUM is the first part of the intestine immediately beyond the stomach, so named because its length is about twelve finger-breadths. (See INTESTINE.)

DUPUYTREN'S CONTRACTURE is a thickening and drawing together of the skin and the underlying tissues in the palm of the hand, which cause gradual and permanent bending of the fingers. The cause of the condition is not known. It is more common among white-collar workers than among manual labourers. The ring and little fingers are most often affected. It is treated in early cases by massage and the occasional wearing of a splint, but the only cure is by means of surgery: by dividing the fibrous bands beneath the skin.

DURA MATER is the outermost and strongest of the three membranes or meninges which envelop the brain and spinal cord. In it run vessels which nourish the inner surface of the skull. (See BRAIN.)

DWARF, or DWARFISM, is a term applied to under-development of the body. The causes are either developmental or due to food insufficient in quantity or unsuitable in quality, or to defects in some of the body secretions which can be corrected. The first-named group includes pituitary dwarfism, the subjects being very small people with normally proportioned parts, also achondroplasic dwarfs (see ACHONDROPLASIA) with large globular head and shortened limbs and stumpy fingers. It is now known that in a certain proportion of children of short stature this can be remedied by administration of the growth hormone of pituitary gland (qv), provided this is given at an early enough age. All children who by the age of 5 years are at least what is technically known as 'three standard deviations below the mean' should be referred for examination by specialists to determine whether or not their lack of height is due to lack of growth hormone and therefore likely to respond to treatment with the hormone. In the class of dwarfism which is partly curable, there are included cretins, whose want of growth in mind and body is attributable to a primary defect of the thyroid gland. (See CRETINISM.) In this class are also included various forms of defective growth associated with defects in the secretions of the digestive organs, especially the pancreas; this type of defect, often known as pancreatic infantilism, is mainly confined to a retardation of physical development, while the mental changes are little marked. Another form of dwarfism, associated with a deformity of the bones, is produced by rickets in early life, such persons showing high forehead, great bending of the leg bones, and deformity of the chest. (See RICKETS.)

DYNAMOMETER is an elliptical ring of steel to which is attached a dial and moving index. It is used to test the strength of the muscles of the forearm, being squeezed in the hand, and registering the pressure in pounds or kilograms.

DYS- is a prefix meaning difficult or painful.

DYSARTHRIA is a general term applied when weakness or inco-ordination of the speech musculature prevents clear pronunciation of words. The individual's speech may sound as if it is slurred or weak. It may be due to damage affecting the centres in the brain which control movements of the speech muscles or damage to the muscles themselves.

Examples of dysarthria may be found in stroke illness, cerebral palsy and the latter stages of Parkinson's disease, multiple sclerosis and motor neurone disease. Whatever the cause a speech therapist can assess the extent of the dysarthria and suggest exercises or an alternative means of communication.

DYSCHEZIA is constipation due to retention of faeces in the rectum. This retention is the outcome of irregular habits, which damp down the normal reflex causing defaecation.

DYSCRASIA means a diseased constitution. (See CONSTITUTION.)

DYSDIADOKOKINESIA means loss of the ability to perform rapid alternate movements, such as winding up a watch. It is a sign of a lesion in the cerebellum.

DYSENTERY, also called bloody flux, is an infectious disease with a local lesion in the form of inflammation and ulceration of the lower portion of the bowels. It occurs in two main forms: bacillary dysentery and amoebic dysentery.

BACILLARY DYSENTERY is found in practically every part of the world.

Cause: The disease may occur sporadically or in epidemics. The causative organism is the dysentery bacillus, or shigella as it is now known, of which there are several strains, named after their discoverers: Shiga, Flexner and Sonne. In England and Wales there were 5003 cases in 1984, with 43,285 in 1960. In Britain in the last two decades the proportion of cases in children has fallen and the seasonal incidence has also changed, with more cases occurring in the summer and autumn. These changes are accounted for by a decrease in the number of cases due to *Shigella sonnei* and an increase in the number of cases due to *Shigella flexneri* because of imported disease. The infection is spread by flies, by direct contact, or by pollution of the water by faeces from infected patients, which contain the bacillus. Epidemics are thus encouraged by overcrowding and insanitary conditions. In the East, uncooked vegetables, especially salads, are a potent source of infection, as are cooks and other foodhandlers who are carriers of the disease. The incubation period is 1 to 7 days. The severity of the disease depends partly upon the strain responsible for the infection. Thus, Shiga infections are usually severe, whilst, except in infants, Flexner and Sonne infections run a more benign course.

The dysentery bacilli affect mainly the large intestine. In mild cases there may be only a catarrh of the intestine with excessive mucoid excretion, whilst in severe cases there may be extensive ulceration involving practically the whole of the large intestine.

Symptoms: These vary from those of a mild attack of diarrhoea to those of an acute fulminating infection. The first symptoms usually consist of colicky pain in the abdomen followed by diarrhoea. There may also be nausea, aching pain in the limbs, and shivery feelings. There is always fever. The number of stools varies, but there may be as many as fifty daily in acute cases. The stools consist mainly of mucus and blood. The duration of the diarrhoea varies from a few days to a fortnight, depending upon the severity of the infection. Diagnosis is established by finding dysentery bacilli in the stools. Complications only occur in severe cases, and consist of perforation of the intestine and severe haemorrhage from the gut. At one time one of the killing diseases of the world, with mortality rates up to 50 per cent during epidemics, the outlook has been entirely altered by the introduction of the sulphonamides, but it is still a serious condition in young infants, old people and the malnourished.

Treatment: PREVENTIVE: This consists of adequate sanitation, the destruction of flies, careful disposal of all garbage, and careful protection of all food from flies. In addition, no carrier of dysentery bacilli should be allowed to handle food.

CURATIVE: Complete rest in bed is essential, and precautions must be taken to ensure that the stools are disposed of without any risk of their spreading the infection. For the first twenty-four hours only water is given. In the case of acutely ill babies or young children it may be necessary to give fluids intravenously, in the form, for example, of 4·3 per cent glucose in 1/5 normal saline, for the first twenty-four hours or so. This is gradually supplemented with milk, milk puddings, and chicken broth, but it is necessary for the diet to be kept light, and to contain as little residue as possible, until the diarrhoea has settled. Purgatives and laxatives are not given. The sheet-anchors of treatment are now the sulphonamides: usually phthalylsulphathiazole, succinylsulpha-thizole or sulphadimidine. Alternatively, neomycin may be used. If there is much abdominal pain, morphine may be given during the first day, but usually the application of heat in some form to the abdomen is sufficient.

AMOEBIC DYSENTERY is almost entirely confined to tropical and sub-tropical countries. Around 200 new cases occur annually in England and Wales.

Cause: The causative organism is the *Entamoeba histolytica.* Infection occurs as a result of food, eg. uncooked vegetables, or drinking water which has been contaminated either by a carrier of the disease or by flies. The amoebae settle in the wall of the large intestine, where they cause first of all inflammatory changes and then ulceration. These ulcers then tend to become infected with other organisms. From the ulcers the amoebae may spread through the portal vein, where they cause abscesses. An amoebic abscess of the liver is not infrequent. More rarely, the amoebae may spread elsewhere, eg. to the lungs or brain, and cause abscesses. In the latter it may cause meningitis (qv) or meningoencephalitis (qv). Occasionally a mass may be formed in the colon, known as an amoeboma.

Symptoms: These may appear within a week of infection or be delayed for months or even years. The onset of the disease is usually gradual, with the passage of several stools daily, which ultimately contain blood. Occasionally there may be an acute sudden onset as described for bacillary dysentery. Even in the cases with gradual onset there is loss of weight, with dyspepsia and anaemia. Complications which may occur include perforation of the intestine, haemorrhage from the gut, and abscess formation in the liver, brain, bones or testes. The condition is liable to run a chronic course. Any individual who has been in the tropics and who complains of abdominal pain and dyspepsia should have the stools examined for the presence of *Entamoeba histolytica*, even though there is no history of dysentery.

Treatment: PREVENTIVE: This consists of the protection of food from flies, the avoidance of contamination of water and uncooked vegetables, and steps to ensure that those handling food are not carriers of the amoeba.

CURATIVE: Emetine, for long the great standby in the treatment of amoebic dysentery, has now been largely replaced by the nitroimidazole group of drugs. These include metronidazole, tinidazole, and ornidazole. While these drugs are being taken alcoholic drinks are forbidden as these may produce a psychotic state. A course of one or other of these drugs is followed by a course of diloxamide furoate. In severe cases these drugs may be supplemented with tetracycline. Cure is assessed by the disappearance of symptoms, the return of normal stools and the absence of parasites from the stools on three separate occasions. If an amoebic abscess has formed in the liver this is treated by aspiration following a course of one of the nitroimidazole group of drugs. Aspiration is performed through a wide-bore needle under local anaesthesia.

DYSIDROSIS means disturbance of sweat secretion.

DYSLEXIA is difficulty in reading or learning to read. It is always accompanied by difficulty in writing and particularly by difficulties in spelling correctly. It is a condition which is attracting increasing attention, particularly the form known as specific dyslexia. This is the name given to difficulties in learning to read and write which affect a minority of children exposed to normal educational processes who do not show backwardness in other school subjects. Four per cent of children are said to be affected by it in a severe form, and it is three times more common in boys than in girls.

Parents of such children would be well advised to get in touch with the British Dyslexia Association, Church Lane, Peppard, Oxfordshire RG9 5JN (049 17 699).

DYSMENORRHOEA means painful menstruation. (See MENSTRUATION.)

DYSPAREUNIA means painful or difficult coitus.

DYSPEPSIA is merely another, somewhat old-fashioned, name for indigestion. In other words, it describes a condition in which the individual is complaining of pain or discomfort, usually in the upper part of the abdomen or the lower part of the front of the chest, which may, or may not, be associated with other disturbances such as heartburn (qv), flatulence (qv), or nausea (qv). It may be due to a multiplicity of causes, such as gastritis, peptic ulcer, hiatus hernia, cancer of the stomach, all of which involve the stomach, and all of which are discussed in the appropriate section. In some it may be due to disease of the gall-bladder or pancreas, or it may be due to disease in some other part of the body, such as heart failure, uraemia, or diabetes mellitus. In all of these conditions the relief of the dyspepsia is dependent upon the treatment of the underlying cause.

Nervous dyspepsia: There is one form of dyspepsia, in which the name is still retained, and that is nervous dyspepsia. This is the form of indigestion that is brought on by psychological or emotional stress. It occurs in the anxious, worrying, highly strung, 'nervous' type of individual. Whenever such individuals get worked up, become unduly tense or excitable, and find life is proving too complicated whether this be due to difficult conditions in the home or at work, illness or death in the family, they develop rather vague, but nevertheless disturbing signs of indigestion. These may take the form of loss of appetite, pain, flatulence or heartburn. Although in some the manifestations of indigestion may be constant, in others – and these constitute the majority – they vary from time to time. Once the stress or strain is relieved or eased, the indigestion disappears, and the individual is able to eat a normal diet –and enjoy it. Among the features characteristic of this form of dyspepsia are the tendency for it to be accompanied by attacks of sweating, weakness, palpitations, a feeling of tenseness, and insomnia. The inability to sleep is not due to the indigestion, which as a rule does not tend to be troublesome at night. Rather is the insomnia due to the stress or strain that is responsible for the dyspepsia.

Treatment is based upon finding the cause of the emotional or psychological disturbance and trying to alleviate this. In some this may be difficult as it is basically the nature of the individual's make-up and cannot be changed. These are the unfortunates of this world who are quite convinced that they have a 'weak' or 'delicate' stomach. Even they, however, benefit if they can be reassured that there is no 'organic' cause for their dyspepsia. If the individual is suffering from an exceptional spell of stress or strain, a holiday may do a world of good. No dietetic restrictions are necessary, except that the diet should be nutritious, attractive and reasonably bland. Excessive smoking, often a feature of these cases, should be curtailed, and, particularly in the case of the harassed business person, a restriction on 'homework' and work at weekends should be imposed.

DYSPHAGIA is the medical term for difficulty in swallowing.

DYSPHASIA is the term used to describe the difficulties in understanding language and in self-expression, most frequently after stroke (see STROKE), or other brain damage. When there is a total loss in the ability to communicate through speech or writing, it is known as *global aphasia*. Many more individuals have a partial understanding of what is said to them. They are also able to put their own thoughts into words to some extent. The general term for this less severe condition is *dysphasia*. Individuals vary widely, but in general there are two main types of dysphasia. Some people may have a good understanding of spoken language but have difficulty in self-expression; this is called *non-fluent dysphasia*. Others may have a very poor ability to understand speech, but will have a considerable spoken output consisting of jargon words; this is known as *fluent dysphasia*. Similar difficulties may occur with reading, and this is called *dyslexia* (a term more commonly encountered in the different context of children's reading disability). Adults who have suffered a stroke or another form of brain damage may also have difficulty in writing, or *dysgraphia*. The speech therapist can assess the finer diagnostic points. (See SPEECH THERAPY.)

No case is too severe or too mild to be referred to a speech therapist for an assessment. The victim, his relatives and other visitors may be anxious about the effects of the stroke and may find it helpful to have the details of the dysphasic problem explained to them. The speech therapist can help them adjust to the effects of the stroke on communication. Treatment may be conducted on an individual or group basis according to the needs of the individual. It is important for people who come into contact with the dysphasic person to treat him just as they would have done before the stroke: to be patient rather than patronizing.

Dysphasia may come on suddenly and last only for a few hours or days, being due to a temporary block in the circulation of blood to the brain. The effects may be permanent, but although the individual may have difficulty in understanding language and expressing himself, he will be quite aware of his surroundings and may be very frustrated by his inability to communicate with others.

Further information may be obtained from Action for Dysphasic Adults, 37 Royal Street, London SE1 7LN; and the Chest Heart and Stroke Association, Tavistock House North, Tavistock Square, WC1H 9JE (01-387 3012).

DYSPNOEA means difficulty in breathing (see BREATHLESSNESS; ORTHOPNOEA).

DYSTOCIA means slow or painful birth of a child.

DYSTONIA refers to a type of involuntary movement characterized by a sustained muscle contraction, frequently causing twisting and repetitive movements or abnormal postures, and caused by inappropriate instructions from the brain. It is sometimes called torsion spasm, and may be synonymous with athetosis when the extremities are involved. Often the condition is of unknown cause (idiopathic), but an inherited predisposition is increasingly recognized among some cases. Others may be associated with known pathology of the brain such as cerebral palsy or Wilson's disease. The presentation of dystonia may be focal (usually in adults) causing blepharospasm (forceful eye closure), oromandibular dystonia (spasms of the tongue and jaw), cranial dystonia/Meige syndrome/Brueghel's syndrome (eyes and jaw both involved), spastic or spasmodic dysphonia/laryngeal dystonia (strained or whispering speech), spasmodic dysphagia (difficulty swallowing), spasmodic torti/latero/ante/retrocollis (rotation, sideways, forward or backward tilting of the neck), dystonic writer's cramp or axial dystonia (spasms deviating the torso). Foot dystonia occurs almost exclusively in children and adolescents. In adults, the condition usually remains focal or involves at most an adjacent body part. In children, it may spread to become generalized. The condition has always been considered rare, but commonly is either not diagnosed or mistakenly thought to be of psychological origin. It may, in fact, be half as common as multiple sclerosis. Similar features can occur in some subjects treated with major tranquillizing drugs, in whom a predisposition to develop dystonia may be present.

DYSTROPHY means defective or faulty nutrition, and is a term generally applied to some developmental change in the muscles occurring independently of the nervous system. The best-known forms are those known as *progressive muscular dystrophy*, in which groups of muscles, especially those of the calves and buttocks, undergo a fatty degeneration associated with increase in size but weakness in power; and *adiposogenital dystrophy* associated with defect of the pituitary gland. (See MYOPATHY.)

DYSURIA means difficulty or pain in urination.

E

E ADDITIVES (see ADULTERATION OF FOOD).

EAR: The ear is concerned with two functions. The more evident is that of the sense of hearing; the other is the sense of equilibration and of motion. The organ is divided into three parts: (*a*) the external ear, consisting of the auricle on the surface of the head, and the tube which leads inwards to the drum; (*b*) the middle ear, separated from the former by the tympanic membrane or drum, and from the internal ear by two other membranes, but communicating with the throat by the Eustachian tube; and (*c*) the internal ear, comprising the complicated labyrinth from which runs the vestibulocochlear nerve into the brain.

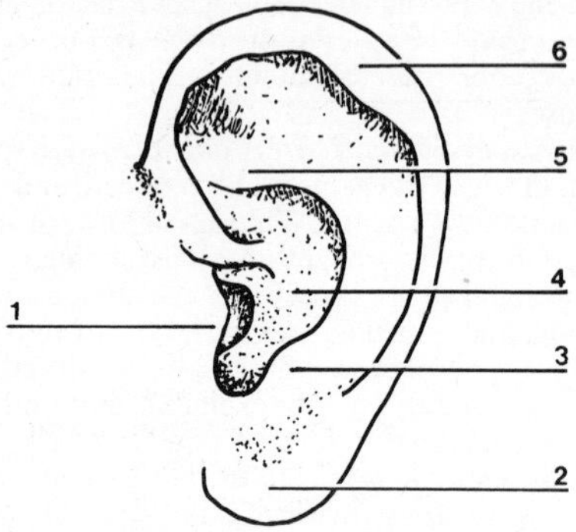

1 tragus
2 lobule
3 antitragus
4 concha
5 antihelix
6 helix

The auricle.

External ear: The auricle or pinna, shaped in man something like a crumpled-up funnel, is not essential to the sense of hearing, although in animals it appears to play an important part. It consists of a framework of elastic cartilage covered by skin, the lobule at the lower end being a small mass of fat. From the bottom of the concha the external auditory (or acoustic) meatus runs inwards for 25 mm (1 inch), to end blindly at the drum. This passage is short in young children, in whom the drum is almost at the surface, and it lengthens as the skull bones develop. The outer half of the passage is surrounded by cartilage, lined by skin, on which are placed fine hairs pointing outwards, and glands secreting a small amount of wax. In the inner half, the skin is smooth and lies directly upon the temporal bone, in the substance of which the whole hearing apparatus is enclosed. The two parts meet at a slight angle, so as to give the whole passage a curve, which can be straightened by pulling the auricle upwards and backwards, when the drum can often be clearly seen by a good light.

Middle ear: The tympanic membrane, forming the drum, is stretched completely across the end of the passage, being placed rather

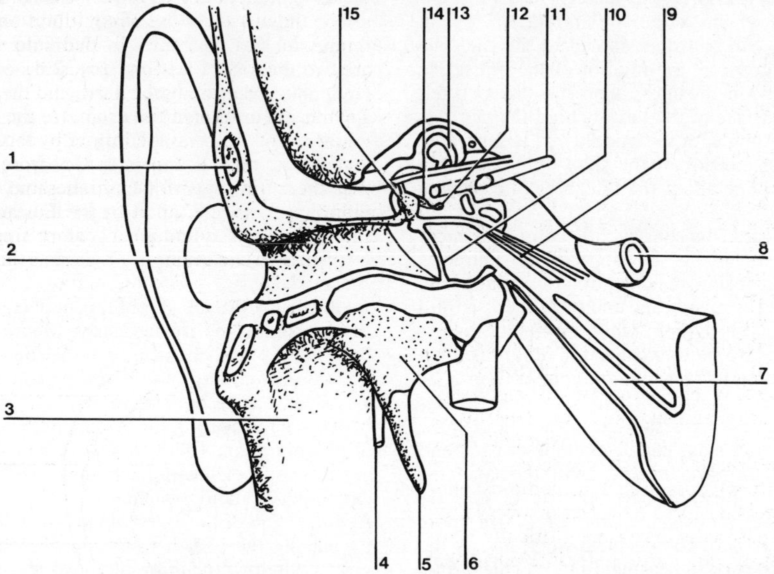

1 cartilage of auricle
2 external acoustic meatus
3 mastoid process
4 facial nerve
5 styloid process
6 sheath of styloid process
7 auditory tube
8 internal cartoid artery
9 tensor tympani
10 tympanic membrane
11 facial nerve
12 stapes
13 superior semicircular duct
14 incus
15 head of malleus

The external and middle portions of the right ear from the front.

obliquely, so that it makes an angle of about 60° with the floor. It is about 8 mm (one-third of an inch) across, very thin, and white or pale pink in colour, so that it is partly transparent, and some of the contents of the middle ear shine through it. From this description it can be readily understood how easily it is torn, and how dangerous are blows on the side of the head, and rough manipulations to remove wax. The cavity of the middle ear is about 8 mm (one-third of an inch) wide and 4 mm (one-sixth of an inch) in depth from the tympanic membrane to the inner wall of bone. Although important structures, like the facial nerve which runs down behind it, lie close around, its only important contents are three small bones, the malleus (hammer), incus (anvil), and stapes (stirrup), collectively known as the auditory ossicles, with two minute muscles which regulate their movements, and the chorda tympani nerve which runs across the cavity. The auditory ossicles are of great importance. The malleus has a long spicule of bone, the handle, embedded in the substance of the drum, while its head is in contact with the incus. The incus, suspended by one process of bone, has another affixed to the stapes, and the latter fits, by what would in a real stirrup be the footpiece, into one (fenestra vestibuli) of the two openings which lead through the inner wall of the middle ear into the internal ear. Accordingly these three bones form a chain across the middle ear, connecting the drum with the internal ear. Their function is to convert the air-waves, which strike upon the drum, into mechanical movements which can affect the fluid in the inner ear, because air-waves produce little effect upon fluid directly.

The middle ear has two connections which are of great importance as regards disease: in front, it communicates by a passage 37 mm (1½ inches) long, the Eustachian (or auditory) tube, with the upper part of the throat, behind the nose; behind and above, it opens into a cavity known as the mastoid antrum. The Eustachian tube admits air from the throat, and so keeps the pressure on both sides of the drum fairly equal. Serious deafness is produced by its closure, and it also, unfortunately, forms a channel by which acute inflammation, as in measles, can and does spread to the ear. The antrum occupies the interior of the projecting mass of bone, the mastoid process, which is felt on the surface of the head behind the ear; this cavity, along with the middle ear, is separated from the interior of the skull only by a thin plate of bone about the thickness of a playing card.

Internal ear: This consists of a complex system of hollows in the substance of the temporal bone enclosing a membranous duplicate. Between the membrane and the bone is a fluid known as perilymph, while the membrane is distended by another collection of fluid known as endolymph. This membranous labyrinth, as it is called, consists of two parts. The hinder part, comprising a sac, the utricle, and three short semicircular canals opening at each end into it, is the part concerned with the balancing sense; the forward part consists of another small bag, the saccule, and of a still more important part, the cochlear duct, and is the part concerned in hearing. In the cochlear duct is placed the spiral organ of Corti, on which the sound-waves are finally received and by which the sounds are communicated to the cochlear nerve, a branch of the vestibulocochlear nerve, which ends in filaments to this organ of Corti. The essential parts in the organ of Corti are a double row of rods and several rows of cells furnished with fine hairs of varying length. Different musical notes are perhaps appreciated by different rods and hair cells.

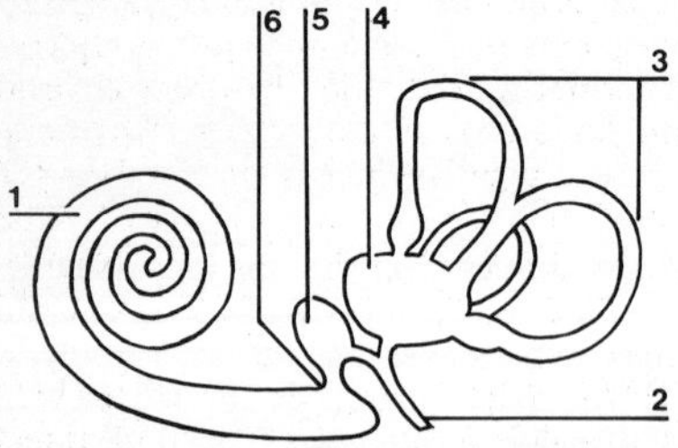

1 cochlear duct
2 ductus endolymphaticus
3 semicircular canals
4 utricle
5 saccule
6 ductus reuniens

The membranous labyrinth.

The act of hearing: When sound-waves in the air reach the ear, the drum is alternately pressed in and pulled out, in consequence of which a to-and-fro movement is communicated to the chain of ossicles. The foot of the stapes communicates these movements to the perilymph. Finally these motions reach the delicate filaments placed in the organ of Corti, and so affect the nerve of hearing, which conveys impressions to the centre in the brain. There are two theories of hearing. The first is that of Helmholtz, who compared the organ of Corti to a piano and presumed that each sound caused a vibration of a corresponding part of Corti's organ. The second and later theory assumes that the entire organ of Corti is thrown into vibration by sounds, and that the nature of the sound is analysed and perceived by the hearing-centre in the brain.

EAR, DISEASES OF: Troubles connected with the ear should be treated early. Mention has been made of the importance of the connection between throat and middle ear by way of the Eustachian tube, both as regards the maintenance of good hearing and as regards the spread of inflammation. There are several simple procedures connected with the management of the ear which demand explanation.

Examination of the external ear is carried out by placing the person's head in a good light near a window, inclining the head away from the window a little, pulling the auricle upwards and backwards, and if a conical speculum is at hand, introducing this with a gentle screwing movement. The drum and deeper part of the external ear may then be viewed. If available, an electric auriscope is a much more satisfactory means of carrying out the examination.

Syringing is done with a large-sized glass or metal syringe provided with a short blunt point (not longer than 25 mm (1 inch), so that no damage to the drum can result). The auricle is pulled gently up and back, while a steady stream from the syringe is directed along the upper wall, and flows out along the lower one. In syringing the ear of a child the point of the syringe should not be inserted within the shallow passage at all.

Inflation of the middle ear is performed for cases in which the Eustachian tube is partly blocked and the drum indrawn. A catheter is passed along the floor of the nose into the opening of the Eustachian tube in the throat, and forcible inflation made through this by means of a rubber bag (Politzer's bag). Or the bag is used to blow up one nostril, the other being closed, while the Eustachian tube is kept open by one of the following devices. The person swallows a mouthful of water, or pronounces some guttural, such as 'Huck', so as to raise the soft palate and close the opening between the nose and throat; and at this moment the bag is suddenly squeezed. The Eustachian tube may also be inflated by forcibly expelling air from the chest while the mouth and nose are closed. The fact of whether air enters the middle ear becomes plain to the person himself by a click followed by a slight ringing in the ear, and often by improved hearing, as so many people nowadays have learned from experience by clearing their ears while coming in to land in an aircraft. *Tuning-fork test* is used to test the internal ear. When a vibrating fork is placed on the centre of the forehead it is heard equally in both ears, the sound being conducted through the bones of the head. If one ear is closed, it is heard better in that ear. Accordingly, if one ear is deaf, and the sound of the fork placed on the forehead is heard better in that ear, the deafness is due to middle ear disease. While if the ear is deaf to the fork when placed on the forehead, as well as when held near the ear, the internal ear or nerve mechanism is at fault.

General symptoms: The following are some of the chief symptoms of ear disease:

DEAFNESS (see DEAFNESS).

EARACHE is most commonly due to acute inflammation in the middle ear, but may also be due to chronic inflammation, or to acute inflammation of the external ear, boils, eczema, wax, or neuralgia affecting the outer ear. Pain in this region may also be caused by carious teeth. The treatment varies with the cause, but the pain may generally be relieved to some extent by applying hot flannel or a hot-water bag to the side of the head. For subsequent treatment see later in this section.

RINGING in the ear, or TINNITUS, is sometimes a very annoying symptom. It may take various forms, but is in general accompanied by catarrh of some part of the ear. Pulsating or throbbing in the ear is sometimes due to bloodlessness, or to large doses of quinine or sodium salicylate, and passes off as the bloodlessness is treated or the drugs producing it are discontinued. Blowing, hissing, and whistling noises, like those made by an escape of steam or by a boiling kettle, are the most common and most annoying forms. Usually they are associated with middle-ear catarrh, but they are often associated with high blood-pressure, and diminish as the general disease is treated. Accompanied by deafness, ringing is not infrequently due to wax. Musical tinnitus sometimes occurs, in which the sound of bells, or of short passages of music, is repeated constantly. It is due to similar causes. A high crescendo musical note, followed by giddiness, is one of the symptoms of Menière's disease (qv).

DISCHARGE from the ear may arise in the external ear as the result of eczema, boils, or the irritation caused by a plug of wax or foreign body, but, in the absence of these, comes in the great majority of cases from suppuration in the middle ear through a perforation in the drum. There are two common fallacies regarding this condition. One is that a discharge from the ear is a trifling thing. In reality the presence of suppuration is accompanied usually by increasing deafness, and is attended always by the risk of an abscess in the mastoid antrum, or even within the skull. The other fallacy is that a perforation in the drum necessarily entails great deafness. As a matter of fact, unless the perforation is so large as to interfere with the tension of the drum, it causes little interference with hearing, the real cause of deafness in suppurative middle-ear disease being adhesions which bind down the ossicles and prevent their movements. Treatment depends upon whether the cause of the discharge is in the outer or the middle ear.

OTITIS EXTERNA, or infection of the outer ear, is commonest in tropical countries with a high humidity. Hence the names of 'Singapore ear' and 'Hong Kong ear' that it has been given. It is not uncommon, however, in Britain. Many factors may cause it, including scratching or poking the ears with dirty fingers or with contaminated objects. Badly fitting and infrequently cleaned hearing-aid earpieces are another cause. In some it is the result of spread of infection from the middle ear, whilst quite a number of cases are allergic in origin, the allergic factor often being some ear-drops that have been prescribed in the past. It may be due to a boil, which is discussed elsewhere in this section. It manifests itself by pain in the ear accompanied by a discharge. There is usually also a considerable degree of itching. Deafness develops if the discharge from the infection blocks the meatus.

Treatment consists of careful syringing out of the meatus with normal saline (see ISOTONIC) at a temperature of 38°C, followed by careful packing of the external ear with some soothing lotion, such as 10 per cent ichthammol in glycerin, or 8 per cent aluminium acetate. Once the acute phase is over, the meatus may be painted with an alcoholic solution of gentian violet or crystal violet. For the pain in the initial stages hot packs or hot applications may be applied to the ear or, simpler and often just as effective, a rubber hot-water bottle. Ear-drops are seldom used nowadays. If the itching is particularly intense at night – which it tends to be – it may be advisable to cover the ear with a gauze bandage, or to wear cotton gloves, to prevent scratching, which may well make the condition worse.

OTITIS MEDIA, or infection of the middle ear, usually occurs as a result of infection spreading up the Eustachian tubes from the nose, throat or one of the sinuses. In other words, it may occur as a complication of a cold, tonsillitis, sinusitis or adenoids. It is above all a disease of children: 1·5 million cases occur every year in Britain. It is not uncommon at the beginning of the swimming season every year, due to the fact that diving and underwater swimming force infected secretions from the nose or throat up through the Eustachian tube into the middle ear. This is most likely to occur after jumping into swimming pools without holding the nose. Pain is always present and, particularly in acute cases of sudden onset, it may be intense and throbbing or sharp in character. It is accompanied by deafness and often tinnitus (qv), and the temperature rises. In infants, crying, for which there is no obvious cause, may be the only sign that something is wrong, though this is usually accompanied by some localizing manifestation such as shaking of the head or the infant putting his hand to the ear. Examination of the ear is difficult because it is so tender but when it is carried out it reveals redness, and sometimes bulging, of the ear drum. In the early stages there is no discharge, but in the later stages there may be a discharge from perforation of the ear drum as a result of the pressure created in the middle ear by the accumulated pus.

Treatment consists of the immediate administration of an antibiotic, and the one of choice is usually one of the penicillins: eg. amoxycillin. While it is taking effect the pain may be eased by the use of heat in the form of a rubber hot-water bottle. If the antibiotic does not quickly bring relief, then it may be necessary to perform the minor operation of myringotomy, or incising the ear drum. This gives immediate relief in those cases in which the middle ear is full of pus; the moment the ear drum is incised, the pus pours out, and the pressure in the middle ear, which has been causing the pain, is relieved. The main complication of otitis media is mastoiditis, which is discussed later in this section. It cannot be too strongly emphasized that, if otitis media is treated immediately with ample doses of the appropriate antibiotic, the chances of any permanent damage to the ear or to hearing is reduced to a negligible degree, as is the risk of any complications such as mastoiditis.

SECRETORY OTITIS MEDIA, or GLUE EAR, is a form of otitis that has come to the fore as the commonest inflammatory condition of the middle ear in children, and one of the commonest causes of the form of deafness known as conduction deafness. (See DEAFNESS.) It is due to a persisting sticky (hence the name of 'glue ear') exudation in the middle ear. It is often associated with enlarged adenoids. If removal of these does not clear the condition, further treatment is needed. If this fails, in bad cases it may be necessary to remove the ossicles and the remains of the ear drum, and so to convert the middle ear into a simple cavity, which can be easily kept clear of infection.

OTOMYCOSIS is infection of the external ear by fungi such as Aspergillus (qv) or Candida (qv). It is a common condition in tropical and subtropical countries, but is occurring more often in Britain. It is characterized by persisting irritation in the ear and rapid reaccumulation of discharged material in spite of this being repeatedly removed. Treatment consists of cleansing of the external ear by dry mopping, and the application of an anti-fungal agent such as nystatin (qv). Drops of 2 per cent salicylic acid in alcohol are sometimes helpful.

WAX in the ear is the commonest cause of deafness, sometimes even of several years' standing. It is removed by syringing with warm water (37°C) containing two teaspoonfuls of baking soda to a tumblerful of water. If the wax is very hard it should be softened by making the person lie down on his side for half an hour with the affected ear upwards, into which is poured some of this solution, or a few drops of warm olive or castor oil. At the end of half-an-hour the syringing is repeated. In some cases it may be necessary to insert the drops several nights running in order to soften the wax sufficiently. If there is a perforation of the drum, the removal of wax should only be carried out by a specialist.

FOREIGN BODIES, such as peas, gravel, beads or bits of rubber, are often pushed by children into the ear, and are extremely difficult to remove. No attempt to remove such a foreign body should be made until it is known whether it is vegetable in nature (eg. a pea) or not. The reason for this is that syringing causes a pea to swell up or to become wedged in the ear, difficult to remove and causing exquisite pain. Non-vegetable foreign bodies such as beads, can be removed by syringing or forceps. No attempt should be made by unskilful persons with hairpins, bent wires, or the like, to remove the object, which is apt by such means to be pushed through the ear-drum.

BOILS in the skin lining the outer ear give rise to intense pain. This pain is much relieved by packing the ear lightly with a piece of gauze dipped in a 10 per cent solution of ichthammol glycerin, or in 8 per cent aluminium acetate. Relief is also gained by applying heat to the ear by means of a rubber hot-water bottle. The essential of treatment, however, is a five-day course of penicillin given intramuscularly.

ECZEMA, consisting of a cracked condition of the skin in the ear, with watery discharge and intense irritation, is common, as an acute affection in infants, and as a chronic one in gouty and rheumatic adults and as a sequel to, or accompaniment of, chronic otitis externa. In children, syringing with Goulard's water affords relief. In adults, weak nitrate of mercury ointment, or tar ointment applied several times daily, does good.

TUMOURS in the ear are mostly either outgrowths from the surrounding bone or soft polypi. The former may block the passage and interfere with hearing, but have often a narrow neck, so that they can be easily removed. Polypi usually develop as a result of the irritation set up by a chronic discharge, and shrivel up as the discharge is cured, though a large one may have to be removed in order to get to the drum.

MASTOIDITIS is a serious complication of inflammation in the ear, the incidence of which has been dramatically reduced by the introduction of the sulphonamides and penicillin.

The mastoid antrum and its connection with the middle ear have been mentioned under EAR. As a rule, inflammation in this cavity arises by direct spread of a long-standing suppuration from the middle ear, sometimes in consequence of neglect to keep the ear clean and prevent discharge from accumulating. The signs of this condition include swelling and tenderness of the skin behind the ear, redness and swelling inside the ear, pain in the side of the head, feverishness, and a discharge from the ear. Current expert opinion is divided as to the best method of treatment: whether this should be by antibiotics, or by antibiotics plus operation. On the whole, the majority opinion today probably is to reserve operation for those cases which do not respond to a full course of penicillin.

EBOLA VIRUS DISEASE is another name for VIRAL HAEMORRHAGIC FEVER (qv).

EBURNATION is a process of hardening and polishing which takes place at the ends of bones, giving them an ivory-like appearance. It is caused by the wearing away, in consequence of osteoarthrosis, of the smooth plates of cartilage which in health cover the ends of the bones.

ECBOLICS are drugs which cause contraction of the womb, such as ergot.

ECCHYMOSIS means the discoloured patch resulting from escape of blood into the tissues just under the skin, often from bruising.

ECHINOCOCCUS is the immature form of a small tapeworm, *Taeniaechinococcus*, found in dogs, wolves, and jackals from which human beings become infected, so that they harbour the immature parasite in the form known as hydatid cyst. (See TAENIASIS.)

ECHOCARDIOGRAPHY is the use of ultrasonics (qv) for the purpose of examining the heart. By thus recording the echo (hence the name) from the heart of ultra-sound waves it is possible to study, for example, the movements of the heart valves (see HEART), as well as the state of the interior of the heart.

ECHOLALIA is the meaningless repetition, by a person suffering from mental degeneration, of words and phrases addressed to him.

ECHOVIRUSES, of which there are more than 30 known types, occur in all parts of the world. Their full name is Enteric Cytopathogenic Human Orphan (hence the abbreviation, ECHO). They owe their cumbersome full name to the fact that they were originally found in the stools of children without disease. Practically all of them, however, have now been identified with definite diseases. They are more common in children than in adults, and have been responsible for outbreaks of meningitis, common-cold-like illnesses, gastro-intestinal infections, and infections of the respiratory tract. They are particularly dangerous when they infect premature infants, and there have been several outbreaks of such infection in neonatal units, in which premature infants and other seriously ill small babies are nursed. The virus is introduced to such units by mothers, staff and visitors who are unaware that they are carriers of the virus.

ECLAMPSIA is the name applied to convulsions arising in pregnancy. This condition is said to occur in around 50 out of every 100,000 cases of pregnancy. It occurs especially in the later months and at the time of delivery, but a certain proportion of cases are manifest only after delivery has taken place. The cause of the condition is not known. In practically all cases the kidneys are profoundly affected.

Symptoms: There are several warning symptoms, such as dizziness, headache, vomiting, and the secretion of urine which is found to contain albumin. These symptoms may be present for some days or weeks before the seizure takes place. The seizure consists of rigidity of the body, with unconsciousness, followed by twitching in the face and limbs lasting for one or two minutes and then passing into a state of deep unconsciousness with stertorous breathing. In mild cases there are a few fits at long intervals and the patient recovers consciousness between them, but in severer cases the fits succeed one another so rapidly that there is no appreciable interval. In cases which progress to a fatal termination, the pulse and temperature rise, and cerebral haemorrhage, uraemia or pneumonia may supervene, or the breathing may gradually cease. It accounts for one in 12 of all maternal deaths. Among 43 cases of eclampsia delivered in Cardiff maternity units during 1969–74, none of the mothers died, but 10 of the 47 babies were lost.

Treatment: The treatment of the seizures is that generally applicable to convulsions of any kind, morphine and chloral being especially used as sedatives. This is usually supplemented with thiopentone sodium (qv) given intravenously. Alternatively a combination of chlorpromazine (qv) and pethidine (qv) may be used. Some obstetricians recommend controlling the initial fit by the inhalation of chloroform, and then switching on to the other drugs mentioned. Magnesium sulphate given intramuscularly sometimes helps to control the fits.

A common presentation of eclampsia is an epileptic fit in the home. The patient should be turned on her side and the airway cleared. An intravenous injection of morphine should be given and the Flying Squad called for urgent hospital admission. The most effective drugs to control eclampsia are intravenous diazepam given slowly or chlormethiazole (Heminevrin) intravenously, slowly. When the patient is in hospital she should be kept quiet as any stimulus, be it auditory, visual or tactile, may provoke a further epileptiform convulsion. The hypertension should be controlled and urgent Caesarean section undertaken.

ECSTASY is a term applied to a morbid mental condition in which the mind is entirely absorbed in the contemplation of one dominant idea or object, and loses for the time its normal self-control. This condition usually presents itself as a kind of temporary religious insanity, and has frequently appeared as an epidemic.

ECTHYMA is the term applied to a pustular eruption accompanied by surrounding inflammation. The pustules burst and discharge, leaving pigmented scars.

ECTO- is a prefix meaning on the outside.

ECTOPIC means out of the usual place. For example, in congenital displacement of the heart outside the thoracic cavity it is said to be ectopic, while an 'ectopic gestation' means a pregnancy outside of the womb.

ECTROMELIA means the absence of a limb or limbs, from congenital causes.

ECTROPION (see EYE, DISEASE AND INJURIES OF).

ECZEMA is a term that trips much too lightly off the tongue of doctors and patients alike. So much so that it is sometimes difficult to know what exactly a dermatologist (a skin specialist) means by the term. The confusion is not alleviated when terms such as eczematous dermatitis are used. For ease of description a relatively simplified form of classification will be used here.

Eczema is a reaction of the skin to a wide range of stimulants or irritants, some known, many unknown. In some cases, if not all, there is apparently some constitutional factor that renders the skin vulnerable, so that it responds in this abnormal manner to stimuli which have no effect upon the skin of normal individuals. The two classical criteria of the eruption in eczema are that it itches and that it causes vesication, or blistering, of the skin. Its first manifestation is erythema, or reddening of the skin. This is due to dilatation of the blood-vessels in the skin. The next stage is the formation of vesicles (qv) or papules (qv); these gradually break down and there is then oozing from the affected area of skin. If the condition persists, the skin tends to become thickened and to start scaling off.

NUMMULAR ECZEMA, or DISCOID ECZEMA as it is sometimes known, consists of coin-shaped areas of eczema, usually on the limbs, which, like all forms of eczema, tend to itch intensely. It is not uncommon in girls when they first start doing manual work, occurring on the back of the hands and fingers, the probability being that the eczema is due to trauma to the skin at work. It also occurs in middle-aged men, usually on the shins, being often aggravated by too frequent hot baths. The outlook for cure is poor, but lotions or pastes containing coal tar are often helpful.

INFECTIVE ECZEMA is a form of eczema that appears on a burn or cut. It comes on suddenly and spreads rapidly. In some cases it is due to sensitivity to the antiseptic that has been applied to the burn or cut. In some instances the eruption may be so severe that admission to hospital may be necessary. Treatment consists of the local application of a corticosteroid (qv) combined with an antibiotic. Alternatively, the application of wet dressings of quarter-strength Dilute Hypochlorite Solution, BPC is often effective. Calamine lotion is a soothing local application.

ATOPIC ECZEMA is one of the most widespread and worrying forms of eczema. Atopy means an inherited state of hypersensitivity which may manifest itself as asthma, hay fever or eczema. Hence the name given to this form of eczema. It is also known as INFANTILE ECZEMA as it starts in infancy at about the age of 3 or 4 months. There is a family history of asthma, hay fever or eczema in about 70 per cent of these infants, and it has been estimated that 3 per cent of all infants suffer from moderate eczema, and that many more probably suffer from a mild degree of it. The condition appears first as red areas or papules on the edge of the scalp, spreading to the face, which soon erupt and start oozing or weeping. In some cases the eruption spreads all over the body and, as it is intensely itchy, the unfortunate infant or child is often worked up into a frenzy and scratches himself until he is bleeding all over. Cold, frosty weather aggravates the condition, as does exposure to heat. Fortunately, parents can console themselves that the outlook is not too gloomy. Many of the children start improving around the age of 2 years, and in one series of 500 cases, only 10 per cent had any appreciable eczema at the age of 10 years. A late appearance of the eczema tends to mean a poor outlook, as does a bad family history of atopy.

Treatment: Local treatment consists of the application of a 1 per cent hydrocortisone ointment (see HYDROCORTISONE). If crusts have formed, these are removed by the application of equal parts of lead diachylon plaster and soft paraffin, applied thickly in strips of lint, and left on for twenty-four hours. Local treatment, however, is only part of the treatment. Equally important is it that parents should not over-protect a baby or child with eczema. He or she must be allowed to lead a perfectly normal life, without any pampering or unnecessary restrictions. The vast majority of children with this form of eczema can eat a normal diet. Only occasionally does such a child prove to be allergic to some particular food. Whether or not soap should be used in washing the baby is an open question. In the more severe cases soap should probably be avoided, and the skin cleaned with Emulsifying Ointment, BP. In cold weather, if there is a tendency for the skin to become dry and crack easily, Oily Cream, BP, may be gently rubbed into the skin at bedtime. If a soap is used for washing, then one of the less alkaline soaps should be used. Adding a processed oatmeal, such as Aveeno Oilated (half a cup per bath of tepid water), to the bath water may help to relieve the itching.

People with eczema and their relatives can obtain advice from the National Eczema Society, Tavistock House East, Tavistock Square, London WC1H 9SR (01–388 4097).

EFFERENT is the term applied to vessels which convey away blood or a secretion from a part, or to nerves which carry nerve impulses outwards from the nerve-centres.

EFFLEURAGE is a form of massage by gentle stroking movements.

EFFORT SYNDROME, also known as Da Costa's syndrome, is a condition in which symptoms occur, such as palpitations and shortness of breath, which are attributed by the patient to disorder of the heart. There is no evidence, however, of heart disease, and psychological factors are thought to be of importance. (See PSYCHOSOMATIC DISEASES.)

EFFUSION means a pouring out of fluid from the vessels in which it is naturally enclosed into the substance of the organs, or into cavities of the body, as a result of inflammation or of injury: for example, pleurisy with effusion, effusions into joints, and effusion of blood.

EGG is a term applied to any animal ovum.

ELBOW is the joint formed between the humerus above and the radius and ulna below. The humerus has at its lower end a rounded surface, against which the head of the radius moves, and a deep groove to which a saddle-shaped surface at the upper end of the ulna fits. The head of the radius rests upon a projection of the ulna and is bound to it by a stout annular ligament, within which it can rotate. Two important movements take place at this joint: a flail-like backward and forward movement of the radius and ulna moving together upon the humerus, and a rotary movement of the radius on the ulna, by which the lower end of the radius is crossed over the ulna and again brought side by side with it, according as the hand is turned palm downwards and palm upwards. The joint is secured at the sides by strong lateral ligaments, and at the back and front is covered by powerful muscles. The ulnar nerve as it passes down to the forearm has an exposed position behind the inner edge of the humerus at its lower end; this is popularly known as the 'funny-bone'. The elbow is seldom dislocated, but a not uncommon accident consists in the chipping off, through a fall on the elbow, of the olecranon process which forms the point behind the joint.

Miner's Elbow, or *Beat Elbow*, is the term applied to an inflammatory condition of the bursa over the point of the elbow, caused by resting the weight of the body on the elbow in hewing coal. The condition corresponds to housemaid's knee in the lower limb, and occurs not only in miners but sometimes in school children and other people who lean upon or bruise the point of the elbow. (See BURSITIS.)

Tennis Elbow is a term applied to a pain over the elbow due to mild inflammation in the tendons of the muscles that extend, or straighten, the elbow, caused by strains and jars in playing tennis and similar games. It is not uncommon in the left elbow of right-handed golfers who catch the head of their club in the ground when making a duff shot. Also known as enthesitis, the condition generally clears up spontaneously if games such as tennis, badminton and squash, or clothes wringing, are avoided, though this may be a somewhat slow process, taking up to a year or longer. A quicker result may be obtained by an injection of hydrocortisone (qv) into the affected area. The local application of ultrasonics (qv) may also be helpful. *Pulled Elbow* is the name applied to a painful condition of the elbow in young children, constituting a slight dislocation of the head of the radius from beneath the ligament which should bind it to the ulna, caused by a jerk of the arm. It is most likely to occur in 1- and 2-year-olds. The condition, which is usually accompanied by loss of power of the arm, may be induced in a variety of ways; by being pulled up when sitting on the floor, when being swung between their parents when walking, when being held firmly by the arm, when in an obstreperous, recalcitrant mood. The pain may occur in the wrist or shoulder. It responds well to manipulation.

ELECTRICAL INJURIES are usually caused by the passage through the body of an electric current of high voltage owing to accidental contact with a live wire or to a discharge of lightning. The general effects produced are included under the term electric shock, but vary greatly in degree. The local effects include spasmodic contraction of muscles, fracture of bones, and in severe cases more or less widespread destruction of tissues which may amount simply to burns of the skin or may include necrosis of masses of muscle and internal organs. Fright due to unexpectedness of the shock and pain due to the sudden cramp of muscles are the commonest symptoms and in most cases pass off in a few minutes or less. In more severe cases, especially when the person has remained in contact with a live wire for some time or has been unable to let go of the electrical contact owing to spasmodic contraction of his muscles, the effects are more pronounced and may be those of concussion of the brain or of compression of the brain. (See BRAIN, DISEASES OF.) In still severer cases, death may ensue either from paralysis of the respiration or stoppage of the heart's action. In either instance, the condition may be at first one of suspended animation, and death may not ensue if prompt measures are taken for treatment.

With regard to the after-effects of an electric shock, recovery in slighter cases is almost immediate, but in cases in which the discharge of current has been prolonged the process of recovery may be prolonged. The more permanent effects depend upon the extent to which tissues have been destroyed. Fractures and splitting of bones are often caused by very powerful currents. Dislocation of a joint is sometimes produced by violent muscular spasm. Masses of muscle and areas of skin may be destroyed, and if these injuries are extensive, a long time may be required for the absorption or sloughing away of the dead tissues and for healing. Electrical injuries show little tendency to become septic as compared with similar injuries due to other causes, and while loss of a part of the body may take place, healing is in the end usually satisfactory.

With regard to the amount of current necessary to produce serious results, this varies enormously according to circumstances. Alternating current is more dangerous than direct current, the risk of death being greatest at 50 cycles per second. So far as voltage is concerned, the lowest recorded fatal shock voltage in Britain is 60; few deaths occur at voltages below 100. Contact with high-tension currents (1000 volts or more) of the alternating type is immediately fatal. Physical factors are important in regard to the effects produced by a given strength of current; after a shock is received through dry shoes or dry clothing, the effect may be negligible as compared with that of contact made with a bare part of the body, especially when the skin is damp or perspiring, or of contact through wet feet. This is why electrical apparatus should never be allowed in a bathroom unless it is out of all possible contact with individuals using the bathroom. Water is a good conductor of electricity. Therefore if an individual touches an electrical heater or fire with wet hands, he may receive a severe shock. If the contact occurs while the individual is still in his bath the result will probably be fatal. Even touching a faulty switch with dripping hands may prove fatal.

In Britain there are an average of 110 deaths a year from electrocution, half of these occurring in the home. (See ACCIDENT PREVENTION IN THE HOME.)

Treatment: No electrical apparatus or switch should be touched by anyone who is in metallic contact with the ground, such as through a metal pipe, especially, for example, from a bath. The first necessity in regard to a person through whose body a powerful electric current is passing is to break the current. This can sometimes be done by turning off a switch. If the victim is grasping or in contact with a live wire, the contact may be severed with safety only by someone wearing rubber gloves or rubber boots, but as these are not likely to be immediately available, his hands may be protected by a thick wrapping of dry cloth, or the live wire may be hooked or pushed out of the way with a long wooden stick. If the injured person is unconscious, and especially if breathing has stopped, *artificial respiration should be applied and continued even for hours*, as described under DROWNING, RECOVERY FROM. When the patient begins to breathe again, he must be treated for shock: ie. put to bed and given hot-water bottles and hot drinks. Electrical burns are treated on the same lines as ordinary burns. If the patient shows undue excitement and restlessness, sedatives may be necessary. The local destructive effects of a powerful current, including burns, fractures, and sloughing of large masses of tissue, are treated later by ordinary surgical means, but strong and irritating antiseptics should be avoided. Bleeding from damaged blood-vessels is liable to occur a few days after a severe injury, and is treated by the ordinary means for arrest of haemorrhage.

ELECTRICITY IN MEDICINE: Electricity is generally spoken of as existing in different forms, but these differ in pressure, in amount, and in duration, rather than in any essential quality. They are named as follows: (*a*) Static, or Frictional, or Franklinic; (*b*) Galvanic or Voltaic; (*c*) Faradic or Induced; (*d*) Alternating or Sinusoidal; (*e*) High Frequency or D'Arsonvalism.

Static electricity has been recognized, by some of its simplest phenomena, from the earliest times. The name electricity is derived from the Greek word, meaning amber, because it is said that Thales of Miletus first discovered this force by noticing that a piece of amber, rubbed with a dry cloth, had the power of attracting small bodies to itself. Subsequently it was found that other bodies, such as sulphur, wax and glass, have similar properties, and a treatise, *De Magnete*, was published on the subject by William Gilbert, physician to Queen Elizabeth, in 1600. This form of electricity is often called Franklinic, after Benjamin Franklin, who, in the middle of the eighteenth century, experimented much with it in the United States.

When a glass rod is rubbed with a piece of dry flannel, the two gain certain properties. If the glass rod is brought near a light pith-ball or piece of paper hanging by a dry silk thread, the pith-ball is attracted towards the rod, but if the two are allowed to touch for a moment, the pith-ball is now as energetically repelled when the rod is brought near it. If, however, the piece of flannel is brought near the ball, the latter is attracted to it. To express these facts conveniently it is said that there are two 'kinds' of electricity, positive and negative, the glass rod becoming positively electrified by the rubbing, the flannel negatively electrified, and further, that like electricities repel one another. Accordingly, when the positively electrified glass rod is brought near the pith-ball, the negative electricity in the latter is supposed to separate from the positive (the ball having till now been uniformly charged with the two) and to collect on that side of the ball nearest to the rod, while the positive electricity is repelled to the point farthest off. When the rod and ball touch, the negative electricity escapes to the rod, leaving the ball positively electrified, so that it is now repelled by the positive electricity of the rod and attracted by the negative electricity of the flannel. Positive electricity is designated shortly by the sign +, and negative by the sign –, while the power possessed by the electricity of passing from pith-ball to glass rod, carrying the ball with it, is known as potential, or pressure, or electromotive force (EMF). All bodies have these properties, developing, when suddenly separated or broken, this difference of potential, the amount and nature of the force produced depending on the nature of the bodies in question. But while in the case of certain bodies called non-conductors, such as glass, plastic, sealing-wax, rubber, dry wool, silk, and amber, the electricity remains upon the surface where it is produced, in the case of others, known as conductors, such as metals, salt solutions, and the bodies of animals and plants, it flows away through the body as soon as formed, and therefore does not show its presence. Static electricity is closely related to magnetism, a set of properties possessed only by iron, steel, nickel, cobalt, and an iron-ore called lodestone.

Static electricity may be stored up in large amounts by means of the Leyden jar. This consists of two conducting surfaces, such as tinfoil, placed one outside, the other inside, a glass jar, so that they are everywhere separated by a thin plate of glass. The outer one simply rests in contact with the earth, the inner is connected to a metal rod ending in a knob. Electrified bodies, like a rubbed glass rod, may be brought up to the knob time after time till the inner sheet of tinfoil becomes highly charged with positive electricity, which attracts negative electricity from the earth into the outside sheet. If the knob of a charged Leyden jar be connected with the outside sheet of foil the two electricities combine suddenly, and if this contact be made through the human body, a severe momentary shock is felt.

For practical medical purposes, static electricity is produced by an influence machine consisting of several pairs of circular glass or vulcanite plates, which are driven in opposite directions. Each plate carries at starting a small amount of electricity; and, as they revolve, the alternate plates generate increasing quantities of + and – electricity, which are drawn off to opposite sides of the machine by fine metal brushes. The electricity can be stored in Leyden jars, or used directly to electrify the body. For the latter purpose, the person sits upon a chair or couch, carefully insulated from the earth by glass legs, rubber mats, or other non-conductors, and becomes charged positively or negatively according to the manner in which he is connected with the machine. During the process of charging, a peculiar tingling over the skin is felt and the hair stands upright; the breathing becomes more rapid, and during a session of fifteen to twenty minutes the chemical changes which accompany bodily activity are markedly increased. The electricity is discharged by bringing a metal point or ball gradually towards the charged person, when, in the former case, a spray of air or 'souffle' passes towards the point as the charge passes off, in the latter case sparks are drawn. Either form of discharge, especially the latter, has a stimulating effect. The atmosphere, both upon high wooded mountains and in the neighbourhood of breaking waves, has, as Lord Kelvin demonstrated, a different electric state from the quiet air of inland plains, so that it is quite possible that some of the advantage derived from summer change to mountain and seaside resorts may be due to stimulation from this cause.

Galvanic electricity is so named after Galvani, professor at Bologna, who published researches upon what he called 'animal electricity' in 1791. It also received the name 'voltaic', after Volta, professor at Pavia, who in 1799 published researches showing that this type of electricity is really due to chemical action. He found that dissimilar metals, moistened and brought in contact, became electrified, so that, when parts of these metals not in contact are connected by a conductor, such as copper wire, a constant current passes through the wire. As chemical action proceeds almost continuously, this current is also continuous; and for this reason, added to the fact that it is of moderate potential or pressure and is easily produced, it is the most convenient for general medical use.

The choice of metals depends upon the fact that one must be very liable to chemical action, the other as little affected as possible by an oxidizing agent. The principal metals may be arranged in a series, thus:

+Sodium	Iron
Magnesium	Copper
Zinc	Silver
Lead	Gold
Tin	Platinum
	–Carbon

– of which each one is more oxidizable than that following it, and becomes positively electrified when brought into contact with one of those lower down in the series. Zinc and carbon, or zinc and copper, on account of their distance apart in this scale, and their comparative cheapness, are the metals usually selected. A vessel containing two metal plates, for example, zinc and copper, immersed in a fluid which maintains chemical action, for example, sulphuric acid in water, is known as a galvanic cell. A collection of such cells is called a battery. When the plates are joined by a conducting wire an electric current passes along it from the copper (+ pole) to the zinc (– pole). At the same time there is set free, on the surface of the zinc plate, oxygen, which acts upon the zinc, and also produces sulphuric acid; while hydrogen is set free at the surface of the copper plate and escapes.

It is important to bear in mind also that if the current passing along the wire is passed for some distance through a moist decomposable substance, such as the tissues of the human body, a similar chemical action is produced at the points where the wire enters and leaves the substance, which are called the electrodes. Thus oxygen is set free and acids formed at the electrode connected to the + pole (the anode), while hydrogen is set free and alkalis developed at the other, or – electrode (the cathode). This action, known as electrolysis, is much used in medicine for removing hairs, destroying naevi or birthmarks, and reducing the size of certain tumours, unsuitable for removal by the knife. There is a great difference between the action of the two electrodes, because the substances formed at the anode are caustic and germicidal in action, whilst those produced at the cathode have no such action. Accordingly, the anode (+ pole) is generally applied to the structure which it is desired to destroy.

Another important property of electric currents, the fact that a powerful current passing through a circuit heats any part which is a poor conductor, is utilized to heat cauteries for delicate surgical work, especially about the nose and throat, and also to light small incandescent lamps for internal examinations. The cautery consists of a piece of platinum (low conducting power), joining the ends of two large copper wires (high conducting power), so that, when the current passes, the former immediately becomes red or white hot, according to the intensity of the current.

Another method in which the galvanic current is employed is in order to carry drugs through the unbroken skin by the process known as iontophoresis (qv).

Faradic electricity dates only from 1831, when it was discovered by Faraday that if two coils of wire be placed near one another, and if a galvanic current is suddenly passed through one of them and again stopped, a current is induced in the second coil at the moments of closing and of opening the first circuit. This secondary current differs from the continuous galvanic current in two important particulars: (1) it is only momentary in duration; (2) it has a much higher potential or pressure, and is therefore much more capable of traversing poor conductors like the human body. The currents induced in the secondary coil at opening and closing the primary coil run in opposite directions; accordingly, if the primary current be very rapidly closed and opened, as, for example, by the vibration of a steel spring, an almost continuous series of alternating currents is obtained in the secondary circuit.

A faradic current sufficient for medical purposes can be obtained from an apparatus consisting of the following: a single galvanic cell connected to a primary coil, with an appliance to make and break the circuit; a secondary coil, which is connected by wires with two electrodes provided with handles, by which the electrodes can be applied to the surface of the body; and a core of iron which fits inside the primary coil, and which, becoming magnetized as the current passes through this coil, increases the effect upon the secondary coil. Such an apparatus can be obtained in the small compass of a box 4 or 5 inches (10 or 12 cm) each way.

The faradic current can be administered to the surface of the body generally by immersion of the patient in a warm bath into which two electrodes dip.

For certain purposes, such as X-ray work, secondary coils with an enormous length of wire are used, the potential or pressure of the faradic current increasing with the number of turns taken by the wire in the secondary coil.

The potential of faradic currents is high: in medical coils it may reach 20,000 or 100,000 volts.

Alternating or sinusoidal currents differ from the faradic current in the fact that the latter consists of a rapid series of sudden impulses or shocks, while with the sinusoidal or alternating current the strength gradually rises from nothing to a maximum, and falls away again to be followed immediately by a current in the reverse direction, which also grows to a maximum and wanes in the same manner. These currents rapidly succeed one another, so that the effect on the body is very much the same as that produced by the faradic current. Most systems of public distribution of electrical energy are carried out by alternating currents of this type, and by means of transformers they can be readily converted into forms of electricity more suitable for medical use. The sinusoidal current, suitably reduced by apparatus, may be used for the electric bath, or may be used for stimulating nerves or muscles, especially when the current is rhythmically cut off and restored by an instrument known as a rhythmic interrupter. Sinusoidal currents on a small scale can be produced by bringing a magnet rapidly up to and away from a secondary coil, or making the coil move while the magnet remains fixed. The sinusoidal form of current generally has a very stinging effect on sensory nerves, and in this way is somewhat unpleasant for use.

High-frequency currents: By apparatus constructed on the principle of the induction coil, but with other complicated arrangements designed to make and break the primary current several hundred thousand times a second, currents, huge in pressure but minute in duration, can be produced which have an action similar to that of a discharge of static electricity. The sensation is merely one of slight tingling when sparks are drawn, and there is no stimulation of muscles or nerves. This may possibly be explained by the currents being confined to the surface, and not passing through the substance of the body at all, or more probably by the theory of D'Arsonval, that the nerve endings are incapable of perceiving such extremely short vibrations. These high-frequency currents formed at one time a very popular mode of stimulating treatment.

The apparatus by which these currents are produced consists essentially of Leyden jars, whose outer coats are united through a solenoid or spiral of thick copper wire. The jars are rapidly charged and discharged by some source of high potential electricity; and, since the discharges from a Leyden jar have the property of taking place in an oscillatory manner, they induce in the solenoid corresponding secondary currents, which are of immensely rapid frequency. A second coil of thick wire, known as a resonator, is in general connected to the solenoid with the purpose of allowing of variations in the potential of the high-frequency discharges.

The currents are applied to the patient in various ways. (*a*) He may be connected to the two ends of the solenoid by thin wires provided with ordinary flat electrodes, from which the currents are simply passed through his body (direct application). (*b*) He may lie upon a couch connected with one end of the solenoid, while the cushion of the couch isolates him from a metal plate connected with the other end; he then becomes rapidly charged and discharged (condensation). (*c*) He may stand or lie within a wide secondary coil, and have currents induced in his body (auto-conduction). (*d*) One end of the solenoid may be connected to earth, while to the other end is attached an electrode, which is cautiously approached to any desired part (local application). (*e*) The method of diathermy or thermo-penetration may be used to produce heat within the body. (See DIATHERMY.)

As already stated, the passage of high-frequency currents through the body produces no stimulation of muscles and no sensation, apart from that of heat caused by the resistance. There is a powerful effect, lasting many minutes, in diminishing the sensitiveness of the skin; the fullness of the blood-vessels in the skin, the output of body heat and of carbon dioxide by the lungs are increased, and the quantity of urine passed becomes much greater.

Applications of electricity: The galvanic and faradic currents are of value as a means of *diagnosis* in many conditions affecting nerves and muscles. In their natural condition nerves react to faradic or to interrupted galvanic currents, muscles to the latter. When excitability by faradization is lost, it shows that the nerves in question are degenerating. The sudden initiation of a weak galvanic current should produce a contraction of muscles to which the cathode is applied, but, if a much stronger current be required, or if a contraction be obtained more readily with the anode, it shows that the muscles in question are also in process of degeneration. This is expressed by the statement that when the anodal closing contraction is stronger than the cathodal closing contraction the reaction of degeneration is present, or, put briefly, ACC>KCC=RD. PAIN, whether headache, neuralgia, sciatica, a chronic rheumatic condition, or due to several other causes, is almost always relieved temporarily, and sometimes, after a protracted course of treatment, severe pain is entirely removed by one of the following. The static breeze may be tried, applied to the seat of pain for some minutes every day. In painful nerve conditions like neuralgia, greater benefit is often derived from the galvanic current, a strong current of 20-30 milliamperes being used, and the anode (+ electrode) being placed over the course of the affected nerve. In most cases of vague but severe pain the faradic current ectrode) being placed over the course of the affected nerve. In most cases of vague but severe pain the faradic current is the simplest of application, and very effective. A small button electrode or wire-brush is applied to the seat of pain, the other electrode, moistened with common salt solution, to the neck, back, or other convenient part. The séance lasts, perhaps, a quarter of an hour, and is repeated several times daily.

SPASMODIC CONDITIONS of all sorts, such as writer's cramp, are relieved or lessened by the static breeze, and still more by a strong galvanic current arranged so that the anode is close to the nerve or nerves connected with the spasmodically acting muscles. The anode decreases the conducting power of nerves for motor impulses as well as for painful sensations.

PARALYSIS, such as poliomyelitis, or that following a stroke or apoplexy, or injury to a nerve, calls specially for the application of interrupted galvanic currents. The muscles in these and similar cases, where the nervous control usually exerted over them is lost, tend to waste. The application of interrupted galvanic currents of about 10 milliamperes strength, or of these combined with faradization, and assisted in every case by massage, and movements of the neighbouring joints, not only keeps up the nourishment of the paralysed muscles and prevents stiffness and wasting, but actually assists recovery. So far as possible, treatment should be daily, and must extend over very long periods.

DESTRUCTION OF HAIRS is almost painlessly accomplished by electrolysis.

BIRTH-MARKS, consisting of masses of blood-vessels beneath the skin (naevi), are successfully destroyed, without leaving a scar, by electrolysis. The electrodes consist of two needles which are pushed through the skin into the mass, and an anaesthetic is usually given during the process.

STRICTURES of the gullet, bowel, and urethra may, it is claimed, also be painlessly dilated by electrolysis, though the process must be repeated several times at intervals of a fortnight or thereabout, in sessions of fifteen minutes.

REMOVAL OF STEEL PARTICLES which have penetrated the eye may often be effected by a powerful electro-magnet consisting of a soft iron core round which is wound an electric coil, through which a heavy current can be passed.

X-RAYS AND ULTRA-VIOLET RAYS are produced by the aid of electricity, and used in the treatment of many skin and other diseases. (See under LIGHT TREATMENT; X-RAYS.)

ELECTROCARDIOGRAM is a record of the variations in electric potential which occur in the heart as it contracts and relaxes. Any muscle in use produces an electric current, but when an individual is at rest the main muscular current in the body is that produced by the heart. This can be recorded by connecting the outside of the body by electrodes with an instrument known as an electrocardiograph. The patient is connected to the electrocardiograph by leads from either the arms and legs or different points on the chest. The normal electrocardiogram of each heart-beat shows one wave corresponding to the activity of the atria and four waves corresponding to the phases of each ventricular beat. Various readily recognizable changes are seen in cases in which the heart is acting in an abnormal manner, or in which one or other side of the heart is hypertrophied. This record therefore forms a useful aid in many cases of heart disease. The main applications of the electrocardiogram are in the diagnosis of myocardial infarction and of cardiac arrhyrthmias.

ELECTROCAUTERY (see CAUSTICS and CAUTERIES).

ELECTROCOCHLEOGRAPHY is a method of recording the activity of the cochlea, the part of the inner ear concerned with hearing. (See EAR.)

ELECTRO-ENCEPHALOGRAPHY: In the brain there is a regular, rhythmical change of electric potential, due to the rhythmic discharge of energy by nerve cells. These changes can be recorded graphically and the 'brain waves' examined. These records – electro-encephalograms – are useful in diagnosis. For example, the abnormal electro-encephalogram occurring in epilepsy is characteristic of this disease. The normal waves, known as alpha waves, occur with a frequency of 10 per second. Abnormal waves, with a frequency of 7 or less per second, are known as delta waves and occur in the region of cerebral tumours and in the brains of epileptics.

ELECTRON is one of the subatomic particles. (See RADIOTHERAPY.)

ELECTRO-OCULOGRAPHY is a method of recording movements of the eyes, which is proving of value in assessing the function of the retina (qv).

ELECTROPHORESIS means the migration of charged particles between electrodes. A simple method of electrophoresis, known as paper electrophoresis, has been introduced which is proving of value in examining the proteins in body fluids. This method consists in applying the protein-containing solution as a spot or a streak to a strip of filter paper which has been soaked in buffer solution and across the ends of which a potential difference is then applied for some hours.

ELECTRORETINOGRAM: An electroretinogram is the record of an electrical response of visual receptors in the retina (qv), which can be measured with corneal electrodes.

ELECTUARY, or CONFECTION, is a soft paste containing drugs mixed with sugar or honey. (See CONFECTIONS.)

ELEPHANTIASIS (synonyms, ELEPHANTIASIS ARABUM, BARBADOS LEG, BOUCNEMIA) is a term applied to a disease which is characterized by gross overgrowth of the skin and subjacent textures. This condition arises from repeated attacks of inflammation of the skin and subcutaneous tissue, and concurrent obstruction of the lymphatic vessels. The common cause in the tropics is infection with certain parasitic worms (filariae) which invade the lymphatic vessels. (See FILARIASIS.) These worms are conveyed to man by mosquitoes. They may attack any portion of the body, but most commonly the leg, which becomes so enlarged and disfigured by the great thickening of its textures as to resemble the leg of an elephant, whence the name of the disease is derived. The thickening is due to excessive increase in the connective tissue, which results from the inflammatory process, and which by pressure on the muscles of the limb causes them to undergo atrophy or degeneration. Hence the limb becomes weak. When affecting the scrotum it often produces a tumour of enormous dimensions. The health ultimately suffers, and serious constitutional disturbance is apt to arise. In elephantiasis of the leg much relief is obtained from the use of elastic bandaging, massage, rest, and elevation of the limb. Prevention must be carried out by destruction of mosquitoes. Promising results are being reported from the use of diethylcarbamazine in the early stages of the disease.

ELIXIR is a liquid preparation of a potent or nauseous drug made pleasant to the taste by the addition of aromatic substances and sugar. The name was specially applied to several preparations greatly used in the Middle Ages, which had the effect of acting as a tonic to the stomach and relieving constipation, and which were known, for example, as the elixir of Paracelsus, the elixir of long life. The main constituent of all of these was tincture of aloes.

EMACIATION means pronounced wasting, and is a common symptom of many diseases, particularly of those which are associated with a prolonged or repeated rise of temperature, such as tuberculosis. It is also associated with diseases of the alimentary system in which digestion is inefficient, or in which the food is not fully absorbed: for example, in diarrhoea of long-standing, whatever its cause. It is also a marked feature of malignant disease.

EMBALMING (see DEAD, DISPOSAL OF THE).

EMBOLISM means the plugging of a small blood-vessel by material which has been carried through the larger vessels by the blood stream. It is due usually to fragments of a clot which has formed in some vessel, or to small portions carried off from the edge of a heart-valve when this organ is diseased; but the plug may also be a small mass of bacteria, or a fragment of a tumour, or even a mass of air bubbles sucked into the veins during operations on the neck. The result is usually more or less destruction of the organ or part of an organ supplied by the obstructed vessel. This is particularly the case in the brain, where softening of the brain, with aphasia or apoplexy, may be the result. If the plug is a fragment of malignant tumour, a new growth develops at the spot; and if it is a mass of bacteria, an abscess forms there. Air-embolism occasionally causes sudden death in the case of wounds in the neck, the air bubbles completely stopping the flow of blood. Fat-embolism is a condition which has been known to cause death, masses of fat, in consequence of such an injury as a fractured bone, finding their way into the circulation and stopping the blood in its passage through the lungs.

EMBROCATIONS are mixtures, usually of an oily nature, intended for external application in cases of rheumatism, sprains, and other painful conditions. Their action is due partly to the massage employed in rubbing in the embrocations, partly to the counter-irritant action of the drugs which they contain. (See LINIMENTS.)

EMBRYO means the foetus in the womb prior to the end of the second month. (See FOETUS.)

EMBRYO TRANSFER is the process whereby the initial stages of procreation are produced outside the human body and completed in the uterus or womb. The procedure is also known as EMBRYO TRANSPLANTATION and IN VITRO FERTILIZATION. It consists of extracting an ovum (or egg) from the prospective mother's body and placing this in a dish where it is mixed with the male partner's semen and special nutrient fluids. After the ovum is fertilized by the sperm it is transferred to another dish containing a special nutrient solution. Here it is left for several days while the normal early stages of development (see FOETUS) take place. The early embryo (qv) as it has then become, is then implanted in the mother's uterus, where it 'takes root' and develops as a normal foetus.

The first 'test-tube baby', to use the popular, and widely used, term for such a child was born by Caesarean section in England on July 25, 1978. A number of other children, conceived in this manner, have been born, and the success rate will undoubtedly improve with experience. Its relative merits, compared with artificial insemination (qv), as a means of dealing with the problem of infertility (qv) have still to be decided. Its potentialities for abuse are not inconsiderable and will obviously require to be carefully watched and controlled if current concepts of human individuality and the integrity of the human race are to be maintained.

EMESIS means vomiting (qv).

EMETICS are drugs or other means which produce vomiting.

Varieties: Emetics are divided into two important classes: (1) direct emetics, which, being taken by the mouth, irritate the stomach and so cause vomiting, and (2) indirect emetics, which will cause vomiting, even when injected into the blood, by action upon the centre in the brain controlling the act of vomiting. Examples of the first type are sulphate of zinc, mustard in water, alum, sal volatile, copper sulphate, and even copious draughts of warm salt water. In the second class we have apomorphine, ipecacuanha, and tartar emetic; to this class also belong such means as tickling the throat, or presenting evil-smelling substances to the nose.

Uses: Emetics are now relatively seldom used except in certain cases of poisoning to remove the poisonous substance as rapidly as possible from the stomach. They must only be given if the victim is conscious, one drink of salty water, containing sodium chloride (common salt), or a dose of Ipecacuanha Syrup USP: 15 millilitres followed by 200 millilitres (a tumblerful) of water, should be given. Emetics in smaller doses than will produce vomiting are often used in cough mixtures, as they render the secretions in the bronchial tubes more fluid and therefore more easily coughed up. Wine of ipecacuanha is used for this purpose.

EMETINE is one of the active principles of ipecacuanha. (See IPECACUANHA; DYSENTERY.)

EMICTORY is a drug which provokes the excretion of urine.

EMMENAGOGUES are drugs which restore the flow at the menstrual periods, when this is scanty or absent. Certain substances, which are mainly dangerous irritant poisons, are credited with the power of producing this effect. Other substances act indirectly by removing the state of ill-health to which the failure is due, such as iron in anaemia. (See MENSTRUATION.)

EMMETROPIA is a term applied to the normal condition of the eye as regards refraction of light rays. In this state when the muscles in the eyeball are completely relaxed the focusing power is accurately adjusted for parallel rays, so that vision is perfect for distant objects.

EMOLLIENTS are substances which have a softening and soothing effect upon the skin. They include dusting powders such as French chalk, oils such as olive oil and almond oil, and fats such as the various pharmacopoeial preparations of paraffin, suet, and lard. Glycerin is also an excellent emollient.

Uses: They are used in various inflammatory conditions such as eczema, when the skin becomes hard, cracked, and painful. They may be used in the form of a dusting powder, an oil or an ointment.

EMPHYSEMA means an abnormal presence of air in certain parts of the body. In its restricted sense, however, it is generally employed to designate an affection of the lungs, of which there are two forms. In one of these there is over-distension of the air-cells of these organs, and in parts destruction of their walls, giving rise to the formation of large sacs, from the rupture and running together of a number of contiguous air-vesicles. This is much the more common of the two forms and is the one which is usually meant when the term 'emphysema' is used. In the other form the air is infiltrated into the connective tissue beneath the pleura and between the pulmonary air-cells, constituting what is known as *acute interstitialemphysema.*

Causes: Where a portion of the lung has become wasted, or its vesicular structure permanently obliterated by disease, without corresponding falling-in of the chest wall, the neighbouring air-vesicles, or some of them, undergo dilatation to fill the vacuum.

In cases of bronchitis, and especially of bronchial asthma, where numbers of the smaller bronchial tubes become obstructed, the air in the pulmonary vesicles remains imprisoned, the force of expiration being insufficient to expel it; on the other hand, the stronger force of inspiration being adequate to overcome the resistance, the air-cells tend to become more and more distended, and permanent alterations in their structure, including emphysema, are the result.

Emphysema also arises from exertion involving expiratory efforts, during which the glottis is constricted, as in paroxysms of coughing, in straining, and in lifting heavy weights. Whooping-cough is well known as an exciting cause of emphysema.

Smoking is an important cause of emphysema. According to the United States Surgeon General's 1984 report, cigarette smoking is the major cause of chronic obstructive lung disease morbidity and 80 to 90 per cent of cases are attributable to smoking.

Symptoms: In the affected portions of the lungs there are loss of the natural elasticity of the air-cells, destruction of many of the pulmonary capillary blood-vessels, and diminution of aerating surface for the blood. As a consequence there is a strain on the heart and the venous system generally, leading to dilatation of the right side of the heart, and so to oedema. The chief symptom in this complaint is shortness of breath, more or less constant but greatly aggravated by exertion, and by attacks of bronchitis, to which people suffering from emphysema are specially liable. The respiration is of a wheezy character. In severe forms of the disease the patient comes to acquire a peculiar bluish and bloated appearance, and the configuration of the chest is altered, assuming the character known as the *barrel-shaped chest.*

Treatment: The main element in the treatment of emphysema consists in attention to the general condition of the health, and in the avoidance of all causes likely to aggravate the disease or induce its complications. Smoking is of particular importance in this context. The same general plan of treatment as that recommended in asthma and bronchitis is applicable in emphysema. During attacks of urgent breathlessness anti-spasmodic remedies should be given, while inhalation of oxygen will often afford marked and speedy relief.
ACUTE INTERSTITIAL EMPHYSEMA, arising from the rupture of air-cells may occur as a complication of the vesicular form, or separately as the result of some sudden expulsive effort, such as a fit of coughing, or, as has occasionally happened, in parturition. Occasionally the air infiltrates the cellular tissue of the mediastinum, and thence comes to distend the integument of the neck and even the whole surface of the body. This air, however, is rapidly absorbed, and the condition soon subsides.
SURGICAL EMPHYSEMA is the term applied when air is present under the skin. It may get there, for example, if the lungs are wounded through the chest wall, or if the windpipe is pierced at any point in its path.

EMPIRICAL treatment is that school of treatment which is founded simply on experience. Because a given remedy has been successful in the treatment of a certain group of symptoms, it is assumed, by those who uphold this principle, that it will be successful in the treatment of other cases presenting similar groups of symptoms, without any inquiry as to the cause of the symptoms or reason underlying the action of the remedy. It is the contrary of 'rational' or 'scientific' treatment. Sometimes a course of treatment must perforce be empirical for want of knowledge.

EMPLASTRUM is the Latin term for a plaster.

EMPORIATRICS is the study of the health of travellers.

EMPROSTHOTONOS is the term applied to the spasm of the belly muscles that occurs in tetanus, making the body arch forwards.

EMPYEMA is an accumulation of pus within a cavity, the term being generally reserved for collections of pus within one of the pleural cavities. The condition is virtually an abscess, and therefore gives rise to the general symptoms accompanying that condition; but, on account of the thick unyielding wall of the chest, it has very little tendency to burst through the surface, and therefore it is of particular importance that the condition should be recognized early, and, as a rule, treated by surgical means.
Causes: The condition most commonly follows an attack of pneumonia. It may also occur in the advanced stage of pulmonary tuberculosis.

Empyema also occurs at times through infection from some serious disease in neighbouring organs, such as cancer of the gullet, or follows upon wounds penetrating the chest wall.

Symptoms: In empyema following a case of pneumonia, symptoms of the former generally appear as the pneumonia is subsiding, and when an ordinary attack of pneumonia does not come satisfactorily to an end after the lapse of eight to ten days, it is usual for the physician to suspect and search for the signs of empyema. A certain amount of inflammation in the membrane lining the pleural cavity always accompanies pneumonia, and the fluid which is thus produced may show any stage between that of clear yellow serous fluid and thick pus of the consistency of cream. When the fluid is clear or merely turbid, absorption generally takes place naturally in course of time, and the mild type of infection which is present is readily overcome by the ordinary powers of the tissues. When, however, a severe infection, due usually either to a virulent pneumococcus or streptococcus, is present, the fluid is of the thicker purulent variety, and active measures of treatment are required. The temperature of the patient, which should revert to normal at the end of the attack of pneumonia, tends to show a daily rise to 39° to 39·5°C (102° or 103°F); there is profuse sweating and the patient presents a flushed appearance. The severity of these symptoms is proportional to the degree of virulence of the infection of the pleural membrane, the symptoms generally being less marked the clearer the fluid. On examination of the chest a dull percussion-note, faint or absent breath sounds, and other characteristic signs of the presence of fluid are found. It is usual for the physician to complete the diagnosis by puncturing the chest by means of a fine needle attached to a small aspiration syringe. A sample of the fluid is thus obtained, and its characteristics as regards the bacteria present, etc., are investigated. The collection of fluid may be very small in size and limited by adhesions to a small portion of the chest, especially in those cases due to the pneumococcus, and it may be necessary in such cases to insert the needle at various points before the purulent fluid is definitely located.

Treatment: In those cases in which the fluid is clear or only slightly turbid, the measures commonly employed for pleurisy (qv) are often sufficient to bring about absorption. In cases in which the fluid is thick and purulent, and especially those following acute pneumonia, it is usually necessary to perform an operation for the drainage of the cavity, an incision being made through the skin and a portion of rib removed. The fluid is thus evacuated, and the lung can then expand naturally against the chest wall, a drainage tube being left in the wound so that the cavity can be irrigated and any fresh fluid which tends to collect can escape freely until the natural closure of the cavity is completed. Penicillin is also given, both intramuscularly and into the cavity. In the great majority of cases the lung ultimately reverts to a normal state.

EMULSIONS are mixtures containing oily substances in a state of very fine division. The division is effected and the oil kept suspended in the fluid by means of alkalis and sticky ingredients such as albumin, glycerin, or mucilage. Milk is an example of a perfect emulsion of fat globules each surrounded by an envelope of albumin. The various preparations of cod-liver oil are usually emulsified by the aid of glycerin. The oil is not only rendered more devoid of taste, but digestion and absorption are also rendered easier by emulsification.

ENAMEL (see TEETH).

ENCEPHALITIS means inflammation of the brain. It is usually a virus infection, and may occur as a complication of the common infectious diseases, including measles (in which it occurs in around 1 in 1000 cases).

ENCEPHALITIS LETHARGICA, also known as SLEEPY SICKNESS and as EPIDEMIC ENCEPHALITIS, and VON ECONOMO'S DISEASE, is a disease that appears from time to time, especially in the spring, in the form of epidemics. There has not been an epidemic in Britain since the late 1920's. It is probably a virus infection, and attacks chiefly the basal ganglia, the cerebrum, and the brain stem. These undergo swelling, haemorrhages, and ultimately destruction of areas of tissue involving both nerve-cells and fibres. The process may involve other parts of the brain, the spinal cord, and even other organs.

Symptoms: The illness begins usually with a rise of temperature and increasing drowsiness or lethargy, which may gradually proceed to a state of complete unconsciousness. In some cases, however, the patient instead of being drowsy passes at first through a stage of restlessness which may amount to maniacal excitement. As a rule the drowsiness deepens gradually over a period of a week or more, and accompanying it there appear various forms of paralysis, shown by drooping of the eyelids, squint, and weakness of one or both sides of the face. The nerves controlling the muscles of the throat are also sometimes paralysed, causing changes in the voice and difficulty in swallowing. In some cases the disease affects the spinal cord, producing severe pain in one or more of the limbs, and it is often followed by partial paralysis. Signs of inflammation are not infrequently found in other organs, and haemorrhages may be visible beneath the skin and may occur in the muscles, or blood may be vomited up or passed in the stools. The effects last usually for many months, the patient remaining easily tired and somnolent or frequently showing rigidity of muscle, mask-like facies, festinant gait (see FESTINATION), and rhythmical coarse tremors, resembling the clinical picture of Parkinsonism (qv).

Treatment: There is no specific treatment for the disease unless the virus responsible is the herpes virus when acyclovir is of benefit. During the acute stage the patient must be kept at rest in bed. After the acute stage is over, physiotherapy in the form of massage, passive movements and exercises should be given to control the muscular rigidity.

JAPANESE ENCEPHALITIS is a disease that occurs on the whole of the eastern seaboard of Asia. It is caused by a virus transmitted by a ricefield-breeding mosquito which also causes encephalitis in horses and abortions in pigs. The duration of the disease is variable and convalescence tends to be prolonged. The death-rate, too, is variable and may be as high as 30 per cent in children, in whom it may also cause permanent damage to the nervous system. There is no known drug treatment or any effective vaccine, though in some areas vaccinating pigs against the disease has proved helpful. Treatment therefore consists simply of efficient nursing and maintaining the patient's strength until he or she has overcome the infection.

TICK-BORNE ENCEPHALITIS is a virus infection which occurs in two forms conveyed by different ticks. The Far Eastern form, occurring particularly in Siberia, is transmitted by *Ixodes persulcatus*, causes a severe paralytic form of disease, and carries a mortality rate of over 30 per cent. The virus responsible for the European form is transmitted by *Ixodes ricinus* as a rule, but occasionally through drinking the unboiled milk of infected goats. It has an incubation period of 4 to 14 days, usually runs a relatively mild course, and has a mortality rate of 1 to 2 per cent. It has a seasonal incidence: May–June, and September–October. It occurs over the greater part of Continental Europe, but especially in Austria, Czechoslovakia and Yugoslavia, where it seems to be on the increase. In Yugoslavia around 1500 cases are reported annually though only 10 per cent of these are virologically confirmed. Being a virus infection, there is no known drug therapy, but promising results are being obtained from a vaccine now under trial.

ENCEPHALOID is the name applied to a form of cancer which, to the naked eye, resembles the tissue of the brain.

ENCEPHALOMYELITIS means inflammation of the substance of both brain and spinal cord.

ENCEPHALOPATHY is the term used to describe certain conditions in which there are signs of cerebral irritation without any localized lesion to account for them. The two best examples are *hypertensive encephalopathy* and *lead encephalopathy*. In the former, which occurs in the later stages of chronic glomerulonephritis, or uraemia (qv), the headache, convulsions, and delirium which constitute the main symptoms are supposed to be due to a deficient blood-supply to the brain. In the latter the symptoms are probably due to spasm of the arteries in the brain.

ENCHONDROMA means a tumour formed of cartilage. (See TUMOURS.)

ENCYSTED means enclosed within a bladder-like wall. The term is applied to parasites, collections of pus, etc., which are shut off from surrounding tissues by a membrane or by adhesions.

ENDARTERITIS means inflammation of the inner coat of an artery. (See ARTERIES, DISEASES OF.)

ENDEMIC is a term applied to diseases which exist in particular localities or among certain races. Some diseases, which are at times epidemic over wide districts, have a restricted area where they are always endemic, and from which they spread. For example, both cholera and plague are endemic in certain parts of Asia.

ENDO- is a prefix meaning situated inside.

ENDOCARDITIS means inflammation of the smooth membrane lining the heart, especially that over the heart valves. (See HEART DISEASES.)

ENDOCRINE GLANDS are organs whose function is to secrete into the blood or lymph substances known as hormones which play an important part in general chemical changes or the activities of other organs at a distance. Some organs have a double function, such as the pancreas, which pours digestive secretions by a duct into the intestine, and, at the same time, has an endocrine or internal secretion (insulin) which is secreted direct into the blood. Various diseases arise as the result of defects or excess in the internal secretions of the different glands. The chief endocrine glands are the thyroid, adrenal, pituitary, parathyroid, pancreas, ovaries, and testicles.

THYROID GLAND: This gland, situated in front of the neck, produces a secretion which has an important effect in regulating the general metabolism of the body. When it is defective, the conditions known as myxoedema and cretinism result; whilst excess of the secretion is associated with thyrotoxicosis. The active principle of this secretion is thyroxine and this is used in patients in whom the secretion is defective.

ADRENAL GLANDS: These two glands, also known as SUPRARENAL GLANDS, lie immediately above the kidneys. The central or medullary portion of the glands forms the secretions known as adrenaline or epinephrine, and noradrenaline. Adrenaline acts upon structures innervated by sympathetic nerves; its action is therefore said to be sympathomimetic. Briefly, the blood-vessels of the skin and of the abdominal viscera (except the intestines) are constricted, and at the same time the arteries of the muscles and the coronary arteries are dilated; systolic blood-pressure rises; blood-sugar increases; the metabolic rate rises; muscle fatigue is diminished. Adrenaline can be synthetically prepared in the laboratory. This substance is widely used in medicine in 1 in 1000 solutions, for the purpose of checking bleeding, relieving congestion of mucous membranes, for the relief of asthma, and in the treatment of anaphylactic shock. The superficial or cortical part of the glands produce a series of chemical substances which have as their basis a complicated steroid nucleus. The best known of these are aldosterone, cortisone, hydrocortisone, and deoxycortone acetate. These substances are essential for the maintenance of life. It is the absence of these substances, due to atrophy or destruction of the suprarenal cortex, that is responsible for the condition known as Addison's disease (qv).

PITUITARY GLAND: This gland is attached to the base of the brain and rests in a hollow on the base of the skull immediately above the hinder part of the throat. The pituitary gland is the most important of all endocrine glands and has been called the conductor of the endocrine orchestra. It consists of two embryologically and functionally distinct lobes. The function of the anterior lobe depends on the secretion by the hypothalamus (qv) of certain 'neuro-hormones' which are carried down the infundibular stalk in the hypophyseal portal system. These neuro-hormones are secreted into the portal venous system flowing from the median eminence of the hypothalamus to the anterior lobe of the pituitary gland and control the secretion of the pituitary trophic hormones. The hypothalamic centres involved in the control of specific pituitary hormones appear to be anatomically separate. Through the pituitary trophic hormones the activity of the thyroid, adrenal cortex and the sex glands is controlled. A reciprocal relationship between the anterior pituitary and the target glands exists. The liberation of trophic hormones is inhibited by a rising concentration of the circulating hormone of the target gland and stimulated by a fall in its concentration. Six trophic hormones are formed by the anterior pituitary. Growth hormone and prolactin are simple proteins formed in the acidophil cells. Follicle-stimulating hormone, luteinizing hormone and thyroid-stimulating hormone are glycoproteins formed in the basophil cells. Adrenocorticotrophic hormone (ACTH), although a polypeptide, is derived from basophil cells. The chromophobe cell, once thought to be inactive, is in fact the stem cell and 50 per cent of chromophobe adenomas secrete prolactin.

All these pituitary hormones are polypeptides. When used therapeutically they cannot be given by mouth, as they would be digested in the gastro-intestinal tract. They are therefore prepared in powder form for intramuscular injection. The powder should be dissolved carefully, and after injection the site should be massaged to ensure efficient absorption.

The posterior pituitary lobe, or neurohypophysis, is closely connected with the hypothalamus by the hypothalmic-hypophyseal tracts. It is concerned with the production or storage of oxytocin and vasopressin (the antidiuretic hormone).

Pituitary Hormones: Rapid advances have taken place in the past decade in the methods of assay of pituitary hormones and in the production and preparation of these hormones for clinical use. Growth hormone, gonadotrophic hormone, adrenocorticotrophic hormone and thyrotrophic hormones can be assayed in blood or urine by radio-immuno-assay techniques. Growth hormone extracted from human pituitary glands obtained at autopsy was available for clinical use until 1985 when it was withdrawn as it is believed to carry the virus responsible for Creutzfeldt-Jakob disease. However growth hormone produced by DNA recombinant techniques is now available as Somatonorm.

Human pituitary gonadotrophins are readily obtained from post-menopausal urine. Commercial extracts from this source are available and are effective for treatment of infertility due to gonadotrophin insufficiency.

The adrenocorticotrophic hormone is extracted from animal pituitary glands and has been available therapeutically for many years. It is used as a test of adrenal function, and, under certain circumstances, in conditions for which cortico-steroid therapy is indicated. The pharmacologically active polypeptide of ACTH has now been synthesized. It is called tetracosactrin, and as it is a pure substance it is prescribed by weight. Thyrotrophic hormone is also available but it has no therapeutic application. Melanocyte-stimulating hormone (MSH) does not occur in the human pituitary.

Hypothalamic Releasing Hormones: Hypothalamic releasing hormones which affect the release of each of the six anterior pituitary hormones have been identified. Their blood levels are only one-thousandth of those of the pituitary trophic hormones. The release of thyrotrophin, adrenocorticotrophin, growth hormone, follicle-stimulating hormone and luteinizing hormone is stimulated whilst release of prolactin is inhibited. The structure of the releasing hormones for TSH, FSH-LH, GH and, most recently, ACTH is known and they have all been synthesized. Thyrotrophin-releasing hormone (TRH) is already in clinical use as a diagnostic test of thyroid function but it has no therapeutic application. FSH-LH-releasing hormone provides a useful diagnostic test of gonadotrophine reserve in patients with pituitary disease and is now used in the treatment of infertility and amenorrhoea in patients with functional hypothalamic disturbance. As this is the commonest variety of secondary amenorrhoea the potential use is great. The therapeutic use of GH-releasing hormone and corticotrophin releasing hormone has yet to be established. Most cases of congenital deficiency of GH, FSH, LH and ACTH are due to defects in the hypothalamic production of releasing hormone and are not a primary pituitary defect, so that the therapeutic implication of this recently synthesized group of releasing hormones is considerable.

Galactorrhoea (qv) is frequently due to a microadenoma of the pituitary and less frequently results from impairment of the tonic inhibition exerted on the pituitary by the hypothalamus. Dopamine is the prolactin-release inhibiting hormone. Its duration of action is short so its therapeutic value is limited. However, bromocriptine is a dopamine agonist with a more prolonged action and is effective treatment for galactorrhoea whether this is due to a prolactin-secreting adenoma or to impairment of the tonic inhibition exerted by the prolactin-release inhibiting hormone.

PARATHYROID GLANDS: These are four minute glands lying at the side of, or behind, the thyroid. They have a certain effect in controlling the absorption of lime salts by the bones and other tissues. When their secretion is defective, tetany occurs.

PANCREAS: This gland is situated in the upper part of the abdomen and, in addition to the digestive ferments which it produces, a substance known as insulin is absorbed from it into the circulating blood. This has the effect of adapting sugary foods for incorporation in the muscles and other tissues that particularly require such foodstuffs. Lack of it is followed by the production of the disease known as diabetes mellitus.

OVARIES AND TESTICLES: In addition to their main function of producing reproductive cells, these organs secrete substances which have a general effect upon the other bodily tissues.

The ovary secretes at least two hormones, known, respectively, as oestradiol (follicular hormone) and progesterone (corpus luteum hormone). Oestradiol develops (under the stimulus of the anterior pituitary lobe) each time an ovum in the ovary becomes mature, causes extensive proliferation of the endometrium lining the uterus, a stage ending with shedding of the ovum about 14 days before the onset of menstruation. The corpus luteum, which then forms, secretes both progesterone and oestradiol. Progesterone brings about great activity of the glands in the endometrium. The uterus is now ready for the nesting of the ovum if it is fertilized. If fertilization does not occur, the corpus luteum degenerates, the hormones cease acting, and menstruation takes place.

The hormone secreted by the testicles is known as testosterone. It is responsible for the growth of the male secondary sex characteristics.

ENDOMETRIOSIS is the condition in which the endometrium (ie. the cells lining the interior of the uterus) is found in other parts of the body. The most common site of such misplaced endometrium is the muscle of the uterus. The next most common site is the ovary, followed by the peritoneum (qv) lining the pelvis (qv), but it also occurs anywhere in the bowel. The cause is not known. It never occurs before puberty and seldom after the menopause. The main symptoms it produces are menorrhagia (qv), dyspareunia (qv), painful menstruation and pelvic pain. Treatment is usually by removal of the affected area, but in some cases satisfactory results are obtained from the administration of progestogens (qv) such as norethisterone (qv), norethynodrel (qv) and danazol.

ENDOMETRITIS means inflammation of the mucous membrane lining the womb. (See UTERUS, DISEASES OF.)

ENDOMETRIUM is the mucous membrane which lines the interior of the uterus.

ENDORPHINS are peptides (qv) produced in the brain which have a pain-relieving action. Hence their alternative name of opiate peptides. Their name is derived from *endo*genous mor*phine*. They have been defined as endogenous opiates or any naturally occurring substances in the brain with pharmacological actions resembling opiate alkaloids such as morphine. There is some evidence that the pain-relieving action of acupuncture (qv) may be due to the release of these opiate peptides. It has also been suggested that they may have an anti-psychotic action and therefore of value in the treatment of major psychotic illnesses such as schizophrenia.

ENDOTHELIUM is the membrane lining various vessels and cavities of the body, such as the pleura, pericardium, peritoneum, lymphatic vessels, blood-vessels, and joints. It consists of a fibrous layer covered with thin flat cells, which render the surface perfectly smooth and secrete the fluid for its lubrication.

ENEMA means an injection of fluid into the bowel.

Uses: PURGATIVE ENEMAS are given generally in large bulk, so as to distend the rectum; they also contain various stimulating substances. For an adult, 450 to 900 ml (1 to 2 pints) are injected, for a young child about 170 ml (6 ounces). The process of injection should be slow, and the person should retain the enema as long as he can, in order to obtain the maximum effect. The water should be tepid: about 38°C (100°F). The usual constituent is soft green soap BP, 14 g (½ ounce) in 450 ml (1 pint) of water. Yellow soap is also satisfactory. In some cases an olive oil enema is preferred, or a glycerin enema of equal parts of glycerin and water). To expel flatulence, two tablespoonfuls of turpentine may be added to each pint of warm water. The frequent use of enemas is unhealthy, as they ultimately increase the constipation.

DISPOSABLE ENEMAS are largely supplanting the traditional soap-and-water enemas – largely on account of their convenience. The ingredients, usually sodium diphosphate and sodium phosphate in the case of a purgative enema, are contained in around 100 ml of solution in a small plastic bag with tube and plug.

MINIATURE ENEMAS are in increasing use. Their great advantage is that they are of a much smaller volume – only 2 millilitres, and therefore much more comfortable for the patient. They are also prepared much more easily and are supplied ready made up in a plastic container with a soft nozzle. They may be self-administered. As a rule, a movement of the bowels occurs within fifteen minutes. A widely used formula for such a miniature enema is: 5 mg of bisacodyl; 0·5 millilitre of glycerin; made up to 2 millilitres with Sulphated Castor Oil BPC.

SEDATIVE ENEMAS are used to quiet spasm, and check excessive action of the bowels. There are two types. A *starch enema* is made by rubbing 8 g of powdered starch to a smooth paste with a little cold water, and then adding 140 ml of boiling water. It is used when it has been allowed to cool. A *starch-and-opium enema* is prepared by adding 0·5 to 2·5 ml of tincture of opium to 60 ml of starch enema.

NUTRIENT ENEMAS are given when the stomach is seriously deranged and cannot retain or cannot digest food, but they are not widely used today. A nutrient enema consists of dextrose, 5 per cent solution in normal saline solution. The enema, which is warmed to 38°C (100°F), must be administered very slowly, and preferably run in through a small funnel and catheter tube. It may be given, to the amount of 230 to 285 ml, every 4 hours, that is five times in 24 hours.

IRRIGATION, or CLEANSING, ENEMAS are used for healing and cleansing purposes. Several pints of warm, weak salt solution (2 teaspoonfuls of salt to every 450 ml (1 pint) of water) or boric acid solution are introduced very slowly, by a douche, into the bowel, and then allowed to run off by lowering the tube, very much in the same way that the stomach is washed out.

Mode of administration: Nutrient enemas are administered by means of a rubber tube 90 to 120 cm (3 or 4 feet) in length, with a funnel at one end, and soft rubber nozzle, with rounded end, at the other. For purgative enemas, the rubber syringe with a ball in the centre may be used, and for small enemas a rubber bag which contains the exact amount required. In all cases the old bone or metal nozzle should be replaced by a soft rubber one, because much pain and injury may be inflicted by a rigid one carelessly or forcibly introduced.

The patient lies upon his left side with the hips raised on a thick pillow, and should remain so after the enema has been given. The nozzle is oiled, introduced forwards and upwards with a screwing motion, and should be passed gently up for 75 or 100 mm (3 or 4 inches). The fluid is now pumped, or, if a tube and funnel is used, allowed to flow gently in by raising the funnel. In the case of nutrient enemas, fully fifteen or twenty minutes should be spent in letting the fluid slowly enter; otherwise the bowels may move and the whole enema be rejected.

ENKEPHALINS are peptides which have the same action as endorphins (qv).

ENOPHTHALMOS is a term applied to abnormal retraction of the eye into its socket: for example, when the sympathetic nerve in the neck is paralysed.

ENSURE (see ENTERAL FEEDING).

ENTAMOEBA (see AMOEBA).

ENTERAL FEEDING: In severely ill patients the metabolic responses to tissue damage may be sufficient to cause a reduction of muscle mass and of plasma proteins. This state of catabolism may also impair the immune response to infection and delay the healing of wounds. It is probable that as many as one half of patients who have had a major operation a week previously show evidence of protein malnutrition. This can be detected clinically by a loss of weight and a reduction in the skinfold thickness and arm circumference. Biochemically the serum albumin falls as does the lymphocyte count. The protein reserves of the body fall even more dramatically when there are sepsis, burns, acute pancreatitis or renal failure.

The purpose of enteral feeding is to give a liquid, low residue food through a naso-gastric feeding tube. It has the advantage over parenteral nutrition that the septic complications of insertion of catheters into veins are avoided. It is also much cheaper. Enteral feeding may either take the form of intermittent feeding through a large-bore naso-gastric tube or continuous gravity feeding through a fine-bore tube.

A number of proprietary enteral foods are available and these avoid the necessity of nursing or dietetic staff making up the preparations. Some of these proprietary feeds contain whole protein as the nitrogen source. Others, and these are called elemental diets, contain free amino acids. Clinifeed, Ensure, Isocal and Triosorbon all contain whole protein whilst Flexical contains 70 per cent amino acids and 30 per cent oligopeptides; Vivonex contains amino acids only. Diarrhoea is the most common problem with enteral feeding and it tends to occur when enteral feeding is introduced too rapidly or with too strong a preparation.

ENTERALGIA is another name for colic.

ENTERIC FEVERS are typhoid fever and paratyphoid fever.

Until the middle of the last century typhoid was not distinguished from typhus fever. Subsequently all doubt upon the subject was removed by the careful clinical and pathological observations made by Sir William Jenner at the London Fever Hospital (1849–51). At the end of the nineteenth century it was noticed that cases of fever resembling typhoid but of shorter duration occurred, and these were found to be due to bacilli resembling the typhoid bacillus and are known as paratyphoid fevers. This group of fevers, again, has a resemblance, both as regards symptoms and as regards the causal bacteria, to cases of food-poisoning and dysentery.

Causes: A bacillus, discovered first by Eberth in 1880, and known as *Salmonella typhi*, is the cause of typhoid fever. (See BACTERIOLOGY.) The bacilli responsible for cases of paratyphoid fever are known as *Salmonella paratyphi A* and *Salmonella paratyphi B*, the latter being the commoner. Other bacilli which do not altogether correspond to either of these are also responsible for mild attacks of fever, sometimes grouped as paratyphoid C.

TYPHOID FEVER: Where the discharges, sheets, etc., from typhoid patients are carefully disinfected, there is little risk of direct spread from person to person. In many hospitals patients with typhoid are therefore treated in the general wards, with little or no risk to the other patients, provided certain precautions are taken.

All insanitary conditions in respect of drainage of houses and localities furnish the most ready means for the spread of the contagion of typhoid fever. The most certain means of preventing its appearance or checking its spread are: the water-carriage system of sewage disposal; prevention of pollution of water-supplies, food, milk, and shell-fish with human excreta; chlorination of drinking water; pasteurization of milk; control of the house-fly; personal cleanliness; detection of carriers of enteric bacilli. The bacillus resides in the stools and urine of typhoid patients. Thus, in badly laid drains, where the contents stagnate, the bacillus may increase indefinitely, and, by the contamination of drinking-water in places where wells or cisterns are exposed to sewage pollution, convey infection to a whole community. Dust may also act as the medium which conveys the bacilli in cases in which the discharges of a typhoid patient or the sewage are allowed to dry, and so get blown into drinking-water or on to food. Milk may readily be contaminated by the bacillus and form the cause of an epidemic, when a case of the fever has occurred in a dairy. The source of an epidemic has also been traced to the eating of oysters taken from oyster-beds near which contaminated sewage is discharged. During an epidemic flies may also form a means of contamination between uncovered stools and uncovered food. It may therefore be said that the spread of typhoid fever depends upon food or drink contaminated by a bacillus which is derived more or less directly from the discharges of previous typhoid cases.

The incubation period is usually ten to fourteen days, but may be as short as five days or as long as twenty-one days.

The chief symptoms will be better understood by a brief reference to the principal changes that take place in the body during the disease. The bowels are chiefly affected, particularly the lower end of the small intestine, where the Peyer's patches on the inner surface of the bowel (see INTESTINES) pass through changes that bear a distinct relation to the symptoms exhibited by the patient during the course of the disease. (1) During the first eight or ten days of the illness these patches, which in health are comparatively indistinct, become enlarged and prominent as the result of inflammation. (2) During the second week of the fever these enlarged patches undergo a process of sloughing, being cast off either in fragments or *en masse*. (3) From the second week onwards during the remainder of the fever, and even into the stage of convalescence, the ulcers formed by this process remain open, though slowly healing. The ulcers vary in size according to the Peyer's patches that have sloughed away, and they may be few or many in number. They are frequently, but not always, oblong in shape, with their long axis in that of the bowel, and they have somewhat thin and ragged edges. They may extend through the thickness of the bowel to the peritoneal coat, and they may perforate this, or may erode blood-vessels in their progress. (4) During convalescence the ulcers usually heal, leaving no contraction in the wall of the bowel.

The mesenteric glands associated with the intestine become enlarged, but usually subside without abscess formation as recovery takes place. The spleen becomes soft and enlarged, this enlargement being a useful guide to the physician in cases which are difficult to diagnose. As in other fevers, the muscular tissues soften and waste, and various complications affecting other organs may arise.

Symptoms: The symptoms at the *onset* of typhoid fever are much less marked than those of most other fevers, and the disease in the majority of instances sets in somewhat insidiously. Indeed, it is no uncommon thing for patients with this fever to go about for a considerable time after it has begun. The most marked of the early symptoms are headache, lassitude, and discomfort, together with sleeplessness and feverishness, particularly at night; this last symptom is that by which the disease is most readily detected in its early stages. Bleeding from the nose is also an early symptom in many cases. The course of *the temperature* is one of the important diagnostic features. During the first week it rises about 1·2°C in the evening and falls 0·7°C in the morning so that by the end of the first week it has reached a plateau of 38·8° to 40°C (102° to 104°F). Because of this feature of rising by steps, so to speak, it is known as a step-ladder temperature.

During the second week the daily range of temperature is comparatively small, a slight morning remission being all that is observed. In the third week the same condition continues more or less; but frequently a slight tendency to lowering may be discerned, particularly in the morning temperature, and the fever gradually dies down as a rule between the twenty-first and twenty-eighth day, although it is liable to recur in the form of a relapse. Although during the earlier days of the fever the patient may be able to move about, he feels languid and uneasy; and usually before the first week is over he has to take to bed, and soon the effects of the attack become more apparent. He is restless, hot, and uncomfortable, particularly as the day advances, and his cheeks show a red flush, especially in the evening or after taking food. The *pulse* in an ordinary case, although more rapid than normal, is not accelerated to an extent corresponding to the height of the temperature, and, at least in the earlier stages of the fever, is rarely above 100 a minute. In severe and protracted cases, where there is evidence of extensive intestinal ulceration, the pulse becomes rapid and weak. The *tongue* has at first a thin whitish fur and is red at the tip and edges. It tends, however, to become dry, brown or glazed-looking, and fissured transversely, while sordes may be present about the lips and teeth. There is much thirst, and, in some cases, vomiting.

From an early period in the disease *abdominal symptoms* show themselves and are often of great help in diagnosis. The abdomen is somewhat distended, and pain accompanying some gurgling sounds may be elicited on light pressure about the lower part of the right side close to the groin – the region corresponding to that portion of the intestine in which the morbid changes already referred to are progressing. *Diarrhoea* is a common but by no means constant symptom. When present, it may be slight in amount, or, on the other hand, extremely profuse, and it corresponds, as a rule, to the severity of the intestinal ulceration, and to the nature of the diet which the patient has been taking. The discharges are highly characteristic, being of light-yellow colour, resembling 'pea soup' in appearance. Sometimes, especially in milder cases, constipation is found instead of diarrhoea. Should intestinal haemorrhage occur, the stools may be dark brown, or composed entirely of blood. Enlargement of the spleen and liver can usually be made out by the physician. The urine is scanty and high-coloured. When the fever is well developed from the second week onwards, the *blood* shows a well-marked feature known as the Widal reaction. (See AGGLUTINATION.)

About the beginning, or during the course, of the second week of the fever, an *eruption* often makes its appearance on the skin. It consists of small isolated spots, oval or round in shape, of a pale pink or rose colour, which are seen chiefly upon the abdomen, chest, and back, and they come out in crops, which continue for four or five days and then fade away. At first they are slightly elevated, and disappear on pressure. In some cases they are very few in number, and their presence is made out with difficulty; but in others they are numerous and sometimes show themselves upon the limbs as well as upon the body. They do not appear to have any relation to the severity of the attack, and in a large proportion of cases (particularly in children) they are entirely absent. Besides this eruption there are often numerous very faint bluish patches or blotches about half an inch in diameter, chiefly upon the body and thighs. When present, the rose-spots, as they are known, continue to come out in crops till nearly the end of the fever, and they may reappear should a relapse subsequently occur.

These various symptoms persist throughout the third week, usually, however, increasing in intensity. The patient becomes prostrated and emaciated; the tongue is dry and brown, the pulse quickened and feeble, and the abdominal symptoms more marked; while nervous disturbance is exhibited in delirium, in tremors and jerkings of the muscles (*subsultus tendinum*), in drowsiness, and occasionally in 'coma vigil'. (See TYPHUS FEVER.) In severe cases the exhaustion reaches an extreme degree, but even in such instances the condition should not be regarded as hopeless. In favourable cases a change for the better may be expected between the twenty-first and twenty-eighth days, although it takes place by a lysis or gradual subsidence of the symptoms (the morning and evening temperatures descending, the pulse becoming stronger, the diarrhoea passing off, the tongue becoming clean, etc.), not by a crisis as in typhus fever or pneumonia. Convalescence proceeds slowly, and relapses are apt to occur (due often to errors in diet). Such relapses may prolong the fever for two or three months, though this is not common.

Abscesses sometimes arise, especially in connection with inflammation in the periosteum of the bones, found after the patient has been convalescent for some time, and these form a troublesome and prolonged complication. Stiff back, known as 'typhoid spine', is an occasional sequel to this disease, due either to inflammation in the spine or more commonly to changes in the muscles with development of fibrous tissue, causing the patient for long, it may be for years, to suffer from severe 'rheumatic' pains. Inflammation of the bile passages, with retention of the bacilli in these and their constant discharge in the stools, is also an occasional sequel; and, although this may cause no trouble to the patient, it renders him a source of danger to others as a 'carrier' of the disease. (See INFECTION.)

When death takes place, it is generally due to one of the following causes: (1) exhaustion in the second or third week or later; (2) haemorrhage from the bowels; (3) perforation of an ulcer and the onset of peritonitis; (4) excessive rise of temperature; (5) complications, such as inflammation of the lungs.

Treatment: The preventive treatment includes all the municipal and domestic measures that aim at securing pure supplies of water and milk and well-laid drains. Inoculation with anti-typhoid vaccine is a precaution which ought to be adopted by people travelling to Africa, Asia, South America, or any country around, or any island in, the Mediterranean, or in the Balkans. It should be repeated every three years. (See VACCINE.)

When an outbreak of typhoid fever occurs in a family, the source of the milk supply especially should be scrutinized. The discharges of a typhoid patient should be mixed so soon as passed with a strong disinfectant. (See DISINFECTION.) Similar care should be taken to sterilize all sheets, towels, etc., soiled by the patient. Special care is necessary on the part of those in attendance on a typhoid-fever patient to cleanse the hands at once after touching the patient, and especially after they have become in any way soiled by contact with his discharges.

The introduction of chloramphenicol has transformed a fever that lasted three to four weeks into a sharp febrile illness of three to four days. This means that diet is not so important as it was, but milk, or milk dishes, are still the great standby.

Ampicillin (qv) is also proving of value, but the relative value of these two antibiotics has not been determined. Whichever is used, however, it is still necessary to keep the patient in bed for three weeks, and to keep him on a bland nutritious diet during this period. Otherwise complications may arise. The patient should be considered infective until six consecutive specimens of stools and urine are found to be negative on bacteriological examination.

In the convalescent stage, and even after apparently complete recovery, the utmost care should be observed by the patient as to diet, all hard and indigestible substances being dangerous from their tendency to irritate or reopen unhealed ulcers and bring on a relapse of the fever or cause a sudden perforation. Lastly, the general health demands careful attention for a length of time.

PARATYPHOID FEVER is a continued fever which closely resembles mild attacks of typhoid and which, like typhoid fever, is due to one or more members of the genus *Salmonella*.

Causes: Paratyphoid fever is due to infection with one of three micro-organisms: *Salmonella paratyphi A*, *B*, or *C*. These organisms closely resemble that of typhoid fever in appearance and some of its reactions. The infection is usually conveyed by a 'carrier' case who has already had the disease, or it is due to contaminated food or water. In the five-year period, 1973-77, there were 509 cases in Britain, one of them a double infection with *S. paratyphi A* and *B*. Of the 158 cases of paratyphoid, 97 per cent were contracted abroad (116 in the Indian subcontinent). Of the 352 cases of paratyphoid B, 57 per cent were contracted abroad (95 in the Mediterranean).

Symptoms resemble those found in a mild case of typhoid fever. The incubation period is shorter (one to ten days), and rose spots are seen less commonly. The onset of the disease is often more sudden than in typhoid fever, but the fever tends to be less prolonged and less severe.

Treatment is the same as for typhoid fever.

ENTERITIS means inflammation of the intestines. (See DIARRHOEA; INTESTINES, DISEASES OF.)

ENTEROBIASIS is infection with *Enterobius vermicularis*, the threadworm, or pinworm as it is known in the USA. It is the most common of all the intestinal parasites in Britain and the least harmful. The male is about 6 mm (¼ inch) in length and the female about 12 mm (½ inch) in length. Each resembles a little piece of thread. These worms live in considerable numbers in the lower bowel, affecting children particularly. They cause great irritation round the anus, especially in the evening when the female worm emerges from the anus to lay its eggs and then die. It lays around 10,000 eggs and these may be found in dust, especially after bedmaking, in the bedclothes and pyjamas, on toys and furniture, and on the fur of cats and dogs, as well as floating in the air. Apart from this irritation around the anus, they seldom cause any symptoms, though in some cases they may cause diarrhoea and, occasionally in girls, they may be responsible for a discharge from the vagina.

Treatment: The most effective form of treatment is either viprynium embonate or piperazine citrate. The former has the advantage of only one dose being necessary repeated twice at 15-day intervals, whereas a 7-day course of piperazine is necessary repeated after a week's interval. Whichever drug is used, a second course should be given after a period of three weeks. If one member of a household is infected, it is necessary to examine all other members of the household and to treat simultaneously all those found infected. During treatment steps must be taken to prevent patients reinfecting themselves or infecting others. This is done by the wearing of drawers day and night to prevent scratching of the anus, and of gloves at night, the daily washing of all infected linen, and scrupulous cleanliness. The local irritation around the anus may be relieved by the application of weak white precipitate ointment.

ENTEROCELE means a hernia of the bowel. (See HERNIA.)

ENTEROGASTRONE is a hormone derived from the mucosal lining of the small intestine which inhibits the movements and secretion of the stomach.

ENTEROKINASE is the enzyme (qv) secreted in the duodenum (qv) and jejunum (qv) which converts the enzyme, trypsinogen, secreted by the pancreas (qv) into trypsin (qv). (See also DIGESTION.)

ENTEROPTOSIS means a condition in which, owing to a lax condition of the mesenteries and ligaments which support the bowels, the latter descend into the lower part of the abdominal cavity. The condition is aggravated by tight lacing and by the lax condition of the abdominal wall which follows repeated child-bearing, and so is commoner in women.
Treatment: Massage of the abdominal muscles, and the wearing of a well-shaped abdominal belt give most relief.

ENTEROSTOMY means an operation by which an artificial opening is formed into the intestine.

ENTEROVIRUSES are a family of viruses which include the poliomyelitis, coxsackie and echo groups of viruses. Their importance lies in their tendency to invade the central nervous system. They receive their name from the fact that their mode of entry into the body is through the gut.

ENTOMOPHOBIA is excessive fear of insects, particularly spiders, mites and other anthropods.

ENTROPION (see EYE, DISEASE AND INJURIES OF).

ENURESIS means the unconscious or involuntary passage of urine. (See NOCTURNAL ENURESIS.)

ENZYME is the name applied to a chemical ferment produced by living cells. The first enzyme was obtained in a reasonably pure state in 1926 and shown to be a protein. Since then several hundred enzymes have been obtained in pure crystalline form. Many more have been purified to less exacting standards and all have been proved to be proteins. They are present in the digestive fluids and in many of the tissues, and are capable of producing in small amount the transformation on a large scale of various compounds. Indeed, they are an integral, essential component of what might be described as the *modus operandi* of the body. Examples of enzymes are found in the ptyalin of saliva and diastase of pancreatic juice which split up starch into sugar, the pepsin of the gastric juice and the trypsin of pancreatic juice which break proteins into simpler molecules and eventually into the constituent amino-acids, the thrombin of the blood which causes coagulation.

EOSINOPHIL is any cell in the body with granules in its substance that stain easily with the dye eosin. About 2 per cent of the white cells of the blood are eosinophils.

EOSINOPHILIA means an abnormal increase in the number of eosinophils in the blood. It occurs in Hodgkin's disease, in asthma and hay fever, in some skin diseases, and in parasitic infestation.

EPHEDRINE is an alkaloid derived from a species of *Ephedra* or prepared synthetically, much used for asthma and other allergic disorders, in doses of 15 to 60 mg. It is similar to adrenaline in pharmacological action.

EPHELIS is a freckle (qv). *Ephelis ab igne* is the dark-brown pigmentation produced on the legs by constant exposure of them to a fire. A similar discoloration of the skin of the abdomen may be produced by constant use of a hot-water bottle.

EPI- is a prefix meaning situated on or outside of.

EPIDEMIC is a term applied to a disease which affects a large number of people in a particular locality at one time. The term is, in a sense, opposed to endemic, which means a disease always found in the locality in question. A disease may, however, be endemic as a rule – for example, malaria in swampy districts, and may become at times epidemic, when an unusually large number of people are affected.

As a rule an epidemic disease is infectious from person to person, but this is not necessarily the case, since many persons in a locality may simply be exposed to the same cause at one time; for example, outbreaks of lead-poisoning are epidemic in this sense.

The laws which govern the outbreak of epidemics are by no means fully understood. Infected food supplies, such as drinking water contaminated by the evacuations of persons sick of cholera or typhoid fever, or milk tainted by the organism of scarlet fever have been traced as the cause of outbreaks of these diseases. The migrations of certain animals, such as rats, are in some cases responsible for the spread of plague, from which these animals die in great numbers. Certain epidemics come with regularity at certain seasons. Thus scarlet fever and diphtheria are autumnal complaints, and produce their epidemics in September, October and November. Whooping-cough, on the other hand, is a spring complaint, and very few cases occur in autumn. Measles produces two epidemics, as a rule, one in winter and one in March. Influenza, the common cold, and other infections of the upper respiratory tract, such as sore throat, occur predominantly in the winter.

These seasonal variations depend largely, no doubt, upon conditions like the amount of sunshine, the rainfall, the temperature of the ground and the aggregation of susceptible individuals.

There is another variation, both as regards the number of persons affected and the number who die in successive epidemics: the severity of successive epidemics rising and falling over periods of five or ten years. Further, scourges like plague and cholera have swept over whole continents at longer periods, and then died down without apparent cause. The reason for these latter variations is still obscure.

EPIDEMIC ENCEPHALITIS is another term for ENCEPHALITIS LETHARGICA (qv).

EPIDURAL ANAESTHESIA (see ANAESTHETICS).

EPIDYDIMIS is an oblong body attached to the upper part of each testicle, composed of convoluted vessels and ducts. It is liable to be the seat of tuberculous and other inflammation. (See TESTICLE.)

EPIGASTRIUM is the region lying in the middle of the abdomen over the stomach. (See ABDOMEN, REGIONS OF.)

EPIGLOTTIS is a leaf-like piece of elastic cartilage covered with mucous membrane, which stands upright between the back of the tongue and the glottis, or entrance to the larynx. In the act of swallowing, it prevents fluids and solids from passing off the back of the tongue into the larynx.

EPIGLOTTITIS: Acute epiglottitis is an acute inflammatory oedema of the epiglottis, due to *Haemophilus influenzae*, which causes laryngeal obstruction due to swelling and immobilization of the epiglottis. It is a disease predominantly of children, occurs usually in the winter, and may prove rapidly fatal.

EPIGNATHUS is a mal-development of the foetus in which the deformed remains of one twin are united to the upper jaw of the other.

EPILATION means the removal of hair by the roots. (See DEPILATION.)

EPILEPSY, or FALLING SICKNESS, is nervous disorder characterized by a fit of sudden loss of consciousness, attended with convulsions. There may, however, exist manifestations of epilepsy much less marked than this, yet equally characteristic of the disease. On the other hand, it is to be borne in mind that many other attacks of a convulsive nature have the term 'epileptiform' applied to them because they resemble epilepsy.

There are two well-marked varieties of the epileptic seizure. To these the terms, *le grand mal* and *le petit mal*, are generally applied. The former of these is that which attracts most attention, being what is generally known as an epileptic fit. In addition to these two forms there is a type known as *Jacksonian epilepsy*, in which the seizure consists of convulsive movements starting in a single muscle or group of muscles, consciousness being in general retained. Cases of this type shade off, however, into *grand mal*, and indeed the subjects of Jacksonian epilepsy may, at a later stage, be affected by typical seizures of severe type.

Incidence: It is estimated that in England and Wales there are around 290,000 epileptics: 190,000 adults and 100,000 children under the age of 16 years. It is also estimated that approximately 33,000 new cases occur every year. Probably one person in 20 has a fit of some sort in the course of a lifetime, but only one in 8 of those who have a fit will suffer from chronic epilepsy: that is, have a continuing liability to fits. The onset of epilepsy occurs before the age of 5 in nearly a quarter of the cases, and before school-leaving age in more than half.

Causes: Epilepsy has many causes. It may be a manifestation of a space-occupying lesion within the cranium such as a cerebral tumour, a cerebral haemorrhage, a scar from a previous cerebral thrombosis or an inflammation such as encephalitis. It may also be a manifestation of a metabolic disturbance, such as hypoglycaemia, hypokalaemia, hypocalcaemia or hypoxia. When it is idiopathic the onset usually occurs during infancy or at puberty. The diagnosis is usually made clinically and is confirmed by an electro-encephalogram (qv) in which characteristic changes are seen in epilepsy.

Symptoms: Although in most instances an epileptic attack comes on suddenly, it is in some cases preceded by certain premonitory indications or warnings. These are of very varied character, and may be in the form of some temporary change in the disposition, such as unusual elevation or depression of spirits, or of some alteration in the look. Besides these general symptoms, there are often peculiar sensations which immediately precede the onset of the fit, and to such the name of *aura epileptica* is applied. The so-called aura, which occurs in over 50 per cent of cases, may be of mental character, in the form of an agonizing feeling of momentary duration; of sensory character, in the form of pain in a limb or in some internal organ, such as the stomach; or an unusual feeling connected with the special senses, such as a strange smell or extraordinary vision; or of a motor character, in the form of contractions or trembling in some of the muscles. The aura may be so distinct and of such duration as to enable the patient to lie down or seek a place of safety before the attack comes on.

The seizure is usually preceded by a loud scream or cry, which is not to be ascribed, as was at one time supposed, to terror or pain, but is due to the convulsive action of the muscles of the larynx, and the expulsion of air through the narrowed glottis. If the patient is standing he immediately falls, and often sustains serious injury. Unconsciousness is complete, and the muscles generally are in a state of stiffness or tonic contraction, which may be found to affect those on one side of the body in particular. The head is turned towards one or other shoulder, the breathing is for the moment arrested, the countenance first pale then livid, the pupils dilated, and the pulse rapid. This, the first stage of the fit, generally lasts for about half-a-minute, and is followed by the state of clonic (ie. tumultuous) spasm of the muscles, in which the whole body is thrown into violent agitation. The eyes roll wildly, the teeth are gnashed together, and the tongue is often severely bitten. The breathing is noisy, and foam (often tinged with blood) issues from the mouth, while even the contents of the bowels and bladder may be ejected. This stage lasts for a period varying from a few seconds to several minutes, when the convulsive movements gradually subside and relaxation of the muscles takes place, together with partial return of consciousness, the patient looking confusedly about him and attempting to speak. This, however, is soon followed by drowsiness and stupor, which may continue for several hours. When he awakes either apparently quite recovered, or fatigued and depressed, he is occasionally in a state of excitement which sometimes assumes the form of mania.

Epileptic fits of this sort succeed each other with varying degrees of frequency, and occasionally though not frequently with regular periodicity. In some people they only occur once in a lifetime, or once in the course of many years, while in others they return every week or two, or even are of daily occurrence, and sometimes there are numerous attacks each day. Occasionally there occurs a constant succession of attacks extending over many hours, and with such rapidity that the patient appears as if he had never come out of the one fit. The term *status epilepticus* is applied to this condition, which sometimes has fatal results. In many epileptics the fits occur during the night as well as during the day, but in some instances they are entirely nocturnal, and in such cases the disease may long exist and yet remain unrecognized either by the patient or by the physician, until observed and described by some other person.

The other variety of epilepsy, to which the name *le petit mal* is given, differs from that just described in the absence of the convulsive spasms. It consists essentially in the sudden arrest of consciousness, which is of short duration, and may be accompanied by staggering or some alteration in position or motion, or may simply exhibit itself in a look of absence or confusion, and, should the patient happen to be engaged in conversation, by an abrupt termination of the act. In general, it lasts a few seconds, and the individual resumes his occupation without perhaps being aware of anything having been the matter. In some instances there is a degree of spasmodic action in certain muscles which may cause the patient to make some unexpected movement, such as turning half round, or walking abruptly aside, or may show itself by some unusual expression of countenance, such as squinting or grinning. There may be some amount of aura preceding such attacks, and also of faintness following them.

There is another sequel of an epileptic fit, particularly *petit mal*, which may have medico-legal implications. This is what is known as *post-epileptic automatism*. In this state, following an attack, an epileptic may carry out or perform some action of which he is entirely unaware when he recovers. Thus, he may proceed to undress himself no matter where he may be, or he may pick up the first thing he lays his hands on, or he may attack someone. An interesting feature of this phenomenon is that the action performed by any one epileptic is stereotype: that is, it is always the same odd action he performs. The possible medico-legal implications of this automatism are obvious.

Treatment: During the fit, little can be done beyond preventing the patient as far as possible from injuring himself while unconsciousness continues. Tight clothing should be loosened, and a cork or pad inserted between the teeth if possible, to prevent biting of the tongue. This, however, should never be done forcibly; otherwise teeth may be broken, and, as has been said, 'broken teeth are worse than a bitten tongue'. Unprotected fingers should never be put in the patient's mouth. When the fit is over, the patient should be allowed to sleep, and have the head and shoulders well raised.

Of medicinal remedies, the most commonly used is phenytoin, which is tending to replace phenobarbitone, either alone or in combination with one of the increasing number of other drugs being introduced for the treatment of epilepsy. The bromides, originally the great standby in the treatment of epilepsy, are seldom used for this purpose at the present day. Other drugs that have proved of value include methoin and primidone. In severe cases which do not respond satisfactorily to one or more of these drugs, there is a further choice of drugs including carbamazepine clonazepam, and sodium valproate. One of the most effective drugs for controlling *petit mal* is troxidone. The secret of success in controlling epilepsy is to remember that every case must be considered individually, and that once a successful means of control has been established, it should not be altered unless there is some special reason for so doing. Alcohol is strictly forbidden. A worrying feature, however, now attracting attention, is the increased rate of congenital malformations in children born to treated epileptic mothers. This is estimated to be about three times the normal rate.

As few restrictions as possible should be placed on the activities of an epileptic. This particularly applies to children. Unless the fits are severe and frequent, the child should be allowed to lead as normal a life as possible. Car driving licences can now be issued in suitable cases to people with epilepsy who, on the basis of medical evidence, have been free from attacks for at least two years, with or without treatment, or who for more than three years have had a history of attacks only during sleep. Heavy goods vehicle driving licences can now be issued to people who have been free from any epileptic attack since reaching the age of five.

Epileptic colonies have been established, where people seriously afflicted in this way can carry out productive work under safe conditions. These colonies are particularly useful for the 20 per cent or so of epileptics who are mentally retarded.

Patients with epilepsy and their relatives can obtain further advice and information from the British Epilepsy Association, Anstey House, 40 Hanover Square, Leeds LS3 1BE (0532–439393); or The Epilepsy Association of Scotland, 48 Govan Road, Glasgow G51 1JL (041–427 4911).

EPILOIA (see TUBEROSE SCLEROSIS).

EPIPHORA (see EYE, DISEASE AND INJURIES OF).

EPIPHYSIS means the spongy extremity of a bone, attached to it for the purpose of forming a joint with the similar process of another bone. An epiphysis is covered on its surface by cartilage, is developed from a distinct centre of ossification, and in a young person is connected with the shaft of the bone by a plate of cartilage that disappears in the adult. Separation of an epiphysis is a form of fracture which sometimes occurs in children, and is apt to be more serious than a break through bony tissue because it involves damage to the plate of growing cartilage, so that, although union takes place readily, the subsequent growth of the bone may be interfered with and the full growth of the limb may afterwards fail to be attained.

EPIPHYSITIS means inflammation of an epiphysis.

EPISIOTOMY is the operation of cutting the outlet of the vagina in childbirth so as to facilitate the birth of the child.

EPISPASTICS are substances which produce blistering of the skin. (See BLISTERS.)

EPISTAXIS means bleeding from the nose. (See HAEMORRHAGE.)

EPITHELIOMA is a tumour of malignant nature arising in the epithelium covering the surface of the body. (See CANCER.)

EPITHELIUM is the cellular layer which forms the epidermis on the skin, covers the inner surface of the bowels, and forms the lining of ducts and hollow organs, like the bladder. It consists of one or more layers of cells which adhere to one another, and is one of the simplest tissues of the body. It is of several forms: for example, the epidermis is formed of scaly epithelium, the cells being in several layers and more or less flattened. (See SKIN.) The bowels are lined by a single layer of columnar epithelium, the cells being long and narrow in shape. The air passages are lined by ciliated epithelium: that is to say, each cell is provided with lashes which

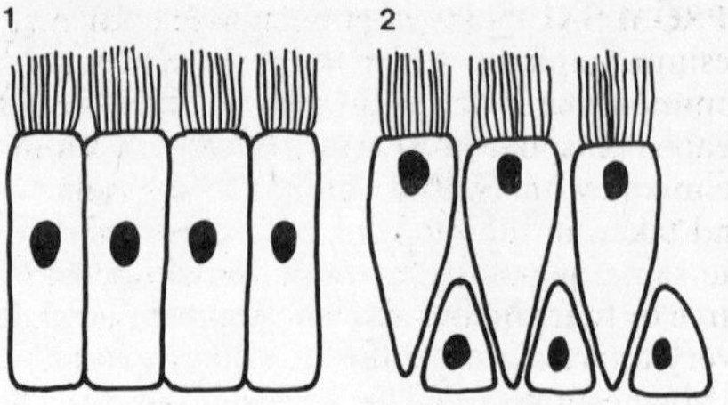

Diagram of ciliated epithelium (1) and pseudostratified columnar ciliated epithelium (2).

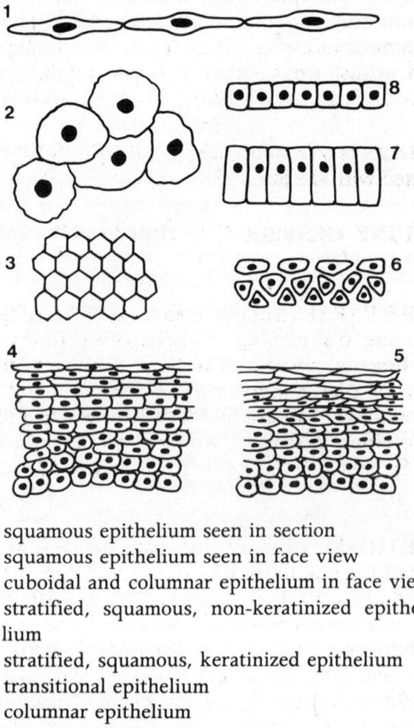

1 squamous epithelium seen in section
2 squamous epithelium seen in face view
3 cuboidal and columnar epithelium in face view
4 stratified, squamous, non-keratinized epithelium
5 stratified, squamous, keratinized epithelium
6 transitional epithelium
7 columnar epithelium
8 cuboid epithelium

Diagram of various types of epithelium.

drive the fluid upon the surface of the passages gradually upwards.

EPIZOOTIC is a term applied to any disease in animals which diffuses itself widely. The term corresponds to the word epidemic as applied to human beings. In plague, for example, an epizoötic in rats usually precedes the epidemic in human beings.

EPSOM SALTS is the popular name for magnesium sulphate, which is perhaps the most commonly used saline purgative. For a dose, a heaped teaspoonful or more of the salt should be mixed with as little water as will dissolve it, and taken in the morning before breakfast, or the same quantity may be taken divided into three or four small doses, one of which is taken every quarter of an hour. (See PURGATIVES.)

Magnesium sulphate is also used for the treatment of inflammatory conditions of the bowels in order to remove by purgation the cause of the irritation. It is sometimes injected through a stomach tube direct into the duodenum in order to produce a copious flow of bile in disorders of the liver and gall-bladder. It has also been used for injection intramuscularly or into the spinal canal in the treatment of tetanus, eclampsia, and other convulsive disorders. External fomentations of 5 to 25 per cent magnesium sulphate solution are applied in cases of rheumatic joints and other forms of inflammation, whilst a paste of magnesium sulphate in glycerin is a useful form of treatment of boils.

EPULIS is a term applied to any tumour connected with the jaws. (See MOUTH, DISEASES OF.)

EQUINE OESTROGENS (PREMARIN) (see OESTROGENS).

ERB'S PARALYSIS is a form of paralysis of the arm due to stretching or tearing of the fibres of the brachial nerve plexus. Such damage to the brachial plexus may occur during birth, and it is found that the arm lies by the side of the body with elbow extended, forearm pronated, and the fingers flexed. The infant is unable to raise the arm.

ERETHISM is the psychic disturbance that is one of the manifestations of chronic mercurial poisoning (qv). It is characterized by irritability, self consciousness, shyness, timidity, embarrassment, lack of concentration, depression and resentment of criticism. It was this condition that gave rise to the phrase, 'mad as a hatter', as chronic mercurial poisoning used to be one of the occupational hazards of the hat-making industry.

ERGOMETRINE is one of the active constituents of ergot (qv). It has a powerful action in controlling the excessive bleeding from the womb wich may occur after childbirth. The official *British Pharmacopoeia* preparation is Ergometrine Maleate.

ERGOSTEROL is a sterol found in yeasts and fungi and in plant and animal fat. Under the action of sunlight or ultra-violet rays it produces vitamin D_2. The substance produced in this way is known as calciferol, and is used for the prevention and cure of rickets and osteomalacia. A similar change in the ergosterol of the skin is produced when the body is freely exposed to sunlight. Calciferol is probably not so active as, and differs chemically from, the vitamin D occurring in fish-liver oils.

ERGOT is the spawn of *Claviceps purpurea*, a fungus which grows in the grain of rye. It contains several active principles, including the alkaloids, ergometrine, ergotoxine and ergotamine. Ergot causes prolonged contraction of unstriped muscle fibres all over the body, particularly the muscle fibres of the blood-vessels and of the womb. This action on the womb makes the drug of great value in midwifery, and it has been in use in midwifery since the 16th century.

Uses: Ergot is used mainly to check haemorrhage, particularly that which is apt to follow upon childbirth. It is also given in small doses for some time after childbirth to reduce the womb to its proper size in cases in which this is not taking place naturally.

ERGOTAMINE is one of the alkaloids in ergot. In the form of ergotamine tartrate it is most effective in the treatment of migraine (qv). It is usually given by mouth. Its continued use is not without risk, occasionally leading to gangrene of the tips of the fingers, so it should only be used under medical supervision. It has also been used for the relief of the itching of the skin which is sometimes such a troublesome feature of uraemia (qv).

ERGOT POISONING or ERGOTISM occasionally results from eating bread made from diseased rye. Several terrible epidemics (*St Anthony's Fire*), characterized by intense pain and hallucinations, occurred in France and Germany during the Middle Ages (cf ERYSIPELAS). Its symptoms are the occurrence of spasmodic muscular contractions, and the gradual production of gangrene in parts like the fingers, toes and tips of the ears.

EROSION means a process of gradual wearing down of structures in the body. The term is applied to the effect of tumours, when they cause destruction of tissue in their neighbourhood without actually growing into the latter: for example, an aneurysm may erode bones in its neighbourhood. The term is also applied to minute ulcers, for example, erosions of the stomach, caused by extreme acidity of the gastric juice.

DENTAL EROSION is the loss of tooth substance due to a cause other than decay or trauma. This is usually due to the presence of acid, eg. frequent vomiting or the excessive intake of citrus fruits. The teeth appear very smooth and later develop saucer-shaped depressions.

ERRHINES are drugs which cause running at the nose; eg. potassium iodide.

ERUCTATION, or belching, is the sudden escape of gas or of portions of half-digested food from the stomach up into the mouth. Many nervous people, and also those people who suffer from acid dyspepsia, have a habit of gulping down mouthfuls of air when digestion is uncomfortable. This air is belched up again after a little while. Some people, especially those in whom dyspepsia occurs from time to time, have at other times the peculiarity of bringing up fragments of food an hour or two after meals. (See FLATULENCE.)

ERUPTION or RASH, means an outbreak, in a scattered form, upon the surface of the skin, usually raised and red, or it may be covered with scales, or crusts, or vesicles containing fluid. The appearance of an eruption depends, to a certain extent, upon the nature of the disease, or other source of irritation, which causes it: for example, the eruption of measles is always distinguishable from that of chickenpox. But the same disease may also produce different eruptions in different people or in the same person in different states of health, or even on different parts of the body at one time.

Eruptions may be acute or chronic. Most of the acute eruptions belong to the exanthemata (qv): ie. they are bright in colour and burst out suddenly like a flower. These are the eruptions of scarlet fever, measles, German measles, smallpox and chickenpox. In general the severity of these diseases can be measured by the amount of eruption, but in cases in which the eruption is suppressed, or, as it is popularly termed, 'goes in', the disease is apt to be serious.

Some eruptions are very transitory, like nettle-rash, appearing and vanishing again in the course of a few hours.

(For chronic eruptions see SKIN, DISEASES OF.)

ERYSIPELAS: (synonyms, *the Rose, St Anthony's Fire*) is a disease characterized by diffuse inflammation of the skin, attended with fever. In the Middle Ages this disease was confused with ergot poisoning.

Causes: It has long been known that the disease is of a highly infectious nature. This contagiousness of erysipelas was often illustrated in the surgical wards of hospitals, where, having once broken out, it was apt to spread with great rapidity, and to produce disastrous results, as well as in lying-in hospitals, where its occurrence gave rise to the spread of a form of puerperal fever of virulent character. The infecting organism is the *Streptococcus pyogenes*. Erysipelas is slightly commoner in women than in men, and is commonest between the ages of 50 and 60.

Symptoms: When erysipelas is of moderate character, there is simply a redness of the skin, which feels somewhat hard and thickened, and upon which there often appear small vesicles. This redness, though at first circumscribed, tends to spread and affect the neighbouring sound skin, until an entire limb or a large area of the body may become involved in the inflammatory process. There is usually considerable pain, with heat and tingling in the affected part. As the disease advances, the portions of skin first attacked become less inflamed, and exhibit a yellowish appearance, which is followed by slight desquamation of the epidermis. Certain complications are apt to arise in erysipelas affecting the surface of the body, particularly inflammation of serous membranes, such as the pericardium, pleura and peritoneum.

Erysipelas of the face usually begins with symptoms of general illness, the patient feeling languid, drowsy and sick, while often there is shivering followed by fever, and the temperature may rise to 40° or 40·5°C (104° or 105°F). Sore throat is sometimes felt, but in general the first indication of the local affection is a red and painful spot at the side of the nose or on one of the cheeks or ears. Occasionally the inflammation begins in the throat, and reaches the face through the nasal fossae. The redness gradually spreads over the whole surface of the face, and is accompanied with swelling, which, in the lax tissues of the cheeks and eyelids, is so great that the features soon become unrecognizable and the eyes quite closed. The spreading edge of the red area is usually sharply marked and raised. Advancing over the scalp, the disease may invade the neck and pass on to the trunk, but in general the inflammation remains confined to the face and head. While the disease progresses, besides the pain, tenderness and heat of the affected parts, the constitutional symptoms may be severe, and delirium may occur. The attack in general lasts for a week or ten days, during which the inflammation subsides in the parts of the skin first attacked, while it spreads onwards in other directions, and after it has passed away there is some slight desquamation of the epidermis.

Although in general the termination is favourable, serious and occasionally fatal results follow from inflammation of the membranes of the brain, and in some rare instances sudden death has occurred from suffocation arising from oedema of the glottis, the inflammation having spread into, and extensively involved, the throat.

A very fatal form occasionally attacks newborn infants, particularly in the first four weeks of life (*erysipelas neonatorum*).

Treatment: The patient must be isolated, and great care must be taken to ensure that the infection is not transmitted to others by those in attendance on the patient. The outlook has changed considerably for the better since the introduction of penicillin, which should be given in full doses as soon as the condition is recognized. For local application the best preparations are either cold compresses of a saturated solution of magnesium sulphate or a 10 per cent solution of ichthyol in water. The patient must be kept in bed until the temperature has settled, and as nourishing a diet as possible should be given.

ERYTHEMA is a general term signifying several conditions in which areas of the skin become congested with blood, and consequently a red eruption appears. The eruption is

accompanied by tingling, and often by itching and pain.
Causes: It may be due to heat, such as exposure to the sun, or the constant exposure, by cooks or iron-workers, of the face, hands or legs to a blazing fire. *Erythema ab igne* is the reddening of the skin of the leg producing a net-like pattern that is found in people who sit huddled over the fire. Another form, known as *erythema pernio*, is due to exposure to cold and wet. (See CHILBLAINS.) A variety, which appears, usually on the front of the legs, in the form of red or livid, tender swellings, often over 2·5 cm in breadth, is known as *erythema nodosum*, and is a hypersensitivity reaction to infection with the streptococcus or mycobacterium tuberculosis. It is also a manifestation of sarcoidosis and may be an allergic reaction to the sulphonamide drugs. Children and young adults, especially women, may also suffer from a severer form, which begins as red blotches on the hands, and, spreading up the arms to the body, produces lumps and vesicles, or even large blebs full of fluid. This form, on account of the diversity of the appearances in different parts, is known as *erythema multiforme*. The cause in some cases is a virus. It also occurs as a drug-rash from the use of such drugs as sulphonamides and barbiturates. *Erythemainfectiosum*, or slapped cheek disease, is characterized by a fiery red rash on the cheeks: hence its alternative name. It occurs in children, in the spring. The rash, which spreads to the rest of the body, lasts for up to three weeks. Although highly infectious, the causative organism, probably a virus, has not been discovered.

ERYTHRASMA is a reddish-brown macular eruption of the skin, caused by a micro-organism known as *Nocardia minutissima*.

ERYTHROBLASTOSIS FOETALIS (see HAEMOLYTIC DISEASE OF THE NEWBORN).

ERYTHROCYTE is another name for a red blood corpuscle.

ERYTHROCYTE SEDIMENTATION RATE (see SEDIMENTATION RATE).

ERYTHROEDEMA: Other terms for this condition are ACRODYNIA and PINK DISEASE. This is a disease of infants with the following features: restlessness, weakness, neuritis and swelling and redness of the face, fingers and toes. In the vast majority of cases it is a manifestation of mercurial poisoning, often due to the infant having been given teething powders containing a mercurial laxative.

ERYTHROMELALGIA, or RED NEURALGIA, is a condition in which the fingers or toes, or even larger portions of the limbs, become purple, bloated in appearance, and very painful. In people suffering from the condition, which is not a common one, the attacks come and go, being worse in summer (unlike chilblains), and worse on exertion or when the affected parts are warmed or allowed to hang down. The condition may appear without apparent cause, but is often associated with vascular diseases, such as hypertension and polycythaemia vera. It aso occurs in association with certain diseases of the central nervous system, and in cases of metallic poisoning: eg. arsenic, mercury and thallium. Treatment is unsatisfactory. Residence in a moderate climate, the wearing of light-weight stockings or socks, and sandals, and the avoidance of excessive heat help to relieve the discomfort. Aspirin also gives marked relief.

ERYTHROMYCIN is an antibiotic derived from *Streptomyceserythreus*. Its antibacterial range of activity is comparable to that of penicillin, and it is effective when taken by mouth.

ERYTHROPOIETIN is the protein, produced mainly in the kidney, that is the major stimulus for the production of erythrocytes, or red blood corpuscles. (See BLOOD.)

ESCHAR is a piece of the body killed by heat or caustics.

ESCHAROTICS are the more powerful varieties of caustics, such as mineral acids, which produce death, to some depth, of tissues with which they come in contact. (See CAUSTICS.)

ESCHERICHIA is the generic name given to the group of gram-negative, rod-shaped bacteria found as normal inhabitants of the lower bowel: eg. *Escherichia coli*.

ESERINE is another name for physostigmine (qv).

ESMARCH'S BANDAGE is a rubber bandage which is applied to a limb from below upwards in order to drive blood from it.

ESSENCES are strong solutions of an active substance. Some of these are made by solution in water, but the aromatic essences are usually solutions of volatile oils (eg. essence of peppermint), in rectified spirit of the strength 1 in 5.

ESSENTIAL HYPERTENSION is the most common form of high blood-pressure. Other causes of a high blood-pressure include kidney disease, especially glomerulonephritis; certain diseases of the endocrine glands; and a congenital abnormality of the aorta known as coarctation of the aorta.
Cause: In spite of its being such a common condition, the cause of essential hypertension is still obscure. It has been recognized for a long time that arteriosclerosis and hypertension often occur together, and at one time it was considered that the arteriosclerosis was the primary lesion and that the raised blood-pressure was a compensatory effort on the part of the

heart to maintain an adequate circulation of blood through the thickened and narrowed arteries. This view is now considered to be wrong, and the general consensus of opinion is that the raised blood-pressure is the cause of the arteriosclerosis in these cases, although it must be remembered that arteriosclerosis can occur without hypertension. At the present moment it is generally believed that the primary lesion in essential hypertension is spasm of the smaller arteries (or arterioles). What is still undecided is what is responsible for this spasm. We know that such spasm can be produced by adrenaline and that adrenaline is produced by emotional, mental and physical strain. On the other hand, it has never been possible to demonstrate an excess of adrenaline in the blood of people with hypertension, nor does this theory explain why only some people exposed to strain develop hypertension. Although we still do not know why this spasm of the arterioles is produced in the first instance, there is now evidence that spasm of the arteries to the kidneys results in the production of a substance called *renin* (qv) which produces a rise in the blood-pressure. It is therefore possible that the course of events in essential hypertension is as follows:
spasm of arterioles→renin→hyper-tension→arteriosclerosis of kidneys. It must be realized, however, that this is a marked simplification of a most complicated problem, but it is useful as a working basis.

The following are among some of the other factors known about essential hypertension. It is much more common among western races than among eastern races. There is a strong hereditary factor. It is more common in males than in females, and it is rare under the age of 40 years. The highest incidence is between the ages of 50 and 60 years. It is also more common among obese individuals than among those who are normal in weight or under-weight. There is no evidence that the consumption of meat has anything to do with essential hypertension.

Symptoms: Essential hypertension may be present without any symptoms whatsoever, and the condition may be discovered accidentally during a routine medical examination. The basis for a diagnosis of hypertension is usually taken to be a systolic pressure which is persistently greater than 150 mm of mercury and a diastolic pressure which is persistently greater than 95 mm of mercury. The emphasis is upon the persistence of the raised pressure, because it is not unusual for the blood-pressure in a normal individual to be raised temporarily by excitement. Even the mere recording of it may be sufficient to raise it quite considerably. From the point of view of prognosis, the height of the diastolic pressure is much more important than that of the systolic pressure.

When essential hypertension is accompanied by symptoms, these usually consist of headache, ringing in the ears (tinnitus) and giddiness. When headache is present, it is often in the back of the head and often worst on wakening in the morning, wearing off during the course of the day, and then becoming worse again towards evening.

When essential hypertension runs its natural course, it usually causes death in the end as a result of heart failure, but a proportion of its victims die of a stroke, or myocardial infarction, whilst some die of failure of the kidneys. To a certain extent it is true to say that the earlier the onset of essential hypertension, the poorer the expectation of life, but many people with this condition live to a ripe old age.

Treatment: As the cause of hypertension is not known there is no specific treatment. However over recent years a large number of drugs which are effective in lowering peripheral resistance and hence lowering blood pressure have been introduced. Most of the newer hypotensive drugs are without serious side effects and so have replaced the old ganglion-blocking drugs such as bretylium tosylate, mecamylamine and the methonium compounds. The first line drugs are probably still the benzothiadiazine diuretics and the beta adreno-receptor blocking drugs. The thiazide diuretics both reduce the circulating blood volume and hence the blood pressure and also, as a result of soldium depletion, render the arterioles less sensitive to the vaso-constrictor effects of nor-adrenaline. They may however cause hypokalaemia and hyperuricaemia, reduce carbohydrate tolerance and pre-dispose to hyperlipidaemia. The beta adreno-receptor blocking drugs are also effective in lowering the blood pressure by reducing peripheral resistance. They are, however, contra-indicated in patients with asthma or obstructive airways disease. The more recently introduced calcium channel blockers such as nifedipine are effective vaso-dilators and hence hypotensive drugs. Alpha-receptor blocking drugs such as prazosin also have a place in the management of hypertension and hydralazine is another effective vaso-dilator independent of any alpha-receptor blockade. The angiotensin converting enzyme inhibitors are potent hypotensive drugs that have been recently introduced. Captopril was the first of these angiotensin inhibitors and enalopril was introduced in 1985.

Since the introduction of these potent hypotensive agents the incidence of cardiac failure, renal disease and strokes complicating hypertension have been drastically reduced. Nevertheless other commonsense measures should still be pursued. The patient who is overweight must reduce weight and life style should be adjusted so that relaxation is possible at weekends. Excess salt intake should be avoided.

ESTER is an organic compound formed from an alcohol and an acid by the removal of water.

ETHACRYNIC ACID (EDECRIN) is a potent diuretic (qv), with a rapid onset, and a short duration (4 to 6 hours), of action. (See BENZOTHIADIAZINES, DIURETICS.)

ETHAMBUTOL is a synthetic drug which is proving of value in the treatment of tuberculosis.

ETHAMIVAN is chemically similar to nikethamide (qv) and has a similar action in stimulating the respiratory centre.

ETHANOL is another name for ethyl alcohol. (See ALCOHOL.)

ETHER is a colourless, volatile, highly inflammable liquid formed by the action of sulphuric acid upon alcohol, with the aid of heat. Ether boils below the body temperature, and so, when sprayed over the skin, rapidly evaporates. It dissolves many substances, such as fats, oils and resins, better than alcohol or water, and is accordingly used in the preparation of many drugs.
Uses: Externally it is used as a cleansing agent before operations. By inhalation it is used as a general anaesthetic. (See ANAESTHETICS.) Internally it is used occasionally for relieving pain such as colic. (For its use as an intoxicant, see DRUG HABITS.)

ETHICS COMMITTEES: It is now generally agreed that research investigations on human beings should be governed by codes, such as those of The World Medical Association (Declaration of Helsinki) and of The Medical Research Council of Britain. Ethics committees developed in this country when the Royal College of Physicians, in 1967, recommended that clinical research investigations should be the subject of ethical review. The Medical Research Council requires ethical review of projects prior to making a grant and some scientific journals require it as a condition of publication. The objectives of ethics committees are to facilitate medical research in the interest of society, to protect subjects of research from possible harm, to preserve their rights and to provide reassurance to the public that this is being done. Ethics committees comprise medical, nursing and lay members. Ethics committees have now been established in most District Health Authorities in this country.

ETHINYLOESTRADIOL (LUNORAL) is a highly active oestrogen (qv), which is about twenty times as active as stilboestrol (qv). It is active when given by mouth. (See OESTROGENS.)

ETHISTERONE is the name approved by the *British Pharmacopoeia* for the orally active analogue of progesterone. It is given in certain cases of menorrhagia and habitual abortion, where a deficient secretion of the corpus luteum is suspected. (See PROGESTERONE.)

ETHMOID is a bone in the base of the skull which separates the cavity of the nose from the membranes of the brain. It is a spongy bone with numerous cavities or sinuses.

Suppuration in the ethmoidal sinuses is sometimes responsible for inflammation in neighbouring parts such as the eye.

ETHOGLUCID is an alkylating agent (qv), which is proving of value in the treatment of cancer.

ETHOSUXIMIDE is a drug that is proving of value in the treatment of the form of epilepsy known as petit mal.

ETHYL CHLORIDE is a gas at ordinary temperatures and pressures, but is liquefied by slight compression. It is extremely volatile, and rapidly produces freezing of the surface, when sprayed upon it. Accordingly it is used to produce insensibility to pain for small and short operations. It is put up in graduated glass or metal tubes, with a fine nozzle. The tube is warmed by the hand and the liquid jets out in a fine spray which evaporates at once and so freezes the skin upon which it is sprayed. At one time it was used by inhalation to produce general anaesthesia for very brief operations, and to induce anaesthesia in patients in whom the anaesthesia is subsequently to be maintained by some other anaesthetic such as nitrous oxide or ether, but is seldom used now for this purpose.

ETHYLENE is a colourless inflammable gas used as an anaesthetic.

ETHYLOESTRENOL (ORABOLIN) (see ANABOLIC STEROIDS).

ETIDRONATE is one of a group of substances known as diphosphonates which are proving of value in the treatment of Paget's disease of bone (qv). One of its practical advantages is that it is taken by mouth, and not by injection as is the case with calcitonin.

ETIOLOGY, or AETIOLOGY, means the group of conditions which form the cause of any disease.

EU- is a prefix meaning satisfactory or beneficial.

EUCALYPTUS, or BLUE-GUM (*Eucalyptus globulus*), is a tree, originally a native of Australia, and now grown all over the world. Its important constituent, oil of eucalyptus, is an oil of pleasant smell and spicy taste, which is obtained by distillation from the leaves of the tree. Similar oils are obtained in varying amount from most species of gum-trees, some of which have peculiar and fragrant odours. Groves of eucalyptus trees exert a marked influence upon the soil and air in their neighbourhood. The trees, which reach a great size, and have wide-spreading roots, remove much moisture from the soil, and have accordingly a powerful action in drying up swampy ground. The oil constantly exhaled from the

leaves has the power of oxidizing and destroying large quantities of the foul gases which emanate from swamps, and of checking to some extent the growth of microbes. Accordingly these trees have a beneficial influence upon unhealthy districts in which they are planted.
Uses: The oil is used as a disinfectant and deodorant. It is also used as an inhalation or internally in bronchitis and in coryza.

EUGENICS is the study and cultivation of conditions that may improve the physical and moral qualities of future generations.

EUPAD is a mixture of chlorinated lime and boric acid, 25 grams of which, dissolved in 1 litre of water, form 'eusol' (qv).

EUSOL, which stands for Edinburgh University Solution, is a solution of 12·5 G of boric acid and 12·5 G of chlorinated lime in 1 litre of water. It was introduced during the 1914–18 War as an antiseptic for the treatment of wounds, and proved to be one of the most valuable antiseptics then available. Although largely replaced by modern antiseptics, and the introduction of the sulphonamides (qv) and antibiotics, it is still a useful dressing for infected wounds. (See EUPAD; HYPOCHLOROUS ACID).

EUPHORIANTS are drugs which induce a state of euphoria or well-being.

EUSTACHIAN TUBES are the passages, one on each side, leading from the throat to the middle ear. Each is about 38 mm (1½inches) long and is large at either end, though at its narrowest part it only admits a fine probe. The tubes open widely in the act of swallowing or yawning. The opening into the throat is situated just behind the lower part of the nose, so that a catheter can be passed through the corresponding nostril into the tube for inflation of the middle ear. (See also EAR; NOSE.)

EUTHANASIA means the procuring of an easy and painless death. It has been advocated in some quarters that a medical practicioner should have the power to put to death painlessly, by means of such drugs as morphine, any person suffering from a painful, distressing and incurable disease the outcome of which is inevitably fatal, the patient or his relatives consenting. Various legal safeguards have been proposed, but there are obvious moral and religious – not to mention medical –objections to the recognition of such a procedure.

EVACUANT is a name for a purgative medicine.

EXANTHEMATA is an old name used to classify the acute infectious diseases distinguished by a characteristic eruption. (See ERUPTION.)

EXCIPIENT means any more or less inert substance added to a prescription in order to make the remedy as prescribed more suitable in bulk, consistence, or form for administration.

EXCISION means literally a cutting out, and is a term applied to the removal of any structure from the body, when such removal necessitates a certain amount of separation from surrounding parts. For example, one speaks of the excision of a tumour, of a gland, of a joint. When an opening is simply made into the body the term incision is used. When a limb, or part of one, is removed, the term amputation is employed.

EXCITEMENT (see DELIRIUM; HYSTERIA; MENTAL ILLNESS).

EXCITING CAUSE of a disease is the direct or immediate cause, as opposed to predisposing causes, which merely render the body more liable to the disease in question. For example, poor expansion of the chest may be a predisposing cause of tuberculosis, but the exciting cause is infection with the tubercle bacillus, or *Mycobacterium tuberculosis* as it is technically known.

EXCORIATION means the destruction of small pieces of the surface of skin or mucous membrane. (See CHAFING OF THE SKIN.)

EXERCISE is a matter of great importance in the maintenance of health at all ages, but particularly for those who are normally engaged in sedentary occupations.
Effects of exercise: The right amount of the right type of exercise results in all parts of the body working at their best. The muscles are firm in tone, strong and working at maximum efficiency, so that the onset of fatigue, with its accompanying aching and soreness, is postponed. The heart, too, works more efficiently, pumping more blood round the body. For instance, when an individual is resting, the output of the heart per minute is 5 litres. When running at 12 km (7½ miles) per hour, this shoots up to around 25 litres: a five-fold increase. This increased volume of blood dealt with by the heart per minute is achieved with increasing efficiency, as is shown by the fact that at each contraction the heart expels 150 millilitres, compared with 70 millilitres at rest. The lungs also function more efficiently. Again taking the example of the individual running at 12 km (7½ miles an hour), the amount of oxygen used up increases twelvefold, although the output of the heart has only increased five-fold. The digestive tract, including the liver, also functions better, partly because it is not being overloaded by unnecessary food. The increased expenditure of energy involved in exercise ensures that the food eaten is metabolized, or used up, immediately to cope with the increased energy demands. The nervous system also works more efficiently, reflexes becoming brisker and the muscles thereby being able to

respond more promptly and more effectively to any special stress or strain. Finally, possibly more imponderable but nevertheless of great practical importance, there is considerable emotional benefit. The individual feels more satisfied with life, is less affected by the normal worries of life in so far as he can forget them in exercising himself –whether this is in some form of athletics or games, or merely tramping the countryside – and when he falls into bed at night his physical tiredness, combined with his emotional peace of mind, allows him to fall asleep – and sleep soundly.

Lack of exercise: Failure to take adequate exercise affects the body adversely at all ages. In children it leads to slouching, faulty posture and flabbiness of the muscles. This leads to the typical round-shouldered child who, in addition, may develop scoliosis (qv), or curvature of the spine. As these children seldom use their lungs to the full in breathing, not only is inadequate oxygen brought to the blood, and therefore to all the cells of the body, which at this period of rapid growth are demanding in their call for oxygen and nutriment, but they render themselves more liable to lung disease. The appetite is poor or capricious, and the skin fails to acquire that healthy, glossy appearance of ebullient childhood. In adolescence these features all become enhanced, associated often with a cigarette hanging out of the corner of the flabby mouth. In adult life, and particularly in middle age, lack of exercise leads to the putting on of weight, with all the hazards to life that this involves (see OBESITY), constipation, not to mention dyspepsia as often as not due to overeating. What is of even more serious import is that there is an increased tendency to atherosclerosis (qv) and coronary thrombosis (qv). The motor car is a lethal weapon, not only because of the accidents it causes, but also because it is the means whereby hundreds of thousands of middle-aged men (and women) are deprived of the useful form of exercise provided by walking to work – or at least part of the way. Cycling to health was the motto of a well-known heart specialist in the United States of America who lived to a ripe old age. It is one which might well be adopted in the United Kingdom.

Over-exercise seldom does any permanent harm except in the rapidly growing adolescent and in the old, provided the individual is healthy. For instance, there is no evidence that a healthy heart can be damaged by exercise. The circulatory system is so adaptable that, if there is any possibility of undue strain being placed upon the heart, certain mechanisms come into play which cause giddiness or fainting, so that the exercise in question is automatically stopped before any real harm is done. On the other hand, should there be any undetected disease of the heart, then undue exercise may produce permanent harm. This is why a careful medical examination is an essential preliminary to any severe form of exercise. This is particularly important, indeed essential, in the case of school children.

The secret of success is moderation. The man in his fifties or sixties must realize that he can no longer do many of the things that he did when he was thirty years younger. If he bears this in mind, there is little chance of his damaging himself by exercise. For instance, if he finds that an afternoon's tennis begins to make him uncomfortably breathless, then he should give up the game for a less exacting one, or alternatively be satisfied with one or two sets instead of several.

In the case of adolescents and young adults, the wise rule is to ensure that the individual, and particularly his heart, is sound, and then to insist upon his undergoing a careful course of training before embarking upon any severe form of exercise such as running or rugger.

EXFOLIATION means the separation, in layers, of pieces of dead bone or skin.

EXOMPHALOS is the term applied to a hernia formed by the projection of abdominal organs through the umbilicus.

EXOPTHTHALMIC GOITRE is a disease in which there is overactivity of the thyroid gland, protrusion of the eyes, and other symptoms. (See GOITRE.)

EXOPHTHALMOS, or PROPTOSIS, refers to forward displacement of the eyeball and must be distinguished from retraction of the eyelids, which causes an illusion of exophthalmos. Lid retraction usually results from activation of the autonomic nervous sytem. Exophthalmos is a more serious disorder caused by inflammatory and infiltrative changes in the retro-orbital tissues and is essentially a feature of Graves' disease (qv), though it has been described in chronic thyroiditis. Exophthalmos commonly starts shortly after the development of thyrotoxicosis but may occur months or even years after hyperthyroidism has been successfully treated. Only 3 per cent of patients with Graves' disease develop severe exophthalmos. The degree of exophthalmos is not correlated with the severity of hyperthyroidism even when their onset is simultaneous. Some of the worst examples of endocrine exophthalmos occur in the euthyroid state and may appear in patients who have never had thyrotoxicosis; this disorder is named ophthalmic Graves' disease. The exophthalmos of Graves' disease is due to auto-immunity. Antibodies to surface antigens on the eye muscles are produced and this causes an inflammatory reaction in the muscle and retro-orbital tissues.

Exophthalmos may also occur as a result of a tumour at the back of the eye, pushing the eyeball forwards. In this situation it is always unilateral.

EXOSTOSIS means an outgrowth from a bone; it may be due to chronic inflammation, constant pressure or tension on the bone, or tumour-formation. (See BONE, DISEASES OF.)

EXPECTANT is a form of treatment in which the cure of the patient is left mainly to nature, while the physician simply watches for any unsatisfactory developments or symptoms, and relieves them if they occur.

EXPECTATION OF LIFE at 1 year of age in England and Wales, based on the figures for 1977, was 70·3 years for men and 76·3 years for women. The comparable figures for Scotland were 68·6 and 74·8, whilst for Northern Ireland they were 67·8 and 74·5. These are all slightly below the best figures recorded in other countries, which are 73·2 for men and 79·5 for women in Iceland. In USA the comparable figures are 69·3 for men and 77 for women. At the other end of the scale is Ethiopia where the expectation of life for men is 37·5 years, and that for women 40·5 years. In all countries for which statistics are available, the expectation of life for women is greater than that for men. There is also a certain variation within socio-economic groups. Thus in England in 1970–72 the expectation of life for men at age 45 was 22 for those in the Armed Forces, 29·3 for farmers on their own account, 28·9 for self-employed professional workers and 26·1 for unskilled manual workers. (See also AGE, NATURAL CHANGES IN.)

EXPECTORANTS are drugs which assist the removal of secretions from the air passages.

Varieties: Most drugs used as expectorants have a complicated mode of action. (1) Some act chiefly by making the secretion in the bronchial tubes more watery, and therefore less sticky; (2) others have exactly the opposite action, drying up the secretion where it is very copious; (3) a third group assists the act of coughing in feeble people, and so helps the removal of secretion; (4) those in a fourth group soothe the lining membrane of the air passages and quiet ineffectual coughing. Some of the chief drugs, arranged as far as possible in the order of these groups, though several have a double action, are as follows: (1) steam inhalations, draughts of hot milk or water, ammonium chloride, potassium iodide, and, generally speaking, all alkalis; (2) volatile oils like anise, eucalyptus, and turpentine, menthol, balsam of tolu and Friars' balsam, syrup of squills, and infusion of senega, inhalation of creosote or tar, and generally speaking, all acids; (3) ipecacuanha, ammonium bicarbonate, sal volatile and tincture of nux vomica; (4) linctuses and codeine.

Uses: These drugs are combined in various ways in bronchitis and other chest conditions. For example, those in the first group are used in the early stages of acute and in chronic bronchitis, those in the next group are better for later stages of acute bronchitis, those of the third group are used for aged persons with pneumonia and bronchitis, and the members of the fourth group are applicable to a constant hacking cough.

EXPECTORATION means either material brought up from the chest by the air passages, or the act by which it is brought up. The term is also used in place of sputum for anything spat out. Expectoration varies considerably in character according to the site in which it is produced, and the disease with which it is associated.

Characters of expectoration: There may be much cough productive of a very small amount of sputum at the start of acute bronchitis or inflammation of the throat, but it must be remembered that young children and some older people swallow their expectoration as soon as they have brought it up instead of spitting it out.

The sputum from the throat in catarrh of this region is usually thick and sticky, speckled with black owing to dust and smoke inhaled and deposited on the throat.

Watery, frothy expectoration is brought up in considerable quantities during the greater part of an attack of acute bronchitis, particularly in old people. A similar fluid is spat up when the lungs are oedematous, as occurs sometimes in the course of heart or kidney disease. At a later stage of an acute bronchitis the sputum becomes more yellow and thicker in consistence.

When cavities are present in the lungs their contents are often expectorated as thick, yellow, oily-looking material, with few air-bubbles in it; and expectoration from this source, when spat into water, flattens out into a round disc resembling a coin, and hence gets the name of nummular sputum (Lat. *nummulus*, money).

Sputum with a 'rusty' tinge, and so sticky that it adheres to the dish into which it is expectorated, when the latter is turned upside down, is characteristic of pneumonia.

Bright red blood in large quantities may be brought up from the lungs. This is the condition known as *haemoptysis* (qv) and usually indicates the presence of pulmonary tuberculosis, carcinoma of the lung or certain forms of heart disease. On the other hand, it must be remembered that spitting of blood may be due merely to bleeding in the nose from which the blood has run backward down the throat: or to the rupture of a small vessel on the wall of the throat in cases in which this part of the air passages is inflamed. Bleeding from the stomach has totally different characteristics from those of lung bleeding. That brought up from the lungs is bright red, frothy and usually comes up with a hawk or with a few suppressed coughs, it may be by mouthfuls. Blood from the stomach is usually dark brown and granular from the action of the gastric juice, and is brought up by a definite act of vomiting. It results generally from some ulcerated or congested state of the stomach.

Expectoration of a 'prune juice' colour occurring in the course of pneumonia is an ominous sign, and indicates usually that softening of parts of the lungs is setting in.

In some diseases the sputum possesses a very foul smell, particularly in gangrene of the lung and in the condition known as bronchiectasis. (See LUNGS, DISEASES OF.)

Microscopic examination of the sputum is of importance in diagnosing the cause of an infection of the lung. Thus the presence of tubercle bacilli, or *Mycobacteria tuberculosis* as they are now known, denotes that the individual is suffering from pulmonary tuberculosis. It is also of importance in determining to which antibiotic the causative micro-organisms are sensitive. In cancer of the lung the microscope may disclose malignant cells in the sputum.

Disposal of expectoration is a matter demanding public attention. The habit of spitting on the ground in public places is one which, in view of the dangerous nature of diseased sputum, should never be tolerated. Where spittoons are provided, these should be washed and disinfected every day.

Most tuberculous patients are supplied with a sputum flask containing a small quantity of some strong antiseptic (eg. carbolic acid solution 1 in 5 or 1 in 20) into which the expectoration is received and by which it is disinfected before it is poured down the drains.

EXTENSION is the process of straightening or stretching a limb. In cases of fractured limbs, extension is employed during the application of splints, in order to reduce the displacement caused by the fracture, and prevent movement of the broken ends of bone. It is effected by gently and steadily pulling upon the part of the limb beyond the fracture. Extension of a more permanent type is used in the after-treatment of some fractures, as well as in diseases of the spine, by placing the patient upon an inclined bed and affixing weights to his lower limbs or to his head by means of adhesive plaster or of straps. A similar procedure is often adopted in tuberculous disease of the knee or hip, to prevent the starting pains, which are apt to occur as the affected person is dropping off to sleep.

EXTRA- is the Latin prefix meaning outside of, or in addition, such as extra-capsular, meaning outside the capsule of a joint, and extrasystole, meaning an additional contraction of the heart.

EXTRACTS are preparations, usually of a semi-solid consistence, containing the active parts of various plants extracted in one of several ways. In the case of some extracts the juice of the fresh plant is simply pressed out and purified; in the case of others the active principles are dissolved out in water, which is then to a great extent driven off by evaporation; other extracts are similarly made by the help of alcohol, and in some cases ether is the solvent.

EXTRASYSTOLE is a term applied to premature contraction of one or more of the chambers of the heart. A beat of the heart occurs sooner than it should do in the ordinary rhythm and is followed by a longer rest than usual before the next beat. In an extrasystole the stimulus to contraction arises in a part of the heart other than the usual. Extrasystoles often give rise to an unpleasant sensation as of the heart stumbling over a beat, but their occurrence is not usually serious.

EXTRAVASATION means an escape of fluid from the vessels or passages which ought to contain it. Extravasation of blood due to tearing of vessel walls is found in apoplexy, and in the commoner condition known as a bruise. Extravasation of urine takes place when the bladder or the urethra is ruptured by a blow on the abdomen or on the crutch (or perineum), or torn in a fracture of the pelvis.

EXUDATION means the process in which some of the constituents of the blood pass slowly through the walls of the small vessels in the course of inflammation, and also means the accumulation resulting from this process. For example, in pleurisy the solid, rough material deposited on the surface of the lung is an exudation.

EYE: The eye is the sensory organ of sight. It is an elaborate photoreceptor detecting information, in the form of light, from the environment and transmitting this information by a series of electro-chemical changes to the brain. The visual cortex is the part of the brain that processes this information (ie. the visual cortex is what 'sees' the environment). There are two eyes, each a roughly spherical hollow organ held within a bony cavity (the orbit). Each orbit is situated on the front of the skull, one on each side of the nose. The eye consists of an outer wall of three main layers and a central cavity divided into three.

The outer coat consists of the opaque *sclera* posteriorly and the clear *cornea* anteriorly; their junction is called the *limbus*.

(a) SCLERA: This is white, opaque, and constitutes the posterior five-sixths of the outer layer. It is made of dense fibrous tissue. The sclera is visible anteriorly, between the eyelids, as the 'white of the eye'. Posteriorly it is covered by Tenons capsule, anteriorly by Tenons capsule, which in turn is covered by transparent conjunctiva. There is a hole in the sclera medial to the posterior pole of the eye through which nerve fibres from the retina leave the eye in the optic nerve. Other smaller nerve fibres and blood vessels also pass through the sclera at different points.

(b) CORNEA: This constitutes the transparent colourless anterior one-sixth of the eye. It is transparent in order to allow light into the eye and is more steeply curved than the sclera. Viewed from in front, the cornea is roughly circular. Most of the focusing power of the eye

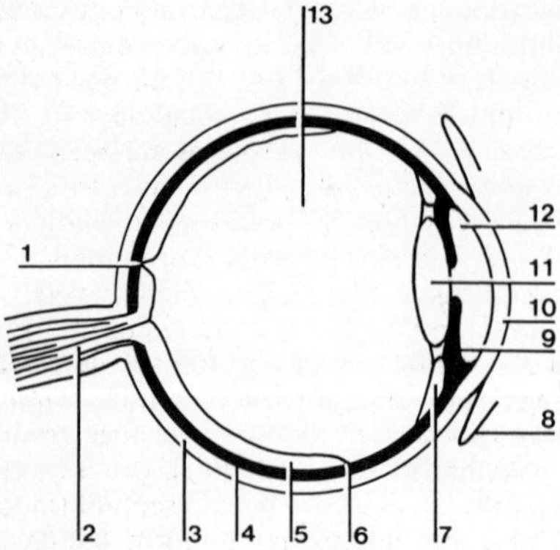

1 fovea
2 optic nerve
3 sclera
4 choroid
5 retina
6 ora serrata
7 ciliary muscle
8 conjunctiva
9 iris
10 cornea
11 lens
12 anterior chamber
13 posterior chamber (vitreous body)

Diagram of the left eye from above.

is provided by the cornea (the lens acts as the 'fine adjustment'). It has an outer *epithelium*, a central *stroma* and an inner *endothelium*. The cornea is supplied with very fine nerve fibres which make it exquisitely sensitive to pain. The central cornea has no blood supply – it relies mainly on aqueous humour for nutrition. Blood vessels and large nerve fibres in the cornea would prevent light entering the eye.

(c) LIMBUS is the junction between cornea and sclera. It contains the *trabecular meshwork*, a sieve-like structure through which aqueous humour leaves the eye.

The middle coat (uveal tract) consists of the *choroid*, *ciliary body* and *iris*.

(a) CHOROID: A highly vascular sheet of tissue lining the posterior two-thirds of the sclera. The network of vessels provides the blood supply for the outer half of the retina. The blood supply of the choroid is derived from numerous *ciliary vessels* which pierce the sclera in front and behind.

(b) CILIARY BODY: A ring of tissue extending 6 mm back from the anterior limitation of the sclera. The various muscles of the ciliary body by their contractions and relaxations are responsible for changing the shape of the lens during accommodation. The ciliary body is lined by cells that secrete aqueous humour. Posteriorly the ciliary body is continuous with the choroid, anteriorly it is continuous with the iris.

(c) IRIS: A flattened muscular diaphragm that is attached at its periphery to the ciliary body and has a round central opening, the *pupil*. By contraction and relaxation of the muscles of the iris the pupil can be dilated or constricted (dilated in the dark or when aroused, constricted in bright light and for close work). The iris forms a partial division between the *anterior chamber* and the *posterior chamber* of the eye. It lies in front of the lens and forms the back wall of the anterior chamber. The iris is visible from in front, through the transparent cornea, as the 'coloured part of the eye'. The amount and distribution of iris pigment determine the colour of the iris. The pupil is merely a hole in the centre of the iris and appears black.

The inner layer: The RETINA is a multi-layered tissue (ten layers in all) which extends from the edges of the optic nerve to line the inner surface of the choroid up to the junction of ciliary body and choroid. Here the true retina ends at the *ora serrata*. The retina contains light-sensitive cells of two types: (i) CONES: Cells that operate at high and medium levels of illumination. They subserve fine discrimination of vision and colour vision. (ii) RODS: Cells that function best at low light intensity and subserve black and white vision.

The retina contains about 6 million cones and about 100 million rods. Information from them is conveyed by the nerve fibres which are in the inner part of the retina to leave the eye in

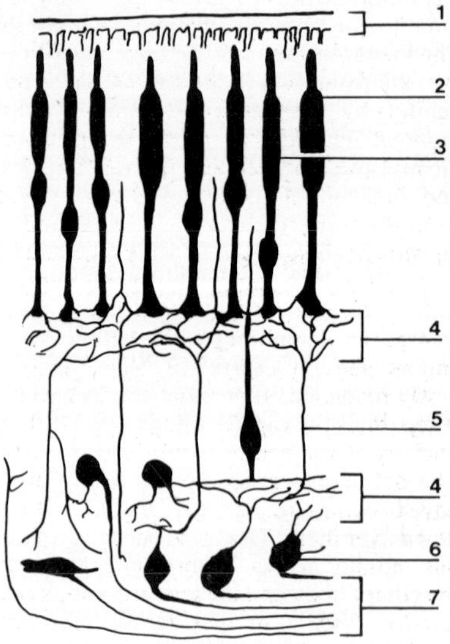

1 pigment cells
2 cone
3 rod
4 felt-work of dendrons
5 axon
6 ganglion cells
7 axon to optic nerve

Diagrammatic section of the retina.

the *optic nerve*. There are no photoreceptors at the *optic disc* (the point where the optic nerve leaves the eye) and therefore there is no light perception from this small area. The optic disc thus produces a physiological blind spot in the visual field.

The retina can be subdivided into several areas: (a) PERIPHERAL RETINA contains mainly rods and a few scattered cones. Visual acuity from this area is fairly coarse. (b) MACULA LUTEA, so called because histologically it looks like a yellow spot. It occupies an area 4·5 mm in diameter lateral to the optic disc. This area of specialized retina can produce a high level of visual acuity. Cones are abundant here but there are few rods. (c) FOVEA CENTRALIS: A small central depression at the centre of the macula. Here the cones are tightly packed, rods are absent. It is responsible for the highest levels of visual acuity.

The chambers of the eye: There are three, *anterior* and *posterior chambers* and the *vitreous cavity*. The ANTERIOR CHAMBER is limited in front by the inner surface of the cornea, behind by the iris and pupil. It contains a transparent clear watery fluid, the *aqueous humour*. This is constantly being produced by cells of the ciliary body and constantly drained away through the trabecular meshwork. The trabecular meshwork lies in the angle between the iris and inner surface of the cornea. The POSTERIOR CHAMBER: A narrow space between the iris and pupil in front and the lens behind. It too contains aqueous humour in transit from the ciliary epithelium to the anterior chamber, via the pupil. The VITREOUS CAVITY: The largest cavity of the eye. In front it is bounded by the lens and behind by the retina. It contains *vitreous humour*. The *lens* is transparent, elastic and biconvex in cross section. It lies behind the iris and in front of the vitreous cavity. Viewed from the front it is roughly circular and about 10 mm in diameter. The diameter and thickness of the lens vary with its accommodative state. The lens consists of (a) *capsule*: a thin transparent membrane surrounding the cortex and nucleus; (b) *cortex*: This is made up of newly made lens fibres that are relatively soft. It separates the capsule on the outside from the nucleus at the centre of the lens; (c) *nucleus*: The dense central area of old lens fibres that have become compacted by new lens fibres laid down over them. The *zonule* consists of numerous radially arranged fibres attached between the ciliary body and the lens around its circumference. Tension in these zonular fibres can be adjusted by the muscles of the ciliary body, thus changing the shape of the lens and altering its power of accommodation. The *vitreous humour* is a transparent clear jellylike structure made up of a network of collagen fibres suspended in a viscid fluid. Its shape conforms to that of the vitreous cavity within which it is contained, ie. it is spherical except for a shallow concave depression on its anterior surface. The lens lies in this depression.

Eyelids: These are multilayered curtains of tissue whose functions include spreading of the tear film over the front of the eye to prevent desiccation, protection from injury or external irritation and to some extent to control light entering the eye. Each eye has an upper and lower lid which form an elliptical opening (the *palpebral fissure*) when the eyes are open. The lids meet at the *medial canthus* and *lateral canthus* respectively. The inner medial canthus is fixed, the lateral canthus is more mobile. An *epicanthus* is a fold of skin which covers the medial canthus in oriental races. Each lid consists of several layers. From front to back they are: very thin skin, a sheet of muscle (*orbicularis oculi* whose fibres are concentric around the palpebral fissure and which produce closure of the eyelids), the orbital septum (modified near the lid margin to form the *tarsal plates*) and, finally, lining the back surface of the lid, the conjunctiva (known here as *tarsal* conjunctiva). At the free margin of each lid are the eyelashes, the openings of tear glands which lie within the lid and the *lacrimal punctum*. Toward the medial edge of each lid in an elevation known as the *papilla*. The lacrimal punctum opens into this papilla. The punctum forms the open end of the *cannaliculus*, part of the tear-drainage mechanism.

Orbit: The bony cavity within which the eye is held. The orbits lie one on either side of the nose, on the front of the skull. They afford considerable protection for the eye. Each is roughly pyramidal in shape, with the apex pointing backwards and the base forming the open anterior part of the orbit. The bone of the anterior orbital margin is thickened to protect the eye from injury. There are various openings into the posterior part of the orbit, namely the *optic canal* which allows the optic nerve to leave the orbit en route for the brain, the *superior orbital fissure* and *inferior orbital fissure* which allow passage of nerves and blood vessels to and from the orbit. The most important structures holding the eye within the orbit are the *extra-ocular muscles*, a *suspensory ligament* of connective tissue that forms a hammock on which the eye rests and which is slung between the medial and lateral walls of the orbit. Finally, the *orbital septum*, a sheet of connective tissue extending from the anterior margin of the orbit into the lids, helps keep the eye in place. A pad of fat fills in the orbit behind the eye and acts as a cushion for the eye.

Conjunctiva: A transparent mucous membrane that extends from the limbus over the anterior sclera or 'white of the eye'. This is the *bulbar* conjunctiva. The conjunctiva does not cover the cornea. Conjunctiva passes from the eye on to the inner surface of the eyelid at the *fornices* and is continuous with the *tarsal* conjunctiva. The *semilunar fold* is the vertical crescent of conjunctiva at the medial aspect of the palpebral fissure. The *caruncle* is a piece of modified skin just within the inner canthus.

Eye muscles (extra ocular muscles): There are six in all, the four rectus muscles (superior, inferior, medial and lateral rectus muscles) and two oblique muscles (superior and inferior oblique muscles). The muscles are attached at various points between the bony orbit and the eyeball. By their combined action they move the eye in horizontal and vertical gaze. They also produce torsional movement of the eye (ie. clockwise or anticlockwise movements when viewed from the front).

Lacrimal apparatus: There are two components, a tear production system, namely the lacrimal gland and accessory lacrimal glands, and a drainage system.

LACRIMAL GLAND is located below a small depression in the bony roof of the orbit. Numerous tear ducts open from it into predominantly the upper lid. *Accessory lacrimal glands* are found in the conjunctiva and within the eyelids. The former open directly on to the surface of the conjunctiva, the latter on to the eyelid margin.

LACRIMAL DRAINAGE SYSTEM consists of (a) *Punctum*: an elevated opening toward the medial aspect of each lid. Each punctum opens into a cannaliculus. (b) *Cannaliculus*: a fine tube-like structure running within the lid, parallel to the lid margin. The cannaliculus from upper and lower lid join to form a common cannaliculus which opens into the lacrimal sac. (c) *Lacrimal sac*: a small sac on the side of the nose which opens into the nasolacrimal duct. During blinking the sac sucks tears into itself from the cannaliculus. Tears then drain by gravity down the nasolacrimal duct. (d) *Nasolacrimal duct*: A tubular structure which runs down through the wall of the nose and opens into the nasal cavity.

Tears keep the front of the eye moist; they also contain nutrients and various components to protect the eye from infection. Crying results from excess tear production. The drainage system cannot cope with the excess and therefore tears overflow on to the face. Newborn babies do not produce tears for the first three months of life.

Visual pathway: Light stimulates the rods and cones of the retina. Electrochemical messages are then passed to nerve fibres in the retina and then via the *optic nerve* to the *optic chiasm*. Here information from the temporal (outer) half of each retina continues to the same side of the brain. Information from the nasal (inner) half of each retina crosses to the other side within the optic chiasm. The rearranged nerve fibres then pass through the *optic tract* to the *lateral geniculate body*, then the *optic radiation* to reach the *visual cortex* in the occipital lobe of the brain.

EYE, DISEASE AND INJURIES: Diseases affecting the eye are numerous and varied. The eye has its own group of disorders that affect one or more of the ocular structures but have no effect on the rest of the body. In addition a wide variety of systemic diseases produce changes in the eye. By careful examination of the eye it is therefore possible to assist diagnosis of many diseases affecting the body as a whole. Some of these disorders are dealt with below. The subjects of ARTIFICIAL EYES (see under ARTIFICIAL LIMBS AND OTHER PARTS); CATARACT; GLAUCOMA; RETINA, DISEASES OF; SPECTACLES; SQUINT; UVEITIS; and VISION, DISORDERS OF, are dealt with under these headings.

Conjunctiva (disorders of)

CONJUNCTIVITIS: An inflammation of the conjunctiva. There are many causes including *bacteria*, *viruses*, *allergy* and *chlamydia*. Symptoms and signs vary depending on the cause. (The conjunctiva may become infected in disorders of the cornea or iris. This is not true conjunctivitis.)

Bacterial conjunctivitis: Almost any bacteria can be involved, the commonest being *streptococci* and *staphylococci*. The patient complains of a mild grittiness or itching, redness of the eye and a yellow discharge (pain and photophobia are *not* features of bacterial conjunctivitis). One eye is involved first but both eyes are invariably affected within a few hours. The conjunctiva is most inflamed in the conjunctival fornices (that area of the 'white of the eye' furthest from the cornea). The disorder is self limiting but recovery can be accelerated with treatment. Topical antibiotic drops (eg. chloramphenicol eye drops) are usually effective within a day or two.

Viral conjunctivitis: There are numerous types of viruses causing conjunctivitis. One of the commonest is the group of *adenoviruses* (there are currently 31 recognized types). Symptoms include redness, watering, discomfort (which may be marked) and photophobia. Usually one eye is affected (although both may be). There is conjunctival swelling (chemosis), subconjunctival haemorrhages (see later), keratitis and pre-auricular lymph node enlargement. There may be an associated upper respiratory tract infection with fever, sore throat, coughing and feeling generally unwell. Adenoviral conjunctivitis is common, highly infectious and occurs in epidemic form (*epidemic keratoconjunctivitis*). Treatment involves the relief of symptoms as there is no active cure. It recovers spontaneously over a variable period of time. It is important that patients keep soap, towels and hairbrushes to themselves and avoid close contact with others in order to limit the chances of spreading the disorder. *Molluscum contagiosum* (see MOLLUSCUM CONTAGIOSUM) is a viral skin infection which usually affects children. Conjunctivitis can occur if the virus affects the eyelids. *Acute haemorrhage conjunctivitis* is caused by a *picornavirus*. It is highly contagious, self limiting and produces sub-conjunctival haemorrhages, keratitis and enlarged lymph nodes in front of the ear.

Allergic conjunctivitis: This includes *Vernal keratoconjunctivitis*. This common disorder affects children and young adults. It is recurrent with most frequent episodes in spring.

Symptoms include itching and watering of the eyes with or without pain, photophobia and discharge. The most marked feature is large flat elevations of the conjunctiva of the upper eyelid, visible on turning the lid inside out. Treatment is with sodium cromoglycate drops or steroid drops. *Hay-fever conjunctivitis* causes a pale swelling of the conjunctiva giving it a jellylike appearance. The condition may be otherwise symptom free or give rise to mild itching. Treatment is with sodium cromoglycate drops.

Chlamydia conjunctivitis: There are various disorders of the conjunctiva produced by chlamydia including (i) *Adult inclusion conjunctivitis*: this occurs two weeks or so following sexual intercourse with an infected partner. There is a mucopurulent discharge from both eyes, and conjunctival follicles (visible with a slit lamp microscope), conjunctival oedema, keratitis and pre-auricular lymph-node enlargement are common. Treatment is with tetracycline tablets for both patient and sexual partners. The patient should also be treated with tetracycline eye drops. (ii) *Trachoma* is caused by *Chlamydia trachomatis*. It is common in the Third World and is the leading cause of preventable blindness worldwide. It is seen in Great Britain in predominantly immigrant populations in its inactive form. The organism is transmitted by flies and causes inflammation of the conjunctiva and cornea with resultant scarring. Treatment of the active disease is with tetracycline tablets and tetracycline eye drops.

Ophthalmia neonatorum: Inflammation of the conjunctiva occurring within the first month of life. It can be caused by *chlamydia* (the commonest cause) or *gonococcal infection* which can result in perforation of the cornea). These two types of infection occur by passage through the mother's infected birth canal. Other causes include *bacteria*, *herpes simplex* or inflammation induced by *eyedrops*. Treatment is of the underlying cause, eg. tetracycline for chlamydia, penicillin for gonorrhoea, and acycloguanosine ointment for herpes simplex.

SUBCONJUNCTIVAL HAEMORRHAGE: Bleeding under the conjunctiva. Because the conjunctiva is transparent, the white of the eye becomes bright red either in part, or totally. Usually it occurs spontaneously in elderly people due to increased fragility of the blood vessels. Subconjunctival haemorrhages can also occur in conjunctival inflammation or as a result of injury. Treatment of the haemorrhage itself is unnecessary as it will disappear over a few days.

Cornea (disorders of):

ARCUS SENILIS: A very common finding in elderly people. Deposits of fat in the peripheral circumference of the cornea appear as a white crescent or a complete ring. It is a normal ageing change (see AGE, NATURAL CHANGES IN). Occasionally an arcus can occur in the young. In this group there may be an association with raised blood lipid levels.

CORNEAL DYSTROPHIES: A group of inherited disorders of the cornea. They are bilateral, usually developing during adolescence and progressing slowly throughout life. They cause opacification of the cornea to a greater or lesser degree. Many do not interfere with vision, those that do may require a *corneal graft* (see CORNEAL GRAFT).

KERATITIS: An inflammation of the cornea. There are numerous causes, only a few of which are dealt with below.

Bacterial keratitis: Bacteria may reach the cornea from an infection of the conjunctiva, the eyelids, lacrimal system, or may be introduced by, for example, a foreign body. For bacterial infection of the cornea to occur there must first be some damage to the corneal epithelium (the exception is *gonorrhoea*). The commonest bacterial causes of keratitis include *staphylococci*, *streptococci*, *pseudomonas* and *enterobacteria*. The eye becomes intensely red and painful with a yellow discharge. There is damage to the corneal epithelium with suppuration of the corneal stroma. The latter results in opacification of the cornea. Blood vessels may grow into the cornea from the limbus. Pus develops within the anterior chamber (*hypopyon* – pus in the anterior chamber). Bacterial keratitis is an extremely serious condition which can rapidly lead to blindness. Treatment is urgent and requires admission to hospital, the administration of intensive antibiotic drops and antibiotic tablets.

Viral keratitis: *Herpes simplex* is a virus that causes infection of the eyes, skin, lips and genitalia. Primary infection occurs during early childhood and thereafter recurrent infection can occur throughout life at variable intervals. Recurrences may be brought on by poor general health, injury, the effect of ultraviolet light on the eye. If the dendritic ulcer involves the central cornea, patients may experience blurred vision. The corneal stroma may also become involved, invariably resulting in blurred vision due to the development of a *disciform keratitis*. Treatment is with acycloguanosine ointment to kill the active virus. Very weak steroids can be used under *strict supervision* by an eye specialist to reduce inflammation in cases of disciform keratitis. Recurrent attacks can lead to dense scarring of the cornea; fortunately this is not common since the introduction of anti-viral drugs. A severely scarred cornea can be replaced with a corneal graft (see CORNEAL GRAFT). Systemic viral illness such as *measles*, *mumps* and *chickenpox* can also affect the cornea.

Exposure keratitis If the front of the eye becomes dry, desiccation and ulceration of the cornea can occur with the possibility of secondary bacterial infection – a potentially blinding condition. During the action of blinking tears are spread over the front of the eye keeping it moist. If the eyelids are prevented from spreading the tear film, exposure of the eye results. Some causes include: (a) *Facial nerve palsy*: the muscles of the face, including orbicularis oculi, are paralysed and unable to close the eyelids. (b) *Scarring*: this can cause distortion and restriction of movement of the eyelids. (c) *Proptosis*, a condition in which the eye is pushed forward for a variety of reasons. The lids cannot then close over the eye.

Peripheral corneal ulceration can occur in a number of conditions including *focal desiccation* (called a *dellen*), *hypersensitivity* to bacteria, or as a complication of one of the *connective tissue disorders*.

KERATOCONUS: The normal symmetrical curve of the cornea is distorted due to abnormal thinning and subsequent forward bulging of the central cornea. This bulging results in deterioration of the vision. Mild forms can be corrected with spectacles, the more severe forms with contact lenses. The most severe forms require corneal grafting because they cannot be corrected either with glasses or with contact lenses – the cornea becomes so distorted that contact lenses fall off.

Eyelids (disorders of):

BLEPHARITIS: A chronic inflammation of the margin of the eyelids. It frequently begins in childhood, although it does not cause much trouble until later life. The cause is a combination of staphylococcal infection, seborrhoeic dermatitis and concurrent dry eyes due to a reduction in the aqueous component of the tear film. The lid margins may become reddened, scales may appear around the lashes, the lashes may point in different directions or may fall out. Less commonly focal ulceration of the skin of the lids can occur. The conjunctiva and cornea may become involved. Treatment is aimed at relieving the symptoms of burning and redness of the eyelids. Cleaning the eyelids with a solution of sodium bicarbonate may help, as does the use of antibiotic eye drops and artificial tear drops. It is difficult to cure but not dangerous.

BLEPHAROSPASM: An involuntary repeated twitching or even full closure of the eyelids due to spasm of the orbicularis oculi muscle (see EYE: EYELIDS). It usually affects the elderly although it may occur as a transient episode in younger people. When marked it is cosmetically unsightly and may even interfere with vision. Some patients improve with drugs, some recover following injections of local anaesthetic into the eyelids, others may require surgery.

CHALAZION (CYST OF MEIBOMIAN GLAND): Meibomian glands are present in the eyelids. A chalazion is a chronic inflammation of these glands. The cysts may be single or multiple. They are slowly enlarging painless non-red swellings in the eyelids. They may become secondarily infected, in which case they become red and painful. A chalazion usually resolves spontaneously over several months or may be removed surgically if infected or cosmetically unsightly. A small incision is made on the under surface of the lid and the contents of the cyst removed. The procedure takes a few minutes and can be done under local anaesthetic.

ECTROPION: The lid turns outwards. It is far more common in the lower than upper lid. Symptoms include watering of the eye and an unsightly appearance. Treatment is surgical.

ENTROPION: The lid turns inwards. Again the lower lid is usually involved. The eyelashes rub against the eye and cause irritation. Treatment is surgical.

PTOSIS: Drooping of the upper lid. This may be minor, or be complete so that the eye is shut. Ptosis may result from damage or weakness of the muscles lifting the lid, or the nerve supply of those muscles, or may be due to mechanical restriction of lid opening, such as by scarring or the presence of a large (and therefore heavy) cyst or lid tumour, pulling the lid down. Treatment depends on the cause of the ptosis. Some patients may benefit from surgery.

STYE: An acute purulent inflammation of an eyelash follicle. A small abscess results. Styes are common and present as a localized red swelling at the lid margin which appears to surround an eyelash. They are often multiple and are usually due to staphylococcal infection. Treatment includes hot compresses, removal of the eyelash to allow the pus to drain and antibiotic drops or ointment (chloramphenicol).

Eye injuries These may be trivial, or so severe as to cause blindness or loss of the eye. Anyone involved in tasks where an eye injury could be expected (eg. welding, grinding, drilling) should wear appropriate protective goggles or visor.

Sub-conjunctival haemorrhage (see above).

Black eye (or periorbital haematoma) is bruising of the skin of the lids due to an injury around the eye, or to the forehead. Most cases occur without any damage to the eye itself and settle within a week or so. No treatment is required for the bruising.

Corneal foreign bodies constitute 25 per cent of eye injuries. They may arise from dust blowing into the eye or from material thrown from mechanical tools such as drills or even a hammer and chisel. Corneal foreign bodies can cause intense irritation, photophobia and watering of the eye. Treatment involves removal of the foreign body, the application of antibiotic drops or ointment and a patch over the eye until the cornea heals (24 hours in most cases).

Sub-tarsal foreign body (ie. a foreign body under the lid): As the lid blinks, the foreign body is dragged across the cornea, scratching it. Causes, symptoms and treatment are the same as for corneal foreign bodies.

Corneal abrasions: These are losses of corneal epithelium due to an injury. They are painful and cause watering and redness of the eye. Most are small and heal quickly, usually with no long-term effects. Treatment consists of the application of antibiotic drops or ointment and wearing a patch until the abrasion heals.

Corneal ulcer: In ophthalmic terms this is an infection of the cornea (see CORNEA, DISORDERS OF).

Blunt injury may result in damage to the interior of the eye. Bleeding from the iris or ciliary body results in blood in the anterior chamber (a *hyphema*). The iris may be torn in a blunt injury. More serious is the possibility of development of a cataract or dislocation of the lens. The retina may become swollen (*commotio retinae*) or detached (see RETINA, DISORDERS OF). Bleeding into the vitreous from the retinal or choroidal vessels can occur. A certain amount of spontaneous recovery will occur but complications such as *cataract*, *retinal detachment* or *glaucoma* may require surgery. These three complications are the commonest long-term problem resulting from eye injury.

Lacerating injury: This is a serious condition, there is initial damage at the time of injury with possible prolapse of the contents of the eye through the laceration (eg. iris, lens, vitreous); in addition infection may gain access to the eye through the penetrating injury. Surgical repair of the injury aims to try and restore the eye to as near anatomically normal as possible and to minimize the risk of infection. This is a matter of some urgency. Foreign bodies within the eye should be removed if they are likely to cause further damage (eg. bits of wood, copper, iron). Other materials (glass and perspex) can be left alone if they are not easily accessible or if their removal would cause further damage.

Chemical injury: Acids coagulate the proteins of the cornea and sclera producing a barrier that can limit the spread of the acid. Alkali are more dangerous in that they destroy normal barriers and can enter the eye resulting in damage that may be progressive for several days after injury. Treatment is immediate and requires copious irrigation of the eye with water with subsequent treatment to try and minimize the complications that can occur.

Radiant energy injuries: *Ultraviolet light* is almost entirely absorbed by the cornea. Excessive exposure to UV light results in a painful watery red eye. On examination there are hundreds of tiny punctate abrasions on the exposed cornea. *Arc eye* and *snow blindness* result from excessive exposure to UV light. *Infra-red* light can result in cataract formation.

Nystagmus: An involuntary rhythmic, oscillatory movement of the eyes. The movements may be horizontal, vertical or torsional. Nystagmus may occur as an isolated finding in a benign form (congenital nystagmus) or may accompany severe disease of the nervous system, or intoxication with certain drugs including alcohol. Some individuals can induce short bursts of voluntary nystagmus. Nystagmus can also be induced by irritation of the middle ear either by disease, or by water in the ear. Nystagmus was previously thought to be associated with poor lighting (hence 'miner's nystagmus'). This is no longer thought to be true.

Sclera and Episclera (disorders of):

EPISCLERITIS: An inflammation of the episclera (the most superficial layer of the sclera). It typically affects young adults, is common, benign and resolves spontaneously. It may be recurrent but is not associated with systemic disease. Treatment is not usually necessary as it recovers spontaneously in a day or two. Steroid eye drops can speed recovery (see EYE DROPS).

SCLERITIS: An inflammation of the sclera. It is uncommon, occurs in middle age and affects women more than men. It can be bilateral and recurrent, may be painful and can result in blindness due to complications of scleritis. Systemic diseases associated with scleritis include *rheumatoid arthritis*, *connective tissue disorders* generally, *sarcoidosis*, *ulcerative colitis*, *ankylosing spondylitis* and *Bechet's disease*. Treatment is with anti-inflammatory drugs (indomethacin, oxyphenbutazone or steroids).

'Watery eye': This may be due to excessive production of tears (lacrimation) as in crying or irritation of the eye. Treatment is aimed at removal of the cause of irritation. It may also be due to inadequate tear drainage so that tears overflow on to the cheek (*epiphora*). Epiphora may result from the punctum of the lower lid turning out from the eye (as in ectropion). Treatment is to turn the lid back inwards so that the punctum is once more in contact with the eye. More commonly epiphora results from an obstruction in the lacrimal drainage system; commonly this occurs because the cannaliculi become narrowed. Occasionally obstruction of the nasolacrimal duct can result in infection of the lacrimal sac (dacryocystitis). A red painful swelling occurs at the side of the nose which may or may not be made smaller (temporarily) by pressing on it. Pressure on the swelling may result in regurgitation of pus through the puncta on to the eyelids. Treatment is to relieve the obstruction. This may be relatively simple if the obstruction can be cleared by dilating the punctum. If infection has occurred, it must first be overcome by antibiotic tablets and drops, followed by surgery to create a channel between the lacrimal sac and the inside of the nose which bypasses the blocked nasolacrimal duct.

Xerophthalmia: A condition in which the conjunctiva and cornea become dry due to a deficiency of vitamin A. It is seen in Third World countries, but is rare in Great Britain. It may present with night blindness and progress to complete blindness.

EYE DROPS (AND OINTMENT) are used extensively in the treatment of eye disease. They should be used as instructed by the prescribing physician. Most can be used for one month after the bottle has been opened but should then be discarded and a repeat prescription obtained if necessary. Any eye drops or ointment can have side effects and any difficulty with them should be referred to the prescribing physician.

EYE STRAIN (see REFRACTION).

F

FACE is that part of the head extending from the forehead to the chin. It is supported by 14 bones: 2 nasal bones. 2 superior maxillae which carry the upper teeth. 2 lacrimal bones, 2 zygomatic bones, 2 palatine bones, 2 nasal bones at the sides of the nose, the vomer, forming a partition between the nostrils, and the mandible carrying the lower teeth. The lower jaw forms a joint of hinge-shape with the temporal bones of the skull, whilst the other bones of the face are firmly fixed together by sutures. The face in man is relatively small, as compared with that in lower animals, on account of the development of the cranium containing the brain. For the same reason, the face has an almost vertical direction instead of being sloped backwards as in animals.

The general character of the features depends chiefly upon the presence of air spaces in the frontal bone, situated immediately behind the eyebrows and in the upper jaw-bones. The varying expressions which are connected with the emotions and the general expression denoting character are chiefly due to the action of numerous thin muscles situated around the openings of the eyes, nose, and mouth. (See MUSCLE.) These are controlled by the 7th cranial nerve, which springs from the hinder part of the brain, passes through the skull to the ear, and, emerging immediately below the latter, passes forward on to the face round the edge of the lower jaw. In this position it is liable to be wounded or injured by such conditions as cold, then giving rise to a flat and expressionless

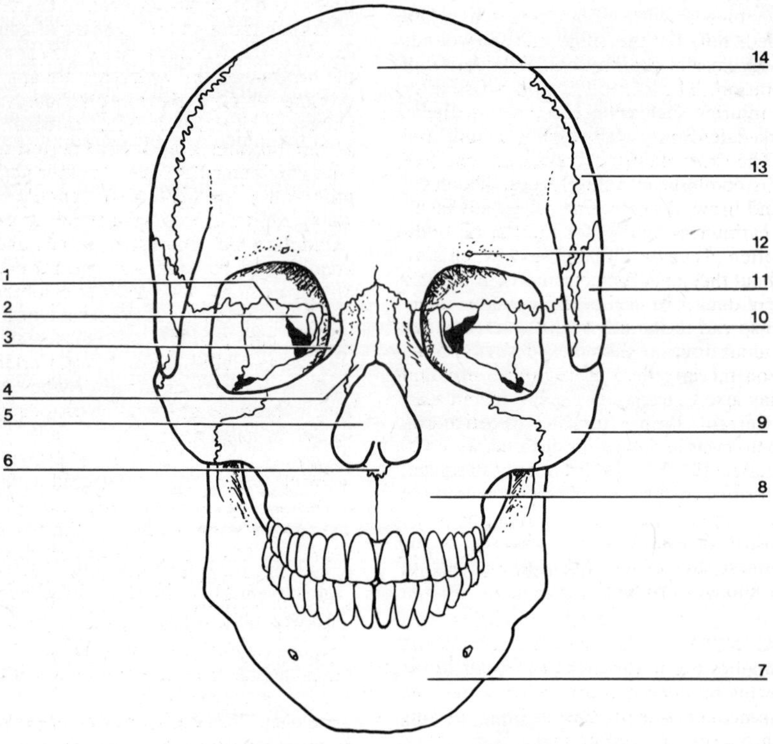

1 greater wing of sphenoid bone
2 lesser wing of sphenoid bone
3 lacrimal bone
4 nasal bone
5 vomer
6 anterior nasal spine of maxilla
7 mandible
8 maxilla
9 zygomatic bone
10 superior orbital fissure
11 squamous part of temperal bone
12 supra-orbital foramen
13 parietal bone
14 frontal bone

The skull from the front.

appearance of one side of the face known as *Bell's palsy* (or *paralysis*) or *facial paralysis*. (See BELL'S PARALYSIS.) The sensory nerve of the face is the 5th cranial nerve, which originates from the neighbouring part of the brain and within the skull divides into three portions called, respectively, ophthalmic, maxillary, and mandibular divisions. Each of these sends branches on to the face through a notch that can be felt near the inner end of the eyebrow, through an opening immediately beneath the eye, and through another opening near the middle of the chin. On their way to the face these nerves supply the parts about the eye, the teeth, and the muscles which move the lower jaw in chewing. The various parts of this nerve are subject to a particularly painful form of neuralgia, known sometimes as tic douloureux. (See NEURALGIA.)

The face is liable to certain deformities, of which hare-lip and cleft palate are the principal. (See PALATE, MALFORMATIONS OF.) The skin of the face, which has an unusually free blood supply, bleeds with great freedom when wounded, but, for the same reason, wounds heal with special rapidity and freedom from suppuration. The contraction of scars after severe injuries, such as burns, sometimes leads to marked deformity of the eyelids, mouth, and nose. The skin condition known as acne (see ACNE) is common in young people about the chin and brow, disappearing as age advances. Boils, carbuncles, and other infectious conditions often occur on the face, and, when situated about the upper lip, present a considerable degree of danger from the liability of the infection to spread to the interior of the head. The tuberculous disease known as lupus is more frequent on the face than in any other situation and may lead to unsightly ulceration and scarring. Certain simple tumours, particularly sebaceous cysts and naevi or birth marks, commonly affect the skin in this region, and cancer, in the form of epithelioma, is not uncommon in the later stages of life about the margins of the lip, nostril, or eyelid. This is also one of the commonest sites of the slow-growing form of cancer known as rodent ulcer.

FACIAL NERVE is the seventh cranial nerve, and supplies the muscles of expression in the face, being purely a motor nerve. It enters the face immediately below the ear after splitting up into several branches. (See BELL'S PARALYSIS.)

FACIES is a term applied to the expression or appearance of the face, which often gives indications of the presence of disease in other parts of the body. Thus the *abdominal facies* is a pinched, anxious expression associated with severe disease in the abdomen. The *cardiac facies* is a condition present in some valvular defects of the heart, showing bright purplish cheeks and lips, with a sallow hue of the rest of the face. The *typhoid facies* is a vacant, bewildered, and apathetic expression seen in typhoid fever and other debilitating diseases. The *Hippocratic facies* is a cast of countenance originally described by Hippocrates, in which the face is drawn, pinched, and livid, indicating approaching death. Anxiety and depression are often reflected in the facial expression.

FAECES is another name for the stools. (See CONSTIPATION; DIARRHOEA; STOOLS.)

FAINTING, or SYNCOPE, is a temporary loss of consciousness.

Causes: The manner in which the loss of consciousness is produced appears to be that temporarily there is an inadequate supply of blood to the brain. If the person who threatens to faint lies down, or, still better, sits and then bends forward so as to bring the head below the knees, the faint is averted. Fainting may occur as part of the general muscular relaxation which takes place in a hot bath. Powerful emotion, generally of a sorrowful nature, but sometimes even great joy, is a cause. Extreme pain, such as that due to the crushing of a limb, and shocks to the nervous system, such as a blow on the head or on the abdomen, are apt to cause fainting, or even the more serious condition known as shock. It is liable to occur on first getting up after a prolonged period of illness with confinement to bed. Another not uncommon cause, particularly in adolescents and young adults, is prolonged standing: eg. on the parade ground. Disgusting smells and sights, breathing of bad air, and general exhaustion are also causes. As a rule, a combination of these causes is necessary, except in hysterical people, and people weak from some illness, who are specially liable to faints. Certain drugs, such as tobacco or alcohol, when taken in excess, produce syncope. Occasionally it may be due to heart disease.

Symptoms are well known. There are certain warning symptoms, such as pallor, feebleness of the pulse, a sinking feeling, and a dullness of sight and hearing. When the faint has occurred, the person lies still, breathing very faintly, with feeble pulse, pallid complexion, and often perspiration standing in drops on the face.

The faint, as a rule, lasts only a few seconds or minutes, but it may last for hours, and hysterical people may pass from one faint, only to fall into another several times.

Treatment: The faint may often be prevented by attending to the cause, as already noted. Sitting down and bending forwards so as to bring the head on a level with the knees, or taking rapid gulps of cold water, is often enough to prevent a threatened faint. The person in a faint should be laid flat on the back, and care should be taken that breathing is unimpeded. If care is not taken to leave the fainting person lying flat, death may ensue, but if this be attended to, nothing more is usually necessary. Stimulants may be applied to the skin in the form of cold compresses on the head, slapping of the hands, pinching of the cheeks; or to the nose in the form of smelling-salts or eau-de-Cologne, or the pungent fumes of burnt feathers. After recovery has taken place from the faint the tendency to its recurrence may be prevented by administration of some stimulant such as sal volatile or brandy.

FALLING SICKNESS is an old name for epilepsy. (See EPILEPSY.)

FALLOPIAN TUBES, or UTERINE TUBES, are tubes, one on each side, which are attached at one end to the womb, and have the other unattached but lying close to the ovary. Each is between 10 to 12·5 cm (4 to 5 inches) long, large at the end next the ovary, but communicating with the womb by an opening which admits only a bristle. These tubes conduct the ova from the ovaries to the interior of the womb. Blockage of them by a chronic inflammatory process resulting from infection is a not uncommon cause of infertility in women.

FALSE MEMBRANE is the name given to the deposit which forms upon the walls of the air passages in cases of diphtheria. It consists partly of fibrin derived from the blood, partly of the destroyed surface of the mucous membrane upon which it rests, and it contains bacteria in enormous numbers. If it is removed, it leaves a raw and bleeding surface upon which new membrane quickly forms.

FAMILY PRACTITIONER COMMITTEE (see NATIONAL HEALTH SERVICE).

FANGO is the name of a kind of mud, derived from thermal springs at Battaglio in Italy, which is applied warm to gouty and rheumatic joints.

FANSIDAR is a combination of pyrimethamine (qv) and sulfadoxine (qv) which is being used for the prevention of malaria (qv). It has the advantage of only needing to be taken once a week, or even only once a fortnight. It should not be taken by pregnant women, nor by those hypersensitive to sulphonamides.

FARCY is another name for glanders. (See GLANDERS.)

FARMER'S LUNG is a form of external allergic alveolitis (see ALVEOLITIS) caused by the inhalation of dust from mouldy hay or straw.

FASCIA is the name applied to sheets or bands of fibrous tissue which enclose and connect the muscles.

FASCIITIS is inflammation of fascia (qv). The commonest site for it is the sole of the foot where it is known as plantar fasciitis. It is characterized by gnawing pain. There is no specific treatment, but it usually clears up spontaneously though over a considerable time. Gentle massage may be helpful in easing the pain. (See POLICEMAN'S HEEL.)

FASCIOLIASIS is the disease caused by the liver fluke, *Fasciolahepatica.* This is found in sheep, cattle and other herbivorous animals, in which it is the cause of the condition known as liver rot. It measures about 35 × 13 mm, and is transmitted to man from the infected animals by snails. In Britain it is the commonest disease found in animal slaughterhouses. The danger to man is in eating vegetables, particularly wild watercress, that have been infected by snails. There have been several outbreaks of fascioliasis in Britain due to eating contaminated wild watercress. Much larger outbreaks of fascioliasis due to eating wild watercress have also been reported in France. The disease is characterized by fever, dyspepsia, heavy sweating, loss of appetite, abdominal pain, urticaria, and a troublesome cough. In the more serious cases there may be severe damage to the liver with or without jaundice. The diagnosis is clinched by the finding of the eggs of the fluke in the stools. The two drugs used in treatment are bithionol and chloroquine. Even though many cases are quite mild and recover spontaneously, prevention is particularly important. This consists primarily of never eating wild watercress, as this is the main cause of infestation. Lettuces have also been found to be infested.

FASTIGIUM means the highest temperature reached in a feverish state.

FASTING means the abstention from, or deprivation of, food and drink.

If food and drink is entirely suspended two results quickly follow: the body becomes thinner and lighter as it draws upon its stored-up nourishment, and also the temperature gradually falls. If water is taken, the process of using up the fat and muscles in order to maintain the activity of the heart, lungs, and other vital organs, proceeds to an extreme extent, and the body becomes very emaciated before death.

After prolonged fasting the return to food should be gradual, and no heavy meal should be taken for a day or two.

FAT as a food has more energy-producing power weight for weight than any other food. Animal fat is a mixture in varying proportions of stearic, palmitic, and oleic acids combined with glycerin. Butter contains about 80 per cent of fat, ordinary cream contains 20 per cent fat, and rich cream 40 per cent, whilst olive oil is practically a pure form of fat. Fat requires, when taken to a large extent in the diet, to be combined with a certain proportion of either carbohydrate or protein in order that it may be completely consumed, otherwise harmful products, known as ketones, are apt to be formed in the blood. Each gram of fat has an energy-producing equivalent of 9·3 Calories.

From the medical point of view, fats are divided into saturated fats, that is, animal fats and dairy produce, and unsaturated fats which include vegetable oils from soya bean, maize and sunflower, and marine oils from fish (eg. cod-liver oil). (See ADIPOSE TISSUE; LIPID; OBESITY.)

FATIGUE is brought about in two ways. In the first place muscles become fatigued by the lactic acid accumulating in them as the result of their activity. For the removal of lactic acid in the recovery phase of muscular contraction oxygen is needed. If the supply of oxygen is not plentiful enough, or cannot keep pace with the work the muscle is doing, then lactic acid accumulates and fatigue results. There is also a nervous element in muscular fatigue: it is diminished by stimulation of the sympathetic nervous system. (See MUSCLE.)

Industrial workers: Many factors enter into the maintenance of efficiency and the avoidance of fatigue, mental and physical. Intensity and direction of illumination, ventilation, temperature and humidity of the air, adequate diet, posture at work, rest pauses, monotony, and, above all, hours of work are among some of these factors. There is a level beyond which the human machine can no longer produce work satisfactorily. If this is exceeded it is shown by a reduction in the quantity and quality of the work done. If work is done under conditions of fatigue, damage to health results and accidents may occur. The shortening of unduly long hours of labour under improved hygienic conditions is followed by increased productive efficiency.

FAT NECROSIS: In injury to, or inflammation of, the pancreas the fat-splitting enzyme in it may escape into the abdominal cavity, causing death of fat-containing cells.

FATTY DEGENERATION: As a result of anaemia, interference with blood or nerve supply, or because of the action of various poisons, body cells may undergo abnormal changes accompanied by the appearance in their substance of fat droplets.

FAUCES is the somewhat narrowed opening between the mouth and throat. It is bounded above by the soft palate, below by the tongue, and on either side by the tonsil. In front of, and behind, the tonsil are two ridges of mucous membrane, the anterior and posterior pillars of the fauces.

FAVISM is a haemolytic anaemia, attacks of which occur within an hour or two of eating broad beans (*Vicia fava*). It is a hereditary disease due to lack of an essential enzyme called glucose-6-phosphate dehydrogenase which plays an important part in the metabolism of glucose and is necessary for the continued integrity of the red cell. This defect is inherited as a sex-linked dominant trait, and the red cells of patients with this abnormality have a normal life span until challenged by certain drugs or fava beans when the older cells are rapidly destroyed, resulting in haemolytic anaemia. Fourteen per cent of American Negroes are affected and 60 per cent of Yemenite Jews in Israel. The perpetuation of the gene is due to the greater resistance against malaria that it carries. Severe and even fatal haemolysis has followed the administration of the antimalarial compounds pamaquine and primaquine in sensitive individuals. These red cells are sensitive not only to fava beans and primaquine but also to sulphonamides, acetanilide, phenacetin, para-aminosalicyclic acid, nitrofurantoin, probenecid and vitamin K analogues.

FAVUS is another name for honeycomb ringworm. (See RINGWORM.)

FAWN-TAIL is the tuft of hair over the lower part of the spine just above the buttocks in infants who have the congenital abnormality of the spine known as diastematomyelia. This consists of a spur of cartilage and bone which interferes with the development of the spinal cord, leading to paraplegia (qv), and loss of control of the bladder and evacuation of the bowels. Surgical removal of the spur, not later than the second year of life, is curative and prevents any neurological complications.

FEEBLE-MINDEDNESS (see MENTAL SUBNORMALITY).

FEEDING (see CEREAL; DIET; DIGESTION; INFANT FEEDING; PROTEIN): The manner and times of administering food are matters of considerable importance in illness. In health appetite forms the usual guide to the amount of food and to meal-times. Most people in health take three meals in the course of the day, one meal being much larger than any of the others and taken either in the middle of the day or in the evening. During the course of a disease or in convalescence, when the digestive powers are weak and a large meal cannot be borne, it is usually found more suitable to feed the patient in small amounts given at frequent intervals. The nature of the food must be such that it is readily digested and the food is usually fluid. Except in certain special cases, milk is the ideal food for this purpose, supplemented by drinks containing glucose. Glucose is given in preference to ordinary sugar (ie. sucrose) because it is not so sweet, and therefore it is possible to give larger amounts without making the dish too sweet. In order to produce variety, and at the same time to ensure an adequate amount of vitamin C, the glucose drinks should be flavoured with fresh fruit juice: eg. orange or lemon. Milk puddings and eggs should be added to the diet as soon as possible. Beef tea, although it has no energy value, adds variety to the invalid diet, as do jellies. Small feeds should be given: two-hourly during the day, and during the night if the patient is awake.

It is sometimes convenient to feed the patient by means of a spoon, but, as a rule, the patient's head being raised by the nurse's arm passed beneath the pillow, the spout of a feeding-cup is introduced into his mouth and the patient is thus able to drink without spilling the fluid. A form of glass from which the patient can drink more naturally consists of a tumbler with an elongated lip on one side, and this is often preferable. Still another method in which the patient may be fed with thin fluids is through a straw or piece of narrow tubing. In this case the straw must be thrown away after use and the tubing carefully boiled before being used again.

Food may be peptonized for administration to invalids. (See PEPTONIZED FOODS; see also MILK, and for preparation of fluid foods for invalids, see ALBUMIN WATER; BARLEY WATER; BEEF-TEA; GRUEL; RICE WATER; TOAST WATER.)

FEHLING'S TEST for glycosuria (see URINE).

FEMUR is the bone of the thigh, and is the longest and strongest bone in the body. As the upper end is set at an angle of about 120 degrees to the rest of the bone, and since the weight of the body is entirely borne by the two femora, fracture of one of these bones close to its upper end is a common accident in old people, whose bones are becoming brittle. The femur fits, at its upper end, into the acetabulum of the pelvis, forming the hip-joint, and, at its lower end, meets the tibia and patella in the knee-joint.

FENBUFEN (LEDERFEN) (see NON-STEROIDAL ANTI-INFLAMMATORY DRUGS).

FENCLOFENAC (FLENAC) (see NON-STEROIDAL ANTI-INFLAMMATORY DRUGS).

FENESTRATION is the operation whereby a new opening is made into the labyrinth of the ear. It has proved most valuable in restoring hearing to patients with otosclerosis (qv), particularly in young people with this disease.

FENFLURAMINE is an anorexiant drug (qv), introduced to aid the slimming process by suppressing or reducing appetite. Although less likely to become a drug of addiction than some of the other anorexiant drugs, it is not without its risks and must only be used under skilled medical supervision. One of its disadvantages is that in some people it induces an increased frequency of dreaming or even nightmares.

FENNEL is the seed-like fruit of *Foeniculum vulgare* used as a carminative: ie. to relieve griping, flatulence, and distension of the stomach. Fennel water used to be a popular remedy for griping.

FENOTEROL is a drug that is proving useful by inhalation in the treatment of asthma.

FEPRAZONE (METHRAZONE) (see ANTI-STEROIDAL ANTI-INFLAMMATORY DRUGS).

FERMENTS are substances which produce chemical changes in other bodies while remaining unchanged themselves.

FERRUM is the Latin name for iron.

FESTER is a popular term used to mean any collection or formation of pus. It is applied to both abscesses and ulcers. (See ABSCESS; ULCER; WHITLOW.)

FESTINATION is the term applied to the involuntary quickening of gait seen in some nervous diseases, especially in PARKINSONISM (qv).

FETISHISM: This is a form of sexual deviation in which the person becomes sexualy stimulated by parts of the body, such as the feet, which are not usually regarded as erotogenic.

FETUS (see FOETUS).

FEVER is the condition of the body characterized by a rise in temperature. It is one of the most common accompaniments of diseases in general, and serves to make the distinction between *febrile* and *non-febrile* ailments.

Causes: The cause of fever is the release of an endogenous pyrogen by phagocytic cells called monocytes and macrophages. The cause of the fever is a small protein which is produced in response to a variety of infectious, immunological and neoplastic stimuli. The lymphocytes play a part in fever production because they recognize the antigen and release substances called lymphokines and these lymphokines promote the production of endogenous pyrogen. The pyrogen then acts on the thermo-regulatory centre in the hypothalamus and this results in an increase in heat generation and a reduction in heat loss, resulting in a rise in body temperature.

In many cases the fever must be regarded as only secondary to, and symptomatic of, the disordered state with which it is found associated. For example, a certain amount of fever may arise in consequence of some nervous shock. But there is a large class of diseases in which fever is the predominant factor, and which arise from the formation in the system of something of the nature of a poison (toxin), upon which all the symptoms depend. To such diseases, the term primary or specific fevers is applied; they include typhoid fever, scarlet fever, diphtheria. These diseases depend on the growth of bacteria in the blood or tissues of the body, the toxins being formed by the activity of these organisms.

In considering the general subject of fever, regard must be had in particular to the two main features of the febrile process: the abnormal elevation of temperature, and the changes affecting the tissues of the body in reference thereto.

The average temperature of the body in health ranges between 36·9° and 37·5°C

(98·4° and 99·5°F). It is liable to slight variations from such causes as the ingestion of food, the amount of exercise, the menstrual cycle, and the temperature of the surrounding atmosphere. There are, moreover, certain appreciable daily variations, the lowest temperature being between the hours of 01·00 and 07·00 hours, and the highest between 16·00 and 21·00 hours, with trifling fluctuations during these periods. (See TEMPERATURE.)

The development and maintenance of heat within the body are generally regarded as depending on the destructive oxidation of all its tissues, consequent on the changes continually taking place in the processes of nutrition. In health this constant tissue disintegration is exactly counterbalanced by the introduction of food, whilst the uniform normal temperature is maintained by the due adjustment of the heat thus developed, and of the processes of exhalation and cooling which take place, especially from the lungs and skin. In the febrile state this relationship is no longer preserved, the tissue waste being greatly in excess of the food supply, while the so-called 'law of temperature' is in abeyance. In this condition the body wastes rapidly, the loss to the system being chiefly in the form of nitrogen compounds (eg. urea). In the early stage of fever a patient excretes about three times the amount of urea that he would excrete on the same diet if he were in health – the difference being that in the latter condition he discharges a quantity of nitrogen equal to that taken in with the food, whilst in the fevered state he wastes the store of nitrogen contained in the tissues and the blood. The amount of fever is estimated by the degree of elevation of the temperature above the normal standard. When it reaches as high a point as 41·1°C (106°F) the term hyperpyrexia (excessive fever), is applied, and is regarded as indicating a condition of danger; while, if it exceeds 41·7° or 42·2°C (107° or 108°F) for any length of time, death almost always results.

Symptoms: The onset of a fever is usually marked by a rigor or shivering, which may exist only as a slight but persistent feeling of chilliness, or, on the other hand, be of a violent character, and, as occasionally happens with children, find expression in the form of well-marked convulsions. Although termed the *cold stage* of fever, in this condition the temperature of the body is really increased. There are, besides, various accompanying feelings of illness, such as pain in the back, headache, sickness, thirst, and great lassitude. In all cases of febrile complaints it is of importance for the physician to note the first occurrence of shivering, which in general fixes the beginning of the attack. This stage is soon followed by the full development of the febrile condition, the *hot stage*. The skin now feels hot and dry, and the temperature, always elevated above the normal standard, will often be found to show daily variations corresponding to those observed in health – namely, a rise toward evening, and a fall in the morning. There is a relative increase in the rate of the pulse and quickness of breathing. The tongue is dry and furred; the thirst is intense, while the appetite is gone; the urine is scanty, of high specific gravity, containing a large quantity of solid matter, particularly urea, the excretion of which, as already stated, is increased in fever; while, on the other hand, certain of the saline ingredients, such as chlorides, are often diminished. The bowels are in general constipated, but they may be relaxed, especially if the gut is the primary site of infection, as in typhoid fever. The nervous system participates in the general disturbance, and sleeplessness and disquietude are common accompaniments, and there may be delirium. The wasting of the muscles, and corresponding loss of strength, may be marked, and continue even although considerable quantities of nutriment may be taken.

The decline of the fever takes place either by the occurrence of a *crisis*, ie. a sudden termination of the symptoms, or by a more gradual subsidence of the temperature, technically termed a *lysis*. If death ensues, this is due to failure of the vital centres in the brain or of the heart, as a result of either the infection or hyperpyrexia. Such terminal failure may be gradual, the patient passing into what is sometimes known as the *typhoid state* (a condition of extreme prostration, associated with low delirium or coma). In other cases death occurs suddenly after slight exertion, as a result of the additional strain on the heart.

Certain well-marked types of fever are recognized. The term *continued fever* is applied to those forms in which the febrile temperature persists for a more or less definite period, uninterrupted by any distinct intermission till the crisis is reached. To this type belong typhus and typhoid fevers, and the eruptive fevers or exanthemata: eg. smallpox, measles, and scarlet fever. *Relapsing fever* is a form of continued fever, the chief characteristic of which is the occurrence in about a week after the crisis of a distinct relapse and repetition of all the symptoms. Occasionally second and third relapses take place.

The term *remittent* is applied to those forms of fever the course of which is interrupted by a short, usually daily, diminution of the fever, followed by a recurrence of all the symptoms. Such fevers are chiefly met in tropical climates, but occasionally continued fevers assume this form, particularly in children.

In *intermittent fever* there is a distinct periodic subsidence of the symptoms, which, according to its duration, characterizes the variety as *quotidian* (where the paroxysm recurs in twenty-four hours), *tertian* (in forty-eight hours), *quartan* (in seventy-two hours).

Treatment: Fever is a symptom, and the correct treatment is therefore that of the underlying condition. Occasionally, however, it is also necessary to try and reduce the temperature by more direct methods. For this latter purpose it will be sufficient to refer to two methods: namely, the external application of cold and the administration of antipyretic remedies. The former of these methods is accomplished by means of baths, in which the patient is placed, the water being somewhat below the febrile temperature and gradually cooled down by the addition of cold water till a temperature of from 15·5° to 21°C (60° to 70°F) is reached. The cooler the bath the longer the effect lasts. Sponging with cold water and the wet pack are other methods used to reduce temperature and exert a soothing influence. (See COLD, USES OF.)

Certain drugs possess the power of reducing the temperature by their action on the heat-regulating centres in the brain, thereby causing an increased loss of heat through dilatation of the blood-vessels in the skin. These drugs include sodium salicylate, aspirin, quinine, and Dover's powder.

FEVERFEW, *Chrysanthemum parthenium*, is a perennial plant which grows throughout Europe, both wild and cultivated. It is one of the old herbal remedies, widely used for the relief of fever. Hence its popular name. It is now being used for the prevention of migraine (qv). The usual dose is one large leaf or three smaller leaves daily, chopped and eaten in a sandwich. Some users sprinkle sugar on it to take away its bitter taste. Its side-effects are not common, but include itching of the skin, ulcers in the mouth and indigestion. It should not be taken by pregnant women.

FIBEROPTIC ENDOSCOPY has transformed the management of gastro-intestinal disease. In chest disease fiberoptic bronchoscopy has now replaced the rigid wide-bore metal tube which was previously used for examination of the tracheo-bronchial tree. The principle of fiberoptics is that a light from a cold light source passes down a bundle of quartz fibres to illuminate the lumen of the gastro-intestinal tract or the bronchi. The reflected light is returned to the observer's eye via the image bundle which may contain up to 20,000 fibres. The tip of the instrument can be angulated in both directions and finger-tip controls are provided for suction, air insufflation and for water injection to clear the lens or the mucosa. The oesophagus, stomach and duodenum can be visualised. Furthermore, visualisation of the pancreatic duct and direct endoscopic cannulation is now possible, as is visualisation of the bile duct. Fiberoptic colonoscopy can visualise the entire length of the colon and it is now possible to biopsy polyps or suspected carcinomas and to perform polypectomy. The flexible smaller fiberoptic bronchoscope has many advantages over the rigid tube and extends the range of view to all segmental bronchi and enables biopsy of pulmonary parenchyma itself. A biopsy forceps can be directed well beyond the tip of the bronchoscope itself and the more flexible fiberoptic instrument causes less discomfort to the patient.

FIBRE, DIETARY (see ROUGHAGE).

FIBRILLATION is a term applied to rapid contraction or tremor of muscles, especially to a form of abnormal action of the heart muscle in which individual bundles of fibres take up independent action. It is believed to be due to a state of excessive excitability in the muscle associated with the stretching which occurs in dilatation of the heart. Fibrillation is distinguished as atrial or ventricular, according as the muscle of the atria or of the ventricles is affected. In atrial fibrillation the heart beats and the pulse become extremely irregular, both as regards time and force. When the atrium is fibrillating there is no significant contraction of the atrial muscle but the cardiac output is maintained by ventricular contraction. In ventricular fibrillation there is no significant contractile force so that there is no cardiac output and the patient is essentially dead. If the ventricular fibrillation takes place in hospital resuscitation and de-fibrillation can be applied and the normal cardiac function restored.

FIBRIN is a substance formed in the blood as it clots. Its formation indeed causes clotting. The substance is produced in threads. After the threads have formed a close meshwork through the blood, they contract, and produce a dense felted mass. The substance is formed not only from shed blood but also from lymph which exudes from the lymph-vessels. Thus fibrin is found in all inflammatory conditions within serous cavities like the pleura, peritoneum, and pericardium, and forms a thick coat upon the surface of the inflamed membranes. It is also found in inflamed joints, and in the lung as a result of pneumonia. (See COAGULATION.)

FIBRIN FOAM is one of a series of absorbable haemostatics introduced into surgical use. A haemostatic is a preparation which arrests bleeding, and the great advantage of an absorbable haemostatic is that it produces no irritation in the tissues into which it is introduced and that it does not need to be removed after the bleeding is arrested, but is gradually absorbed by the tissues. Fibrin foam is a spongy material which is soaked in a solution of thrombin immediately before use. Other absorbable haemostatics now in use include oxidized cellulose which is prepared as a gauze, and calcium alginate (derived from seaweed) which is prepared as a gauze and as wool. These absorbable haemostatics, which constitute a great advance in surgery, are of particular value in operations on the brain and in operations on blood-vessels and nerves.

FIBRINOGEN is the soluble protein in the blood which is the precursor of fibrin (qv), the substance in blood-clot.

FIBROCYSTIC DISEASE OF THE PANCREAS, or MUCOVISCIDOSIS, which is also known as cystic fibrosis, is the commonest serious genetic disease in Caucasian children, with an incidence of about 1 per 2000 births. It is a disorder of the mucus-secreting glands of the lungs, the pancreas, the mouth, and the gastro-intestinal tract, as well as the sweat glands of the skin. It is characterized by failure to gain weight in spite of a good appetite, repeated attacks of bronchitis, and the passage of loose, foul-smelling and slimy stools. A simple, cheap, reliable test for detecting the disease by examination of the stools has now been evolved, which permits the early diagnosis of the disease. As yet there is no reliable method of detecting carriers of the disease or of detecting affected children before birth by antenatal tests. Treatment consists basically of regular physiotherapy and postural drainage (qv), and the taking of pancreatic enzyme tablets and vitamins. The earlier treatment is started, the better the results. Whereas two decades ago, only 12 per cent of affected children survived beyond adolescence, today 75 per cent survive into adult life, and an increasing number are surviving into their 40's. Parents of children with cystic fibrosis, seeking help and advice, can obtain this from the Cystic Fibrosis Research Trust, Alexandra House, 5 Blyth Road, Bromley, Kent BR1 3RS (01–464 7211).

FIBROID is a term sometimes applied to tumours of the womb consisting partly of muscular and partly of fibrous tissue. (See UTERUS, DISEASES OF.)

FIBROMA is a tumour consisting of fibrous tissue. (See TUMOURS.)

FIBROSIS means the formation of fibrous or scar tissue, which is usually due to either infection or deficient blood supply.

FIBROSITIS is another name for muscular rheumatism. (See RHEUMATISM.)

FIBROUS DYSPLASIA is a rare disease in which areas of bone are replaced by fibrous tissue (qv). This renders the bone fragile and liable to fracture. It may involve only one bone, usually the thigh bone, or femur (qv), or several bones. This latter form of the disease may be accompanied by pigmentation of the skin and the early onset of puberty. There is another form of the disease known as cherubism because of the appearance it gives to the face, in which the abnormality of bone is confined to the upper and lower jaw-bones (the maxilla and mandible). The cause of the disease is not known.

FIBROUS TISSUE is one of the most abundant tissues throughout the body. White fibrous tissue consists of fibres of a substance known as collagen, which yields gelatine on being boiled. Between these fibres lie flattened or star-shaped cells, by which the fibres are produced. The fibres, like the cells, are of microscopic size, and are grouped into bundles which are held together by other fibres running round them. Yellow fibrous tissue is a rarer form, and consists of bundles of long yellow fibres, formed from a substance known as elastin. White fibrous tissue is very unyielding and forms sinews, ligaments, the material which binds muscle fibres together, the substance of the true skin. It is also the tissue which is laid down in the repair of wounds, or as a result of inflammation, and so forms the tissue composing a scar. It has the property of contracting and becoming denser as time goes on, and hence the puckering seen in scars, and the contraction resulting from burns and inflammation. Yellow fibrous tissue is highly elastic, and so is found in the walls of arteries, and in ligaments, like that on the back of the neck, which are often stretched. (See also ADHESIONS; SCAR; WOUNDS.)

FIBULA is the slender bone upon the outer side of the leg.

FILARIASIS is the name given to a group of tropical diseases in which minute Nematode worms, called filariae, are found in the blood. The estimated prevalence is 250 million cases. The most widespread of these is Bancroftian filariasis, so called after Dr. Joseph Bancroft. The causative worm is *Wuchereria bancrofti*, also known as *Filaria bancrofti*. This is a threadlike worm which is transmitted by certain mosquitoes. It is named after Wucherer, who discovered microfilariae in the urine of a filarial patient in Brazil in 1866 and Bancroft, who first described the adult worms in Australia in 1876. The adult female worm measures up to 100 millimetres in length. One of the striking features of these worms is that they are found in the circulating blood in large numbers in the evening, whilst during the day they disappear from the blood-stream. Its geographical distribution is widespread in warm countries, but it is most prevalent in India. It is also found in Sri Lanka, South East Asia, China, New Guinea, tropical Africa, Egypt, many Pacific islands, and parts of the West Indies and Central and South America.

The form of filariasis produced by *W. bancrofti* is characterized by inflammation and blockage of the lymphatics. In the early stages this leads to enlargement of the lymphatic glands. There is also involvement of the testicles, which become painful and enlarged, and this is accompanied by the formation of a hydrocele. Repeated inflammation of the lymphatic vessels ultimately leads to their blockage and this is responsible for the most characteristic of the later stages of the disease –elephantiasis, ie. gross enlargement of the lower limbs and the scrotum. This may be so marked that the leg may attain a circumference of several feet, whilst the scrotum may weigh 23kg. Elephantiasis may occur elsewhere in the body, eg. the arms, but not very commonly. (See ELEPHANTIASIS.)

Treatment: Encouraging results are being obtained, particularly in early cases, from the use of diethylcarbamazine. Surgery is required for the treatment of elephantiasis. Prevention consists primarily of (*a*) destroying the mosquitoes which transmit the worm, and (*b*) protection of the individual against mosquito bites by the use of mosquito nets and repellents.

FINGERS consist of three bones called phalanges united by hinge-joints and strong ligaments. The thumb, like the great toe, differs from the others in having only two bones. These are bent or flexed, and straightened or extended by powerful sinews, two in front and two behind, which are brought into action by the contraction of muscles in the forearm. The sinews are enveloped in complicated synovial sheaths, through which they slide without friction, and are attached to the bases of the middle and end phalanges, back and front.

Running up each side of each finger are two small arteries and two small nerves, which supply the various structures and especially the overlying skin. The skin of the fingers is specially strong and particularly sensitive, and the end of the finger has a highly specialized part, the nail (see SKIN). Each finger is set upon a bone, the metacarpal, which lies in the substance of the hand between the finger and the carpus or wrist.

FINSEN LIGHT (see LIGHT TREATMENT).

FIRST AID: Courses of instruction in first aid comprise six to twelve sessions, each of about two hours' duration. Syllabuses of instruction are published by various organizations, the principal ones being the British Red Cross Society, the St. John Ambulance Association, and the St. Andrew's Ambulance Association. For full details reference should be made to the secretary of one of these associations: British Red Cross Society, 9 Grosvenor Crescent, London, SW1X 7EJ (01–235 5454); St. John Ambulance, 1 Grosvenor Crescent, London, SW1X 7EF (01–235 5231. Fax 01–235 0796); St. Andrew's Ambulance Association, Strachan House, 16 Torphichen Street, Edinburgh EH3 8JB (031–229 5915).

(For subjects connected with first-aid, see under BANDAGES; BURNS; CONVULSIONS; DROWNING; FAINTING; FRACTURES; HAEMORRHAGE; INJURED, REMOVAL OF; NURSING; POISONING; WOUNDS.)

FISSURE is a term applied both to clefts of normal anatomical structure and also to small narrow ulcers occurring in skin and mucous membrane. The latter type of fissure occurs especially at the corners of the mouth and at the anus. (See LIPS; RECTUM, DISEASES OF.)

FISTULA is an unnatural, narrow channel, leading from some natural cavity, such as the duct of a gland, or the interior of the bowels, to the surface. Or it may be a communication between two such cavities, where none should exist, as, for example, a direct communication between the bladder and bowel.

Cause: Sometimes a child is born with a fistula, as a result of some defect in development, for example, a fistula from the thyroid gland to the surface; but, as a rule, the cause of the formation is either disease or injury. Often, the blockage of the duct of a gland leads to a fistula and the escape of the secretion from the gland on to the surface. Thus a salivary fistula may form on the face as a result of blockage by a concretion of the salivary duct in the cheek, and saliva then runs out on the cheek instead of into the mouth. Injury may also be the cause. For example, if the pelvis is fractured, the urethra may be torn across, so that urine, instead of being properly voided, passes among the tissues, and, by a process of suppuration, gradually bursts its way out through the skin, forming a permanent urinary fistula. A fistula from the bowel or bladder occasionally arises in women as a result of injury during protracted child-birth. Disease is another cause; thus an abscess may form at the side of the lower end of the bowel, and, bursting into the bowel on one side, and through the skin on the other, forms a fistula. This fistula in ano, as it is known, forms the most important variety of fistula. The abscess which produces the fistula may be tuberculous or an acute abscess due to other micro-organisms. (See ABSCESS, ACUTE.) Sometimes a fishbone or pin, which has been swallowed, travels through the whole digestive canal without doing damage, till it reaches this point, where it lodges and produces a fistula.

Treatment: As a rule, a fistula is extremely difficult to close, especially after it has persisted for some time. The treatment consists in an operation to restore the natural channel, be it salivary duct, or urethra, or bowel. This is effected by appropriate means in each locality, and when it is attained the fistula heals quickly under simple dressings.

Fistula in ano is a very troublesome condition, and is kept from healing by the constant entrance into it of material from the bowel. It is only to be cured by dividing the tissues which separate it from the bowel, and, each day, after the bowels move, packing the wound in such a way as to compel it to heal gradually from its deepest part. The process of healing is therefore a tedious one.

FIT is a popular name for a sudden convulsive seizure, although the term is also extended to include sudden seizures of every sort. During the occurrence of a fit of any sort the chief object should be to prevent the patient from doing any harm to himself by the convulsive movements. The person should therefore be laid flat, and the head supported on a pillow or other soft material. To prevent the tongue from being bitten, some object of moderate hardness may be placed between the teeth. (See APOPLEXY; CONVULSIONS; ECLAMPSIA; EPILEPSY; FAINTING; HYSTERIA; URAEMIA.)

FLAIL CHEST (see FRACTURES).

FLAT-FOOT, or PES PLANUS, is a deformity of the foot in which its arch sinks down so that the inner edge of the foot comes to rest upon the ground. Flat-foot seldom occurs in active, energetic people, and its presence debars people from the public services, or even from engagement in positions where physical activity is needed, for example, as sailors.

Causes: Most cases occur in growing and undernourished young men and young women who have much standing on the feet. The ligaments which support the arch are in these people still soft, the four muscles (two tibial muscles on the inner side, and two peroneal muscles on the outer side) which sling it up become weak or tired, and hence the arch gradually subsides. It also tends to develop in obese middle-aged individuals who have to stand about a great deal without actually exercising the muscles: eg. fat housewives.

Symptoms: There is pain both along the instep and beneath the outer ankle, the foot is stiff and broad, walking is tiresome, and the toes turn far out. The footprints of a flat-foot are broad all the way from toe to heel, instead of being a mere line at the instep. The extent to which the flatness has proceeded may be tested by wetting the bare feet with inky water and causing the person to stand on a piece of clean white paper.

Treatment: Change of occupation to one which allows sitting is sometimes necessary. In early cases the leg muscles may be strengthened by tiptoe exercises performed for ten minutes night and morning, the legs being thereafter bathed with cold salt water and massaged. This may be enough, or a steel sole, with instep to support the arch, may have to be worn inside the shoe. Sponge rubber pads also make an effective, and resilient, support for the arch. In other cases providing the shoe with a sole which is thicker on the inner side of the foot than it is on the outer side may both relieve discomfort in walking and help to remedy the flat-foot by throwing the weight of the body on to the outer edge of the foot. The toes should be habitually turned inwards in walking. In severe cases of long standing it may be necessary either to wrench the foot into position, under a general anaesthetic, and put it in plaster of Paris for a month, or even to remove part of the bone from its inner side, so as to shorten the instep and make a new arch.

FLATULENCE means a collection of gas in the stomach or bowels. In the former case the gas is expelled from time to time in noisy eructations by the mouth; in the latter case it may produce unpleasant rumblings in the bowels, or be expelled from the anus.

Causes: The presence of gas in the stomach has been explained under the heading of ERUCTATION. When gas is found in large amount in the bowels its production is usually due to fermentation set up by bacteria. Marsh gas and hydrogen are formed from the cellulose of vegetables, sulphuretted hydrogen and carbon disulphide from eggs, peas, and other articles of diet containing much sulphur. Many cases of flatulence are much aggravated by a habit of gulping mouthfuls of air.

Treatment: Flatulence in the stomach is treated by relieving the dyspepsia which causes it. It may also be relieved, or eased, by the administration of carminatives (qv). In many cases the flatulence is aggravated by a nervous condition which must receive appropriate treatment. If the flatulence is due to, or aggravated by, the habit of swallowing air, the patient must, by taking a careful note of the occcasions when he does this almost unconsciously, break himself of this habit. When this is done the flatulence often passes off. In cases of intestinal flatulence, articles of diet which tend to decompose, eg. green vegetables and starchy foods, should be avoided, and the food should be light and quickly digestible.

FLAVINE (see ANTISEPTICS).

FLEAS (see INSECTS IN RELATION TO DISEASE).

FLEXIBILITAS CEREA is an abnormal state in which the limbs remain in any position into which they are moved.

FLEXICAL (see ENTERAL FEEDING).

FLEXION means bending, and is a term applied either to the bending of joints or to an abnormal shape of organs.

FLIES (see INSECTS IN RELATION TO DISEASE).

FLOATING KIDNEY (see KIDNEY, DISEASES OF).

FLOCCITATION means the fitful picking at the bed-clothes by a delirious patient, as, for example, in typhoid fever.

FLOODING is a popular name for an excessive blood-stained discharge from the womb. (See MENSTRUATION.) In the majority of cases flooding is the sign of a miscarriage. (See MISCARRIAGE.)

FLUCLOXACILLIN (see PENICILLIN, ANTIBIOTIC).

FLUCTUATION is a sign obtained from collections of fluid by laying the fingers of one hand upon one side of the swelling, and, with those of the other, tapping or pressing suddenly on a distant point of the swelling. The thrill communicated from one hand to the other through the fluid is one of the most important signs of the presence of an abscess, or of effusion of fluid into joints or into the peritoneal cavity.

FLUCYTOSINE is a drug that is proving of value in the treatment of certain fungal infections such as candidiasis (qv) and cryptococcosis (qv).

FLUFENAMIC ACID is a drug with analgesic, anti-inflammatory and anti-pyretic actions which is proving of value in the treatment of osteoarthrosis and rheumatoid arthritis.

FLUKES are a variety of parasitic worms. (See FASCIOLIASIS.)

FLUNITRAZEPAM (ROHYPNOL) (see BENZODIAZEPINES).

FLUOCINOLONE is a corticosteroid for application to the skin as a cream, lotion or ointment. It is more potent than hydrocortisone. It must not be given by mouth.

FLUORESCEIN is a dye which has the special property of absorbing blue-light energy and emitting this energy as green light. This property is made use of in examining the cornea for scratches or ulceration and it is also used to detect abnormally permeable (or leaking) blood vessels in the retina and iris – especially in diabetic retinopathy and diseases of the macula.

FLUORINE, one of the halogen series of elements, is one of the constituents of bone and teeth. During recent years evidence has accumulated that supplementing the daily intake of fluorine diminishes the incidence of dental caries. American and British evidence indicates that people who, throughout their lives, have drunk water with a natural fluorine content of 1 part per million, have less dental caries than those whose drinking water is fluorine free. All the available evidence indicates that this is the most satisfactory way of giving fluorine, and that if the concentration of fluorine in drinking water does not exceed 1 part per million, there are no toxic effects.

FLUOROSCOPE is an apparatus for rendering X-rays visible after they have passed through the body by projecting them on a screen of calcium tungstate. The technique of using it is known as FLUOROSCOPY. It provides a method of being able to watch, for instance, the beating of the heart, or the movements of the intestine after the administration of a barium meal. (See X-RAYS.)

FLUOROURACIL (EFUDIX) is a drug that is proving of value when given intravenously, in the treatment of recurrent and inoperable carcinoma of the colon and rectum, as well as secondaries from cancer of the breast. (See CYTOTOXIC DRUGS.)

FLUPENTHIXOL is a tranquillizer that is proving of value in the treatment of schizophrenia (qv).

FLUPHENAZINE (MODITEN) is one of the phenothiazine derivatives which is proving of value as an anti-psychotic drug. (See ANTI-PSYCHOTIC DRUGS.)

FLURAZEPAM (DALMANE) (see BENZODIAZEPINES).

FLURBIPROFEN (FROBEN) is a drug that is proving of value in the treatment of rheumatoid arthritis and ankylosing spondylitis. (See NON-STEROIDAL ANTI-INFLAMMATORY DRUGS.)

FLUSPIRILENE is a tranquillizer that is proving of value in the treatment of schizophrenia (qv). It is given by intramuscular injection, and the effect of one injection lasts for six to fifteen days.

FLUTTER, or ATRIAL FLUTTER, is the term applied to a form of abnormal cardiac rhythm, in which the atria contract at a rate of between 200 and 400 beats a minute, and the ventricles more slowly. The abnormal rhythm is the result of a diseased heart.

FLUX means an excessive discharge from any of the natural openings of the body. 'Bloody flux' is a popular name for dysentery, 'white flux' or 'whites' for leucorrhoea.

FOETOR OF THE BREATH (see BREATH, DISORDERS OF).

FOETUS, or EMBRYO, is the name given to the child while still within the womb. The human being, like the young of all animals, begins as a single cell, the *ovum*, in the ovary. After fertilization with a spermatozoon the ovum becomes embedded in the mucous membrane of the uterus, its covering being known as the decidua. Increase in size is rapid, and development of complexity is still more marked. The original cell divides again and again to form new cells, and these become arranged in three layers, known as the ectoderm, mesoderm, and endoderm. From the first are produced the skin, the brain and spinal cord, and the nerves; from the second the bones, muscles, blood-vessels, and connective tissues; while the third develops into the lining of the digestive system and the various glands attached to it.

The ovum produces not only the foetus but several membranes and appendages which serve it till birth, and are then cast away. The embryo develops upon one side of the ovum, its first appearance consisting of a groove, the edges of which grow up and join to form a tube, which in turn develops into the brain and spinal cord. At the same time, a part of the ovum beneath this is becoming pinched off to form the body, and within this the endoderm forms a second tube, which in time is changed in shape and lengthened to form the digestive canal. From the gut there grows out very early a process called the allantois, which attaches itself to the wall of the womb, forming later on the navel-string and afterbirth, by which nourishment is gained for growth. (See AFTERBIRTH.)

The remainder of the ovum, which within two weeks of conception has increased to about 2 mm (1/12 inch) in size, splits into an outer and inner shell, from the outer of which are developed two covering membranes, the chorion and amnion, while the inner constitutes the yolk sac, attached by a pedicle to the developing gut of the embryo. From two weeks after conception onward, the various organs and limbs appear and grow, the name of *embryo* being applied to the developing being while almost indistinguishable in appearance from the embryo of other animals, till the middle of the second month, when it begins to show a distinctly human form. After this stage it is called the *foetus*. The property of 'life' is present from the very beginning, although the movements of the foetus are not felt by the mother till the fifth month.

During the first few days after conception the eye begins to be formed, beginning as a cup-shaped outgrowth from the mid-brain, its lens being formed as a thickening in the skin. It is very soon followed by the beginnings of the nose and ear, both of which arise as pits on the surface, which increase in complexity, and are joined by nerves that grow outward from the brain. These three organs of sense have practically their final appearance as early as the beginning of the second month.

As already stated, the body closes in from behind forward, the sides growing forward from the spinal region. In the neck, the growth takes the form of five arches, similar to those which bear gills in fishes. From the first of these the lower jaw is formed, from the second the hyoid bone, all the arches uniting, and the gaps between them closing up by the end of the second month. At this time the head and neck have assumed quite a human appearance.

The digestive canal begins as a simple tube running from end to end of the embryo, but it grows in length and becomes twisted in various directions to form the stomach and bowels. From this tube also the lungs and the liver arise as two little buds, which quickly increase in size and complexity. The kidneys also appear very early, but go through several changes before their final form is reached.

The genital organs appear late. The swellings, which form the ovary in the female and the testicle (or testis) in the male, are produced in the region of the loins, and gradually descend to their final positions. The outward organs are exactly similar in the two sexes till the end of the third month, and the sex is not clearly distinguishable till late in the fourth month.

The blood-vessels appear in the ovum even before the embryo. The heart, originally double, forms as a dilatation upon the arteries which later produce the aorta. These two hearts later fuse into one. (For the circulation in the foetus, see CIRCULATION OF BLOOD.)

The limbs appear about the end of the third week as buds which increase quickly in length and split at their ends into five parts, for fingers or toes. The bones at first are formed of cartilage, in which true bone begins to appear during the third month.

The following table gives the average size and weight of the foetus at different periods:

Age	*Length*	*Weight*
4 weeks	5 mm	1·3 grams
3 months	8 to 9 cm	30 to 60 grams
5 months	15 to 25 cm	170 to 340 grams
7 months	32 to 35 cm	1360 to 1820 grams
Birth	45 to 60 cm	3200 grams

Approximate length and weight of the foetus at different periods.

The foetus is legally viable after the end of the 28th week of pregnancy (see BIRTH), when it weighs around 1400 grams (3 pounds), but the number of babies who survive such premature birth is small. Thus, in England in 1980, of the 4825 babies born with a weight of 1500 grams or less, 1806 died within 28 days of birth. On the other hand, modern methods of dealing with premature infants are so efficient that babies weighing as little as 680 grams (1½pounds) have survived.

FOLIC ACID, one of the constituents of the vitamin B complex, derives its name from the fact that it is found in many green leaves, including spinach and grass. It has also been obtained from liver, kidney, and yeasts. In 1945 it was synthesized by American workers, who proposed that the chemical name should be pteroylglutamic acid. It has proved of value in the treatment of macrocytic anaemias, particularly those associated with sprue and nutritional deficiencies.

FOLIUM is the latin term for leaf: eg. digitalis folium is digitalis leaf. (Plural: folia.)

FOLLICLE is the term applied to a very small sac or gland: eg. small collections of adenoid tissue in the throat and the small digestive glands on the mucous membrane of the intestine.

FOLLICULAR HORMONE (see OESTRADIOL).

FOMENTATION (see also POULTICES) is any warm application to the surface of the body in the form of a cloth. Usually the fomentation cloth is heated by being wrung out of hot water, but the term is also applied to dry applications and to hot cloths upon which various drugs are sprinkled. A fomentation dilates the blood-vessels of the part to which it is applied and has a soothing effect upon the endings of the nerves, so that it both aids the absorption of effusions and relieves pain. In the case of superficial abscesses it softens the skin and helps the abscess to 'point'.

COLD-WATER DRESSINGS are sometimes also known as fomentations because they become gradually warmed by the heat of the body. They are prepared by dipping a piece of lint in saturated boric acid lotion or other weak antiseptic, applying to the part, and then covering with a piece of gutta-percha tissue or oiled silk which is larger than the piece of lint and projects at least half an inch beyond it all round.

DRY FOMENTATION: This is made by toasting a piece of thick flannel in front of the fire and laying it on the part to be fomented, covering with a thick layer of cotton-wool and on the outside a hot-water bag. This does not retain its heat for long, but the heat is retained longer by a flannel bag containing salt or bran which is warmed and applied in a similar manner. Flat rubber bags, 'thermophores', which retain their heat for many hours, contain a mixture of salts which liquefies when the bag is boiled. The bag is boiled for a few minutes in a kettle each time it is required, and then applied and covered with cotton-wool. These dry applications are useful for relieving the pain of colic, neuralgia, and the like. An ordinary rubber hot-water bottle, of course, is often as effective a method of applying heat as any.

FOMITES is a term used to include all articles which have been brought into sufficiently close contact with a person sick of some infectious disease to retain the infective material and spread the disease. For example, clothes, bedding, carpets, toys, books, may all be fomites till disinfected.

FONTANELLE is the term applied to areas on the head on which bone has not yet formed. The chief of these is the anterior fontanelle, situated on the top of the head between the frontal and two parietal bones. In shape it is four-sided, about 25 mm square (1 inch) at the time of birth, gradually diminishing until it is completely covered by bone, which should happen by the age of 18 months. The pulsations of the brain can be readily felt through it. Delay in its closure is particularly found in cases of rickets, as well as in other states of defective development. The fontanelle becomes more tense than usual in acute fevers, whooping-cough, and bronchitis, and tends to bulge in cases of hydrocephalus. It becomes unusually depressed in all cases of diminished vitality, such as that due to diarrhoea or wasting from any cause.

FOOD (see ADULTERATION OF FOODS; BREAD; CANNED FOODS; CEREAL; DIET; DIGESTION; FAT; FEEDING; INFANT-FEEDING; MILK; PROTEIN; FRUIT; VITAMIN).

FOOD INTOLERANCE: Most cases of food intolerance are not due to allergy. The most common cause of an aversion to food is psychological. Patients with a history of neurotic ill health may develop an obsessional aversion first to one food and then to another. Other cases of food intolerance are due to idiosyncrasy, that is a genetic defect in the patient, such as alactasia, where the intestine lacks the enzyme that digests milk sugar with the result that individuals so affected develop diarrhoea when they drink milk. Intolerance to specific foods, as distinct from allergy, is probably quite common and may be an important factor in the aetiology of the irritable bowel syndrome.

For the diagnosis of true food allergy it is necessary to demonstrate that there is a reproducible intolerance to a specific food and then that there is evidence of an abnormal immunological reaction to it. Occasionally the allergic response may not be to the food itself but to food contaminants such as penicillin, or to food additives such as tartrazine. There may also be reactions to foods which have pharmacological effects, such as caffeine in strong coffee or histamine in fermented cheese, or such reactions may be due to the irritant effect on the intestinal mucosa, especially if it is already diseased, by highly spiced curries. Of those patients who believe that their symptoms are provoked by food, probably only two out of every ten can be shown to have a true food intolerance and one in ten to have an immunological basis which would justify the diagnosis of food allergy.

FOOD POISONING is usually characterized by vomiting, diarrhoea, and abdominal pain, the result of eating food contaminated with metallic or chemical poisons, or with bacteria, or with the toxins of bacteria; or as a result of eating poisonous 'foods', such as poisonous mushrooms. (See FUNGUS-POISONING.) One of the characteristics of food poisoning due to chemical or metallic causes is its relatively quick onset – within ten minutes to ten hours of eating the food.

Bacterial food poisoning is now what is commonly meant by the term 'food poisoning'. It comprises those conditions formerly and erroneously described as 'ptomaine poisoning'. The gravest, and fortunately the rarest, form of food poisoning is botulism (qv).

In staphylococcal food poisoning, certain staphylococci produce in the food they contaminate an enterotoxin which after ingestion makes the consumer suddenly ill within a matter of one to six hours, with vomiting, diarrhoea, and abdominal pain. The staphylococci themselves do not act thus on ingestion; it is the preformed toxin which is noxious. Contamination of food with staphylococci can usually be traced to faulty handling and is usually human in origin. Foods, such as meat products (often cold meat served as sandwiches), milk, custard, and egg products, can be contaminated either before or after cooking. As the toxin produced by the *Staphylococcus aureus* is heat resistant, subsequent cooking will not make the toxin-contaminated food safe.

Many cases of food poisoning are caused by infection with one of a group of bacteria belonging to the genus *Salmonella. Salmonella typhimurium* is responsible for 65 to 70 per cent of all outbreaks of food poisoning due to salmonellae. Other salmonellae commonly involved are *Salmonella bredeny, Salmonella enteritidis, Salmonella heidelberg, Salmonella newport, Salmonella stanley*, and *Salmonella thompson. Salmonellae* are found in all foods of animal origin: meats, meat products (such as pies), soups, milk, eggs and foods such as custards and cream cakes in which the egg products are only partially cooked. The onset of food poisoning due to salmonellae occurs twelve to forty-eight hours after eating the contaminated food.

Salmonella infections are common in pigs, sheep, rabbits, cattle, rats, mice, dogs, and cats. If a cow is infected with a *Salmonella* – eg. *S. enteritidis* – the organism may get into the milk, and the consumer of the milk suffers from food poisoning. Of the reported cases of salmonella poisoning where the food responsible has been identified, 7 per cent are associated with the consumption of untreated milk. Food may become infected by the excreta of rats or mice. Ducks are susceptible to *Salmonella* infections, especially *S. typhimurium*, and the organism may get into the duck's egg – an occasional source of human infection. *S. hadar* is found in turkeys. Most types of salmonella are killed by heating to 60°C for fifteen minutes, but a considerably higher temperature is required for much longer to ensure that the temperature is raised throughout the whole of the food being cooked. It is therefore essential to ensure that frozen food is well thawed before being cooked.

In recent years an increasing number of outbreaks of food poisoning have been due to *Clostridium welchii*. This is a common cause of food poisoning in communal feeding establishments, and is usually associated with meat dishes, soups or gravy, which have been cooked the day before consumption. To reduce the incidence of this form of food poisoning, the pre-cooked dish must be rapidly cooled, kept in a refrigerator overnight, and when reheated it must be cooked as thoroughly as if it were raw meat. This type of food poisoning comes on eight to twenty-four hours after eating the contaminated food.

There is increasing evidence that viruses may play a larger part in food poisoning than has hitherto been suspected. Thus in almost a quarter of the outbreaks of gastroenteritis reported to the Public Health Laboratory Service in 1980, as possible food-borne infection, food-poisoning organisms could not be found. The incubation period in a third of this group was longer than for the usual bacterial food-poisoning organisms. Viruses were detected by electron microscopy in 88 per cent of cases associated with shellfish (cockles, oysters) and in 23 per cent of outbreaks associated with other foods.

Food poisoning is now a notifiable disease. In 1983, 11,265 cases were notified in England and Wales, but this is only a fraction of the total number of cases that must occur. Of the 10,856 cases notified in 1980 9540 were due to salmonellae, 1056 to *Clostridium perfringens* and 189 to staphylococci. Most of the outbreaks due to salmonellae were caused by contaminated poultry (turkey or chicken), while most of the outbreaks due to staphylococci were caused by meat other than poultry. Five outbreaks of Campylobacter (qv) enteritis associated with the consumption of raw milk were reported. Twenty-six incidents of scrombotoxin poisoning (qv) were reported. Smoked, canned or soused mackerel accounted for 11 incidents, canned sardine for four, pilchards and raw tuna for one each. Food poisoning is on the increase and in 1986, 23,948 cases were reported, 16,502 of which were formally notified and the other 7,446 ascertained by other means.

Present regulations relate to the construction of, and equipment used in, food premises, the transport of certain foods, the temperature at which food must be stored, and to food handlers in food businesses. Thus, food handlers who suffer from, or are carriers of, a salmonella infection (including typhoid and paratyphoid), or who have a staphylococcal infection likely to cause food poisoning must be reported to the local district community physician. Such individuals can be suspended from work as food handlers and in certain circumstances they can be allowed compensation for loss of wages. (See also SHELLFISH POISONING.)

FOOT is that portion of the lower limb situated below the ankle-joint. Its structure is similar to that of the hand. There are seven tarsal bones, of which the talus, supporting the leg bones, and the calcaneus, forming the heel, are the largest. The others are the navicular, three cuneiform, and the cuboid bones. Then comes a row of five metatarsal bones (known together as the metatarsus), and finally fourteen phalanges contained in the toes, the great toe having two only, while each of the others has three. The arrangement of the arteries and nerves is similar to the found in the hand and fingers.

The arch of the foot is a most important structure. The bones are so arranged that the sole is hollow both from before back and from

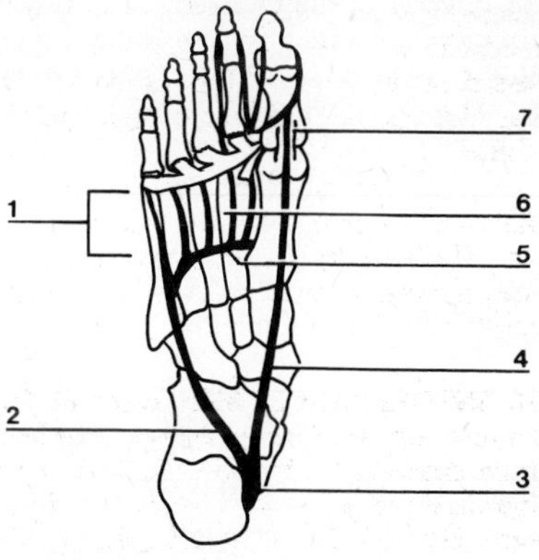

1 perforating branches of plantar arch
2 lateral planta
3 posterior tibial
4 medial plantar
5 plantar arch
6 plantar metatarsal
7 adductor hallucism

Arteries of the foot.

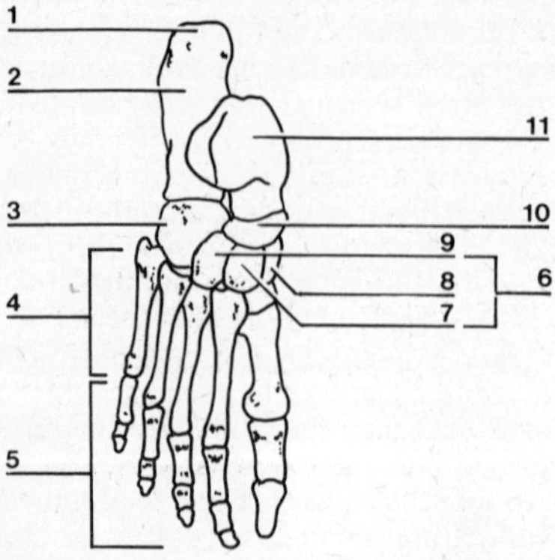

1 calcanean tuberosity
2 calcanus
3 cuboid
4 metatassals
5 5 phalanges
6 cuneiforms
7 intermedial
8 medial
9 lateral
10 navicular
11 talus

Bones of the foot as seen from above (i.e. superior aspect).

side to side. In walking, the outer edge only, at the middle of the sole, should touch the ground. The arch is further supported by a short plantar ligament situated in the hollow of the arch, running from the calcaneus to the cuboid bone, and by a long plantar ligament situated nearer the surface. It is also slung up by two sinews on either side, coming from muscles in the leg, the two tibial muscles on the inner side, and the two peroneal muscles on the outer side. When this arch gives way, flat-foot (qv) is the result.

For diseases of the foot see BONES, DISEASES OF; CHAFING OF THE SKIN; CHILBLAINS; CLAW-FOOT; CLEFT-FOOT; CLUB-FOOT; CORNS AND BUNIONS; DROP-FOOT; FLAT-FOOT; GOUT; HALLUX RIGIDUS; HALLUX VALGUS; KOHLER'S DISEASE; MALLET TOE; METATARSUS VARUS; METATARSALGIA; NAIL.

FORAMEN is the Latin term for a hole. It is especially applied to natural openings in bones, such as the foramen magnum, the large opening in the base of the skull through which the brain and spinal cord are continuous.

FORCED FEEDING (see GAVAGE).

FORGETFULNESS in many people is inborn; in others it arises as the result of some disease. Memory is defined by William James as 'the knowledge of an event or fact, of which meantime we have not been thinking, with the additional consciousness that we have thought or experienced it before'. This process necessitates two things: the retention of an event and the reproduction of it, both depending upon the same process in the nervous system. In this system there are, according to Meynert, some 600,000,000 nerve-cells. These are united together by numberless nerve-fibres into countless combinations. When a sensation affects the brain it influences certain of these groups, and if the sensation is very powerful or very often repeated the groups of associated nerve-cells develop a habit of acting in concert and tend, upon future stimulation by any means, to reproduce this sensation in its entirety. This process is known as association, and the multitudinous fibres which connect cell with cell and group with group, forming the chief bulk of the brain, are known as association fibres.

Sound memory depends upon the rational grouping of ideas of things in the mind, so that one may call up the other. No training will make up for a deficiency of nerve-cells or association fibres, which are inborn characters.

For good memory of important facts, a certain amount of forgetfulness is necessary. Facts in the past should become 'foreshortened', so to speak, and the inability to recount an incident without going over all its petty details forms a type of mental weakness. For this purpose, mental relaxation and change of employment are just as necessary as the quiet pondering over past events that leads to their classification and orderly retention.

According to modern psychological theory, forgetting is often an active process. Painful memories may be repressed out of consciousness, and, buried in the 'unconscious mind', may be the source of anxiety and neurotic behaviour.

There are certain changes in which memory becomes impaired. Chief among these is old age. (See AGE, NATURAL CHANGES IN.) In the old man's memory the events of yesterday are a blank, and only the events of youth, and later of childhood, forgotten in busy middle age, are again brought to light, all, however, crumbling and half rubbed away. When this defect is extreme it is due to degenerative changes in the old man's arteries and brain. Apoplexy is another cause either of permanent impairment (see APHASIA) or, in slighter cases, of frequent losses of memory which occur in old people, and last a few hours or a few days. In hypnotism and various mental diseases, especially dementia, curious vagaries occur. Concussion of the brain, too, may produce at first total unconsciousness, followed by partial loss of memory, lasting for some time. (See BRAIN, DISEASES AND INJURIES OF.)

Treatment: For improving the memory there are three methods.

Judicious methods are those of classification, repeated presentation of facts to be remembered in different guises, and the formation of numerous connecting links between these facts and facts already in the mind.

Mechanical methods are sometimes useful in remembering new facts. For example, little children are taught to read in unison words or figures clearly written on the blackboard, so that ideas of these entering by the channels of eye, ear, and muscular sense may form on the brain deep impressions upon which future memories can be built. Similarly, a person, hearing a new name, repeats it several times, so that it may make a lasting impression upon his brain-cells.

Artificial memories (*memoriae technicae*) are often constructed by people who have either very few facts in mind with which to form new associations, or who wish in a short time, and for a special purpose, such as an examination, to remember certain facts, and then blot out the whole as a useless encumbrance of memory.

FORMALDEHYDE: The *British Pharmacopoeia* preparation, Formaldehyde Solution, also known as FORMALIN, contains 34 to 38 per cent formaldehyde in water. It is a powerful antiseptic, and has also the power of hardening the tissues. The vapour is very irritating to the eyes and nose.

Uses: For disinfection it is largely used in the form of a spray. It can also be vaporized by heat. One of its advantages is that it does not damage metals or fabrics. In 3 per cent solution in water it is used for the treatment of warts on the palms of the hands and the soles of the feet.

FOSSA is a term applied to various depressions or holes, both on the surface of the body and in internal parts, such as the iliac fossa in each lower corner of the abdomen, and the fossae within the skull which lodge the different parts of the brain.

FOXGLOVE (see DIGITALIS).

FRACTURES are breaches in the structure of bones produced by violence.

Varieties: The great division of fractures is into those which are simple and those which are compound. (See also MARCH FRACTURE; STRESS FRACTURES.)

SIMPLE FRACTURES form the commonest variety, consisting of those in which the bone is broken, with or without much laceration of the surrounding parts, but in which there is no wound leading from the fracture through the skin.

COMPOUND or OPEN FRACTURES are those in which the skin is injured, so that a wound leads from the outer air to the broken bone, which may indeed protrude through this wound. The fact that a fracture is compound renders it very much more serious, even though there may be little splintering of the bone or laceration of the soft tissues. The special dangers attending compound fractures are as follows. The injury is apt to be much more serious than in simple fracture, and a large quantity of blood may be lost. The union of the bone is delayed, repair taking place by a much slower process when there is an open wound, and a lengthy illness is the result. The greatest danger, however, is that the wound may become infected with virulent micro-organisms, so that suppuration or blood-poisoning may ensue, and amputation of the limb may even become necessary. For all these reasons the greatest care is necessary in handling a fractured limb, so that a simple fracture may not be converted into a compound one.

COMPLETE FRACTURES are those in which the bone is broken completely across, and no connection left between the pieces.

INCOMPLETE FRACTURES are those in which the bone is broken only partly across, or in which the periosteum, the tough membrane surrounding the bone, is not torn. This variety occurs in children, whose bones contain more fibrous material and less bone earth than those of old people, a fact which renders them tougher and more pliant in earlier life. A child's bone may, like a twig, crack half-way across and then split some distance up its length, suffering in this way what is called a 'greenstick' fracture.

FISSURED FRACTURES are mere cracks in the bone, and are found commonly in the skull.

DEPRESSED FRACTURES occur generally on the skull, and consist of fractures in which a fragment of bone is forced inwards below the general level. This may give rise to interference with the brain, either when the fracture is produced or at a later date from thickening consequent on repair of the bone.

COMPLICATED FRACTURES are those in which, in addition to the fracture, some other serious injury is produced: eg. a dislocation, or tearing of a nerve.

COMMINUTED FRACTURES are those in which there is much splintering.

IMPACTED FRACTURES are those in which, after the break has occurred, one fragment is jammed inside the other, usually at an angle.

UNUNITED FRACTURES are those in which, after the time has elapsed in which the fracture usually mends, it is found that union has not taken place. The failure to unite may be simply due to delayed union, in which the process of repair is proceeding slowly on account of ill-health, or of damage to the chief artery which supplies the bone with blood, or usually in consequence of the fact that the fractured limb is not kept sufficiently at rest. Or there may be actual failure of the healing process to take place. In the latter case the ends of the bone are thoroughly rubbed together under a general anaesthetic, and the fracture again set. If this produces no good effect, an operation is usually performed in order to remove any piece of muscle which may have got between the ends, or to fasten the ends with wire or with metal plates. In some cases the local application of electrical stimulation to the fractured area of the bone appears to be beneficial.

MALUNITED FRACTURES are those which have not been properly set, or in which displacement occurs after setting, so that the bone is twisted, or united with a neighbouring bone, as sometimes happens after fracture of the forearm, or is enlarged and shortened, or does not unite by bone, but forms what is known as a 'false-joint'. Sometimes malunion is unavoidable, owing to spasm of muscles or to production of an excessive amount of new bone.

Causes: Certain causes render some people more liable than others to fracture of bones. Of these, by far the most important is old age. The bones decrease in thickness after middle age, the fibrous tissue composing them becomes less resilient, and there is an increase of the merely earthy part – facts which all tend to produce increasing brittleness. In old age, a fall upon a hard surface, even a moderate strain like that of jumping off a moving vehicle, is apt to be followed by a fracture. Rickets, tuberculosis of bones, osteomalacia, and malignant disease all render the bones more easily broken. Apart from these causes, fractures are due to force, which may be applied in three ways.

DIRECT VIOLENCE may cause a fracture, and in such a case the fracture is apt to be a compound one, or attended by serious complications, such as damage to the brain where the skull is fractured, or to the lungs in fracture of the ribs.

INDIRECT VIOLENCE is the most common cause. In this case the violence is applied at some distance from the seat of the fracture, and whether a fracture or a dislocation occurs depends upon the point which in the circumstances is weakest and exposed to most stress. Thus a fall on the palm of the hand may cause a Colles's fracture at the wrist, or dislocation of the shoulder, or fracture of the collar-bone, according to the position of the arm. Similarly, a twist of the foot may cause fracture of the leg, as well as other injuries.

MUSCULAR ACTION in rare cases produces fracture. The most common example is fracture of the knee-cap, which may be snapped across the end of the thigh-bone in the sudden pull given to recover the balance after missing a step on a flight of stairs. Throwing a cricket ball has also been known to fracture the arm.

Symptoms and signs: *Uselessness of the part* is the main symptom if the fracture affects a limb. If the lower limb is affected, it is useless for support; if the upper limb, the part beyond the fracture cannot be raised. *Pain* is a variable sign. So long as the affected part remains at rest, it is generally slight; movement, however, is apt to be painful. In fracture of the ribs, the moderate movements of tranquil respiration are free from pain, whilst a deep breath or squeezing of the chest causes considerable pain. *The sound of a crack* is sometimes heard, or the sensation of something giving way may be experienced by the injured person at the moment of the accident, but this is not a reliable symptom, because it occurs also when a muscle or sinew is torn. *Deformity* is found at the site of fracture. There is *shortening* of the limb in consequence of contraction of the muscles which pass over the fracture. There is also *swelling*, partly owing to the overlapping of the ends of the bone, partly in consequence of the blood and lymph which are at once poured out from the torn vessels around the injury. *Unnatural mobility* is also found, the limb giving way at a point where it should be rigid. *Crepitus* or grating is the final and only certain sign of fracture, experienced when the ends are rubbed together. It should never be felt for except by skilled hands, since much damage can be done by the sharp broken ends of bone to surrounding structures.

Healing of fractures: When the bone breaks, many vessels both in its substance and in the periosteum are torn, and accordingly a large clot of blood forms around the ends, between them, and for some distance up the inside of the bone. Later, great numbers of white corpuscles find their way into this clot, which becomes organized, blood-vessels and, later, fibrous tissue being formed in it (soft callus). Next lime-salts are gradually deposited in this fibrous tissue, which thus develops into bone (hard callus). In this process a thick ring of new bone forms round the broken ends, filling up all crevices, and when union is complete this thickening is again gradually absorbed, leaving the bone as it was before the injury. When the fragments have not been properly set, but allowed to remain overlapping, considerable thickening remains, the ring of new bone being permanent for the sake of strength.

Treatment: After the fracture has been recognized, a certain amount of temporary treatment is advisable till the broken bone can be properly fixed in place by a surgeon, and in the following descriptions the temporary treatment will be given, short reference being made to the permanent treatment where it differs from the temporary.

A compound fracture is treated first of all as a wound (see WOUNDS) by cleansing and by dressings, and then as a simple fracture. It is particularly necessary that the skin around should be well cleansed; the wound itself is often very dirty. A thorough washing and scrubbing of the wound, under an anaesthetic, is usually necessary, and some surgeons fasten the fragments with silver wire or plates.

For temporary treatment the splints, etc., may be applied above the clothes in the case of simple fractures, and little padding is then necesary. But, for a compound fracture, the limb must be exposed, the wound dressed, and then the splints have to be carefully padded.

For permanent treatment, the fracture must first of all be 'reduced': ie. the broken ends must be brought accurately together; then it must be 'set': ie. the ends firmly fixed in good position; and finally it must be kept at rest, with attention to the patient's general health, until union has taken place. Reduction is effected usually by one person, who pulls gently and steadily upon that part of the limb beyond the fracture (extension), so as to overcome the shortening and bring the ends a little apart from one another, in order to prevent grating, and so avoid pain. At the same time, a second person should steady the limb above the seat of fracture (counter-extension). This he maintains while a third person applies the necessary splints, bandages, etc. For keeping the bone in position, various devices, such as bandages, plaster, cradles, splints of wood, leather, or poroplastic felt, sandbags, and extension by weight and pulley are adopted in different cases. Splints are generally made from strips of wood, about 6 mm (¼inch) thick, but they may be improvised from bundles of twigs, broom-handles, folded-up newspapers, and many other rigid articles. Care must be taken, especially in old people confined to bed for a fracture, that no bed sores form. In the case of fracture of the lower limbs it is a general practice to keep the person in bed with the limb fixed by ordinary splints for two or three weeks, and then to apply a case of plaster of Paris to the whole limb, and allow the patient to get up and go about with crutches.

For bandages to fix splints, one uses either a strip of calico bandage 7·5 cm (3 inches) wide or an Esmarch's triangular bandage folded narrow. The latter is a triangle made by cutting a yard of calico across from corner to corner (so as to form two pieces), and then doubling in the point of the triangle three times, so as to form a sort of flat cravat. (See BANDAGES.)

COLLAR-BONE: This bone is apt to be fractured by falls on the hand, or by blows or falls on the point of the shoulder. As it supports the weight of the arm to a large extent, and gives squareness to the shoulder, when it is broken the shoulder droops downwards, forwards, and inwards towards the chest. On account of the shortness of the bone, splints are useless, and the deformity is remedied by bandages. These are applied in many different ways, of which the following is one of the simplest. A pad of cloth or wool, the size of the fist, is first placed high up in the armpit, and the elbow is bent so that the arm lies across the chest. An unfolded triangular bandage is then placed on the chest with one end over the sound shoulder, the base running down over the elbow of the injured arm, and the point of the bandage lying on the front of the chest. The other end, which is hanging down, is brought up behind the elbow of the injured arm, carried up across the back, and tied as tightly as possible to the first-mentioned end behind the neck. The point of the bandage hanging loose beneath the wrist is folded up round the wrist and pinned to the bandage above it. Finally a triangular bandage, folded narrow, is carried round the chest and elbow of the injured arm and tied tightly, thus levering the shoulder outwards round the pad in the armpit. After this bandage is applied, there is a special necessity to feel that the pulse is not stopped by its tightness. Instead of this sling and narrow-folded bandage, one may use a couple of narrow-folded bandages similarly applied with a pad.

The permanent treatment is usually carried out by a roller bandage applied in somewhat the same way, or by broad strips of plaster, or by a figure-of-eight bandage passing in front of the shoulders and crossing between the shoulder-blades, the arm then being supported by a triangular sling tied over the opposite shoulder.

The fractured bone is fairly strong in three weeks, and the bandage can then be discarded. During this three-week period the fingers, wrist and elbow must be exercised regularly every day. Full activity can usually be resumed within six weeks but body-contact sports should not be resumed until a longer period has elapsed.

UPPER ARM: This fracture is usually due to a direct blow, and is easily recognized. For setting, two splints, 5 to 7·5 cm (2 to 3 inches) wide, and long enough to reach, the one from the armpit, the other from the shoulder, to beneath the elbow, are taken and well padded. The forearm being laid across the chest, one splint is applied to the front of, the other behind, the upper arm, and fixed by two ties, the first above, the second below, the site of fracture. A narrow sling is then applied to support the wrist.

This fracture takes up to ten weeks to mend. The permanent treatment is similar, with the arm splintered by Gooch splintering or a plaster of Paris splint which fixes the elbow. The wrist is supported by a collar and cuff sling.

FRACTURES NEAR ELBOW: These all cause great swelling as they implicate the joint more or less, and it is usually very difficult to recognize the precise nature of the injury. The temporary treatment of all is the same. An L-shaped, or rectangular, splint 7·5 cm (3 inches) wide, and resembling a mason's 'square', is used, one limb being long enough to reach from the tips of the fingers to the elbow, the other from the elbow to the armpit. It is fastened to the inside of the arm and forearm by one tie round the hand and round the forearm, and one round the upper arm. A broad sling is applied to support the forearm.

For permanent treatment, the same plan is very satisfactory and is often adopted, though it is more common to fix the arm in plaster of Paris. Sometimes the elbow is bent as far up as possible and tightly bandaged in this position. When the fracture consists in the chipping off of the olecranon process of the ulna, ie. the point of the elbow, as tends to happen in a fall on the bent elbow, the fragment may be drawn upwards by the triceps muscle, leaving a distinct gap behind the elbow. To correct this an operation is necessary to fix the fragment to the ulna by means of a silver wire or screw. If there is no such displacement, then all that is necesary is a bandage and a sling.

All fractures round the joint are apt to cause some permanent stiffness, and in order to lessen the risk of this the patient is encouraged to move the joint after three or four weeks, in order to prevent adhesions forming.

FOREARM: One or both bones may be broken by a blow or fall, and the condition is easily recognized. For treatment the forearm is laid across the chest with the thumb upwards. Two splints, at least 10 cm (4 inches) wide, and long enough to reach from the elbow to beyond the tips of the fingers, are well padded (especially down the centre) and placed one behind and one in front of the forearm. The splints are fixed by one tie round the hand and wrist, and another above the fracture.

A rectangular splint, similar to that used for fractures about the elbow, is applied to prevent movement at this joint, though not absolutely essential in the temporary treatment, and finally a broad sling to support the forearm.

This fracture is put up for permanent treatment in precisely the same way in plaster of Paris. It takes about the same time to heal as a fracture in the upper arm. There is a danger that the movements of turning the hand palm up and palm down (pronation and supination) may be permanently interfered with by malposition of the bones, unless the fracture be very carefully set.

WRIST: Fracture of the radius close to the wrist, known as Colles's fracture, is a common result of a fall on the palm of the hand. The forearm and hand present a peculiar 'dinner-fork' bend, in consequence of the lower fragment turning upwards and backwards. The temporary treatment is similar to that for fractures of the forearm higher up. For permanent treatment, the forearm is fixed in plaster of Paris with the wrist flexed and the fingers and thumb free. The danger of stiffness, after union has taken place, is even greater here than in fractures near the elbow, and is prevented by similar means.

HAND AND FINGERS: A splint is laid along the palm, reaching from the tips of the fingers to the elbow, and the hand and forearm are bandaged to it, or the fist is closed on a thick pad and tightly bandaged in this position. A sling is then applied. The fingers mend quickly.

THIGH: In all fractures of the upper limb the person is usually allowed to go about while he is wearing the splints, but in all fractures of the lower limb he lies in bed. Fracture of the neck of the thigh-bone, or femur, is a specially common accident in old people, following upon falls on stairs or ice, but in the young this strong bone is broken only by great violence. There are complete inability to move the limb, shortening amounting to 5 to 7·5 cm (2 to 3 inches) on comparison with the other limb, and rotation outwards of the foot. For treatment a long splint, reaching from the armpit down to below the foot, is laid along the side, and three shorter splints reaching from the groin to the knee may be laid, one in front, one on the inner side, and one behind the thigh, but are not essential for treatment. The long splint, if no regular splint be procurable, may be easily improvised from a broom-handle or plank. These splints are fixed by the following ties. One broad band, for example a bolster case, round the chest, with or without a narrow-folded bandage round the hips; two ties round the thigh, one above and one below the fracture, fixing the short splints; two narrow ties round the leg below the knee. Finally, the feet are tied together.

The permanent treatment varies with the site of the fracture. If it is in what is known as the neck of the fracture – ie. at the very upper end of the femur – the usual procedure is to fix the fragments internally by a metallic device. After operation the patient is allowed to move about freely in bed for a few days, and then allowed up on a couch. Walking with a crutch is allowed in a few weeks, but weight-bearing is not allowed for three months. If the fracture is in the shaft of the femur the usual form of treatment is to reduce the fracture –ie. get the two pieces of bone into alignment – and then hold them there by fixing the leg in a Thomas's splint and applying traction to the lower part. Firm union of the fracture takes twelve to sixteen weeks.

KNEE-CAP: This bone is seldom fractured. A long splint is laid along the back of the limb and fixed by ties to thigh and leg. The fragments of the knee-cap may be fixed together by a bandage passing round above the knee-cap, crossing behind the joint, and then passing round below the knee-cap.

It is extremely difficult to get good bony union, and for the permanent treatment most surgeons prefer to cut in to the fracture and unite the fragments with silver wire.

LEG: There is particular need for care in the handling of this fracture, because the tibia, or shin-bone, which lies in its whole length just beneath the skin, usually breaks with a sharp-pointed end, like a pen-nib, that is very readily pushed through the skin, thus making the fracture compound. Two splints, about 10 cm (4 inches) wide, and long enough to reach from a few inches above the knee to beyond the foot, are carefully padded, above and below the knee-joint, and above and below the ankle-joint, so as to prevent them from pressing upon the skin where the bone lies just beneath. They are applied one along the outer, one along the inner side of the leg, and fixed with two ties, one above and one below the fracture. A third tie is applied above the knee to fix this joint, and the feet are finally tied together.

For permanent treatment the leg is encased in plaster of Paris after reduction of the fracture, with the plaster extending half-way up the thigh. Care must be taken to ensure that the foot is fixed in the position of dorsiflexion: ie. bent upwards. The plaster is kept on for eight to twelve weeks but, if all goes well, walking is encouraged after two or three weeks. A careful watch must be kept of the foot, to ensure that the plaster is not interfering with the circulation to the foot.

Fracture of the fibula, the slender bone on the outer side of the leg, may take place in consequence of a kick or twist of the foot, while the tibia is uninjured. If the fracture occurs in the middle or upper part of the fibula the person may be quite able to walk, though with considerable pain. If, however, the fracture occurs at the lower end of the fibula, it is more likely to be due to indirect violence to the foot as a result of severe strains. This injury, which is one of those included under the term, 'Pott's fracture', is accompanied by considerable tearing of the ligaments on the inner side of the ankle-joint. The temporary treatment is as for fracture of both bones. Permanent treatment consists of applying plaster of Paris – from below the knee downwards. In the case of a fracture of the fibula alone this is worn for three weeks. In the case of a Pott's fracture it is worn for six to ten weeks.

PELVIS: The bones of the pelvis are broken only by excessive violence, such as a crush from the wheel of a lorry. For temporary treatment, the injured person should have a broad binder fastened round the hips and be lifted on a rug or shutter. The seriousness depends upon the extent of damage done to internal organs.

RIBS are commonly fractured by a blow or kick on the side. If only one or two be broken and the fracture be simple and uncomplicated, the accident is comparatively trivial but painful. The traditional treatment is by restricting movement of the chest by strips of sticking plaster, using inextensible adhesive plaster such as zinc oxide strapping. To be effective these must be applied well round the chest. The taking of pain-relieving drugs such as aspirin may also be necessary for a few days. If this does not suffice, a local anaesthetic may be injected by a doctor. The ribs usually heal fairly quickly, those above and below the broken ribs acting as splints. No form of body-contact sports should be participated in for at least six weeks. If the injured person spits up blood after the injury the condition is serious, this being a sign that the broken ribs have pierced the pleura and wounded the lung.

FLAIL CHEST is the condition in which a segment of the rib cage is broken loose and moves inward as the patient tries to breathe. As a result, air cannot be drawn into the lungs. It is a crushing injury which is not uncommon in serious car accidents, and is life-threatening unless quickly dealt with. This may be done by applying a firm binder round the chest to provide an artificial rib cage which will not sink in with inspiration.

SPINAL COLUMN: Mere damage to the bone, as in the case of the so-called compression fracture, in which there is no damage to the spinal cord, is not necessarily serious. If, however, the spinal cord is damaged, as in the so-called fracture dislocation, the accident may be a very serious one, the usual result being paralysis of the parts of the body below the level of the injury. Therefore the higher up the spine is fractured, the more serious the consequences. The injured person should not be moved till medical assistance is at hand, or, if he must be removed, this should be done on a rigid shutter or door, not on a canvas stretcher or rug, and there should be no lifting which necessitates bending of the back. In such an injury an operation designed to remove a displaced piece of bone and free the spinal cord from pressure is often necessary and successful in relieving the paralysis. Dislocation or subluxation (qv) of the spine is not uncommon in certain sports, particularly rugby. Anyone who has had such an injury in the cervical spine (ie. in the neck) should be strongly advised not to return to any form of body-contact sport or vehicular sport such as motor or motor-cycle racing.

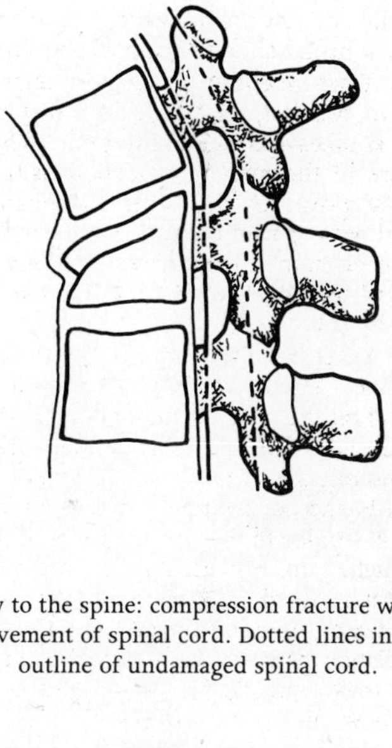

Injury to the spine: compression fracture with no involvement of spinal cord. Dotted lines indicate outline of undamaged spinal cord.

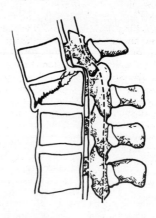

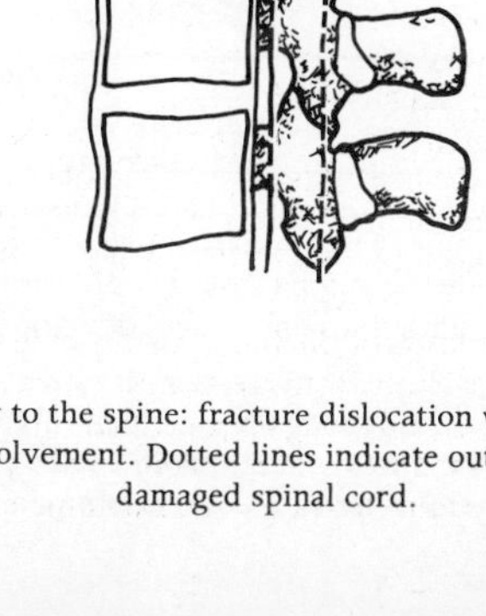

Injury to the spine: fracture dislocation with cord involvement. Dotted lines indicate outline of damaged spinal cord.

SKULL: Simple fissured fractures and depressed fractures of the skull often follow blows or falls on the head, and are not at all serious, as a rule, apart from the damage which may have been done to the brain at the same time.

Compound fractures are attended by risk of suppuration which may spread within the skull, and if the skull is extensively broken and depressed the operation of trephining (qv) is often done in order to cleanse the wound thoroughly. Another risk of fracture is that some of the small arteries on the inner surface of the skull may be torn and may bleed, thus causing compression of the brain. For this reason also the skull is often trephined. Thorough cleansing of the wound, and confinement to bed in a darkened room constitute the treatment.

JAW: The lower jaw is often fractured by a blow on the face. There is generally bleeding from the mouth, the gum being torn. Also there are pain and grating sensations on chewing, and unevenness in the line of the teeth. The treatment is simple, the line of teeth in the upper jaw forming a splint, against which the lower jaw is bound, with the mouth closed. One bandage is passed below the chin and tied on the top of the head; another passes in front of the chin, and is tied on the back of the neck. The two are then prevented from slipping forward and backward, respectively, by tying the one to the other on the crown of the head. If there are multiple fractures of the jaw, there is a risk that the tongue may fall back and choke the victim. He should therefore be kept face down so that there is no risk of obstruction of the airway. It is essential that the victim is seen as soon as possible by a specialist surgeon to ensure that the jaw heals properly with the teeth in correct alignment. The patient must be fed for two or three weeks with liquid food, eg. eggs and milk, poured into the corner of the mouth from a feeding-cup with a spout.

NOSE: The bridge of the nose may be fractured by a fall. The bleeding is copious, and should be arrested by the usual means. (See HAEMORRHAGE.) An operation may later be performed to restore the shape of the nose.

FRAMBOESIA is another name for YAWS (qv).

FRAMYCETIN is an antibiotic derived from *Streptomyces decaris*. It is active against a wide range of organisms, when taken by mouth or applied locally in infections of the skin.

FRECKLES, or SUMMER-SPOTS, are small yellow or brown spots which appear on the exposed parts of the body during hot or windy weather. They appear especially in people with fair skin and red hair. They consist of small pigmented areas in the deeper part of the epidermis, which are stimulated to increased development by exposure.

FREMITUS is a sensation which is communicated to the hand of an observer when it is laid upon the chest in certain diseases of the lungs and heart. Friction fremitus is a grating feeling communicated to the hand by the movements of lungs or heart when the membrane covering them is roughened, as in pleurisy or pericarditis. Vocal fremitus means the sensation felt by the hand when a person speaks; it is increased when the lung is more solid than usual. The 'thrills' felt over a heart affected by valvular disease are also varieties of fremitus.

FRENKEL'S EXERCISES are a series of movements of precision intended to be performed by patients suffering from difficulty of control of the muscles, with a view to regaining lost power of co-ordination. The exercises for the lower limbs of a patient confined to bed begin with such movements as those of raising the foot and carefully bringing it down upon a particular part of the edge of a padded board. At a later stage, the patient, supported if necessary under the armpits, practises walking along a broad strip painted on the floor, later still on a narrow strip, and afterwards tracing out marked patterns with the toes and placing the feet carefully as he walks on marked positions. Similar exercises are devised for re-establishing co-ordination of the muscles in the arms: eg. carefully inserting pegs into small holes in a board, picking up pins from a smooth surface, and similar movements.

FREUD'S THEORY is the term applied to a theory that emotional and allied diseases are due to a psychic injury or trauma, generally of a sexual nature, which did not produce an adequate reaction when it was received and therefore remains as a subconscious or 'affect' memory to trouble the patient's mind. As an extension of this theory Freudian treatment consists in encouraging the patient to tell everything that happens to be associated with trains of thought which lead up to this memory, thus securing a 'purging' of the mind from the original 'affect memory' which is the cause of the symptoms. This form of treatment is also called psychocatharsis or abreaction. The general term, psychoanalysis, is applied, in the first place, to the *method* of helping the patient to recover buried memories by free association of thoughts. In the second place, the term is applied to the body of psychological knowledge and theory accumulated and devised by Sigmund Freud (1856–1939) and his followers. The term 'psychoanalyst' should be applied only to those who have had a strict Freudian training, not to anyone who happens to practise psychotherapy.

FRIARS' BALSAM (see BALSAM).

FRICTION is the name given either to the fremitus felt, or to the grating noise heard, when two rough surfaces of the body move over one another. It is characteristically obtained over the chest in cases of dry pleurisy.

FRIEDREICH'S ATAXIA is a hereditary disease resembling locomotor ataxia, and due to degenerative changes in nerve tracts and nerve cells of the spinal cord and the brain. It occurs usually in children, or at any rate before the twentieth year of life, and affects often several brothers and sisters. Its chief symptoms are unsteadiness of gait, with loss of the knee jerks, followed later by difficulties of speech, tremors of the hands, head, and eyes, deformity of the feet, and curvature of the spine. There is often associated heart disease. The sufferer gets gradually worse, but may live, more of less helpless, for twenty or thirty years.

FROHLICH'S SYNDROME is a condition in children characterized by obesity, physical sluggishness, and retarded sexual development. It is the result of disturbed pituitary function.

FRONTAL BONE is the bone which forms the forehead and protects the frontal lobes of the brain. Before birth, the frontal bone consists of two halves, and this division may persist throughout life, a deep groove remaining down the centre of the forehead. Above each eye is a heavy ridge in the bone, most marked in men, and, behind this, in the substance of the bone, is a cavity on each side, the frontal sinus, which communicates with the nose. Catarrh in these cavities produces the frontal headache characteristic of a 'cold in the head', and suppuration may occur in them, producing discharge from the nose. (See NOSE, DISEASES OF.)

FROSTBITE results from the action of extreme cold. In mild cases, the condition sometimes known as frostnip, the skin on exposed parts of the body, such as the cheeks or nose, becomes white and numb with a sudden and complete cessation of cold and discomfort. In more severe cases blisters develop on the frozen part, and the skin then gradually hardens and turns black until the frozen part, such as a finger, is covered with a black shell of dead tissue. Swelling of the underlying tissue occurs and this is accompanied by throbbing and aching. If, as is often the case, only the skin and the tissues immediately under it are frozen, then in a matter of months the dead tissue peels off, leaving behind it shiny red babyskin, as it is known, which at first is exquisitely tender. In the most severe cases of all, muscles, bone and tendon are also frozen, and the affected part becomes cold, swollen, mottled and blue or grey. There may be no blistering in these severe cases. At first there is no pain, but in time shooting and throbbing pains usually develop.

Prevention: This consists of wearing the right clothing and never venturing on even quite short expeditions in cold weather, particularly on mountains, without taking expert advice as to what should be worn.

Treatment: Frostnip is the only form of frostbite that should be treated on the spot. As it usually occurs on exposed parts, such as the face, each member of the party should be on the look out for it in the other. The moment whitening of the skin is seen, the individual should seek a place sheltered from the wind, or turn his back on the wind, and warm the affected part by covering it with his warm hand or a glove until the normal colour and consistency of the affected part are restored. In more severe cases treatment should only be given in hospital or a well-equipped camp. In essentials this consists of warming the affected part, preferably in a container filled with water at 44°C. This temperature must not be exceeded. If there is no thermometer available, the alternative is a normal unfrostbitten finger. If the water is too hot for comfort, then cold water should be added. If no container is available, the alternative is hot water poured over towels or a cloth wrapped round the affected part. Rewarming should be done for spells of twenty minutes at a time. If facilities are not available for warming in this way, the alternative is to place the affected part in contact with a warm abdomen or armpit, or held in warm air. It should never be placed near an open fire. Generalized warming of the whole body may also be necessary, and this is achieved by giving hot drinks, and putting the victim in a sleeping bag. Extra heat may be supplied by his companions lying alongside him – either in their own sleeping bags, or by one getting into the same sleeping bag. After rewarming, the part should be very gently cleaned. Blisters should not be pricked. Antibiotics may be given to reduce the risk of infection. An important point to bear in mind is that no-one should be allowed to walk on a thawed, or partly thawed, foot, as this will almost certainly do irreparable damage. On the other hand, walking on frostbitten feet for a period does not appear to increase the liability to further damage.

The treatment of frostbite which has resulted in gangrene is given under GANGRENE.

FROZEN SHOULDER is a painful condition of the shoulder accompanied by stiffness and considerable limitation of movement. The usual age-incidence is between 50 and 70. The cause is not known. There is no specific treatment, but there is practically always complete recovery, even though this may take twelve to eighteen months.

FRUCTOSE is another name for laevulose, or fruit sugar, which is found along with glucose in most sweet fruits. It is sweeter than sucrose (cane or beet sugar) and this has led to its use as a sweetener.

FRUIT: Almost all fresh fruits contain about 80 per cent of water, and the nutritive material, consisting chiefly of starch and sugar, does not exceed one-fifth of the fruit. The banana is the most nutritious of the fresh fruits, followed by grapes, plums, and apples. In addition to their food value, fruits contain vegetable acids, such as tartaric, citric, and malic acids, which have an agreeable flavour, a mildly laxative action, and are beneficial to the kidneys. Oranges, lemons, and grapefruit are specially useful in this way. The importance of fruits lies in the fact that they are the chief source of vitamin C, especially the citrus fruits and black-currants. The odour and flavour of fruits, which depend upon volatile oils and ethereal bodies, render them an agreeable article of food and improve appetite and digestion.

Dried fruits, such as apples, figs, dates, prunes, and grapes (raisins), form a highly nutritious form of diet, containing 60 or 70 per cent of starch, gum, and sugar; thus dried dates, figs, or raisins are more nourishing than an equal weight of bread. They are also a relatively rich source of iron and calcium, but a poor source of vitamin C.

FRUSEMIDE (ALUZINE, DIURESAL, DRYPTAL, FRUSETIC, FRUSID, LASIX) is a potent diuretic (qv) with a rapid onset (30 minutes), and short duration, of action. (See BENZOTHIADIAZINES, DIURETICS.)

FUGUE literally means flight and it is used to describe the mental condition in which an individual is suddenly seized with an unconscious motivation to flee from some intolerable reality of everyday existence. This usually involves some agonizing interpersonal relationship. As a rule, it lasts for a matter of hours or days, but may go on for weeks or even months. During the fugue the individual seldom behaves in a particularly odd manner though he may be considered somewhat eccentric. When it is over there is no remembrance of events during the fugue.

FULLER'S EARTH is a grey powder free from all grittiness. It consists mainly of aluminium silicate, but differs from kaolin in containing traces of iron. It is a valuable dusting powder for tender, moist skins, such as those of infants.

FUMIGATION is a means of disinfection by the vapour of powerful antiseptics. (See DISINFECTION).

FUNCTIONAL DISEASES (see PSYCHOSOMATIC DISEASE).

FUNGUS-POISONING: Several diseases are due to the growth of minute fungi in the tissues of the body; for example, actinomycosis (caused by the ray-fungus), ringworm, and Madura foot of India. As to the large fungi, or mushrooms as they are often called, although they grow in dead and decaying material, they do not infest the living body, but many of them contain a poisonous alkaloid known as muscarine, others a body called phallin, both of which are poisons when swallowed. About 2000 of these larger fungi grow in England, of which 200 are edible. There are about a dozen which are classified as poisonous, but several of these cause no more than indigestion. The most poisonous of all is the 'death cap' or *Amanita phalloides*. In the USA it is responsible for over 90 per cent of deaths from mushroom poisoning. The fatal dose is three mushrooms (50 grams), and one in three cases proves fatal. The distinguishing features of this fungus are that it has a yellowish green cup, the gills are white and at the base of the stem, or stalk, there is a cup, or volva. These features distinguish it from the common edible mushroom (*Psalliota campestris*), which has brownish purple gills and no cup at the base of the stem. Other poisonous mushrooms include *Amanita virosa, Amanita vernu*, and *Amanita muscaria*. Deaths from mushroom poisoning are rare in England. They are much more common in Continental Europe.

Symptoms: There is usually a latent period of 8 to 12 hours before the onset of symptoms. Initially these consist of severe abdominal pain, vomiting and violent diarrhoea. These usually respond to treatment but in serious cases are followed in 2 or 3 days by the onset of jaundice, circulatory failure, failure of the kidneys, and widespread haemorrhage, leading on in fatal cases to liver failure and death.

Treatment: The first thing to do is to wash out the stomach. A duodenal tube is then passed into the duodenum, the contents of which are aspirated every hour. This is done as it has been shown that the poisonous toxins accumulate here for up to 36 hours. Addition of charcoal to the washing-out fluid is useful as it binds the toxins. For this reason haemodialysis (qv) over charcoal is also useful. Ample fluids must be given to compensate for the fluid lost in the vomiting and stools. Drugs that are given to counteract the effect of the toxins include thiotic acid, penicillin, and silymarin which is prepared from milk thistle (*Silybum marianum*). In all serious cases atropine should be administered, since it forms a direct antidote to muscarine. There is also an antiphallinic serum which is sometimes of value.

FURAZOLIDONE is a drug used in the treatment of bacterial diarrhoea, bacterial food-poisoning and typhoid fever.

FURFURACEOUS is a term applied to skin diseases which produce scaliness of the surface, resembling bran.

FURUNCLE is another name for a boil. (See BOILS.)

FUSIDIC ACID is an antibiotic derived from the fermentation products of the fungus, *Fusidium coccineum*. It is particularly active against staphylococci, including those which are resistant to penicillin.

G

GAIT is an important sign of health and disease. Children, as a rule, begin to walk between the ages of twelve and eighteen months, having learned to stand before the end of the first year. If a good-sized child shows no ability to make movements by this time the possibility of his being mentally retarded must be borne in mind, and if the power of walking is not gained by the time the child is a year and a half old, he is probably the subject either of rickets, cerebral palsy, or a malformation of the hip-joint. (See RICKETS; PARALYSIS.)

Lameness in later life may be due to flat-foot (qv), when the spring of the foot is lost and the person walks with his toes turned out at right angles; or to the stiffness following disease of the knee-joint (see JOINTS, DISEASES OF), when the limb is carried forward like a rigid bar; or to the stiffness following hip-joint disease, when the person walks in a lop-sided manner, alternately taking a long step with the sound limb and swinging the whole pelvis round with the lame leg, as well as bending over to one side.

In **hemiplegia**, or paralysis down one side of the body following apoplexy (qv), the person drags the paralysed leg, and carries the paralysed side as if it were, so to speak, hung upon the healthy one. There is a tendency for this walk to improve gradually, the paralysed leg regaining power almost completely even when the arm remains helpless and bent stiffly across the body.

Steppage, or heather-step, gait occurs in certain cases of alcoholic neuritis and other conditions where the muscles that raise the foot are weak and the toes in consequence droop. The person bends the knee and lifts the foot high, so that the toes may clear obstacles on the ground, much as a person steps in going through heather or long grass. (See DROP-FOOT.)

In **locomotor ataxia** (qv) the sensations derived from the lower limbs are blunted, and consequently the movements of the legs are uncertain and the heels planted on the ground with unnecessary force. When the person tries to turn or stands with the eyes shut he is apt to fall over. When he walks he feels for the ground with a stick or keeps his eyes constantly fixed upon it.

In **spastic paralysis** the limbs are moved with jerks. The foot first of all clings to the ground (the person being very apt to trip over small objects), and then leaves it with a spasmodic movement, being raised much higher than necessary.

In **trembling palsy**, paralysis agitans, or Parkinsonism (qv) as it is now known, the movements are tremulous, and as the person takes very short steps, he has the peculiarity of appearing constantly to fall forward, or to be chasing himself, being, in advanced cases, unable to stop himself till he brings up against some object of which he can lay hold.

In **St. Vitus's dance (chorea)** (qv) the walk is bizarre and jerky, the affected child often seeming to leave one leg a step behind him, and then, with a screwing movement on the other heel, go on again.

GALACTAGOGUES are drugs which increase the flow of milk in nursing women. The normal stimulus of an infant's lips is the most powerful agent in producing milk, and a mother who has little or no milk should nevertheless hold her infant to the breast. Good food and the hormone, prolactin, from the pituitary gland increase the quantity and improve the quality of milk.

GALACTOCELE is a cyst-like swelling in the breast which forms as a result of obstruction in the milk-duct draining the swollen area.

GALACTORRHOEA is a recurrent or persisting discharge of milk from the breast.

GALACTOSAEMIA is a hereditary disease due to the lack of the enzyme which normally converts galactose, the sugar derived from lactose, or sugar-milk, into glucose. The incidence is around 1 in 75,000 births. Soon after birth the affected baby becomes jaundiced and lethargic. If he survives and is not treated, he becomes mentally retarded. Treatment consists basically of a diet free of lactose. Special lactose-free milks are now available.

GALENICAL PREPARATIONS are preparations of drugs sanctioned by the pharmocopoeia, the list of drugs and remedies published under government regulations. The term, official, is more commonly used in the same sense; official means drugs procurable in ordinary shops.

GALL is another name for bile. (See BILE.)

GALL-BLADDER (see LIVER).

GALL-BLADDER, DISEASES OF: The bile ductules begin as minute passages scattered throughout the liver, and lying between its rows of cells, from which they collect the bile secreted by the latter. They unite into larger and larger vessels just as do the tributaries of a river, and finally a single, large hepatic duct emerges from the right lobe and another from the left lobe of the liver. (See LIVER.) The connection of these with the gall-bladder is somewhat complicated. The right and left ducts unite first into one vessel, the common hepatic duct, which meets the cystic duct coming from the gall-bladder, and the two unite to form the bile duct, which opens into the small intestine a few inches below the outlet of the stomach. The importance of this arrangement lies in two facts: first, the entrance to the gall-bladder is a cul-de-sac, bile in entering it from the liver running down the hepatic and up the cystic duct; and, secondly, if the gall-bladder or its cystic duct becomes blocked, the bile can still escape from the liver down the common hepatic and bile ducts, into the bowel.

The size and condition of the gall-bladder can be determined in many cases by X-ray examination. A substance which is opaque to X-rays, such as iopanoic acid, when taken by mouth is excreted in the bile and passed into the gall-bladder. If an X-ray is taken some sixteen hours afterwards, the gall-bladder and any stones that it may contain are seen outlined as a shadow in the plate. Inflammation of the gall-bladder is known as cholecystitis. The condition characterized by the presence of gall-stones is known as cholelithiasis.

CHOLECYSTITIS: Catarrh, or inflammation, may occur in the gall-bladder and bile passages as in other cavities lined by mucous membrane. It may either arise in the bile-ducts themselves, or may follow upon a catarrhal condition in the bowels, spreading up from the point where the bile duct opens into the small intestine. Cholecystitis may be either acute or chronic. Both forms are more common in women than in men, and are more liable to occur in the obese than in the thin. The condition is more liable to occur in middle age. Since the bile is expelled from the liver largely by the movements of breathing, any condition which impedes this causes stagnation of the bile, and favours catarrh. Pigments are deposited from the bile in the finer vessels, producing 'bile-sand', and thick, stringy mucus collects in these passages and in the gall-bladder, the irritation caused by these deposits still further aggravating the catarrh. Finally, this bile-sand may collect into small masses in the larger ducts or gall-bladder, and, chemical changes in the mucus taking place, a crystalline substance incorporating cholesterol encrusts them in a gradually thickening layer, so that finally large gall-stones may be produced.

Symptoms: An acute attack of cholecystitis causes, in general, pain and tenderness to touch beneath the margin of the ribs on the right side: ie. over the edge of the liver and the gall-bladder. This may be followed by a certain degree of jaundice (qv). In chronic catarrh there is general ill-health and indigestion, associated with a dark, sallow skin, and occasional attacks of 'biliousness'. There is often, too, a vague, uneasy feeling in the region mentioned above, and in advanced cases there may be recurring attacks of gall-stone colic.

Treatment: The treatment of acute cholecystitis consists of rest in bed, the administration of antibiotics and pain-relieving drugs and a diet containing ample carbohydrate and protein but a minimum of fat. The patient should be encouraged to drink as much bland fluid as possible: eg. glucose drinks flavoured with fruit juice. If the condition does not settle quickly, an operation may be necessary.

Even in cases which settle satisfactorily, the possibility of an operation at a later date must be considered. Such elective operation, as it is known, is recommended by most surgeons today. Removal of the gall-bladder, the operation known as cholecystectomy, is the only satisfactory treatment for chronic cholecystitis. It is the most commonly performed major operation at the present, some 50,000 being performed in England every year. If, however, surgical treatment is not carried out for any reason, the regime followed should be based upon a simple life, with not more than three meals daily, the avoidance of alcoholic drinks and highly spiced food, and the taking of more exercise together with the practice of deep breathing. The administration by mouth of a concentrated solution of magnesium sulphate one hour before breakfast is sometimes of value by virtue of the fact that it helps to drain the biliary passages.

SUPPURATION is a rarer but much more serious condition which occasionally appears in the course of a chronic cholecystitis. Its symptoms are an exaggeration of those of catarrh along with shivering, high fever, and often delirium. The treatment is an operation to drain the gall-bladder of its suppurating contents, after which recovery often ensues, though the outlook is serious.

GALL-STONES: The formation of these has been already described. The smaller stones consist of a combination of bile-pigment with lime (bilirubin-calcium), and are deep brown in colour; the larger ones have a core of this surrounded by cholesterol, and are lighter or even white in colour. The size varies from that of small gravel, in which case several hundred stones may be present, to the size of a large egg, when the stone is single. When there are several stones they are faceted so as to fit against one another. Gall-stone disease, or cholelithiasis, is a major affliction in modern society, and operations on the gall-bladder are now the commonest form of major abdominal surgery in the United Kingdom. They are equally common in the USA, where approximately 16 million of the inhabitants are said to have gall-stones.

Symptoms: To begin with, there are the symptoms described under the heading of cholescystitis, which causes the formation of the stones. Apart from these, stones may lie for years in the gall-bladder and give no trouble, being found accidentally on X-rays, at an operation or after death. But as a rule they produce symptoms in one of three ways.

(1) The mere presence of stones in the gall-bladder may give rise to much irritation, and the tenderness and pain over the region of the gall-bladder then become very marked. These symptoms are specially liable to become aggravated during digestion, so that the condition is taken for a form of dyspepsia, although the pain is at the right side of the body. When bacteria find an entrance from the bowel, high temperature, shiverings, and sweating develop, and suppuration may come on.

(2) The usual way in which gall-stones show their presence is by passing out of the gall-bladder along with the bile. If the stone is small, it reaches the bowel and is voided, without

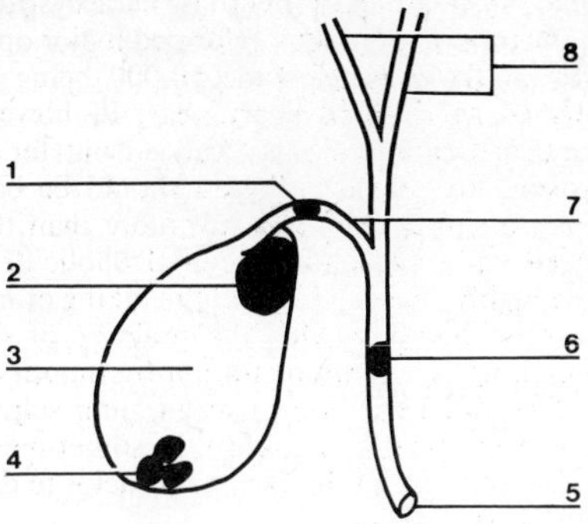

1 stone in cystic duct
2 stone in Hartmann's pouch
3 gall-bladder
4 silent stones
5 ampulla of Vater
6 stone in common bile duct
7 bile duct
8 hepatic ducts

Diagram showing various positions of gall-stones.

attracting attention beyond perhaps passing discomfort in the upper part of the abdomen, after a meal. If the stone be large enough to stick in the cystic or bile-duct, and particularly if it is angular, it sets up great spasm of the muscle fibres in the wall of the duct, causing the most agonizing pain shooting up to the right shoulder. It comes on, as a rule, very quickly, and is accompanied by collapse, cold sweat, and vomiting. It lasts usually several hours, and often ceases quite suddenly as the stone passes into the bowel or back to the gall-bladder. Next day there is usually some jaundice, which may last for a week or two.

(3) Sometimes the stone remains jammed or impacted in one of the ducts, passing neither up nor down. In this case, the pain passes slowly off as the muscle fibres of the ducts become tired out, only to return again and again, till, in a milder degree, it becomes almost constant. Gradually increasing jaundice may develop till the skin becomes even a dark olive brown.

Treatment: To prevent gall-stones, what has been said in the section on cholecystitis holds good, and if the accompanying cholecystitis is cured, even after large gall-stones have been formed, they may be comparatively harmless. Many substances, which will dissolve gall-stones outside the body, have been recommended in the hope that, taken into the system for long periods, they may gradually dissolve the stones in the gall-bladder – for example, ether, turpentine, and olive oil, but they are of no practical value. The exceptions to this are chenodeoxycholic acid and ursodeoxycholic acid which will dissolve cholesterol gall-stones in about one in five patients, but must be given for a relatively long period – even up to a year. Fortunately they are relatively safe drugs. They are taken by mouth. The gall-stones must be completely radiolucent as even the thinnest rim of calcium salts prevents dissolution. Pigment stones are also resistant to oral drug therapy. If the gall bladder is non-functioning this is a contra-indication to drug treatment of gall-stones. These drugs are teratogenic so should not be given to patients who could possibly become pregnant. The treatment usually takes at least six months and probably only 50 per cent of stones will dissolve completely. The rate of stones returning after complete dissolution is around 50 per cent. Cholelitholytic therapy is of value in elderly or unfit patients but cholecystectomy (see below) is usually the treatment of choice. Certainly oral drug treatment has not made a significant effect on the cholecystectomy rates in the United Kingdom.

When an attack of gall-stone colic occurs, hot fomentations should be at once applied to the abdomen. Morphine sulphate, 15 mg, with or without atropine, 0·6 mg, should be given hypodermically. Inhalations of amyl nitrite are also useful. A hot bath sometimes gives great relief.

If a person suffers from constant catarrh and repeated attacks of gall-stone colic, it is well that he should undergo the comparatively simple operation of having the gall-bladder removed (cholecystectomy), which may relieve both conditions. In cases in which a gall-stone is impacted, an operation is practically always essential. Sometimes, as when the duct is permanently closed, a fistula follows upon operation, and the bile drains away permanently through a wound in the abdomen. In this case, the jaundice and colic at least are alleviated, and the fistula can be closed at a later operation by the surgeon, who makes an opening between the gall-bladder and adjacent bowel.

GALLS, or NUTGALL, is the name of an excrescence growing upon oaks and containing a large quantity of tannic acid which gives the galls a strongly astringent action. Galls are chiefly used in the form of ointment of galls, and ointment of galls with opium, for application to bleeding piles.

GALL-STONES (see GALL-BLADDER, DISEASES OF.)

GALTON'S WHISTLE is a metallic whistle producing extremely high notes which is used in testing the sense of hearing.

GALVANOCAUTERY means a cautery (see CAUSTICS and CAUTERIES) made by a wire heated by a galvanic current.

GAMETE is a sexual or germ cell: for example, an ovum (qv) or spermatozoon (qv).

GAMGEE TISSUE is a surgical dressing composed of a thick layer of cotton-wool between two layers of absorbent gauze, introduced by the Birmingham surgeon, Sampson Gamgee (1828–1886).

GAMMA BENZENE HEXACHLORIDE is a drug that is used in the treatment of pediculosis (qv) and scabies (qv).

GAMMA-GLOBULIN: It has been known for a long time that the protective antibodies of the body are closely associated with the proteins of the blood. Gamma-globulin is a concentrated solution of the antibody fraction of human blood which has proved of great value in providing immunity against certain infectious diseases, particularly measles. It is of little value once the disease is begun but, if given before the disease manifests itself, it either prevents its onset or modifies its severity very considerably.

GAMMEXANE is the proprietary name for a synthetic insecticide which is a formulation of benzene hexachloride. It is active against a large range of insects and pests, including mosquitoes, fleas, lice, cockroaches, house-flies, clothes moths, bed-bugs, ants, and grain pests.

GANGLION is a term used in two senses. In anatomy, it means an aggregation of nerve-cells found in the course of certain nerves (see NERVES). In surgery, it means an enlargement of the sheath of a tendon, containing fluid. The latter occurs particularly in connection with the sinews in front of, and behind, the wrist.

Causes: The cause of these dilatations on the tendon-sheaths is either some irregular growth of the synovial membrane which lines them and secretes the fluid that lubricates their movements, or the forcing out of a small pouch of this membrane through the sheath in consequence of a strain. In either case a bag-like swelling forms, whose connection with the synovial sheath becomes cut off, so that synovial fluid collects in it and distends it more and more.

Symptoms: A soft, elastic, movable swelling forms, most often on the back of the wrist. When noticed first it is perhaps the size of a pea, and its connection with a tendon can easily be made out. It may remain this size for many years and occasion no trouble at all, but generally a ganglion gives a peculiar feeling of weakness to the wrist, and on account of its size or position it may be very inconvenient. A ganglion which forms in connection with the flexor tendons in front of the wrist sometimes attains a large size, and extends down the sinews to form another swelling in the palm of the hand.

Treatment: Sudden pressure with the thumbs may often burst a ganglion and disperse its contents beneath the skin, after which it should be prevented from refilling by bandaging the part tightly, a very efficient pad being made by wrapping up a large coin in a piece of lint. If it cannot be burst, there only remains the opening of the ganglion, with scraping of its interior. As the ganglion may disappear spontaneously there should be no rush to remove it unless it is causing inconvenience or pain.

GANGRENE, or MORTIFICATION, means the death of a part of the body sufficiently large to be seen. When the process is slow and superficial, only microscopic parts dying in succession, the process is called ulceration, whilst the term necrosis is usually restricted to the death of internal parts, particularly of bones. There are two varieties of gangrene, dry and moist, dry gangrene being a process of mummification, in which, as a rule, the circulation simply stops, and the part, so to speak, withers up; whilst in moist gangrene there is inflammation accompanied by putrefactive changes. The dead part, when formed of soft tissues, is known as a slough, and, when part of a bone, is called a sequestrum.

Causes: Certain diseases which lessen the strength and vitality of the tissues throughout the body render them more liable to die when subjected to injury. Chief among these is diabetes mellitus. The nervous system, too, exerts an important influence over the nutrition and repair of the body, so that where it is diseased a quite trifling injury may produce gangrene of the injured part: for example, in paralysis bed sores are apt to form, owing to the mere pressure of the body on the bed.

Direct injury is perhaps the commonest cause. If a limb is badly crushed, or frozen, or burned by heat or powerful chemicals, it may not recover.

Interference with the nutrition of a part by the gradual closure of the arteries, which may occur in old age; by their sudden closure in Raynaud's disease, or after the eating of diseased rye (see ERGOT POISONING); or by prolonged mechanical compression, may also cause it.

Infection by bacteria is another, and the most serious, cause, although fortunately it is rare and seldom occurs save in people of very low vitality. The hospital gangrene, so much dreaded by surgeons last century, belonged to this type, but is now practically unknown, thanks to aseptic surgery.

Symptoms: DRY GANGRENE usually comes on in old people with diseased arteries, and is preceded by pain in the affected limb, which gradually becomes a dusky red colour and later brown and black. The line between the dead and living tissues is quite sharp (line of demarcation), and marked by a red ring, where a slight degree of inflammation is going on. There is some smell, especially if care is not taken to keep the foot or other affected part absolutely dry. There is little or no pain after gangrene has occurred, nor any fever, and the red ring gradually deepens till the gangrenous part drops off in the course of some months.

MOIST GANGRENE is the more common form, and is accompanied by putrefaction. The part becomes swollen, livid, and covered with blebs; later it turns bluish-green and black in places. The smell is very offensive, and much fluid is effused from the decaying tissues, speedily soaking the dressings applied. There is not much pain, but the general symptoms are apt to be very serious, and there is then high fever. In the latter case the person may die of blood-poisoning, and in any case the line of demarcation is not definite, and the gangrene is apt to extend up the limb.

GAS GANGRENE is a form which may occur when wounds are infected with soil from highly cultivated fields. Gas-producing bacilli (eg. *Clostridium welchii*) from the soil then grow with great rapidity in the wound, and the gas spreads along the spaces in the muscles and connective tissues. Some of these bacilli grow only in the absence of oxygen, so that incisions to admit the air, together with application of oxidizing agents, and the use of gas-gangrene antitoxin, check their spread. In this form speedy amputation may be necessary. Experience gained in the 1939–45 War clearly demonstated the value of penicillin, in conjunction with surgery, in the treatment of this condition.

Treatment: The dry form must be kept dry by wrapping in cotton-wool, and, when the line of demarcation has distinctly formed, amputation may be performed close above it. In the moist form, which is not spreading quickly, the surgeon also waits till he can see clearly how much is to become gangrenous, and an attempt is made to control any infection by means of antibiotics. The gangrenous area is left dry. When small parts, like the fingers, become gangrenous after frostbite, they may be treated by applying on lint some simple antiseptic ointment, such as boric acid ointment, containing a small amount of eucalyptus or other volatile oil, to subdue the smell. (See also FROSTBITE.)

GARGLES: Gargling is a process by which various substances in solution are brought in contact with the throat without being swallowed. The watery solutions used for the purpose are called gargles.

Gargles are used in the treatment of infections of the throat: ie. 'sore throat', pharyngitis, and tonsillitis. They are also of value in the treatment of the condition known as 'relaxed throat' or 'clergyman's sore throat' (qv). A gargle consists of either (*a*) a solution (in warm water) of an antiseptic, eg. potassium permanganate; or (*b*) a concentrated solution of common salt or glycerin in warm water. It exerts its beneficial action in throat infections by virtue of one or more of the following properties: (1) the mechanical effort of gargling induces a hyperaemia in the throat which has a beneficial effect on the infection. (2) The heat of the gargle has the same effect and is also soothing to the inflamed tissues. (3) A strong solution of common salt, or glycerin, induces a hyperaemia. (4) If the gargle contains an antiseptic, this may help to control the infection.

One of the simplest and most effective gargles is common salt: sufficient should be added to a tumblerful of warm water to give it a strong salty flavour. Potassium chlorate is also a satisfactory gargle: 800 mg to a tumblerful of warm water. Another simple and effective gargle is one containing sufficient potassium permanganate to give it a faint pink colour. A more elegant gargle consists of: sodium bicarbonate, 4 grams; compound thymol solution, 57 ml; glycerin, 57 ml. A tablespoonful of this mixture is added to a cup of warm water. Another useful glycerin gargle is: boric acid, borax, glycerin (4 grams of each); water, 170 ml.

An aspirin gargle (600 mg to a cupful of warm water) is sometimes useful in relieving local discomfort, especially following tonsillectomy.

Mode of use: About a tablespoonful of the warm solution is taken into the mouth after the person has drawn a deep breath. The head is then tilted far back and a constant stream of bubbles is blown up through the fluid, so as to prevent it from running down the larynx and to send fine drops in every direction about the throat. When the throat is much inflamed gargling is painful. The gargle is then allowed to pass back as far as possible into the throat and kept there as long as the breath can be held.

GARGOYLISM, or HURLER'S SYNDROME, is a rare condition due to lack of a specific enzyme (qv). It is a progressive disorder usually leading to death before the age of 10 years. The affected child is usually normal during the first few months of life. Mental and physical deterioration then set in. The characteristic features include coarse facial features (hence the name of the condition), dwarfism, chest deformity, stiff joints, clouding of the cornea, enlargement of the liver and spleen, deafness, and heart murmurs, with mental deterioration. It occurs in about 1 in 100,000 births.

GAS (see ANAESTHETICS; CARBON MONOXIDE; NITROUS OXIDE GAS; DAMP).

GAS GANGRENE (see GANGRENE).

GASTRALGIA means pain in the stomach. (See DYSPEPSIA.)

GASTRECTOMY is an operation for removal of the whole or part of the stomach.

GASTRIC means anything connected with the stomach, such as gastric ulcer.

GASTRIC ULCER (see STOMACH, DISEASES OF).

GASTRITIS is inflammation of the stomach. (See DYSPEPSIA.)

GASTROCNEMIUS is the large double muscle which forms the chief bulk of the calf, and ends below in the tendo calcaneus.

GASTROENTERITIS is inflammation of the stomach and intestines. Its main symptoms are vomiting and diarrhoea. (See DIARRHOEA.)

GASTROENTEROSTOMY is an operation performed usually in order to relieve some obstruction to the outlet from the stomach, and consists in making one opening in the lower part of the stomach, another in a neighbouring loop of the small intestine, and stitching the two together.

GASTROPTOSIS is the condition in which the stomach occupies an abnormally low position in the abdomen. (See STOMACH, DISEASES OF.)

GASTROSCOPE is an instrument for viewing the interior of the stomach, by means of a special arrangement of light and mirrors attached to a hollow tube, which is introduced into the stomach via the mouth and gullet. A special camera attachment makes it possible to photograph the interior of the stomach. (See FIBROSCOPE.)

GASTROSTOMY is an operation on the stomach by which, when the gullet is blocked by a tumour or other cause, an opening is made from the front of the abdomen into the stomach, so that fluid food can be passed into the organ.

GATHERING is a popular term applied to an abscess.

GAUCHER'S DISEASE is a disease characterized by abnormal storage of lipoids, particularly in the spleen, bone marrow, and liver. This results in enlargement of the spleen and the liver, particularly the former, and anaemia. It runs a chronic course. There is no curative treatment, but splenectomy (removal of the spleen) is often helpful.

GAULTHERIA, or WINTERGREEN, is an American evergreen plant (*Gaultheria procumbens*) containing an oil with peculiar smell and aromatic taste. The oil consists almost entirely of methyl salicylate. Externally, oil of wintergreen is applied by rubbing on painful joints, in cases of acute and chronic rheumatism, often giving great relief.

GAVAGE means forced feeding by a soft rubber tube in cases when a person cannot swallow owing to weakness or other cause, or when an insane person refuses food. The tube, in the former case, is passed through the mouth into the stomach, and in the latter case a small tube is often simply passed through one nostril into the back of the throat, from which the person must automatically swallow food. By this means only liquid food, like strong soup, whipped eggs, or milk, can be administered. (See ENTERAL and PARENTERAL NUTRITION.)

GEL is the term applied to a colloid substance which is firm in consistence although it contains much water: eg. ordinary gelatin.

GELATIN is derived from collagen (qv), the chief constituent of connective tissue. It is a colourless transparent substance which dissolves in boiling water, and on cooling sets into a jelly. Such a jelly is a pleasant addition to the invalid diet, especially when suitably flavoured, but it is of relatively little nutritive value as not more than 1 ounce can be taken in the day: ie. the amount required to make one pint of jelly. Although it is a protein, it is lacking in several of the vital amino-acids. The ordinary household 'stock' made from boiling bones contains gelatin. Mixed with about two and a half times its weight of glycerin, gelatin forms a soft substance used as the basis for many pastilles and suppositories.

GELSEMIUM is the root of the yellow jasmine, *Gelsemiumsempervirens*, a climbing plant of the Southern United States. Its action upon the body is to dull the central nervous system. It must be used with caution, because in larger doses it is a dangerous poison. Its main use is in the relief of migraine, when it is given in the form of tincture of gelsemium combined with other drugs. (See GOWERS'S MIXTURE.)

GENERAL PARALYSIS OF THE INSANE, also known as GPI, GENERAL PARALYSIS, DEMENTIA PARALYTICA, is a disease in which both bodily and mental powers degenerate; though in some cases the bodily symptoms are for a time most marked, whilst in others the mental change appears first.

Causes: The disease is a late manifestation of syphilis, usually beginning eight to twenty years after infection: ie. it usually begins between the ages of 30 and 50 years. It is much commoner among males than among females. Occasionally it is found in adolescents, when it is due to congenital syphilis.

When a person dies in an advanced stage of the disease, certain very marked changes are found in the brain and its membranes. There is inflammatory thickening of the latter, and they are more or less adherent to the brain, in the superficial part of which the blood-vessels show various signs of chronic inflammation, while the brain tissue of nerve cells and fibres has to a great extent disappeared. The cells of the neuroglia or supporting tissue of the brain are found increased in size ('spider cells') and numbers, on microscopic examination.

Symptoms come on insidiously, as a rule, and the disease is often far advanced before it is recognized, although it may now and then be ushered in by convulsive seizures, by a sudden maniacal attack, or by a rapid nervous breakdown.

The first stage is characterized by slight physical symptoms, which generally escape the notice of the affected person's friends. These are tremors of the tongue and facial muscles in speaking, transient paralysis of eye muscles producing slight squint and double vision for a time, stammering over difficult words and, later on, increasing feebleness in walking and disinclination for exertion of all sorts. The handwriting degenerates greatly, and this is often the first symptom that excites remark. All these physical signs are apt to be masked by the peculiar state of mental exaltation which sometimes ushers in the disease. The person often feels himself to be stronger and better than usual, and is never tired of stating that he is 'all right', or 'as strong as an elephant', or that he 'could jump over a house'. But these are delusions, and, if he is actually put to the proof, his weakness is discovered. Often these delusions go further and he believes himself to be very rich, or embarks upon great commercial schemes, or identifies himself with some well-known personality; but however grand his dreams may be, there is in them an element of foolishness. Sometimes the first sign of the malady is a squandering of money on useless trifles; or foolish and criminal actions may be done which bring the incipient general paralytic into conflict with the law. In other cases the first mental symptoms consist of depression with delusions of poverty or of personal unfitness, the type of delusion being largely a matter of temperament. Great emotionalism is another feature, and the affected person is easily excited to tears or to laughter while the memory at the same time fails and the patient gets notably absent-minded. Important early signs, in addition to the mental excitement or mental enfeeblement, are diminished reaction of the pupil of the eye to light, and alteration of the knee-jerks and other reflexes.

In the second stage the physical weakness becomes more and more marked. The sight grows bad, and the affected person loses his power to feel pleasure or sorrow. Gradually, too, he loses feeling for actual physical pain, so that he is liable to get bruised and cut. The mind, too, becomes quite clouded, and unfit to sustain the simplest exercise.

In the third stage the mental failure is profound, and the sufferer cannot recognize even his nearest relatives. Speech degenerates to a series of meaningless noises. The paralysis becomes complete, and the person lies oblivious to all around him, and unable even to control his bladder and bowels. In this stage he becomes a ready prey to any infectious disease, and large bed sores.

The whole course of the disease lasts usually only two to three years, and, though occasional remissions take place, which may prolong life to ten years or more, a genuine case of general paralysis must be regarded as affording little ground for hope, unless effective treatment is instituted at as early a stage as possible.

Treatment: Recognition of general paralysis at a very early stage is of the greatest importance for two reasons. In the first place, treatment at this stage affords considerable prospect of stopping the progress of the disease. In the second place, the person suffering from an early stage of this disease is liable through mental weakness to transact his business affairs badly and lose his means, although still regarded by his friends as merely slightly peculiar or eccentric. The most effective form of treatment is penicillin, particularly if given early enough.

In the late stages of GPI the patient's mental condition is such that admission to a mental hospital is either desirable or necessary.

GENES, of which there are more than 100,000 in a human being, are the biological units of heredity. They are arranged along the length of the chromosomes (qv). (See HEREDITY.)

Dominant Genes: A dominant characteristic is an effect which is produced whenever the gene is present. If a disease is due to a dominant gene those affected are heterozygous, that is they only carry the gene in one of the pair of chromosomes concerned. Affected people married to normal individuals transmit the gene directly to one half of the children. In the ABO blood group system A and B are dominant over O. Huntington's chorea is due to the inheritance of a dominant gene, as is neurofibromatosis. Another dominantly inherited condition is multiple polyposis of the colon. Haemolytic disease of the newborn, due to Rhesus (Rh) incompatibility, is the commonest genetically determined disease in this country. The Rh antigen is a dominant characteristic which in haemolytic disease of the newborn is inherited from the father. The mother, being Rh negative, may develop antibodies against antigen present in the foetal red cells if they enter the maternal circulation and these antibodies may give rise to the disease in the foetus.

Achondroplasia is an example of a dominant mutation, for the majority of affected people have normal parents and siblings. However the chances of the children of a parent with achondroplasia being affected are one in two, as with any other dominant characteristic. Other diseases inherited as dominant characteristics include spherocytosis, haemorrhagic telangiectasia and polycystic kidney. Further examples are listed below:

Recessive Genes: If a disease is due to a recessive gene, those affected must have the gene on both members of the chromosome pair (ie. be homozygous). The possession of a single recessive gene does not result in overt disease and the bearer usually carries this potentially unfavourable gene without knowing it. If he marries another carrier of this recessive gene there is a one in four chance that their children will receive the gene in double dose and so have the disease. If an individual sufferer from a recessive disease marries an apparently normal person who is a heterozygous carrier of the same gene, one half of the children will be affected and the other half will be carriers of the disease. The commonest of such recessive conditions in Britain is fibrocystic disease of the pancreas, which affects about one child in two thousand. It can be calculated that 5 per cent of the population must carry the gene.

Most of the inborn errors of metabolism, such as phenylketonuria, galactosaemia and congenital adrenal hyperplasia, are due to recessive genes. Further examples are listed above. There are characteristics which may be incompletely recessive, that is, neither completely dominant nor completely recessive and the heterozygote, who bears the gene in a single dose, may have a slight defect whilst the homozygote, with a double dose of the gene has a severe illness. There are certain mild bony defects in the heterozygote such as the shortening of the middle phalanx of the second finger and toes in brachy-phalangia which results in gross deformity of the skeleton in the homzygote. The sickle cell trait is a result of the sickle cell gene in single dose and sickle cell anaemia is the consequence of a double dose. Thalassaemia minor and major demonstrate a similar incompletely recessive characteristic.

Sex-linked genes: If a condition is sex-linked, affected males are homozygous for the mutated gene as they carry it on their single X chromosome. The X chromosome carries many genes while the Y chromosome bears few genes, if any, other than those determining masculinity. The genes on the X chromosome of the male are thus not matched by corresponding genes on the Y chromosome. There is thus no chance of the Y chromosome neutralizing any recessive trait on the X chromosome. A recessive gene can therefore produce disease since it will not be suppressed by the normal gene of the homologous chromosome. The same recessive gene on the X chromosome of the female will be suppressed by the normal gene on the other X chromosome. Such sex-linked conditions include haemophilia, Christmas disease, the severe form of Duchenne type of muscular dystrophy and nephrogenic diabetes insipidus. If the mother of an affected child has another male relative affected she is a heterozygote carrier; half her sons will have the disease and half her daughters will be carriers. The sister of a haemophiliac thus has a 50 per cent chance of being a carrier. An affected male cannot transmit the gene to his son because the X chromosome of the son must come from the mother; all his daughters however will be carriers as the X chromosome of the father must be transmitted to all his daughters. Hence sex-linked recessive characteristics cannot be passed from father to son. Sporadic cases may be the result of a fresh mutation in which case the mother is not a carrier and is not likely to have further affected children. It is probable that one third of haemophiliacs arise as a result of mutation and these patients will be the first in their families to be affected. Sometimes the carrier of a sex-linked recessive gene can be identified. A proportion of haemophilia carriers reveal haematological abnormalities and carriers of the sex-linked variety of retinitis pigmentosa can be detected by ophthalmoscopic examination.

A few rare disorders are due to dominant genes carried on the X chromosome. An example of such a condition is familial hypophosphataemia with vitamin D resistant rickets. Glucose phosphate dehydrogenase deficiency is due to a sex-linked incompletely dominant gene.

Many hundreds of conditions are due to mutations of genes on the autosomes and more than sixty conditions are due to gene mutations on the X chromosomes. Gene mutations duplicate themselves at cell division in the same way as normal genes. As a result of these mutations a number of alternative forms for a given gene exist and these are called allenes. In many inherited conditions the disease is due to the combined action of several genes and the genetic element is then called multi-factorial. In this situation there will be an increased incidence of the disease in the families concerned but it will not follow the Mendelian ratio. The greater the number of independent genes involved in determining a certain disease, the more complicated will be the pattern of inheritance. Furthermore, many inherited disorders are the result of a combination of genetic and environmental influences. Diabetes mellitus is the most familiar example of such multifactorial inheritance. The predisposition to develop diabetes is an inherited recessive character although the gene is not always able to express itself: this is called incomplete penetrance. Whether or not the individual with the genetic predisposition towards the disease actually develops diabetes will also depend on environmental factors. Diabetes is more common in the relatives of diabetic patients and even more so amongst identical twins. However as the incidence of diabetes amongst the children of marriages between diabetic patients is well below 100 per cent, the gene does not receive complete functional expression. Non-genetic factors which are of importance in precipitating overt disease are obesity, excessive intake of carbohydrate foods and pregnancy. The influence of diet was made apparent during the two world wars when the mortality rate for diabetes mellitus showed a fall throughout Europe.

Schizophrenia is another example of the combined effects of genetic and environmental influences in precipitating disease. The risk of schizophrenia in a child, one of whose parents has the disease, is one in ten, but this figure is modified by the early environment of the child.

The capacity of genes for replication has recently been explained in terms of the structure of the deoxyribonuceic acid (DNA) molecule, which consists of a long double spiral with thousands of mononucleotides, each containing sugar, phosphoric acid and bases. A single change in the base sequence causes a permanent change in genetic information and provides a chemical explanation of mutations.

Genes control the production of specific proteins. The proteins are either structural proteins in the cell and thus a definitive product of the gene or they act as enzymes and are thus a link in the biochemical reaction in the body.

GENETIC CODE: A human being originates in the union of two gametes, the ovum and the sperm. These two cells contain all that the new individual can inherit from his parents. The hereditary elements or genes are carried on the chromosomes, which are present in the cell nucleus. Man has 46 chromosomes, comprising two sex chromosomes and 44 autosomes. The autosomes, which are somatic or non-sex chromosomes, can be matched according to their size and shape and arranged in 22 homologous pairs. In the female the pair of sex chromosomes are equal in size and are called XX. In the male the pair are unequal and are called XY. Every somatic cell of the male contains 44 autosomes and one X and one Y chromosome; every somatic cell of the female contains 44 autosomes and two X chromosomes. The hereditary elements themselves are the genes and are arranged in a linear manner along the length of the chromosomes. The chromosomes are long filaments, which during division become coiled and interwoven like spiral springs. Genes are responsible for the protein synthesis of the cell. They instruct the cell how to make a particular polypeptide chain for a particular protein.

Genes carry in coded form the detailed specifications for the thousands of kinds of protein molecules the cell requires for its existence, for its enzymes, for its repair work and for its reproduction. These proteins are synthesised from the 20 natural amino acids, which are uniform throughout nature and which exist in the cell cytoplasm as part of the metabolic pool. The protein molecule consists of amino acids joined end to end to form long polypeptide chains. An average chain contains 100 to 300 amino acids. The sequence of bases in the nucleic acid chain of the gene corresponds in some fundamental way to the sequence of amino acids in the protein molecule, and hence it determines the structure of the particular protein. This is the genetic code. Deoxyribonucleic acid (DNA) is the bearer of this genetic information.

DNA has a long backbone made up of repeating groups of phosphate and the sugar deoxyribose. To this backbone four bases are attached as side groups at regular intervals. These four bases are the four letters used to spell out the genetic message. They are adenine, thymine, guanine and cystosine (A, T, G and C in the figure below). The molecule of DNA is made up of two chains coiled round a common axis to form what is called a double helix. The two chains are held together by hydrogen bonds between pairs of bases. Since adenine only pairs with thymine and guanine only with cystosine, the sequences of bases in one chain fixes the sequence in the other. Several hundred bases would be contained in the length of DNA of a typical gene. If the message of the DNA base sequence is a continuous succession of thymine, the ribosome will link together a series of the amino acid phenylalanine. If the base sequence is a succession of cytosine the ribosome will link up a series of prolines. Thus each amino acid has its own particular code of bases. In fact each amino acid is coded by a word consisting of three adjacent bases. In addition to carrying genetic information, DNA is able to synthesise or replicate itself and so pass this information on to daughter cells.

All DNA is part of the chromosome and so it remains confined to the nucleus of the cell. Proteins are synthesised by the ribosomes which are in the cytoplasm. DNA achieves control over protein production in the cytoplasm by directing the synthesis of ribonucleic acid (RNA). Most of the DNA in a cell is inactive, otherwise the cell would synthesise simultaneously every protein that the individual was capable of forming. When part of the DNA structure becomes 'active' it acts as a template for the riboneucleic acid (RNA) which itself acts as a template for protein synthesis when it becomes attached to the ribosome. Ribonucleic acid exists in three forms. Firstly 'messenger RNA' carries the necessary 'message' for the synthesis of a specific protein, from the nucleus to the ribosome. Secondly, 'transfer RNA' collects the individual amino acids, which exist in the cytoplasm as part of the metabolic pool, and carries them to the ribosome. Thirdly, there is RNA in the ribosome itself.

RNA has a similar structure to DNA, but the sugar is ribose instead of deoxyribose, and uracil replaces the base thymine. Before the ribosome can produce the proteins, the amino acids must be lined up in their correct sequence on the messenger RNA template. This alignment is carried out by transfer RNA, of which there is a specific form for each individual amino acid. Transfer RNA can not only recognise its specific amino acid but also identify the position it is required to occupy on the messenger RNA template. This is because each transfer RNA has its own sequence of bases and recognises its site on the messenger RNA by pairing bases with it. The ribosome then travels along the chain of messenger RNA and links the amino acids, which have thus been arranged in the requisite order, by peptide bonds and the protein is released.

Proteins are important for two main reasons. Firstly, all the enzymes of living cells are made of protein. One gene is responsible for one enzyme. Genes thus control all the biochemical processes of the body and are responsible for the inborn difference between human beings. Secondly, proteins also fulfil a structural role in the cell so that genes controlling the synthesis of structural proteins are responsible for morphological differences between human beings.

During ordinary somatic or mitotic division each chromosome divides longitudinally, duplicating itself with an exact copy of all the genes it bears. When the cell divides, each double chromosome separates, one half passing to each of the two daughter cells, so that the two daughter cells contain exact replicas of the 23 pairs of chromosomes of the mother cell. In the formation of the gametes (ovum and sperm) a special kind of cell division takes place, called meiosis or reduction division, in which two divisions of the nucleus occur and only one division of the chromosomes so that the number of chromosomes in the gametes is half that of the somatic cells. The gamete thus receives only one member of each pair of chromosomes from the parent cell.

It was not until 1956 that the number of chromosomes in the human cell was established as 46. The morphology of the human chromosomes has only been appreciated since the discovery that colchicine has the property of stopping mitosis at the stage of the metaphase when the chromosomes assume their most visible form. Tissue culture provides a source of dividing cells, whose mitosis may be arrested by colchicine. The cells used are white blood cells which are incubated in their plasma with an added synthetic culture medium. There is as yet no known way of producing meiosis artificially. Chromosomes can be seen quite clearly under a microscope and arranged in order of decreasing size. Variations in size, the position of the centromere and specific characteristics of shape enable the 22 pairs of autosomes to be identified and numbered from 1–22. The paired sex chromosomes are of equal length in the female (XX) but of unequal length in the male (XY). The longest chromosome is 7–8 microns in length and the shortest about 1–5 microns.

In 1949 it was discovered that cells of females had a nucleolar satellite, which stains readily with certain dyes, whereas no such body could be detected in the cells from males. This is because the two X chromosomes in the female contain more chromatin than the XY pair in the male and are therefore more visible when stained. It is believed that one X chromosome remains condensed and physiologically inactive when a cell is not dividing and this forms the sex chromatin characteristic of female cell nuclei. The sex chromatin is not a complete index of sexual genetic makeup. All that can be inferred is whether an individual does or does not carry two X chromosomes. It does not indicate whether the normal Y chromosome is present. This sex chromatin body can be identified in 30 to 60 per cent of cells in the female. Buccal smears and biopsies of skin are the most favoured sources of cells as these cells have an open nucleus, though polymorphonuclear granulocytes can also be used. As the chromatin body (or drumstick of the polymorph) is formed from part of the X chromosome of the female cell, it is not present in cells, which carry only one X chromosome, such as those of normal males or patients with Turner's syndrome (XO). If a cell carries three X chromosomes two chromatin bodies will be visible in the cells.

Recently it has become possible to identify the Y chromosome. The anti-malarial drug quinacrine has been shown to be extremely useful for staining chromosomes with a fluorescence that is clearly visible through an ultraviolet microscope. The Y chromosome fluoresces intensely and this fluorescence is even visible in non-dividing (interphase) cells. Quinacrine is thus a reliable way of sexing human cells whether they are resting or dividing.

GENETIC COUNSELLING is the procedure whereby advice is given to couples wishing to have children, as to the likelihood of their having congenitally abnormal children. It is a procedure which is assuming enhanced value now that by means of antenatal diagnosis it is possible in certain cases to tell in the early stages of pregnancy whether or not the unborn child is abnormal: for example, whether or not he or she has Down's syndrome. There are now over twenty genetic advisory centres in the United Kingdom, to which patients can be referred by their family doctors.

GENETIC ENGINEERING, or genetic manipulation, has only developed in the past decade; it is the process of changing the genetic material of a cell. Genes from one cell, for example a human cell, can be inserted into another cell, usually a bacterium, and made to function. It is now possible to insert the gene responsible for the production of human insulin, human growth hormone and interferon from a human cell into a bacterium. Segments of DNA for insertion can be prepared by breaking long chains into smaller pieces by the use of restriction enzymes. The segments are then inserted into the affecting organism, usually the bacteria *Escherichia coli* by using plasmids and bacteriophages. Plasmids are small packets of DNA that are found within bacteria and can be passed from one bacterium to another. Already genetic engineering is contributing to easing the problems of diagnosis. At the present time beta-thallassaemia can be diagnosed antenatally by obtaining a sample of foetal blood at 15 weeks gestation.

GENETICS is the science which deals with the origin of the characteristics of an individual or the study of heredity.

GENITALIA are the organs of reproduction.

GENITO-URINARY MEDICINE (see VENEREAL DISEASES).

GENITO-URINARY TRACT consists of the kidneys, ureters, bladder, and urethra and, in the male, the genital organs.

GENOME is a complete set of chromosomes derived from one parent, or the total gene complement of a set of chromosomes.

GENTAMICIN is an antibiotic derived from a species of micro-organisms, *Micromonospora purpurea*. Its main value is that it is active against certain micro-organisms such as *Pseudomonas pyocyanea*, *E. coli* and *Aerobacter aerogenes* which are not affected by other antibiotics, as well as staphylococci which have become resistant to penicillin.

GENTIAN is the root of the yellow gentian (*Gentiana lutea*), a European plant. Preparations made from it are very bitter. It is one of the most commonly used bitters (qv) in dyspepsia and loss of appetite.

GENTIAN VIOLET, or CRYSTAL VIOLET, is a dye belonging to the rosaniline group. Gentian violet is a good superficial antiseptic. It is used in the treatment of burns, either alone or in conjunction with brilliant green and proflavine. Applied to a burn, gentian violet forms a tough pliable film.

GENU VALGUM is the medical term for knock-knee (qv).

GENU VARUM is the medical term for bow leg (qv).

GERIATRICS is that branch of medicine which treats of the disorders and diseases associated with old age.

GERMAN MEASLES, or RUBELLA, is an acute infectious disease of a mild type, which may sometimes be difficult to differentiate from mild forms of measles and scarlet fever. It is also known by the name of rötheln. The term, 'german', has no geographical significance. It comes from 'germane' meaning akin to. Rubella comes from the Latin, *rubellus* meaning red.

Cause: The cause of infection is a virus. It is spread by close contact with infected individuals, and is infectious for a week before the rash appears and at least four days afterwards. It occurs in epidemics every three years or so, predominantly in the winter and spring. Children are more likely to be affected than infants. One attack gives permanent immunity. The incubation period is usually 14 to 21 days.

Symptoms are very mild, and the disease is not at all serious. On the day of onset there may be shivering, headache, slight catarrh with sneezing, coughing and sore throat, very slight fever, not above 37·8°C (100°F), and at the same time the glands of the neck become enlarged. These symptoms are usually slight. Within 24 hours of the onset a pink, slightly raised eruption appears, first on the face or neck, then on the chest, and the second day spreads all over the body. The appearance of the rash is intermediate between that of measles and scarlet fever, being less blotchy, and remaining more as minute pink spots than the rash of measles, and the spots being more definite than the fairly uniform redness of scarlet fever. The rash is very bright on some parts of the body, while other parts are almost entirely free. The duration of the rash is variable. It may last for the greater part of a week, and, as it disappears, fine bran-like scales separate from the surface. The most distinguishing feature of this disorder is a well-marked but transient enlargement of the glands in the neck.

An attack of German measles during the early months of pregnancy may be responsible for congenital defects in the foetus, and it is for this reason that the disease has assumed such great importance in recent years. The incidence of such defects is not precisely known, but probably around 20 per cent of children, whose mothers have had German measles in the first three months of the pregnancy, are born with congenital defects. These defects take a variety of forms, but the most important ones are: low birth weight with retarded physical development; malformations of the heart; cataract, and deafness. Parents of such handicapped children can obtain help and advice from the National Association for Deaf, Blind and Rubella Handicapped.

Treatment: The only treatment necessary is confinement to bed so long as there are any symptoms. Infectivity ceases within four days provided there are no symptoms. Children who develop the disease should not return to school until they have recovered, and in any case not before four days have passed from the onset of the rash. In view of the mildness of the disease, contacts are seldom kept in quarantine, but they should be carefully watched from the tenth to the twenty-first day from exposure to infection.

In view of the possible effect of the disease upon the foetus, particular care should be taken to isolate pregnant mothers from contact with infected subjects. As the risk to the foetus is particularly high during the first sixteen weeks of pregnancy, any pregnant mother exposed to infection during this period should be given an intramuscular injection of gamma-globulin (qv). Female members of school staff who have not had the disease or been vaccinated against it, who might probably become pregnant should be recommended not to attend the school until the risk of infection is over. A vaccine is now available which should make it possible to give a girl an immunity to the disease before she attains adult life, and it is now officially recommended that such vaccination should be offered to all girls between 11 and 14 years of age. It is also recommended that all women of childbearing age, who have been shown by a simple laboratory test not to have had the disease, should be vaccinated, always provided the woman is not pregnant at the time and has not been exposed to the risk of pregnancy during the previous eight weeks.

GERMS (see BACTERIOLOGY).

GESTATION is another name for pregnancy.

GIARDIASIS is a condition caused by a parasitic organism known as *Giardia lamblia*, which is found in the duodenum (qv) and the upper part of the small intestine. This organism is usually harmless, but is sometimes responsible for causing diarrhoea. Over 3000 cases a year are reported in Britain. In most of these the infection has been acquired from drinking untreated water in the Middle East or Russia. The illness develops one or two weeks after exposure to infection, and usually starts as an explosive diarrhoea, with the passage of pale fatty stools, abdominal pain and nausea. It responds well to metronidazole or mepacrine.

GIDDINESS (see VERTIGO).

GIGANTISM (see ACROMEGALY).

GIGGLE MICTURITION is characterized by sudden, involuntary, complete emptying of the bladder during laughing. This is in contrast to the dampness of the pants which may occur with excessive laughter and which is not uncommon. The cause of giggle micturition is not known. It occurs in childhood and may persist into adult life. A sympathetic discussion of the problem may right it, supplemented by an atropine-like drug such as propantheline (qv). In some cases it can be prevented by sitting down on starting to laugh.

GINGER is the root of *Zingiber officinale*, a plant which grows in India, Jamaica, and other tropical countries. The tincture and syrup of ginger act like preparations of other volatile oils, and are given in doses of about a teaspoonful. They are used in cases of flatulence to stop griping, and are added to purgatives for the same purpose. The powder, in gelatin capsules, is of value in the treatment of travel sickness.

GINGIVITIS means inflammation of the gums. (See TEETH, DISEASES OF.)

GIPPY TUMMY (see TRAVELLER'S DIARRHOEA).

GLANDERS, or EQUINIA, is a specific infectious disease to which certain animals, chiefly those possessing an undivided hoof – such as horses, asses, and mules – are liable, and communicable by them to man. The term farcy is also used to designate a variety of the disease in which the lymphatic glands are first and chiefly affected. Glanders is a rare form of disease in man. It occurs chiefly among those who from their occupation are in contact with horses and seems to be produced either by direct inoculation of the organism from a diseased animal into the broken skin or by inhalation. The

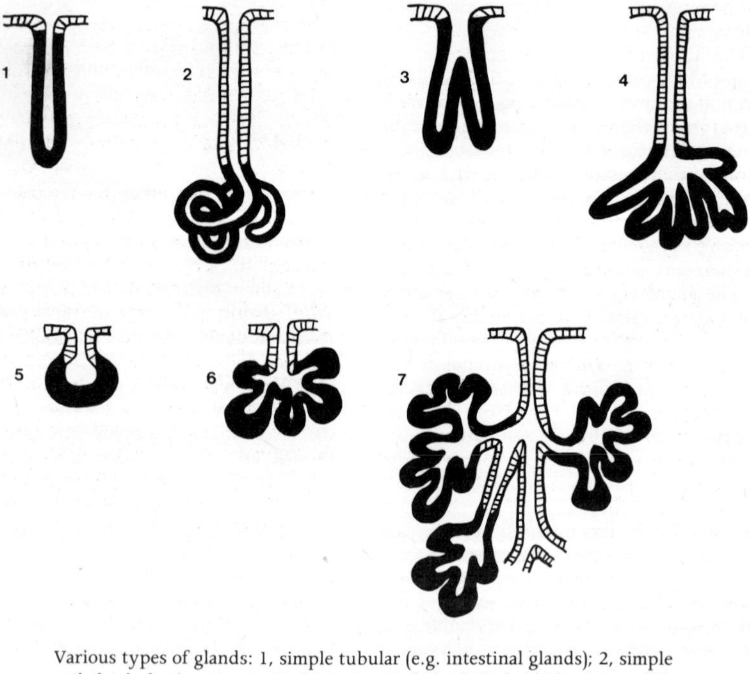

Various types of glands: 1, simple tubular (e.g. intestinal glands); 2, simple coiled tubular (e.g sweat glands); 3, 4, simple branched tubular (eg. gastric glands); 5, simple alveolar; 6, simple branched alveolar (eg. sebaceous glands); 7, compound (eg. salivary and mammary glands). The secretory part of the gland is black.

cause of glanders is a short rod-shaped organism, known as the *Loefflerella mallei*. It has been eradicated from Britain, but still occurs in Eastern Europe and Asia.

In the untreated acute form of the disease, the case generally terminates fatally in a period varying from two or three days to as many weeks. A chronic form of glanders and farcy is more common, in which the symptoms advance much more slowly, and are attended with relatively less constitutional disturbance. Around 30 to 50 per cent of patients with chronic glanders survive without treatment. Promising results have been reported from the use of sulphonamides, penicillin and streptomycin.

GLANDS are divisible into several classes. In the first place, the term is applied to organs like the liver, pancreas, and kidneys, which produce a secretion; but in general the term is limited to smaller structures concerned in the production of some excretion from the body, or of some substance needful to its working. These latter are divided into two quite distinct groups: (1) glands which produce some form of secretion or excretion; (2) lymphatic glands.

(1) SECRETING AND EXCRETING GLANDS comprise glands in almost all parts of the body, which vary much in appearance, in size, and in the character of the substances they produce. The skin, for example, is richly supplied with sebaceous glands, which secrete an oily material, and with sweat glands, which are placed in rows whose openings can be seen with a weak magnifying lens upon the ridges of the palms and soles. The lining membrane of the stomach is made up of long tubular glands set closely side by side, and in these the gastric juice is formed. The structure of the mucous membrane in the intestine is much the same. In all these mucous membranes there are situated other glands, generally formed each of a small mass of twisted tubes, which secrete a clear shining fluid known as mucus, that gives to these membranes their soft, smooth appearance and their name. The glands so far mentioned are all of microscopic size, but there are many of large dimensions. The parotid gland, situated just in front of the ear, the submaxillary gland, which can be easily felt, of the size of a chestnut beneath the jaw, and the sublingual gland, which can be seen beneath the tongue, are occupied in producing saliva, and known as salivary glands. The breasts or mammary glands are a pair of large glands situated in the skin over the front of the chest, and secrete milk. The thyroid gland, situated in front of the neck, has no outlet to the exterior, but produces an important secretion which is absorbed by the blood and carried throughout the body. The suprarenal glands situated immediately above the kidneys act under similar conditions. Many of the glands which have an outlet through which one secretion comes, such as the pancreas and testes, also produce what is called an internal secretion that is absorbed by the blood, and exerts a profound effect upon general nutrition and metabolism.

Glands which produce an internal secretion are known as endocrine glands. (See ENDOCRINE GLANDS.)

(2) LYMPHATIC GLANDS are scattered all through the body in connection with the system of lymphatic vessels. They vary much in size, from that of microscopic masses to that of large beans, but they have essentially the same structure everywhere. Round each gland is a fibrous tissue capsule, from which partitions and bands run into the gland to join one another and give it cohesion. In the meshes of these lie enormous numbers of lymph corpuscles in the circulating blood. These corpuscles are arranged in masses round which the lymph circulates freely. Numbers of lymph-vessels (afferent vessels) pierce the capsule of the gland, and the lymph, after passing from them, percolates through the gland and leaves its central part, carrying with it many corpuscles, by a few larger lymph-vessels (efferent vessels). The vessels leaving one gland pass on to enter another, the glands being, as a rule, arranged in chains.

In the limbs the lymph-vessels pass from the foot and hand up to the knee and elbow, respectively, before they encounter glands. A few glands are situated in the bend of each of these joints, and the vessels passing from these reach large chains of glands in the groin and armpit, respectively. The chains of glands beneath the jaw and down each side of the neck are known to everyone from the frequency with which they become inflamed and swollen. Inside the abdomen small lymph vessels known as lacteals collect certain parts of the food from the intestine, and pass their contents through mesenteric glands, situated deep in the abdominal cavity. Deep in the chest, too, lie many large bronchial glands, receiving lymphatics from the lungs. The lymph-vessels from the lower limbs and abdomen, after passing through numerous glands, unite into a single trunk, about the size of a quill, called the thoracic duct, which passes upwards through the chest, collecting the lymphatics of the chest, left arm, and left side of the neck, to open into the veins on the left side of the neck. A shorter lymphatic vessel collects the lymphatics from the right side of the chest, right arm, and right side of the neck, opening into the veins of the right side. The point where the lymphatic system on each side opens into the venous system is at or close to the point of union of the subclavian vein with the internal jugular vein. By means of these connections the lymph corpuscles formed in the glands may reach the blood. Beyond forming these corpuscles, the glands have another function, acting as a species of filters upon the lymph circulation, and keeping back micro-organisms and other dangerous impurities from entering the blood circulation.

GLANDS, DISEASES OF: The diseases of the chief secreting glands are described under various headings, and reference is made here only

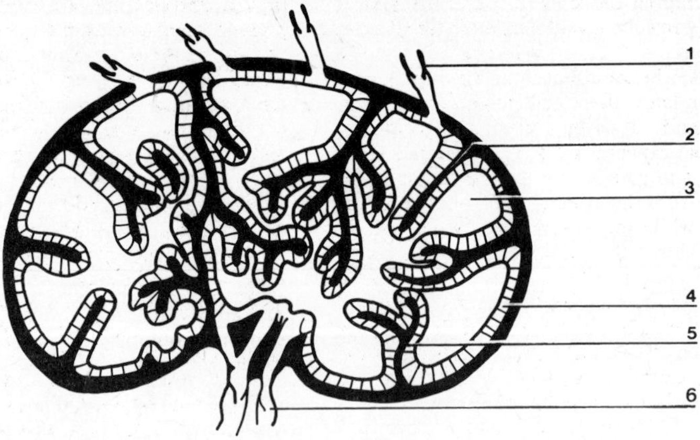

Structure of a lymph gland: 1 afferent lymphatic; 2 capsule; 3 cortical lymph follicle; 4 lymph sinus; 5 trabecula; 6 efferent lymphatic.

to diseases of the lymphatic glands. Most of the diseases which affect these glands are of an inflammatory nature, various poisonous substances lodging in them in the attempt to pass through the system by way of the lymphatic vessels. (See also ENDOCRINE GLANDS.)

SIMPLE ENLARGEMENT AND SUPPURATION OF A GLAND is the commonest condition. This is generally the result of a wound or other source of infection in the area drained by the lymphatic vessels going to the gland. For example, any source of irritation about the head, such as lice or eczema, is apt to produce swelling of the glands behind the ear and down the neck; or a wound of the foot or hand to cause inflammation of the glands in the groin or armpit, respectively.

Treatment: The object at first is to prevent suppuration of the enlarged and inflamed gland. For this purpose the source of irritation must be removed by opening the gumboil, cleaning the head, dressing the wound of the foot, etc. If the infection is due to a penicillin-sensitive organism, penicillin should also be given unless the infection is very mild. The gland itself is best left entirely alone, or at most kept supported and at rest by a pad and flannel bandage. If the swelling becomes soft and the skin over it reddened, suppuration is taking place, and the condition must be treated as an acute abscess. (See ABSCESS, ACUTE.)

TUBERCULOUS GLANDS, or SCROFULA, is a disease of childhood, especially in the neck. In many cases the glands become infected by the tubercle bacillus, *Mycobacterium tuberculosis*, through the tonsils. The chain of glands under the jaw and that running up and down the neck become affected in most cases, whilst in others the glands inside the abdomen are diseased, producing the condition of wasting known as tabes mesenterica. The condition progresses very slowly, as a rule, the glands enlarging for some months, then becoming matted together, to form an irregular mass, which softens, reddens here and there, and finally bursts through the skin to produce sinuses, which may go on discharging for years, healing finally with red, puckered, unsightly scars.

Treatment: Tuberculous glands are often the result of infection with the bovine tubercle bacillus. Therefore, one of the most important preventive measures is to see that children drink only milk that has been pasteurized. In the first stage, while the glands are simply enlarging, general treatment to improve the constitution is required, as well as the administration of anti-tuberculous drugs.

The introduction of the anti-tuberculous drugs has meant that in many cases the infection can be brought under control without any of the procedures about to be described, but there is still a certain number of cases in which they are necessary. A bandage or other appliance is often used in order to keep the part where the enlarged glands are situated more effectually at rest. This form of treatment may be persevered with so long as the glands are not becoming matted together. When the latter change takes place it is usually best to have the whole mass removed by operation, after which healing is usually immediate, and a narrow, barely visible scar is left. When a chronic abscess has formed but has not burst, it is treated like a chronic abscess in other sites. (See ABSCESS, CHRONIC.) If suppuration be allowed to take place, and the abscess to burst of itself, it is almost impossible to avoid an unsightly scar. When this accident has occurred, and a discharging sinus is present, the best that can be done, in general, is for the surgeon to aid healing by scraping the sinus out and dressing it frequently in such a way that it may heal from the bottom.

CANCER, when it is present in any organ, may sooner or later affect the neighbouring lymphatic glands. It is by way of the lymphatic system that cancer usually spreads to parts at a distance, and glands in a part of the body far removed from the original cancer may become affected, while the intervening tissues remain healthy. This is the chief reason for the recurrence of cancer after apparently complete removal. As an example of this, it may be noted that the glands on the left side of the neck are prone to be diseased as a result of cancer in the stomach; those in the armpit may become affected early in cancer of the breast.

OTHER CONDITIONS which produce enlargement of glands are the venereal diseases, leukaemia, and the disease known as lymphadenoma, or Hodgkin's disease. (See also BUBO.)

GLANDULAR FEVER, or INFECTIOUS MONONUCLEOSIS, is an acute virus infection which occurs predominantly among older children, adolescents and young adults. The incubation period is variable and may be as long as seven weeks. The glands of the neck become, in the course of a day or two, much enlarged and tender. This is accompanied by fever and a sore throat, and the patient loses all appetite for food. Jaundice may occur in a few cases. One of the characteristics of the disease is the presence in the blood of a large number of mononuclear, non-granular white cells. There is also a specific test for the disease known as the Paul-Bunnell Test (qv). Children recover fairly quickly but in adults convalescence may be prolonged.

Treatment: The patient should be confined to bed until the temperature has settled or the patient feels fit to get up. Analgesics, such as aspirin or paracetamol, should be given to relieve pain and discomfort, and the neck should be kept warm and still by a flannel bandage and cotton-wool.

GLAUBER'S SALT, or SULPHATE OF SODA, is used as a saline purgative.

GLAUCOMA is a term used to describe a group of disorders characterized by the intra-ocular pressure being so high as to damage the nerve fibres in the retina and optic nerve as it leaves the eye. Glaucoma is usually classified as being either open-angle glaucoma or narrow-angle glaucoma. *Open-angle glaucoma* is a chronic, slowly progressive, usually bilateral disorder. It occurs in 1 in 200 of people over 40 and amounts for 20 per cent of those registered blind in Great Britain. Symptoms are virtually non-existent until well into the disease, when the patient may experience visual problems. It is not painful. The characteristic findings are that the intra-ocular pressure is raised (normal pressure is up to 21 mm Hg) causing cupping of the optic disc and a glaucomatous visual-field loss. The angle between the iris and the cornea remains open. Treatment is aimed at decreasing the intra-ocular pressure initially by drops and tablets. Surgery may be required later. A *trabeculectomy* is an operation to create a channel through which fluid can drain from the eye in a controlled fashion in order to bring the pressure down. *Narrow-angle glaucoma* affects 1 in 1000 people over 40 years of age and is more common in women. Symptoms may start with coloured haloes around street lights at night. These may then be followed by rapid onset of severe pain in and around the eye accompanied by a rapid fall in vision. One eye is usually affected first; this alerts the surgeon so that action can be taken to prevent a similar attack in the other eye. Treatment must be started as an emergency with intensive drops and tablets to bring the pressure down. This is followed by surgery to prevent recurrence. Acute narrow-angle glaucoma occurs because the peripheral iris is pushed against the back of the cornea. This closes off the angle between iris and cornea through which aqueous humour drains out of the eye. Since the aqueous humour cannot drain away, it builds up inside the eye causing a rapid increase in pressure.

GLEET means a chronic form of gonorrhoea.

GLENOID is the term applied to the shallow socket on the shoulder-blade into which the humerus fits, forming the shoulder-joint.

GLIBENCLAMIDE (DAONIL, EUGLUCON) is a drug which stimulates the beta cells of the pancreas to liberate insulin, and is thereby proving of value in some cases of diabetes mellitus (qv). (See SULPHONYLUREAS.)

GLIBORNURIDE (GLUTRIL) (see SULPHONYLUREAS).

GLICLAZIDE (DIAMICRON) (see SULPHONYLUREAS).

GLIOMA is a tumour which forms in the brain or spinal cord, composed of neuroglia, which is the special connective tissue that in these organs supports the nerve-cells and nerve-fibres.

GLIPIZIDE (GLIBENESE, MINODIAB) (see SULPHONYLUREAS).

GLIQUIDONE (GLURENORM) (see SULPHONYLUREAS).

GLOBULIN is a class of proteins which are insoluble in water and alcohol and soluble in weak salt solution. (See also GAMMA-GLOBULIN.)

GLOBUS is a term applied generally to any structures of ball shape, but especially to the sensation of a ball in the throat causing choking, which forms a common symptom of hysteria.

GLOMERULONEPHRITIS describes a bilateral non-suppurative disease of the kidneys, affecting primarily the glomerulus. Usually all the glomeruli are involved. On the rare occasions when only a limited number of glomeruli are affected the disorder is known as focal or segmental glomerulonephritis. When the disease presents abruptly the term acute glomerulonephritis is used.

Cause: The disease is the result of the depositing of immune complexes in the capillary wall of the glomerulus. The activation of complement as a result leads to a combination of inflammation and coagulation which damages the glomeruli. This may resolve completely or it may lead to progressive scarring and obliteration of the glomeruli as occurs in chronic glomerulonephritis.

By studying the histology of the kidney from renal biopsy specimens three histological varieties have been recognised. These are: (a) minimal change glomerulonephritis; (b) proliferative glomerulonephritis, and (c) membranous glomerulonephritis. These three varieties are dependent on the differing ways in which the glomerulus reacts to injury. The most common antigen responsible for the development of soluble immune complexes is the streptococcus. This is the bacteria which causes acute tonsillitis and scarlet fever. Rarer forms of glomerular disease caused by immune complexes occur in systemic lupus erythematosis and polyarteritis and in the course of some tumours which provoke circulating antibodies.

Symptoms and Treatment: Glomerulonephritis can present in a number of different ways. The syndrome of acute nephritis following a streptococcal throat infection is the most common. It usually presents with swelling of the face and the eyelids and to a less extent the rest of the body. The urinary output is reduced and the urine contains blood and albumin. There is nearly always a rise in the blood pressure. The disease most commonly occurs in children and adolescents and the onset is abrupt with malaise, fever and sometimes pain in the loins. Ninety per cent of children with this form of acute nephritis make a complete and permanent recovery. A few patients will develop a rapidly progressive nephritis leading to renal failure. Some patients appear to make a good initial recovery but continue to pass protein in the urine although they may feel well within themselves. If the protein loss in the urine exceeds the liver's ability to produce the protein the plasma level will fall and a nephrotic syndrome will result. The rationale of medical treatment of this disorder is to maintain the water and electrolyte balance of the body and to provide adequate calories until the spontaneous recovery of renal function occurs. In view of the hypertension it is important to restrict the intake of salt. Initially when the patient is oliguric the amount of fluids taken by mouth must be restricted. As the urinary output increases the fluid intake can also be increased. The amount of fluid allowed is estimated as 500ml plus a volume equal to the amount of urine passed in the previous 24 hours. Penicillin is probably advisable to clear streptococci from the throat. No other drug influences the course of acute glomerulonephritis. As has been mentioned acute nephritis may be a manifestation of systemic lupus erythematosis, polyarteritis nodosa, anaphylactic purpura or Goodpasture's syndrome and then the treatment is that of the primary disorder.

When nephritis is due to the minimal change lesion or membraneous glomerulonephritis the onset is more insidious. Because these conditions are associated with an increase in the permeability of the glomerulus and hence proteinuria the clinical presentation is usually as a nephrotic syndrome. This is a syndrome characterised by a heavy proteinuria, hypoalbuminaemia and peripheral oedema. The nephrotic syndrome may be the result of a primary nephritis or it may occur secondary to diabetic renal damage, amyloid disease, malaria or systemic lupus erhythematosis. The management of the oedema is by diuretics.

When the nephrotic syndrome is secondary to other diseases the management is the control of those diseases. When it is the result of primary renal disease corticosteroids are often of benefit, especially in the minimal change lesion. Immunosuppressive drugs such as azathioprine may also be indicated. If hypertension is present it will require treatment in its own right.

Chronic glomerulonephritis results when proliferative glomerulonephritis becomes progressive and in most cases of membraneous glomerulonephritis. The clinical symptoms are those of chronic renal failure, usually associated with hypertension, polyuria, loss of energy, nausea and vomiting: anaemia is usually present. Muscle and bone pain frequently result due to osteomalacia. The disease progresses relentlessly as a rule and the only effective treatment is dialysis or renal transplantation.

GLOMERULUS is a small knot of blood-vessels about the size of a sand grain, of which around 1,000,000 are found in each kidney, and from which the excretion of fluid out of the blood into the tubules of the kidney takes place.

GLOSSITIS means inflammation of the tongue.

GLOSSOPHARYNGEAL nerve is the ninth cranial nerve, which in the main is a sensory nerve, being the nerve of taste in the posterior third of the tongue and the nerve of general sensation for the whole upper part of the throat and middle ear. It also supplies the parotid gland and one of the muscles on the side of the throat.

GLOTTIS is the narrow opening at the upper end of the larynx. The glottis is made up of the true vocal cords. (See AIR PASSAGES; CHOKING; LARYNX.)

GLUCAGON is a hormone secreted by the alpha cells of the islets of Langerhans in the pancreas, which increases the amount of glucose in the blood. This it does by promoting the breakdown of liver glycogen (glycogenolysis). It is secreted in response to a lowered blood sugar and is used therapeutically to treat hypoglycaemia (qv).

GLUCOCORTICOIDS is the group of steroid hormones produced by the adrenal cortex, which includes cortisol and cortisone (qv), and which particularly affect protein, fat and carbohydrate metabolism.

GLUCONEOGENESIS means the formation of sugar from amino-acids in the liver.

GLUCOSE (DEXTROSE; GRAPE SUGAR) is the form of sugar found in honey and in grapes and some other fruits. It is also the form of sugar circulating in the blood stream and the form into which all sugars and starches are converted in the small intestine before being absorbed. Glucose is a yellowish-white crystalline substance soluble in water and having the property of turning the ray of polarized light to the right. It is often given to patients as an easily assimilated form of carbohydrate. It has the further practical advantage in this context of not being nearly as sweet-tasting as cane sugar and therefore relatively large amounts can be consumed without sickening the patient. For patients unable to take food by the mouth, glucose is sometimes administered in the form of an enema consisting of 5 per cent of glucose in normal saline fluid, or 28·5 grams (1 ounce) of glucose to 570 ml (1 pint) of water. The same fluid, when carefully sterilized, may be injected beneath the skin or directly into the veins, and is quickly absorbed. (See SUGAR; URINE.)

GLUCOSIDE is a glycoside (qv) formed from glucose.

GLUE EAR is another name for secretory otitis media. (See EAR, DISEASES OF.)

GLUE SNIFFING has become increasingly widespread, especially among children and adolescents, during the last two decades. It is four times more common among boys than among girls. The precise number indulging in the habit is not known, but it has been estimated as running into the tens of thousands. In some of the deprived areas of the country, as many as one in three children aged 13 to 15 are experimenting with it, and children under the age of 10 have been found practising it. Only 5 per cent of those indulging in it become addicts. In 1980–81 it was responsible for 54 deaths in the United Kingdom, 12 of them in Scotland. The fumes are inhaled from plastic bags containing glue or thinner containing the solvent, toluene. Dry-cleaning products, aerosols, petrol, lighter fuels, typewriter correcting fluids, and camping gas are also used. Included in the use of substances thus inhaled are Evostick, Chemico, UHU, Britifix, Bostik and Thiofix.

The following are some of the common solvents and their toxic constituents:

Common solvents	*Toxic constituents*
Cleaning fluid-spot remover	Carbon tetrachloride Trichlorethane Trichlorethylene
Fingernail polish remover	Acetone Alcohol Aniphatic acetates Benzene
Household cements	Acetone Isopropanol Methyl ethyl ketone Methyl isobutyl ketone Toluene
Lacquer thinners Methyl, Ethyl	Aliphatic acetate Propyl alcohol Toluene
Lighter fluid	Carbon tetrachloride Naphtha (petroleum origin) Perchlorethylene Trichlorethylene
Model cements	Acetone Naphtha (petroleum origin) Toluene
Plastic cements	Acetone Aliphatic acetate Cyclohexane Hexane Toluene

The immediate, and sought for, effect is a sensation of happiness. This is followed by drowsiness and dizziness. There may be hallucinations. The after-effects include nightmares, depression and breathing difficulties. The habit can be recognized from the strong smell of the chemicals involved, and the suspicious stains on the skin around the mouth, nose and hands. Running noses and eyes, nausea and loss of appetite should also arouse the suspicion of parents.

GLUTAMIC ACID is an amino-acid with the formula $C_3H_5(NH_2)(COOH)_2$. It has been used in the treatment of epilepsy.

GLUTEAL is the name applied to the region of the buttock and the structures situated in it, such as the gluteal muscles, arteries, and nerves.

GLUTEN is the constituent of wheat-flour which forms an adhesive substance on addition of water, and allows the 'raising' of bread. It can be separated from the starch of flour, and being of a protein nature is used to make bread for those diabetics who are debarred from starchy and sugary foods.

It is also responsible for certain forms of what is now known as the malabsorption syndrome (qv). In these cases an essential part of treatment is a gluten-free diet.

GLUTETHIMIDE is a non-barbiturate hypnotic, which induces sleep fairly rapidly, and whose effects last about six hours.

GLYCERIN, or GLYCEROL, is an alcohol, $C_3H_8O_3$, which occurs naturally in combination with organic acids in the form of fats of triglycerides. It is a clear, colourless, thick liquid of sweet taste. It dissolves many substances, and it has a great power of absorbing water, in consequence of which, in the pure state, it diminishes congestion in surfaces with which it is brought in contact.

Uses: Glycerin has many varied uses. Numerous substances, such as carbolic acid, tannic acid, alum, borax, boric acid, starch, are dissolved in it for application to the body. It is frequently applied along with other remedies to inflamed areas for its action in extracting fluid and thus diminishing inflammation.

Mixed with an equal quantity of water it forms a useful mouth-wash when the tongue and gums are furred or dry, and, as a spray, is one of the best ways of relieving the discomfort of laryngitis. It is also useful for application to the skin in order to prevent chapping in cold weather, and to protect and heal all sorts of small abrasions.

Internally, pure glycerin, in doses of 1 or 2 teaspoonfuls, acts as a laxative, administered either by the mouth or as an enema. For its pleasant taste it is added to various medicines. It is mixed with gelatin to form a basis for pastilles. (See GELATIN.)

GLYCERITE is a mixture of glycerin with a medicinal substance. The principal glycerites are those of alum, borax, boric acid (known as boroglycerin), gallic acid, subacetate of lead, carbolic acid, starch, and tannic acid. These are used as applications, especially to the mucous membrane of the mouth and throat, for the action of the various medicinal substances contained.

GLYCEROL is another name for glycerin (qv).

GLYCEROPHOSPHATES are compounds of glycerin and phosphates, supposed by some to be beneficial as tonics in debility, because glycerophosphoric acid is a constituent of nerve tissue.

GLYCERYL TRINITRATE is a drug which is used in the treatment of angina pectoris (qv). Also known as TRINITRIN and NITROGLYCERIN, it is a thick oily liquid of sweet taste and explosive properties. When a small quantity is taken internally it produces marked effects in about two minutes, relaxing the smaller arteries, capillaries (qv) and veins so as to cause the skin to flush visibly, quickening the pulse, and causing a sense of fullness all over the body and throbbing in the head. It greatly lessens the blood pressure and temporarily relaxes all muscle, whether striped or unstriped.

Uses: This sudden action in relaxing muscle fibres and lessening blood-pressure proves very valuable in conditions where serious effects are produced by spasm, particularly in angina pectoris, but also in bronchial asthma (due in part to spasm of the small bronchial tubes), in gall-stone and renal colic, and in the vomiting of seasickness. In these it diminishes the spasmodic condition and gives relief.

It is used in the form of glyceryl trinitrate tablets B.P., each containing 500 micrograms made up with chocolate. These should not be swallowed intact, but allowed to melt in the mouth before being swallowed. As these tablets quickly lose their strength, they are prescribed in a special glass bottle tightly sealed with a foil-lined cap, and it is essential that the cap is screwed tightly back on to the bottle each time after a tablet is removed. The tablets must not be transferred to any other container. They must not be kept for longer than eight weeks. There is usually a date on the bottle label, and any tablets remaining on this date must be flushed down the lavatory or returned to the pharmacist and a fresh supply be obtained of fresh tablets. (See ANGINA PECTORIS.)

Other substances have a similar action. Sodium nitrite and potassium nitrite are used in doses of 200 to 500 mg, and have the advantage of producing their effect more slowly and more permanently. Erythrol tetranitrate has a similarly prolonged effect. Amyl nitrite, on the other hand, produces its effect in a few seconds, and, being volatile, may be inhaled as well as swallowed. For this purpose small thin glass perles are prepared, and are carried in the pocket by those liable to angina pectoris or other sudden convulsive seizure. Immediately the spasm comes on, one of these perles is crushed between the finger and thumb and held to the nostrils.

GLYCO- is a prefix meaning of the nature of, or containing, sugar.

GLYCOGEN, or ANIMAL STARCH, is a carbohydrate substance found specially in the liver, as well as in other tissues. It is the form in which carbohydrates taken in the food are stored in the liver and muscles before they are converted into glucose as the needs of the body require.

GLYCOPYRRONIUM BROMIDE is an anticholinergic, or atropine-like, agent which is used in the treatment of duodenal ulcer.

GLYCOSIDE is a compound of a sugar and a non-sugar unit. Glycosides are widespread throughout nature and include many important drugs such as digoxin.

GLYCOSOLATED HAEMOGLOBIN (HBA1): Normal haemoglobin on chromatography separates into the major component HBA, which accounts for 94 per cent of the total, and HBA1. HBA1 has the same structure as HBA except that a glucose group is attached to the terminal amino-acid of the beta chain. The rate of synthesis of HBA1 is a function of the blood glucose concentration. The red blood cell lives for 120 days and as HBA1 accumulates throughout the life of the erythrocyte its concentration is related to the mean blood glucose concentration over the previous three months. It is thus a very useful test for the overall control of the blood glucose in diabetes mellitus (qv).

GLYCOSURIA means the presence of sugar in the urine. By far the most common cause of glycosuria is diabetes mellitus, but it may also occur as a result of a lowered renal threshold for sugar when it is called renal glycosuria, and is not indicative of disease.

GLYCYRRHETINIC ACID is the active principle of liquorice (qv) and has been shown to have an anti-inflammatory action resembling, though much weaker than, that of cortisone. (See CARBENOXOLONE.)

GLYMIDINE (GONDAFON) is one of the oral hypoglycaemic agents: that is, a drug which, when taken by mouth, is able to control certain milder cases of diabetes mellitus without the help of insulin. (See SULPHONYLUREAS.)

GOA POWDER (see CHRYSAROBIN).

GOITRE is a term applied to a swelling in the front of the neck caused by an enlargement of the thyroid gland. The thyroid lies between the skin and the front of the windpipe and in health is not large enough to be seen. The four main varieties of goitre are the simple goitre, the nodular, the lymphadenoid goitre and the toxic goitre.

SIMPLE GOITRE is a benign enlargement of the thyroid gland with normal production of hormone. It is a physiological response to maintain the synthesis of thyroid hormone. It may occur sporadically, but in certain geographical areas of the world it is found more frequently and it is then referred to as 'endemic'. It may be the result of a deficiency of iodine, which is essential for thyroid hormone production. If iodine intake is deficient and the production of thyroid hormone is threatened, the anterior pituitary secretes increased amounts of thyrotrophic hormone with consequent hyperplasia of the thyroid gland. The prevalence of endemic goitre can be, and has been, reduced by the iodinization of domestic salt in many countries. Simple goitres commonly occur at puberty, during pregnancy and at the menopause, which are times of increased demand for thyroid hormone. They may also result from defective utilization of iodine in the synthesis of thyroxine. The immediate cause of simple goitre is increased production of thyrotrophic hormone by the pituitary. The only effective treament is thyroid replacement therapy to suppress the enhanced production of thyrotrophic hormone.

NODULAR GOITRES do not respond as well as the diffuse goitres to thyroxine treatment. They are usually the result of alternating episodes of hyperplasia and involution which lead to permanent thyroid enlargment. The only effective way of curing a nodular goitre is to excise it and thyroidectomy should be recommended if the goitre is causing pressure symptoms or if there is a suspicion of malignancy.

LYMPHADENOID GOITRES are due to the production of antibodies against antigens in the thyroid gland. They are an example of an auto-immune disease. They tend to occur in the 3rd and 4th decade and the gland is much firmer than the softer gland of a simple goitre. Lymphadenoid goitres respond to treatment with thyroxine.

TOXIC GOITRES are usually the result of Graves' disease (qv), though much less frequently autonomous nodules of a nodular goitre may be responsible for the increased production of thyroxine and render the patient hyperthyroid (toxic). Graves' disease is also an auto-immune disease in which an antibody is produced that stimulates the thyroid to produce excessive amounts of hormone, making the patient thyrotoxic.

GOLD SALTS are used in the treatment of rheumatoid arthritis. Gold may be administered in various forms, such as sodium aurothiomalate. It is injected in very small doses intramuscularly and produces a reaction in the affected tissues which leads to their scarring and healing. If gold is administered in too large quantities skin eruptions, albuminuria, metallic taste in the mouth, jaundice, and feverishness may be produced, so that it is necessary to prolong a course of this remedy over many months in minute doses. Routine blood and urine tests are also necessary in order to detect any adverse or toxic effect at an early stage.

GOLDEN OINTMENT is another name for yellow oxide of mercury ointment, which is used for inflammation of the eyelids.

GOLFER'S ELBOW is a term applied to a condition comparable to tennis elbow. It is not uncommon in the left elbow of right-handed golfers who catch the head of their club in the ground when making a duff shot. (See ELBOW.)

GONAD is a gland which produces a gamete; an ovary or a testis. There are four stages of sexual development: (1) gonadal differentiation, (2) development of internal genitalia, (3) external genital differentiation, (4) puberty.

The testis and ovary both develop from the undifferentiated gonad which appears in the fourth week of gestation. This indifferent gonad has a cortex and a medulla. In the presence of a Y chromosome the medulla of this structure evolves into a testis and the cortex regresses. In the presence of two X chromosomes the cortex differentiates into an ovary and the medulla regresses. (See GENETIC CODE.)

The internal genitalia also develop from separate primitive structures that transiently coexist in embryos of both sexes. In the male the Wolffian ducts give rise to the vas deferens, the seminal vesicles and the epididymus, and the Mullerian ducts regress (the prostatic utricle is a remnant). In the female the Mullerian ducts fuse to produce the Fallopian tubes, the uterus and the upper vagina, and the Wolffian ducts regress. The development of the Wolffian ducts and the suppression of the Mullerian ducts requires the presence of a functioning foetal testis from which an 'inducer' diffuses locally to both suppress the Mullerian ducts and stimulate the development of the Wolffian ducts. This inducer is not androgen which is unable to suppress the Wolffian ducts. In the absence of this substance the duct system differentiates along feminine lines irrespective of the genetic sex. Thus if there is no gonad, as in gonadal agenesis, the ducts will develop along female lines. Jost showed in 1947 that surgical castration of the animal foetus before the time of sexual differentiation prevented masculinisation and all the litters grew up as apparent females. The developing testis was thus essential for masculinity but the ovary was not essential for feminity. The female form, both internal and external, was that of the neuter sex.

The third stage of sexual development, namely the differentiation of the external genitalia, also involves development from primitive structures common to both sexes. In the female the genital folds become the labia minora, the genital swellings the labia majora and the genital tubercule the clitoris, whilst in the male under the influence of androgens the shaft of the penis, the glans penis and the scrotum are resectively developed. Failure of the genital folds to fuse correctly in the male results in hypospadias. Thus both in the development of the internal genitalia and the external genitalia differentiation to the male form requires a positive influence, otherwise development follows the female pattern.

The final stage of sexual development is puberty when pituitary gonadotrophin production increases to adult levels, and secondary sex characteristics appear.

GONADOTROPHINS, or GONADOTROPHIC HORMONES, are hormones that control the activity of the gonads (ie. the testes and ovaries). In the male they stimulate the secretion of testosterone and the production of spermatozoa. In the female they stimulate the production of ova and the secretion of oestrogen (qv) and progesterone (qv). There are two gonadotrophins produced by the pituitary gland. *Chorionic gonadotrophin* is produced in the placenta and excreted in the urine.

GONAGRA means an attack of gout affecting the knee. (See GOUT.)

GONORRHOEA is an inflammatory disease affecting especially the mucous membrane of the urethra in the male and that of the vagina in the female, but spreading also to other parts. It is the most common of the venereal diseases (qv). According to the World Health Organization, 200 million new cases are notified annually in the world. In 1986, there were 46,000 cases.

Causes: The disease is directly contagious from another person already suffering in this manner, usually by sexual intercourse, but occasionally it is conveyed by the discharge on sponges, towels or clothing as well as by actual contact. The infecting agent is the gonococcus or *Neisseria gonorrhoeae*. This is found in the discharge expressed from the urethra, which may be spread as a film on a glass slide, suitably stained, and examined under the microscope; or a culture from the discharge may be made on certain bacteriological media and films from this, similarly examined under the microscope. Since discharges resembling that of gonorrhoea accompany other forms of inflammation, the identification of the organism is of great importance.

Symptoms: These differ considerably, according to whether the disease is in an acute or a chronic stage. In *men*, after an incubation period of between two and ten days, irritation in the urethra, scalding pain on passing water, and a viscid yellowish-white discharge appear; the glands in the groin often enlarge and may suppurate. The urine when passed is hazy and is often found to contain yellowish threads of pus visible to the eye. After some weeks, if the condition has become chronic, the discharge is clear and viscid, there may be irritation in passing urine, and various forms of inflammation in neighbouring organs may appear, the testicle, prostate gland and bladder becoming affected. At a still later stage the inflammation of the urethra is apt to lead to gradual formation of fibrous tissue around this channel. This contracts and produces narrowing, so that the passage of water becomes difficult or may be stopped for a time altogether (the condition known as stricture). Inflammation of some of the joints is a common complication in the early stage, the knee, ankle, wrist, and elbow being the joints most frequently affected, and this form of 'rheumatism' is very intractable and liable to lead to permanent stiffness. The fibrous tissues elsewhere may also develop inflammatory changes, causing lumbago, pain in the foot, etc. In occasional cases, during the acute stage, a general blood-poisoning results, with inflammation of the heart-valves (endocarditis) and abscesses in various parts of the body. The infective matter occasionally is inoculated accidentally into the eye producing a very severe form of conjunctivitis. In the newly born child this is known as *ophthalmia neonatorum* and until recently was one of the chief causes of blindness. (See EYE DISEASES.)

In *women* the course and complications of the disease are somewhat different. It begins with a yellow vaginal discharge, pain on passing water, and very often inflammation or abscess of the Bartholin's glands, situated close to the vulva or opening of the vagina. The chief seriousness, however, of the disease is due to the spread of inflammation to neighbouring organs, the uterus, Fallopian tubes, and ovaries, causing permanent destructive changes in these, and leading occasionally to peritonitis through the Fallopian tube, with a fatal result. Many cases of prolonged ill-health and sterility or recurring miscarriages are due to these changes.

Treatment: The chances of cure are better the earlier treatment is instituted. The treatment of gonorrhoea was revolutionized by the introduction of the sulphonamides. These, in turn, have now been replaced by the antibiotics. Penicillin is now the antibiotic of choice: a single injection of 2·4 or 4·8 mega units of procaine penicillin. Unfortunately, the gonococcus is liable to become resistant to penicillin. In patients who are infected with penicillin-resistant organisms, one of the other antibiotics is used. In all cases it is essential that bacteriological investigation should be carried out at weekly intervals for three or four weeks, to make sure that the patient is cured.

GOSSYPIUM is the Latin word for cotton.

GOULARD'S WATER is the popular name for the dilute solution of subacetate of lead, which is employed in the treatment of sprains, bruises, and localized inflammations. It is commonly mixed with laudanum in the proportion of 4 ml of laudanum to 28·5 ml of the Goulard's water, and the mixture, known as lead and opium lotion, is applied on a piece of moist warm flannel, and covered with waterproof cloth.

GOUT is a constitutional disorder connected with excess of uric acid in the blood, and manifesting itself by inflammation of joints with deposition therein of urate of soda, and also by morbid changes in various important organs.

Causes: The cardinal feature of gout is the presence of an excessive amount of uric acid, and its deposition in the joints in the form of sodium monourate. The cause of this excess of uric acid is not known. Uric acid is formed in the system in the processes of nutrition, and is excreted by the kidneys, the amount passing off in the urine being 0·1 to 2 grams daily. In the healthy human subject the blood contains 3 to 6 mg per 100 millilitres, but in gout it is increased, both before and during the acute attack, while in chronic gout the amount in the blood and elsewhere in the body is always above the normal level.

Gout is in a marked degree hereditary. A family history of the disease is obtained in from 50 to 80 per cent of cases. Gout is said to affect the sedentary more readily than the active, but this cannot be taken as a constant rule. On the other hand, inadequate exercise, habitual over-indulgence in animal food and rich dishes, and especially in alcoholic drinks, are undoubtedly important precipitating factors in the production of the disease. These, however, are no more than precipitating factors, and the disease can occur in vegetarians and teetotallers.

Gout is more common in mature age than in the earlier years of life, being infrequent before the age of 40, but it may occasionally affect very young people in whom there is a strong family history. About 95 per cent of patients are males. In women it most often appears after the cessation of the menses.

Symptoms: An attack of gout may appear without warning, or there may be premonitory symptoms. On the night of the attack, the patient retires to rest apparently quite well, but about two or three o'clock in the morning is awakened by a painful feeling in the foot, most commonly in the ball of the great toe, but it may be in the instep or heel, or in the thumb. With the pain there often occurs a distinct shivering, followed by feverishness. The pain soon becomes of an agonizing character.

When the affected part is examined it is found to be swollen and of a deep red hue. The skin is tense and glistening, and the surrounding veins are more or less distended. After a few hours there is a remission of the pain, slight perspiration takes place, and the patient may fall asleep. The pain, however, returns next night, and these nocturnal exacerbations occur with greater or less severity during the continuance of the attack, which generally lasts for a week or ten days. As the symptoms decline, the swelling and tenderness of the affected joint abate, but the skin over it pits on pressure for a time, and with this there is often associated slight desquamation of the skin. It is rare that the first is the only attack of gout, although by care and treatment recurrences may be warded off. In the earlier recurrences the same joints as were the original seat of the gouty inflammation suffer again, but in the course of time others become implicated, until in advanced cases scarcely any joint escapes, and the disease becomes chronic. When gout assumes this form, the frequently recurring attacks are usually attended with less pain, but chalk-stones, or tophi, are gradually formed round the affected joints. These deposits, which are highly characteristic of gout, at first occur in the form of a semi-fluid material, consisting for the most part of bi-urate of soda, which gradually becomes more dense, and ultimately quite hard. In some cases of chronic gout the deposit is so slight as to be barely appreciable externally, but on the other hand it occasionally causes great enlargement of the joints, and fixes them in a flexed or extended position which renders them entirely useless. Any of the joints may be thus affected, but most commonly those of the hands and feet. The deposits occur in other structures besides those of joints, such as along the course of tendons, underneath the skin and periosteum, in the sclerotic coat of the eye, and especially on the cartilages of the external ear. When bi-urate of soda is largely deposited in joints the skin sometimes gives way, and the concretion is exposed.

A variety of urinary calculus – the uric acid stone –formed by concretions of this substance in the kidneys is a not infrequent occurrence in connection with gout; hence the well-known association of this disease and gravel (qv).

Treatment: During the acute attack the affected part should be kept at perfect rest, and be enveloped in cotton-wool covered with oil-silk. The medicinal agent upon which most reliance was placed was colchicum. The first known record of the use of this drug, which is said to derive its name from Colchis in Asia Minor, is in the Eber papyrus of around 1500 BC. The mode of action of colchicum is uncertain, but it is probable that it has simply a special sedative action upon the gouty inflammation without affecting the excretion of uric acid. It is usually administered as colchicine, which is the active principle of the drug and was first isolated in 1820. In cases which do not respond satisfactorily to colchicine, one of the non-steroidal anti-inflammatory drugs such as Indomethacin should be used. For the long-term management and prevention a uricosuric agent such as probenecid should be used or an xanthine oxidase inhibitor such as allopurinol which prevents the formation of uric acid.

GOWERS'S MIXTURE was introduced, in 1888, by Sir William Gowers for the treatment of migraine. It contains sodium bromide, solution of glyceryl trinitrate, dilute hydrobromic acid, tincture of nux vomica, tincture of gelsemium, and syrup of lemon. It is still widely and successfully used for the purpose for which it was introduced.

GRAFT is the term applied to a piece of tissue removed from one person or animal and implanted in another, or the same, individual in order by its growth to remedy some defect. Skin grafts are commonly used. Bone grafts are also used to replace bone which has been lost by disease: for example, a portion of rib is sometimes removed in order to furnish support for a spine weakened by disease, after the disease has been removed. Also, the bone of young animals is used to afford additional growth and strength to a limb bone which it has been necessary to remove in part on account of disease or injury. Vein grafts are used to replace stretches of arteries which have become blocked, particularly in the heart and lower limbs. The veins most commonly used for this purpose are the saphenous veins of the individual in question provided they are healthy. An alternative is specially treated umbilical vein. (See SKIN GRAFTING.)

GRAM, or GRAMME, is the unit of weight in the metric system and is equal to a little over 15·4 grains. For purposes of weighing food, 30 grams are usually taken as approximately equal to 1 ounce.

GRAM'S STAIN, named after the bacteriologist, H. C. J. Gram, who first described it in 1884, is one of the most valuable methods of differentiating certain micro-organisms. The principle involved depends upon the fact that certain bacteria, when treated with a dye such as gentian violet and then with iodine, fix the dye, whereas other bacteria do not. Those bacteria, such as the pneumococcus, that fix the dye are known as Gram-positive, whilst those that do not fix it, eg. the gonococcus, are said to be Gram-negative.

GRAND MAL is the name applied to a convulsive epileptic attack, in contrast to petit mal, which includes the milder forms of epilepsy (qv).

GRANULAR KIDNEY is the name given to the state of the kidney in chronic glomerulonephritis (qv), which often occurs in association with chronic arterial disease.

GRANULATIONS are small masses of formative cells containing loops of newly formed blood-vessels which spring up over any raw surface, as the first step in the process of healing of wounds. (See ULCER; WOUNDS.)

GRANULOMA is a tumour or new growth made up of granulation tissue. This is caused by various forms of chronic inflammation, such as syphilis and tuberculosis.

GRAVEL is the name applied to any sediment which falls down in the urine, but particularly to small masses of uric acid. It produces various unpleasant symptoms. (See BLADDER, DISEASES OF; GOUT; URINE.)

GRAVES' DISEASE is a syndrome consisting of diffuse goitre, hyperthyroidism and eye signs and is due to the production of various auto-antibodies. The hyperthyroidism is due to the production of antibodies to the TSH receptor which stimulate the receptor with resultant production of excess thyroid hormones. The goitre is due to antibodies that stimulate the growth of the thyroid gland. The exophthalmos is due to another immunoglobulin called the ophthalmopathic immunoglobulin which is an antibody to a retro-orbital antigen on the surface of the retro-orbital eye muscles. This provokes inflammation in the retro-orbital tissues which is associated with the accumulation of water and mucopolysaccharide which fills the orbit and causes the eye to protrude forwards.

Although Graves' disease may affect any age group the peak incidence is in the 3rd decade. Females are affected ten times as often as males. The prevalence in females is one in 500. As with many other auto-immune diseases, there is an increased prevalence of auto-immune thyroid disease in the relatives of patients with Graves' disease. Some of these patients may have hypothyroidism and others thyrotoxicosis. Patients with Graves' disease may present with a goitre or with the eye signs or, most commonly, with the symptoms of excess thyroid hormone production. Thyroid hormone controls the metabolic rate of the body so that the symptoms of hyperthyroidism are those of excess metabolism. Patients thus lose weight despite a good appetite. They become intolerant of heat and sweat more than previously. The heart rate is rapid so that patients may be aware of palpitations or shortness of breath. There is excess stimulation of the central nervous system so that patients become irritable, hyperactive and develop tremor. They commonly also develop muscle weakness due to a myopathy. This tends to affect the girdle muscles so that patients may have difficulty getting out of chairs or climbing stairs or combing their hair. In addition to the prominence of the eyes due to exophthalmos there may also be swelling of the eyelids and congestion of the conjunctiva, and paralysis of the eye muscles leading to double vision. Some patients with exophthalmos also develop pretibial myxoedema. This is a localised involvement of the skin with infiltration of muco polysaccharide which occurs in the front of the shins but may extend to the dorsum of the foot and even to the toes.

The diagnosis of Graves' disease is confirmed by the measurement of the circulating levels of the two thyroid hormones, thyroxine and tri-iodothyronine.

Treatment: There are three effective treatments for Graves' disease. (1) Antithyroid drugs: these drugs inhibit the iodination of tyrosine and hence the formation of the thyroid hormones. The most commonly used drugs are carbimazole, propylthiouricil and methimazole. They will control the excess production of thyroid hormones in virtually all cases. Once the patient has been rendered euthyroid the dose can be reduced to a maintenance dose and is usually continued for two years. The disadvantage of antithyroid drugs is that even after two years' treatment nearly half the patients will relapse and will then require more definitive therapy.

(2) Partial thyroidectomy: removal of three-quarters of the thyroid gland is effective treatment of the hyperthyroidism of Graves' disease. It is the treatment of choice in those patients with large goitres. The patient must however be rendered euthyroid before surgery is undertaken, or thyroid crisis and arrhythmias may complicate the operation.

(3) Radioactive iodine therapy: this has been in use for more than 30 years. It is an effective means of controlling hyperthyroidism and does not require admission to hospital but merely the taking of a tasteless, colourless drink. One of the disadvantages of radioactive iodine is that the incidence of hypothyroidism is much greater than with other forms of treatment. The incidence of hypothyroidism increases as the years pass and after 20 years the incidence approaches 80 per cent of patients. However the management of hypothyroidism is simple and requires only the taking of thyroxine tablets, so that, provided the patients are followed up and the hypothyroidism is diagnosed, this presents little problem. There is no evidence of any increased incidence of cancer of the thyroid or leukaemia following radio-iodine therapy over the 30 years that it has been used. It has been the pattern in Britain to reserve radio-iodine treatment to those over the age of 35 or those whose prognosis is unlikely to be more than 30 years as a result of cardiac or respiratory disease.

GRAVID means pregnant.

GREEN SICKNESS is a popular name for chlorosis. (See ANAEMIA.)

GREENSTICK FRACTURE is an incomplete fracture, in which the bone is not completely broken across. It occurs in the long bones of children and is usually due to indirect violence. (See FRACTURES.)

GREGORY'S MIXTURE or POWDER is a powder of light-yellow colour containing rhubarb, magnesia, and ginger. In doses of 0·6 to 4 grams it is used as an antacid and purgative.

GRENZ RAYS are very soft, poor penetrating X-rays which are used in the treatment of certain skin diseases. (See X-RAYS.)

GREY POWDER is a powder composed of mercury and chalk. It was at one time much used as an ingredient of powders intended to check infantile diarrhoea, but is not used now for this, or any other, purpose in children because of the risk of inducing mercurial poisoning. (See ERYTHROEDEMA.)

GRINDELIA is an American plant used as an asthma remedy. The leaves are generally used soaked in nitre, dried, and then either burned on a plate, from which the fumes are inhaled, or rolled in a cigarette and smoked.

GRINDER'S ROT is the term applied to a disease of the lung in steel-grinders caused by inhaling particles of the metal.

GRIPES is a popular name for the colic of infants, generally due to irregular feeding. (See COLIC.)

GRIPPE is a popular name for influenza. (See INFLUENZA.)

GRISEOFULVIN is an antibiotic obtained from *Penicilliumgriseofulvum Dierckse*, which is proving of value in the treatment of various forms of ringworm.

GROIN is the region which includes the upper part of the front of the thigh and lower part of the abdomen. A deep groove runs obliquely across it, which corresponds to the inguinal ligament, and divides the thigh from the abdomen. The principal diseased conditions in this region are enlarged glands (see GLANDS), and hernia (qv).

GROMMET is a small bobbin-shaped tube used to keep open the incision made in the ear drum in the treatment of secretory otitis media. It acts as a ventilation tube by allowing the Eustachian tube to recover its normal function. (See EAR, DISEASES OF; EUSTACHIAN TUBES.)

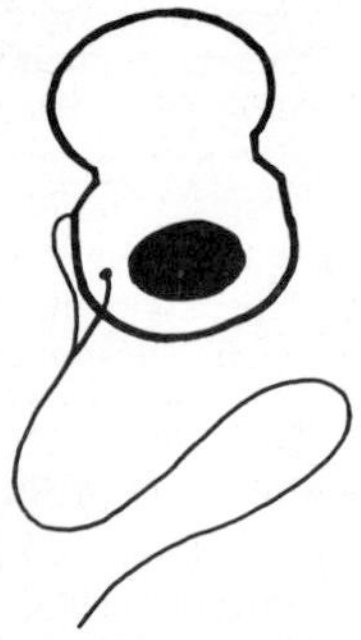

A grommet.

GROWING PAINS occur in children during the course of development most commonly in the legs and back. As often as not they are of no significance, but they must not be entirely ignored because they may on occasion be the first manifestation of rheumatic fever. Severe pains in young children are occasionally due to actual disease in a bone, either of tuberculous nature or caused by acute inflammation (osteomyelitis), and special attention is required in such cases.

GROWTH is a popular term applied to any new formation in any part of the body. (See CANCER; CYST; GANGLION; TUMOUR.) For growth of children, see WEIGHT AND HEIGHT.

GUAIAC is a resin obtained from the wood of *Guaiacum officinale* or *Lignum vitae*, a West Indian tree. It is seldom used now, except in the form of guaiac lozenges, which are sometimes of value in the treatment of sore throats.

GUANETHIDINE is one of the hypotensive drugs which act by inhibiting the action of the sympathetic nervous system (qv).

GUINEA-WORM (see DRACUNCULIASIS).

GULLET, or OESOPHAGUS, is the tube down which food passes from the throat to the stomach. (See OESOPHAGUS.)

GUM is a complex viscid substance which exudes from the stems and branches of various trees, and consists principally of arabin or bassorin. The two best-known gums are gum acacia and gum tragacanth. Gum-resins such as asafoetida, galbanum, and myrrh also contain resin. For gum-saline, see ACACIA.

GUMBOIL is a condition of inflammation, ending generally as an abscess, situated about the root of a carious tooth.
Symptoms: One tooth becomes a little painful and seems a little raised above the others, but the pain is at first relieved by clenching the teeth tightly, although after a day or more the affected tooth becomes extremely tender. A thickening forms at the side of the tooth, which is also at first relieved by pressure, as by holding a pad of cotton-wool, or similar soft mass between gum and cheek. After some days the pain lessens, and either the swelling gradually subsides, or an abscess forms and bursts, generally between gum and cheek, but it may be on the cheek.
Treatment: If there is any cavity in the tooth it should be stopped with cotton-wool soaked in a volatile oil, such as oil of cloves, or with a mixture of zinc oxide and oil of cloves, and if the pain and swelling do not speedily abate, the tooth should be pulled. Relief of the inflammation in the early stages is often gained by painting the gum freely with tincture of iodine. These, however, are only first-aid remedies, and expert dental advice should always be sought as soon as possible.

GUMMA means a hard swelling situated usually in connective tissue, although it may be in internal organs, muscle, or brain, and resulting from syphilis. The swelling is usually painless but it may produce very marked symptoms by interference with the organ in which it is situated. A gumma generally disappears speedily when the treatment appropriate to syphilis is administered.

GUMS, DISEASES OF (see MOUTH, DISEASES OF; TEETH, DISEASES OF).

GUTTA PERCHA is used in the preparation of some varieties of sticking plaster, but its main use is, rolled out in thin films, known as gutta-percha tissue, to keep surgical dressings moist by preventing evaporation.

GYMNASTICS (see EXERCISE; CHEST DEVELOPMENT).

GYNAECOLOGY is the branch of medical science which deals with diseases peculiar to women.

GYNAECOMASTIA is the term used for describing an abnormal increase in size of the male breast.

GYRUS is the term applied to a convolution of the brain.

H

HABIT SPASM (see CRAMP).

HABITS (see DRUG HABITS; also CHILDREN, PECULIARITIES OF).

HAEMANGIOMA is a benign tumour composed of tortuous dilated blood-vessels.

HAEMARTHROSIS denotes bleeding into, or the presence of blood in, a joint.

HAEMATEMESIS means vomiting of blood. Blood brought up from the stomach is generally dark in colour, and is often so far digested as to form small brown granules resembling coffee grounds. Vomiting of blood is one of the chief symptoms of peptic ulcer, but it may also occur in gastritis, especially when this is due to the action of irritant poisons or alcohol, and cancer of the stomach. It should always be remembered that the blood may come from the nose or throat, and, after being swallowed, provoke vomiting. (See HAEMORRHAGE.)

HAEMATOCELE means a cavity containing blood. Generally as the result of an injury which ruptures blood-vessels, blood is effused into one of the natural cavities of the body, or among loose cellular tissue, producing a haematocele.

HAEMATOCOLPOS is the condition in which menstrual blood is held up in the vagina as a result of an imperforate hymen.

HAEMATOCRIT is a graduated capillary tube for estimating the concentration of red corpuscles in the blood. The blood, made non-coagulable, is drawn into the tube; this is placed in a centrifuge and revolved at a speed of 3000 revolutions per minute for 30 minutes. The red corpuscles will then congregate at the end of the tube. Above this will be a clear layer of plasma. Normally, plasma occupies 55 divisions of the tube, and the red corpuscles 45 divisions.

HAEMATOIDIN and HAEMIN are crystalline bodies derived from the blood when it is allowed to clot and dry up. The former is produced where blood is effused in internal haemorrhages and then partly absorbed, for example, in cases of apoplexy. Chemical analysis proves it to be the same substance as bilirubin, the chief colouring matter of the bile. It produces the yellow colour noticed in a bruise as the blood is being absorbed and the bruise fading away. *Haemin* is of great medico-legal importance, because it can be obtained from long-dried stains on clothing, knives, etc., its discovery proving such stains to be due to blood. To obtain it, one scrapes off a few particles of the stain upon a microscopic slide, adds a drop of strong acetic acid, and a small crystal of sodium chloride. The drop is heated until it dries up and then examined under the microscope. Haemin appears as minute, dark brown plates and prisms.

HAEMATOLOGY is the study of diseases of the blood.

HAEMATOMA means a collection of blood forming a definite swelling. It is found often upon the head of new-born children after a protracted and difficult labour. It may occur as the result of any injury or operation.

HAEMATOXYLON, or LOGWOOD, is the wood of *Haematoxylon campechianum*, which is used as a dye in staining tissues in histology. As it has a mildly astringent action, it is used for checking diarrhoea.

HAEMATURIA means the condition of blood in the urine. (See URINE.) The blood may come from any part of the urinary tract. When the blood comes from the kidney or upper part of the urinary tract, it is usually mixed throughout the urine, giving the latter a brownish or smoky tinge. This condition is usually the result of acute or subacute glomerulonephritis, or it may be present in persons suffering from high blood-pressure or pyelitis (qv). Blood may also appear in the urine from time to time in considerable quantites when a stone or gravel is present in the pelvis of the kidney setting up irritation, especially when the person undergoes unwonted exercise. The blood may also originate from the bladder in cases in which this is inflamed, and is then present in smaller quantities as a rule. The presence of a stone in the bladder is also productive of blood, and in either of the latter cases the urine is generally turbid from admixture with pus. A condition which leads to the passage of bright red blood at occasional intervals is the presence of a species of warty growth (papilloma) on the wall of the bladder. Blood may also be derived from the urethra following some inflammatory condition in this passage, or injury to it as by a fracture of the pelvic bones. Occasionally the bleeding may be due to purpura.

The recognition of the site of the haemorrhage is important in relation to the measures to be adopted for its treatment. This can often be made out by the character of the blood, whether intimately mixed with the urine or in the form of clots, also by the shape of the clots, and by the presence of other abnormal constituents in the urine. For the final diagnosis, examination of the interior of the bladder by the cystoscope and the passage of fine catheters up the ureters to the kidneys is often of importance.

HAEMIC MURMUR is a term applied to unusual sounds heard over the heart and large blood-vessels in severe cases of anaemia. They disappear as the condition is recovered from. Murmurs of this type are to be distinguished from 'organic murmurs', which are due to some disease of the heart-valves or vessel walls.

HAEMOCHROMATOSIS, or BRONZED DIABETES, is a disease in which cirrhosis of the liver, enlargement of the spleen, pigmentation of the skin, and diabetes mellitus are associated with the abnormal and excessive deposit in the organs of the body of the iron-containing pigment, haemosiderin.

HAEMOCYTOMETER is an instrument for counting corpuscles in the blood.

HAEMODIALYSIS is the principle used in the artificial kidney (see KIDNEY, ARTIFICIAL), whereby the patient's blood is circulated through a cellophane tube, on the other side of which is a dialysing solution containing electrolytes in the concentration they should be in normal blood, but no urea. In this way the patient's blood is restored to its normal state as it would were it passing through normally functioning kidneys. (See also DIALYSIS.)

HAEMOGLOBIN is the colouring material which produces the red colour of blood. It is a chromoprotein, made up of a protein called globin and the iron-containing pigment, haemin. When separated from the red blood corpuscles, each of which contains about 600 million haemoglobin molecules, it is crystalline in form. It exists in two forms: simple haemoglobin, found in venous blood, and oxyhaemoglobin, which is a loose compound with oxygen, found in arterial blood after the blood has come in contact with the air in the lungs. This oxyhaemoglobin is again broken down as the blood passes through the tissues, which take up the oxygen for their own use. This is the main function of haemoglobin: to act as a carrier of oxygen from the lungs to all the tissues of the body. When the haemoglobin leaves the lungs it is 97 per cent saturated with oxygen. When it comes back to the lungs in the venous blood it is 70 per cent saturated. The oxygen content of 100 millilitres of blood leaving the lungs is 19·5 millilitres, and that of venous blood returning to the lungs is 14·5 millilitres. Thus each 100 millilitres of blood delivers 5 millilitres of oxygen to the tissues of the body. Human male blood contains 13 to 18 grams of haemoglobin per 100 millilitres. In women, there are 12 to 16 grams per 100 millilitres. A man weighing 70 kilograms (154 pounds) has around 770 grams of haemoglobin circulating in his red blood corpuscles.

HAEMOGLOBINOPATHIES: Haemoglobin (qv) is a pigment composed of an iron protoporphyrin complex combined with a protein globin. It is the globin portion which varies in different types of haemoglobin. Impairment of adult haemoglobin formation is the characteristic abnormality of the haemoglobinopathies, which are hereditary haemolytic anaemias, genetically determined and related to race. The haemoglobin may be abnormal because: (1) there is a defect in the synthesis of normal adult haemoglobin and this occurs in thalassaemia when there may be an absence of one or both of the polypeptide chains characteristic of normal adult haemoglobin, or (2) an abnormal form of haemoglobin such as haemoglobin S, that of sickle-cell disease, is formed instead of adult haemoglobin. This abnormality may involve as little as one amino acid of the 300 in the haemoglobin molecule. In sickle-cell haemoglobin one single amino acid molecule, that of glutamic acid, is replaced by another, that of valine, and this results in such a deficient end product that the ensuing disease is frequently rapidly fatal.

HAEMOGLOBINURIA means the presence of blood pigment in the urine caused by the destruction of blood corpuscles in the blood-vessels or in the urinary passages. It produces in the urine a dark red or brown colour. In some people this condition, known as intermittent haemoglobinuria, occurs from time to time, especially on exposure to cold. It is also produced by various poisonous substances taken in the food. It occurs in malarious districts in the form of one of the most fatal forms of malaria: blackwater fever (qv). (See also MARCH HAEMOGLOBINURIA.)

HAEMOLYSIS means the breaking up of blood corpuscles by the action of poisonous substances, usually of a protein nature, circulating in the blood, or by certain chemicals. It occurs, for example, gradually in some forms of anaemia and rapidly in poisoning by snake venom.

HAEMOLYTIC DISEASE OF THE NEWBORN (also known as ERYTHRO-BLASTOSIS FOETALIS and ICTERUS GRAVIS NEONATORUM) is a serious disease of the newborn characterized by severe haemolytic anaemia and jaundice. There is also some oedema, and when this is severe, with excess fluid in the pericardial, pleural, and peritoneal cavities, the condition is known as HYDROPS FOETALIS. The fundamental cause is the haemolysis (or breakdown) of the red blood cells, and this is due to a Rhesus-negative mother bearing a Rhesus-positive child. Such a mother becomes sensitized to the Rhesus-positive factor in her unborn child, thereby producing agglutinins (or antibodies) to it, and these pass through the placenta into the foetus and destroy its red blood cells. (See BLOOD GROUPS.)

Treatment consists of blood transfusion: either a simple transfusion or an exchange transfusion. (See TRANSFUSION OF BLOOD.) The efficacy of treatment is largely dependent upon the awareness of the fact that the baby may be born with haemolytic disease, and that all the necessary steps have been taken to start treatment immediately after birth. This is the reason why so much importance is attached nowadays to the careful blood-grouping of all mothers early in pregnancy. All Rhesus-negative expectant mothers are now given a 'Rhesus card' showing that they belong to the rhesus-negative blood group. This card they should always carry with them. As a result of modern treatment the mortality for this condition has dropped from around 75 per cent to around 5 per cent. The number of stillbirths and infant deaths in England and Wales ascribed to haemolytic disease of the newborn fell from 750 in 1968 to 123 in 1978 and to 12 in 1984.

Two advances have gone far towards reducing the incidence of this disease. One is the method whereby the Rhesus-negative mother can be prevented from developing antibodies should the child she bears be Rhesus-positive. This is done by giving her gamma-globulin (qv) which contains antibodies, or anti-D immunoglobulin as it is known, that will destroy the Rhesus-positive cells from the foetus. Thus these cells are destroyed before they can induce the production of antibodies in the mother's tissues. The injection of gamma-globulin is given within forty-eight hours of delivery as it is usually during delivery that most of the child's cells pass into the mother's bloodstream. The other preventive measure is to give the Rhesus-positive foetus an intra-uterine transfusion of Rhesus-negative blood. In skilled hands this is a perfectly feasible procedure, the blood being injected directly into the peritoneal cavity of the foetus any time from the 20th week onwards.

The current practice in the United Kingdom is that when a woman attends for ante-natal care her blood group is tested. If she is Rh-negative anti-D antibody is then tested. If she has anti-D antibody the foetus, if Rh-positive, is at risk of developing haemolytic disease of the new born and the pregnancy is managed to anticipate this. If the mother has no anti-D antibody she is usually re-tested at 28 and 34 weeks and at delivery. After delivery the baby's blood group is tested. If the baby is Rh-positive the mother is given anti-D immunoglobulin. This should be given for vaginal and Caesarean delivery and for abortion and stillbirth. Significant foeto-maternal transfusion may also occur ante-natally after major abdominal trauma or threatened abortion. Prophylaxis should be given at the time.

HAEMOPHILIA is a hereditary disease, confined almost entirely to males, and characterized by a tendency to uncontrollable haemorrhage even after quite slight wounds. The victims are popularly known as 'bleeders'.

Causes: The defect is in the blood and is one of clotting, or coagulation. The coagulation time may be prolonged up to 12 hours or even longer, compared with a normal of 4 to 10 minutes. The cause of the prolonged coagulation time is deficiency of the antihaemophiliac factor, or Factor VIII as it is known, which is part of the globulin fraction of plasma. The most characteristic feature of the disease is its manner of hereditary transmission, this being through the mother, who is not a bleeder, although her brother may be. In other words, the males of the affected family are bleeders but do not transmit the disease to their male offspring, whilst the females are not bleeders but their male children may be.

The disease occurs predominantly in white races, and it has been estimated that the overall incidence of the disease is 8 per 10,000 of the population, the incidence of severe cases being 3 to 4 per 100,000. Correlated with births, the incidence is thought to be 1 haemophiliac in every 3000 to 4000 live births. There are around 3000 haemophiliacs in Britain. At one time probably only around 10 per cent of bleeders survived beyond puberty. Today advances in treatment have so altered the outlook that few bleeders die of the disease. As a result of this longer survival, the number of bleeders, or haemophiliacs, in the community will steadily rise.

Symptoms: The characteristic feature of haemophilia is the slow, persistent oozing of blood from any wound or injury that, untreated, may go on for hours or even days despite all attempts to stop it by local pressure or by the application of haemostatics (qv). Even when the bleeding does stop, it is liable to start again some days later. On the other hand, contrary to popular belief, superficial cuts and scratches do not cause much trouble with bleeding unless they involve mucous membranes, such as that of the mouth. Neither do haemophiliacs bleed rapidly to death from deep cuts unless, of course, as in the case of non-bleeders, they involve a major artery or vein. One of the major risks a haemophiliac runs is a large haemorrhage into a muscle or joint. Recurrent bleeding into the joints is one of the commonest features of the disease, the symptoms starting as soon as the child begins to walk. By the age of 10 years, 80 per cent of severe haemophiliacs have abnormal joints. This is why it is so important to try and reduce such bleeding into the joints as much as possible and so reduce the amount of crippling. Bleeding from the kidney is quite common, manifesting itself by the passage of blood in the urine. (See HAEMATURIA.)

Treatment: The fundamental treatment of bleeding in a haemophiliac is the intravenous administration of Factor VIII. This is now available in various forms, including fresh frozen plasma, freeze-dried human antihaemophiliac globulin concentrate (AHG),

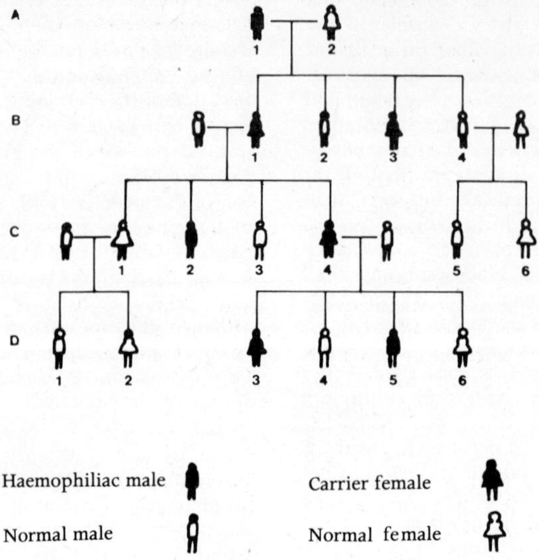

Mode of inheritance of haemophilia. Transmission through an affected male (A,1) and carrier females (B,1 and C,4).

and cryoprecipitate (qv). Cryoprecipitate, which is prepared from human plasma, can be prepared by most blood transfusion centres, and is proving a most useful source of Factor VIII. It will soon be possible to prepare Factor VIII by genetic engineering. If any operation has to be performed on a haemophiliac, even such a minor one as the extraction of a tooth, the patient must be carefully prepared by having adequate amounts of Factor VIII. As always, of course, prevention is better than cure, and, in the case of the teeth, this means that every care should be taken with the teeth of a haemophiliac, whether child or adult, by ensuring that he should see a dentist at regular intervals so that preventive action can be taken that will reduce the possibility of dental extraction to a minimum. To facilitate treatment and ensure that the best possible care is available to every haemophiliac, a National Haemophilia Register has been established in Great Britain, and some thirty Haemophilia Centres have been set up throughout the country where expert treatment can be obtained at any time. Every haemophiliac whose name is on this Register is provided with a card which gives full details about his condition.

It is now realized that the general management of the haemophiliac is just as important as the actual treatment of the bleeding episode. He must be allowed to lead as normal a life as possible, going to an ordinary school and participating in sport. In this last respect, body-contact games such as rugby should be avoided, but there is no reason why a haemophiliac should not go in for cycling, running, or swimming, for instance. In planning such a social life parents and relatives can obtain advice, not only from the Haemophilia Centres, but also from the Haemophilia Society, 123 Westminster Bridge Road, London, SE1 7HR (01–928 2020).

HAEMOPTYSIS means the spitting up of blood from the lower air passages. The blood is usually coughed or gently hawked up, it may be in mouthfuls at a time, and is bright red and frothy, thus differing from the blood brought up from the stomach. Generally the condition results from some disease of the heart or lungs. It should be remembered, however, that in elderly people haemoptysis may be due to a varicose condition of the small veins in the throat, not to haemorrhage in the lungs; while in young people this condition is often due to bleeding from the nose, in which, owing to the position of the head, the blood happens to run backwards instead of forwards through the nostrils. (See HAEMORRHAGE; TUBERCULOSIS.)

HAEMORHEOLOGY is the study of the dynamics of the blood.

HAEMORRHAGE means any escape of blood from the vessels which naturally contain it. It may occur from a wound of the skin, in which case it escapes externally, or into some internal cavity such as the stomach or bowels, or may simply be poured out into the tissues in consequence of a blow or similar injury; but, in all cases alike, the blood escaping from the vessels is lost to the circulation. Haemorrhage is classified according to the vessels from which it occurs, as *(a) arterial*, in which case the blood is bright and appears in jets or spurts, corresponding to the heart-beats; *(b) venous*, when it comes from veins, is dark, and wells up gradually into the wound; *(c) capillary*, when it flows merely from torn capillaries, and comes in a gentle ooze out of the general surface of the wound. The immediate result of a severe haemorrhage is great anaemia, so that in extreme cases the bodily organs may be unable to continue their functions, and the person dies in consequence, with symptoms of shock.

In general, arterial haemorrhage is the most serious, and if a large artery, such as the femoral, is wounded, the person concerned may bleed to death in a few minutes. Venous haemorrhage is so easily checked by slight pressure, and the valves in the veins so effectively prevent blood from running backwards in these vessels, that this form is not dangerous to life except in the case of ruptured varicose veins of the leg, or when a serious internal injury is received. Capillary haemorrhage stops so quickly, that only in the case of the disease known as haemophilia (qv) is it of serious import. The following terms are applied to haemorrhage from special sites: *haematemesis*, bleeding from the stomach; *haemoptysis*, bleeding from the lungs; *epistaxis*, bleeding from the nose; and *haematuria*, bleeding from the kidney or urinary passages. (See these headings.) Haemorrhage is also classed as primary, reactionary, and secondary. (See WOUNDS.)

Natural arrest: When a small artery is cut across, the bleeding stops in consequence of changes in the wall of the artery on the one hand, and in the constitution of the blood on the other. Every artery is surrounded by a fibrous sheath, and when cut, the vessel retracts some little distance within this sheath, in consequence of the shortening of its muscle fibres; and further, by the same process the end contracts so as to form an opening of smaller size than the rest of the vessel. In the space between the end of the vessel and its sheath, and afterwards for some distance up the interior of the narrowed artery, blood-clot quickly forms by the following process, and rapidly blocks the open end of the vessel. When blood is shed so as to come in contact with any surface other than the smooth lining of blood-vessels, the fibrinogen which is dissolved in its fluid becomes converted into threads of fibrin through combination with the lime salts of the blood, and the action of a ferment given off probably by the blood platelets. These threads of fibrin slowly contract and develop into a dense felt-work, in the meshes of which the corpuscles are held, and in this way a blood-clot of increasing hardness is produced, within and round the ends of the injured vessels. When an artery is only partially severed it is evident that contraction and retraction within the sheath cannot take place, and accordingly bleeding is apt to be more serious than when the vessel is completely cut across. Again, if an artery is torn across or twisted instead of cut, the opening at its end is still more narrowed, and the blood clots more rapidly on the ragged surface than it would do upon a clean cut, so that haemorrhage from a torn or bruised wound is in general much smaller in amount than from a stab or cut. The natural arrest of bleeding is usually described therefore as depending upon four factors: *(a)* the retraction, and *(b)* the contraction of the cut artery: *(c)* the external, and *(d)* the internal clot formed by the blood. For the means by which circulation is subsequently carried on after an artery is cut, see ANASTOMOSIS.

Control of external haemorrhage: Four main principles are applicable in the control of a severe external haemorrhage: *(a)* direct pressure on the bleeding point or points; *(b)* elevation of the wounded part; *(c)* pressure on the main artery of supply to the part; and *(d)* application of substances known as styptics, which contract the vessels or aid the coagulation of the blood.

(a) DIRECT PRESSURE may be made with the finger, which is the best method, when a definite bleeding point is seen in a gaping wound. This is the method adopted at an operation by the surgeon, who places his finger at once upon any bleeding point, afterwards seizing the cut artery with forceps and tying a piece of silk or catgut tightly round its end. If the artery lies between the skin and a hard surface, as in the case of scalp wounds, a wedge-shaped pad and tight bandage (known as a graduated compress) may be substituted for pressure with the finger, the edges of the wound being compressed between the pad and skull.

(b) ELEVATION of the bleeding member is an important method, the blood running off more readily by the veins, and a smaller quantity being driven into the limb the higher it is raised. This method is applicable, of course, only in cases of bleeding from the hand or foot.

(c) PRESSURE UPON THE MAIN ARTERY of supply to the injured limb is a certain method of stopping the circulation and consequently all bleeding, much after the manner of stopping the water supply of a district by closing the main pipe. At certain points where the arteries lie close to bones and near the surface, the pulsation of the vessel may be felt, and *pressure with the finger* over the artery serves to obliterate it against the bone, the points where this may be adopted being as follows. In cases of bleeding from the upper part of the scalp, the temporal artery may be felt and compressed immediately in front of the upper part of the ear, while for wounds at the back of the head the occipital artery can be felt and compressed a short distance behind the mastoid process, the bony prominence at the back of the ear.

Bleeding from the face may be checked by pressure on the facial artery, which passes on to the face about 2·5 cm in front of the angle of the jaw, across the jaw-bone, against which it is to be pressed.

All bleeding from the head and neck may be lessened by pressure upon the common carotid artery in the neck a short distance below the prominent Adam's apple, and between it and the edge of the large sternocleidomastoid muscle. In this groove the artery is pressed straight back against the transverse processes of the spinal column.

Bleeding from the region of the shoulder and armpit is checked by pressure on the subclavian artery, the pressure being applied with the thumb directly downwards in the hollow behind the middle part of the collar-bone, so as to press the artery down upon the first rib.

Bleeding from the region of the elbow or forearm may be controlled by feeling for the brachial artery on the inner side of the upper arm, behind the biceps muscle, and pressing it against the humerus.

Bleeding from the hand is checked by pressure on the radial artery, where it lies between the skin and radius in front of the wrist, and on the ulnar artery just before it enters the hand near its inner margin.

In the lower limb the arteries lie deeply among the muscles, but bleeding from any part of the limb may be checked by pressure backwards on the femoral artery, which is to be felt pulsating in the centre of the groin, and which is compressed backwards against the head of the thigh-bone.

Bleeding from the sole of the foot may be controlled by pressure on the posterior tibial artery, which lies about 1·5 cm behind the inner ankle.

A second method for applying pressure on the main artery consists in *forced flexion* at the elbow, hip, or knee, as the case may be. A pad is placed in the bend of the joint, which is then flexed as completely as possible and firmly bound in this position, the artery being thus sharply bent upon itself.

A third method for control of the main blood supply is by the *tourniquet*, which consists of an elastic band or ligature passed round a fleshy part of any of the limbs, and pulled or twisted tight. A surgical tourniquet consists of a rubber cord or band with an arrangement for fixing the ends together, or of a strap with buckle and a screw appliance for tightening it up. A tourniquet may, however, be improvised from a piece of rope, or a handkerchief folded cravatwise, tied round the limb and then twisted up tight by a piece of wood, large key, or similar object introduced beneath it. The handle of such a tourniquet is prevented from untwisting by passing a second band round the limb and including the end of the handle within it before tying. A tourniquet may be applied to the fleshy part of the thigh, leg, upper arm, or forearm. It is most important to note on a label the time of appliction of a tourniquet. No tourniquet should ever be left on longer than an hour. It must be loosened every fifteen minutes, to be tightened again if bleeding restarts. (See TOURNIQUET.)

Occasionally, when bleeding is continuous or when it occurs from a deep-seated wound like a stab, or injury to the root of the tongue, it is impossible to get at the bleeding point, and permanent control of the bleeding is only to be achieved by the surgeon, who cuts down upon the main artery of supply and ties a ligature round it.

(d) STYPTICS are applied when the bleeding is a general ooze from a wound, or when the bleeding comes from an inaccessible position, such as the interior of the nose or a wound in the side. The most important styptics are heat and cold. Although moderate warmth greatly increases bleeding, ice-cold water and also water between 46° and 49° C (115° and 120° F) (ie. a temperature which the hand can hardly bear) both favour clotting and contract the blood-vessels. Heat is much more effectual than cold, if applied directly to the wound. Various drugs, such as perchloride of iron (steel drops) and hazeline, act similarly. Cayenne pepper has a traditional reputation as a styptic in controlling superficial bleeding when applied locally: eg. from a bleeding lip. Adrenaline has a powerful local action in contracting vessels and stopping bleeding. Russell-viper venom is most effective as a local application in cases such as bleeding from a tooth socket. Other styptics include oxidized cellulose, gelatin by-products, calcium alginate, and thrombin powder.

Control of internal haemorrhage is not to be so certainly achieved as in the case of bleeding from the vessels of the limbs. There are certain general principles to which it is most important to adhere. Chief among these is the maintenance of the recumbent position, since the heart beats less forcibly and the blood-pressure is consequently lowered as soon as the injured person lies down. For the same reason, all excitement must be avoided, and the mind of the sufferer quieted as far as possible. The patient must also be kept warm. Stimulants must be avoided. Ice-bags or compresses wrung out of cold water may be laid over the chest or stomach, according to the origin of the haemorrhage. The most valuable drug in the treatment of internal haemorrhage is morphine given hypodermically. In the haemorrhage which sometimes follows child-birth, the source of bleeding is usually the uterus. This is controlled by the injection of ergometrine, the removal of the placenta if this has not already come away, and then compression of the uterus. This may need to be supplemented by plugging of the vagina with sterile gauze.

It should be mentioned that in operations on internal organs or other highly vascular tissue, in the case of which bleeding would be very difficult to stop, the cautery is often used instead of the knife, and not only removes the part desired, but, by its heat, prevents all bleeding.

Treatment of bleeding from special sites:

NOSE: Keep quiet, lying or sitting; loosen collar; no blowing of nose; cold key or sponge to neck; if these are not successful, plugging of nostrils with lint soaked in tincture of perchloride of iron or adrenaline.

TONGUE: Ice to suck; pressure with the fingers; if serious, compression of carotid artery.

FACE OR SCALP: Direct pressure with fingers or bandage and pad on wound; if bleeding be severe, pressure in addition on facial, temporal, or occipital artery.
NECK: Pressure on carotid artery.
ARMPIT OR SHOULDER: Pressure on subclavian artery.
FOREARM: Pressure on brachial artery by fingers, tourniquet, or forced flexion at elbow.
HAND: Elevation and direct pressure with pad and bandage; if bleeding severe, pressure on radial and ulnar arteries, or tourniquet to forearm.
THIGH: Pressure on femoral artery at groin; tourniquet, if low down.
LEG: Tourniquet to thigh, or forced flexion at knee. In the case of ruptured varicose veins, a pad and bandage round leg extending above and below wound with elevation of limb suffice.
FOOT: Direct pressure and elevation; if bleeding severe, forced flexion at knee, or pressure on posterior tibial artery.

HAEMORRHOIDS (see PILES).

HAEMOSTATICS are any means, whether of the nature of mechanical appliances or drugs, used to control bleeding. (See FIBRIN FOAM; HAEMORRHAGE.)

HAEMOTHORAX means an effusion of blood into the pleural cavity.

HAIR DISEASES (see BALDNESS).

HAIR (see SKIN; WHITE HAIR).

HAIR, REMOVAL OF (see DEPILATION).

HALIBUT-LIVER OIL is the oil expressed from fresh, or suitably preserved, halibut liver. It is a particularly rich source of vitamin A (30,000 international units per gram), and also contains vitamin D (2300 to 2500 units per gram). Because of the relatively small volume required, it is often used as a means of giving vitamin D: either as drops of the oil or in capsules. Care must be taken to ensure that the child is receiving at least 700 international units of vitamin D daily. (See VITAMIN.)

HALISTERESIS is the term applied to softening of a bone resulting from the disappearance of lime salts from it.

HALITOSIS is another term for bad breath. (See BREATH, DISORDERS OF.)

HALLUCINATIONS are errors in perception, affecting some sense organ to such an extent that a person imagines he perceives something for which there is no foundation. For example, a person may fancy he hears himself called during perfect stillness, or may see lights in pitch darkness. *Illusions* are misinterpreted sensations: for example, a person may constantly mistake an article of furniture for the figure of some friend, or of an animal. Both these errors occur in sane people, and may indicate some slight brain derangement, due to sleeplessness, overwork, feverishness, or other cause. They are usually, however, a symptom of insanity. (See MENTAL ILLNESS.)

HALLUCINOGENS are compounds characterized by their ability to produce distortions of perception, emotional changes, depersonalization, and a variety of effects on memory and learned behaviour. They include lysergic acid diethylamide (qv) and mescaline (qv). (See also DRUG ADDICTION.)

HALLUX is the anatomical name of the great toe.

HALLUX RIGIDUS is stiffness of the joint between the great toe and the foot which induces pain on walking. It is usually due to a crush injury or stubbing of the toe. Such stubbing is liable to occur in adolescents with a congenitally long toe. If troublesome it is treated by an operation to create a false joint.

HALLUX VALGUS is outward displacement of the great toe and is always associated with a bunion. It is due to the pressure of footwear on an unduly broad foot. In adolescents this broad foot is inherited; in adults it is due to splaying of the foot as a result of loss of muscle tone. The bunion is produced by pressure of the footwear on the protruding base of the toe. In mild cases the wearing of comfortable shoes may be all that is needed. In more severe cases the bunion may need to be removed, while in the most severe the operation of arthroplasty (qv) may be needed. (See also CORNS AND BUNIONS.)

HALO is a coloured circle seen round a bright light in some eye conditions. When accompanied by headache it is specially likely to be caused by glaucoma (qv).

HALOPERIDOL is one of the butyrophenone group of drugs that is proving useful in the treatment of mania and schizophrenic excitement. It is also of value in some cases of stuttering, intractable hiccups and uncontrollable sneezing.

HALOTHANE is a non-inflammable anaesthetic, the chemical formula of which is $CF_3CHClBr$. Patients recover rapidly from its effects.

HAMAMELIS (see WITCH-HAZEL).

HAMARTOMA: These are benign tumours, usually in the lung, containing normal components of pulmonary tissue such as smooth muscle and connective tissue.

HAMMER-TOE is the deformity in which there is permanent flexion, or bending of the middle joint of the toe. The condition may affect all the toes as in claw-foot (qv). More commonly it affects one toe, usually the second. It is due to a relatively long toe and the pressure on it of the footwear. A painful bunion usually develops on it. In mild cases relief is obtained by protecting the toe with adhesive pads. If this does not suffice operation is necessary. (See CORNS AND BUNIONS.)

HAMSTRINGS is the name given to the tendons at the back of the knee, two on the inner side and one on the outer side, which bend this joint. They are attached to the tibia below.

HAND is the section of the upper limb below the wrist. The hand of man is more highly developed in its structure and in its nervous connections than the corresponding part in any other animal. Indeed the possession of a thumb which can be 'opposed' to the other fingers for grasping objects is one of the distinguishing features of the human race. Of all the parts of the body, the hand, which is connected with a large area on the surface of the brain, is capable of the highest degree of education, and in cases in which the brain degenerates, as in general paralysis, the uses of the hand deteriorate particularly early; while in those cases in which part of the brain is destroyed by apoplexy, the hand is apt to suffer more permanently than either face or leg.

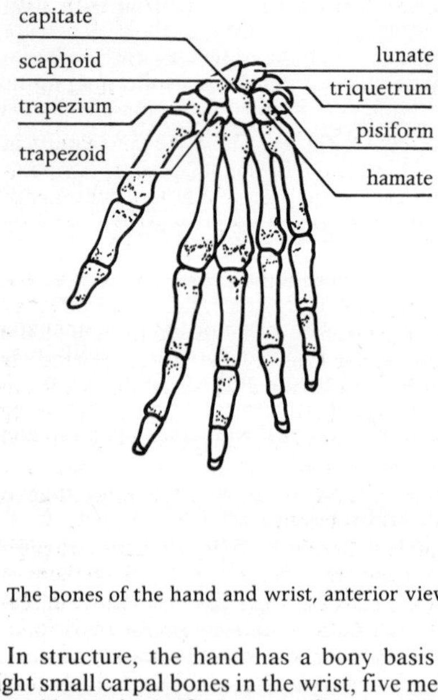

The bones of the hand and wrist, anterior view.

In structure, the hand has a bony basis of eight small carpal bones in the wrist, five metacarpal bones in the fleshy part of the hand, and three phalanges in each finger, two only in the thumb. From the muscles of the forearm twelve strong tendons or sinews run in front of the wrist. Of these, nine go to the fingers and thumb and are bound down by a strong band, the flexor retinaculum, in front of the wrist. They are enclosed in a complicated synovial sheath, and pass through the palm and down the fingers. (See FINGER.) Behind the wrist twelve tendons likewise cross from forearm to hand.

Forming the ball of the thumb and that of the little finger, and filling up the gaps between the metacarpal bones, are other muscles, which act to separate and bring together the fingers, and to bend them at their first joints (knuckles).

Deep in the palm the ulnar artery makes an arch across the hand, giving off branches which run down the sides of the fingers; while the radial artery makes an arch across at a still deeper level, lying in close contact with the bones.

The skin of the hand is richly supplied with nerve filaments, in accordance with its highly specialized sense of touch, the outer three and a half digits being supplied in front by the median, behind by the radial nerve, whilst the inner one and a half fingers have their nerve supply both back and front from the ulnar nerve.

In addition to the diseases mentioned above, certain nervous diseases affect the hand early. Thus in multiple sclerosis and in chorea there are tremors; in alcoholic neuritis and in lead-poisoning, drop-wrist; in progressive muscular atrophy one of the first signs is wasting of the small muscles belonging to the thumb and little finger; in syringomyelia there is loss of sensation for pain and for change of temperature in the fingers.

Deformities of the hand, in the shape of chalk-stones, may occur in gout; rheumatoid arthritis affects the joints of the hand and all too often causes crippling disabilities; and acromegaly is characterized by great enlargement of the hands. Swellings on the back or front of the wrist are usually due to collection of fluid in the tendon sheaths (see GANGLION). Deep abscesses on the front of the fingers are serious, because of the ease with which the infection spreads up the synovial sheaths of the tendons into the palm of the hand. (See WHITLOW.) A condition in which the fingers, especially the ring and little fingers, are gradually flexed up into the palm follows sometimes on a severe strain of the palm or long-continued pressure of a tool. (See DUPUYTREN'S CONTRACTURE.)

Special terms are applied to deformities of the hand. Claw hand (qv) or *main en griffe* is applied to a condition in which the hand is atrophied and the fingers bent in paralysis of the ulnar nerve; cleft hand (qv), or *lobster hand*, is a rare congenital defect characterized by the absence of one or more fingers and a deep central cleft that divides the hand into two; monkey hand or *main en singe* is applied to a condition in which the muscles of the thumb are wasted; obstetrician's hand is a condition in which the thumb and fingers are held together in a kind of cone in tetany and other conditions; and skeleton hand is a condition in which the muscles of the hand are generally wasted, as in progressive muscular atrophy. (See also DROP-WRIST.)

HAND, FOOT AND MOUTH DISEASE is a disease characterized by an eruption of blisters on the palms of the hands, on the feet (often the toes) and in the mouth. It is most common in children and is due to infection with coxsackie A16 virus. The incubation period is three to five days.

HANGING is a form of death due to suspension of the body from the neck, either suddenly, as in judicial hanging, so as to damage the spinal column and cord, or in such a way as to constrict the air passages and the blood-vessls to the brain. Death is, in any case, speedy, resulting in two or three minutes, if not instantaneous, although in bygone days criminals who were shored-up, or supported by their friends, have come round after half-an-hour's suspension. The mark of the noose on the neck is oblique in hanging, which serves to distinguish this form of death from strangling, in which the mark is circular. Apart from judicial hanging, and in the absence of any signs of a struggle, hanging is usually due to suicide. The resuscitation of people found hanging is similar to that for drowning. (See DROWNING.)

HANG-NAIL means a splitting of the skin at the side of the finger-nail. It is often a painful condition and difficult to heal. This is best effected by wearing constantly for several days a wet boric dressing covered by a rubber finger-stall.

HARD METAL DISEASE is a disease that occurs in those involved in tungsten carbide grinding. Tungsten carbide is a hard metal (hence the name of the disease) that has revolutionized metal machining and metal working. It is made from tungsten and carbon with cobalt as a binder. The disease is characterized by cough, expectoration (spitting), shortness of breath and tightness in the chest. In most cases the manifestations of the disease are mild and disappear on withdrawal from exposure to the risk. In some they may be severe enough to involve giving up working with tungsten.

HARDNESS is a term applied to water that contains a large amount of calcium and magnesium salts (lime salts) which form an insoluble curd with soap and thus interfere with the use of the water for purposes of washing. Hard water is especially found in districts where the soil is chalky. Temporary hardness, which is due mainly to the presence of bicarbonates of lime, can be remedied by boiling, when the lime is precipitated as carbonate of lime. Permanent hardness is not remedied by boiling, and is due to the presence of a large amount of sulphate of lime. It may be removed by the addition of sodium carbonate (washing soda) or by the Permutit process which involves the use of various combinations of silicate of alumina and soda. In the past hard water was often blamed for many ills – without any convincing evidence. Today medical statisticians are suggesting that the drinking of soft water may lead to heart disease.

HARE-LIP (see PALATE, MALFORMATIONS OF).

HARTMANN'S SOLUTION is a solution commonly used as a means of fluid replacement in dehydrated patients. Each litre contains 3·1 grams of sodium lactate, 6 grams of sodium chloride, 0·4 gram of potassium chloride, and 0·7 gram of calcium chloride.

HARTSHORN is a popular name for ammonia. (See AMMONIA.)

HARVEST MITE, or HARVEST BUG (see BITES AND STINGS).

HASHIMOTO'S DISEASE is a condition in which the whole of the thyroid gland is diffusely enlarged and firm. It is one of the diseases produced by auto-immunity (qv). The enlargement is due, not to increase of colloid, but to diffuse infiltration of lymphocytes and increase of fibrous tissue. This form of goitre appears in middle-aged women, does not give rise to symptoms of thyrotoxicosis, and tends to produce myxoedema.

HAUNCH-BONE is the bone which encloses the lower part of the abdomen on each side. (See PELVIS.)

HAUSTUS is the Latin word for a draught.

HAVERSIAN CANALS are the fine canals in bone which carry the blood-vessels, lymphatics, and nerves necessary for the maintenance and repair of bone. (See BONE.)

HAY FEVER, otherwise known as SUMMER CATARRH, and in North America as AUTUMN CATARRH, means an allergic condition of the mucous membranes of the eyes, nose, and air passages, which year after year affects certain individuals during the summer and early autumn. It is estimated that around 3,000,000 people in Britain suffer from it, and that 500,000 of these are so severely affected as to need medical treatment.

Causes: Hay fever is an allergic reaction in individuals who are hypersensitive to the pollens of grasses, weeds or trees. This explains the seasonal distribution of the disease. In Britain, where grass pollens are the commonest cause, it occurs from the middle of May to the end of July. In North America it occurs over a longer period: in April and May, due to tree pollens; in June and July, due to grass pollens; in August and September, due to weed pollens. The inhalation of such a pollen to which the individual is hypersensitive results in the production of an excessive amount of histamine (qv) and it is the histamine which is responsible for the manifestations of hay fever.

The tendency to develop hay fever runs in certain families. It is due to the inheritance of a reagin antibody that attaches itself to the mast cells in the mucosa. Exposure to the antigen then results in an immunological reaction on the cell surface with the release of histamine. Only some members of these families will develop hay fever, whilst others may develop other allergic manifestations, such as asthma, eczema, or food allergy.

The age of onset ranges from infancy to the 60's but is most common in late adolescence. Spontaneous cures are not uncommon, but there may be a remission later in life.

Symptoms: The malady recurs with regularity during the summer months in those susceptible to it. It begins with an itching of the eyes and nose, followed by symptoms of a severe cold or influenza, such as headache, violent sneezing, and profuse watery discharge from the eyes and nose, together with dry, hard cough, and occasionally severe asthmatic paroxysms. The attack usually runs a course of several weeks. During rainy weather the symptoms may subside. Susceptible people who move to the seaside early in May, or to a place where vegetation is scanty, rarely suffer.

Treatment: The most effectual method of treatment in hay fever is to avoid the exciting cause, namely, the neighbourhood of grass fields, during the summer season. Removal to the seaside often succeeds in putting an end to an attack. A course of vaccines either immediately before the hay fever season, or spread out over the preceding winter, sometimes provides relief. Of recent years a number of antihistamine preparations (qv) have been produced which practically always bring relief. In those cases in which they fail to give adequate relief, corticosteroids (qv), usually in the form of a spray, may be used for a short period to tide over an emergency: eg. examinations. In cases in which there is some nasal defect, cauterization of the turbinate process or an operation to straighten a distorted nasal septum sometimes helps. If the watering of the eyes is particularly severe, relief may be obtained from the use of eye-drops containing 1 per cent of ephedrine in saline, and sun-glasses should be worn out of doors.

Susceptible people living in the country should sleep with their bedroom windows shut. Ionization of the nasal mucosa with zinc sulphate may help.

1. Never walk through long grass – even after you have had benefit from treatment.
2. During June and July sleep with bedroom windows closed.
3. During June and July do not go for country holidays or outings and do not go camping.
4. During June and July, if you have to travel by train, keep the windows closed.
5. You can only do yourself harm by neglecting these principles.
6. If you have injection treatment for pollen allergy, it is usually necessary for it to be continued for at least 3 years.

Instructions issued by University College Hospital, London, to patients with hay fever.

HAZELINE, or HAMAMELIS WATER, is an extract made from the leaves or bark of *Hamamelis virginiana*, the witch-hazel. It is a useful astringent in checking bleeding and excessive mucous discharges. (See WITCH-HAZEL.)

HEAD (see BRAIN; FACE; SCALP; SKULL).

HEADACHE is very common, but its significance varies tremendously. Thus, at one extreme it may denote the presence of a tumour of the brain or meningitis, whilst at the other extreme it may only be a sign of tiredness. In spite of being such a common finding, the precise mechanism whereby it is produced is still somewhat obscure. The brain itself is insensitive to pain, but the arteries supplying it and the membranes of the brain in relationship to these arteries are sensitive to pain. The general view at the moment is that headache is usually due to dilatation of these arteries or pressure (or traction) on them. This dilatation of the intracranial arteries may be due either to a lesion in the brain or it may be caused reflexly: ie. by a stimulus somewhere else in the body which through the nervous system (often the vagus nerve) causes such dilatation. In other cases the headache arises in the scalp or in the muscles of the back of the neck. The following are some of the more important, or more common, conditions in which headache is present.

ANXIETY: One of the most common forms of headache is that which occurs in individuals when they are worried, anxious, or overworked. In some cases it may be a manifestation of what is known as the anxiety state or of emotional instability, but quite often it occurs in individuals who are emotionally stable. On the other hand, it seldom occurs in the phlegmatic type of person. Manual workers and those who live an out-of-door life seldom complain of headache, and there can be little doubt that the stress and strain under which the modern town-dweller lives have much to do with its incidence. Aggravating factors are inadequate ventilation of offices and excessive smoking. In women it is liable to occur during or shortly before menstruation.

MIGRAINE: This is one of the most characteristic forms of headache. For further details the section on migraine should be consulted.

REFRACTIVE ERRORS OF THE EYE are not as common a cause of headache as is sometimes thought. It occurs in the region of the brow and tends to be worse in the evening, particularly if much reading or close work has been done during the course of the day. It is sometimes accompanied by a sensation of grittiness in the eye. The remedy in such cases is the wearing of spectacles which correct the faulty vision.

INFECTION OF THE SINUSES is a common cause of headache. The location of the pain depends upon which sinus is involved. If the maxillary antrum, which lies in the cheek-bone, is infected, the pain is usually over the cheek, although it may be referred elsewhere in the head. In the case of involvement of the frontal sinuses the pain is over the eyes, whilst in the case of the deeper-lying ethmoidal sinuses the pain appears to be deep-seated behind the eyes. In such cases there is usually a history of a cold in the head followed by a discharge from the nose. The pain is usually worse about midday and tends to wear off towards evening. It is usually made worse by coughing and even sometimes by change of position.

DENTAL SEPSIS: Septic teeth may sometimes be responsible for headache. Usually, of course, there is also the classical toothache, but occasionally the pain of septic teeth is referred to the head.

INDIGESTION AND CONSTIPATION: Any form of dyspepsia due to disordered function of the stomach and which is liable to be accompanied by nausea (ie. a feeling of sickness), may be responsible for headache. On the other hand, individuals with a duodenal ulcer are not particularly liable to headache. Constipation is quite a common cause of headache, especially in children, but the old theory that the headache is due to absorption of toxic material from the gut has now been discarded. The headache is relieved so rapidly by the passing of a stool that it must be due to distension of the lower part of the bowel.

FEVER: Any infection, such as pneumonia or measles, causing a rise in temperature is liable to be accompanied by headache. This is probably due to dilatation of the blood-vessels in the brain resulting from the fever itself and from the infecting organism or its toxins.

URAEMIA: This is the terminal stage of glomerulonephritis (qv) and it is often accompanied by severe headache, which is due partly to the high blood-pressure which is always present and partly to the toxic substances which are retained in the body as a result of the failure of the kidneys.

HIGH BLOOD-PRESSURE: Although many people with a high blood-pressure are not unduly troubled with headache, the headache when it does occur is characteristic. It tends to occur at the back of the head and to be worse in the morning, wearing off during the course of the day.

RHEUMATIC CONDITIONS: Many rheumatic subjects are subject to aches and pains about the head. These are due to rheumatic changes in the muscles of the head and the back of the neck, and can usually be easily recognized by the fact that they are accompanied by tender spots elicited by pressure on the affected parts.

SUNSTROKE AND HEAT-STROKE: Headache is the prominent feature in these conditions, and its occurrence after undue exposure to the sun or to exceptionally hot conditions renders easy its recognition.

DISEASES OF THE BRAIN: Finally, there are the conditions in which a headache indicates the presence of some disturbance or disease of the brain. This may take the form of infections of the brain or its membranes: eg. encephalitis, brain abscess, meningitis. There is seldom any difficulty in determining the presence of these conditions, as there are practically always other signs of involvement of the brain: eg. rigidity of the neck and squint in meningitis. In young children meningitis must always be considered when a febrile illness is accompanied by severe headache. In tumours of the brain severe headache develops sooner or later, but here again there are other manifestations, such as giddiness and apparently causeless vomiting, which indicate the cause of the headache. In middle-aged or old people headache may be due to arteriosclerosis or thrombosis of the arteries in the brain. A relatively uncommon, but very acute, type of headache, usually in the back of the head, is caused by rupture of a small aneurysm (qv) in the circle of Willis, a network of arteries at the base of the brain. Headache is one of the main manifestations of concussion, whether or not this is accompanied by a fractured skull. The persistence of this headache after the individual has otherwise recovered from the concussion is sometimes most troublesome. If the concussion is due to an accident for which the victim considers he should receive compensation, this post-concussion, or post-traumatic, headache is one of the manifestations of a compensation neurosis. Once the case is settled, whether favourably or unfavourably to the claimant matters little, the headache usually clears up.

Treatment: It will be clear from this outline that in the majority of cases the treatment of headache is the treatment of the underlying cause. The main exception to this is migraine (qv). When the headache is associated with anxiety, worry or overwork, the same principle holds true. In these cases there may be an associated general debility, and for this the best remedy is a holiday with complete change of environment, adequate rest, and plenty of good food. If the headache is associated with sleeplessness, the administration of a mild sedative is helpful provided it is not continued indefinitely. Similarly with aspirin; this will relieve many headaches, but its continued use by an increasing number of the population is not in the interest of the health of the community. Used sensibly for short periods aspirin has its uses, but its repeated and continued use is to be deprecated. Local soothing applications to the forehead are often of value in relieving headache. For this purpose there is much to be said for eau-de-Cologne. If the individual is lying down, a moist handkerchief on the forehead is sometimes just as effective.

HEALING (see WOUNDS).

HEALTH: The state of health implies much more than freedom from disease, and good health may be defined as the attainment and maintenance of the highest state of mental and bodily vigour of which any given individual is capable. People vary in the degree of strength and activity which they are capable of attaining. For the maintenance of this individual standard it is essential that each person should recognize his capabilities and limitations, and also that he should be aware of any defects of body or mind to which he is liable, either as the result of heredity or of previous disease. The recognition of, and allowance for, these in the conduct of daily life is of immense importance in maintaining health in other respects. Many people have some inborn hereditary defect or tendency, eg. a neurotic temperament or a liability to disease of some special organ of the body, such as the heart or lungs, and the maintenance of health in such people should be particularly directed towards avoiding conditions which lead to disorders common in their family. (See, for example, HEART DISEASES; HEREDITY; LUNG DISEASES.)

Environment is another matter with an important bearing upon health. This involves such considerations as the choice of an occupation suited to the individual's capabilities and temperament and the avoidance in dangerous occupations of the influences which are specially deleterious to health. (See OCCUPATIONAL DISEASES.) The social surroundings also involved in environment play an important part with many persons in the development of nervous affections. (See NEURASTHENIA.) Speaking generally, it may be said that the majority of people, long before middle life is reached, have contracted some defect of body or constitution arising from their surroundings, and the maintenance of health depends largely upon making appropriate allowance for this.

The preservation of health should begin early in life, and as infants are more prejudicially affected by improper feeding than by any other physical influence, the care of the child in this respect is of the greatest importance. (See INFANT FEEDING.) Equally important is it to nurture the child's emotional development by providing a home in which security and mutual trust and loving kindness are the keynotes. Children display at an early age peculiarities and tendencies which, if unchecked, sometimes develop into undesirable habits, and these form a matter for careful education. (See CHILDREN, PECULIARITIES OF; MENTAL SUBNORMALITY; SCHOOL CHILDREN.)

At a later stage the most important factor in the due care of body and mind consists in attention to the natural functions of the body. Of these, the question of food that is proper in quality and in amount is one of the most important. (See DIET.) Careful attention to the proper care of the teeth (see TEETH, DISEASES OF) is important. In regard to the care of the skin and the maintenance of its functions, see BATHS; SKIN; and CLOTHING. A due maintenance of the relation between the exercise of the body and the amount of rest is of great importance (see EXERCISE; FATIGUE; SLEEP), whilst the correction of bad habits in regard to the posture of the body, especially while at work, is also of importance in maintaining good health. (See CHEST DEVELOPMENT; SPINE, DISEASES OF.) Various habits in regard to eating and drinking, and the practice of smoking, require to be carefully studied in order that due moderation may be exercised. (See ALCOHOL; OBESITY; TOBACCO.)

Despite all the ordinary precautions that may be taken in regard to matters of everyday life, such as those already mentioned, people become, especially in the earlier years of life, exposed to accidents and diseases; these may, however, with care be avoided to a large extent. (See INFECTION; SANITATION.) Certain diseases and influences are particularly liable to affect the health in different parts of the world. (For the influences exerted by climate upon health, see CLIMATE IN RELATION TO DISEASE, and for reference to the diseases which are liable to be contracted by persons in tropical countries, see references under TROPICAL DISEASES.)

All of which may be summed up in seven rules of health prescribed by a team of investigators in the USA:

(1) Do not smoke cigarettes.
(2) Get seven hours of sleep.
(3) Eat breakfast.
(4) Keep your weight down.
(5) Drink moderately.
(6) Exercise daily.
(7) Do not eat between meals.

According to the propagators of these rules, those who follow all seven rules are healthier than those who follow six, six more than five, and so on. Their investigations also showed that the health status of those over the age of 75 who obeyed all the rules was about the same as that of those aged 35–44 who obeyed less than three. Further a person who followed at least six of the rules has an 11-year longer expectancy of life at the age of 45 than someone who has followed less than four.

HEALTH SERVICE SUPERVISORY BOARD (see NATIONAL HEALTH SERVICE).

HEARING (see DEAFNESS; EAR).

HEARING AIDS have been in use for many years. In the pre-electronic era they took the form of horns, ear trumpets, speaking tubes and the like. These acted by collecting the sound waves and reflecting them along a conducting tube to the ear. In other words, they were the equivalent of bringing the speaking voice close to the listener's ear. Such aids had much to be said for them, but today they would be socially unacceptable to the vast majority of the deaf.

Their place has been taken by electronic amplifiers, an adaptation which became a practical proposition when radio valves were developed, though these in turn have been superseded by transistors. Basically an electronic hearing aid consists of three elements: (1) a microphone, (2) an amplifier, (3) a miniature earphone. From the practical point of view there are three basic types of hearing aids. (1) *Body-worn aid*: In this type of aid the microphone and amplifier are housed in a small case worn on the body (eg. in a breast pocket), and the sound receiver is attached to the amplifier by a cord and situated at or near the ear. (2) *Ear-level aid*: This is a very small aid mounted in the vicinity of the ear; often behind the ear, but sometimes mounted in spectacle frames. (3) *Within-the-ear aid*: This is a very small aid mounted, together with the receiver, directly at the outer entrance to the ear.

From the point of view of hearing aids there are two types of hearing loss, or deafness. (1) *Conductive loss* is due to a defect in the conducting mechanism of the ear, usually in the middle ear. This is the type of deafness that responds particularly well to hearing aids, as the actual hearing part of the ear in the inner ear is functioning well, and the amplification produced by the hearing aid compensates almost completely for the defect. (2) *Sensorineural loss* is due to a defect in the mechanism of the inner ear, either the cochlea (see EAR) or the cochlear nerve, and the conducting mechanism is quite satisfactory. This is the type of hearing loss, or deafness, that occurs in old age. The response to hearing aids is not as satisfactory as in the case of conductive hearing loss, but in many it is satisfactory enough to justify the use of hearing aids. Part of the trouble is that the use of a hearing aid does not actually increase the ability of the affected ear to discriminate, but it may improve hearing by bringing the sound into an intensity range where a degree of discrimination is possible. Thus, the deafness sometimes takes the form of inability to recognize the sounds spoken by a very quiet speaker. By amplifying the quiet speaker's voice a hearing aid allows the deaf person to discriminate more words, and thus much of his deaf disability is overcome.

In the planning, and choice, of hearing aids it is too often forgotten that they are needed for old people who, in addition to being deaf, are also suffering from short-sightedness and are not as nimble-fingered as they were in their younger days. This means that the switches and controls on the aid must be easily managed by the elderly, and not too small. The same applies to children. So-called automatic volume control can also be an advantage in these cases as it helps to maintain a steady level without the need to make manual adjustments. With body-worn aids a polished metal case to diminish clothes rustle is helpful. An important practical point is the contact between the ear-piece and the ear. The ear-piece usually consists of a moulded insert made of special plastic resins and moulded for the individual wearer. The insert is drilled and the earphone (receiver) is fitted to it. A snugly fitting insert is essential; otherwise the aid will oscillate, producing an all too familiar howling or whistling sound. This can be a very difficult problem in the case of young children.

One final word of warning is necessary. Modern hearing aids are masterpieces of modern technology, including, as they do, transistors, miniature circuitry and lightweight batteries; and variations of output and response characteristics, as well as automatic volume control, are provided in many of them. Fundamentally, however, these requirements are relatively marginal benefits, which are only of real value to a minority of more sophisticated individuals. To the generality of elderly who provide so many of the deaf people in our midst, what is required, as has already been noted, is the less sophisticated, more robust, easily managed hearing aid, an essential element of which is ample power output. In making a choice therefore from the large range of effective hearing aids now available, including the Medresco hearing aid supplied under the National Health Service, the expert advice of an ear specialist must be obtained. The Royal National Institute for the Deaf, 105 Gower Street, London, WC1E 6AH, provides a list of clinics where such a specialist can be consulted. It also gives reliable advice concerning the purchase and use of hearing aids.

A behind-the-ear hearing aid weighing 7·65 grams (about ¼ounce) is now available under the National Health Service for all who will benefit from it.

HEART is a hollow muscular pump with four cavities, each provided at its outlet with a valve, whose function is to maintain the circulation of the blood. The two upper cavities are known as atria, the two lower ones as ventricles. The term auricle is applied to the ear-shaped tip of the atrium on each side.

Position: The heart lies in the chest between the two lungs, but projecting more to the left side than to the right. On the left side its apex reaches out in the adult between 8 and 9 cm (3½and 4 inches), almost to the nipple, and lies beneath the fifth rib, while its right border extends only a short distance, at most 2·4 cm, beyond the margin of the breast-bone. Its lower border rests upon the diaphragm, by which it is separated from the liver and stomach, and this close connection has an important influence upon the heart in several disorders of the stomach. Above, the heart extends to the level of the second rib, where the great vessels, the aorta on the right side and the pulmonary artery on the left, lie behind the breast-bone.

Shape and size: The heart of any individual was described by Laennec as, roughly, of the size and shape of the clenched fist. Its weight in the male varies from 280 to 340 grams, and in the female from 230 to 280 grams. It continues to increase in weight and size up to a ripe old age, more so in men than in women. One end of the heart is pointed (apex), the other is broad (base), and is deeply cleft at the division between the two atria. One groove running down the front and up the back shows the division between the two ventricles; a circular, deeper groove marks off the atria above from the ventricles below. The capacity of each cavity is somewhere between 90 and 180 ml.

Structure: The heart lies within a strong fibrous bag, known as the pericardium, and since the inner surface of this bag and the outer surface of the heart are both covered with a smooth, glistening membrane faced with flat cells and lubricated by a little serous fluid (around 20 millilitres), the movements of the heart are accomplished almost without friction. The main thickness of the heart wall consists of bundles of muscle fibres, which run, some in circles right round the heart, others in loops, first round one cavity, then round the corresponding cavity of the other side. Within all the cavities is a smooth lining membrane, continuous with that lining the vessels which open into the heart. The investing smooth membrane is known as epicardium, the muscular substance as myocardium, and the smooth lining membrane as endocardium.

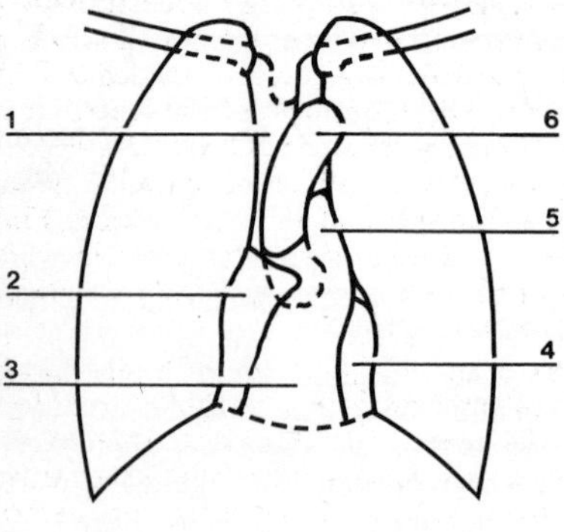

1 superior vena cava
2 right atrium
3 right ventricle
4 left ventricle
5 pulmonary artery
6 aorta

Diagram of the heart as seen using X-rays.

For the regulation of the heart's action there are important nervous connections, especially with the vagus nerve and with the sympathetic system. In the hinder part of the atria lies a collection of nerve cells and connecting fibres, known as the sinuatrial node, which forms the starting-point for the impulses that initiate the beats of the heart. Hence its alternative name of the pacemaker of the heart. In the groove between the ventricles and the atria lies another collection of similar nerve tissue, known as the atrioventricular node. From it there runs downwards into the septum between the two ventricles a band of special muscle fibres, known as the atrioventricular bundle, or the bundle of His. This splits up into a right and a left branch for the two ventricles, and the fibres of these distribute themselves throughout the muscular wall of the ventricles and control their contraction.

Openings: There is no direct communication between the cavities on the right side and those on the left; but the right atrium opens into the right ventricle by a large circular opening, and similarly the left atrium into the left ventricle. Into the right atrium open two large veins, the superior and inferior venae cavae, with some smaller veins from the wall of the heart itself, and into the left atrium open two pulmonary veins from each lung. One opening leads out of each ventricle, to the aorta in the case of the left ventricle, to the pulmonary artery from the right.

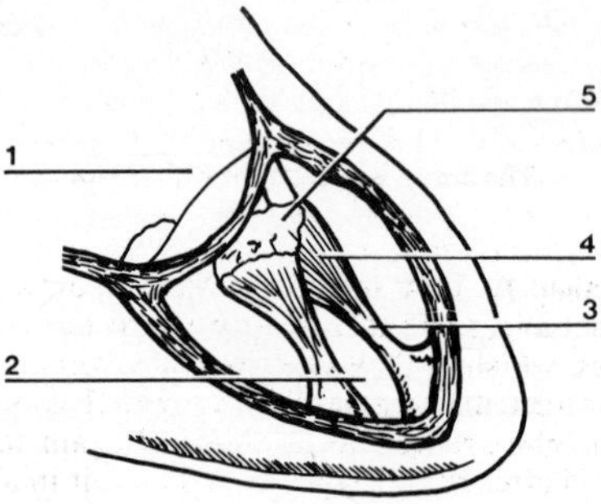

1 left atrium
2 left ventricle
3 papillary muscle
4 chordae tendinae
5 mitral valve, anterior cusp

Interior of the left ventricle, showing structure of mitral valve.

Prior to birth there is an opening (*foramen ovale*) from the right into the left atrium through which the blood passes; but when the child first draws air into his lungs this opening closes and is represented in the adult only by a depression (*fossa ovalis*).

Valves: As stated above, there are four valves. The mitral valve consists of two triangular cusps, the tricuspid valve of three smaller cusps. The aortic and pulmonary valves each consist of three semilunar-shaped segments. The structure of a valve is a double layer of the lining membrane of the heart (endocardium) strengthened by fibrous tissue between. Two valves are placed at the openings leading from atrium into ventricle, the tricuspid valve on the right side, the mitral valve on the left, so as completely to prevent blood from running back into the atrium when the ventricle contracts. Two more, the pulmonary valve and the aortic valve, are at the entrance to these arteries, and prevent regurgitation into the ventricles of blood which has been driven from them into the arteries. The noises made by these valves in closing constitute the greater part of what are known as the heart sounds, and can be heard by anyone who applies his ear to the front of a person's chest. Murmurs heard accompanying these sounds indicate defects in the valves, and form one of the chief signs of heart disease.

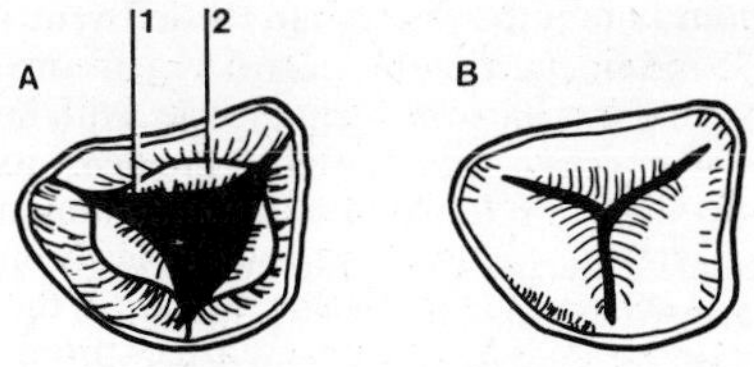

1 cavity of left ventricle
2 valve cusp

The aortic valve: (A) open, (B) closed.

Action: At each heart-beat the two atria contract and expel their contents into the ventricles, which at the same time they stimulate to contract together, so that the blood is driven into the arteries, to be returned again to the atria after having completed a circuit in about fifteen seconds through the body or lungs as the case may be. The heart beats from sixty to ninety times a minute, the rate in any given healthy person being about four times that of the respirations. The heart is to some extent regulated by a nerve centre in the medulla, closely connected with those centres which govern the lungs and stomach, and nerve fibres pass to it in the vagus nerve. By some of these fibres its rate and force can be diminished, by others increased, according to the needs of the various organs of the body. If this nerve centre is injured or poisoned, for example, by lack of oxygen, the heart stops beating in human beings, although in some of the lower animals – eg. frogs, fishes, and reptiles – the heart may under favourable conditions go on beating for hours even after its entire removal from the body.

HEARTBURN means a burning sensation experienced in the region of the heart and up the back to the throat. It is caused by an excessive acidity of the gastric juice, and is relieved temporarily by taking alkaline substances, such as 1 · 2 grams of bicarbonate of soda or a similar amount of bismuth carbonate or carbonate of magnesia in water. It is also relieved by the chewing of aluminium-containing antacid tablets such as Aluminium Hydroxide Tablets, BP.

HEART DISEASES belong to that class of diseases which can be recognized only by the trained observer, although their presence may occasion severe symptoms and evident signs of general illness perceptible to every one. Their treatment, and a true appreciation of their slightness or gravity, belong still more to the specialist.

Varieties: Many general diseases affect the heart; but, considering the arduous work which this organ constantly performs (see EXERCISE), and the fact that it never rests completely from the time of its formation till death ensues, it is subject to wonderfully few disorders. Its diseases are classified according to the part of the heart affected, or the nature of the changes produced. *Inflammatory affections* are divided into pericarditis, myocarditis, and endocarditis, according as the pericardium or enveloping membrane, the myocardium or muscular substance, and the endocardium or lining membrane is affected. *Valvular diseases* form one of the most important groups; any of the four valves may be stenosed: ie. the aperture between its flaps narrowed, or a valve may be incompetent, so that some blood leaks back through the opening in the wrong direction. *Hypertrophy*, in which the heart is enlarged and its wall thickened, and *dilatation*, in which one or more of the cavities is dilated, form another group often associated with the valvular diseases. *Degeneration* of the muscular tissue, producing enfeeblement of the heart's action, may occur usually as a result of inadequate blood supply to the heart muscle. Then there is a class of disorders characterized by *disturbances of rhythm*, such as palpitation, irregularity, rapidity, or slowness, of the heart action. Finally, there is *congenital heart disease*, in which a child is born with a malformed heart. (See also CARDIOMYOPATHY.)

Causes: In 1984, what are officially known as 'circulatory diseases' accounted for more than 40 per cent of all deaths in England. Circulatory diseases include diseases of the heart and of the blood-vessels. In this group, by far the commonest cause of death was ischaemic heart disease, or coronary artery heart disease, which was responsible for more than one-quarter of all deaths in that year. Deaths from ischaemic heart disease numbered 158,667 in 1986.

The main causes of heart disease are disease of the coronary arteries, the arteries which nourish the heart muscle (see CORONARY THROMBOSIS), and high blood-pressure, followed by acute rheumatism, and syphilis. One of the most important causes of coronary artery disease is cigarette smoking. The Royal College of Physicians in its report 'Smoking For Health' (1983) stated that 30 per cent of heart disease deaths are attributable to smoking. The United States Surgeon General in 1983, stated that cigarette smoking is the most important of the known modifiable risk factors for coronary artery disease. Acute rheumatism is predominantly a disease of childhood, and most cases of heart disease occurring between the ages of 5 and 40 years of age are of rheumatic origin. High blood-pressure and coronary-artery disease are predominantly diseases of middle age, and their incidence has increased markedly during the last fifty years. Syphilitic heart disease also occurs in later life as a result of infection acquired during early adult life.

Other causes of heart disease include diphtheria, disease of the thyroid gland (thyrotoxicosis), and certain chronic forms of disease of the lungs. A small, but important group of cases of heart disease are those due to congenital abnormalities of the heart: ie. developmental errors in the heart which occur before the birth of the child. These account for 1 to 2 per cent of all cases of organic heart disease. Certain deficiency diseases involve the heart, particularly gross deficiency of vitamin B_1, which causes the condition known as beri-beri (qv).

General Symptoms: The heart possesses a remarkable power, known as compensation, by which it adapts itself to new conditions. Thus if a person takes up some more arduous employment than usual the heart beats more powerfully and becomes larger, in order to overtake the extra strain; and, in a similar way, disease in one part of the organ, such as a valve, may be so compensated that not only do no symptoms arise, but the person may pass through a long life without suspecting the existence of any such defect. The establishment of this compensation is one of the chief objects of the gradual training which is necessary before undertaking any strenuous athletic exercise. It is a common mistake to suppose that disease of the heart ends always in sudden death, for only disease of the aortic valve and coronary-artery disease are associated with this accident, which even in these conditions is infrequent. If, however, the defect is so great that it cannot be remedied by compensation, or if general ill-health or the debility of age come on, the pumping power of the heart weakens and symptoms appear, some of which are referable to the organs in which the circulation is defective, others, like pain and palpitation, to the heart itself. For example, breathlessness and lividity are due to bad circulation in the lungs; faintness and giddiness to want of blood in the brain; dyspepsia, swelling of the abdomen, and oedema of the feet, to impeded circulation in the veins of the lower part of the body.

PERICARDITIS is an inflammation of the membrane covering the exterior of the heart. It may be dry, in which case the two opposing surfaces of the membrane are covered by a layer of fibrin (qv) worked up by the movements of the heart into ridges; or effusion may accompany this condition, when the pericardial bag becomes much distended by fluid. The causes include a virus infection (the condition known as acute benign pericarditis); rheumatic fever; uraemia; tuberculosis; spread of infection from the lungs, as in pneumonia, though this is remarkably rare considering the close relationship between the lungs and the heart; injury to the chest; any acute infection in the body, such as septicaemia; neoplasm. Pericarditis with effusion generally follows the dry form, unless the latter is very slight in extent, and the amount of fluid may reach as much as one litre (2 pints). If the amount of fluid becomes excessive it may so compress the heart as to produce the condition known as cardiac tamponade. This is a dangerous condition characterized by a rapid, weak pulse and a low blood-pressure. Pain over the heart, high fever, rapid and feeble pulse, restlessness and difficulty in breathing, mark the presence of this serious condition.

The characteristic finding in dry pericarditis is the appearance of a friction, or superficial scraping, sound on auscultation (qv) over the heart.

Treatment during the acute stage, apart from treatment of the underlying infection by an antibiotic, consists of rest in bed, good nursing, and the relief of pain should this be present. Occasionally it becomes necessary to tap the pericardial cavity and draw off some of the fluid which is embarrassing the heart's action.

ENDOCARDITIS is an inflammatory condition of the membrane lining the heart, and since the part most subjected to friction and strain is that covering the valves, so these valves are the most commonly affected parts, those on the left side of the heart being affected much more often than those on the right side. The inflammatory process consists in the appearance of small groups of nodules upon the valves. These unite to form wart-like growths, upon which fibrin is deposited from the blood to form pendants, often of some length. The condition just described is known as simple endocarditis, and occurs most commonly in connection with rheumatic fever in childhood. Tonsillitis and scarlet fever may also be complicated by simple endocarditis. Simple endocarditis arises especially in those cases of rheumatic fever which are not allowed to rest during the attack, and although the endocarditis may give no symptom of its presence, it may leave the heart with serious valvular disease. Palpitation and a slight increase of temperature may often form the only warning of the onset of endocarditis during an attack of rheumatic fever.

Another form of endocarditis is known as bacterial, or infective, endocarditis. In 40 per cent of cases there is a previous history of rheumatism or chorea, whilst in 15 per cent of cases it is superimposed on a congenitally deformed valve. It has declined in incidence in young people, associated with the decrease in rheumatic heart disease, but there has been an increase among older people with degenerative disease of the aortic valve. The annual incidence in England and Wales is 19 per million, with a mortality of 30 per cent, depending upon the causative micro-organism. When this is *Streptococcus viridans*, the mortality may be as low as 10 per cent. The essential feature is a progressive microbic infection of the heart valves or the endocardium of the heart wall. It is of much more serious import than the simple type, since fragments of the ulcerating valves may be carried by the blood-stream all over the body and set up abscesses in diverse organs, this form at one time resulting almost always in death. There is, however, no hard and fast dividing line between simple and ulcerative endocarditis, and various grades of intermediate severity are found. Treatment consists of full doses of an antibiotic to which the causative micro-organism is sensitive – usually one of the penicillins.

CHRONIC VALVULAR DISEASES form the most common and most important group of heart disorders. Although, in consequence of the power of compensation the heart may become more powerful and so neutralize the ill-effects of a narrowed or leaking valve, it is not possible to predict how far this change will be affected by ill-health or the strain of a laborious life, and consequently the detection of valvular disease may render a person unfit for public service, and renders him subject, if he becomes a candidate for life assurance, either to refusal or to a heavily increased premium. The commonest cause of valvular disease is rheumatic endocarditis, which, instead of passing off with the disease that produced it, has become chronic, leading ultimately either to thickening and contraction of the valves, so that they become unable to close their respective openings, or to adhesion of the segments of the valves to one another at their margins, so that the opening is very much narrowed. The former condition is known as incompetence, the latter as stenosis, and the two are found either separately, or together affecting the same valve. The valves on the left side of the heart are more often affected than those on the right side, in the proportion of about 18 to 1.

AORTIC DISEASE: Of all the valvular defects, incompetence of the aortic valve is the most serious, and next to it in importance comes stenosis of the mitral opening. Aortic incompetence leads to hypertrophy of the heart. Although aortic disease in young people follows upon rheumatic endocarditis, and may produce a rapidly fatal issue, on the other hand it may give rise to few symptoms directly referable to the heart until later in life. Stenosis at the aortic valve is much rarer than incompetence and is due either to rheumatic endocarditis or a congenital lesion. Syphilis is especially apt to lead to a degenerative and hardened condition of the aortic valve, which renders it incompetent. Angina pectoris is not infrequently associated with this condition, in consequence of the spread of the degenerative process to the coronary arteries which supply the muscle of the heart itself with blood. (See ANGINA PECTORIS.) When compensation begins to fail, throbbing of the arteries becomes very noticeable, and headache, giddiness, faintness on rising quickly, and dull pain about the heart appear. Later, shortness of breath causing inability to lie down, and oedema of the feet and legs appear. Sudden death may occur in a case of aortic stenosis, but death may also come on gradually, ushered in by increasing oedema, great difficulty of breathing, and mental excitability.

MITRAL DISEASE is of two types. In one case the valve itself is at fault, owing almost always to endocarditis, which produces incompetence, or stenosis, or both. In the other, the left ventricle is dilated so that the two segments of the valve are held apart by their attachments to its walls, and consequently a state of temporary, secondary, or functional incompetence is produced. It is of great importance to recognize this distinction, because, whilst the former is permanent and organic, the latter, which is due to weakness of the heart muscle, as a result, for instance, of an acute infection such as diphtheria, or anaemia, may end in complete recovery. Mitral incompetence unaccompanied by stenosis may be of relatively little importance, and people with this defect sometimes live to an advanced age. In defects of this valve, the symptoms relate chiefly to the lungs, breathlessness on exertion being one of the most common, and the lips and ears becoming of a bluish tint, in consequence of the slow passage of blood through the lungs. Bronchitis and spitting of blood are common, particularly in cases in which stenosis is present. When compensation is failing, these symptoms become more marked, the liver and stomach get congested, producing a jaundiced tint of the skin, together with dyspepsia, and congestion of the kidneys develops, shown by the presence of albumin in the urine. All these symptoms pass off under treatment, to be renewed again and again at intervals. When the valve is stenosed, there is a tendency to the formation of small clots in the atrium; these may be carried away and lodged in various organs: eg. in the brain, causing apoplexy. Sudden death in mitral disease is rare. Cases of mitral disease, and especially cases in which marked stenosis is present, are often, as time goes on, associated with a state of dilatation of the atria, and the condition of disordered action in these cavities is known as atrial fibrillation. This leads to great irregularity in the time and force of the heart-beats, with corresponding irregularity felt in the pulse.

ENLARGEMENT OF THE HEART is of two types: HYPERTROPHY of the walls, and DILATATION of the walls. The first takes place as the result of simple, constant strain, as in professional runners and other athletes. It also arises from the increased difficulty in the circulation that results from a diseased valve, and it produces compensation of the valvular disease. It also occurs in consequence of high blood-pressure. To this extent, and while general health lasts, hypertrophy is an altogether good thing, the only sign of its presence being a large heart with an extra-powerful beat. But in the later years of life there is a special tendency for the muscle of these hypertrophied hearts to degenerate. DILATATION of the heart, with thinning of its walls, is always a bad thing, leading to feeble action of the organ. It occurs also as the result of strain when the heart has not sufficient reserve force to hypertrophy. Sometimes it occurs suddenly, the heart becomes unable to contract upon the blood which accumulates in it, and death results in a few minutes or hours, in consequence of some extraordinary effort by a feeble person, or in consequence of injudicious exercise too soon during convalescence from a fever.

Treatment is much the same as for valvular heart disease where compensation is failing.

DEGENERATION OF THE HEART occurs principally in old people, the most common form being a change of the muscle fibres, in scattered patches, into fat. In another form of degeneration a deposition of fibrous tissue gradually takes place between the muscle fibres, which at the same time waste away. Less common forms of degeneration consist in a granular change in the fibres, producing great softening in the course of some fatal fevers; and a condition known as brown atrophy, in which the heart-muscle wastes as old age advances, and contains much brown pigment.

DISEASE OF THE VALVES ON THE RIGHT SIDE is relatively rare. The tricuspid valve may be incompetent in consequence of far advanced mitral disease, which increases the difficulty of circulation through the lungs and so leads to dilatation of the right side of the heart. Stenosis of the pulmonary valve sometimes forms a congenital condition in children.

Treatment of valvular diseases: When a valvular defect is accidentally discovered, even though it be perfectly compensated and give rise to no symptoms, it is well that the person should take certain precautions in his daily life, and he should therefore, unless of a particularly nervous and highly strung temperament, be informed by his medical adviser of the condition found in his heart. When compensation begins to fail, and this is usually manifest by increasing exertional dyspnoea and peripheral oedema, the physical activity of the patient must be reduced. Treatment with diuretics will also be required (see DIURETICS). If the patient is in atrial fibrillation control of the ventricular rate by Digoxin is indicated. There are now many surgical procedures available for the correction of stenosed or incompetent valves. When all else fails heart transplantation may be indicated.

FATTY DEGENERATION: In stout people a deposit of fat takes place upon the heart (fatty infiltration), interfering with its action and causing shortness of breath upon slight exertion, but this is not so serious as true degeneration, in which the change involves a gradual destruction of the actual muscle. Fatty degeneration arises as a senile change, most commonly in people addicted to alcohol, in whom it may appear early in middle life; and also as a sequence to hypertrophy of the heart. In general, in devitalizing diseases, or when the coronary arteries, which supply the heart itself with blood, are narrowed by disease, fatty degeneration of the heart-muscle is common. It may come on acutely in infective diseases like pneumonia or influenza. If it comes on gradually, it causes attacks of pain in the centre of the chest and left arm (see ANGINA PECTORIS), with great irregularity and palpitation of the heart on exertion. Unusual torpor in the early part of the day following on very slight exertion, is also a sign of its presence. Other symptoms are occasional fainting fits and great loss of mental activity, and there is a special danger of sudden death in people affected by this degenerative process.

FIBROID DEGENERATION of the muscular wall of the heart is usually a result of gradual and extensive blocking in branches of the coronary arteries, due to patches of atheromatous thickening in their walls. The muscle fibres waste or die in patches as a result of defective nourishment, and are replaced by useless fibrous tissue. Dilatation of the cavities, clotting of the blood on the fibroid patches, followed, it may be, by angina pectoris or by sudden death, take place. This condition of the heart is often associated with advanced disease in the kidneys. The symptoms are much the same as those due to fatty degeneration. In the treatment, the same drugs are used as for valvular disease, though more sparingly. Careful regulation of daily life with simple diet is of great importance. The person should beware of any excessive physical strain.

CORONARY ARTERY DISEASE, or ISCHAEMIC HEART DISEASE: This is the most important form of heart disease at the present day because it is the most killing. (See CORONARY THROMBOSIS; ANGINA PECTORIS.)

DISTURBANCES OF RHYTHM: Several varieties of abnormal action of the heart are recognized. Some of these are due to a definite organic disease of the heart, but in many there is no discoverable disease, and the abnormal action is then described as of functional nature. Some of these conditions are due to disease affecting the mechanism in the heart which controls the regular sequence of contraction of the different cavities, but such disease is only recognizable during life by the abnormal action which it sets up.

Many troublesome irregularities of the heart are now known to be caused by defective action of the conduction mechanism. The site of these defects can be analysed by means of elaborate modern instruments. Of these the chief is the *electrocardiograph* (qv), which by means of a galvanometer registers photographically the electrical changes that take place as the heart beats.

The heart-muscle has in itself, independently of nervous control, the power of contracting rhythmically when excited to do so, of conducting the impulse to contract from one part of the muscle to another, and of maintaining itself in a moderate state of tension or tone. When any of these properties is affected by disease some change in the force or rhythm of the heart-beat is apt to appear.

PALPITATION is a condition in which the heart beats fast and the person becomes conscious of its beating. (See PALPITATION.)

SINUS ARRHYTHMIA is a condition of irregular action in which the heart speeds up during inspiration and slows again during expiration. It is a normal phenomenon, but may occasionally be so accentuated that the individual becomes aware of it, when it may give rise to anxiety.

ATRIAL (or AURICULAR) FIBRILLATION is the commonest form of persistent irregularity of the heart's action, accounting for about one-half of all the cases of irregular pulse. It may be due to ischaemic or hypertensive heart disease, or disease of the mitral valve, and is recognized by great irregularity in time and force of the pulse (what has been described as an 'irregular irregularity'). In this type of irregularity the atria do not empty themselves by the normal regular waves but shiver, and in consequence the ventricles do not receive the normal rhythmic stimulus to contract, and they accordingly contract irregularly. This is a serious irregularity.

EXTRASYSTOLES form a common cause of irregular action in irritable states of the heart; the extrasystole is a premature beat followed by a pause of the heart for rest. This is not a serious form of disorder, and it may come and go for many years in certain individuals.

HEART-BLOCK is a serious condition in which the conducting mechanism between atrium and ventricle is impaired (incomplete heart-block), or destroyed (complete heart-block) so that the atrium and ventricle beat at different rates independently of one another. During the incomplete stage the pulse is irregular, but when the heart-block becomes complete and the ventricles contract independently of the atria, the pulse becomes regular and very slow, and the individual is liable to fainting or convulsive attacks (Stokes-Adams attacks). (See also CARDIAC PACEMAKER.)

PULSUS ALTERNANS, or ALTERNATING PULSE, is a condition in which there are regularly alternating strong and weak beats of the heart, forming a persistent type of irregularity, which is caused by degeneration of the heart-muscle. It is of serious import.

RAPID HEART (*tachycardia*) with a pulse considerably above 100 per minute is found in a large variety of conditions. In its most benign form it may be due to emotional disturbance, whether excitement, fear, or pleasure. In other cases it may be due to overactivity of the thyroid gland as in thyrotoxicosis (qv). A more common cause is fever. A rise in temperature is always accompanied by a rise in heart rate. The most common cause of all is a failing heart.

SLOW HEART (*bradycardia*) is a natural phenomenon in some individuals, the heart beating only forty, fifty, or sixty times per minute instead of the normal seventy or eighty times. Slowness of the heart-beat is also a character of complete heart-block.

CONGENITAL HEART DISEASE accounts for 1 to 2 per cent of all cases of organic heart disease. Its incidence is 6 to 7 per 1000 live births. The cause is variable. In a small minority of cases it is hereditary, but in the majority it is due to some illness of the mother, such as German measles, or some other adverse factor, such as certain drugs, affecting her during the early period of pregnancy. The abnormality may take almost an infinite variety of forms, such as an abnormality of the valves of the heart, the heart lying on the right side of the chest instead of the left, a patent ductus arteriosus (see DUCTUS ARTERIOSUS), a defect in the septum separating the chambers of the heart, or coarctation of the aorta (qv). These last three have become of great interest in recent years, in view of the satisfactory results which have been obtained with surgical treatment.

HEAT: (see also BURNS; HEAT-STROKE.) The curative uses of heat as applied by hot water and hot air are mentioned under BATHS. Hot-air applications are much used in the treatment of rheumatic conditions in the joints and muscles, and a more powerful application of heat for the same purpose is obtained by the use of high frequency electricity. (See DIATHERMY.) Excessive heat, in the form of the cautery, is also used in order to destroy diseased tissues. (See CAUSTICS AND CAUTERIES.)

HEAT-CRAMPS are painful cramps in the muscles occurring in workers, such as stokers, who labour in hot conditions. The cramps are the result of loss of salt in the sweat, and can be cured by giving salty water to drink. (See HEAT-STROKE.)

HEATING: People vary tremendously in what they consider to be a comfortable temperature in which to sit or do sedentary work, and this individual reaction is partly dependent upon other factors such as the efficiency of the ventilation of the room. Thus, by and large, a stuffy room will tend to feel uncomfortably hot to many people even though the temperature may be within the recognized limits of comfort. These levels are usually taken to be 15·5° to 19·8°C (60° to 65°F). In nurseries, sick-rooms and rooms for old people a higher range of 18·3° to 21°C (65° to 70°F) is usually aimed at.

HEAT SPOTS is a vague term applied to small inflamed and congested areas which appear especially upon the skin of the face, neck, and chest or other parts of the body in warm weather.

HEAT-STROKE is the term applied to the effects produced on the body by exposure to excessive heat. Although most commonly observed in tropical regions, it may occur also in temperate climates during hot weather. A moist condition of the atmosphere, which interferes with cooling of the overheated body, greatly increases the liability to suffer from this ailment.

Causes: The fundamental cause of the condition is exposure of the body to amounts of radiant energy for which it cannot compensate. This inability to compensate for excessive exposure to heat results in overheating of the body and loss of fluid. In any given case one or other of these factors, or both, may come into play (see table below). In the more acute cases the condition is characterized by failure of the sweating mechanism: these are the cases which are rapidly fatal unless treatment is instituted immediately. When excessive sweating occurs, in the early stages this loss of fluid is accompanied by a corresponding loss of salt (sodium chloride), resulting in a disturbance of the electrolyte balance of the body fluids. Unless this loss of water and sodium chloride is compensated for, one of three things may occur: (i) the individual may be seized with severe cramp in the muscles: ie. heat cramps; (ii) the blood volume is diminished and the circulation of the body is seriously disturbed, resulting in a condition analogous to surgical shock; (iii) the sweating mechanism may break down, with resultant further rise in the temperature of the body, leading to a fatal termination.

Dilatation of blood-vessels of skin
Sweating
Dilution of blood
Decreased muscle tone
Inclination to reduced activity
Stretching, or extension, of body to increase loss of heat
Decrease in volume of urine
Thirst
Loss of chloride leading to heat-cramps
Difficulty in maintaining blood supply to brain, leading to dizziness, nausea and heat-exhaustion
Rising body temperature
Impairment of heat-regulating centre in brain
Cessation of breathing

Effects of exposure to high temperatures.

Predisposing factors are bad living or working conditions, lack of acclimatization to tropical conditions, unsuitable clothing, poor health, and dietetic and alcoholic indiscretions.

Symptoms: The symptoms, which obviously depend upon the disorganization of the normal heat-regulating mechanism as well as of the functions of circulation and respiration, vary in their intensity and to some extent in their form. Four chief types of the disease are usually described.

(1) HEAT COLLAPSE: This is the mildest form of the condition. It is characterized by fatigue, giddiness, and temporary loss of consciousness. The blood-pressure is low and the pulse is slow. In the more severe cases there is a state of collapse, with cold, clammy skin and a subnormal temperature. Vomiting is not uncommon and there may be muscular cramps. The urine is much diminished in volume, is highly coloured and has a high specific gravity: eg. over 1020. This type of case practically always recovers.

(2) HEAT EXHAUSTION: The mild case of heat exhaustion is similar to one of heat collapse. The more severe case tends to occur towards the end of the hot season in the tropics. The onset is charcterized by increasing weakness, dizziness, and insomnia, and this is accompanied by defective sweating in the majority of cases. Cramps and vomiting seldom occur, but large volumes of urine are voided. The temperature is usually about 37·8°–38·3°C (100°–101°F), the pulse rate is within normal limits, and there are seldom signs of dehydration, the skin usually having quite a good colour.

(3) HEAT CRAMPS: These have been recognized for many years and occur in individuals who perform hard physical work in high temperatures. Hence the many different names by which they have been known: eg. miners' cramps, stokers' cramps, bakers' cramps. The characteristic feature is agonizing cramp, usually in the legs, arms, or back. Occasionally the abdominal muscles are involved, and in these cases the intensity of the pain may suggest some acute condition of the stomach or gut. The cramps are accompanied by sweating, pallor of the skin, and a feeling of intense anxiety. There may be headache and giddiness. The temperature is seldom raised very much.

(4) HEAT HYPERPYREXIA: This is the most serious type of all. The initial manifestations are loss of energy and irritability. Then follow mental confusion and diminution or cessation of sweating. Gradually, or sometimes with startling suddenness, this passes into restlessness and then coma and the temperature rises rapidly to 41·7°C (107°F) or even higher. Unless treatment is instituted immediately, there is soon a fatal termination.

Prevention: Careful selection of personnel who have to perform hard physical work under tropical conditions or in high temperatures is essential. Even in the case of such selected individuals acclimatization is necessary and they should not be allowed to perform severe physical exertion at high temperatures until a period of several weeks' training has elapsed. In the tropics elderly people should move to a cool area during the hot season. Personal hygiene is important. Only light clothing should be worn, with a minimum of constrictions such as tight belts.

Diet should be light and nourishing and ample fluids should be taken. Salads and fruit should constitute an important part of the diet, and fluids should be bland: eg. fruit drinks, tea, iced coffee. Alcoholic drinks should be taken in moderation, and only after sundown. In the case of individuals performing hard physical exertion at high temperatures, water containing salt (ie. sodium chloride) should be drunk freely. Unless the water contains a certain amount of salt, there is an increased tendency to develop cramps. In industries where men work under such conditions, they are now provided with salt and water flavoured with lemon to disguise the salty flavour. Attention to ventilation and air-conditioning is also essential. In the tropics, when air-conditioning is not available, houses should be closed up in the early morning and opened up again at sundown. This reduces the amount of hot air entering the house during the day and allows free circulation of the cool night air. Fans are also of value,

and, in hot, dry conditions, sprinkling the compound with water during the afternoon sometimes helps to keep the house cool.
Treatment: In the case of *heat cramps, heat collapse*, and *heat exhaustion*, treatment consists of removal of the affected individual to a cool place and the administration of normal saline (see ISOTONIC). In severe cases this can be given intravenously, but it can usually be given by mouth. *Heat hyperpyrexia* is an emergency which requires immediate attention with a view to reducing the temperature. The individual should be placed in the shade, stripped, and drenched with water. To increase the cooling property of the water the surface of the body should be fanned. The patient is then wrapped in a sheet soaked in as cool water as possible (see WET PACKS), and the fanning is continued. This treatment must be stopped when the rectal temperature falls to 38·9°C (102°F) and the patient is then wrapped in a dry blanket. The reason for stopping at this temperature is that the temperature continues to fall after treatment ceases and therefore if treatment was continued until the temperature became normal, the further fall in temperature might have serious consequences. As soon as the patient is conscious he should be given normal saline to drink, and this usually provokes sweating – a favourable sign. Whenever possible, further treatment should be carried out in hospital, as there is always a risk of circulatory collapse occurring. Convalescence may be prolonged, and the advisability of the affected individual returning permanently to a cooler climate must always be given careful consideration.

HEBEPHRENIA is a form of mental disorder coming on in youth and marked by depression and gradual failure of mental faculties with egotistic and self-centred delusions. It is one of the forms of schizophrenia.

HEBERDEN'S NODES are little hard knobs which appear at the sides of the last phalanges of the fingers in people who are the subject of osteoarthrosis.

HEBETUDE is mental dullness, especially the temporary dullness which arises in the course of fevers.

HECTIC is a type of fever which may occur in certain severe forms of tuberculosis or septic poisoning. The temperature rises during the day to 39° to 40°C (102° to 104°F), and falls during the night almost to normal or even to below normal, 35·6° to 36·1°C (96° to 97°F), with profuse sweating. (See TUBERCULOSIS.)

HEEL is the hinder part of the foot formed by the calcaneus and the specially thick skin covering it. It is not subject to many diseases. Severe pain in the heel is sometimes a sign of gout or rheumatism.

HEIGHT (see WEIGHT AND HEIGHT).

HELIOTHERAPY is treatment of disease by exposing the body to the sun's rays. It has been widely used in the treatment of tuberculosis of the bones and joints. (See LIGHT TREATMENT.)

HELIUM is the lightest gas known, with the exception of hydrogen. This property renders it of value in anaesthesia (qv), as its addition to the anaesthetic means that it can be inhaled with less effort by the patient. Thus it can be used in the presence of any obstruction to the entry of air to the lungs.

HELLEBORE (see VERATRUM).

HELMINTHS is a name for worms.

HEMERALOPIA is the term for describing the condition of day-blindness, in which the patient can see better in a dull light than in bright daylight.

HEMIANAESTHESIA means loss of touch-sense down one side of the body.

HEMIANOPIA, HEMIANOPSIA, and HEMIOPIA are terms meaning loss of half the usual area of vision. The affected person may see everything clearly to the left or to the right, the field of vision stopping abruptly at the middle line, or he may see things only when straight in front of him, or thirdly, he may see objects far out on both sides, although there is a wide area straight in front for which he is quite blind. The position of the blind area is important in localizing the position in the brain of the disease responsible for the condition.

HEMIATROPHY is atrophy of one side of the body, or of part of the body on one side: for example, facial hemiatrophy, in which one-half of the face is smaller than the other either in the course of development or as a result of some nervous disorder.

HEMIBALLISMUS are involuntary movements similar to choreiform movements but of much greater amplitude and force. They are violent throwing movements of the limbs which are usually unilateral. They tend to occur acutely as a result of vascular damage to the mid-brain.

HEMICRANIA means a headache limited to one side of the head. (See MIGRAINE.)

HEMIMELIA: This consists of defects in the distal part of the extremities such as the absence of a forearm or hands. This is a congenital defect and large numbers of cases resulted from the administration of Thalidomide during pregnancy.

HEMIPLEGIA means paralysis limited to one side of the body. (See PARALYSIS.)

HEMLOCK, or CONIUM, is used in the form both of the leaves and fruit of *Conium maculatum*. Its action depends upon the property which it possesses of paralysing the endings of the motor nerves. It therefore diminishes spasmodic conditions of all sorts, producing at the same time muscular weakness and confusion of vision. In large amount it causes complete paralysis and acts as a narcotic. The action depends upon an alkaloid, coniine.
Uses: It is seldom used in medicine now. At one time it was considered to be of value in the treatment of spasmodic or convulsive conditions such as chorea, whooping-cough, and epilepsy.

HENBANE (see HYOSCYAMUS).

HEPARIN is a substance, first obtained from the liver, which prevents coagulation of the blood. It is present chiefly in liver, muscle, and lung. It is thought to act by neutralizing thrombin. (See FIBRIN.) Heparin has a complicated chemical structure and has been prepared in crystalline form. It is carbohydrate in nature, and contains amino and sulphuric acid groups. It is used for the prevention of clot formation in the blood or to prevent the spreading of this process once it has occurred. It is not active when given by mouth and must therefore be given by injection – usually intravenously. (See also ANTICOAGULANTS.)

HEPATECTOMY is the operation for removal of the liver, or part of it.

HEPATITIS means inflammation of the liver. (See LIVER.)

HEPATITIS, ACUTE INFECTIVE, is an acute infection of the liver, caused by a virus known as virus A. The disease is an intestinal infection, the virus passing from the stools of one patient to the mouth of the next. In temperate climes it tends to occur in late summer, with a peak in winter or early spring. In England in 1983, 6316 cases were notified. These included all cases of infective jaundice, whether caused by virus A or virus B. In the tropics and subtropics there is no seasonal incidence. The incubation period varies from 15 to 50 days (commonly 28). The disease may come on suddenly or gradually. In many patients, there is no jaundice, the patient merely feeling 'liverish', off his food and complaining of some abdominal discomfort. When jaundice does occur it usually appears about the 7th or 9th day, and may persist for 2 or 3 weeks. As already noted, it is spread by the stools of the infected individual. The duration of infectivity of the patient is uncertain, but is probably from 7 to 14 days before, to 7 days after the onset of jaundice. Treatment in the majority of cases consists simply of rest in bed, and a high-protein, low-fat diet, washed down with ample glucose drinks flavoured with lemon or orange juice. Alcohol is forbidden, and this ban should be maintained for three months after recovery. Those who have had the disease should not return to work until at least seven days following the disappearance of jaundice or until complete clinical recovery. The prognosis is good, and the vast majority of patients make a satisfactory recovery, but some often feel unwell for several weeks after all signs of the disease have disappeared and liver function tests have returned to normal. They complain of tiredness, nausea and dyspepsia which may be quite severe. The disease is notifiable in Britain.
SERUM HEPATITIS is a closely allied disease, which differs in three respects. It has a longer incubation period (up to 100 days or even longer). It is transmitted by the transfusion of contaminated blood or by the use of contaminated syringes or needles. It is a more fatal disease, the mortality ranging from 6 to 20 per cent, compared with 1 to 2 per 1000 for acute infectious hepatitis. It is due to a different virus, known as virus B. The virus may remain in the blood stream for many years, so making them carriers of the disease. It is thus becoming a disease of increasing significance as larger volumes of blood and blood products are being used. This particular danger is slight in Britain, where all blood for transfusion is now routinely checked for the presence of the virus before it is released for use. What is a real danger, however, is the transmission by contaminated needles in tattooing and drug addicts.
CHRONIC ACTIVE HEPATITIS is defined as an inflammation of the liver of more than six months duration with characteristic microscopic appearances. Chronic hepatitis B infection and auto-immune disease of the liver are the major causes. It may, however, also result from non-A, non-B hepatitis, Wilson's disease and Alpha one antitrypsin deficiency. Drugs such as methyldopa, isoniazid and oxyphenisatin may also cause chronic active hepatitis, as may alcohol. The importance of non-A, non-B hepatitis as a cause of acute and chronic inflammation of the liver is becoming increasingly recognised. It is almost certainly another virus. It can be transmitted by the gastro-intestinal tract or parenterally by transfusion. Although the acute illness is often mild, 36 to 100 per cent of parenterally affected patients develop chronic hepatitis. Although this may be relatively benign, some patients do progress to cirrhosis.

HEPATOLENTICULAR DEGENERATION (see WILSON'S DISEASE).

HEREDITY is the principle on which various peculiarities of bodily form or structure, or of physical or mental activity are transmitted from parents to offspring. (See GENES.)

HERMAPHRODITE is an individual in whom both ovarian and testicular tissue is present. Hermaphrodites may have a testis on one side and an ovary on the other, or an ovotestis on one side and an ovary or testis on the other, or there may be an ovotestis on both sides. Both gonads are usually intra-abdominal. The true hermaphrodite usually has a uterus and at least one fallopian tube on the side of the ovary. On the side of the testis there is usually a vas deferens. Most true hermaphrodites are raised as males but external virilisation is not usually complete. Even when significant phallic development is present hypospadias and cryptorchism are common. At puberty gynaecomastia devlops and menstruation is common, as ovarian function is usually more nearly normal than testicular function.

HERNIA means the protrusion of any organ, or part of an organ, into or through the wall of the cavity which contains it. Thus hernia of the brain may occur because of a severe injury to the skull, hernia of the lung from a wound of the chest wall, but these are uncommon, and the most common form is hernia of the bowel, the popular term for which is rupture.

Varieties: Although far the commonest organ found in a hernia is part of the bowel, any of the abdominal structures, such as stomach, kidney, ovary, womb, bladder, or omentum, may be found projecting through an opening in the wall of the abdomen and lying close beneath the skin. Probably the only two organs exempt are the liver and pancreas, by reason of their position and connections. The projecting organ carries in front of it, and is enveloped by, a sac of peritoneum, the smooth membrane lining the interior of the abdomen. It is separated from the surface at least by this sac and by the skin. A hernia is usually described according to the position at which it protrudes. There are certain natural openings in the region of the groin on either side: one, known as the inguinal canal, through which the testicle descends in early life, and which the spermatic cord keeps always more or less open; the other, known as the femoral canal, which lies to the inner side of the large femoral vessels that pass from the abdomen to the thigh. The inguinal canal ends just above the pubic bone, its exit, known as the external abdominal ring, being large enough to admit the tip of the finger. The femoral canal is smaller and is separated from the former only by the inner end of the inguinal ligament, a strong band which lies beneath the oblique groove that can be seen on the surface to separate the abdomen from the thigh. A hernia emerging from the former is known as an *inguinal hernia*, and tends to descend along the spermatic cord into the scrotum. A hernia emerging through the femoral canal comes forwards on the front of the thigh, and is called a *femoral hernia*. A weak spot exists in the centre of the abdomen at the navel, and here, not infrequently in young children of poor development, a hernia may appear, which is then known as an *umbilical hernia*. A hernia which protrudes at some accidental opening on the abdomen, as, for example, through the scar of an operation wound, is known as a *ventral hernia*. A rare form of hernia is one which passes through the gap in front of the pelvis between the ischial and pubic bones; it is known as an *obturator hernia*. Finally, there are various forms of *internal hernia*, the protruded organ passing up into the chest, or into some other region where it does not show itself on the surface. (See HIATUS HERNIA.)

A hernia may also be considered as *congenital*, that is, existing at birth, or *acquired* later on in life. The only positions in which congenital hernia is found are in the umbilical and inguinal regions. In the latter case the hernia descends along with the testicle towards the scrotum, the hernia being inside the tubular process of peritoneum which descends with the testicle in order to provide it with a smooth tunic.

An important classification of hernia is made according to the condition of the protruding organ. A *reducible hernia* is one which is so freely movable that it may be pressed back into the abdomen, although it comes down again by the same opening unless this is blocked up. An *irreducible hernia* is one which cannot be returned, either because it has become adherent to its new surroundings, because it has enlarged after emerging, because much fat has been deposited inside the abdomen, or for some similar reason. An *obstructed hernia* is one in which, a part of the bowel being protruded, some of its contents become caught inside, and cannot for a time pass on, a state of costiveness arising in fact inside the hernia. A *strangulated hernia* is by far the most important variety, because of its immediate danger to life. In this form, the circulation of blood in the protruded bowel becomes cut off by the margin of the opening through which the loop of bowel has passed; and, if an operation is not immediately performed for its relief, the bowel will become gangrenous, and the patient may die within a few days. The great danger attending all forms of hernia is that they may at any time become strangulated.

Causes: Two factors come into play in causing hernia. First, some defect or injury of the abdominal wall; and, secondly, some increase of pressure within the cavity. With regard to the hernia at the umbilicus of young children, there is usually some defect in the closure of the opening through which the navel-string passes before birth, and through this opening a loop of bowel is forced by excessive crying or the like. In inguinal hernia, which is far commoner in men than in women, the defect consists in some failure of the inguinal canal through which the testicle descends before birth to close completely. There may, in congenital hernia, be a completely open passage leading out of the abdomen, or there may be simply a small pocket in the peritoneum which, by a sudden strain or by long-continued pressure, such as coughing, gets torn or stretched in front of a protruded organ. Femoral hernia is commoner in women than in men, probably on account of the special shape and inclination of the pelvic bones, and arises in a manner similar to inguinal hernia. Both in these and in ventral hernia, the occurrence of marked changes in size of the abdomen, such as great increase in stoutness, great loss of fat, and repeated child-bearing, has the effect of greatly weakening the abdominal wall and predisposing to the formation of hernia. All laborious occupations involving great efforts, and bodily conditions involving frequently repeated strains, such as chronic cough or constipation, conduce to hernia of all sorts. Accordingly hernia is much more common in the male sex – who lead a more strenuous physical life –than among females.

Symptoms: The symptoms vary considerably, depending upon the particular organ which is protruded, upon the size of the opening, which may or may not compress the hernia, and upon the condition of the latter. In the great majority of cases the hernia consists of one or more loops of the small intestine, and, if the hernia is small and readily reducible, the symptoms are somewhat as follows. If the hernia is produced quite suddenly, as during the lifting of a heavy weight, the person affected may hear or feel a distant crack, and be conscious that something has given way, but, as a rule, suffers no sharp pain. More usually the hernia develops gradually, and the symptoms have then no definite onset, but simply increase till they attract attention. An undefinable sense of weakness, and occasionally pain, are felt in the region of the hernia. When any great effort is made, such as coughing, or straining at stool, or lifting a weight, a swelling appears with a gurgling feeling at the seat of the hernia, although this can be made to disappear by pressure when the person lies down. Even if the hernia does not come far down, a distinct impulse on coughing is communicated to the hand laid upon the swelling, which is situated usually at the inner end of the groin. When the hernia has become irreducible, the swelling does not vary in size, but the impulse on coughing is still to be felt. The presence even of a small hernia may occasion some interference with digestion, and constipation is a common accompaniment. A dragging sensation in the back is another frequent symptom.

When a hernia becomes strangulated, as the result of stoppage of its circulation by the pressure of the margin of the ring through which it comes, a marked set of symptoms ensues. The hernia first becomes inflamed, acutely painful, and then in a few hours turns gangrenous, producing general peritonitis and death if not relieved. At the same time, all passage of contents through the bowel is stopped, and as a result the bowels do not move, although some of their contents pass in the reverse direction, up to the stomach, whence they are vomited. Accordingly the onset of abdominal pain, accompanied by stoppage of the bowels and vomiting in a person possessed of a hernia, forms an ominous sign, and, even if no hernia is known to exist, the appearance of these three symptoms calls for immediate examination of the region of the groin by a medical practitioner.

Treatment: When a hernia is present, it may be treated in a palliative manner, so as to relieve unpleasant symptoms and diminish the risk of strangulation, or an attempt may be made to cure it.

PALLIATIVE TREATMENT: If the hernia is reducible, it is pushed back through the opening into the abdomen by manipulation known as taxis, and is then retained by an artificial support known as a truss. The truss in its simplest form may consist merely of a pad of lint or folded handkerchief kept in position by a spica bandage. In infants, a very simple truss may be improvised from a skein of worsted, which is carried round the waist, one end passed through the other end over the site of the hernia, and the loose end carried down between the legs, and pinned to the circular part behind the back. For adults, the usual truss consists of a pad which fits over the opening, a spring to run round the pelvis and a strap to pass between the legs and prevent the truss from sliding upwards. The pad for an inguinal hernia is differently shaped from, and should be much larger than, that for femoral hernia. In getting a truss the particulars required are: *(a)* the girth round the pelvis below the crests of the haunch-bones; *(b)* the variety of hernia; *(c)* the side on which it is situated; *(d)* the age and sex of the patient; *(e)* the strength desired in the spring. No pains should be spared to get a correctly fitting truss. (See TRUSS.)

If the hernia is irreducible, a different type of truss designed merely to protect the hernia must be used.

CURATIVE TREATMENT: The danger of strangulation, involving an immediate operation with great risk to life, is present as long as a hernia exists, and, except in old people with a very wide opening, the chance of radical cure and removal of the danger offered by an operation deserve to be carefully considered. The operation, known as the radical cure, is not in itself a dangerous one, and the period of enforced idleness consequent on it amounts only to a few weeks. Many operations are performed by different surgeons, but all consist briefly in this, that an opening is made over the hernia and, after the hernia has been returned into the abdomen, the sac is cut off, bunched up, turned aside, or otherwise disposed of, and the margins of the opening united by strong sutures. Almost all cases operated upon in this way result in complete cure.

When a hernia is irreducible, some special diet or other treatment is often required before the operation, in order to diminish the amount of fat in the abdomen, reduce the size of the hernia, and so forth.

When a hernia becomes strangulated, an operation becomes urgently necessary. The first object of this operation is to set free the hernia from the margin of the opening, tight band, or other cause that is impeding the circulation in it. This having been achieved, if the bowel is not too much damaged by the pressure it has received, it is returned to the abdomen, and the radical cure performed. Sometimes, however, the bowel has been so much damaged by several hours of pressure, that it would be too dangerous to replace it, and then, the compression having been relieved, either the damaged portion is completely cut out and the ends united by stitching, or the bowel is simply left in the wound for a few days, and the operation completed at a subsequent stage, if the bowel recovers its vitality. If the damaged loop of bowel does not recover, but sloughs away, then either the patient dies, or a fistula is left, from which the contents of the bowel escape to the exterior. This can, however, be closed by subsequent operation.

HEROIN, also known as DIAMORPHINE HYDROCHLORIDE, is a white crystalline powder of slightly bitter taste derived from morphine. It is a much more potent pain killer, or analgesic, than morphine but also a much more dangerous drug from the point of view of addiction. (See DRUG ADDICTION.)

HERPANGINA is a short febrile illness in which minute vesicles or punched-out ulcers develop in the posterior parts of the mouth. It is due to infection with the group A Coxsackie viruses (qv).

HERPES SIMPLEX is an acute infectious disease, characterized by the development of groups of superficial vesicles, or blebs, in the skin and mucous membrane. It is due to a virus, and infection can occur at any time from birth onwards, but the usual time for primary infection is between the second and fifteenth year. Once an individual is infected, the virus persists in the body for the rest of the individual's life. It is one of the causes of scrum-pox (qv).

Symptoms: The symptoms vary with the age of infection. In young infants it may cause a generalized infection which may prove fatal. In young children the infection is usually in the mouth, and this may be associated with enlargement of the glands in the neck, general irritability and fever. The condition usually settles in seven to ten days. In adults the vesicles may occur anywhere in the skin or mucous membranes. The more common sites are the lips, mouth and face where they are known as cold sores. The vesicles may also appear on the genitalia, or in the conjunctiva or cornea and the brain may be infected, causing encephalitis (qv) or meningitis. The first sign is the appearance of small painful swellings. These quickly develop into vesicles (qv), containing clear fluid, and surrounded by a reddened area of skin. Some people are particularly liable to recurrent attacks, and these often tend to be associated with some debilitating condition or infection, such as pneumonia.

Except in the case of herpes of the cornea, the eruption clears completely unless it becomes contaminated with some other organism. In the case of the cornea, there may be residual scarring, which may impair vision.

Treatment: The most effective local treatment, if the skin is involved, is idoxuridine. Grenz rays and soft X-rays are also used. In the case of cold sores the local application of the oily form of vitamin E is said to be of value in speeding up the healing process. Should the eye be involved the patient must be referred immediately to an eye specialist. In those cases in which the eye or the brain is involved, the antiviral agent, adenine arabinoside, and acyclovir, are proving of value. The only preventive measure that is worth consideration is the administration of gamma-globulin (qv) in the case of infants under the age of 3 months who are in close contact with a case. This is particularly applicable if the infant suffers from eczema.

HERPES ZOSTER, or SHINGLES, is a skin eruption of acute nature, closely related to chickenpox, consisting in the appearance of small yellow vesicles (qv), which spread over an area, dry up, and heal by scabbing. It receives its name from the Greek word, ζωστηρ, a 'circingle', or girdle, because it spreads in a zone-like manner round half the chest. Herpes of the face also occurs, particularly on the brow and round the eye.

Causes: It is due to a virus identical with that of chickenpox. This invades the ganglia of the nerves, particularly the spinal nerves of the chest and the fifth cranial nerve which supplies the face. In spite of its being due to the same virus as chickenpox, it is rare for herpes zoster to occur as a result of contact with a case of chickenpox. On the other hand, it is not unusual for a patient with herpes zoster to infect a child with chickenpox. It is a disease of adults rather than children, and the older the person the more likely is he to develop the disease. Thus in adults under 50 the incidence is around 2·5 per 1000 people a year. Between 50 and 60 it is around 5 per 1000, whilst in octogenarians it is 10 per 1000. Most adults who acquire the disease have had chickenpox in childhood. Occasionally it may be associated with some serious underlying disease such as leukaemia, lymphadenoma, or multiple myeloma.

Symptoms: The first symptoms of herpes are much like those of any feverish attack. The person feels unwell for some days, has a slight rise of temperature, and vague pain in the side or in various other parts. The pain finally settles at a point in the side, and, two or three days after the first symptoms, the rash appears. Minute yellow blebs or vesicles as they are known are seen on the skin of the back, of the side, or of the front of the chest, or simultaneously on all three, the points corresponding to the space between one pair of ribs right round. These blebs increase in number for some days, and spread till there is often a complete half girdle round one side of the chest. The pain in this stage is severe, but it appears to vary a good deal with age, being slight in children and very severe in old people, in whom indeed herpes sometimes forms a serious illness. After one or two weeks, most of the vesicles have dried up and formed scabs, which finally drop off, leaving the skin just as it was before, or covered with small scars. Occasionally the little vesicles run together into large blebs, which leave ulcers difficult to heal, and followed by marked scars. The skin is generally healed completely in two or three weeks, but a distressing peculiarity about the pain is that, in old people especially, it may not pass off when the eruption disappears, but may remain for weeks or even months: a condition known as post-herpetic neuralgia.

Treatment: In the very early stage, before the vesicles have formed, cocaine or atropine ointment rubbed into the side eases the pain and seems to prevent to some extent the outbreak of the eruption. Later, when the vesicles have formed and are discharging, a dusting-powder of starch, zinc oxide, and bismuth subnitrate gives much relief, or the side may be painted with glycerin jelly containing menthol or with a mixture of chloral, camphor, and menthol in equal parts. Alternatively, the lesions may be dabbed with calamine lotion. In any case, the part should be kept warm by a dressing of cotton-wool. Analgesics may be required for relief of the pain.

Should post-herpetic neuralgia persist, the administration of analgesics is essential. Acupuncture is also said to be helpful.

HERTZ is the SI (International System of Units) unit of frequency. It indicates the number of cycles per second (c/s). The abbreviation for hertz is Hz.

HESPERIDIN is a glycoside (qv) derived from the rind of citrus fruit, which is believed to control the permeability of capillaries.

HETEROGRAFT is a transplant from one animal to another of a different species. It is also known as a xenograft.

HEXACHLOROPHANE is a widely used antiseptic which is active against a range of micro-organisms, including Gram-positive and Gram-negative organisms, *Shigella dysenteriae*, and *Salmonellatyphi*. One of its advantages is that it retains its activity in the presence of soap, and it is therefore often used in soaps and creams in a concentration of 1 to 2 per cent. It must be used with caution in babies as it can be absorbed through the skin and prove harmful.

HEXAMINE is a substance which, when excreted by the kidneys, sets free formaldehyde, that has an antiseptic action. It is given in cases of cystitis when the urine decomposes within the bladder, and it exerts its beneficial action very speedily. It acts only in urine with an acid reaction, and, if the urine is alkaline, acid phosphate of soda is usually taken along with the hexamine. The dose of each of these is 0·6 to 2 grams several times daily.

HEXOESTROL (see OESTROGENS).

HIATUS HERNIA is a displacement of a portion of the stomach through the opening in the diaphragm through which the oesophagus passes from the chest to the abdominal cavity.

HICCUP is a spasmodic indrawing of air to the lungs, ending with a click, due to sudden closure of the vocal cords. The cause is some irritation of the nerves which go to the diaphragm, producing sudden contractions of the latter. Most cases, especially those recurring habitually about the same hour of the day, are due to indigestion. The symptom also occurs in some serious general diseases, like uraemia and typhoid fever, being in such cases a grave sign. Hiccup lasting over some days or weeks is in some cases a symptom of mild encephalitis lethargica.

Treatment: If the condition is due to dyspepsia, it is often relieved by a copious draught of cold water or by some aromatic like a few drops of spirit of chloroform, a teaspoonful of Hoffmann's anodyne, or a tablespoonful of peppermint water or cinnamon water. When continuous and excessive it is usually controlled by the inhalation of carbon dioxide. The popular remedy of breathing in and out of a paper bag is probably successful because of the accumulation of carbon dioxide in the bag. If persistent, and resisting all these traditional measures, more potent drugs may need to be resorted to. In this respect, chlorpromazine (qv) has achieved a certain reputation for efficacy in bringing it under control. Haloperidol has also been used with success in such persistent cases. There are a number of time-honoured cures which do not necessitate drug therapy. One of these is to take a deep breath; then take seven sips of water; take another deep breath and hold for the count of seven.

HIERA PICRA, popularly known as 'hickory pickory', is a powder composed of aloes and canella (the bark of *Canella alba* or white cinnamon), used as an aperient and emmenagogue.

HIGH FREQUENCY (see ELECTRICITY IN MEDICINE).

HILUM is a term applied to the depression on organs such as the lung, kidney, and spleen, at which the vessels and nerves enter it and round which the lymphatic glands cluster. The hilum of the lung is also known as its root.

HIP-JOINT is the joint formed by the head of the thigh-bone and the deep cup-shaped hollow on the side of the pelvis which receives it (acetabulum). The joint is of the ball-and-socket variety, is dislocated only by very great violence, and is correspondingly difficult to reduce to its natural state after dislocation. The joint is enclosed by a capsule of fibrous tissue, strengthened by several bands, of which the principal is the ilio-femoral or Y-shaped ligament placed in front of the joint. A round ligament also unites the head of the thigh-bone to the margin of the acetabulum.

For hip-joint disease see under JOINTS, DISEASES OF; DISLOCATIONS.

HIPPUS is a tremor of the iris which produces alternating contraction and dilatation of the pupil. This is often a sign of hysteria.

HIRSCHSPRUNG'S DISEASE, or MEGACOLON, is a condition in childhood which is characterized by great hypertrophy and dilatation of the colon.

HIRSUTISM, or HYPERTRICHOSIS, is the growth of hair of the male type and distribution in women. It is either due to the excess production of androgens or to undue sensitivity of the hair follicle to normal female levels of circulating androgens. The latter is called idiopathic because the cause is unknown. The increased production of androgens in the female may come from the ovary and be due to the polycystic ovary syndrome or an ovarian tumour, or the excess androgen may come from the adrenal cortex and be the result of congenital adrenal hyperplasia, an adrenal tumour or Cushing's syndrome. However there is a wide range of normality in the distribution of female body hair. It varies with different racial groups. The Mediterranean races have more body hair than Nordic women and the Chinese and Japanese have little body hair. Many normal women, especially those with dark hair, have hair apparent on the upper lip and a few coarse hairs on the chin and around the nipples are not uncommon. Extension of the pubic hair towards the umbilicus is frequently found in normal women. Dark hair is much more apparent than fair hair and this is why bleaching is of considerable benefit in the management of hirsutism.

The treatment of hirsutism is that of the primary cause. When it is idiopathic hirsutism it must be managed by simple measures such as bleaching the hair and the use of depilatory waxes and creams. Coarse facial hairs can be removed by electrolysis, although this is time consuming. Shaving is often the most effective remedy and neither increases the rate of hair growth nor causes the hairs to become coarser.

HISTAMINE is an amine (qv) derived from histidine (qv). It is widely distributed in the tissues of plants and animals, including man. It is a powerful stimulant of gastric juice, a constrictor of smooth muscle including that of the bronchi, and a dilator of arterioles and capillaries. It is this last action which is responsible for the eruption of nettlerash (qv).

HISTIDINE is an amino-acid from which histamine is derived by bacterial decomposition.

HISTOLOGY is the study of the minute structure of the tissues.

HISTOPLASMOSIS is a disease due to a yeast-like fungus known as *Histoplasma capsulatum*. Most cases have been reported from USA. In infants it is characterized by fever, anaemia, enlargement of the liver and spleen, and involvement of the lungs and gastro-intestinal tract. In older children it may resemble pulmonary tuberculosis, whilst in adults it may be confined to involvement of the skin.

HIVES is a popular term applied to eruptions of the nature of nettle-rash (qv).

HLA ANTIGENS are antigens (qv) which we inherit on the surfaces of cells throughout the body. They are known as Human Leucocyte Antigens (HLA) because they were first identified on leucocytes (qv). It is these HLA antigens which are responsible for the body rejecting a transplanted organ such as a kidney. This is because the body into which the organ is transplanted recognizes the organ as a 'foreign body' if its HLA antigens are different and immediately starts producing antibodies to destroy it. In some ways they are comparable to the ABO blood groups (qv). They are, however, far more complicated. Over fifty of them have already been recognized, and most people have four of them. This means that matching those of the donor kidney and the recipient body is much more difficult than in the case of blood. Hence the high proportion of transplanted organs that are rejected by the recipient body. (See also TRANSPLANTATION.)

HODGKIN'S DISEASE, so called after Thomas Hodgkin (1798–1866), the Guy's Hospital pathologist who first described it, or LYMPHADENOMA, is a condition in which the lymphatic glands all over the body undergo a gradually progressive enlargement. The cause is not known. The glands affected may reach a great size. The patient often runs a characteristic form of fever (Pel-Ebstein fever), in which bouts of fever alternate with several days with no fever. Along with these changes a considerable degree of anaemia arises, and the affected person becomes gradually weaker. Treatment consists of radiotherapy when the disease is relatively localized. When it is more widespread, however, chemotherapy is the treatment of choice. This is now given in the form of a combination of drugs, rather than one single drug. The most commonly used combination at the moment is: mustine, vinblastine, procarbazine and prednisone. The results of treatment are now such that over 80 per cent treated by radiotherapy, and 78 per cent of those treated by combined chemotherapy, are still alive after five years.

HOMATROPINE is an alkaloid derived from atropine, which is used to produce dilatation of the pupil and to paralyse accommodation temporarily for the purpose of examining the interior of the eye. It is used in 1 per cent solution, and its effects pass away in the course of a few hours.

HOMOCYSTINURIA is a congenital disease due to the inability of the affected individual to metabolize, or utilize properly one of the essential amino-acids (qv) known as methionine. The main features of the condition are abnormality of the lens of the eye, mental retardation, fair complexion and fair hair and a high cheek colour.

HOMOEOPATHY is a system of medicine founded by Hahnemann at the end of the eighteenth century. It is based upon the theory that diseases are curable by those drugs which produce effects on the body similar to symptoms caused by the disease (*similia similibus curantur*). In administering drugs, the theory is also held that their effect is increased by giving them in minute doses obtained by diluting them to an extreme degree.

HOMOGRAFT is a piece of tissue or an organ, such as a kidney, transplanted from one animal to another of the same species: eg. from man to man. It is also known as an allograft.

HOMOSEXUALITY is preferential or exclusive sexual activity with a member of the same sex. There has been considerable debate among psychiatrists as to whether homosexuality should be regarded as a normal sexual variant or as a psycho-pathological development or deviation. Although homosexuality is found in virtually every society and culture there is no society in which it is the predominant or preferred mode of sexual activity. Various attempts have been made to link homosexuality to hormonal factors, particularly lowered testosterone levels but there is no convincing evidence that this is so. Nor is there any evidence in favour of a genetic explanation. Psycho-analytic theories link homosexuality to early child-rearing influences, in particular the close binding and intimate mother.

The number of homosexual men in the UK is unknown. There has never been a representative population survey. Re-analysis of the Kinsey report suggests that only 3 per cent of adult men have exclusively homosexual leanings and a further 3 per cent have extensive homosexual and heterosexual experience. Homosexuality seems to be less common among women. Most homosexual men have a high number of sexual partners each year and very few are in stable, faithful relationships with other men. Homosexual men have higher levels of anxiety and depression than heterosexual men but those who are in stable relationships seem content. It would seem that the lack of a stable relationship is the factor responsible for higher levels of anxiety and depression.

There are still differences in the way homosexuals and heterosexuals are treated in British law. The age of consent for homosexuals is 21 while for heterosexuals it is 16.

HONEY is the viscid sweet fluid produced by bees from the nectar they collect from flowers. It contains around 75 per cent of sugars, mostly fructose and glucose. Its traditional reputation as an antiseptic has been confirmed in recent years, and it has been shown to be active against a wide range of micro-organisms, including haemolytic streptococci, staphylococci, *Proteus mirabilis, E. coli*, and *Candida albicans*. (See also MOLASSES; SYRUP.) It is also widely used as a demulcent (qv) and as a sweetening agent in tinctures and cough mixtures.

HONKING is the term applied to a persistent cough of emotional origin which occurs in emotionally disturbed children. It is of an explosive brassy character and has been compared to the call of the Canada goose. When coughing the child grimaces and tends to hold the chin close to the chest. One of its major characteristics is that it never occurs at night. Quite often it follows on a cold or sore throat. No specific treatment is needed. It disappears when the cause of the emotional upset, such as, for example, difficulties at school, is dealt with and removed.

HOOKWORM (see ANCYLOSTOMIASIS).

HOPS have been used in medicine as the powder obtained from the dried fruit of *Humulus lupulus*. The plant contains an alkaloid, lupuline, which has a weak sedative action. A poultice made from crushed hops is a household sedative in cases of localized pains, and hop pillows have been used for nervous insomnia.

HORDEOLUM: An outdated term meaning a stye, occasionally a chalazion.

HOREHOUND is the dried leaves and tops of *Marrubium vulgare*, which are used for coughs, either mixed with sugar as a syrup in doses of 2 to 4 ml or as fluid extract in doses of 4 to 8 ml.

HORMONE REPLACEMENT THERAPY (see MENOPAUSE).

HORMONES are substances which, on absorption into the blood, influence the action of tissues and organs other than those in which they are produced. The internal secretions of the ovary, pancreas, thyroid, pituitary and suprarenal bodies afford examples of this action. (See ENDOCRINE GLANDS.)

HORNER'S SYNDROME: This is the description given to a combination of changes resulting from paralysis of the sympathetic nerve in the neck. They are: small pupil, a drooping upper lid and an apparently (though not actually) sunken eye.

HORNETS (see BITES AND STINGS).

HORRIPILATION is another term for goose-flesh, due to contraction of the small muscles in the skin which make the hairs erect.

HORSESHOE KIDNEY (see KIDNEYS, DISEASES OF).

HOSPITAL is a building intended for receiving sick or injured persons. The introduction of the National Health Service Act in 1948 completely changed the organization of the hospitals in Great Britain. Under this Act all hospitals in the country, with the exception of private hospitals and a few which insisted on remaining outside the National Health Service, passed under the control of the Minister of Health. With the exception of the teaching hospitals, these hospitals in the National Health Service passed to the control of Regional Boards appointed by the Minister of Health. These Regional Boards further subdivided the hospitals in their areas into units under the control of Hospital Management Committees. The endowments of the voluntary hospitals were transferred to a Hospital Endowments Fund, and the income from this is used for purposes outside the official budget. Hospitals are no longer allowed to appeal for funds. In the case of old age pensioners a small (lodging) deduction is made from their pensions. Hospitals are allowed to have special blocks of private wards for patients who wish to pay for the additional comforts of such private wards. Teaching hospitals were given a larger measure of independence. They were allowed to keep their own Boards of Governors and they retained control over their endowments.

Hospitals are also classified according to the type of case with which they deal, as follows: (*a*) GENERAL HOSPITALS admit both cases of disease requiring treatment by diet, drugs and other non-operative procedures (medical cases), and cases of disease and injury requiring operation (surgical cases). Most of the larger general hospitals also possess special departments (for eye diseases, diseases of ear, nose and throat, diseases peculiar to women, etc.). *Teaching Hospitals* form a special subdivision of the general hospitals, which are connected with a medical school, and are attended by medical students. (*b*) SPECIAL HOSPITALS are reserved for one special kind of case. Of these, the best known types are *Children's Hospitals, Eye Hospitals, Maternity Hospitals*, and *Mental Hospitals*. (*c*) CONVALESCENT HOSPITALS are usually situated in a rural or seaside district where light and fresh air are abundant. They receive patients, usually from general or special hospitals, who require little in the shape of treatment, but whose bodily powers are still enfeebled after serious illness or operation.

Under the National Health Service Reorganization Act 1973, a complete overhaul of the Service came into effect on April 1, 1974, bringing into a single administrative structure the hospital services previously administered by Regional Hospital Boards, Boards of Governors and Hospital Management Committees, the local authority health services and the family practitioner services. (See NATIONAL HEALTH SERVICE.)

HOUR-GLASS STOMACH is the term given to the X-ray appearance of a stomach which is constricted in its middle part because of either spasm of the stomach muscle or contraction of scar tissue from a gastric ulcer.

HOUSEMAID'S KNEE is an inflammation of the bursa in front of the knee-cap, often mistaken for some disease in the joint itself (see BURSITIS).

HUMAN LEUCOCYTE ANTIGEN (HLA): HLA antigens are found in most tissues of the body. They are genetically determined by genes on chromosome 6. They are the antigens that result in rejection of tissues from other individuals, such as skin, kidney, heart and liver. They are similar to the blood-group antigens that are situated on red blood cells. There are four groups of HLA antigen: A, B, C and DR. If they are well defined, they are given a number such as HLA A1 and, if they are poorly defined, they are given a letter, for example HLA AW. If the HLA groups between two individuals are identical, graft rejection is unlikely. There are associations between HLA types and certain diseases. For example, ankylosing spondylitis tends to occur only in individuals who are HLA B27. Rheumatoid arthritis tends to occur in individuals that are HLA DR4 and thyrotoxicosis in those that are HLA B8.

HUMAN MILK BANKS (see INFANT FEEDING).

HUMERUS is the bone of the upper arm. It has a rounded head, which helps to form the shoulder joint, and at its lower end presents a wide pulley-like surface for union with the radius and ulna. Its epicondyles form the prominences at the sides of the elbow.

HUMIDIFICATION of the air we breathe is essential for the efficient working of the lungs. (See RESPIRATION.) This is achieved largely by the nose (qv) which acts as an air-conditioner, warming, moistening, and filtering the 10,000 litres of air which we inhale daily, in the process of which, incidentally, it produces around 1·5 litres of secretion daily. Humidity is expressed as relative humidity (RH). This is the amount of moisture in the air expressed as a percentage of the maximum possible at that temperature. If the temperature of a room is raised without increasing the moisture content, the RH falls. The average outdoor RH in Britain is around 70 to 80 per cent. With central heating it may drop to 25 per cent or lower.

This is why humidification, as it is known, of the air is essential in buildings heated by modern heating systems. The aim should be to keep the RH around 30 to 50 per cent. In houses this may be achieved quite satisfactorily by having a jug or basin of water in the room, or some receptacle that can be attached to the heater. In offices some more elaborate form of humidifier is necessary. Those suffering from chronic bronchitis are particularly susceptible to dry air. (See also VENTILATION.)

HUMIDIFIER FEVER is a form of alveolitis (qv) caused by contamination of the water used to humidify, or moisten, the air in air-conditioning plants. The breathing of the contaminated air results in infection of the lung, which is characterized by fever, cough, shortness of breath and malaise, worse on Monday and tending to improve during the course of the week.

HUMOUR is a term applied to any fluid or semi-fluid tissue of the body: eg. the aqueous and vitreous humours in the eye. The term, humour, is also associated with a theory regarding the causation of disease, which originated with Pythagoras and lasted in a modified form until the early part of the nineteenth century. According to this theory diseases are due to an improper mixture in the body of blood, bile, phlegm and black bile.

HUNGER is a craving for food or other substance necessary to bodily activity. Hunger for food is supposed to be directly produced by strong contractions of the stomach which occur when it is empty or nearly so. (See also THIRST.)
AIR HUNGER is an instinctive craving for oxygen resulting in breathlessness, either when a person ascends to great heights where the pressure of air is low, or in some diseases such as pneumonia and diabetes mellitus.

HUNTINGTON'S CHOREA is a hereditary disease characterized by involuntary movements and dementia. Each child of a parent with the disease has a 50:50 chance of developing it. The usual time of onset is between 35 and 45, but 10 per cent of cases occur under the age of 20. Some patients show more severe mental disturbance, others more severe disturbances of movement, but in all it pursues an inexorable downward course over a period of ten to twenty years to a terminal state of physical and mental helplessness. It is estimated that there are around 6000 cases in Britain. The cause is not known and there is no effective treatment. People with Huntington's chorea and their relatives can obtain help and guidance from The Association to Combat Huntington's Chorea, 34a Station Road, Hinckley, Leicestershire LE10 1AP (0455 615558).

HURLER'S SYNDROME (see GARGOYLISM).

HUTCHINSON'S TEETH is the term applied to the narrowed and notched permanent incisor teeth which occur in congenital syphilis. They are so named after Sir Jonathan Hutchinson (1828–1913), the London physician who first described them.

HYALINE MEMBRANE DISEASE is a condition found in premature infants and infants born by Caesarean section, characterized by the onset of difficulty in breathing a few hours after birth. It is also known as the respiratory distress syndrome. About half the affected babies die, death usually occurring before the third day. At post-mortem examination the alveoli and the finer bronchioles of the lungs are found to be lined with a dense membrane. The cause of the condition is obscure. Administration of corticosteroids (qv) to the mother at least twelve hours before delivery seems to reduce its incidence in white boys, but not in black boys or in girls. More promising results are now being reported from the instillation into the trachea of surfactant (qv).

HYALURONIDASE is an enzyme (qv) which hydrolyzes hyaluronic acid. The latter is a gel-like substance which is widely distributed throughout the body and which helps to bind together the tissue cells and also acts as a lubricant in joints. By virtue of its action in hydrolyzing hyaluronic acid, hyaluronidase is now used in subcutaneous injections of fluid as it facilitates the spread of the injected fluid and therefore its absorption.

HYDATID is a cyst produced by the growth of immature forms of a tapeworm. (See TAENIASIS.)

HYDATIDIFORM MOLE, or VESICULAR MOLE as it is sometimes known, is a rare complication of pregnancy, in which there is tremendous proliferation of the epithelium of the chorion (the outer of the two foetal membranes). It seldom occurs during a first pregnancy. Treatment consists of immediate evacuation of the womb.

HYDRADENITIS SUPPURATIVA is a chronic inflammatory disease of the apocrine sweat glands (see PERSPIRATION). It is more common in women, in whom it usually occurs in the armpit, than in men in whom it is most common in the perineum of the drivers of lorries and taxis. It occurs in the form of painful, tender lumps underneath the skin, which burst often in a week or so. Treatment consists of removal by operation.

HYDRAEMIA is a condition in which the blood contains an excess of water.

HYDRAGOGUE is a drug that produces a watery stool. (See PURGATIVES).

HYDRALLAZINE is a hypotensive drug. (See ESSENTIAL HYPERTENSION.)

HYDRAMNIOS is the condition characterized by excess of fluid in the amniotic cavity. (See AMNION.)

HYDRARGYRUM is another name for mercury.

HYDROCELE is a collection of fluid connected with the testicle or spermatic cord. It is sometimes due to inflammation of the sac in which these structures are enclosed, but in many cases the cause cannot be discovered. It develops usually in middle life, although it may appear at any time, increases gradually in size, and is usually devoid of pain. The condition presents some resemblance to hernia, and there is occasionally some doubt in distinguishing between them, particularly when the hydrocele communicates with the abdominal cavity. In infants and young children the hydrocele disappears spontaneously. When treatment is required it takes one of three forms. It may take the form of aspirating, or withdrawing, the fluid with a needle and syringe. The fluid is liable to recur and further aspirations have to be carried out. In these cases it is more satisfactory to remove the fluid and replace it with sclerosing agent that seals off the cavity. Some surgeons prefer to operate and remove the sac.

HYDROCEPHALUS is the condition in which there is abnormal accumulation of cerebrospinal fluid within the skull. It is due to one or more of three main causes: (i) excessive production of spinal fluid (qv); (ii) defective absorption of cerebrospinal fluid; (iii) blockage to the circulation of cerebrospinal fluid. The causes of these disturbances of circulation of cerebrospinal fluid may be congenital (most commonly associated with spina bifida (qv), meningitis, or a tumour.

Symptoms: In children the chief symptoms observed are the gradual increase in size of the upper part of the head, out of all proportion to the face or the rest of the body. The head is globular, with a wide anterior fontanelle and separation of the bones at the sutures. The veins in the scalp are prominent, and there is a 'crackpot' note on percussion. The normal infant's head should not grow more than 2·5 cm (1 inch) in each of the first two months of life and much more slowly subsequently. Growth beyond this rate should arouse suspicions of hydrocephalus. Another useful rule is that the circumference of the head should not exceed that of the chest. In chronic hydrocephalus, the head of an infant 3 months old has been known to measure 72·5 cm (29 inches); and in the well-known case of the man, Cardinal, who died in Guy's Hospital, the head measured 82·5 cm (33 inches).

The cerebral ventricles are widely distended, and the convolutions of the brain flattened, while occasionally the fluid escapes into the cavity of the cranium, which it fills, pressing down the brain to the base of the skull. As a consequence of such changes, the functions of the brain are interfered with, and in general the mental condition of the patient is impaired. The child is dull and listless, irritable and sometimes suffers from severe mental subnormality. The special senses become affected as the disease advances, especially vision, and sight is often lost, as is also hearing. Towards the end paralysis is apt to occur.

The outlook for children with hydrocephalus is not as gloomy as was at one time thought to be the case. Such a child has a 50 per cent chance of survival with the disease arrested. He then has a 75 per cent chance of being educable. Almost one-third of arrested cases can be expected to enjoy normal intelligence with little or no physical disability.

Treatment: Numerous ingenious operations have been devised for the treatment of hydrocephalus. The most satisfactory of these utilize the Holter or Pudenz unidirectional valves, whereby the cerebrospinal fluid is bypassed into the right atrium of the heart or the peritoneal cavity, but it is only in a proportion of affected children that these operations produce a satisfactory result. The choice of operation and of the children likely to benefit is a highly skilled one that can only be made by an experienced surgeon.

HYDROCHLORIC ACID is a colourless, pungent, fuming liquid. It is present in the gastric juice to the extent of 2 parts in 1000. (See DIGESTION.) In large quantities it is a corrosive poison.

Uses: Its chief use is in cases in which the gastric juice is deficient: ie. in cases of achlorhydria (qv). The Dilute Hydrochloric Acid of the *British Pharmacopoeia* is given in doses of 0·5 to 4 millilitres, or in some such mixture as Acid Gentian Mixture BPC, Acid Gentian Mixture with Nux Vomica BPC, or Acid Nux Vomica Mixture BPC in doses of 10 to 20 millilitres.

HYDROCHLOROTHIAZIDE (ESIDEX, HYDROSALURIC) (see BENZOTHIADIAZINES).

HYDROCORTISONE, or compound F, has the chemical formula, 17-hydroxycorticosterone. It is closely allied to cortisone (qv) both in its structure (cortisone is an oxidation product of hydrocortisone) and in its action. Its anti-rheumatic potency is said to be 50 per cent greater than that of cortisone. Its main use to date in rheumatoid arthritis has been for local injection into affected joints. It is also used as a local application to the skin in the form of a cream or lotion in the treatment of certain skin diseases.

HYDROCYANIC ACID (see PRUSSIC ACID).

HYDROFLUMETHIAZIDE (HYDRENOX) is a derivative of chlorothiazide (qv). It is a powerful diuretic which acts by causing an increased urinary excretion of sodium and chloride. On a weight for weight basis it is about ten times as potent a diuretic as chlorothiazide. (See BENZOTHIADIAZINES.)

HYDROGEN PEROXIDE is a syrupy, colourless, odourless liquid which differs in chemical composition from water by containing two atoms of oxygen (H_2O_2) to every one in water (H_2O). It has the property of readily giving up its extra oxygen and being reduced to water, and this renders it of value in medicine for antiseptic, deodorant, and other purposes. It is most commonly employed as a solution in water of such a strength that any quantity will give off twenty times its bulk of oxygen gas; this is known as 20-volume strength, or as Hydrogen Peroxide Solution BP. It is also prepared as Strong Hydrogen Peroxide BP, also known as 100-volume strength as it gives off one hundred times its volume of oxygen. This strong solution must never be used undiluted. When added to ether the mixture is known as ozonic ether. Volatile oils which have become oxidized contain a considerable quantity of peroxide of hydrogen, and to this substance the power they possess of destroying foul odours is largely due.

Uses: The solution of hydrogen peroxide is applied externally to ulcers, and by sprays or swabs to cavities like the nose and throat, in order to act as an antiseptic, and also for the valuable property possessed by the little bubbles of oxygen that it gives off in breaking up and causing the separation of discharges. It is used to remove surgical dressings that are very adherent. Internally, it is sometimes used to wash out the stomach in cases of chronic gastritis, in a strength of 14 ml to 570 ml. It is also used to bleach hair and to remove superficial stains from teeth; for this purpose it is mixed with an equal volume of water. A hydrogen peroxide cream is also available for local application to leg ulcers and other skin disorders. It has the practical advantage of having a more prolonged action (several hours) than the solution.

HYDROGEN SULPHIDE, or SULPHURETTED HYDROGEN, is a potential hazard in petroleum refining, the gas industry, tanning and the chemical industry. It is found in sewers and coalmines (stink damp), and can be given off during the vulcanization of rubber containing sulphur. It is also a fishing hazard as it is given off in trawlers' holds containing what is known as 'trash' fish, the fish used for making fish-meal. Its well-known 'rotten egg' smell is detectable at as low a concentration as 0·025 part per million (p.p.m.), and by the time the concentration attains 30 p.p.m. it is intolerably unpleasant. Unfortunately, in prolonged exposure to it the smell rapidly disappears, which explains why it can be such a dangerous poison as the exposed individual has no idea that he is breathing it. Exposure to 150 to 300 p.p.m. leads to headache, spasm of the eyelids, with pain and redness of the eyes, blurred vision and coloured haloes round lights (gas eye). It may be several hours before these effects appear and they usually take several days to go. Serious effects appear above concentrations of 500 p.p.m.: mental confusion, convulsions, and oedema of the lungs with cyanosis (qv).

There is no specific antidote, and treatment consists of the usual first-aid measures for asphyxia (qv), the patient having first been removed well away from the contaminated area. If artificial respiration (qv) is started as soon as breathing stops, recovery is usually complete.

HYDROLYZED PROTEIN is protein (qv) which has been broken down into its constituent amino-acids. (Hydrolysis means the reaction of a large molecule with one or more molecules of water, with the production of two or more smaller molecules.) This is the process which normally occurs in the course of digestion of protein, but in certain conditions, such as marasmus and severe liver disease, where the process of digestion is badly upset, it is sometimes of value to give the patient protein that has already been hydrolyzed.

HYDRONEPHROSIS is a chronic disease in which the kidney becomes greatly distended with fluid. It is caused by obstruction to the flow of urine at the pelvi-ureteric junction. If the ureter is obstructed the ureter proximal to the obstruction will dilate and pressure will be transmitted back to the kidney to cause hydronephrosis. Obstruction may occur at the bladder neck or in the urethra itself. Enlargement of the prostate is a common cause of bladder-neck obstruction. This would give rise to hypertrophy of the bladder muscle and both dilatation of the ureter and hydronephrosis. If the obstruction is not relieved progressive destruction of renal tissue will occur. As a result of the stagnation of the urine infection is probable and cystitis and pyelonephritis may occur.

HYDROPHOBIA is another name for RABIES (qv).

HYDROPS FOETALIS (see HAEMOLYTIC DISEASE OF THE NEWBORN).

HYDROTHERAPY, or HYDROPATHY, is the name for all those curative measures in which water is the agent employed. (See BATHS; COLD DOUCHES; FOMENTATIONS; WET PACK.)

HYDROTHORAX means a collection of fluid in the pleural cavities.

HYDROXOCOBALAMIN, or vitamin B_{12}, has now replaced cyanocobalamin (qv) in the treatment of pernicious anaemia. (See ANAEMIA.) It has the practical advantage that fewer injections are required than in the case of cyanocobalamin. Like cyanocobalamin it belongs to the group of substances known as cobalamins which have an enzyme (qv) action in practically every metabolic system in the body and are essential for normal growth and nutrition.

HYDROXYUREA is a drug that is proving of value in the treatment of chronic myeloid leukaemia.

HYDROXYZINE PAMOATE is a tranquillizer that is proving of value in the treatment of anxiety states. (See BENZODIAZEPINES.)

HYGIENE is the science of preserving health.

HYMEN is the thin membranous fold partially closing the lower end of the virginal vagina.

HYOID is a U-shaped bone at the root of the tongue. It can be felt from the front of the neck, lying about 2·5 cm above the prominence of the thyroid cartilage.

HYOSCYAMUS, or HENBANE, is a plant that grows commonly in the United States and in Europe. The preparations are made from the leaves, and have an effect in quieting pain and relieving spasm. In large quantities it is a narcotic poison.
Uses: In spasmodic and painful conditions, particularly in colic and in irritable states of the bladder, the tincture of hyoscyamus is used with good effect. Hyoscine, an alkaloid obtained from hyoscyamus, is used in very small doses to quiet raving mania and in some nervous diseases, eg. Parkinsonism. It is also used for the production of 'twilight sleep', and for the prevention of travel sickness.

HYPERACUSIS means an abnormally acute sense of hearing.

HYPERAEMIA means congestion or presence of an excessive amount of blood in a part.

HYPERAESTHESIA means over-sensitiveness of a part, as found, for example, in certain nervous diseases. (See TOUCH.)

HYPERALGESIA means excessive sensitiveness to pain. (See PAIN; TOUCH.)

HYPERCALCIURIA means an abnormally large amount of calcium in the urine. It is the most common single cause of stones in the kidneys in Britain.

HYPERALIMENTATION (see ENTERAL AND PARENTERAL NUTRITION).

HYPERCAPNIA means an abnormal increase in the amount of carbon dioxide in the blood or in the lungs.

HYPERCHLORHYDRIA is the condition in which there is an excessive production of hydrochloric acid in the stomach. It is a characteristic finding in certain forms of dyspepsia, particularly that associated with a duodenal ulcer. It causes heartburn (qv) and waterbrash (qv). (See DUODENAL ULCER; DYSPEPSIA; STOMACH, DISEASES OF.)

HYPEREMESIS is a term applied to excessive vomiting, especially that which occurs in pregnancy.

HYPERGLYCAEMIA means excess of sugar in the blood, the condition accompanying diabetes mellitus. The amount of sugar normally present in the blood is dependent upon how much sugar has been consumed, but in the fasting state it runs around 80 to 100 milligrams per 100 millilitres of blood. A fasting blood level of sugar above this is regarded as hyperglycaemia; in diabetes mellitus (qv) the sugar may rise to four or five times that amount.

HYPERIDROSIS, or HYPERHIDROSIS, means excessive sweating. (See PERSPIRATION.)

HYPERLIPIDAEMIA means an excess of fat in the blood. The two most important fats circulating in the blood are cholesterol and triglycerides. Raised blood levels of cholesterol predispose to atheroma and coronary artery disease and raised triglycerides predispose to pancreatitis. Some of the hyperlipidaemias are familial and some are secondary to other diseases such as hypothyroidism, diabetes mellitus, nephrotic syndrome and alcoholism. There is evidence that therapy which lowers the lipid concentration reduces the progression of premature atheroma, particularly in those who suffer from the familial disorder. There are a number of drugs available for lowering the lipid content of the plasma but these should be reserved for patients in whom severe hyperlipidaemia is inadequately controlled by weight reduction. Clofibrate (Atromid S), bezafibrate (Bezalip), nicotinic acid and nicofuranose (Bradilan) lower plasma cholesterol and plasma triglyceride concentration through their effect on reducing the hepatic production of lipoproteins. Cholestyramine (Questran) and colestipol (Colestid), both of which are resins, bind bile salts in the gut and so decrease the absorption of the cholesterol that these bile salts contain and hence lower plasma cholesterol concentrations. Probucol (Lurselle) lowers plasma cholesterol concentrations by increasing the metabolism of low-density lipoproteins.

HYPERMETROPIA or HYPEROPIA, is a term applied to long-sightedness, in which the eye is too flat from front to back and rays of light are brought to a focus behind the retina. (See VISION; SPECTACLES.)

HYPERNEPHROMA is a term applied to a tumour resembling the tissue of the suprarenal gland and occurring in the kidney.

HYPERPIESIS is another term for high blood-pressure. HYPERPIESIA is another term for ESSENTIAL HYPERTENSION (qv).

HYPERPLASIA means an abnormal increase in the number of cells in a tissue.

HYPERPYREXIA means an excessive degree of fever. (See FEVER; TEMPERATURE.)

HYPERSENSITIVITY is the abnormal immunological reaction produced in certain individuals when re-exposed to antigens that are innocuous to normal individuals. An antigen or allergen stimulates an allergic response. This produces a state of altered re-activity or an allergic state. Such a state of altered re-activity may be beneficial to the host, as in establishing a state of immunity, or it may be harmful to the host and produce a state of disease. Hypersensitivity is thus an allergic reaction in an individual sensitised by previous exposure to the antigen and in whom the allergic process constitutes the disease.

HYPERTELORISM or TOTEM-POLE HEAD, is a rare congenital deformity of the head and face. The forehead is broad and low and the orbits are large and set widely apart. The divergence of the eyes is such that focusing on near objects is impossible. Strabismus (qv), or squint, is common.

HYPERTENSION is another term for high blood-pressure. (See ESSENTIAL HYPERTENSION; MALIGNANT HYPERTENSION.)

HYPERTHERMIA means abnormally high body temperature. It is also the name given to the treatment of disease by the artificial production of fever. This can be achieved by various methods, such as radiation heat cabinets boosted with radio frequency (RF); immersion in a hot wax bath; heated suits or blankets; techniques using electromagnetic waves (eg. RF, microwaves (qv)); ultrasound (qv) of appropriate frequencies. It is sometimes of help as an adjunct to surgery, chemotherapy, or radiotherapy in the treatment of cancer.

HYPERTHYROIDISM is excessive activity of the thyroid gland: eg. Graves' disease. (See GOITRE.)

HYPERTROPHY means the increase in size which takes place in an organ as the result of an increased amount of work demanded of it by the bodily economy. For example, when valvular disease of the heart is present, compensation occurs by an increase in thickness of the heart-muscle, and the organ, by beating more powerfully, is able to overtake the strain thrown upon it. Similarly, if one kidney is removed, the other hypertrophies or grows larger to overtake the double work.

HYPERVENTILATION, or overbreathing, is a common reaction to stress or anxiety. Overbreathing lowers the amount of carbon dioxide in the arterial blood and increases its acidity. These changes cause a wide variety of symptoms such as dizziness, feelings of unreality, pins and needles and numbness, tremor, choking, chest pain and palpitations: these unpleasant sensations cause the patient further anxiety and frequently provoke fears of heart attacks or sudden death. Hyperventilation has also been implicated in agoraphobia. The treatment consists of training to respond to stress or anxiety with slow breathing.

HYPNO-ANALYSIS is a method of treating certain neuroses by first releasing the patient's repressed fear under hypnosis, and then helping the patient to the necessary adjustment by suggestion.

HYPNOTICS are measures, including drugs, which produce sleep.

Varieties: As certain conditions are necessary for the onset of sleep, even a slight departure from these may be sufficient to keep people who are not in good health awake. Thus a diminution of the circulation in the brain, and freedom from pain or irritation in any bodily organ are essential, whilst quiet and darkness are desirable, though many people can adapt themselves to noise and there are not a few who can sleep equally well whether it is light or dark. Often some trivial alteration of the daily life or diet is enough to relieve habitual insomnia; in other cases the quieting of pain is alone necessary; in other cases drugs must be used which have a light dulling effect upon the brain itself. For the relief of pain the drugs known as anodynes (qv) are used. Of the hypnotics, which dull the brain without much other effect, there is a large variety.

Uses: Simple remedies should always receive a fair trial first of all. Thus a person may be kept awake by severe mental labour or worry just before retiring to rest. The activity of the brain continues and sleeplessness results. Some quiet employment for the latter part of the evening, or a light meal, may relieve this. In other cases sleeplessness is often due to difficulty of digestion through a meal having been taken shortly before retiring to rest, and this may be relieved by abstaining from the last meal at night. In old people insomnia may be due to cold feet, and in such cases the best hypnotic is a pair of warm sleeping socks. A condition of anaemia of the brain occurs in old men whose arteries are unhealthy, and this also debars sleep, unless the head is kept warm or a small quantity of alcohol is taken at bedtime: ie. a night cap literally or metaphorically. Occasionally sleep can be obtained by purely external applications. Massage of the head, the wet pack, and electrical (especially high frequency) applications are all used in different cases. Should these measures fail, and a hypnotic is required, the choice of which to use can only be made satisfactorily by the family doctor.

HYPNOTISM is the process of producing a state of mind known as hypnosis. Although a process which has been known for hundreds of years, its precise nature is still unknown. One modern writer has defined hypnosis as 'a temporary condition of altered attention, the most striking feature of which is greatly increased suggestibility'. There is no evidence, as has been claimed, that women can be more easily hypnotized than men. Children and young adults are the more easily hypnotized, middle-aged people being more resistant. There are various methods of induction of hypnosis, but the basis of them is some rhythmic stimulus accompanied by the repetition of carefully worded suggestions. The most commonly used method is to ask the patient to fix his eye on a given spot, or light, and then keep on repeating to him, in a quiet soothing voice, that his eyes will gradually become tired and that he will want to close them. There are various levels of hypnosis, usually classified as light, medium, and deep, and it has been estimated that 10 per cent of people cannot be hypnotized, 35 per cent can be taken into light hypnosis, 35 per cent into medium hypnosis, and 20 per cent into deep hypnosis.

Although in the past, hypnotism has often been frowned upon by orthodox medicine, largely because of its prostitution by charlatans, at the present day it is recognized to be a most useful method of therapy. Like all effective forms of therapy, however, it is not without its dangers, and this is why it should only be practised by those who have been adequately trained. Thus, under deep hypnosis suggestion can induce the person concerned to perform some prescribed automatic action when he awakes from the hypnotic state. Although there is good evidence that no-one can be hypnotized to perform acts which are fundamentally contrary to his moral or ethical principles and which he does not want to do, this is only reassuring if one has sound evidence that the hypnotized subject has conventional moral or ethical principles.

Apart from its use in psychiatry, it is of value in the treatment of many psychosomatic conditions: that is, conditions in which physical manifestations, such as skin lesions, headaches and other forms of pain, are primarily due to some psychological or emotional disturbance. It is also being used to an increasing extent in obstetrics for the relief of pain during labour, and for the relief of pain in dentistry. Asthma is another condition that sometimes responds well to it. Another condition in which it is proving most valuable is as part of the treatment of alcoholism.

HYPOCALCAEMIA is the condition of the blood in which its content of calcium is below normal. (Normally there are between 9 mg and 11 mg of calcium in 100 ml of serum.)

HYPOCHLORHYDRIA means an insufficient secretion of hydrochloric acid from the digestive cells of the stomach lining.

HYPOCHLOROUS ACID is a powerful antiseptic which both kills organisms and neutralizes the poisons they produce. It forms the active principle of the powder known as eupad and of its solution eusol. The powder is produced by mixing equal weights of boric acid and bleaching powder. The solution is prepared by adding 25 grams of this powder to 1 litre of water, and filtering. The clear solution so produced is eusol, and should contain 0·5 per cent of hypochlorous acid. Popularized during the 1914–1918 War, eusol has now been displaced to a great extent by the newer antiseptics, such as the acridine derivatives, the sulphonamides and penicillin, but it is still of value in the treatment of septic wounds.

HYPOCHONDRIASIS is a chronic mental condition in which the affected person's mind is constantly occupied with a delusion that he is seriously ill. As a rule, the ailments are referred to the stomach or the liver, and very often some trivial derangement of these exists to give colour to the person's views. Along with these complaints, there is a self-centred and gloomy turn of mind that prevents the patient from doing much of his proper work. Not uncommonly this mental trouble is hereditary, and passes gradually at a later stage into melancholia. The condition, apart from the affected person making a strong effort of will and taking up some active work which may distract his thoughts, is very difficult to treat.

HYPODERMIC means of, or pertaining to, the region immediately under the skin. Thus, a hypodermic injection means an injection given underneath the skin. A hypodermic syringe is a small syringe which, fitted with a fine needle, is used to give such injections. A hypodermic injection is given for one of three main reasons: (1) because the substance administered cannot be given by mouth on account of its being destroyed in the stomach before it can be absorbed, eg. insulin; (2) because it is not possible or it is inadvisable to give anything by mouth to the patient, eg. because of vomiting; (3) because a quick action is necessary, eg. morphine in cases of severe pain.

HYPODERMOCLYSIS is injection of a fluid under the skin: for example, of a solution of glucose or of saline as a method of restoring fluids to the circulation of a person who is dehydrated.

HYPOGASTRIC means pertaining to the lower middle part of the abdomen just above the pubis.

HYPOGLOSSAL NERVE is the twelfth cranial nerve, and supplies the muscles of the tongue, together with some others lying near it.

HYPOGLYCAEMIA is a deficiency of sugar in the blood. It may occur in states of starvation, or after the administration of insulin in too large doses, causing symptoms of weakness, tremors, nervousness, breathlessness and excitement, followed sometimes by unconsciousness. These symptoms are relieved by taking sugar or by an injection of adrenaline, which antagonises the action of insulin.

HYPOGLYCAEMIC AGENTS: There are two groups of oral hypoglycaemic drugs, the sulphonylureas and the biguanides. Both have been used in the treatment of diabetes for about 30 years. The sulphonylureas act on the beta cell to stimulate insulin release and on peripheral tissues to increase sensitivity, though the latter is a less important action. Chlorpropamide and glibenclamide have a higher ceiling of potency than tolbutamide and this is associated with a considerably longer half life in the body. A newer arrival, gliquidone, claims to have the hypoglycaemic power of the second generation and the short biological half life of tolbutamide and may therefore be more suitable for those who require protection from nocturnal hypoglycaemia. The biguanides reduce carbohydrate absorption and facilitate the action of insulin on peripheral tissues. In the obese diabetic in whom increased insulin production is better avoided metformin alone may be used to reinforce the dietary treatment.

HYPOGONADISM is the condition characterized by deficient production of the hormones secreted by the gonads: that is, the ovaries and testes.

HYPOMANIA is a slight degree of mania.

HYPOPHOSPHITES of lime, iron, etc., are administered in combination as 'a tonic'.

HYPOPHYSECTOMY means surgical excision of the pituitary gland.

HYPOPHYSIS is another name for the pituitary gland.

HYPOPIESIS is the condition, or state, characterized by abnormally low blood-pressure.

HYPOPLASIA means excessive smallness of an organ or part, arising from imperfect development.

HYPOPYON: A collection of pus in the anterior chamber of the eye. It usually appears as a white fluid level in the inferior part of the anterior chamber, obscuring the iris (see EYE, DISEASE AND INJURIES OF).

HYPOSPADIAS is a developmental abnormality in the male, in which the urethra opens on the under-surface of the penis or in the perineum (qv).

HYPOSTASIS is the term applied to the condition in which blood accumulates in a dependent part as a result of a feeble circulation. Congestion of the base of the lungs in old people from this cause, and infection, is called hypostatic pneumonia.

HYPOTENSION means abnormally low blood-pressure. *Postural hypotension* is the abnormal fall in blood-pressure which may occur on suddenly standing up. It is more liable to occur in old folk.

HYPOTHALAMUS is that part of the forebrain situated beneath the thalamus on each side and forming the floor of the third ventricle. The hypothalamus contains collections of nerve cells believed to form the controlling centres of (1) the sympathetic and (2) the parasympathetic nervous systems. The hypothalamus is the nervous centre for primitive physical and emotional behaviour. It contains nerve centres for the regulation of certain vital processes: the metabolism of fat, carbohydrate and water; sleep; body temperature and genital functions.

HYPOTHERMIA means low temperature. This is a term that is used in three different contexts.

(1) It is being widely used in conjunction with operations on the heart and on the brain. The rationale of its use is that it lowers the requirements of the tissues for oxygen. This means that the cells of the brain, which are particularly susceptible to lack of oxygen, can be safely deprived of their blood supply for a longer period than at normal temperature. In practice this means that in operations on the heart, for instance, the action of the heart can be arrested for a few minutes while the surgeon actually operates on the heart.

Two methods are used to produce hypothermia. In one the blood of the patient is circulated through a special cooling machine. In the other the body temperature is lowered by the use of ice packs, iced water or a special cooling mattress. (See also CRYMOTHERAPY.)

(2) The term is also used to describe the condition which may develop, especially in old people and in infants, if they are exposed to abnormally low temperatures. The effects of exposure to low temperatures are as follows:

Constriction of the blood-vessels of the skin; increased muscle tone, and shivering.

Each winter in the British Isles old people die at home as the result of cold. Accidental hypothermia occurs in apparently fit old people and has been described as 'a common domestic disorder of the elderly'. It is defined as a deep body temperature (that is, a temperature recorded in the rectum or by a thermistor (qv) in the ear) below 35°C (95°F), and it has been estimated that around half a million old people in Britain are at risk of hypothermia. One of the main causes is that old people cannot maintain their body temperature because they lose heat through the skin. Normally on exposure to cold the blood-vessels of the skin are reflexly constricted through the autonomic nervous system (qv). This is a powerful mechanism for conserving heat as it greatly reduces the heat conductivity of the skin.

As many old people cannot conserve the heat they make because they lose it through the skin, the obvious treatment is that they should wear adequate insulating clothing indoors as well as outdoors. As half the heat loss from a clothed adult is from the head, there is much to be said for the elderly reviving the old fashion of wearing nightcaps, smoking caps and mutches. They should wear long underwear, or combinations, and gloves or mittens by day, and bed socks and extra warm blankets at night. In this last respect the metallized 'space blankets' on sale for mountaineers are light and efficient. Basic to all these measures, however, is an adequately heated house. For those who cannot afford to keep their homes adequately heated, additional supplementary benefits are available for extra heating. Details of these benefits can be obtained from local offices of the Department of Health and Social Security.

(3) There is a third important context in which hypothermia may occur: on immersion in water, usually the sea. This is the form known as immersion hypothermia. (See DROWNING, RECOVERY FROM.)

HYPOTHYROIDISM means the condition produced by defective action of the thyroid gland. (See MYXOEDEMA.)

HYSTERECTOMY is the operation of removing the uterus. HYSTERO-OOPHORECTOMY is the term applied to removal of the uterus and ovaries.

HYSTERIA is a condition or set of conditions which it is difficult to define. The condition is also known as PITHIATISM because many of its symptoms appear to be due to auto-suggestion and are readily relieved by suggestion from another person. Hysteria manifests itself by over-action of some parts of the nervous system, or by failure of other parts to perform their necessary work. In consequence, there follow mental changes, convulsive seizures, spasms and contractions of limbs, paralyses, loss of sensation over areas of the body, affections of various internal organs, derangements of joints and combinations of these which closely mimic various organic diseases. Hysterical manifestations are among the most difficult affections upon which the specialist is called to give an opinion.

Causes: The condition is far more common in women than in men. It used to be supposed that the origin of the disease, as its name indicates, lay in trouble of the womb, but, though sexual disturbances often occur in the condition, they should more probably be classed as symptoms. Heredity is of importance, as is upbringing.

Symptoms: MENTAL CHANGES are almost always observable in hysterical cases, although the other symptoms in different cases may differ widely from one another. The affected person becomes whimsical, dominated by ideas, and incapable of the same work and concentration as before. She becomes easily excitable, and is either morbidly sensitive, feeling slight rebuffs keenly, or unusually demonstrative, bursting into fits of laughter or paroxysms of weeping upon slight provocation. In marked cases, hysterical subjects become morally unhinged, deceiving everyone around them, so that little credence can be given to their statements.

CONVULSIVE HYSTERIA is the most marked form. An attack may begin upon some excitement, with laughter or weeping, or may give no warning sign. The person falls in an unconscious or half-conscious condition, but whereas the fall in epilepsy is downright, the hysterical person subsides gently in general upon a couch or chair, and rarely or never so as to hurt herself, and seldom without an audience. She may then lie still, or more generally moans or talks incoherently, rolls the head from side to side, and tosses the hands and feet about. In serious attacks, known as hystero-epilepsy, the onset resembles epilepsy and may be followed by curious posturing, the sufferer placing herself in attitudes which suggest powerful emotions of fear, ecstasy or joy. In this state visions are seen, voices heard, and conversations held with imaginary persons. This forms one of the most perverted types of hysteria and one of the least hopeful as regards a cure.

LOSS OF SENSATION over some part of the body is one of the commonest symptoms. This loss may affect a limb, or may be irregularly distributed in patches, or may affect some special sense organ, causing, for example, failure of taste, blindness for all objects to one side of the field of vision, or for objects of some special type repugnant to the patient, or deafness in one ear. Sometimes there is complete loss of the sense of pain, so that pricks, pinches, and other painful stimuli are borne without wincing.

SPASMS AND CONTRACTIONS of muscles also form a common manifestation of hysteria without any other sign save mental hebetude (qv). If this contraction exist in the muscles of the body wall, it may, and often does, give rise to the idea that the person is the subject of a tumour. Such spasms may also lead to the drawing up of an arm or foot, so that the limb in time becomes permanently deformed. Or when the mind becomes powerfully impressed by some person or idea, the spasm may pass off, and gradual or sudden recovery takes place.

PARALYSIS is perhaps the most troublesome symptom of all to overcome. It may extend over one-half of the body, and is then very difficult to differentiate from the effects of apoplexy. Most commonly the foot is affected and the person declares herself unable to walk. As the paralysis sometimes lasts for years unimproved, and then suddenly vanishes, these cases are eminently suited for successful ministration by the faith-healer or by wonder-working shrines. Such people, when the paralysis affects both legs, and is accompanied by pain in the back, have again and again been confined for years to bed or couch as cases of spinal disease, only to recover suddenly when some new interest has come into their lives, or force of circumstances has rendered an active life imperative. The muscles of the larynx are often affected, and the person may be deprived of speech for years, till some powerful influence forces her to exert her will and the organ of voice again comes into play.

CHANGES IN INTERNAL ORGANS take place in some cases and produce such signs as constant hiccup, barking noises, excessive vomiting, diarrhoea, absolute loss of appetite, and profound changes in the circulation. Among the features of the last-named may be mentioned the appearance of swollen and congested areas in the skin, and, showing the power which the mind may exert over bodily functions, there is recorded the case of Louise Lateau, who, after meditating for many days upon the Crucifixion, developed on hands and feet 'stigmata' or bleedings beneath the skin.

JOINT AFFECTIONS are among the most remarkable physical changes. A joint, especially the hip or knee, becomes swollen, stiff, and painful, and may remain so for months. (See PAIN.)

MASS HYSTERIA is a phenomenon characterized by extreme suggestibility. It most commonly occurs when large numbers of girls are massed together under conditions, such as fêtes and competitions, which induce emotional tension and excitement. Under such conditions the girls often feel faint or giddy, or sick. If one of them actually faints or is sick in the presence of the others, then they may start following her example, and faint or vomit. In this way a chain reaction is started, and large numbers may be affected. It is a well-recognized hazard in girls' schools, particularly among the older girls. Recovery quickly ensues when the affected girls are separated from each other. (See also NEUROMYASTHENIA.)

Treatment: In acute hysterical attacks rest and quiet are chiefly necessary. For symptoms such as vomiting, joint affections, loss of sensation, and spasms, removal from home and from the attention of sympathetic friends to strict isolation, where the patient sees nobody but a nurse and eats only the simplest of food, is a useful form of treatment. For the severest forms of hysteria isolation and absolute rest in bed are employed. Further, massage takes the place of exercise, and the patient is encouraged to eat large amounts of readily digestible food. In all cases of hysteria psychotherapy forms an important element in treatment. This is carried out especially by suggestion, but in other cases it may take the form of persuasion, psychoanalysis, or education and employment.

I

IATRIC means anything pertaining to a physician.

IATROGENIC DISEASE is disease induced by a physician: essentially a drug-induced disease.

IBUPROFEN (BRUFEN) is a drug which is proving of value as an anti-inflammatory agent and as an analgesic in the treatment of rheumatoid arthritis and other forms of rheumatism. (See NON-STEROIDAL ANTI-INFLAMMATORY DRUGS.)

ICE is used as a convenient form of applying cold, both externally and internally. For external application the most convenient form of application is by placing chopped ice in a rubber bag, known as an ice-bag. The bag is closed by a screw cap and is laid upon the head, abdomen, or other part to which it is desired to make the cold application, a layer of flannel or a garment being placed between the bag and the skin to prevent a direct freezing action on the surface. Iced water is sometimes applied by means of a coiled tube, especially in cases of inflammation of the head. The iced water is allowed to percolate slowly from a jug placed above the bed through the coiled tube laid on the affected part.

For internal application ice is seldom used now. (See also COLD, USES OF; CRYMOTHERAPY.)

ICHOR is the thin fluid, yellowish or bloody, which issues from a sore or a wound.

ICHTHAMMOL, ICHTHYOL, is ammonium ichthosulphonate, an almost black, thick liquid of fishy smell, prepared from a bituminous shale. It is used in several chronic skin diseases.

ICHTHYOSIS is a skin disease in which the surface is very rough and presents a dry, cracked appearance, resembling fish-scales. The peculiarity is generally hereditary, and persists through life, the skin being permanently hard, and deficient in oily material. The appearances differ considerably according to the part affected and the surrounding conditions. Thus the knees and elbows when affected become black from the collection of dirt in the deep crevices, and in winter the skin becomes specially hard and the condition still more marked.

Treatment: There is no specific internal treatment, but improvement sometimes follows the administration of vitamin A. Those who suffer from the disease should live, if possible, in a warm sunny climate. External treatment is most important and consists of daily warm baths with bran or starch, followed by the application of 20 to 50 per cent glycerin in water, olive oil, or equal parts of salicylic acid ointment (2 per cent) and glycerin. An alternative form of treatment is to add the *British Pharmacopoeia* Emulsifying Ointment to the bath: 28·5 grams (1 ounce) is added after preliminary creaming in a jug of hot water. This is followed by the application to the skin of the *British Pharmacopoeia* Hydrous Ointment as often as is required. Another promising line of treatment is the use of a urea cream. (See UREA.)

ICTERUS is another name for jaundice (qv).

ICTERUS GRAVIS NEONATORUM (see HAEMOLYTIC DISEASE OF THE NEWBORN).

ICTUS is another term for a stroke.

IDIOCY is a term no longer used. Those who were described as idiots are now included in the category of 'severe subnormality' as defined in the Mental Health Act, 1959. (See MENTAL SUBNORMALITY.)

IDIOGLOSSIA means the continued utterance of meaningless sounds, the afflicted person 'speaking' a language intelligible to no-one.

IDIOPATHIC is a term applied to diseases to indicate that their cause is unknown.

IDIOSYNCRASY implies an inherent abnormal qualitative reaction to a drug that is primarily the result of a constitutional defect in the patient. The abnormal sensitivity of patients with porphyria to barbiturates and sulphonamides is an example. Hereditary biochemical defects of red blood cells are responsible for many drug-induced haemolytic anaemias and for favism. Drug-sensitive red cells are deficient in the enzyme glucose phosphate dehydrogenase which plays an important part in the metabolism of glucose and is necessary for the continued integrity of the cell. When patients with porphyria are given certain drugs, particularly barbiturates and sulphonamides, they are liable to develop acute neurological episodes with peripheral and respiratory paralysis which may result in death. Porphyria variegata, the South African variety of porphyria, is an example of an inborn error of metabolism which was without serious symptoms until the advent of barbiturate drugs. Taking these drugs can precipitate total paralysis and death. A metabolic error is inherited as a dominant characteristic and there are now 8,000 affected people in South Africa, all of whom can be traced to a single couple who married in the seventeeth century.

IDOXURIDINE: An antiviral agent still widely used in the treatment of cases of herpes simplex involvement of the cornea of the eye (see EYE, DISEASE AND INJURIES OF).

IFOSFAMIDE (MITOXANA) (see CYTOTOXIC DRUGS).

ILEITIS means inflammation of the ileum. REGIONAL ILEITIS, or CROHN'S DISEASE, is the term applied to a condition in which there is an inflammation of an area of the small intestine. This is accompanied by colicky abdominal pain, irregularity of the bowels, loss of weight and slight fever. The abdomen is distended and the thickened intestine may be felt. The narrowed intestinal canal may become obstructed, necessitating immediate operation. The cause is unknown. The primary lesion is hyperplasia (qv) of the lymph tissue in the submucosa of the intestine and in the lymph glands.

As the cause is not known, there is no specific treatment. In the early stages, treatment is medical, including a high-vitamin, low-residue diet, sulphonamides and antibiotics. Promising results have been reported from the use of corticosteroids in some cases. Operation, consisting of removal of the damaged section of gut, is reserved for cases which do not respond to medical treatment. Even in cases apparently successfully operated on, recurrence tends to occur in 15 per cent or more of cases.

Patients and their relatives can obtain help and guidance from the National Association for Colitis and Crohn's Disease, 3 Thorpefield Close, St. Albans, Hertfordshire AL4 9TJ.

ILEO-CAECAL is the term applied to the region of the junction between the small and large intestines in the right lower corner of the abdomen. The ileo-caecal valve is a structure which allows the contents of the intestine to pass onwards from the small to the large intestine, but, in the great majority of cases, prevents their passage in the opposite direction.

ILEOSTOMY is the operation by which an artificial opening is made into the ileum. It is most often performed as part of the operation for cancer of the rectum, in which the rectum has usually to be removed. An ileostomy is then performed which acts as an artificial anus. Distressing though this may at first be, the vast majority of people with an ileostomy learn to lead a fully active and normal life. Help and advice in adjusting to what can be described as an 'ileostomy life' can be obtained from the Ileostomy Association of Great Britain and Ireland, Amblehurst House, Black Scotch Lane, Mansfield, Notts NG18 4PF (0623–28099). (See STOMA.)

ILEUM is the lower part of the small intestine. (See INTESTINE.)

ILEUS is a paralysis of the bowel muscle. (See INTESTINE, DISEASES OF.)

ILIUM is another name for the haunch-bone, the uppermost of the three bones forming each side of the pelvis. (See BONE; PELVIS.)

ILLUSIONS (see HALLUCINATIONS).

IMBECILITY is a term no longer used. What used to be known as imbecility is now included in the category of 'severe subnormality', as defined in the Mental Health Act, 1959. (See MENTAL SUBNORMALITY.)

IMIPRAMINE (PRAMIL, TOFRANIL) is one of the so-called tricyclic antidepressants which is proving of value in the treatment of depression. (See ANTIDEPRESSANTS.)

IMMERSION FOOT is the term applied to a condition which develops as a result of prolonged immersion of the feet in cold or cool water. It was a condition commonly seen during the 1939–45 War in shipwrecked sailors and airmen who had crashed in the sea and spent long periods before being rescued. Such prolonged exposure results in vasoconstriction of the smaller arteries in the feet, leading to coldness and blueness of the feet, and finally, in severe cases, to ulceration and gangrene.

IMMUNITY (from *immunus*, Latin for exempt) is a principle by which the body is protected from the invasion of certain diseases, or the action of certain poisons. It is a well-recognized fact that some people expose themselves again and again to the risk of infection and are not affected, whilst others seem prone to contract any disease with which they are brought into contact. The immunity so enjoyed is of several types. Natural immunity is one which is inborn; but immunity may also be acquired in the course of life, or it may be produced artificially by inoculation, or by injection of the blood serum of immune individuals.

Natural immunity: Certain animals seem to be little affected by poisons which to others are very deadly. Thus the snake-killing mongoose of India is said to be highly immune to cobra poison. Pigeons are little affected by large doses of morphine; rabbits and other animals eat freely the leaves of the deadly nightshade plant. (See IDIOSYNCRASY.) The rat is little affected by tuberculosis, to which other creatures, including particularly man and the guinea-pig, are very susceptible. Man, on the other hand, is unaffected by swine fever, and some other diseases which are very infectious and fatal among the lower animals, while no animal, so far as is known, contracts cholera, a disease which is so disastrous to man. Other examples are found in the fowl and the alligator, which are peculiar in being exempt from lockjaw, and white rats, which are not affected by anthrax. There is probably no such thing as absolute immunity, however, since animals are affected by any poison if their health is very low or if the amount of poison is very great.

Acquired immunity is that which is gained by passing through an attack of some disease. Protection is probably given by all infectious diseases for a longer or shorter period against a second attack of the same disease. In the case of some, such as smallpox, typhoid fever, scarlet fever, the protection appears to last throughout life, or, at all events, for many years. Recovery from a disease is in fact a process of immunity, the poison of the disease being destroyed by antagonizing substances, known as antibodies, produced in the tissues of the body, so that the disease comes to an end after a definite period. Some individuals acquire these antibodies by coming in contact with the infecting organisms without ever actually showing signs of the disease or possibly by having it in such a mild form that it is not recognized.

Artificial immunity is of two kinds, known as active and passive immunity.

(*a*) ACTIVE IMMUNITY is produced by injecting beneath an animal's skin, or administering by the mouth in some cases, a small dose of some particular poison insufficient to produce death. This has the effect of stimulating the animal's powers of resistance, so that next time it can withstand a larger dose. The process is repeated over and over, the dose each time increasing, till finally the animal is unaffected by many times the dose which would have originally killed it. This applies to snake poisons also, and the snake-charmers of India appear to render themselves indifferent to cobra-bites by a similar process.

With regard to disease-producing bacteria and the toxins or poisons which they form, immunity is reached by injecting small quantities of bacteria, or of their toxins, which have been weakened by mixing with antiseptics, by drying in air, by passing through the bodies of partially immune animals, or by other highly technical processes. The best-known practical

Vaccine	*Age at which to give*
BCG	Within first week of life if any contact likely with anyone with tuberculosis
Diphtheria, tetanus and whooping-cough (one injection of Triple vaccine) and poliomyelitis vaccine by mouth	3 months Repeated 6 weeks later and again after a further 6 months
Measles	During 2nd year
Diphtheria and tetanus (one injection) and poliomyelitis vaccine by mouth	On going to school
BCG if child is Mantoux-negative	10 to 13 years
German measles (girls only)	11 to 13 years
Diphtheria and tetanus (one injection), poliomyelitis vaccine by mouth	On leaving school

Timetable for routine immunization of children. – *The Practitioner.*

example of this treatment is vaccination against smallpox, in which cowpox, a modified form of the disease, is produced in persons so as to render them immune to the far severer smallpox. Another is Pasteur's preventive treatment for rabies, in which, during the long incubation period before the disease has had time to appear, the person is treated by increasing doses of the poison, taken from rabbits that have been killed by the disease. (See RABIES.)

The principle of this method, then, consists in stimulating the power of the body to resist the action of poisons. Great success in preventing diphtheria has been achieved by injecting one to three doses of diphtheria toxoid (inactivated toxin). Other common diseases against which protection can be provided in this way include typhoid fever, whooping-cough, tetanus, measles, German measles and poliomyelitis. A summary of current practice of immunization for children is shown in the table on page 354. (See also VACCINE.)

(*b*) PASSIVE IMMUNITY is that form of artificial immunity obtained by injecting into the body of one person, whom it is desired to render immune, blood serum drawn from an already rendered immune by the active method. (See SERUM THERAPY.)

IMMUNOGLOBULINS: Antibody globulin is now called immunoglobulin. In man there are five different types of immunoglobulin and differences in structure between these groups coincide with variations in biological behaviour. Most antibodies have a molecular weight of about 160,000 and when their rate of sedimentation is measured they have a sedimentation constant of about 7 Svenberg units (7s). There is, however, another group of antibodies which move faster on electrophoresis, have a greater molecular weight (900,000) and have a sedimentation constant of 19 Svenberg units (19s). Immunoglobulin G, or IgG, constitutes three-quarters of the protein within the electrophetically-defined gamma area of serum. It is a 7s antibody and constitutes the majority of the acquired antibacterial and antiviral antibodies. It is distributed equally between the blood and interstitial tissues and it is the only immunoglobulin which passes across the placenta to reach the foetal circulation. This transfer is not due to simple filtration but to an active cellular process. IgM of macroglobulin is so named because of its high molecular weight (900,000), and is predominantly intravascular. It is a 19s globulin and includes the blood-group antibodies.

IgG and IgM antibodies combine with antigen to form either soluble complexes or precipitates, depending on the relative proportion of antigen to antibodies. They activate complement and this enables them to neutralize toxins, bacteria and viruses and to promote phagocytosis. If the reaction occurs across a vascular membrane the result will be an Arthus reaction consisting of oedema and haemorrhage. Complement consists of nine different substances which act as a cascade analogous to the clotting mechanism. Some of the substances making up the complement are only present in trace quantities; others can be measured in milligrams. Two of these substances (C3 and C5) release histamine from mast cells, another (C5) is chemotactic to polymorphs, and others cause damage to cells by forming micelles in the surface layer of cells (C8 and C9).

IgA is a 7s gamma globulin synthesized by plasma cells at mucosal surfaces and appearing in secretions in which its concentration is often much higher than that of IgG. IgA antibodies do not activate the complement system: they are mainly protective and are not involved in hypersensitivity reactions. They have been aptly described as an antiseptic paint. The immunological function of the IgD group of antibodies is unknown. IgE possesses reagin activity and is the anaphylactic antibody in man.

Each immunoglobulin consists of four polypeptide chains. Each has a basic molecular unit of two heavy chains (molecular weight 50,000) joined to light chains (molecular weight 25,000). The heavy chains are specific to the type of immunoglobulin but there are two light chains (k and λ) which are common to all classes of immunoglobulin. The specificity of different antibodies is due to differences in the sequence of amino acids in those parts of the polypeptide chains which form the antibody-combining sites. In normal antibody-forming cells immunoglobulin synthesis is so well balanced that none of these peptide chains escapes from the cells. In myelomatosis, however, the malignant proliferation of plasma cells results in an imbalanced production of the heavy and light chains of immunoglobulin molecules and the excess of free light chains escapes into the circulation and is filtered through the renal glomeruli as Bence-Jones protein. Such incoordinate production of immunoglobulin is a manifestation of the greater malignancy of the cell and hence augurs a worse prognosis for the disease. It must however be realised that rarely are humoral factors solely responsible for protection against infection, as the scavenger action of cells such as polymorphs and macrophages is also necessary.

IMPACTION is a term applied to a condition in which two things are firmly lodged together. For example, when after a fracture one piece of bone is driven within the other, this is known as an impacted fracture; when a tooth is firmly lodged in its socket so that its eruption is prevented, this is known as dental impaction.

IMPERIAL DRINK (for composition see under CREAM OF TARTAR).

IMPERSEX is another name for infantilism (qv) or imperfect sexual development.

IMPETIGO is an infectious skin disease often found in schools and also in rugby football players (see SCRUMPOX), and caused usually by the *Staphylococcus aureus*. It consists of vesicles which appear here and there, on the face particularly, and dry up, leaving yellowish-brown scabs from which the discharge is infectious. These scabs fall off, leaving no scars, but the disease spreads from place to place over the skin, and may last for months if untreated. When it occurs in very young children, it is liable to run a severe course unless treatment is initiated immediately. This form of the disease is known as pemphigus neonatorum (see PEMPHIGUS) because of the marked blistering of the skin that tends to occur.

Treatment: Affected children should be off school and use separate washing and eating utensils. Infected crusts are removed by washing with saline or cetrimide lotion. Starch poultices may be necessary where the crusts are extensive. Infection can be caused by *Staphylococcus Aureus* or *Streptococcus* and both are sensitive to synthetic penicillins.

When nits are present on the hair, treatment is ineffective until these have been removed. (See PEDICULOSIS.)

IMPLANTS, DENTAL. To allow false teeth to be held more firmly in the mouth a number of methods have been devised to embed a framework in the bone to which the denture can be fixed. This has been partly successful, but the ideal material, which will not be rejected, is still being sought. Titanium is the most promising.

IMPOTENCE is the inability to perform the sexual act. It may be partial or complete, temporary or permanent. Of the many classifications of this not uncommon condition, the most satisfactory is probably that which divides it into two main groups: *organic* and *psychological*. Among organic causes are lesions of the external genitalia, eg. a tight foreskin; disturbances of the endocrine glands, such as diminished activity of the gonads, thyroid gland or pituitary gland; diseases of the central nervous system, eg. tabes dorsalis; any severe disturbance of health, such as diabetes mellitus, addiction to alcohol and the like. Among the psychological factors are ignorance, fear, weakness of sexual desire or abnormality of such desire.

INCISION means a cut or wound and is a term specially applied to surgical openings.

INCISOR is the name applied to the four front teeth of each jaw. (See TEETH.)

INCOMPATIBILITY is a term applied to unsuitability in a prescription owing to the fact that its different contents either cannot be mixed, or that when mixed they undergo chemical changes, or that their actions are opposed to one another.

INCOMPETENCE is a term applied to the valves of the heart when, as a result of disease in the valves or alterations in size of the chambers of the heart, the valves become unable to close the orifices which they should protect. (See HEART DISEASES.)

INCONTINENCE is a term applied to the inability to retain the evacuations of the bowels and bladder. It occurs in diseases of these organs, injuries and diseases of the spinal cord, etc.

INCO-ORDINATION is a term applied to irregularity of movements produced either by loss of the sensations by which they are governed or by defects in the muscles themselves or their nerves.

INCUBATION means the period elapsing between the time when a person becomes infected by some agent and the first appearance of the symptoms of the disease. Most acute infectious diseases have fairly definite periods of incubation, and it is of great importance that people who have run the risk of infection should know the length of time which must elapse before they can be sure whether or not they are to contract the disease in question. A person who has been exposed to infection is, during the incubation period, technically known as a contact. By isolating and watching contact cases medical officers can often successfully check a threatened epidemic. It must be noted that diseases are not communicated to others by a person while passing through the stage of incubation. Some diseases, however, such as measles, become infectious as soon as the first symptoms set in after the incubation period is over; others, like scarlet fever and smallpox, are not so infectious then as in their later stages. The incubation period for any given disease is remarkably constant, although in the case of a severe attack the incubation is usually slightly shortened, and if the oncoming attack be a mild one, the period may be lengthened. So far as schools are concerned, children who have been contacts should not be allowed to return to school till several days beyond the maximum incubation period has elapsed since exposure to infection. All of these may, however, take a few days longer than the time stated to show themselves. (See INFECTION.)

	days
Chickenpox	14–21
Diphtheria	2–5
German measles	14–21
Measles	10–15
Mumps	18–21
Poliomyelitis	3–21
Smallpox	10–16
Typhoid fever	7–21
Whooping-cough	7–10

Incubation periods of the commoner infectious diseases.

Several also, and especially whooping-cough, may be difficult to recognize in their early stages.

INDAPAMIDE (NATRILLIX) (see BENZOTHIADIAZINES).

INDIAN HEMP (see CANNABIS INDICA).

INDIGESTION (see DYSPEPSIA).

INDOMETHACIN is a drug that is used in the treatment of gout and rheumatoid arthritis. It is said to be of particular value in the relief of night pain and morning stiffness. It is also proving of value in the treatment of the congenital abnormality of the heart known as patent ductus arteriosus. (See DUCTUS ARTERIOSUS.)

INDOPROFEN (FLOSINT) (see NON-STEROIDAL ANTI-INFLAMMATORY DRUGS).

INDORAMIN is an alpha-adreno-receptor-blocking drug which is proving of value in the treatment of high blood-pressure. (See ADRENERGIC RECEPTORS.)

INDUSTRIAL DISEASES (see OCCUPATIONAL DISEASES).

INFANT FEEDING: An infant may either be breast-fed or bottle-fed.

Breast feeding: Unless there is some definite contraindication, every new-born child should be breast-fed. The advantages are clear cut and definite. The milk is specially prepared in composition for the human baby. It is at the right temperature. It is available at any time no matter where the mother may be. It is most unlikely to be infected or contaminated, and it provides protection against infection at an age when the baby is particularly vulnerable in this respect. Further, breast feeding helps the womb to return to its normal shape more quickly and helps to prevent the mother from putting on weight. It also reduces the risk of the baby becoming too fat, and there is evidence that fat babies are more likely to have chest infections and to grow up into fat adults. Finally – but by no means least – breast feeding offers the most intimate contact between a mother and her new-born baby. A point to be borne in mind, however, is that many drugs taken by a nursing mother are excreted in her milk and may therefore affect her babe. These include antibiotics, barbiturates, tranquillizers, corticosteroids, vitamins, alcohol, and nicotine. Doctors can obtain from their local Drug Information Centre a list of drugs which could be potentially harmful to breast-fed babies.

The baby should be put to the breast six to eight hours after birth, and thereafter every three or four hours. Whether the baby is fed three-hourly or four-hourly depends upon how he progresses, but in the majority of healthy babies who weigh 3·2 kg (7 pounds) or more at birth, four-hourly feeding is sufficient. Five feeds are usually sufficient in the twenty-four hours, a useful time-table being feeds at 6 am., 10 am., 2 pm., 6 pm., and 10 pm. There is no reason why a healthy infant should not go through the night without a feed, although it may sometimes be found more convenient to give the first feed in the morning somewhat earlier. This undisturbed night is invaluable to the nursing mother. Both breasts should be used at each feed, and it is an advantage to start each feed on alternate breasts. For the first feed of all, one minute at each breast is sufficient, and this time should be gradually increased until by the end of the first week the baby is having seven to ten minutes at each breast every feed.

The main guide as to whether an infant is being adequately fed is the weight. During the first few days of life a healthy infant loses weight, but this he should have regained by the tenth day of life. Thereafter he should gain 28 grams (1 ounce) daily. All the known vitamins are present in breast milk. The amount is closely associated with the vitamin status of the mother, and is sufficient for the baby's requirements provided the mother has a plentiful supply. To be on the safe side, however, the official recommendation is that from the age of 1 month until at least 2 years of age, and preferably until 5 years of age, infants and children should be given five drops daily of the Children's Vitamin Drops available under the Welfare Foods Scheme in the United Kingdom. Each drop contains: 200 micrograms of vitamin A, 20 milligrams of vitamin C and 7 micrograms of vitamin D. Any alternative proprietary vitamin preparation may be used.

The fluid secreted by the breasts during the first few days of lactation is known as colostrum. It has a high content of protein, but a smaller amount of sugar and fat than mature milk. The precise function of colostrum is not known, but it is of value in helping to establish the immunity to certain infectious diseases which the breast-fed baby so often possesses. In addition, it has of course a certain nutritional value, but it is doubtful whether it has any more aperient action on the bowels than any other form of liquid food.

Human Milk Banks are now being set up in hospitals throughout the country to provide milk for babies with special needs who are unable to feed at the breast. The milk is collected from mothers who have a supply in excess of their own babies' needs and who are willing to donate the surplus. Such milk may be stored in a domestic refrigerator for up to twenty-four hours or should be deep-frozen before being transported to the hospital milk bank.

	Protein per cent	*Fat per cent*	*Sugar per cent*	*Calories per cent*
Human milk	1·1	4·2	7·0	70
Cow's milk	3·5	3·9	4·6	66

Composition of human and cow's milk.

Artificial feeding: If breast feeding is not possible, then some substitute for human milk must be used, and the most satisfactory is cow's milk. Cow's milk differs in certain important aspects from human milk: it contains less sugar, more protein, and about the same amount of fat. In addition, however, there are important qualitative differences. Milk contains two types of protein – casein and albumin. The albumin in milk is known as lactalbumin; it forms a finer clot and is more digestible than casein. In addition it contains larger amounts of two amino-acids, cystine and lysine, which are of special importance for growth. Breast milk has a higher proportion of lactalbumin than cow's milk. The fat in cow's milk also differs from that in human milk in that its globules are larger and coarser.

The other drawback to cow's milk is that in the liquid form it is a potentially dangerous food for infants unless it is boiled. Dangerous diseases such as tuberculosis can be conveyed by milk, and the only safe rule for infants is to boil all milk. The results of infection in infants can be so disastrous that up to the age of two years all milk should be boiled. After the age of two years pasteurization is reliable and therefore above this age children should be given pasteurized milk. The simplest way of boiling milk is in a double saucepan, and it is only necessary to bring the milk up to the boil. Prolonged boiling is not necessary. Statements are sometimes made that boiling adversely affects the nutritious qualities of milk. There is no evidence in favour of this, except in the case of the vitamin C content, and this deficiency can readily be overcome by giving orange juice. What has been said here, of course, only applies to liquid milk. The processes whereby dried and condensed milks are made ensure that these are safe from all infection.

GENERAL PRINCIPLES: Feeding times depend upon the weight of the infant. If the weight is over 3·2 to 3·6 kg (7 to 8 pounds), feeds are given every four hours from the tenth day, ie. at 6 am., 10 am., 2 pm., 6 pm., and 10 pm. If the weight is less than this, three-hourly feeds should be instituted, ie. 6 am., 9 am., 12 noon, 3 pm., 6 pm., and 10 pm. In all cases four-hourly feeds are sufficient after the age of three months or after the weight is 4·5 kg (10 pounds).

Absolute cleanliness is essential. This is achieved by effective sterilization of the bottle and teat – either by boiling or a sterilizing solution. With both methods, the bottle and teat must first be thoroughly cleaned. Immediately after a feed, before the film of milk hardens, they are rinsed under running water. They are then thoroughly washed in warm water and detergent, using a bottle brush. After sterilization the bottle and teat are left in the boiled water or sterilizing solution covered with a lid until needed again. If chemical sterilization has been used, the excess fluid should be drained from bottle and teat before use but there is no need to rinse off the remaining drops of fluid. The hands of the mother or nurse must be carefully washed before handling the bottle, teat or feed. The teat must be as big as the baby can cope with, and the hole in it must be so adjusted that the feed drips freely through it (about 1 drop per second). This ensures that the baby is able to take each feed in ten to fifteen minutes.

The amount of each feed depends upon the daily caloric requirements of the infant, which can be taken to be 75 ml (2½ fluid ounces) of human milk or its equivalent per 455 grams (1 pound) of body weight.

INFANT FOODS: Artificial feeds to replace human milk are manufactured as what are technically known as infant formulae. These may be powders, or concentrated liquids, some of which are already constituted as 'ready-to-feed'. The powders and concentrated liquids are reconstituted with water. Amidst the brands on the market are three main types: (1) Cow's milk with added carbohydrate. Examples of this type are Cow and Gate Baby Milk, Improved Ostermilk No. 2, and Ostermilk Complete Formula. (2) Skimmed cow's milk with added carbohydrate and mixed fats. Examples of this type are Milumil and SMA. (3) Skimmed cow's milk with demineralized whey and mixed fats. Examples of this type are Cow and Gate Premium, Osterfeed, and SMA Gold Cap. The protein in type 3 formulae is cow's milk protein which has been modified so that the ratio of whey proteins (including lactalbumin) to casein resembles human milk fat more closely (as is also the case with type 2 preparations). The carbohydrate is lactose from skimmed milk and demineralized whey. The use of demineralized whey permits the mineral content to be less than in types 1 and 2

Age	Height				Weight			
	Boys		Girls		Boys		Girls	
	Inches	*Centimetres*	*Inches*	*Centimetres*	*Pounds*	*Kilograms*	*Pounds*	*Kilograms*
Birth	20·0	50·9	19·5	49·5	7·5	3·4	7·3	3·3
2 weeks	20·3	51·7	20·1	51·0	7·5	3·4	7·3	3·3
3 months	23·7	60·2	23·2	58·8	12·9	5·8	12·0	5·5
6 months	26·2	66·7	25·6	65·0	17·4	7·9	16·4	7·4
9 months	28·0	71·2	27·4	69·6	20·4	9·2	19·2	8·7
1 year	29·6	75·1	29·1	73·9	22·8	10·3	21·7	9·8
2 years	34·0	86·4	33·7	85·5	27·0	12·2	25·7	11·6
3 years	37·8	95·9	36·9	93·8	31·5	14·3	30·4	13·8
4 years	40·6	103·0	40·0	101·6	35·6	16·2	34·5	15·7
5 years	43·1	109·5	42·9	108·9	40·2	18·3	39·4	17·9

Mean height and weight of infants and young children. *Thomson.*

	Human Milk per 100 millilitres	Cow's Milk per 100 millilitres
Vitamin A	170 international units	
Summer		150 international units
Winter		100 international units
Vitamin D	1 international unit	
Summer		1·5 international units
Winter		0·5 international unit
Thiamine	23 micrograms	60 micrograms
Ascorbic Acid (Vitamin C)	5·4 milligrams	3 milligrams

Vitamin content of human and unboiled cow's milk.

and to approach more nearly the average concentration in human milk. All three types contain added minerals, including iron, and added vitamins A, C and D.

The formulae named above, all satisfy the criteria laid down in the report, *Present Day Practice in Infant Feeding*, of a Working Party of the Panel on Child Nutrition Committee on Medical Aspects of Food Policy issued by the Department of Health and Social Security in 1974, a revised edition of which was published in 1980. These criteria were: (1) That milk feeds should contain a concentration of phosphate, sodium and protein which is lower than that of cow's milk and nearer to that of human milk. (2) That artificial feeds should be so manufactured that they are either liquids which are ready to feed, or liquids or powders that require the addition only of water and no other substance. (3) That artificial feeds should be so manufactured that the dilution required to reconstitute the milk should be independent of the age of the baby and that instructions about dilution should thus apply to feeds from birth onwards.

Detailed instructions about the preparation of feeds are provided by the manufacturers. All that need be added here is that many of the factors discussed in connection with breast feeding are just as important in the case of artificial feeding, such as contact between mother and baby. In some ways this is even more important in the case of artificial feeding, a process which can so easily become an impersonal, mechanical routine, thus depriving the baby of his (or her) full quota of mother love and the constant reminder that it really exists.

Weaning: It is usual to start weaning about the fifth month or when the infant weighs about 7·8 kg (17 pounds), though the modern tendency is to start even earlier than this. Provided the process is carried out gradually, there is seldom any difficulty in having the child completely off the breast by the end of the ninth month. It is essential to remember that all cow's milk given to the baby must be boiled. The amount of milk, including that used for cooking, should be about 850 ml (1½ pints) daily. From the age of six months the baby should be given a crust to chew every day. Vitamin drops containing A, C and D are, of course, continued.

No hard and fast rules can be laid down for the process of weaning. If the baby has been breast-fed, then it is usually a mistake to switch on to an intermediate stage of bottle feeding. It is better, and usually not difficult, to teach baby to drink from a teaspoon or a feeding cup. The consistency of the food is important in the early stages of weaning. In the initial stage it should be semi-fluid, and for quite a long time it must be pulpy in consistency without any lumps. The large variety of powdered cereals and purées of vegetable and meat now available make the weaning process much simpler than it used to be – and much more pleasant for the baby. From a very early stage of weaning the aim should be to get baby on to a programme of three meals a day, with the meat, fish and vegetables given at the mid-day meal.

Digestive disturbances: These are much more likely to occur with artificial feeding than with breast feeding. Only mild digestive upsets associated with feeding will be mentioned here. Any serious digestive disturbance in an infant should be referred immediately to a medical practitioner. (See also DIARRHOEA.) In the case of breast feeding, overfeeding may cause vomiting, colic and diarrhoea, whilst underfeeding is accompanied by constipation. Sometimes, however, underfeeding may be accompanied by a special type of diarrhoea characterized by the passage of small, dark-green stools containing an excess of mucus – usually during or just after a feed. In the case of artificial feeding the most common digestive disturbances are colic and diarrhoea. These may be due to either dirty feeding utensils or an unsuitable feeding mixture.

Treatment: It is important to remember that in a breast-fed baby vomiting, occurring immediately or soon after a feed, is usually of no significance provided there is no loss of weight. Should it be due to overfeeding (and this can be checked by test feeding) and should it persist, it can often be remedied by reducing the time at each breast and also by giving the infant a little boiled water before each feed. If underfeeding on the breast is confirmed by test feeding, the first essential is to reassure the mother and to ensure that she is taking sufficient diet, adequate fluid, and adequate rest. Other measures which help are to institute three-hourly feeding instead of four-hourly and to give an extra feed at night. If these fail, then complementary feeding may be used: ie. a bottle feed after one or more breast-feeds. In the case of artificial feeding, the first essential is to ensure that the feeding utensils are all being adequately sterilized by boiling and that there is no contamination of the feed. The next step is to change to some other food. Should all these measures fail, it may then be necessary to treat the milk in some special way. This may be done by adding 60 mg of sodium citrate to each 28·5 ml of milk mixture, or peptonized milk may be used. If all else fails, it must never be forgotten that human milk is the best food for human infants and that it is possible to obtain supplies from maternity hospitals which maintain a human milk bank.

General rules for feeding young children:

1. Take ample time; do not hurry the child in sucking or chewing.

2. If a child is disinclined to eat he should not be coaxed or forced to do so. If a child is losing weight, or off his food, he should be examined for signs of disease; otherwise the regulation of the amount of food should be left to his appetite.

3. Although all food given to a child should be simple, it ought to be varied from day to day, well cooked, and attractively served.

4. Highly seasoned food, much dressed food, and food with a large indigestible residue should not be given to children.

5. If a child is feverish, food should be reduced in strength and quantity. In very hot weather a young child often eats less food than usual and drinks more water.

6. The basis of a child's diet should be pasteurized milk (up to 1 litre (2 pints) a day); brown, wholemeal, or wheatmeal bread; butter or vitaminized margarine; eggs; cheese; fruit; salad vegetables; green leafy vegetables; potatoes and other root vegetables; meat; fish; sugar (but not too much); and water to drink. This should be supplemented with a daily intake of vitamins A, C and D in the form of Children's Vitamin Drops (see under **Breast feeding** above) or a comparable proprietary vitamin preparation.

INFANT MORTALITY is the number of deaths of infants under one year of age. The infant mortality rate in any given year is calculated as the number of deaths in the first year of life in proportion to every 1000 registered live births in that year. Along with perinatal mortality (qv), it is accepted as one of the most important criteria for assessing the health of the community and the standard of the social conditions of a country.

The improvement in the infant mortality rate has occurred mainly in the period from the second month of life. There has been much less improvement in the neonatal mortality rate: ie. the number of infants dying during the first four weeks of life, expressed as a proportion of every 1000 live births. During the first week of life the main causes of death are asphyxia, prematurity, birth injuries and congenital abnormalities. After the first week the main cause of death is infection.

Social conditions also play an important rôle in infant mortality. In England and Wales the infant mortality rate in 1930–32 was: Social Class I (professional), 32·7; Social Class III

Cause		1911–1920	1931–1939	1970
Whooping-cough	M	3·31	1·35	0·0166
	F	3·85	1·64	
Tuberculosis	M	2·88	0·80	0·0013
	F	2·26	0·65	
Measles	M	2·57	0·78	0·0115
	F	2·21	0·66	
Bronchitis and pneumonia	M	21·33	13·62	2·95
	F	16·43	10·28	
Gastro-enteritis	M		6·22	0·0013
	F		4·31	
Congenital malformations	M	4·29	6·03	3·72
	F	3·56	5·22	
Immaturity	M	21·48	16·40	2·01
	F	17·48	13·32	
All causes	M	111·70	66·17	18·19
	F	88·66	51·03	

Infant mortality rates per 1000 live births in England and Wales in 1911–20, 1931–1939, and 1970. M = Male. F = Female.

(skilled workers), 57·6; Social Class V (unskilled workers), 77·1. The comparable figures for Scotland for 1939-45 were: Class I, 30·9; Class III, 53·4; Class V, 78·6. Many factors come into play in producing these social variations, but overcrowding is undoubtedly one of the most important. For instance, in 1936 the infant mortality rate in Bournemouth, where only 0·3 per cent of working class families were overcrowded, was 78 per cent of that for the entire country, compared with 145 per cent in Newcastle-upon-Tyne where 10·7 per cent of working-class families were overcrowded. The same discrepancy persists to the present day as shown by a comparison of the Standardized Mortality Ratios in the areas covered by the North Western (which includes Lancashire) and the East Anglian Regional Health Authorities. In 1976–78 for children under the age of 1 year these were 110·2 for boys and 110·7 for girls in the former and 86 for boys, and 69·5 for girls in East Anglia.

1838–39	146	1946–50	36·4
1841–50	153	1951–55	26·9
1851–60	154	1956–60	22·6
1861–70	154	1961–65	20·6
1871–80	149	1968	18·3
1881–90	142	1970	18·2
1891–1900	153	1971	17·5
1901–05	138	1972	17·2
1906–10	117·1	1973	16·9
1911–15	108·1	1974	16·3
1916–20	90·9	1975	15·7
1921–25	74·9	1976	14·2
1926–30	67·9	1977	13·7
1931–35	62·2	1978	13·1
1936–40	55·3	1979	12·7
1941–45	49·8	1980	12·0

Infant mortality rate in England and Wales (1838–1968) and England 1970–1980.

It is thus evident that for a reduction of the infant mortality rate to the minimum figure the following conditions must be met. The mothers and potential mothers of the country must be housed adequately amid surroundings which permit adequate fresh air and healthy exercise. The pregnant and nursing mother must be ensured an adequate diet. Effective antenatal supervision must be available to every mother, as well as skilled supervision during labour. The new-born infant must be adequately nursed and adequately fed. This means that all possible steps must be taken to encourage breast feeding. Mothers must be instructed in the proper care and feeding of their children, particularly during the first year of life. This in itself would reduce the mortality rate, but in addition adequate public-health measures must be taken to ensure a clean milk supply and full availability of such protective measures as immunization against diphtheria, measles, poliomyelitis and whooping-cough. (See also PERINATAL MORTALITY.)

INFANTILE PARALYSIS is an old name for POLIOMYELITIS (qv).

INFANTILISM is the condition characterized by imperfect sexual development at puberty. It may or may not be associated with small stature. It may be due to lack of development of certain of the endocrine glands: ie. the gonads (qv), pituitary gland or the adrenal glands. In other cases it may be associated with a generalized disease such as diabetes mellitus, asthma, ulcerative colitis and rheumatoid arthritis.

INFARCTION means the changes which take place in an organ when an artery is suddenly blocked, leading to the formation of a dense, wedge-shaped mass in the part of the organ supplied by the artery. It occurs as the result of embolism or of thrombosis. (See EMBOLISM.)

INFECTION is the process by which a disease is communicated from one person to another.

All diseases so communicable are called infectious. There is, in the case of all such diseases, some micro-organism produced in the body of the diseased person which, on being transmitted to a second person, is capable of reproducing itself in larger quantity and causing a particular disease.

This micro-organism may be a bacterium, a Rickettsia, a virus, a protozoon, or a metazoon. Invasion of the body by a metazoon (eg. by an intestinal worm) is more often known as an infestation.

The germs of disease may be grouped into those which will not flourish except about the temperature of the body, and those which are capable of maintaining their existence in decaying animal or vegetable matter, making only occasional migrations into the body and setting up disease. Speaking generally, bacteria of the first group are consistently much more deadly in their action, whilst those in the second group vary much in the severity of the disease they produce, causing a severer type if they have come direct from an infected person than if they have been germinating in drains, in the soil or floating on dust particles in the air. This principle is of immense practical importance. In the course of a surgical operation many bacteria must fall from the air into the wound, but this does not appear to be any drawback, unless the bacteria are derived direct from suppurating wounds or like virulent source. Similarly diphtheria or pneumonia bacteria of a mild type may be found in the mouth of people who are, nevertheless, quite healthy, if certain conditions, necessary to render the bacterium virulent, are not present.

The same bacterium may produce very different types of disease, not only on account of its previous life-history, but even according to the channel by which it enters the body. The *Mycobacterium tuberculosis*, for instance, produces a very different picture, depending upon whether it invades the lungs, the intestines, the joints, the glands or the skin. A certain amount of protection against the entrance of infective matter into the tissues of the body is afforded by the horny layer of the skin, by the acid of the gastric juice, and by the movements of the intestine, and a still greater measure of protection is afforded by the factors which ensure immunity against diseases. (See IMMUNITY; SERUM THERAPY.)

Modes of infection: The infective material may be transmitted to the person by direct contact with a sick person, when the disease is said to be contagious, although such a distinction is purely artificial. Different diseases are specially infectious at different periods of their course; and the practical question of guarding against infection is rendered much more difficult by the fact that some diseases are infectious at a stage even before they are clearly recognizable. This applies particularly to the early stage of measles before the rash appears, when the infected child is showing symptoms merely resembling those of catarrh or a cold in the head.

Infection may be conveyed on dust driven by the wind, in drinking-water, food, particularly milk, evacuations with which the healthy person's hands have become contaminated, crusts and scabs from the infected person's body, or even clothes and linen which have been in contact with him.

In this connection what are termed carriers are of great importance. Some people who have suffered from a disease, or who have simply been in contact with an infectious case, harbour the germ of the disease. This is particularly the case in typhoid fever, the bacillus continuing to develop in the gall-bladder of some people, who have had the disease, maybe for years after the symptoms have passed away; it is estimated that 2 to 5 per cent of patients with typhoid fever become permanent typhoid carriers and where a cook or food purveyor is affected, he is apt to start an epidemic unless he exercises the most scrupulous cleanliness. In the case of cholera, which is endemic in some localities of the East, 80 per cent or more of the population may harbour the bacillus and spread infection when other circumstances favour this. Similarly in the case of dysentery, people who have completely recovered may still be capable of infecting dust and drinking-water by their stools. Diphtheria is similarly liable to be carried by people in whose throat the germ remains after recovery from the disease. Cerebrospinal meningitis, which is particularly liable to infect children, appears to be transmitted through the germ being carried in the nose of people who may not develop any symptoms.

Flies pass from garbage heaps to unprotected food, and are especially dangerous as regards the infection of milk and other food with the organisms causing typhoid fever and food poisoning. Mosquitoes convey from sick to healthy the germs of malaria and yellow fever, these undergoing part of their development in the body of the mosquito. Fleas convey the germ of plague from rat to man, lice are responsible for inoculating typhus fever and one form of relapsing fever by their bite. A tick is responsible for spreading another form of relapsing fever, and kala-azar (or leishmaniasis) is spread by the bites of sandflies.

Notifiable diseases: Certain of the common and most serious infectious diseases were scheduled in the Infectious Diseases Act of 1889 as notifiable in Great Britain. That is to say that any medical practitioner, attending or called in to visit a person suffering from one of these, must immediately, on becoming aware that the patient is suffering from it, send a notice to the local medical officer for environmental health as he is now known. The current list of notifiable infectious diseases in England and Wales is:

Acute encephalitis
Acute meningitis
Acute poliomyelitis
Anthrax
Cholera
Diphtheria
Dysentery
Infective jaundice
Lassa fever
Leprosy
Leptospirosis
Malaria
Marburg disease
Measles
Ophthalmia neonatorum
Paratyphoid fever
Plague
Rabies
Relapsing fever
Scarlet fever
Smallpox
Tetanus
Tuberculosis
Typhoid fever
Typhus
Viral haemorrhagic fever
Whooping-cough
Yellow fever

Food poisoning and suspected food poisoning are also notifiable.

In Scotland the following diseases are also notifiable in addition to the above list:

Cerebrospinal fever
Encephalitis lethargica
Erysipelas
Pneumonia (influenzal and acute primary)
Puerperal fever
Puerperal pyrexia

In Northern Ireland gastroenteritis (under 2 years of age) is notifiable.

Anthrax and toxic jaundice are notifiable as industrial diseases. Similar regulations are found in other countries.

Prevention of infection: The various channels of infection are mentioned under the heading of the different infectious diseases, and also briefly under SANITATION. As children are much more liable to contract infectious diseases than adults, attempts to prevent the spread of these diseases are specially directed towards separating affected people from healthy children. The measures taken apply particularly to schools, which form the places of dissemination in a large proportion of cases, but the rules applicable to children may well be practised with regard to people of any age and in respect of any public institution. If, in opposition to medical advice, a patient with a communicable disease refuses to go to an infectious disease hospital, the local authority has compulsory powers to insist on such transfer provided the medical officer for environmental health certifies that there is a risk of infection, and that the sufferer should be detained in an isolation unit until he is certified as no longer likely to spread the disease in question. (See also IMMUNITY; INCUBATION.)

INFECTIOUS MONONUCLEOSIS (see GLANDULAR FEVER).

INFERTILITY: Some 10 to 15 per cent of all marriages in Britain are said to be infertile. The inability of a couple to have children may be the fault of either partner, or both. As one or more of many factors may be involved, it is essential, if success is to be achieved, that the problem should be approached in an unemotional and systematic manner. Nothing is more likely to lead to failure than mutual recrimination.

In the first place it must be remembered that the fertility, or ability to have children, of couples varies considerably. This means that many a couple must have patience. Some couples may find that the woman becomes pregnant almost immediately, whilst others may have to wait months – or even years. Speaking generally, there is no need to become worried until at least a year has elapsed. Among the first factors to be looked into are the frequency and timing of intercourse and the technique. The main point about timing is its relationship to menstruation, taking this as a guide to the time of ovulation: that is, the release of the ovum from the ovary. It is in the early days of marriage that psychological factors can play a strong inhibitory part, particularly if there is inadequate mutual trust and understanding. If, after a year, there is still no evidence of pregnancy, or earlier if undue anxiety is being aroused, then advice should be sought from some reliable source, such as the family doctor, or the Marriage Guidance Council (qv).

If further investigations are called for, then it is essential that these should include both partners unless it is initially clear which is responsible. The man is usually examined first, as male infertility is probably the main factor in infertile marriages in 15 per cent of cases. Both partners must have a general medical examination to make sure that it is not their general health that is at fault. If there is no such fault, the frequency, timing and technique of intercourse are investigated, and corrected if necessary. If the man is impotent, this is investigated and can often be corrected provided full cooperation of both partners is obtained. A careful examination of the semen is then carried out to decide whether or not the man is sterile. Many factors can be responsible for absolute or relative sterility of the man, and for some of these nothing can be done. Great care and experience are required in the interpretation of sperm counts obtained from an examination of semen but, if there is absolute sterility (that is, total and permanent absence of sperms), then there is nothing left that can be done to render the marriage fertile – except artificial insemination from a donor. (See ARTIFICIAL INSEMINATION.)

In the case of the woman, infertility may be due to some obstruction to the sperm reaching the ovum or to the ovum reaching the uterus. Alternatively, it may be due to some disturbance of the woman's hormones so that she is unable to produce ova or to release them into the uterus at regular monthly intervals. Modern methods of investigation can usually reveal which of these factors is responsible. If there is some physical obstruction, say, in the Fallopian tubes (qv), it may be possible to remove this. Alternatively, if there is some factor that is destroying the sperm before it can reach the uterus, this may be counteracted. If the defect is in the hormonal make-up of the woman, the so-called fertility drugs may right the matter.

Anovulatory infertility may be associated with normal menstruation or with amenorrhoea. The disorders that cause infertility are essentially the same as those that cause amenorrhoea, but there are in addition a number of anatomical and pathological abnormalities in the genital tract, particularly obstruction of the fallopian tube. It is important to exclude primary ovarian failure because if the ovary is unresponsive to gonadotrophins there is no point in giving them as treatment. This can be established by determining the serum level of the follicular stimulating hormone which is raised in primary ovarian failure. Hyperprolactinaemia is a common cause of female infertility and the serum prolactin concentration must be estimated in all infertile patients. Patients with hyperprolactinaemia will respond to bromocriptine treatment. If there is no evidence of hyperprolactinaemia or of primary ovarian failure and the serum gonadotrophin levels are detectable, though low, ovulation may be established by treatment with clomiphene. Patients who fail to respond to clomiphene should be treated with human menopausal gonadotrophins. Human gonadotrophins can be extracted from menopausal urine and are available commercially (Pergonal and Humergon). The major hazards of HMG treatment are ovarian hyperstimulation and the risk of multiple pregnancies. This is due to the fact that the sensitivity of the ovaries to FSH stimulation varies widely in different women and often in the same women at different times. The aim of treatment is to develop a single mature graafian follicle. Various treatment schedules have been advocated but the most favoured is the three-injection schedule, giving injections of HMG intramuscularly on days 1, 3 and 5. Biochemical monitoring is carried out by measurement of urine or plasma oestrogen levels. When the required oestrogen level is achieved ovulation is produced by the intramuscular injection of chorionic gonadotrophin (Pregnyl).

If after full investigation it appears that the woman should be capable of becoming pregnant, and her male partner is capable of producing healthy semen, but the relationship remains childless, artificial insemination may be considered. If artificial insemination is not congenial to both partners –and it is certainly a practice that should not be embarked upon except after very careful thought and the obtaining of the best possible advice – and both partners are anxious to have children, there is always the well-established practice of adoption.

INFESTATION is a term applied to the occurrence of animal parasites in the intestine, hair or clothing. (See INSECTS IN RELATION TO DISEASE.)

INFLAMMATION is the reaction of the tissues to any injury, short of one sufficiently severe to cause their immediate death. The term is limited sometimes to the changes which take place when bacteria enter the body, but the changes in the latter case, though specially severe, are essentially the same as those produced by any other source of irritation. There are four cardinal symptoms of inflammation: redness, heat, pain and swelling, all of which, and particularly the last, are present in greater or less degree, so that these are also made a basis for defining the condition.

The first sign of inflammation consists in a dilatation of the arteries and veins of the affected part, so that the blood circulates in it more quickly and in larger quantity than before, thus causing heat and redness. Very soon, however, and apparently as the result of some change in the walls of the smaller blood-vessels, the circulation becomes gradually slower, and the white corpuscles of the blood are seen to adhere to the inner surface of these vessels. Later, these corpuscles push their way in great numbers through the walls of the smaller veins and capillaries, migrating into the surrounding tissues along with large quantities of the fluid material of the blood and a few red corpuscles, a process known as DIAPEDESIS. Hence the swelling, which is the most characteristic sign of inflammation. These white corpuscles subserve many functions. In the first place, they have been shown to attack the bacteria which have invaded the tissues, to envelop them in their own substance, and, apparently by a process of digestion, to break them up. They also remove tissues which are dead or useless. Other corpuscles, at a later stage, when the source of irritation has been removed, play a part in producing the new tissues to repair the damage done, although the greater part of this repair is effected by cells from the surrounding tissues.

One of two results may follow inflammation. Either *resolution* may take place, when the white corpuscles, having played their part, find their way back into the circulation after the process of repair has been started at the site of injury, and the circulation proceeds as before, or *abscess-formation* results, the circulation comes to a complete standstill in the affected part, an excessive number of white corpuscles migrate from the vessels, an area of tissue becomes destroyed, and the process ends by a discharge of pus through the surface of the body, after which repair proceeds. (See ABSCESS, ACUTE.)

Symptoms: As already mentioned, redness, heat, pain and swelling are the classical symptoms of inflammation, and there are usually general symptoms of feverishness, varying with the severity of the inflammation. Various special symptoms are set up in special localities: for example, inflammation of the mucous membranes of the stomach and bowels leads to a copious excretion of mucus; inflammation of outlying parts, if very severe, may cause death of these parts, and are then called gangrenous inflammation; intense inflammation limited to a surface may destroy patches of the surface and convert them into a leather-like membrane, such types being known as croupous inflammations. Inflammation may become chronic, and in this case not only does the process described proceed in a minor degree, but there is an exaggerated process of repair leading to the formation of much fibrous or scar tissue, which may come to replace almost entirely the organ in which the chronic inflammation is proceeding, thus rendering the organ small, hard and irregular in outline.

Treatment: This depends upon different factors, such as the type of organism responsible, the site of infection and the severity of the infection. Thus, if the inflammation is due to tuberculosis, treatment will be by means of a combination of two, or more, anti-tuberculosis drugs. If, on the other hand, it is in the appendix, immediate removal of the appendix is called for, whilst in the case of superficial inflammation of the skin, all that may be required is careful cleansing of the skin and the application of some antiseptic preparation.

Two general principles, however, apply to the treatment of all forms of inflammation: rest and the maintenance of the general health of the patient.

INFLUENZA is an acute infectious disease, characterized by a sudden onset, fever and generalized aches and pains, which usually occurs in epidemics and pandemics.

Cause: The disease is caused by a virus of the influenza group. There are at least three types of influenza virus, known respectively as A, B and C. One of their most characteristic features is that infection with one type provides no protection against another type. Equally important is the ease with which the influenza virus can change its character. It is these two characteristics which explain why one attack of influenza provides little, if any, protection against a subsequent attack, and why it is so difficult to prepare an effective vaccine against the disease.

Epidemics of influenza due to virus A occur in Britain at two- to four-year intervals, and outbreaks of virus B influenza in less frequent cycles. Virus A influenza, for instance, was the prevalent infection in 1949, 1951, 1955 and 1956, whilst virus B influenza was epidemic in 1946, 1950, 1954 and, along with virus A, in 1958–59. The pandemic of 1957, which swept most of the world, though fortunately not in a severe form, was due to a new variant of virus A – the so-called Asian virus –and it has been suggested that it was this variant that was responsible for the pandemics of 1889 and 1918. Since 1957, variants of virus A have been the predominating causes of influenza accompanied on occasions by virus B.

Symptoms: The incubation period of influenza A and B is two to three days and the disease is characterized by a sudden onset. In most cases this is followed by a short, sharp febrile illness of two to four days' duration, associated with headache, prostration, generalized aching and respiratory symptoms. In many cases the respiratory symptoms are restricted to the upper respiratory tract, and consist of signs of irritation of the nose, pharynx and larynx. There may be nose-bleeds, and a dry hacking cough is often a prominent and troublesome symptom. The fever is usually remittent and the temperature seldom exceeds 39·4°C (103°F), tending to fluctuate between 38·3° and 39·4°C (101° and 103°F).

The most serious complication is infection of the lungs. This infection is usually due to organisms other than the influenza virus. It is a complication which can have serious results in elderly people.

The very severe form which tends to occur during pandemics – and which was so common during the 1918–19 pandemic – is characterized by the rapid onset of broncho-pneumonia and severe prostration. Because of the toxic effect on the heart there is a particularly marked form of cyanosis, known as heliotrope cyanosis.

Convalescence following influenza tends to be prolonged. Even after an attack of average severity there tends to be a period of weakness and depression.

Treatment: Expert opinion is still divided as to the real value of influenza vaccine in preventing the disease. Part of the trouble is that, as already pointed out, there is no value in giving any vaccine until it is known which particular virus is causing the infection. As this varies from winter to winter, and as the protection given by vaccine does not exceed one year, it is obviously not worth while attempting to vaccinate the whole community. The general rule therefore is that, unless there is any evidence that a particularly virulent type of virus is responsible, only those should be vaccinated who are particularly vulnerable, such as children in boarding schools, elderly people, pregnant women, and people who suffer from chronic bronchitis. In the face of an epidemic, people in key positions, such as doctors, nurses and those concerned with public safety, transport and other public utilities should be vaccinated.

For an uncomplicated attack of influenza, treatment is symptomatic: that is, rest in bed, analgesics to relieve the pain, sedatives, and a light diet. A linctus is useful to sooth a troublesome cough. The best analgesic is aspirin – either alone, or combined with paracetamol and codeine. None of the sulphonamides or the known antibiotics has any effect on the influenza virus. On the other hand should the lungs become infected, antibiotics should be given immediately, because, as has already been pointed out, such an infection is usually due to other organisms. If possible, a sample of sputum should be examined to determine which organisms are responsible for the lung infection. The choice of antibiotic then depends upon which antibiotic the organism is most sensitive to.

INFUSIONS are preparations of vegetable drugs made by steeping them for some time in water and straining. In order that an infusion may keep well it is usually concentrated and mixed with spirit, being diluted just before it is dispensed.

Infusion is also the term applied to the injection into blood-vessels or subcutaneous tissues of warm normal salt solution, glucose solution or gum acacia solution, in the case of persons who are in a feeble state from loss of blood, loss of fluid by diarrhoea, etc. The infusion is sometimes administered in an amount of about 570 ml (1 pint) at a time, or is often used by a drip method in which the warm fluid is suspended at a height and allowed to pass drop by drop for several hours into a vein.

INGUINAL REGION (see ABDOMEN, REGIONS OF).

INHALATION is a method of applying drugs in a finely divided or gaseous state, so that, on being breathed in, they may come in contact with the nose, throat and lungs. There are two chief means by which drugs are mingled with the air and so taken in by breathing. These are:

(*a*) Steam inhalations. Steam itself, or hot moist air, has a soothing effect upon the mucous membrane of the air passages, and the steam may be impregnated with many moderately volatile drugs. This type of inhalation is used especially in bronchitis and inflammatory conditions of the throat and larynx. If it be desired to surround the patient constantly with a steamy atmosphere, the most convenient mode of doing so is by a kettle placed over a spirit lamp or electric heater, from which a long funnel leads in beneath a tent formed by a blanket over the upper half of the patient's bed. In cases of chronic bronchitis, one teaspoonful of the following mixture may be usefully added to the hot water: pinewood oil 28·5 ml, eucalyptus oil 28·5 ml, creosote 14 ml. Or in acute cases, where a soothing effect is specially necessary, a teaspoonful of the following: compound tincture of benzoin 28·5 ml, menthol 600 mg, spirit of chloroform 14 ml. Either of these formulae may be used by simply adding it to a jug half full of boiling water, over which the mouth is held, the head being enveloped in a towel that falls down round the sides of the jug. The same remedies may be added in similar quantity to a Nelson's inhaler with mouthpiece, and the mouth directly applied to the tube leading from it.

(*b*) The most recent form of inhalation consists of a fine spray or cloud driven off from a fluid by a stream of compressed air. By this means, various medicaments can be made to reach the farthest recesses of the lungs. The smaller of these nebulizers or atomizers are worked by a hand-ball of rubber, which drives a strong stream of air across the mouth of another tube dipping into the liquid. In various spas, larger nebulizers worked by force pumps are employed to fill whole rooms with medicated vapour, which patients sit and inhale for hours.

INHIBITION means arrest or restraint of some process effected by nervous influence. The term is applied to the action of certain inhibitory nerves: eg. the vagus nerve which contains fibres that inhibit or control the action of the heart. It is also applied generally to the mental processes by which instinctive but undesirable actions are checked by a process of self-control.

INJECTIONS (see ENEMA; HYPODERMIC INJECTIONS).

INJURED, REMOVAL OF: Careless or unskilful handling or moving of injured people may produce much pain and may aggravate the bodily damage already done.

Precautions before removal: In the case of some injuries, such as that of the brain in apoplexy, or the perforation of the bowels caused by a bullet-wound of the abdomen, the less movement of the patient that takes place at first the better are the chances of recovery, and it is sometimes advisable that treatment should be carried out for some time near the spot where the injury has been sustained. When a bone has been broken it is essential that the fragments should be temporarily supported and made rigid by suitable devices before any attempt is made to change the patient's position (see FRACTURES). In other cases, as, for example, those of faintness, shock, immersion in water, some other form of first-aid treatment or the administration of stimulants is urgently necessary prior to removal. (See COLLAPSE; FAINTING; DROWNING, RECOVERY FROM; HAEMORRHAGE.) During removal an attendant must be constantly with the injured person, or at least the latter must be carried in such a way that one of the bearers constantly sees his face.

Position in removal: Severely injured people, or those with any tendency to faintness, bleeding, shock or other general symptoms, should be carried lying at full length with the head slightly supported on a low pillow; a similar position should be adopted in the case of those who have sustained any injury to the bones or joints of the lower limb, or of the shoulder-joint, or severe wounds of the head, chest or abdomen. On the other hand, injuries of the hand or forearm when properly supported, no matter how severe they may be, slight injuries of the foot, and uncomplicated wounds to the head, face or upper part of the body, permit generally the patient to walk or to be removed in the sitting posture, as by one of the forms of hand seat.

In wounds of the head care should be taken that the injured part does not press upon the stretcher.

In severe injuries to the back the greatest care must be exercised in lifting the patient, and some rigid though well-covered form of stretcher is to be preferred, upon which the patient is placed face downwards.

In fractures of the leg or thigh the patient should lie upon his back inclined slightly towards the injured side and supported thus by a pillow, folded coat, or the like; in this position there is least jarring of the injured part.

In fractures of the upper limb, if the patient has to lie down, which is not usual, he should incline slightly towards the sound side, so that there is no risk of the body pressing the injured part.

In wounds or diseases of the chest there is often difficulty in breathing, which is relieved by propping the patient half up and turning him towards the affected side.

In painful conditions of the abdomen, or in the case of transverse or punctured wounds of this region, the patient should lie upon his back with the knees drawn well up and supported. In the case of a vertical wound of the abdomen the legs are kept straight.

The patient is usually carried feet first, but in going uphill or upstairs this position is reversed; in all cases, however, in which there is a fracture of the lower limb, the patient's head is kept lowest on a hill or stair so that the weight of the body may not press down upon the helpless and motionless part of the limb below the fracture. The taller bearer should be the farther down on the hill or stair.

No attempt should be made by inexperienced bearers to carry a stretcher over a wall or ditch, and on no account should a stretcher be carried upon the bearers' shoulders, because a fall may do very serious injury to the patient.

The stretcher should be carried at the full length of the bearers' arms, as horizontal as possible, and the bearers, though walking at an equal rate, must be careful not to keep in step, which causes the stretcher to swing painfully.

Care of unconscious patient: The unconscious patient must not be allowed to lie on his back. In this position he may suffocate. This is particularly likely to occur if he should vomit or if there is any bleeding into the mouth or throat. The unconscious patient is unable to swallow properly and any blood or vomited material in the mouth drains into the lungs and interferes with breathing. Even if the patient does not actually suffocate, if such material as blood gets into the lungs it may have serious results. This means that the patient who is bleeding into the mouth or throat, as a result, for example, of a blow to the head or neck, should be treated in this respect as an unconscious patient.

Once the unconscious patient has been removed from danger he should be placed in what is known as the semi-prone, or recovery, position. In this position the body lies on its side with the face turned towards the ground. To prevent the body rolling right over, both arms are bent at the elbows, and the upper, or top, leg is bent slightly at the hip and knees so that it falls forward over the lower, or under, leg.

Before rolling the patient into the semi-prone position it is essential to make sure that there are no fractures, especially of the spine. If there are, then the fractured part must be carefully supported as the patient is rolled over gently but firmly. In the case of the patient suspected of having a fractured spine, the whole body should be rolled over in one piece, without bending or twisting. If the unconscious patient has to be removed he should be placed on the stretcher in the semi-prone position.

There are certain other important rules to be observed in the management of the unconscious patient. No attempt should be made to move him in the first instance if he is in no danger. If he wears false teeth, these should be removed, and any tight clothing, especially round the neck or waist, should be loosened. Under no circumstances should he be given any fluid by mouth, as he cannot swallow, and any fluid forced into his mouth will probably be breathed into the lungs, with serious consequences.

Method of removal depends upon (1) how many persons are available as bearers, and (2) the degree of assistance required by the patient, as already stated.

I. BY ONE BEARER: When an arm is injured the patient is usually quite able to walk, and the arm being suitably supported, the bearer draws the patient's sound arm *over his shoulders* and places his own arm round the patient's waist.

If the bearer is strong and the patient seriously incapacitated, the latter may be carried *in the bearer's arms*, the right one passing beneath the patient's shoulder blades, the left beneath the upper part of the thighs; in this case the patient should be carried high and supported as much upon the bearer's chest as by his arms. In other cases the patient may be carried *upon the bearer's back*, his arms round the bearer's neck and his legs under the bearer's arms.

In cases of complete unconsciousness, where the dead-weight of the patient's body must be raised and borne by one bearer, the method known as the *Fireman's Lift* is applicable. The patient is turned on his face, arms by the sides; the bearer stands at the patient's head, and passing his hands beneath the latter's shoulders, raises him to a kneeling posture. The bearer next slides his hands under the patient's armpits and raises him still farther; then stooping and pushing his head between the patient's right arm and his body, he allows the patient's body to fall over his right shoulder upon his back, while the patient's right arm comes round the bearer's neck and is steadied temporarily by his left hand. Finally, the bearer, passing his right arm round one or both thighs of the patient, grasps the patient's right wrist with his right hand, and bringing the weight of the body well on to the centre of his own back, rises to the erect position.

II. BY TWO BEARERS WITH HAND SEATS: If the patient is suffering from such a condition as an injured foot and is able to give some assistance, and if there are two bearers, the bearers divide his weight by means of one of the forms of hand seats, of which the two-handed seat is the most useful. If the patient is more seriously injured, some form of stretcher must be obtained or improvised as described below.

For the *two-handed seat* the bearers face one another, the one on the right interlocking the fingers of his right hand with those of the left hand of the other bearer; each places his disengaged hand behind the patient or on the other bearer's hip or shoulder. In lifting the patient, they kneel at his sides, each upon the knee nearest to his feet, and, forming the seat beneath his thighs, they rise together supporting him, while he assists if possible by putting his arms round their necks.

For the *three-handed seat* the right-hand bearer grasps his own left forearm. The left-hand bearer places his right hand upon the shoulder of the other, and grasps the right forearm of the other with his left hand, his left forearm at the same time being grasped by the left hand of the other bearer.

For the *four-handed seat* each bearer grasps his own left wrist with his right hand; each then clasps the disengaged right wrist of the other with his left hand. To carry a patient by the three-handed or four-handed seat the patient must stand up, and the bearers, stooping, form the seat behind him.

If a patient is absolutely helpless and it is urgently necessary to carry him quickly for a short distance only, the *fore-and-aft carry* may be used. One bearer stands at the patient's head and passes his hands behind the shoulders into the armpits, while the other bearer stands between the patient's legs facing towards his feet and takes one leg under each arm.

III. BY HELP OF A STRETCHER: If the patient is unable to walk or to sit upright in the conditions described, a stretcher must be obtained. If no regular canvas stretcher be at hand, a satisfactory one may be improvised from a pair of poles and a couple of coats with the sleeves turned outside in. The coats are buttoned over the sleeves, through which the poles are then passed. Various other articles, such as a light sofa or a window-shutter, or a blanket supported by four people, one at each corner, may also be used.

The patient having received suitable first-aid treatment is lifted on to the stretcher as follows:

(a) When there are four bearers, which is the ideal, one acts as leader. The others place themselves on one side of the patient, kneeling on the knee farthest from the head of the patient. They then place their hands and forearms under the patient. When all are ready, at the word of command they simultaneously and carefully lift the patient on to their bent knees, taking care not to jolt the patient and to keep him absolutely straight. The leader then slips the stretcher under the patient and gives the order for the patient to be lowered on to it.

(b) If only three bearers are available, the same technique is used but, when the three bearers are all set with their arms under the patient, they then lift him directly – but just as carefully – on to the stretcher.

(c) When only two bearers are available the stretcher is placed close to the patient's head and in line with his body. The bearers then straddle the patient facing his head. One passes his arms under the shoulders, at the same time supporting the head. The other passes one arm under the buttocks and the other under the legs. When both are ready they gently lift the patient, walk over the stretcher and then gently lower the patient on to it.

INOCULATION is the process by which infective material is brought into the system through a small wound in the skin or in a mucous membrane. Many infectious diseases and blood-poisoning are contracted by accidental inoculation of microbes. Inoculation is now used as a preventive measure against many infectious diseases. (See VACCINE.)

INOSITOL is one of the components of the vitamin B complex. Deficiency in mice produces baldness, but little is known yet about its rôle in human nutrition.

INSANITY (see MENTAL ILLNESS).

INSECT REPELLENTS (See DIBUTYL PHTHALATE; DIMETHYL PHTHALATE.)

INSECTICIDES are substances which kill insects. Since the discovery of the insecticidal properties of DDT in 1940, a steady stream of new ones has been introduced, and their combined use has played an outstanding part in international public health campaigns, such as that of the World Health Organization for the eradication of malaria.

Unfortunately, insects are liable to become resistant to insecticides, just as bacteria are liable to become resistant to antibiotics, and it is for this reason that so much research work is being devoted to the discovery of new ones.

It is against this beneficial background that must be viewed the increasing evidence that the indiscriminate use of some of these potent preparations is having an adverse effect, not only upon human beings, but also upon the balance of nature.

The following are some of the more common insecticides now in use, brief notes on which will be found under the name of the substance: benzene hexachloride, chlordane, DDT, dieldrin, parathion, malathion.

INSECTS IN RELATION TO DISEASE: Many insects play an important part in the transmission of infectious diseases. Thus, flies by their feet and their feeding habits carry the organisms which cause typhoid fever, the tsetse fly spreads sleeping sickness, mosquitoes transmit the germs of malaria and yellow fever, fleas convey plague germs and lice convey typhus fever and one form of relapsing fever. In addition, these creatures are nuisances as well as dangers.

HOUSE-FLY (*Musca domestica*): This fly lays its eggs in manure, or in moist, fermenting vegetable matter. The maggot is hatched in eight hours to two days, feeds on the manure, passes through the pupa stage in anything from a few days to four weeks, and, becoming a fly, is capable of egg-laying about three weeks from its own appearance as an egg. As 120 to 150 eggs are laid in a batch by each female fly, this fly is capable, under the most favourable conditions, of producing over half-a-million progeny within her life of three months. The fly gorges on fluid food which it sucks up by means of its proboscis, and it has the habit of repeatedly vomiting and re-swallowing the contents of its crop as it feeds. It walks in filth habitually, and being provided with hairy legs and body it is apt to carry off portions of this, in which are entangled numbers of bacteria. The fly has been well described as a 'winged sponge', and its immense power to distribute disease germs over the surface of uncovered food is evident.

BLOW-FLY, or BLUE-BOTTLE (*Calliphora erythrocephala*), lays its eggs (450 to 600 in number) on meat, fish or decaying animal matter. The maggot hatches out within a day, passes through the pupa stage and becomes a full-grown fly in about three weeks. Its habits are similar to those of the house-fly, though in numbers it is much less plentiful.

Treatment of flies: The most important measure is to destroy their breeding grounds near human dwellings. No kitchen refuse should be left exposed so that flies may deposit their eggs in it. Stable litter and manure must be disposed of, or kept covered and shut up in outhouses, not allowed to accumulate in the open air and sunshine near houses. Adult flies may be destroyed in a great extent by proper protection and storage of all food. DDT (qv), which may be used as a powder, a spray or a paint, has established itself as a most efficient means of treatment, but care must be exercised that it does not come in contact with food.

LICE: There are three lice which infest man: the body louse (*Pediculus corporis*), the head louse (*Pediculus capitis*) and the crab louse (*Pediculus pubis*). The head louse is by far the most common in Britain and adults. Infestation is most common in children under school age, but it is not unusual in adults. In schoolchildren it seems to be ineradicable: a recent survey in England showed that 9 per cent of 12,000 schoolchildren were infested. It used to be much commoner in girls than boys, but this sex difference is disappearing. Head lice spread by close human contact. (See also PEDICULOSIS.)

As already noted, lice convey the causative micro-organisms of typhus fever, one form of relapsing fever, and trench fever, and it has been estimated that in this way the louse is responsible for more human deaths than any other insect barring the malaria mosquito (see RELAPSING FEVER; TRENCH FEVER; TYPHUS)

Treatment of lice: In individuals infested with the body louse the clothing should be dusted with 10 per cent DDT, packed in a bag and then sent for washing or storing. A temperature of 54°C (129°F) is rapidly lethal to both lice and their eggs. At a temperature of -20°C (-4°F) lice are killed in half-an-hour and eggs are killed in five hours. As the lice tend to congregate into the seams, hot ironing these is a useful measure.

For body lice, the body should be coated with malathion cream or 1 per cent dusting powder. This may need to be repeated for several days. Calamine lotion containing 1 per cent phenol eases the itching. For crab, or pubic, lice, the affected area is rubbed with either Dicophane Application BPC, or Malathion dusting powder which is left on for two days, and the process then repeated. Alternatively, carbaryl or malathion may be used.

For head lice, a lotion containing 0·5 per cent Malathion in 10 ml should be rubbed with the fingers into the hair and its roots and left for twenty-four hours. The hair is then washed. This may need to be repeated twice or three times. The hair is then carefully combed with a fine comb to remove the nits. Removal may be easier if the hairs are rubbed previously with a swab soaked in vinegar. Unfortunately the head louse is becoming resistant to gamma benzene hexachloride, which is therefore being replaced by malathion (qv) or carbaryl. Malathion is applied in a 0·5 per cent solution in spirit until the scalp is thoroughly moist. The hair is then allowed to dry naturally without the use of any heat. After twelve hours the hair is shampooed and combed with a fine metal comb while wet to remove the dead nits. Only one such treatment is usually necessary, but all close contacts including the parents of the infested child should be examined and treated forthwith with malathion if infested. Only in this way can the infestation be eradicated from the family. Carbaryl is available as a shampoo and a lotion. The lotion is the preparation of choice. It is rubbed gently into the hair. The hair is then left to dry naturally and washed with a shampoo the next day. After the shampoo, the hair, while still wet, is combed with a fine metal comb to remove the dead lice and eggs (nits).

FLEAS: *Pulex irritans* is the common flea that afflicts mankind. *Xenopsylla cheopis* is the rat flea that conveys *Pasteurellapestis*, the causative organism of plague, from rat to man. The flea lays its eggs singly. They take two to four days in summer, two weeks in winter, to hatch into larvae which are fully grown in a fortnight. The larva then becomes a pupa from which the adult emerges two weeks later. The flea can survive for a long time without food.

Treatment of fleas: Human beings vary tremendously in their susceptibility to flea bites. For those who are susceptible the best preventive is dimethyl phthallate sprayed on the trousers or socks where it is effective for several days. In the absence of dimethyl phthallate, alternative methods of prevention are the smearing of the skin with oil of pennyroyal, oil of lavender, or 10 per cent crotamiton cream or lotion, or dusting the socks and underclothing with pyrethrum powder, menthol or camphor. For disinfestation of buildings, a 5 per cent solution of DDT in kerosene is effective. For bedding a powder containing 10 per cent DDT, or 0·5 per cent gamma benzene hexachloride, is effective. Other anti-flea agents are pyrethrum, flaked naphthalene, or parachlorbenzene.

BED BUGS (*Cimex lectularius*) are best got rid of by a 5 per cent solution of DDT in kerosene, with or without the addition of pyrethrum. (See BED BUG.)

MOSQUITOES: One of these (*Anopheles gambiae*) is responsible for conveying the parasite of malaria, another (*Aedes aegypti*) for distributing the infection of yellow fever.

Treatment of mosquitoes: See under MALARIA; YELLOW FEVER.

INSOLATION is a term applied both to treatment by exposure to the sun's rays (see LIGHT TREATMENT) and to fever caused by excessive heat (see HEAT-STROKE).

INSOMNIA (see SLEEP; HYPNOTICS).

INSPISSATION is the process of the drying or thickening of fluids or excretions by evaporation.

INSUFFLATION means the blowing of powder or vapour into a cavity, especially through the air passages, for the treatment of disease.

INSULIN is the internal secretion of the pancreas formed by groups of cells called the islands of Langerhans in this organ. Its existence was indicated by Sharpey-Schafer in 1909, and it was successfully isolated in a pure form by McLeod, Banting and Best in 1921. It acts by enabling the muscles and other tissues which require sugar for their activity to take up this substance from the blood. When it is deficient, the sugar derived from the food accumulates in the blood and is wastefully excreted in the urine. Insulin is administered by hypodermic (subcutaneous) injection in cases of diabetes mellitus (qv), and thus enables the sugar in the circulation to be utilized so that its excretion in the urine ceases. Each unit of insulin administered to a diabetic patient enables him to utilize somewhere between one and two grams of additional carbohydrate material. The appropriate dose of insulin in any given case depends upon its severity.

Twenty-seven insulin preparations are listed in the *British National Formulary*. These differ in their speed of onset, and duration, of action.

Hitherto insulin has been obtained from the pancreas of oxen and pigs. Human insulin is now available. This is made either by genetic manipulation of the micro-organism, *Escherichia coli*, or by enzymatic manipulation (see ENZYME) of pig insulin. Beef, pig, and human insulin differ in the number of amino-acids (qv) they contain. Hitherto insulin has been available in three strengths: of 20, 40 and 80 units per millilitre. These are now being replaced by one strength of 100 units per millilitre, known as U100 insulin. This is being accompanied by the issue of a U100 syringe in two sizes: 0·5 and 1 millilitre, graduated in units of insulin.

INTELLIGENCE QUOTIENT, or IQ as it is usually known, is the ratio between the mental age and chronological age multiplied by 100. Thus, if a boy of 10 years of age is found to have a mental age of 12 years, his IQ will be: 120.

On the other hand, if he is found to have a mental age of 8 years his IQ will be: 80.

The mental age is established by various tests, the most widely used of which are the Stanford-Binet Scale, the Wechseer Adult Intelligence Scale, and the Mill Hill Vocabulary Test.

Average intelligence is represented by an IQ of 100, with a range of 85 to 115. For practical purposes it is taken that the intellectual level reached by the average 15-year-old is indistinguishable from that of an adult.

INTERCOSTAL is the term applied to the nerves, vessels and muscles that lie between the ribs, as well as to diseases affecting these structures.

INTERFERON: It has been known for many years that one virus will interfere with the growth of another. In 1957, workers at the National Institute for Medical Research in London isolated the factor that was responsible for the phenomenon. They gave it the name of interferon. There are now known to be three human interferons. They are glycoproteins and are released from cells infected with virus or exposed to stimuli which mimic virus infection. They not only inhibit the growth of viruses. They also inhibit the growth and reduplication of cells. This is the basis for their investigation as a means of treating cancer. Hitherto the major difficulty has been obtaining sufficient supplies, but methods have now been evolved which promise to provide adequate amounts of it. The most promising of these is by means of what is known as genetic engineering, or manipulation, whereby a portion of DNA (qv) from interferon is inserted into the micro-organism known as *Escherichia coli* (see ESCHERICHIA) which thus becomes a source of almost unlimited amounts of interferon as it can be grown so easily. The evidence to date indicates that interferon is of value in treating certain virus infections, particularly different forms of herpes. The case for its value in the treatment of cancer is still not proven.

INTERLEUKINS: Interleukins are lymphokines, that is polypeptides produced by activated lymphocytes. There are two varieties called interleukin 1 and interleukin 2. Interleukin 1 is produced as a result of inflammation and antigenic stimulation from both T and B lymphocytes. They enhance the immune response by stimulating other lymphocytes and activating dormant T cells. Interleukin 2 has anti-cancer effects as it is able to activate T lymphocytes to become killer cells which destroy foreign antigens such as cancer cells. Cancers of the skin and kidney are particularly sensitive *in vitro* to the effects of these killer cells. There are serious side-effects when interleukin 2 is used in individuals with cancer and it is uncertain whether this will become an effective way of treating patients with malignant disease.

INTERMITTENT is a term applied to fevers which continue for a time, subside completely and then return again. The name is also used in connection with a pulse in which occasional heart-beats are not felt, in consequence of irregular action of the heart.

INTERMITTENT CLAUDICATION is a condition occurring in middle-aged and elderly people, which is characterized by pain in the legs after walking a certain distance. The pain is relieved by resting for a short time. It is due to arteriosclerosis (see ARTERIES, DISEASES OF) of the arteries to the leg, which results in inadequate blood supply to the muscles. Drugs have little effect in easing the pain, but useful preventive measures are to stop smoking, reduce weight (if overweight) and to take as much exercise as possible within the limits imposed by the pain.

INTERSEXUALITY is the condition resulting from faulty sex differentiation during the development of the foetus. Although not a common condition, it is one that is now recognized should be diagnosed as early as possible in life in order that an early decision may be reached as to the sex of the child, or at least the sex he (or she) is to be brought up as. Equally important is it that any treatment that may be possible should be instituted at the optimum moment.

INTERSTITIAL is a term applied to indifferent tissue set among the proper active tissue of an organ. It is generally of a supporting character and formed of fibrous tissue. The term is also applied to the fluid always present in this in a small amount, and to diseases which specially affect this tissue, such as interstitial keratitis. (See EYE, DISEASES OF.)

INTERTRIGO is a term applied to a chafed or abraded condition between two surfaces of skin that rub together: eg. under the breast, between the toes, or the armpit. (See ATHLETE'S FOOT; CHAFING OF THE SKIN.)

INTESTINE is the whole of the alimentary canal situated below the stomach. In it most digestion is carried on, and through its walls all the food material is absorbed into the blood and lymph streams. (See DIGESTION.) The length of the intestine in man is about 8·5 to 9 metres (28 to 30 feet), and it takes the form of one continuous tube suspended in loops in the abdominal cavity.

Divisions: The intestine is divided into small intestine and large intestine. The former comprises that part of the tube which extends from the stomach onwards for 6·5 metres (22 feet) or thereabout, and at its broadest point is about 35 mm (1½ inches) in width. The large intestine is the second part of the tube, and though shorter (about 1·8 metres (6 feet) long) is much wider than the small intestine, reaching in places a width of 65 mm (2½ inches). The *small* *intestine* is divided rather arbitrarily into three parts: the *duodenum*, consisting of the first 25 or 30 cm (10 or 12 inches), into which the ducts of the liver and pancreas open; the *jejunum*, which is generally found empty after death, and comprises the next 2·4 or 2·7 metres (8 or 9 feet); and finally the *ileum*, which at its lower end opens into the large intestine.

The *large intestine* begins in the lower part of the abdomen on the right side. The first part is known as the caecum, and into this opens the *appendix vermiformis*. The appendix is a small tube, about the thickness of a quill, from 2 to 20 cm (average 9 cm) in length, which has much the same structure as the rest of the intestine. At one end it is closed, at the other it opens into the caecum, and although it appears to play little or no part in digestion, it is of great importance because of the frequency with which serious inflammation takes place in it. (See APPENDICITIS.) The caecum is continued into the colon. This is subdivided into: the *ascending colon* which ascends through the right flank to beneath the liver; the *transverse colon* which crosses the upper part of the abdomen transversely to the left side; the *descending colon* which bends downwards and descends through the left flank into the pelvis where it becomes the *sigmoid* colon. The last part of the large intestine is known as the *rectum*, which passes straight down through the back part of the pelvis, to open to the exterior through the *anus*.

Structure: The intestine, both small and large, consists of four coats, which vary slightly in structure and arrangement at different points, but are of the same general nature throughout the entire length of the bowel. On the inner surface there is a mucous membrane; outside this is a loose submucous coat, in which blood-vessels run; next comes a muscular coat in two layers; and finally a tough, thin peritoneal membrane. The total thickness of all four coats amounts to about 3 mm.

MUCOUS COAT: The interior of the bowel is completely lined by a single layer of pillar-like cells placed side by side. These rest upon a smooth, fine membrane, beneath which is a loose network of connective tissue and muscular fibres, richly supplied with blood-vessels and lymphatic-vessels. There are two arrangements by which the surface in the small intestine is much increased for the purposes of digestion and absorption. Countless ridges with deep furrows between them run across the upper part, and the whole surface is thickly studded with short hair-like processes called villi. As blood- and lymph-vessels run up to the end of these villi, the digested food passing slowly down the intestine is brought into very close relation with the circulation. Between the bases of the villi are set little openings, each of which leads into a simple, tubular gland lined by cells, which are similar to those covering the surface, and which produce a fluid with digestive powers. In the small intestine, cells here and there produce mucus, and, in the large intestine, a great number of cells are devoted to the production of this substance for lubricating the

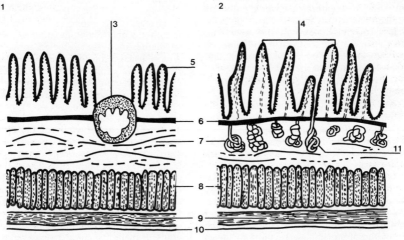

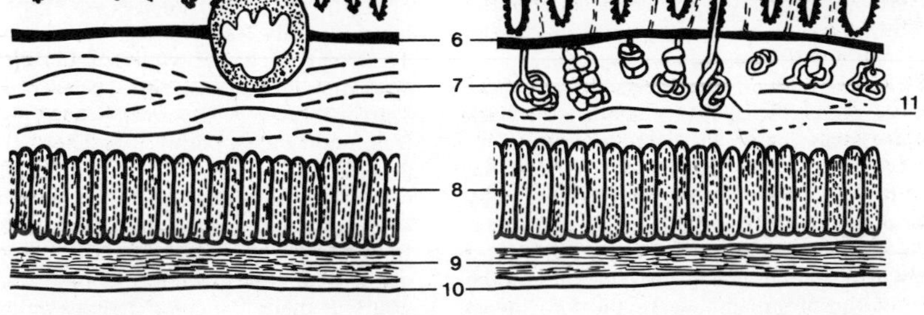

1 small intestine
2 duodenum
3 lymph follicle
4 villi
5 intestinal gland
6 muscularis mucosae
7 submucous coat
8 circular muscles
9 longitudinal muscles
10 peritoneum
11 duodenal gland

Diagram of intestine.

passage of the food through the bowel. A large number of minute masses, called lymph follicles, similar in structure to the tonsils and lymphatic glands, are scattered over the inner surface of the intestine. In the lower part of the small intestine these are grouped into patches of 2·5 square centimetres or thereabout in size, known as Peyer's patches, which are of special interest, because the inflammation and ulceration of the bowels that occur in typhoid fever are limited to them and to the scattered follicles. The large intestine is bare both of ridges and of villi, and, as already stated, its mucous membrane produces mucus in large amount.

SUBMUCOUS COAT: This consists of a loose connective tissue which allows the mucous membrane to play freely over the muscular coat. The blood-vessels and lymphatic-vessels which absorb the food in the villi pour their contents into a network of large vessels lying in this coat.

MUSCULAR COAT: The muscle in the small intestine is arranged in two definite layers, in the outer of which all the fibres run lengthwise with the bowel, whilst in the inner they pass circularly round it. The muscular coat is of immense importance, because by its contraction and relaxation the food is slowly squeezed down the bowel, the process being known as peristalsis. In the large intestine the only departure from this arrangement is that the fibres which are placed lengthwise are collected into three thick bands upon the outward surface of the bowel, and these bands, being slightly shorter than the other coats of the bowel, cause it to present a puckered appearance.

PERITONEAL COAT forms the outer covering for almost the whole intestine except parts of the duodenum and of the large intestine. It is a tough, fibrous membrane, covered upon its outer surface with a smooth layer of cells, which in the movements of the bowel rub against a similar surface upon the peritoneum lining the general cavity of the abdomen, and so cause a minimum of friction. From the peritoneal coat of the intestine of animals catgut is prepared.

Support: The duodenum and greater part of the large intestine are covered only in front by the peritoneum which lines the abdominal cavity, and this tough membrane serves to bind these parts of the intestine firmly against the back wall of the abdomen. The jejunum and ileum, the transverse colon, and the first part of the rectum are not only completely surrounded by peritoneum, but a double layer of this membrane suspends these parts of the bowel at a distance of several inches from the lines on the back of the abdomen, where the two layers become continuous with the rest of the peritoneum. In this way freedom is given to the movements of these parts of the bowels. These suspending structures are known as mesenteries. That of the small intestine is the largest, being shaped like a fan, 200 mm (8 inches) long at its attached margin, and spreading out to 6·5 metres (22 feet) at its frilled border, where it meets the intestine. The vessels and nerves which supply the intestine run between the two layers of the mesentery.

INTESTINE, DISEASES OF: The principal signs of trouble which has its origin in the intestines consist of pain somewhere about the abdomen, sometimes vomiting, and irregularity in movement of the bowels in the direction either of stoppage or of excessive action.

Several diseases are treated under separate headings. (See APPENDICITIS; CHOLERA; COLITIS; CONCRETIONS; CONSTIPATION; DIARRHOEA; DYSENTERY; ENTERIC FEVER; HERNIA; ILEITIS; INTUSSUSCEPTION; IRRITABLE BOWEL; PERITONITIS; PILES; RECTUM, DISEASES OF.)

INFLAMMATION of the bowel may affect either its outer or its inner surface. The outer surface is covered by peritoneum, and peritonitis is a serious disease. (See PERITONITIS.) Inflammation of the inner surface is known generally as enteritis, inflammation of special parts receiving the names of colitis, appendicitis, and the like. Enteritis may form the chief symptom of certain infective diseases due to special organisms: for example in typhoid fever, cholera, dysentery. Again, it may be acute, though not connected with any definite organism, when, if severe, it is a very serious condition, particularly in young children. Or it may be chronic, especially as the result of dysentery, and then constitutes a less serious though very troublesome complaint. Indiscretions in diet, such as the eating of unripe fruit, are a not uncommon cause. A very serious type results from the action of irritant poisons. In some people inflammation of the stomach and bowels is liable to result from exposure to cold and damp.

Symptoms: Diarrhoea is the most common and most marked symptom, and in chronic cases usually the only symptom, although, when the small intestine alone is affected, constipation is a more usual result than diarrhoea. Pain, particularly of a griping nature, which comes and goes, is also common. The temperature in acute cases is raised, and there is restlessness, even delirium. If the diarrhoea is very profuse, collapse speedily comes on.

Treatment: Each case requires special handling, according to the cause and the severity. Where diarrhoea is very severe this requires special treatment. (See DIARRHOEA.) There are a few general principles which are applicable to all cases. The diet should be light, bland, non-irritating and containing a minimum of roughage. In more acute cases only milk and glucose drinks should be given for the first twenty-four hours. If there is much diarrhoea ample fluids should be given to prevent dehydration. Rest in bed is essential. Considerable quantities of warm water, containing bicarbonate of soda, have a beneficial action by flushing out the bowel and removing irritating substances. In general, water is given by the mouth, but in some cases it is introduced by an enema to irrigate the lower bowel. Various drugs which have a mildly astringent and soothing action, of which the chief are bismuth carbonate and kaolin, are given by the mouth. When the inflammation is not the result of a chemical or physical irritant, but the result of an infection, as in dysentery, treatment with a sulphonamide drug absorbed only slowly from the intestine is indicated. Phthalylsulphathiazole, succinylsulphathiazole and sulphadimidine have proved particularly useful in the treatment of dysentery.

ULCERATION of the bowels arises in a manner similar to the production of ulcers on the skin surface, although probably these internal ulcers heal much more rapidly than others. Typhoid fever regularly produces ulcers in the lower part of the small intestine, this variety arising in the patches of lymphatic tissue found in this region. Tuberculous ulcers arise late in the course of tuberculosis, and produce a diarrhoea which is always a serious sign. Ulceration also occurs in amoebic dysentery.

Symptoms of ulceration are much the same as those of enteritis, and the formation of ulcers is simply an advanced stage of this condition. In addition, the ulcerated surface is apt to bleed, and, if the ulcer is situated high up in the bowel, this blood is voided as black or brown material; if it comes from near the lower end of the bowel the blood is red and unchanged. The healing of these ulcers leads, in the case of all save those of typhoid fever, to the formation of scars, and, as these scars contract there is a tendency to narrowing of the bowel and obstruction. This is particularly apt to follow tuberculous ulcers, if these should heal, because they often run circularly round the inside of the bowel.

Treatment in cases of ulceration is similar to that for inflammation.

PERFORATION of the bowel may take place as the result either of injury or of disease. Stabs and other wounds which penetrate the abdomen may damage the bowel, and severe blows or crushes may tear it without any external wound. Ulceration, as in typhoid fever, or, more rarely, in tuberculosis, may cause an opening in the bowel-wall also. Again, when the bowel is greatly distended above an obstruction, faecal material may accumulate and produce ulcers, which rupture with the ordinary movements of the bowels. Whatever the cause, the symptoms are much the same.

Symptoms: The contents of the bowel pass out through the perforation into the peritoneal cavity, and, making their way between the coils of intestine, set up a general peritonitis. In consequence, the abdomen is painful, and after a few hours becomes extremely tender to the touch, as a result of the peritonitis. The abdomen swells, particularly in its upper part, owing to gas having passed also into the cavity. Vomiting is a symptom, and the person passes into a state of collapse. Such a condition is almost invariably fatal in two, or at most three, days, if not promptly treated. Occasionally, however, the perforation is preceded by a certain amount of peritonitis, which forms adhesions in the neighbourhood of the ulcerated part, so that when perforation finally takes place a localized abscess, instead of general peritonitis, may result, and the person may recover.

Treatment: All food should be withheld, because whatever is taken into the stomach is either vomited or is liable to pass out of the perforation into the peritoneal cavity. An operation is urgently necessary, the abdomen being opened in the middle line, the perforated portion of bowel found, and the perforation stitched up. If the bowel is damaged badly, a part is often cut out and the divided ends joined together. Finally, the peritoneal cavity is thoroughly washed out, and a drainage tube left for some days in the abdominal wound. The local application of penicillin or sulphonamides to the peritoneum during operation has effected a marked reduction in the mortality rate.

OBSTRUCTION of the bowels means a stoppage to the passage down the intestine of the partially digested food. Obstruction may be due either to some cause within the abdomen or to the thrusting of a loop of bowel through an opening in the wall of this cavity. The latter class of cases has been referred to under HERNIA. Obstruction may be acute when it comes on suddenly with intense symptoms, or it may be chronic, when the obstructing cause gradually increases and the bowel becomes slowly more narrow till it closes altogether, or when slight obstruction comes and goes till it ends in an acute attack. In chronic cases the symptoms are much the same as those of the acute variety, although they are milder in degree and more prolonged.

Causes: Obstruction may be due to causes outside the bowel altogether, for example, the pressure of tumours in neighbouring organs, the twisting round the bowel of bands produced by former peritonitis, or even the twisting of a coil of intestine round itself so as to cause a kink in its wall. Chronic and partial forms of obstruction are sometimes due to such kinks near the end of the small intestine, sometimes to the pressure of the mesentery on the upper end of the small intestine. Chronic causes of the obstruction may exist in the wall of the bowel itself: for example, a tumour, or the contracting scar of an old ulcer. The condition of intussusception (qv), where part of the bowel passes inside of the part beneath it, in the same way as one turns the finger of a glove outside in, causes obstruction and other symptoms. Finally some body, such as a concretion, or the stone of some large fruit, or even a mass of hardened faeces, may become jammed within the bowel and stop up its passage.

Symptoms: There are four chief symptoms of this condition, and any case in which these are combined demands immediate treatment. These are pain, vomiting, constipation and swelling of the abdomen. The *pain* is of a griping character, and may be very severe although it comes and goes, getting now stronger and again for a time less marked. When the small intestine is the seat of obstruction the pain is almost always referred to the region round the navel; when the large intestine is affected the pain may be more accurately referred to the part from which it arises. In addition to this, acute cases are marked by great tenderness of the abdomen to touch. The *vomiting* is peculiar in character. It begins with the first onset of pain, and consists of the contents of the stomach. Later it is yellow or green, bitter, and contains much bile, while, after several hours have elapsed, it becomes brown and ill-smelling, and is then known as faecal vomiting. The *constipation* in acute cases comes on suddenly, whilst in chronic cases it may be preceded by a state in which constipation and diarrhoea alternate, or by one in which the stools gradually get smaller and smaller in size, possibly over a period lasting for several months. In chronic cases of obstruction to the large intestine, it is not uncommon for the sufferer to possess a constant desire to go to stool with straining pain, although he can pass nothing (tenesmus). In some conditions, particularly that due to intussusception, though there is constipation in the ordinary sense, the excessive straining produces a copious discharge of blood-stained mucus. The *swelling of the abdomen* varies in different cases. In acute cases the whole belly is blown up with gas, much increasing the pain of the condition. The constipation is so complete as to prevent even flatus from being passed – a very important sign of its gravity. Another grave sign is the absence of the sounds of intestinal movement which can be heard on auscultation over the normal abdomen. In chronic cases, in which the wall of the intestine is thickened, individual loops stand out now and then and become visible on the surface in their attempts to force their contents past the obstruction. When the small intestine is affected, its loops stand out one over the other, resembling the rungs of a ladder; whilst obstruction low down in the large intestine causes a bulging in the flanks and across the upper part of the abdomen.

In addition to these abdominal symptoms, in the later stages there is generally collapse, although consciousness is retained till the end. If the condition is not relieved by operation, death almost always results: in acute cases, in the course of three to six days.

Treatment: As a rule the surgeon opens the abdomen, finds the obstruction and relieves it or if possible removes it altogether. The task of the surgeon is rendered specially hard by the difficulty of determining, before he opens the abdomen, where the obstruction is, by the fact that the intestine is inflamed, and by its distension with gas and faeces. He has generally to open the abdomen in the middle line, examine the usual sites of obstruction, and, failing to find any cause at these points, to pass the whole length of intestine carefully through his hands till he finds the obstruction. Even after this is found, if it is of the nature of a tumour, it may be impossible to remove. If the obstruction is successfully removed, something must next be done, by puncturing the bowel or other means, to relieve the collection of gas and faeces, and this adds to the operation the great risk of sepsis. The introduction of the sulphonamides and antibiotics, however, has diminished this risk considerably. In all these manipulations care must be taken, by warm towels and the like, to prevent unnecessary exposure and chilling of the bowel.

TUBERCULOSIS of the intestine is a relatively uncommon disease in the United Kingdom today, where it is encountered predominantly in Asian immigrants. Treatment consists of the administration of ethambutol, rifampicin and isoniazid, as in the case of pulmonary tuberculosis, but for a longer period: 18 months. In order to prevent the risk of obstruction occurring, the use of corticosteroids (qv) has also been recommended for two months. As these patients are often debilitated and anaemic, they must be put on a high-protein diet with ample vitamins, and the anaemia must be energetically treated. This may require a blood transfusion in the initial stages.

TUMOURS are relatively uncommon in the small intestine and, when they do occur, they are usually benign. Conversely, they are relatively common in the large intestine where they are usually cancerous. The most common site for cancer of the large intestine is the rectum, with the sigmoid, caecum and ascending colon next in order of frequency. It is a disease of the older age-groups, and occurs with equal frequency in men and women. A history of altered bowel habit, in the form of increasing constipation or diarrhoea, or an alternation of these, or of bleeding from the anus, in a middle-aged person is an indication for taking medical advice. If the condition is cancer, then the sooner it is operated on, the better the result.

INTIMA is the innermost coat lining the arteries and the veins.

INTOXICATION is a term applied to states of poisoning. The poison may be some chemical substance introduced from outside, eg. alcohol (see ALCOHOLISM), or it may be due to the products of bacterial action, the bacteria either being introduced from outside or developing within the body. The term auto-intoxication is applied in the latter case.

INTRACRANIAL is the term applied to structures, diseases, and the like, contained in or rising within the head.

INTRATHECAL means within the membranes or meninges which envelop the spinal cord. The intrathecal space, between the arachnoid and the pia mater, contains the cerebrospinal fluid.

INTRA-UTERINE DEVICES (see CONTRACEPTION).

INTROSPECTION is the observation of one's own thoughts or feelings. It is generally applied to this process when it occurs to an abnormal extent in association with melancholia.

INTUBATION is a simple operation consisting in the introduction, through the mouth into the larynx, of a tube designed to keep the air passage open at this point.

INTUSSUSCEPTION is a form of obstruction of the bowels in which part of the intestine enters within that part immediately beneath it. This can best be understood by observing what takes place in the fingers of a tightly fitting glove as they turn outside in when the glove is pulled off the hand. The people affected are almost always infants. The cause is not known. The point at which it most often occurs is the junction between the small and the large intestines, the former passing within the latter. The symptoms are those of intestinal obstruction in general, and in addition there is often a discharge of blood-stained mucus from the bowel. The treatment consists – unless the symptoms rapidly subside, when it may be assumed that the bowel has righted itself – of either hydrostatic reduction by means of a barium enema, or an operation. At operation the intussusception is either reduced or, if this not possible, the obstructed part is cut out and the ends of the intestine then stitched together. If treated adequately and in time, the mortality is now reduced to around 1 per cent.

INUNCTION is a method of administering drugs by rubbing them into the skin mixed with oil or fat. The method is not often used now.

IN VITRO is a term commonly used in medical research and experimental biology. Literally 'in a glass', it refers to observations made outside the body: eg. on the action of drugs on bacteria. The opposite term is IN VIVO, which refers to observations of processes in the body.

INVOLUCRUM is the term applied to the sheath of new bone which is formed round a piece of dead bone in, for example, osteomyelitis.

INVOLUTION is the process of change whereby the uterus returns to its resting size after parturition. The term is also applied to any retrograde biological change, as in senility.

IODIDES are salts of iodine; those which are especially used in medicine being the iodide of potassium and iodide of sodium.
Action: Iodides have a threefold action. They are excreted in the mucus secretions, as well as in the urine, saliva and sweat, and have an action in liquefying the mucus secretion of the bronchial tree. They are therefore used in expectorant mixtures. Their second action is in assisting to absorb diseased tissue, particularly in syphilis. Finally, they are used to assist in providing a supply of iodine in patients with goitre, or in individuals who live in an area where goitre is liable to occur because of a deficiency of iodine in the drinking water. They may be given in the form of iodised salt. (See GOITRE.)

Over-dosage of iodides results in iodism (qv).
Uses: At one time the chief use of the drug was to cause absorption of the unhealthy tissues in syphilis. It is used for a similar reason in chronic forms of rheumatism. Iodides are given in chronic lead-poisoning, because they dissolve the lead deposited in the tissues and so permit its excretion from the body. They are also a common constituent of expectorant mixtures. Iodide is administered over long periods in small doses to children living in districts where goitre is common, with the object of preventing the onset of this disease.

IODINE is a non-metallic element which is found largely in seaweed. It is prepared in the form of dark violet-brown scales. It has a pleasantly pungent smell and a burning taste. It has a highly irritating action and when applied to the skin, stains the latter dark brown and causes it to peel off in flakes, while internally it is a violent irritant poison in large doses.
Uses: Externally iodine is used as an antiseptic. Its only drawback in this respect is that it is fixed by protein, which reduces its antiseptic efficiency in open wounds. Its main use in this sphere therefore is for sterilizing the unbroken skin, as before an operation. For this the Weak Iodine Solution BP, which contains 2·5 per cent iodine, is used. This solution is also used as a preventive of chilblains, applied while the hands are still red before the skin has begun to crack.

In the form of Mandl's paint (ie. dissolved with potassium iodide in glycerin) iodine is a useful remedy in inflammatory conditions of the throat and tonsils. Small doses of the weak iodine solution (2 to 5 drops) often control vomiting when other measures fail; for this purpose it is usually given in milk. Iodine – often as Aqueous Iodine Solution BP, or Lugol's solution as it is sometimes known (5 per cent iodine and 10 per cent potassium iodide in water) – is given internally in the treatment of goitre, especially before the operation of thyroidectomy for Graves' disease.

IODISM is the condition which is produced by an over-dose of iodides, but in some susceptible individuals iodism may be produced by very small amounts of iodides. It is characterized by running of the eyes and nose, sore throat, a heavy, dull feeling over the eyes, increased secretion of saliva and a typical skin eruption. These manifestations usually disappear rapidly upon the drug being withdrawn.

IODOFORM is a mild antiseptic made by the action of iodine upon a mixture of alcohol and

potash. It has a most penetrating, not unpleasant odour and strong taste. It relieves pain when applied to a raw or mucous surface, and has the property of preventing putrefaction when brought in contact with discharges. When applied in large quantities to a raw surface it is apt to be absorbed and to cause symptoms of poisoning, consisting of a red rash over the body, fever, loss of appetite and, it may be, delirium.
Uses: Because of its combined analgesic and antiseptic properties, it is a useful application for ulcers and granulating wounds. In the form of Bipp (qv) it was a popular wound dressing in the 1914–18 War. It is also sometimes used as an insufflation in the treatment of ozaena and ulcers of the mouth.

ION EXCHANGE RESINS are synthetic organic substances which have the power of exchanging ions. Chemically, they are closely related to plastics. They are divided into two groups: *cation exchange resins*, which take up and liberate cations, eg. sodium, potassium, hydrogen ions; *anion exchange resins*, which take up and liberate anion, eg. chloride, hydroxyl ions. The former are used in the treatment of oedema, and the latter in the treatment of peptic ulcers.

IONIZATION means the breaking up of a substance in solution into its constituent ions.

IONTOPHORESIS is the process by which various substances are made to pass through the skin into the underlying tissues by means of the electric current. This is also called iontherapy, galvano-ionization and medical ionization. Only those drugs can be used for ionization which are soluble in water and can be dissociated when dissolved. They include inorganic salts and similar organic compounds such as salts of the alkaloids and salts of organic acids like sodium salicylate. The form of electricity used for ionization is the continuous current. Iontophoresis is largely restricted nowadays to its use as a means of alleviating rheumatic pains. Among the substances used for this purpose are sodium chloride, sodium salicylate and histamine. Zinc ionization is sometimes used for the treatment of nasal allergy.

IOPANOIC ACID is an organic iodine preparation which is radio-opaque and is used to visualize the gall-bladder on X-rays, as it is excreted in the bile. It is given by mouth.

IPECACUANHA, IPECAC, or HIPPO, is the root of *Cephaëlis ipecacuanha*, a Brazilian shrub. It contains an alkaloid, emetine, which acts as an irritant when brought in contact with the interior of the stomach, producing vomiting. This effect is also brought about after its absorption into the blood by its action on the vomiting centre in the brain. In small doses it acts, not as an irritant, but as a gentle stimulant to the mucous membrane of the stomach, bowels and respiratory passages. Emetine was for long the great stand-by in the treatment of amoebic dysentery.
Uses: Ipecacuanha is a constituent of many expectorant mixtures given in the treatment of bronchitis. It is of value in this connection because of its action in liquefying the thick mucous secretion which occurs in bronchitis. It is also a constituent of Dover's Powder (qv), which is one of the most efficient diaphoretics for use in febrile conditions, such as the common cold. Syrup of ipecacuanha is the treatment of choice for evacuating the stomach in young children who have swallowed a poison.

IPRINDOLE (PRONDOLE) is a drug that is proving useful in the treatment of depressive illness. (See ANTIDEPRESSANTS.)

IPRONIAZID (MARSILLID) is a drug which inhibits monoamine oxidase (qv), an enzyme which plays an important part in the metabolism of the brain. It was originally introduced into medicine for the treatment of tuberculosis. It proved too toxic for this purpose, however. It is now being used in the treatment of depressive states. (See ANTIDEPRESSANTS.)

IPROTROPIUM is a drug that is proving of value in the treatment of asthma.

IRIDECTOMY: The operation by which a hole is made in the iris, as, for example, in the treatment of glaucoma (qv) or as part of cataract surgery (qv).

IRIDENCLEISIS was an operation formerly used in the treatment of glaucoma. It has now been replaced by trabeculectomy (see GLAUCOMA).

IRIDOLOGY is the study of the iris (qv). It is an old practice dating back to the days of Aristotle, which has been revived in recent days as one of the more exotic branches of what is popularly known as 'fringe medicine'. By its exponents it is defined as 'diagnosis through photography of the iris', and extravagant, as yet unsupported, claims are made for its validity.

IRIS (see EYE).

IRISH MOSS (see CARRAGEEN).

IRITIS (see UVEITIS).

IRON is a metal which is an essential constituent of the red blood corpuscles, where it is present in the form of haemoglobin. It is also present in muscle, myoglobin, and in certain respiratory pigments which are essential to the life of many tissues in the body. Iron is absorbed principally in the upper part of the small intestine. It is then stored: mainly in the liver; to a lesser extent in the spleen and kidneys, where it is available, when required, for use in the bone marrow to form the

haemoglobin in red blood corpuscles. The daily iron requirement of an adult is 15 to 20 milligrams. This requirement is increased during pregnancy. Iron salts also have an astringent action, especially the chloride, and this property is sometimes made use of when it is used as a styptic to check bleeding.
Uses: The main use of iron is in the treatment of iron-deficiency anaemias. (See ANAEMIA.) The main form in which it is used is ferrous sulphate. Iron preparations sometimes cause irritation of the gastro-intestinal tract, and should therefore always be taken after meals. They sometimes produce a tendency towards constipation. Whenever possible, iron preparations should be given by mouth. It is a very small proportion indeed of cases of iron-deficiency anaemia which will not respond satisfactorily to iron given by mouth. For the occasional cases in which oral administration is not suitable, a preparation of iron is now available which can be given intravenously.

IRRADIATION is treatment by various forms of light and radiant activity.

IRRIGATION is the method of washing out wounds, or cavities of the body, like the bladder and bowels. (See DOUCHES; ENEMA.)

IRRITABLE BOWEL SYNDROME is a motility disorder of the gut. It is not confined to the large intestine so that the terms spastic colon or irritable colon are inaccurate. Some of the symptoms of the irritable bowel syndrome affect more than 10 per cent of the normal adult population, but most people accept these symptoms as a minor nuisance. Only those with severe symptoms or those who worry about their symptoms consult a doctor.
Symptoms: Abdominal pain is the commonest symptom and it frequently moves from one area of the abdomen into another. A disturbed bowel habit is also common and this may alternate between diarrhoea and constipation. A feeling of abdominal distension is common, as is heartburn. Some patients suffer from painless, watery diarrhoea. The symptoms are either due to abnormal motility of the gut or to increased intestinal sensitivity to distension. The pain can, in fact, often be produced in patients by balloon inflation within the colon or other parts of the gut. The symptoms frequently start after an acute intestinal infection, and acute psychological stresses can also influence the activity of the bowel.
Treatment requires reassurance and explanation of the functional nature of the disorder. Anticholinergic drugs inhibit colonic motor activity and mebeverine has a direct relaxant effect on intestinal smooth muscle. Antidiarrhoeal drugs such as codeine phosphate reduce the frequency and urgency of defaecation. Lomotil is an effective alternative. Bulking agents speed colonic transit and allow the passage of softer, bulkier motions. High-fibre diets are beneficial.

ISCHAEMIA means bloodlessness of a part of the body, due to contraction, spasm, constriction or blocking (by embolus or by thrombus) of the arteries: for example, of the heart.

ISCHAEMIC HEART DISEASE (see CORONARY THROMBOSIS).

ISCHIO-RECTAL ABSCESS is an abscess arising in the space between the rectum and ischial bone and often resulting in a fistula.

ISCHIUM is the bone which forms the lower and hinder part of the pelvis. It bears the weight of the body in sitting.

ISCHURIA means insufficiency in the amount of urine passed, due either to suppression of excretion or retention in the bladder.

ISHIHARA TEST (see VISION).

ISOCAL (see ENTERAL FEEDING).

ISOCARBOXAZID (MARPLAN) (see ANTIDEPRESSANTS).

ISO-IMMUNIZATION is the immunization of one member of a species by an antigen lacking in himself but present naturally in other members of the species, as, for example, the immunization of an Rh-negative mother by an Rh-positive foetus, the mother as a result producing anti-Rh agglutinins which injure the foetus. (See also HAEMOLYTIC DISEASE OF THE NEWBORN; RH FACTOR.)

ISOLATION in infectious diseases is an important procedure, applied both to people who are themselves sick and to those who have come in contact with them, technically known as contacts or suspects, and who may later develop the disease. (See INCUBATION; INFECTION; QUARANTINE.)

ISONIAZID is one of the anti-tuberculous drugs. It has the advantages of being relatively non-toxic and of being active when taken by mouth. Unfortunately, like streptomycin, it may render the *Mycobacterium tuberculosis* resistant to its action. This tendency to produce resistance is considerably reduced if it is given in conjunction with streptomycin and/or para-aminosalicylic acid.

ISOPRENALINE is a bronchodilator drug that is widely and successfully used in the treatment of asthma, mainly as an aerosol for inhalation. In view of its action on the heart it must be used with caution.

ISOTONIC is a term applied to solutions which have the same power of diffusion as one another. An isotonic solution used in medicine is one which can be mixed with body fluids without causing any disturbance. An isotonic *saline solution* for injection into the blood, so that it may possess the same osmotic pressure as the blood serum, is one of 0·9 per cent strength or containing 9 grams of sodium chloride to 1 litre of water. This is also known as *normal* or *physiological salt solution*. An isotonic solution of *bicarbonate of soda* for injection into the blood is one of 1·35 per cent strength in water. An isotonic solution of *glucose* for injection into the blood is one of 5 per cent strength in water.

Solutions which are weaker, or stronger than, the fluids of the body with which they are intended to be mixed are known as hypotonic and hypertonic, respectively.

ISOTOPES: There are four fundamental atomic particles: the proton, the neutron, the electron and the positron. The proton has mass and a unit positive electrical charge. The neutron has mass and no charge. The electron has very small mass compared with the proton and neutron, and has unit negative electrical charge. The positron is the positively charged counterpart of the electron, having equal mass and unit positive charge.

The atom is composed of a positively charged central nucleus surrounded by a number of electrons. The nucleus is made up of protons and neutrons. The number of protons determines the positive charge and is known as the atomic number. The number of protons plus the neutrons is the atomic mass number and determines the atomic weight. The number of orbital electrons surrounding the nucleus of an atom is equal to the number of protons in the nucleus. Hence the atom is electrically neutral. Since chemical reactions concern only interactions between the outer electrons the chemical properties of an atom are determined by the number of orbital electrons–that is, they are characterised by the atomic number.

An element is matter consisting of atoms having the same atomic number. The number of neutrons in the atom of an element may vary and therefore its atomic mass number may vary. A nuclide is a species of atom characterised by its atomic number, atomic mass number and nuclear energy state. Isotopes are nuclides having the same atomic number but different mass number. For example hydrogen with atomic number one occurs in nature as a mixture of the nuclides hydrogen-1 with mass number one (that is, one proton in its nucleus), and hydrogen-2 (deuterium or heavy hydrogen) with mass number two–that is, one proton and one neutron is its nucleus.

Hydrogen-1 and hydrogen-2 are both isotopes of hydrogen and are chemically indistinguishable. The terms isotope and radioactive isotope are frequently used when nuclide and radioactive nuclide would be more accurate. Atomic weight is not quite synonymous with atomic mass number. The atomic weight for a given specimen of an element is the mean weight of its atoms expressed in atomic mass units, for many elements consist of a mixture of different nuclides of that element.

Isotopes may be stable or radioactive. In stable isotopes the relative number of protons and neutrons are found to lie within quite close limits. In radioactive isotopes this balance is upset owing to an excess or deficiency of neutrons, with the result that the nuclei become unstable. They tend to change into stable configurations by processes known collectively as radioactive decay. This involves spontaneous disintegration with emission of radiation.

The artificially produced radioactive isotopes may be grouped roughly in two categories: those produced in a nuclear reactor and those produced in a cyclotron. In nuclear reactors the target elements are bombarded with neutrons. The nuclides produced, therefore, are usually isotopic with the stable target elements, and have more neutrons in their nuclei. The radioactive isotope of hydrogen, tritium, has a mass number of 3 and the ratio of neutrons to protons is 2 : 1. Isotopes with excess neutrons in the nuclei tend to decay by the emission of beta rays. In the process of producing isotopes in a cyclotron the target material in bombarded with protons, deuterons, or alpha particles. The radioactive products are thus isotopes of a different element from the target. They are deficient in neutrons, and therefore tend to decay by emission of positrons.

Each radioactive substance, whether naturally occuring, produced in a nuclear reactor, or in a cyclotron, is characterised not only by the type and energy of radiation given off but also by the rate of disintegration. The half-life is the time taken for one-half of the original number of unstable atoms to disintegrate. Half-lives of different isotopes vary enormously. For example, carbon-14 has a half-life of over 5,000 years, while silver-109 has a half-life of only 39 seconds. The unit of radioactivity is the curie, which may be defined as that activity in which the number of disintegrations per second is 3·7 × 10.

Within the atomic nucleus the particles are in constant motion, and therefore they collide frequently. In these collisions energy transfers take place, so that all particles do not have the same kinetic energy. In a stable nucleus no particle ever acquires sufficient energy to overcome the potential barrier and to escape from the nucleus. In an unstable nucleus, owing to the presence of an excess number of neutrons, there is an excess of energy among the particles, so that there is a probability that one particle will acquire sufficient kinetic energy to overcome the barrier and to escape from the nucleus.

Types of Radiation: The type and energy of radiation given off by radioactive substances is the same for any one nuclide. The primary radioactive decay process is always either the emission of a charged particle (alph particle, beta particle, or positron) or the capture by the nucleus of an orbital electron. These processes alter the charge on the nucleus, giving rise to a chemically different element. Any one of these may be accompanied by gamma rays or X-rays. In medical diagnosis the beta particles and gamma rays are the most commonly encountered forms of radioactivity.

Beta particles are electrons and have limited tissue penetration dependant on their energy. Even energetic beta particles are only able to penetrate about 1 cm of tissue, so they are not suitable for the study of deep organs. Gamma rays are not particulate, but are electromagnetic radiations of the same nature as light, though of much shorter wavelength, and therefore of much higher energy. They may be considered as being made up of discrete amounts of energy or photons. They have a much greater power of penetration than beta particles and this power is dependent on their energy.

Isotopes having an excess of neutrons usually decay by emission of negative beta particles. Decay of an isotope by emission of a beta particle may be thought of as the conversion of a neutron into a proton and electron, with the immediate ejection of the electron from the nucleus. The loss of a unit of negative charge means that the nucleus has effectively gained a proton in place of a neutron, and the resulting nucleus is that of the next higher element in the periodic system. To maintain electrical neutrality the atom must acquire an extra orbital electron. The decay of radioactive isotopes has thus fulfilled the dream of the alchemist. Radioactive carbon decays by emission of a beta particle and become stable nitrogen. Similarly phosphorus-32 disintegrates with the emission of a beta particle, and thereupon becomes stable sulphur.

The beta particles from a particular isotope have varying energies up to a maximum characteristic of that isotope. Phosphorus-32, sulphur-35, carbon-14 and hydrogen-3 are beta emitters. In some isotopes the available energy in the radioactive nucleus is not accounted for completely by beta decay. The excess energy is then emitted as a gamma ray. This occurs with such isotopes as iodine-131, iodine-132, sodium-24 and potassium-42.

Measurement of Radioactivity: Radioactive substances are detected by virtue of the radiation they emit. Ionization and excitation of the atoms is produced in the absorbing medium through which they pass. The beta rays produce ionization directly by their electrical charge. The gamma rays, by interaction with the atoms in the absorbing medium, produce so-called secondary electrons which behave in the same way as beta particles. Some radiation detectors–namely the ionization chamber, the proportional counter and the Geiger counter–depend on the ionization produced in a gas. Essentially each of these instruments consists of two electodes in a chamber filled with gas, across which a potential difference is maintained. The passage of ions between the electrodes gives rise to an electric current or a series of pulses, both of which may be measured.

The scintillation detector consists of a phosphor, such as a sodium iodide crystal, photo-multiplier tube and associated electronic equipment. When radiation energy is absorbed in the phosphor each quantum absorbed gives rise to a number of light quanta (photons). These cause emission of electrons from the photocathode of the photo-multiplier tube, which in turn gives rise to a pulse at its output. The size of these pulses is proportional to the energy of the absorbed radiation and the number of pulses to the intensity of the absorbed radiation. The pulses are measured and counted by the associated electronic equipment.

Ionization chambers are the least sensitive of detectors. The Geiger counter and the scintillation counter are equally sensitive to beta radiations, but the scintillation counter has much greater sensitivity to gamma radiation than the Geiger counter.

Applications of Radioactive Isotopes to Diagnosis: The use of radioactive isotopes in diagnosis is based on the fact that it is possible to tag many of the substances normally present in the body with a radioactive label. Because it is possible to detect minute quantities of radioactive material, only very small doses may be given. The body pool of the material is therefore not appreciably altered, and metabolism is not disturbed. Thus in studies of iodine metabolism the ratio of radioactive atoms administered to stable atoms in the body pool is of the order of 1 to 1,000 million. By measuring radioactivity in the body, in blood samples, or in the excreta it is possible to gain information about the fate of the labelled substance, and hence of the chemically identical inactive material. Hence it is theoretically possible to trace the absorption, distribution and the excretion of any substance normally present in the body, provided that it can be tagged with a suitable radioactive label.

If the investigation necessitates tracing the path of the material through the body by means of external counting over the body surface it is obviously essential to use an isotope that emits gamma radiation or positrons. If, however, only measurements on blood sample or excreta are required it is possible to use pure beta emitters. Recently whole-body counters have been introduced which measure the total radioactivity in the body, and these are of great value in absorption studies. Another development has been that of more sensitive scanning devices, which are used in studying the distribution of radioactive isotopes in various organs and tissues. Furthermore, the recent production of isotopes with shorter lives has made it possible to give higher radioactive doses without increasing the radiation hazard. This is of particular advantage to the scanning techniques which now enable most organs of the body to be visualized.

Five main groups of diagnostic uses may be defined:

1. *Metabolic Studies*: The use of radioactive materials in metabolic studies is based on the fundamental property that all isotopes of an

element are chemically identical. The radioactive isotope is used as a true isotope tracer–that is, when introduced into the body (in whatever form) it behaves in the same way as the inactive element. Thus isotopes of iodine are used to measure thyroid function, and isotopes of calcium enable kinetic studies of bone formation and destruction to be performed. The distribution of iron-59 from the serum to the bone marrow, liver and spleen may be followed and its incorporation into the haemoglobin of the red cell used as a measure of bone marrow function. Orthoiodohippurate (Hippuran) labelled with iodine-131 may be used to assess renal vascularity and to detect differences in renal blood supply due to such conditions as renal artery stenosis.

2. *Absorption and Distribution Studies*: The fate of labelled substances given by mouth can be followed to assess their absorption, utilization and excretion. In most of these studies the isotope is a true isotope tracer. For example, iron absorption can be measured with radioactive iron; vitamin-B absorption may be investigated with vitamin B tagged with radioactive cobalt. In studies of fat absorption, on the other hand, triolein labelled with iodine-131 may be used, but this is not a true isotopic tracer.

3. *Body Composition by Dilution Studies*: By introducing an isotope into a compartment, such as the blood or extracellular space, it is possible to measure the volume of that compartment by determining the dilution of readioactivity when equilibrium has been reached. In this way iodine-131-labelled human serum albumin is used to estimate the plasma volume; chromium-51-labelled red cells to measure the red-cell volume; and bromine-82 to determine the extracellular water. The total body exchangable potassium can be measured with potassium-42 and total exchangable sodium with sodium-24 or sodium-22.

4. *Physical Tracing Studies*: In this type of study the isotope is not necessarily used as a true isotopic tracer. In other words, it does not trace the path of the corresponding inactive isotope. For example, xenon-133 is used in measurements of blood flow in muscles, and in lung-funtion studies; krypton-85 is used to detect intracardiac shunts. Neither of these elements is normally present in the body. The survival of red cells may be followed and the organ of sequestration revealed by labelling red cells with radioactive chromium. Though chromium is normally present in the body, it does not take part in the metabolic process of the red cell, and the labelling of cells with chromium-51 is simply used as a convenient tag to trace their fate.

5. *Scanning of Organs and Tissues*: Scanning is a technique which is used to determine the distribution of radioactive isotopes within the body or within one particular organ. In the conventional scanner the radiation detector, which is a scintillation counter, 'sees' only a small cross-sectional area of the body at a time. The activity 'seen' at each point is registered, and a 'map' of the activity seen over the scanned area is recorded. Various methods of presentation have been used, and the recently improved display systems present the information gathered by the scanner more effectively. Mechanical printing of blacks, which are closer together for higher count rates, has been followed by photoscanning and by 'colour print-outs', where the colour of the mark is selected by the count rate. A pictorial representation of the degree of radioactivity is thus achieved. This is advantageous, as the eye can detect quite small variations in colour pattern from point to point much more easily than in monochrome. More recent developments are stationary detectors such as the gamma camera, autofluoroscope, and other devices which can view the whole of the area simultaneously. Thus when selective concentration of an isotope in a tissue occurs it is possible to examine the distribution of that isotope by means of scanning. A toxic nodule in the thyroid may be identified by its selective concentration of iodine-131. Areas of absent function on the radioactive scan ('cold' areas) suggest the presence of tumours, abscesses, and similar lesions. Iodine-131 may be used to localize tumours of the thyroid, and chlormerodrin labelled with mercury-197 to delineate tumours of the kidneys. Of even greater practical application is the localising of brain tumours with human serum albumin labelled with iodine-131 or with radioactive technetium.

Treatment: Radioactive isotopes are also used in medical treatment. The overactivity of the thyroid gland in thyrotoxicosis can be treated by the ingestion of radioactive iodine. The ingested iodine is taken up by the thyroid gland where local irradiation of the gland takes place, reducing its activity. Radioactive phosphorus is used in the treatment of polycythemia rubra vera. It is largely taken up in bone as this is the main source of body phosphate and irradiation of the bone marrow results, controlling the overactivity that is characteristic of polycythemia rubra vera. In cobalt teletherapy the isotope cobalt 60 is used to deliver 1·2–1·3-million-volt radiation which is equivalent to X-rays generated at a peak voltage of 3–4-million-volts. (See RADIOTHERAPY.)

ISSUE is an old term for a suppurating sore.

ITCH is a popular name for scabies (qv).

ITCHING, or PRURITUS, is an unpleasant condition of the skin surface which in some cases is so constant as to become unbearable.

Causes: It is due to many different conditions, some of which are local and can be easily removed. Some are general, while occasionally the condition becomes so chronic and the skin so changed by scratching, that it is incurable. Itching is produced by slight mechanical irritation, such as contact with rough woollen underclothing, also by parasites such as lice, or scabies ('the itch'), and these mechanical causes being removed the itching speedily vanishes. There is often a large psychological factor and this must always be borne in mind. (See NEURODERMATITIS.)

Various skin diseases, of which eczema is the chief, have itchiness as one of their main symptoms. In old age, when the skin is becoming thin and inelastic, itching sometimes becomes a troublesome complaint. In these and other conditions, a habit of scratching, which in course of time renders the skin rough and thickened, is apt to be acquired and this of itself aggravates and keeps up the itchiness. Among the general diseases which set up itchiness, the chief is diabetes mellitus. In fact, any one who is much troubled by itchiness, especially if this is situated about the genital organs, should have his urine examined for the presence of sugar. Jaundice caused by various liver derangements, and glomerulonephritis, are often accompanied by itchiness in a milder degree. Food allergy is not uncommonly the cause of nettle-rash, which may be of an itching type and appear soon after the food has been taken. Some people are much troubled by itching of the body when changes in size of the blood-vessels in the skin take place, as occur upon getting warm in bed or at the start of spring and autumn. A similar condition, which affects people on going to the tropics, is known as prickly heat (qv).

Cold weather itch is a common form of itching in cold weather when the skin tends to become dry. It is commonest and most marked on the legs of old people.

A special and often very aggravated form of itching occurs sometimes at the anus, known as *pruritus ani*. In all cases of irritation in or around the anus, a careful search should be made for threadworms. (See RECTUM, DISEASES OF.) An equally troublesome form of itching occurs round the vagina, known as *pruritus vulvae*. It may be associated with excessive vaginal discharge. (See WHITES.)

Treatment: The use of detergents should be avoided, and as little soap as possible should be used for cleansing purposes. Warm baths, alkaline or containing bran, are among the most soothing applications for general itching. The addition of an ounce or two (30 to 60 grams) of the *British Pharmacopoeia* Emulsifying Ointment is often beneficial. Calamine lotion is the most efficient local application, but talcum powder is often useful. In the treatment of cold weather itch some such preparation as E45 Cream or *British Pharmacopoeia* Emulsifying Ointment should be applied regularly, especially after a bath. Overwashing with soap should be avoided, and a non-alkaline substitute such as *British Pharmacopoeia* Aqueous Cream used instead of soap. Rough winter underclothing should not be used next the skin. It is essential that a proper examination should be made as to the functions of the internal organs in cases in which itching is a chronic complaint. In diabetic cases the surest remedy to prevent the itching is to treat the diabetes. In pruritus ani attention to anal hygiene is important, and the anal region should be washed twice a day, using a soft sponge, and, if possible, every time the bowels move. Talcum powder should be applied after the washing and careful drying. In persistent cases of pruritus ani and pruritus vulvae the application of a corticosteroid (qv) ointment is often helpful. If there is a psychological cause, this must always be dealt with.

-ITIS is a suffix added to the name of an organ to signify any diseased condition of that organ.

IVORY, or DENTINE, is the hard material which forms the chief bulk of the teeth. (See TEETH.)

J

JACKSONIAN EPILEPSY (see EPILEPSY).

JAIL FEVER is another term for typhus fever.

JALAP is the tuber of *Iopmoea purga*, a Mexican plant, which contains two resins of irritating properties. It is a potent purgative which is seldom used now except in combination with milder purgatives in certain pills. On the relatively few occasions on which a powerful purgative action is required, compound jalap powder may be used, in a dose of 2·4 to 4 grams.

JANICEPS is a foetal monstrosity characterized by one combined head and two faces.

JAUNDICE is a yellow discoloration of the skin due to the deposition of bile pigment in its deeper layers. (See also HEPATITIS, ACUTE INFECTIVE.)

Causes: Jaundice is divided into two main classes: *hepatogenous jaundice*, arising from the absorption of bile formed by the liver, and *haemolytic jaundice*, arising from the formation of a yellow pigment in the blood, derived from the breaking down of red blood corpuscles. The former is the usual type, and is described below; the latter is found in such conditions as pernicious anaemia, haemolytic anaemia, acholuric jaundice and snake poisoning.

When the bile cannot escape into the intestine in the usual way, it is absorbed by the blood- and lymph-vessels, and some of its constituents are deposited in the various tissues throughout the body. Some obstruction to the outflow of bile is therefore a necessary condition, and this obstruction may either exist in the bile-ducts, which convey the bile from liver to intestine, or it may be caused by some disorganization in the liver (eg. hepatitis) which prevents the bile, formed by the liver-cells, from finding its way to the bile-ducts at all. The tint of the jaundice has not necessarily any direct relation to the severity of the cause. Obstruction may be due to gall-stones, and the resulting jaundice is then a symptom of this condition. (See GALL-STONES.) Obstruction may be due to some cause quite outside the liver and bile-ducts, for example, enlarged glands lying near the liver or cancer of the pancreas, the seriousness of the jaundice depending then upon the seriousness of the disease responsible for the pressure. In elderly people, who are likely to be the subject of cancer, long-continued jaundice is for this reason a serious symptom. Cirrhosis of the liver, in which the small branches of the bile-duct become compressed by the formation of fibrous tissue, may also be a cause of chronic jaundice. (See CIRRHOSIS.)

Among the causes which disorganize the liver, one finds many poisons which are carried to it in the blood – for example, phosphorus, mercury, and snake poison, as well as a number of widely used drugs. Much more common as a cause of jaundice are two inflammatory conditions of the liver, known as infective hepatitis and serum hepatitis (qv). They are both due to viruses but they differ in that the former has a shorter incubation period. Infective hepatitis, which is much the more common of the two, is the condition which used to be known as catarrhal jaundice. Certain infective diseases are also prone to produce this effect: eg. yellow fever, malaria, typhoid fever and pyaemia. A serious but uncommon condition, accompanied by rapid and often fatal jaundice, is that known as acute yellow atrophy of the liver. Another form of jaundice is known as spirochaetal jaundice or *spirochaetosis icterohaemorrhagica* (qv). These conditions cause such changes in the liver that the bile is unable to escape except by reabsorption into the blood.

Neonatal jaundice is a form of jaundice not uncommon in the newborn infant. It is due to temporary inability to deal with the normal metabolism of bilirubin and usually passes off in a few days. If it should persist, however, or become severe, it requires treatment. The most effective form of treatment is exposure of the infant to blue light. This converts bilirubin into the harmless bile pigment known as biliverdin (qv). (See also BILIRUBIN; HAEMOLYTIC DISEASE OF THE NEWBORN; KERNICTERUS.)

Symptoms: Yellowness, appearing first in the whites of the eyes and later over the whole skin, is the symptom that attracts notice. This tint varies from a pale sulphur-yellow through all gradations to a deep olive or bronze colour, according to the completeness of the obstruction and the length of time the jaundice has lasted. The urine passed during the time the jaundice lasts is of a dark greenish-brown colour, owing to the excretion of bile by the kidneys. Various digestive disturbances are present: the tongue is furred, the appetite poor, and a feeling of sickness is often felt, and is aggravated by eating fats. The stools are of a grey or white colour, owing to the want of bile in the intestine, and for the same reason constipation, relieved occasionally by diarrhoea, is present, and the stools have an excessively offensive smell. A bitter taste in the mouth is generally felt by the jaundiced person, due, as it is supposed, to the presence in the saliva of salts of the bile-acids; and the same or other substances in the sweat lead to itching of the skin. Slowness of the pulse, and, in long-continued cases, mental confusion and dullness, are other less evident accompaniments of jaundice.

Treatment: The first essential is to treat the underlying cause if possible: for instance, gall-stones, if these be the cause of the jaundice. For the actual treatment of the jaundice the patient must be kept in bed. The diet should contain as much protein and carbohydrate as possible and a minimum of fat. The diet to be aimed at should contain 3000 Calories daily, including 100 to 120 grams of protein and supplemented with vitamins. Such a diet should not be forced in its entirety in the early days of treatment when the appetite is poor and the mere thought of food nauseating. For the pruritus, or itching, which may be very severe, calamine lotion containing 2 per cent phenol should be used. This may need to be supplemented with analgesics: eg. aspirin or a tablet containing aspirin, paracetamol and codeine. Sedatives may also be required.

As the jaundice clears, the amount of protein may be reduced, and if there is much residual indigestion this is best treated by a modified peptic ulcer diet.

JAW is the name applied to the bones that carry the teeth. The two upper jaw-bones, the maxillae, are firmly fixed to the other bones of the face. The lower jaw, the mandible, is shaped somewhat like a horseshoe, and, after the first year of life, consists of a single bone. It forms a hinge-joint with the squamous part of the temporal bone, immediately in front of the ear. Both upper and lower jaw-bones possess deep sockets, known as alveoli, which contain the roots of the teeth. (See DISLOCATIONS; FRACTURES; GUMBOIL; MOUTH; TEETH.)

JEJUNUM is part of the small intestine. (See INTESTINE.)

JELLY (see GELATIN).

JIGGER is a popular term used to denote a parasite also known as the sand-flea. The term is also used to denote the small worm-like masses of fatty material which can be squeezed out of the sebaceous glands on the face of those suffering from acne (qv).

JOINT-MOUSE is a popular term for a loose body in a joint. It is found especially in the knee. (See JOINTS, DISEASES OF.)

JOINTS: A joint or articulation is the meeting-place between different parts of the skeleton, whether bones or cartilages.

Structure: The great division of joints is into those which are fixed or relatively fixed (*fibrous* and *cartilaginous joints*), and those at which free movement can take place (*synovial joints*). In the former, a layer of cartilage or of fibrous tissue intervenes between the bones and binds them firmly together. This type of joint is exemplified by the sutures between the bones that make up the skull. Among these fixed joints, some have a thick disc of fibro-cartilage between the bones, so that, although the individual joint is really capable of very little movement, a series of these, like the joints between the bodies of the vertebrae, gives to the spinal column, as a whole, a flexible character (amphiarthrodial joint).

Into the formation of every *movable joint* four structures enter. These are the bones whose junction forms the joint; a layer of cartilage covering the end of each of these and rendering the ends smooth; a sheath of fibrous tissue known as the capsule, thickened at various points into bands or ligaments, which hold the bones together; and, finally, a membrane known as synovial membrane, which lines this capsule and produces a synovial fluid to lubricate the movements of the joint. Further, the bones are kept in position at the joints by the various muscles passing over them and by atmospheric pressure. This type of joint is known as a synovial joint.

Some joints possess subsidiary structures, such as discs of fibro-cartilage, which adapt the ends of the bones more perfectly to one another in places where these do not quite correspond. In others, movable pads of fat under the synovial membrane fill up larger cavities and afford additional protection to the joint.

Varieties: Apart from the main division of joints into those which are fixed and those which are movable, the movable joints fall into several groups. Gliding joints are those in which, like the wrist and ankle, the bones have flat surfaces capable of only a limited amount of movement. In hinge-joints, like the elbow and knee, the chief movement takes place round one axis. The ball-and-socket type is exemplified by the shoulder and hip, in which free movement is possible in any direction. There are other subsidiary varieties, named according to the shape of the bones which enter into the joint.

JOINTS, DISEASES OF: The larger joints, on account of their exposed position, are subject to constant injuries, and this, together with the wear they suffer and the richness of their blood supply, renders them liable to a number of serious diseases. The knee is the joint most often diseased, and after it, in order, the hip, ankle, and elbow. Although minor injuries may be followed by serious diseases, it is an important fact that very severe injuries, in which the skin remains unbroken, such as dislocations of, and fractures into, the joints rarely occasion any serious disease beyond stiffness and other direct results of the injury. On the other hand, penetrating wounds of joints are among the most serious injuries, and require immediate and expert treatment. The following are some of the conditions from which joints suffer.

SYNOVITIS is the name given to any inflammation of the membrane lining the joint cavity. It may be acute, subacute or chronic.

Causes: The joints being much exposed to blows, wounds and strains, some injury often precedes the onset of inflammation. In many cases, the condition is due to some rheumatic

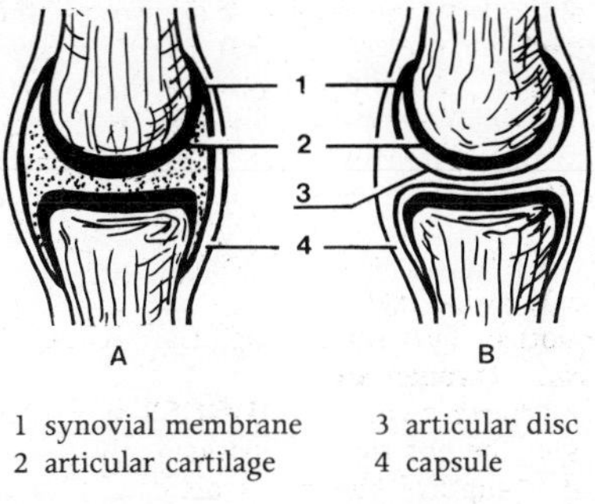

(A) diagram of a simple synovial joint. (B) diagram of a synovial joint with an articular disc.

condition such as rheumatoid arthritis, osteoarthrosis (see RHEUMATISM), gout (qv), or tuberculosis.

Symptoms: In acute synovitis, following usually upon some injury, the synovial membrane becomes inflamed, thickened, and secretes an excessive amount of fluid into the joint. As a result, the joint becomes painful, red, swollen and hot to touch. It is usually kept more or less bent, and is painful to straighten and to handle. If the synovitis remains of a simple nature, these symptoms last some days and then gradually subside. Or the condition may persist for a long time, getting better for a little and then relapsing; or it may become chronic, and, whilst the heat and redness disappear, the joint remains stiff and distended with fluid. This condition most frequently affects the knee, and is then popularly known as water on the knee. On the other hand, in occasional cases which have begun in the simple form, and in cases due to a penetrating wound of the joint to which bacteria have gained entrance, a very serious inflammation occurs. Suppuration then takes place in the joint, an abscess forms with fever, great pain and other aggravated symptoms of abscess. A joint cavity is very difficult to render free from suppuration, and may even necessitate amputation of the limb in order to save life.

Treatment: In the early stages, complete rest of the joint, the limb being placed on a splint, together with the application of cold or of warm fomentations to soothe the pain, is alone necessary. Later, massage and compression of the joint by a bandage aid the absorption of the fluid and dispel the stiffness. When the condition becomes chronic, counter-irritation by iodine, blisters, etc., is necessary, and the joint is often punctured to draw off the fluid. Suppuration is, as already stated, a serious matter, and is treated like an abscess elsewhere by opening, irrigation with antiseptics, drainage and the administration of antibiotics.

SYNOVITIS OF THE HIP in a transient form is not uncommon in children. The precise cause is not known, but it tends to follow a cold or sore throat or an injury, and is more common in fat children. It occurs more often in boys than girls, and the commonest age is around six. The child suddenly complains of pain in the hip or is seen to be limping. No treatment is required except to prevent weight-bearing during the acute phase. The condition usually lasts for about a fortnight, and recovery is complete within a couple of months.

EPIPHYSITIS is an inflammation situated at the end of a long bone just outside the joint. An important point regarding this type of inflammation in children is that if the inflammation is severe it may permanently damage the plate of cartilage, situated close to the end of the bone, from which increase in length takes place, so that the child's limb may be seriously impaired in growth.

TUBERCULOUS DISEASE of a joint begins in the synovial membrane or in the end of the bone, and is popularly known as white swelling, on account of the characteristic appearance of the affected joint, particularly when the knee is involved. In many cases there are other manifestations of the disease, the lungs, for example, being affected, or the glands of the neck enlarged. Tuberculosis of the joints is commoner in children than in older persons. A proportion of cases, especially in children, are due to the drinking of tuberculous milk.

Symptoms: The condition is usually chronic, begins insidiously, sometimes being dated from a slight accident, and progresses slowly. Slight stiffness, wasting of the muscles in the affected limb, and pain and tiredness brought on by slight exertion, are the earliest symptoms. The joint later on assumes its characteristic appearance, becoming enlarged, losing the natural hollows about it, and appearing white and glistening, with large veins showing through the skin. The wasting of muscle above and below the joint causes it to look still more enlarged than it really is. Gradually the use of the limb is lost, and the general health deteriorates. Later in the disease, when the joint is becoming thoroughly disorganized, starting-pains at night, which waken the sufferer as he is dropping off to sleep, become troublesome. If the condition remains untreated after this stage is reached, an abscess forms in the joint and bursts through the skin, and hectic fever develops.

Treatment: As in all other forms of tuberculosis the outlook has been revolutionized by the excellent results which have been obtained from the use of chemotherapy, giving combined therapy for at least six months. The use of chemotherapy has not only reduced the time of treatment by one-half, but has resulted in a much larger number of patients being left with almost full range of movement of the diseased joints.

STIFFNESS OF JOINTS may be due to various causes. It may result from spasm of the muscles around the joint in cases of early tuberculous disease and of hysterical joints, or it may be due to permanent shortening in these muscles or contraction of the skin, due, for example, to a burn. Often a severe injury to the joint itself, such as a fracture of one of the bones that form it, or a dislocation, is followed by some stiffness. A large number of slight injuries, which set up a mild degree of inflammation, are followed by some adhesions in the joint, often of a painful nature. These limit the use of the joint considerably, but, when they are broken by forcible movements of the limb, recovery and relief are immediate.

LOOSE BODIES IN JOINTS result from inflammation of various types, the bodies being developed as projections on the synovial membrane or on the cartilages of the joint, and later pulled off by its movements. They bring on repeated attacks of synovitis, and often cause sudden locking of the joint, so that for a time it is immovable. They are removed by operation.

GOUT, RHEUMATISM AND RHEUMATOID ARTHRITIS are diseases of a constitutional nature which affect joints. (See under these headings.)

SPRAIN is a vague popular term indicating the result of any slight wrench to a joint. A sprain consists generally of a mild attack of synovitis, or of tearing of ligaments with effusion of fluid into or round the joint. At the ankle, a twist of the foot inwards is followed by some tearing of the outer lateral ligament of the joint constituting a severe sprain, but a more serious accident, consisting of fracture at the lower end of the fibula, is apt to follow a wrench or twist of the foot outwards. (See FRACTURES.) In the knee, a sudden twist is occasionally responsible for loosening and rumpling up the inner of the two fibro-cartilages found in that joint. This accident has the awkward consequence of producing at subsequent times attacks of synovitis, or of sudden locking of the knee-joint. Behind the wrist and at the ankle, a sprain results sometimes in the displacement of some of the tendons which should be bound firmly to the bone, leading to occasional pain and a sense of weakness till the tendon happens to get replaced by another twist.

Treatment: When a sprain is of inflammatory character, the treatment is of the nature described under synovitis, and in the case of a bad sprain rest for a week or two may be essential. A sprain consisting in tearing of the ligaments round a joint, accompanied by effusion of blood beneath the skin, may be treated at the very beginning by applying wet compresses, or by holding the joint in a stream of cold water, which materially checks the effusion. After some time has elapsed, this form of treatment is of little use, and compression by a moderately tight, or by an elastic, bandage over the injured joint, together with elevation of the limb, forms a better line of treatment. The immediate application of an ointment containing heparinoid may also be of value. Massage is of great assistance in cases of sprain to prevent stiffness of the affected joint and to aid repair of injured tissues. Strapping (qv) of the affected joint is of use in the later stages of treatment and, in the case of sportsmen, may be retained during training, but should never be used, it has been said, 'as an excuse to allow an unfit joint back to competitive activity. Joints which are not strong enough to stand competition without strapping are not strong enough to stand competition at all'.

DISLOCATION (see DISLOCATIONS).

BURSITIS often occurs over the region of a joint. The prominences of several joints are protected by large bursae, and inflammation of these structures is sometimes mistaken for inflammation of the joint. (See BURSITIS.)

JOULE is the unit of energy in the International System of Units. The official abbreviation is J. 4186·8 J = 1 Calorie (or kilocalorie). (See also CALORIE; WEIGHTS AND MEASURES.)

JUGULAR is a general name for any structure in the neck, but is especially applied to three large veins, the anterior, external and internal jugular veins, which convey blood from the head and neck regions to the interior of the chest.

JUNKET is the name of a food consisting of milk which has been acted upon by rennet. This forms a soft curd of the casein which is more easily digested than the curd which would naturally form in the stomach. Junket therefore forms a more easily digestible food than natural milk. If the curd is strained through muslin, whey is obtained which contains simply the water, sugar and albuminous materials of the milk and is very easily digestible. It is therefore used in the treatment of gastric ulcer and similar conditions. 300 ml of whey has an energy value of about 65 Calories.

K

KAHN REACTION is a substitute for the *Wassermann reaction* in the diagnosis of syphilis.

KALA-AZAR is another name for visceral leishmaniasis. (See LEISHMANIASIS.)

KANAMYCIN is an antibiotic derived from *Streptomyceskanamyceticus*. It is active against a wide range of organisms, including *Staphylococcus aureus* and *Mycobacterium tuberculosis*.

KAOLIN or CHINA CLAY, is a smooth white powder consisting of natural white aluminium silicate resulting from the decomposition of minerals containing felspar. It is used as a dusting powder for eczema and other forms of irritation in the skin. It is also used internally in cases of diarrhoea. The dose is 10 ml of Kaolin Mixture, BPC, best taken in water or milk before meals. Talc, French chalk and Fuller's earth are similar silicates.

Kaolin poultice contains kaolin, boric acid, glycerin and various aromatic substances.

KAOLINOSIS is a form of pneumoconiosis (qv) caused by the inhaling of clay dust.

KATA-THERMOMETER is a thermometer, invented by Sir Leonard Hill, which shows the rate of loss of heat, or cooling power, of the air. It is a spirit thermometer with a large bulb and marks on the stem at 95°F and 100°F. The thermometer, having been warmed up to above 100°F, is suspended in the air and the time taken in cooling from 100°F to 95°F is observed. Each instrument has marked on the stem a factor proportional to the total heat lost per square centimetre of the bulb in cooling from 100°F to 95°F. Dividing this factor by the number of seconds taken to cool gives a figure called the 'cooling power'.

KAWASAKI DISEASE is a disease of childhood of unknown origin, which was first described in Japan but has now spread to Europe. It most commonly occurs between the ages of 6 months and 2 years, and is characterized by high fever, conjunctivitis (qv), skin rashes, and swelling of the glands in the neck. In most cases there is complete and spontaneous recovery. Arteritis is however a common complication and results in the development of coronary artery aneurysms in 20 to 60 per cent of cases. These aneurysms and myocardial infarction are commonly detected after the second week of the illness.

KELOID is an overgrowth of fibrous tissue, usually on the site or scar of a previous injury. It gets its name from its claw-like off-shoots which pucker up the surrounding skin. It is sometimes painful, sometimes painless. It is much commoner in coloured than in white people. The most effective form of treatment is by injection of corticosteroids (qv) directly into the abnormal tissue. If this fails, surgical excision is performed.

KERATIN is the substance of which horn and the surface layer of the skin are composed.

KERATITIS (see EYE, DISEASE AND INJURIES OF).

KERATOMALACIA: Softening of the cornea due to a severe vitamin A deficiency (see EYE, DISEASE AND INJURIES OF).

KERATOPLASTY: Technical term for corneal graft.

KERATOSIS is a disease of the skin characterized by overgrowth of the horny layer of the skin (qv). It is induced by exposure to sunshine and in temperate climates usually develops in older people. In sunnier areas it may develop much earlier particularly in sun-bathing enthusiasts who repeatedly over-expose their skin to the sun. It takes the form of firm, dry adherent scales with redness of the surrounding skin and patchy pigmentation of the skin exposed to sunlight. Treatment, and prevention, consist of avoiding over-exposure to the sun.

KERION is a suppurating form of ringworm (qv).

KERNICTERUS is the staining with bile of the basal nuclei of the brain, with toxic degeneration of the nerve cells, which sometimes occurs in HAEMOLYTIC DISEASE OF THE NEWBORN (qv).

KERNIG'S SIGN is a sign found in cases of meningitis, consisting in the fact that, whereas a healthy person's thigh can be bent to a right angle with the body when the knee is straight, in cases of meningitis the knee cannot be straightened when the thigh is thus bent, or intense pain is caused to the patient by doing so.

KETAZOLAM (ANXON) (see BENZODIAZEPINES).

KETOCONAZOLE is an imidazole antifungal drug available for both oral and topical use. It also has an anti-androgen effect which may give rise to gynaecomastia and impotence in men. In view of its potential hepatotoxicity it should not be given orally for trivial infections but reserved for systemic fungal infections.

KETOGENIC DIET is one containing such an excess of fats that acetone and other *ketone bodies* appear in the urine. It is sometimes used in the treatment of epilepsy and chronic infections of the urinary tract by *Escherichia coli*. In this diet, butter, cream, eggs and fat meat are allowed, whilst sugar, bread and other carbohydrates are cut out as far as possible.

KETONE is another name for acetone or dimethyl ketone. The term, ketone bodies, is applied to a group of substances closely allied to acetone, especially beta-hydroxybutyric acid and acetoacetic acid. These are produced in the body from imperfect oxidation of fats and protein foods, and are found in specially large amount in severe cases of diabetes mellitus. KETONURIA is the term applied to the presence of these bodies in the urine.

KETOPROFEN (ORUDIS) (see NON-STEROIDAL ANTI-INFLAMMATORY DRUGS).

KHELLIN is a crystalline principle which has been isolated from the fruit of *Ammi visnaga*, an umbelliferous plant indigenous to the Mediterranean area, which has for long had a local reputation for the relief of renal colic. Khellin has been introduced to western medicine for the treatment of angina pectoris.

KIDNEY, ARTIFICIAL, is the term applied to an instrument which has been introduced to take over the function of the kidneys in cases of renal (kidney) failure. Such failure of the kidneys may be acute or chronic. In the acute form it may occur in a number of circumstances, including severe accidents such as the crush syndrome (qv), incompatible blood transfusions, mercury poisoning and severe haemorrhage in the later stages of pregnancy. It is also used in the treatment of chronic renal failure, and with increasingly satisfactory results. As recently as twenty years ago, patients with chronic renal failure were not expected to survive. Today, as a result of progress in dialysis and kidney transplantation, a young patient with chronic renal failure and no complicating features has a better that 90 per cent chance of living ten years and more. In most patients accepted for such treatment, the survival rate over five years exceeds 50 per cent.

The principle of the artificial kidney is that the patient's blood circulates through it and there comes in contact with a dialysing membrane, on the other side of which is a specially prepared dialysing fluid. In this way the biochemical balance of the blood is restored to normal, just as it would have been had the kidneys been functioning normally. (See DIALYSIS; HAEMODIALYSIS; TRANSPLANTATION.)

KIDNEYS are a pair of glands situated close to the spine in the upper part of the abdomen. They are on a level with the last dorsal and upper two lumbar vertebrae, and each is, to a great extent, covered behind by the twelfth rib of its own side. They are kept in this position by a quantity of fat and loose connective tissue, in which they are embedded, by the large vessels which supply them with blood, and by the peritoneal membrane stretched over their front surface.

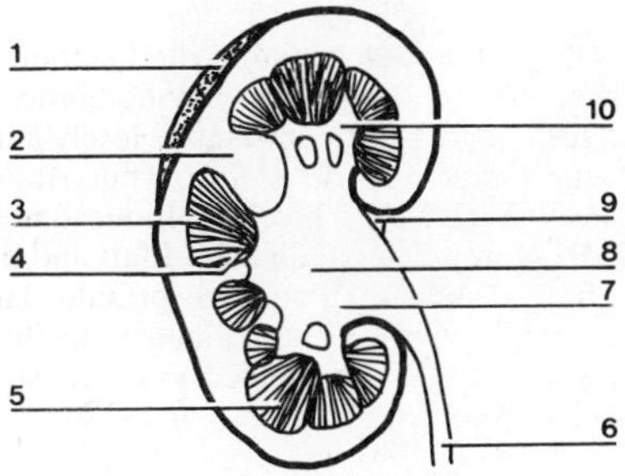

1 fibrous capsule
2 cortex
3 pyramid
4 papilla
5 medulla
6 ureter
7 calyx major
8 pelvis
9 hilum
10 calyx minor

Vertical section through the kidney.

Structure: In size each is about 10 cm (4 inches) long, 6·5 cm (2½ inches) wide, 5 cm (1½ inches) thick and weighs around 140 grams (5 ounces). The size, however, varies a good deal with the development, and probably with the habits of the individual. Kidney mass maintains a remarkably constant ratio to body weight. The left kidney is slightly longer and narrower, and lies a trifle higher in the abdomen than the right.

The kidney in adults presents a smooth exterior, although in early life (as in many animals) it is divided up into distinct lobes, corresponding to the pyramids found in the interior. Enveloping it is a tough fibrous coat, which, in the healthy state, is bound to the kidney only by loose fibrous tissue and by a few blood-vessels that pass between it and the kidney. The outer margin of the kidney is convex, the inner is concave, presenting a deep depression, known as the hilum, where the vessels enter its substance. At the hilum the renal vein lies in front of the renal artery, the former joining the inferior vena cava, and the latter springing from the aorta almost at a right angle. Here, too, is attached the ureter, which conveys urine down to the bladder. The ureter is spread out into an expanded, funnel-like end, known as the pelvis, to which the capsule of the kidney is firmly attached, and which further divides into little funnels known as the calyces. On splitting open a kidney, one finds it to consist of two distinct parts: a layer on the surface, about 4 mm thick, known as the cortex, and a part towards the hilum known as the medulla. The latter consists of pyramids, arranged side by side, with their base on the cortex and their apex projecting into the calyces of the ureter. The apex of each pyramid, of which there are about twelve, is studded with minute holes, which are the openings of the microscopic uriniferous tubes.

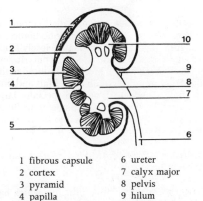

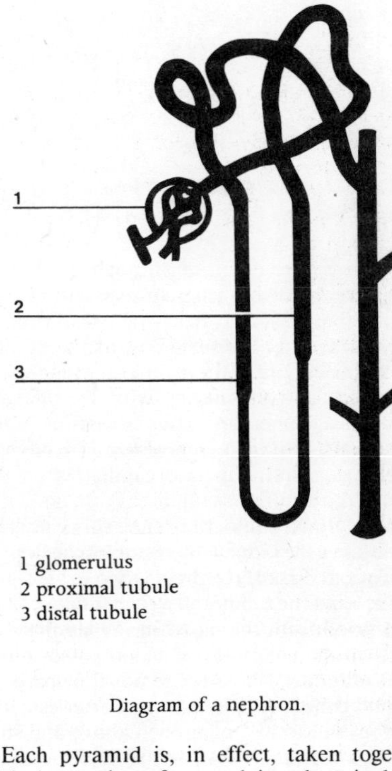

1 glomerulus
2 proximal tubule
3 distal tubule

Diagram of a nephron.

Each pyramid is, in effect, taken together with the portion of cortex lying along its base, an independent little kidney. About a score of small tubes open on the surface of each pyramid, and these, if traced up into its substance, divide again and again so as to form bundles of convoluted tubules, known as medullary rays, passing up towards the cortex. If one of these is traced still farther back, it is found, after a very tortuous course, to end in a small rounded body: the Malpighian corpuscle or glomerulus. Each glomerulus and its convoluted tubule is known as a nephron, which constitutes the functional unit of the kidney. Each kidney contains around one million nephrons.

If the blood-vessels are now traced through the kidney their course is found to be as follows. The renal artery splits up into branches, which form arches at the line of junction of cortex and medulla, and from these again

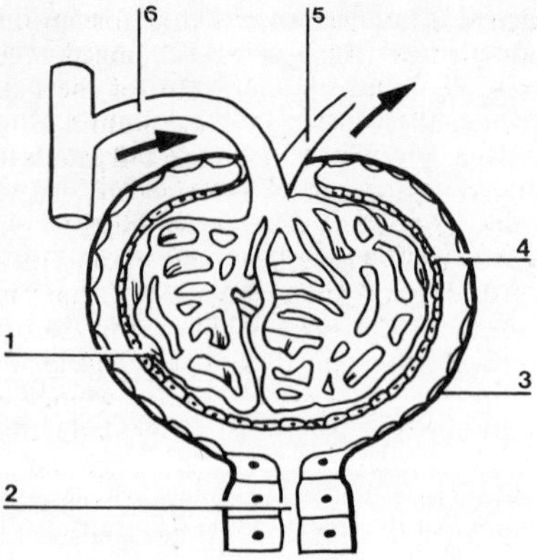

1 capillary tuft
2 tubule
3 capsule
4 glomerular capsule
5 efferent vessel
6 afferent vessel

Diagram of glomerulus.

spring vessels that run up through the cortex, giving off small branches in every direction. Each of these last ends in a little tuft of capillaries enclosed in a capsule (Bowman's capsule) that forms the end of the uriniferous tubule just described, and capillaries with capsule are known as a glomerulus. After circulating in the glomerulus, the blood emerges by a small vein, which again splits up into capillaries on the walls of the uriniferous tubules. From these it is collected finally into the renal veins and by them leaves the kidney. By means of the double circulation, first through the glomerulus and then around the tubule, a large amount of fluid is removed from the blood in the glomerulus, and then the concentrated blood passes on to the uriniferous tubule for removal of parts of its solid contents. Other straight arteries come off from the arches mentioned above and supply the medulla direct, the blood from these passing through another set of capillaries and also finally into the renal veins. Although the circulation just described is confined entirely to the kidney, it has certain small connections both by arteries and veins which pass through the capsule and, joining the lumbar vessels, communicate direct with the aorta.

Function: The chief function of the kidneys is to separate fluid and certain solids from the blood. Briefly, the glomeruli filter from the blood the non-protein portion of the plasma. As this filtrate passes through the convoluted tubules, varying parts of it are reabsorbed. It is estimated that in 24 hours the total human glomeruli will filter between 150 and 200 litres, 99 per cent of which is reabsorbed by the tubules. The constituents of the filtrate may be grouped according to the extent to which they are reabsorbed by the tubules: (1) substances actively reabsorbed, such as amino-acids, glucose, sodium, potassium, calcium, magnesium and chlorine; (2) substances passing through the tubular epithelium by a simple process of diffusion when their concentration in the filtrate exceeds that in the plasma, such as urea, uric acid, phosphates; (3) substances not returned to the blood from the tubular fluid: eg. creatine.

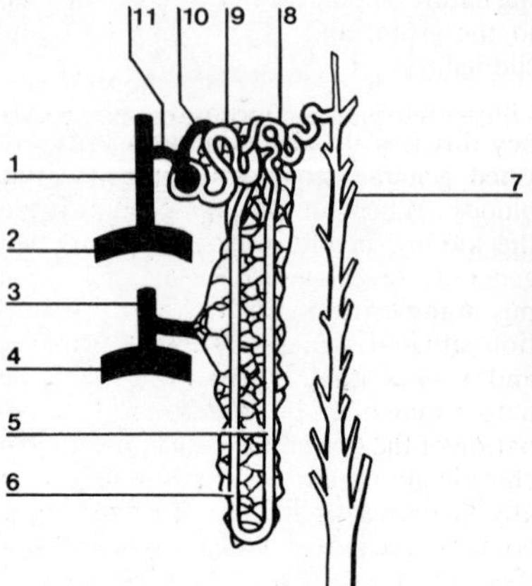

1 interlobular artery
2 arcuate artery
3 interlobular vein
4 arcuate vein
5 ascending limb of Henle's loop
6 descending limb of Henle's loop
7 collecting tubule
8 distal convoluted tubule
9 proximal convoluted tubule
10 efferent arteriole
11 afferent arteriole

Diagram of renal tubules and blood supply of the kidney.

When the kidneys are diseased and the number of glomeruli and tubules decreased in consequence, this alternating action is not so readily carried out, and therefore the work of the diseased kidney becomes increasingly embarrassed. When the blood-vessels of the kidney are partially closed by disease (arteriosclerosis), the general blood-pressure rises with the object of forcing more blood through the kidneys; in consequence, marked changes are produced upon the heart in this type of renal disease.

When the kidneys fail to act, these solid waste substances accumulate in the blood. The general 'poisoning' resulting from failure of renal functions produces the clinical condition known as uraemia (qv).

KIDNEYS, DISEASES OF: The kidneys, being deeply buried in the abdomen, give little direct sign even when seriously diseased, although many of the effects upon the general constitution are sufficiently marked and serious.

General symptoms: The following are some of the general symptoms common to various types of kidney disease.

PAIN, of an aching nature, situated high up in the loins, is occasionally a symptom of inflammation of the kidneys, but pain in the lower part of the back is found in so many other diseases, and is so generally absent in serious kidney affections, that it is of little importance as a symptom. When a stone lodges in the ureter, however, there is a very definite type of pain known as renal colic. This pain is of an agonizing nature, shoots down from the kidney region to the groin, and usually appears with great suddenness.

URINE almost invariably shows changes in kidney diseases. In acute conditions it is diminished, generally contains albumin, and may be bloody. When unusual material is present in the kidney, careful examination of the urine generally reveals evidence of it: for example, pus in the urine points to a suppurative condition situated somewhere in the urinary tract; and when a stone is present in the kidney, its nature may often be conjectured by an examination of the crystalline deposit in the urine. In chronic glomerulonephritis the urine is generally increased in amount, pale and, as a rule, contains greater or less amounts of albumin. (See ALBUMINURIA.)

OEDEMA, though due to many other conditions than glomerulonephritis, is a most important symptom of this and other kidney troubles. When dependent upon some defect in the kidneys, it appears generally in the morning after sleep, and affects the loose tissues of the body, such as the skin beneath the eyes and that on the back of the hands, which become swollen and puffy.

URAEMIA is a condition which is present in all cases in which the function of the kidneys is seriously impaired. It is a general poisoning of the system by waste products which the kidneys have failed to excrete, and may be acute or chronic in type. (See URAEMIA.)

The most important class of diseases affecting the kidneys is that comprising the changes grouped together as glomerulonephritis, in which albumin is excreted in the urine and oedema is often present. (See GLOMERULONEPHRITIS.) The following are some of the other important affections of the kidney. (See also PYELITIS.)

GRAVEL and STONE are produced by the deposit in the urinary passages of solid substances which are naturally present in the urine, and whose deposition depends upon their presence in excessive amount, or upon the failure of some condition which in general keeps them in solution. The most common constituents of such stones are ammonium phosphate, calcium phosphate and calcium carbonate, calcium oxalate, and uric-acid and urates.

Among many factors responsible for the formation of stones in the kidneys is alteration in the reaction of the urine. Thus an excessive acid reaction may be accompanied by the formation of uric-acid stones, whilst phosphate stones form in alkaline urine. Other factors which are associated with the formation of stones in the kidneys are prolonged recumbency, eg. following a fracture of the femur; infection of the kidney; lack of vitamin A in the diet; over-action of the parathyroid glands (qv); a high level of calcium in the urine; excessive sweating, as in hot climates, leading to a persistently concentrated urine; gout; and leukaemia. The most common cause in Britain is an abnormally high level of calcium in the urine: the condition known as hypercalciuria. They are more common in men than in women, and may occur at any age and particularly among sedentary workers. In cases in which the presence of a stone is suspected, X-ray examination is an important procedure in diagnosis.

Treatment: This depends upon the size of the stone. If it is large, it has usually to be removed by operation. If it is small, it may be passed out in the urine following medical treatment. This consists of ensuring a large volume of urine by drinking large amounts of bland fluids. It is also helpful to alter the reaction of the urine. Thus, in the case of a uric-acid stone, the excessively acid urine is made alkaline by giving large doses of alkali: eg. 2 grams of sodium bicarbonate four times daily. In the case of stones associated with a high level of calcium in the urine, promising results are being obtained from the administration of: bendrofluazide, one of the benzothiazines (qv); cellulose phosphate (qv); a combination of the two; unprocessed bran. In the case of phosphate stones the excessively alkaline urine is made acid by the taking of 1 gram of ammonium chloride four times daily. If there is any infection of the kidney, this must be fully treated. The latest development is the use of ultrasonics to smash the stone into minute pieces which can then be passed in the urine. The efficacy and safety of this technique are under investigation. (See LITHOTRIPSY.)

RENAL CARBUNCLE is an abscess within the kidney. At one time the commonest cause was *Staphylococcus aureus* which reached the kidney via the blood-stream from staphylococcal infection elsewhere in the body. It is now more commonly due to infection spreading from the ureter or bladder. Patients debilitated by drug addiction and diabetes mellitus are especially at risk. The condition is characterized by pain in the loin and fever. The onset may be sudden with all the manifestations of septicaemia, or more gradual. Treatment consists of withdrawal of the pus and injection of the appropriate antibiotic into the abscess cavity.

TUBERCULOSIS of the kidneys is more common in adults than in children, and more common in men than in women. For a long time it may give rise to no symptoms or signs. It must therefore always be considered a possible diagnosis in cases in which urinary symptoms arise for which no cause can be found. Diagnosis partly depends upon the finding of *Mycobacterium tuberculosis* in the urine. As in other forms of tuberculosis, treatment has been revolutionized by the introduction of the anti-tuberculosis drugs: eg. rifampicin, ethambutol and isoniazid. It is only in a minority of cases that surgical removal of the kidney is required.

MOVABLE KIDNEY is commoner in women than in men. The undue mobility of the kidney is part of a general visceroptosis (qv), and treatment should be directed to this. One risk of an abnormally mobile kidney is hydronephrosis (qv) from kinking of the ureter. Occasional kinking of the ureter may cause what are known as Dietl's crises: sudden attacks of intense abdominal pain radiating down the ureter, shivering, nausea, vomiting, fever, collapse. They are not common. If hydronephrosis develops, operation may be necessary.

INJURIES OF THE KIDNEY are very serious, although one of these organs may be completely shattered without a necessarily fatal result if the other kidney is healthy and uninjured. The kidney may be ruptured by a blow in the small of the back or when a person is run over, and death may result from the consequent loss of blood, which may appear in the urine.

TUMOURS of the kidney are not common. In 1980 they were responsible for 1606 deaths in England. As a rule, they give little or no trouble till they have reached a large size. If growing in the pelvis of the kidney, large quantities of blood may be passed now and then in the urine with, however, no pain or other symptom referable to the kidney. *Congenital cystic kidney* is a form of tumour in the kidney which may last for many years with little trouble to the person in whom it occurs. *Hypernephroma* is a tumour that occasionally develops in the kidney, being composed of cells resembling the suprarenal gland in appearance. *Nephroblastoma* (or *Wilms' tumour*) is the commonest kidney tumour in infancy. It is a malignant tumour, which occurs in around 1 per 10,000 live births. The survival rate with modern treatment (removal of the kidney followed by radiotherapy and chemotherapy) is now around 80 per cent.

HORSESHOE KIDNEY: Around 10 per cent of all live-born infants are born with malformations of the kidneys. Horseshoe kidney, so called because of its shape, is among the commonest of these. It results from a partial fusion of the two kidneys, and is more common in males than females. In quite a number of cases, ranging from one-quarter to one-half according to different reports, the kidneys function normally. In the others the complications that are liable to occur are hydronephrosis (qv), pyelonephritis (see PYELITIS) and stones. Such kidneys are also more liable to develop cancer than normal kidneys. (See also TRANSPLANTATION.)

KINAESTHETIC SENSATIONS is a term used to describe those sensations which underlie muscle tension and position of joint and muscle. These sensations send impulses along nerves to the brain, and thus inform it of the position of the limb in space and of the relative position to each other of individual muscles and muscle-groups and of joints.

KING'S EVIL is an old name for scrofula, which was supposed to be curable by the touch of the royal hand. (See TUBERCULOSIS; SCROFULA.)

KININS are substances present in the body which are powerful vasodilators (qv). They also induce pain and are probably involved in the production of the headache of migraine. In addition, they play a part in the production of allergy (qv) and anaphylaxis (qv).

KINO is the dried juice of *Pterocarpus marsupium*, an Indian tree. It contains an astringent principle, and its powder is useful in the treatment of diarrhoea, the tincture being also used as a gargle for relaxed throat.

KISS OF LIFE (see RESUSCITATION).

KLEPTOMANIA is a psychological disorder in which the person afflicted has an irresistible compulsion to steal things, without necessarily having any need for the object stolen.

KLINEFELTER'S SYNDROME: The original syndrome described by Klinefelter consisted of gynaecomastia, testicular atrophy and infertility. Intelligence was unimpaired. Cases have been described with associated mental defects and striking tallness of stature but the only constant feature of the syndrome is testicular atrophy with resulting azoospermia and infertility. The atrophy of the testis is the result of a peritubular fibrosis which begins to appear in childhood and progresses until all the seminiferous tubules are replaced by fibrous tissue. Gynaecomastia, mental retardation and eunuchoidism may be associated but the first is inconstant and the two last are infrequent. Most patients with Klinefelter's syndrome have 47 chromosomes instead of the normal 46. The extra chromosome is an X chromosome so that the sex chromosome constitution is XXY instead of XY. Klinefelter's syndrome is one of the most common chromosome abnormalities and occurs in 1 in 300 of the male population. Patients with this syndrome show that the Y chromosome is strongly sex determining. Thus a patient who has an XXY chromosome constitution may have the appearance of a normal male and the only incapacity is infertility. However the loss of a Y chromosome leads to the development of a bodily form which is essentially feminine, (XO, Turner's syndrome).

KNEE is the joint formed by the femur, tibia and patella (knee-cap). It belongs to the class of hinge-joints, although movements are much more complex than the simple motion of a hinge, the condyles of the femur partly rolling, partly sliding over the flat surfaces on the upper end of the tibia, and the acts of straightening and of bending the limb being finished and begun, respectively, by a certain amount of rotation. The cavity of the joint is very intricate: it consists really of three joints fused into one, but separated in part by ligaments and folds of the synovial membrane. The ligaments which bind the bones together are extremely strong, and include the popliteal and the collateral ligaments, a very strong patellar ligament uniting the patella to the front of the tibia, two cruciate ligaments in the interior of the joint, and two fibro-cartilages which are interposed between the surfaces of tibia and femur at their edge.

All these structures give to the knee-joint great strength, so that it is seldom dislocated. Its exposed position and the intricacy and consequent difficulty in cleansing its cavity, render this joint liable to be wounded, and make wounds of it very serious. The knee may also be affected by tuberculous disease.

A troublesome condition often found in the knee consists of the loosening of one of the fibro-cartilages lying at the head of the tibia, especially of that on the inner side of the joint. The cartilage may either be loosened from its attachment and tend to slip beyond the edges of the bones, or it may become folded on itself. In either case, it tends to cause locking of the joint when sudden movements are made. This causes temporary inability to use the joint until the cartilage is replaced by forcible straightening, and the accident is apt to be followed by an attack of synovitis, which may last some weeks, causing a certain amount of lameness with pain and tenderness especially felt at a point on the inner side of the knee. This condition can be relieved by wearing for a prolonged period of some months a bandage with pad or knee-truss which presses upon the inner side of the joint, or it may be more quickly remedied by an operation to remove the loose portion of the cartilage. (See also JOINTS, DISEASES OF.)

KNEE JERK (See REFLEX ACTION).

KNOCK-KNEE, or GENU VALGUM, is a deformity of the lower limbs in such a direction that when the limbs are straightened the legs diverge from one another. As a result, in walking the knees knock against each other. The amount of knock-knee is measured by the distance between the medial malleoli of the ankles, with the inner surfaces of the knee touching and the knee-caps facing forwards.

Causes: The condition is so common in children between the ages of 2 to 6 years that it may almost be regarded as a normal phase in childhood. When marked, or persisting into later childhood, it is usually due to faulty muscular tone. The condition is aggravated in children who are overweight or debilitated. At one time rickets was a common cause, but this is seldom the cause today in Great Britain.

Treatment: If rickets is the cause this must be treated. If, as is usually the case, there is no obvious cause, no treatment is required for knock-knee up to 75 mm (3 inches) in a child under 7 years of age. In the vast majority of cases it will have righted itself by this age. If the degree of knock-knee is more severe than this splints may be necessary, or even operation. When there is established bony deformity with over 100 mm (4 inches) of separation at the age of 4 years, or when there is still a considerable degree of knock-knee at the age of 9 years, operation should be performed. This may consist of cutting away the prominent part of the inner side of the lower end of the femora.

KOHLER'S DISEASE is a not uncommon condition of the foot in younger schoolchildren, characterized by osteochondritis (qv) of the navicular bone. Treatment consists of immobilization of the foot in plaster of Paris for six to eight weeks. Healing takes place spontaneously, but return to the playing of games must be gradual over a period of many months. (See FOOT.)

KOILONYCHIA is the term applied to nails that are hollow and depressed like a spoon, a condition sometimes associated with chronic iron deficiency.

KOLA is the nut of *Kola acuminata*, a tree growing in various parts of Africa. It contains caffeine, upon which its action mainly depends, and also an astringent principle. Its action is a stimulating one, almost identical with that of tea or coffee. (See COFFEE.)

KOPLIK SPOTS are bluish-white spots appearing on the mucous membrane of the mouth in cases of measles about the third day, and forming the first part of the rash in this disease.

KORSAKOW'S SYNDROME is a form of mental disturbance occurring in chronic alcoholism and other toxic states, such as uraemia, lead poisoning and cerebral syphilis. Its special features are talkativeness with delusions in regard to time and place, the patient, although clear in other matters, imagining that he has recently made journeys or been in distant places.

KUMMELL'S DISEASE is a condition resulting from undiagnosed crush fracture of a vertebra, due to injury. The patient complains of backache, persistent rigidity of the spine and deformity.

KUPFFER CELLS are the star-shaped cells present in the blood-sinuses of the liver (qv). They form part of the reticulo-endothelial system (qv) and are to a large extent responsible for the breakdown of haemoglobin into the bile pigments.

KURU is a slowly progressive fatal disease due to degeneration in the central nervous system, particularly the cerebellum (qv). It is confined to the Fore people in the Eastern Highlands of New Guinea. It is believed to be due to a slow virus infection acquired from the cannibalistic rite of eating the organs, particularly the brains, of deceased relatives (out of respect). This origin of the disease was suggested by the fact that originally it was a disease of women and children, and it was they who practised this rite. Since the rite was given up, the disease has largely disappeared in children, but still occurs in women as it has an incubation period of up to 20 years.

KWASHIORKOR is one of the most important causes of ill health and death among children in the tropics. It is predominantly a deficiency disease due to a diet deficient in protein. There is also some evidence that there may also be a lack of the so-called essential fatty acids. It affects typically the small child weaned from the breast and not yet able to cope with an adult diet, or for whom an adequate amount of first-class protein is not available, and it is mainly found in the less well-developed countries.

The onset of the disease is characterized by loss of appetite, often with diarrhoea and loss of weight. The child is flabby, the skin is dry, and the hair is depigmented, dry, sparse and brittle. At a later stage oedema develops and the liver is often enlarged. In the early stages the condition responds rapidly to a diet containing adequate first-class protein, but in the later stages this must be supplemented by careful nursing, especially as the child is very liable to infections.

KYPHOSIS is the term applied to curvature of the spine in which the concavity of the curve is directed forwards. (See SPINE, DISEASES OF.)

L

LABETALOL is an alpha- and beta-adrenoceptor blocker (see ADRENOCEPTOR BLOCK) which is proving of value in the treatment of high blood-pressure.

LABIUM is the Latin word for a lip or lip-shaped organ.

LABORATORY ANIMAL ALLERGY (see ALLERGY).

LABOUR, or PARTURITION, often popularly spoken of as the confinement, is the act of bringing forth young, and forms the end of the period of gestation or pregnancy during which the new individual is nourished from the maternal body.

It is difficult to define an absolutely *normal labour* because individual labours differ so much in small details. Generally speaking, however, a normal labour is one in which the vertex of the child's head is born first, and the whole process ends favourably to mother and child within twenty-four hours, and without any operative interference. In the case of a first baby the confinement usually lasts from eight to sixteen hours, whilst the births of second and subsequent children tend to become progressively shorter processes. There are, of course, considerable variations in individual cases from these general statements. The majority of confinements end between midnight and 6 am. In 96 per cent of all cases the vertex of the child's head presents (that is, leaves the womb and descends through the vagina to the exterior first). In some cases, owing to a faulty position of the head or to the presentation of the child's face, the labour is considerably delayed, while for various reasons operative assistance may be necessary, in which case the labour is known as an instrumental one. The child may present quite another part than the head, the second most common presentation being the breech or buttocks. A rarer and more serious presentation is a transverse presentation or cross-birth, where the child lies obliquely across the womb. In these abnormal presentations skilled assistance is specially necessary for the sake of both mother and child, and in the case of a cross-birth, assistance is imperative if the mother's life is to be saved. Finally, various complications, such as deformities of the mother and child, an excessive amount of bleeding, the birth of twins, and various general conditions of the mother, such as heart or kidney disease or convulsions, may influence the progress of the labour to an extreme degree.

Stages of labour: The process of labour is naturally divided into three stages. The *first stage* is that of dilatation of the neck of the womb to permit the subsequent descent of the child. This is ushered in by the onset of the pains caused by the powerful intermittent contractions of the muscular wall of the womb. At first the pains come at considerable intervals – ten to twenty minutes – but as time passes the intervals become shorter and the pains become stronger. This stage is much the longest, particularly in the case of a first baby, when it may last for seven to fourteen hours. It is sometimes accompanied by sickness and vomiting. The full dilatation of the mouth of the womb is usually accompanied by the rupture of the amnion, the membrane containing the fluid in which the foetus moves, and the sudden escape of the amniotic fluid or 'waters'. The two events, however, do not necessarily take place at the same time, and sometimes the amnion ruptures at a much earlier, and sometimes at a later, period.

The *second stage* is the stage of expulsion of the child, during which the child's head, followed by the body and limbs, descends through the bony girdle of the pelvis and passes down through the vagina to the exterior. This process usually occupies two hours in a first labour, but, in the case of a woman who has had several children before, it may occupy a much shorter time. During this passage through the pelvis, the child's head goes through certain movements by which it adapts itself to the alterations in the shape of the pelvic canal as it passes down. The size of the head of an average child is such that there is just room for it to pass through the pelvis and no more. Accordingly the head is liable to be considerably pressed upon during this stage of labour, and this pressure manifests itself in the moulding of the child's skull. This moulding, which is rendered possible by the softness of the bones and by the presence of spaces between the bones enables the head to pass down with the minimum of damage to the child and to the mother. In most cases the moulding disappears in the first day or two after birth. The second stage is one of strenuous muscular exertion, as not only the muscular wall of the womb, but the abdominal muscles and the diaphragm are all involuntarily called into play to aid the expulsion of the child. Pains are more severe, but at the same time the patient has a consciousness that she is making progress and this sometimes makes them more easily tolerated than the pains of the first stage. It is towards the end of the second stage that an anaesthetic is often administered, the actual birth of the head being the time of greatest pain. Immediately thereafter there is a pause for a moment or two, and then the child's body is born, thus completing the second stage of labour. As soon as he is born the child usually cries loudly and in doing so establishes the function of respiration. The tying and cutting of the umbilical cord (see AFTERBIRTH) finally sever the child's vital connection with the mother.

The *third stage* is the stage of delivery of the afterbirth. It begins immediately the child is born and rarely lasts more than half an hour. It is associated with the loss of a certain amount of blood: on average about 280 ml (10 fluid ounces). The great danger is from excessive haemorrhage associated with the separation of the afterbirth from the wall of the womb, and although the stage is much the shortest, yet this danger makes it imperative that it should be conducted with the greatest care.

Management of labour: In the absence of skilled assistance a normal labour will in all probability conduct itself to a successful issue, but it is always desirable that trained assistance should be obtained, both for the comfort as well as for the safety of the mother and the child. Obstetrical complications have a habit of arising suddenly and sometimes unexpectedly.

Where trained assistance is not at once available, the untrained person can still do much to help the prospective mother. As soon as the labour begins the mother should, if possible, have the lower bowel washed out with a soap-and-water enema, and if there is time it is advisable for the mother to have a warm bath, or at least to have the genital regions thoroughly washed with soap and water. The bed upon which she is to be delivered should be prepared with a mackintosh sheet if possible, or failing that, one or two sheets of glazed brown paper, placed across the middle of the bed and drawn well over the right-hand edge of it. A draw-sheet should be placed over this which can be changed afterwards. The clothing for the infant should be hung before the fire to be aired and warmed, and provision should be made for an ample supply of hot water and clean basins for the doctor or nurse, who should have been sent for. Ligatures should be prepared for tying the umbilical cord and these are best made of 3-ply linen thread twisted together and knotted at the ends so as to form a ligature of about 25 cm (10 inches) in length. Two of these are required, and should be sterilized by being boiled. The mother may, with advantage, remain up, either sitting or moving about her room as may be most comfortable for her, during the first stage; but when she feels fatigued and desires to lie down, and in any case when the membranes rupture and the 'waters' escape, she should lie down on the bed on her back.

During the second stage the mother will tend involuntarily to hold her breath and press down during the pains, and this down-bearing, as it is called, is helpful and should be encouraged, as it will expedite delivery. It is a mistake to urge a woman to bear down during the first stage, as it does no good and merely exhausts her strength. It helps the mother to be given something to hold on to during the down-bearing pains of the second stage, and it is a customary thing to tie a roller towel to the head of the bed and give her that to pull upon. This enables her to fix her abdominal muscles and to use her strength to the greatest advantage.

As soon as the child's head is born the eyes should be gently wiped clean with a pledget of cotton-wool or a clean soft linen handkerchief moistened in clean boiled water. After the child is born the cord should not be ligatured for two or three minutes until the pulsation in it is beginning to cease. One of the linen ligatures should then be tied tightly round the umbilical cord at a distance of about 5 cm (2 inches) from the child's navel. The other should be applied a few inches nearer the mother. With a clean pair of scissors which has been boiled, the cord should then be divided between the two ligatures. It is essential to make sure that there is no bleeding from the child's end of the cut umbilical cord. The infant should then be wrapped in a soft flannel or shawl and laid aside in some warm place until arrangements can be made for bathing. After the delivery of the child there will be an interval of some minutes before the uterine contractions start once more, and as a rule only a few contractions are needed to bring about the expulsion of the after-birth or placenta. This should be placed in a basin with some clean water and kept for inspection by the doctor or nurse.

All that now remains to be done is to clean the mother by gently swabbing her with pledgets of cotton-wool wrung out of clean boiled water, the hands of anybody who comes in contact with the patient having been previously most carefully and scrupulously scrubbed. The swabbing must be done from above downwards. A clean pad of cotton-wool, preferably scorched in front of a hot fire to sterilize it, should then be placed over the genitals and a firm binder drawn round the hips and over the lower part of the abdomen. After the confinement is over, the mother should be encouraged to sleep, or at least to rest quietly, and anything in the nature of excitement is to be avoided. For this reason friends and neighbours should as far as possible be excluded until the patient has had a good sleep.

Abnormalities and dangers of labour: These may arise in connection with the presentation or position of the child, with the uterus or maternal pelvis, or from the mother's health.

ABNORMAL PRESENTATIONS are relatively uncommon. The most frequent is a *breech presentation* (3 per cent of all labours). Here the labour is apt to be slow, but while there should be no increased risk to the mother (unless the labour happens to be a first labour), there is considerably greater danger to the child. Skilled assistance should always be obtained, but in its absence the labour should be allowed to conduct itself without interference, until the lower limbs are born. These should then be wrapped in a warm flannel and gently supported, while steady pressure is applied to the top of the womb through the mother's abdominal wall. The after-coming head is thus gently pressed down into and through the pelvis. The main risk to the child is pressure on the umbilical cord during this stage, as it lies between the head of the child and the hard, bony pelvis. If this pressure is sufficient to impede the child's circulation for more than 8 or 10 minutes, the probability is that the child will be suffocated before he is born. (Until the head is born, the child obtains the necessary oxygen by interchanges taking place between his blood and the blood of the mother in the placenta or after-birth, and that pressure on the cord prevents the passage of the foetal blood between the body of the foetus and the placenta.)

Face presentations are rare (0·4 per cent of all labours). Usually the mother is able to deliver herself after a prolonged and tedious labour. The outlook is tolerably good for the child and should be satisfactory for the mother. There are, however, possibilities of serious danger, and medical help should always be sought.

The most dangerous mal-presentation is a *cross-birth*, where the child lies across the womb and the pelvis. None but an extremely premature child can be born in this position. If the condition is not corrected, the womb goes on trying to expel the child until it either becomes utterly exhausted and ceases to contract, or else it ruptures. In the former event, sufficient time may be gained – before the womb starts to contract again – in which to obtain skilled assistance to change the position of the child. In this way the mother's life may be saved, although the child will almost certainly have succumbed. In the second event, the shock and internal bleeding from the ruptured womb involve very grave risk to the mother's life, and delivery is impossible except by skilled assistance.

DEFORMITIES AND CONTRACTIONS of the mother's pelvis create great difficulty and may make natural labour impossible. The pelvis of every woman pregnant for the first time should be measured by a medical practitioner prior to labour with a view to the exclusion of any such possibility. Sometimes labour has to be induced early in these cases; in others, operative delivery at full time has to be arranged. (See CAESAREAN SECTION.)

HAEMORRHAGE during the last three months of pregnancy, or during labour, is always fraught with serious possibilities. It is due to the premature detachment of some portion of the placenta, which in many cases is situated too low down in the womb (*placenta praevia*). In the absence of skilled assistance, all that can be done is to keep the patient quite quiet in bed with the head low. No alcoholic stimulants should be given.

Bleeding during the third stage of labour or immediately after (*post-partum haemorrhage*) can be alarming and even fatal. In the absence of skilled assistance an attempt should be made to compress the womb forcibly by grasping it through the abdominal muscles. The foot of the bed may be raised and the patient provided with ample fresh air. No alcoholic stimulants should be given, as these only serve to increase the bleeding. Very hot applications to the vulva may help, and the doctor or nurse may administer a hot vaginal douche. (See DOUCHE.)

CONVULSIONS in association with pregnancy or labour, or occurring immediately after labour (*eclampsia*), constitute one of the most grave complications. Medical advice should be obtained without fail, and in the absence of such the patient should be kept absolutely quiet in a darkened room. No food, either solid or liquid, should be given. The actual convulsion should be treated on the ordinary lines, and if labour ensues, it also should be treated on the ordinary lines. (See ECLAMPSIA.)

PUERPERAL INFECTION is one of the most serious complications of labour. This is, in essence, the same as the infection of a wound, there being always a large, raw surface in the interior of the uterus (the placental site), and in most cases innumerable small lacerations of the birth canal. All or any of these may be invaded by bacteria which subsequently tend to invade the blood-stream of the mother and give rise to acute septicaemia. About half the puerperal infections are due to the haemolytic streptococcus and about half to other organisms. The haemolytic streptococcus reaches the genital tract from the doctor, nurse, or midwife, from one of the patient's own household, or from the patient's own nasopharynx. The swabbing of throats, the exclusion from the patient's presence of streptococcal carriers and of anyone with a cold or sore throat, and strict aseptic precautions during labour, will all help to diminish the incidence of haemolytic streptococcal puerperal infections. If infection occurs in spite of all precautions, then the sulphonamide drugs and penicillin are remedies. (See PUERPERAL FEVER.)

MATERNAL DEATHS: The number of mothers who die during pregnancy or childbirth, or the maternal mortality rate, is falling steadily in Britain. Thus, in the three-year period 1967–69, out of a total of 2,457,000 deliveries only 455 mothers died. This gives a rate of 18·5 deaths per 100,000 maternities, compared with a rate of 22·3 for the three years, 1964–66, and 53·3 for the three years, 1952–54. In England in 1980, the maternal mortality rate was 10 per 100,000 total births, there being 68 deaths, 3 due to abortion.

LACHESINE is a mydriatic: ie. it dilates the pupil of the eye. It is sometimes used for this purpose instead of atropine, as its action is of shorter duration.

LACRIMAL: Gland, duct, apparatus (see EYE, DISEASE AND INJURIES OF).

LACTATION is the period during which an infant is suckled on the mother's breast. (See BREASTS, DISEASES OF; INFANT FEEDING.)

LACTEAL is a lymphatic vessel that transmits chyle (qv) from the intestine. (See LYMPH.)

LACTIC ACID is a colourless, syrupy, sour liquid, which is produced by the action of a bacterium upon lactose. The growth of this organism and consequent formation of lactic acid causes the souring of milk, and the same change takes place to a limited extent when food is long retained in the stomach.

Lactic acid (CH_3.CHOH.COOH) is produced in the body during muscular activity, the lactic acid being derived from the breakdown of glycogen. Muscle fatigue is associated with an accumulation of lactic acid in the muscle. Recovery follows when enough oxygen gets to the muscle, part of the lactic acid being oxidized and most of it then being built up once more into glycogen.

LACTIC ACID BACILLI were introduced by Metchnikoff to prepare milk as a special article of diet. The bacilli, which are issued in various forms, are added to fresh milk, allowed to act on it in a warm place for several hours (according to the degree of sourness desired), and the milk is then consumed with the active bacilli. These, after a course of such treatment, come to replace the bacteria naturally found in the intestines, and are supposed to be less injurious to the system. The bacilli, which are harmless, have, in some cases of intestinal disease or of rheumatism, a beneficial action. Buttermilk has a similar effect. (See YOGHURT.)

LACTOSE is the official name for sugar of milk. (See SUGAR.)

LACTOSE INTOLERANCE is a form of indigestion which is much more common in certain coloured races than in white races. It is due to lack in the intestine of the enzyme (qv) known as lactase which is responsible for the digestion of lactose, the sugar in milk. In individuals the taking of milk is followed by nausea, a sensation of bloating, or distension, in the gut, abdominal pain and diarrhoea. Such disturbances after taking milk may also be due to the individual being allergic to milk. Treatment is by means of a low-lactose diet. Foodstuffs high in lactose, such as fresh or powdered milk, and milk puddings should be avoided. Most people subject to it can tolerate fermented milk products and the small amounts of milk used in baking and added to margarine and sausages. In Britain it is said to occur in up to 80 per cent of non-white adults but only 5 per cent of white adults.

LACUNA means a small pit or depression.

LAEVULOSE is a sugar which forms one of the constituents of invert sugar. (See SUGAR.)

LAGOPHTHALMOS is the condition in which the eye cannot be completely closed.

LAMBLIA (see GIARDIASIS).

LAMELLA is a small disc of glycerin jelly, 3 mm (⅛inch) in diameter, containing an active drug for application to the eye. It is applied by insertion behind the lower lid.

LAMENESS (see GAIT; JOINTS, DISEASES OF).

LAMINECTOMY is an operation in which the arches of one or more vertebrae are removed so as to expose a portion of the spinal cord for removal of a tumour, relief of pressure due to a fracture, or disc protrusion.

LANOLIN is a fat derived from the wool of the common sheep. It is much used for ointments because it does not become rancid, and because it is supposed to have a special power of penetrating the skin. It is very sticky, and for use is mixed generally with an equal quantity of petroleum jelly to make it softer. Lanolin also possesses the valuable property of being able to mix with and absorb water to a considerable extent.

LAPAROTOMY is a general term applied to any operation in which the abdominal cavity is opened.

LARYNGECTOMY is the operation for removal of the larynx.

LARYNGISMUS STRIDULUS: This condition is not universally recognized in all classifications but has the following characteristics: recurrent attacks, attacks commencing without prodromal features, often at night. The majority of cases do not require any form of airway intervention. Children suffering these bouts of spasmodic croup or so-called laryngismus stridulus usually grow out of the condition spontaneously and in most cases no further treatment is necessary.

LARYNGITIS, or inflammation of the mucous membrane of the larynx, may be either acute or chronic. This may be due to an infectious cause, most commonly viral but also bacterial, or may be due to voice abuse.

ACUTE LARYNGITIS: **Causes**: This complaint is usually a concommitant feature of an upper-respiratory-tract infection, usually viral in origin. It may accompany any form of infection of the upper respiratory tract. Excessive use of the voice, as in loud and prolonged speaking, singing or shouting, may also produce an acute laryngitis. Inhalation of irritating particles in vapours may also lead to acute laryngitis.

Symptoms: The main sympton is of hoarseness but there may also be pain in the throat. If there is marked swelling this may narrow the channel for the entrance of air leading to a noisy form of breathing called stridor. There may be some constitutional disturbance in the form of fever, malaise, generalized aches and pains and there may also be some difficulty in swallowing. A cough is a common accompanying symptom. The cough may be dry or may be productive of purulent sputum. The voice is hoarse and the breathing stridulous. The majority of cases of acute laryngitis require early voice rest, perhaps some steam inhalation and symptomatic treatment. Antibiotics are seldom necessary, although these would be prescribed if a bacterial infection were thought to supervene. Acute airway obstruction is an unusual event following laryngitis but, if the airway becomes threatened in any way, immediate specialist referral should be sought.

Treatment: Bed rest may be indicated if severe constitutional symptoms are present. The voice should be rested and smoking forbidden. Steam inhalations and warm gargles are often soothing and help reduce mucosal oedema or swelling. Antibiotics should be prescribed if indicated. Some form of airway intervention, either endotracheal intubation or tracheostomy may have to be performed on rare occasions if severe obstruction results.

CHRONIC LARYNGITIS: This may occur as a result of repeated attacks of acute laryngitis or may arise independently due to such causes as habitual exposure, especially when, along with this, there is an over-indulgence in alcohol and the habitual over-use of the vocal cords. Patients are often smokers. Chronic laryngitis may be caused, or exacerbated, by nasal obstruction, leading to excessive mouth breathing. The changes taking place in the vocal cords are more permanent than in the acute form, consisting mainly in thickening of the mucous membrane of the vocal cords. Rarely, chronic laryngitis is due to tuberculosis, syphilis or other chronic inflammatory diseases. These are apt also to produce ulceration of the vocal cords and other parts of the larynx with gradual destruction of its cartilages. The symptoms are similar to those of acute laryngitis except more prolonged. Any doubts as to diagnosis on initial examination would require examination under anaesthetic using a direct laryngoscope by which a view of the affected parts can be obtained and the proper treatment instituted.

Treatment: Voice rest is essential. Any aggravating factors should be removed. Antibiotics are indicated if bacterial infection has supervened. The assistance of a speech therapist is of immense value. Smoking should be forbidden and alcohol preferably avoided. In resistant cases of chronic laryngitis a surgical procedure may be required in which the mucous membrane of the vocal cords is stripped in the hope that a more normal mucous membrane may be generated.

TUBERCULOUS LARYNGITIS practically always occurs as the result of infection spreading from the lungs. This is fortunately a rare disease in developed countries and the treatment involves the administration of anti-tuberculous drugs. It is always necessary to distinguish tuberculous laryngitis from carcinoma of the larynx.

TUMOURS and various inflammatory growths are often met with in the larynx and may give rise to hoarseness. Such growths may be benign or malignant. Benign tumours or small nodules, such as singer's nodules, may be dealt with by speech therapy or may be removed at the operation of direct laryngoscopy. This is usually performed under general anaesthetic. Cancer of the larynx may be treated either by radiotherapy or by surgery, depending on the extent of the disease. Hoarseness may indeed be the only symptom of vocal cord disturbance or of carcinoma of the larynx and any case of hoarseness which has lasted for 6 weeks should be referred for a specialist opinion, so that the larynx can be viewed to exclude the presence of carcinoma. The earlier the diagnosis is made, the more successful the results of treatment are. Laryngectomy clubs are now being established throughout the country to advise and help patients who have had laryngectomy. Details of these can be obtained from the National Association of Laryngectomee Clubs, 39 Eccleston Square, London SW1V 1PB. An important feature of patients who have undergone laryngectomy is the rehabilitation of their speech and the assistance of a speech therapist is fundamental to performing such surgery with the aim of the patient's producing some form of voice following surgery.

Other abnormalities of voice may be caused by paralysis of either of the vocal cords. This may be a congenital problem or may be the result of pressure upon the recurrent laryngeal nerve by aneurysm or tumour or the nerve may be damaged in operations on the chest and neck. The symptom in this condition is one of weakness of the voice rather than actual hoarseness. *Aphonia* is a condition in which there is no voice at all. This is usually of psychological origin and the diagnosis is made after excluding any local pathology. Once again, the assistance of a speech therapist is invaluable.

LARYNGOLOGY is that branch of medical science concerned with disorders and diseases of the larynx.

LARYNGOSCOPE: Examination of the larynx may be performed indirectly with use of a laryngeal mirror, or directly by use of a laryngoscope. The direct examination is usually performed under general anaesthetic.

LARYNGO-TRACHEO-BRONCHITIS (CROUP) is an acute infection of the respiratory tract in infants and young children. It is usually a virus infection or may be caused by *Haemophilus influenzae*. The onset is variable but the croupy cough and stridulous breathing usually occur a few days after the onset of a viral upper-respiratory-tract infection. The harsh barking cough is typical of the condition. The majority of children with this condition can be treated with humidification and antibiotics if necessary, but they should always be referred for specialist assessment and hospitalization is preferable in all cases. Rarely, some form of intervention is necessary and this will either be in the form of endotracheal intubation or of a tracheostomy.

LARYNX is the organ of voice and also forms one of the higher parts of the air passages. It is placed high up in the front of the neck and there forms a considerable prominence on the surface. It is covered in front by the skin, a layer of fibrous tissue and a thin layer of muscles, whilst its sides are protected by the lateral lobes of the thyroid gland and by the large sternocleidomastoid muscles.

The larynx is almost 5 cm or 2 inches in height and forms a sort of box, well protected in front by cartilages, rather more open behind and communicating above with the pharynx at the root of the tongue and below the windpipe or trachea. The larynx is enclosed by five large cartilages: the thyroid cartilage, whose prominent pointed front forms the Adam's apple; the cricoid cartilage, a ring placed below it; the epiglottis, a leaf-like cartilage projecting above the thyroid cartilage into the interior of the throat at the root of the tongue; and a pair of arytenoid cartilages jointed to the top edge of the cricoid cartilage behind, where the thyroid cartilage is deficient. There are also four small nodules of cartilage above the arytenoids. The edges of the laryngeal cartilages do not fit closely together, and the spaces between are filled up by membranes. Certain of the ligaments which bind the cartilages together are of great importance. These pass along each side of the larynx, from the arytenoid cartilage behind to the thyroid cartilage in front, two bands of elastic fibres covered by the mucous membrane which lines the whole larynx. One pair of these bands lies directly above the other, the upper pair being known as the false vocal cords; the lower pair are the true vocal cords. The latter are capable of various degrees of tenseness and slackness and of approximation and separation, these results being achieved by several small muscles, which are attached to the arytenoid cartilages and governed in their movements through branches of the vagus nerves. Between the true and false cord is a deep depression on each side known as the ventricle

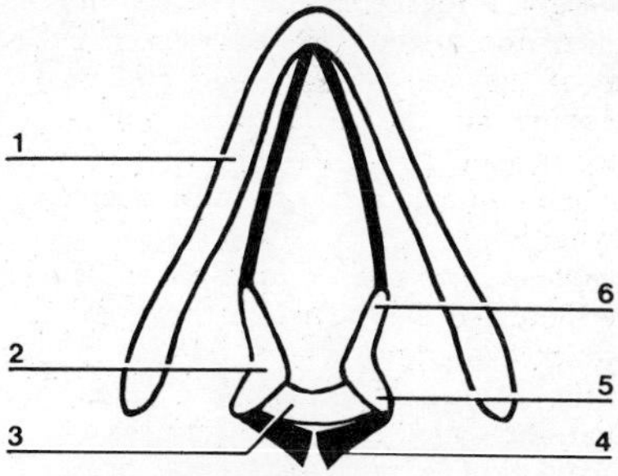

1 thyroid cartilage
2 arytenoid cartilage
3 upper border of cricoid cartilage
4 posterior crico-arytenoid muscles
5 muscular processes
6 vocal processes

Diagram of the opening of the larynx to show the action of the muscles. A horizontal section has been made at the level of the true vocal cords. The two cords are widely separated by the action of 4.

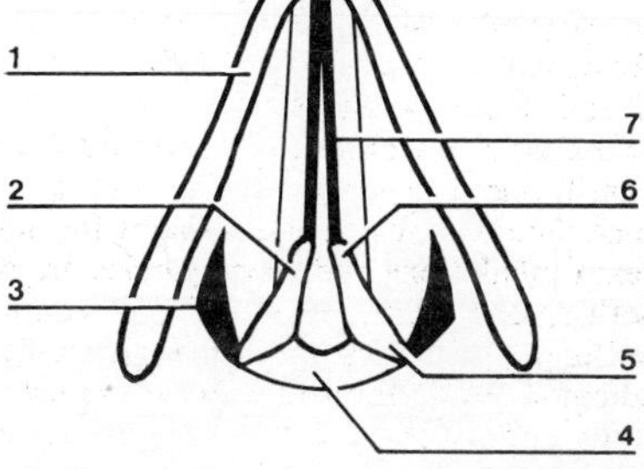

1 thyroid cartilage
2 arytenoid cartilage
3 lateral aryttenoid
4 arytenoid muscles
5 muscular processes
6 vocal processes
7 thyroartenoid

Diagram of the opening of the larynx to show the action of the muscles. The cords are now held together by the action of 3, 4 and 7.

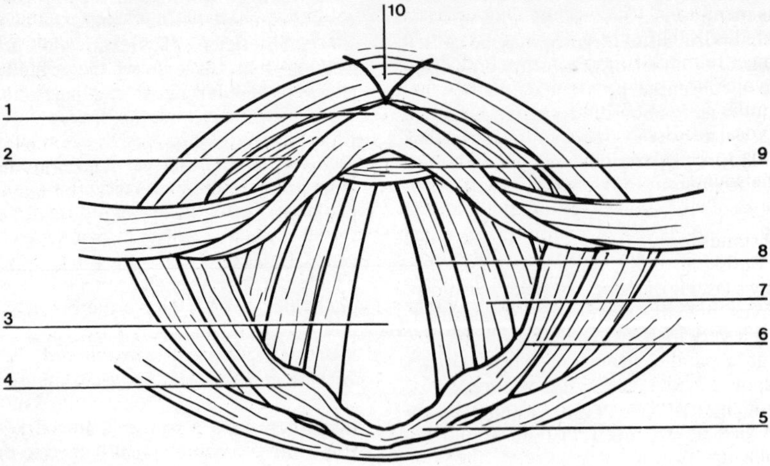

1 epiglottis
2 vallecula
3 trachea
4 cuneiform cartilage
5 corniculate cartilage
6 aryepiglottic fold
7 vestibular fold
8 vocal fold
9 tubercle of epiglottis
10 glossoepiglottic fold

A laryngoscopic view of the interior of the larynx.

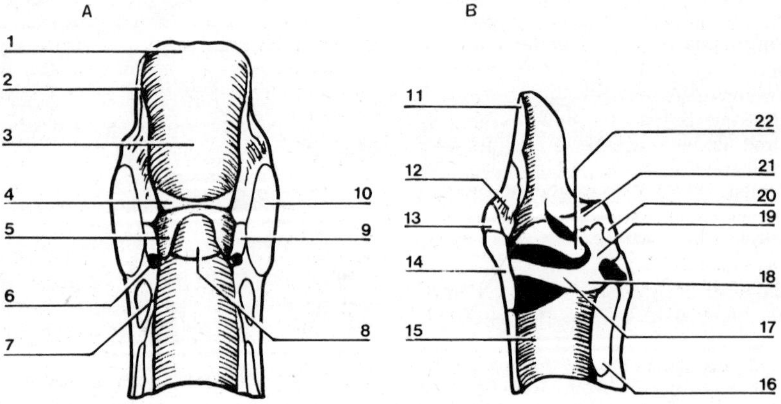

1 epiglottis
2 aryepiggottic fold
3 tubercle
4 ventricular fold
5 vocal fold
6 interior thyro-arytenoid muscle
7 cricoid membrane
8 cricothyroid membrane
9 ventricle of larynx
10 thyroid cartilage
11 epiglottis
12 adipose tissue
13 ventricle
14 thyroid cartilage
15 cricothyroid membrane
16 cricoid cartilage
17 vocal cord
18 respiratory glottis
19 artyenoideus muscle
20 corniculate cartilage
21 cuneiform cartilage
22 false vocal cord

Vertical section of larynx: (A) from behind, (B) from left side.

of the larynx. The larynx is lined throughout by mucous membrane, which generally is covered by ciliated cells; but over the true cords, which are subject to much friction in the production of the voice, the surface consists of flattened cells similar to those of the skin.

The vocal cords vibrating in different notes, according to their tenseness and the like, produce the sounds of voice and speech (qv).

LASER stands for Light Amplification by Stimulated Emission of Radiation. The light produced by a laser is of a single wavelength and all the waves are in phase with each other, allowing a very high level of energy to be projected as a parallel beam or focused onto a small spot. Various gases, liquids and solids will emit light when they are suitably stimulated. A gassed laser is pumped by the ionising effect of a high voltage current. This is the same process as that used in a flourescent tube. Each type of laser has a different effect on biological tissues and this is related to the wavelength of the light produced. The wavelength determines the degree of energy absorption by different tissues and because of this different lasers are needed for different tasks. The argon laser produces light in the visible green wavelength which is selectively absorbed by haemoglobin. It heats and coagulates tissues and it is thus possible to seal bleeding blood vessels and to selectively destroy pigmented lesions. The carbon-dioxide laser is the standard laser for cutting tissue. The infra-red beam it produces is strongly absorbed by water and so vapourises cells. Thus by moving a finely focused beam across the tissue it is possible to make an incision.

The two main uses of the laser in surgery are the endoscopic photocoagulation of bleeding vessels and the incision of tissue. Lasers have important applications in ophthalmology in the treatment of such disorders of detachment of the retina and the diabetic complication of proliferative retinopathy. Lasers have three great advantages. They are potent, they act speedily and they can be focused on a small area, even an area as small as one micrometer.

LASSA FEVER, which derives its name from the fact that it was first reported in Lassa in Nigeria, is a disease due to an arenavirus (qv). This may be transmitted by rodents or direct from an infected person to those around him. The incubation period is three to twenty-one days. It is characterized by headache, lethargy and severe muscular pains, and there is often a rash due to bleeding into the skin and mucous membranes. Sore throat is often present. It may carry a high mortality rate, particularly in pregnant women. As it is a virus infection, there is no specific treatment, and all that can be done is careful nursing, with rest in bed.

LASSAR'S PASTE, officially known as Zinc and Salicylic Acid Paste, BP, is a preparation used as a remedy for eczema. It has a combined softening, antiseptic, astringent, and soothing action. It is made up of zinc oxide 24 grams; salicylic acid 2 grams; starch 24 grams; white soft paraffin 100 grams.

LATHYRISM is the disease in which stiffness, pains in, and trembling and paralysis of, the legs are caused by varieties of lathyrus pea (chick-pea).

LAUDANUM is the popular name for tincture of opium. (See OPIUM.)

LAUGHING-GAS is a popular name for nitrous oxide (qv).

LAUREL is the name applied to two plants. From the leaves and berries of *Laurus nobilis* or bay tree an oil is extracted which is used for application in rheumatic and similar pains. From *Prunus laurocerasus* or cherry laurel, cherry laurel water is produced, containing a small quantity of hydrocyanic acid, and is used for making up soothing solutions.

LAVAGE is the name applied to the washing out of the stomach.

LAXATIVES (see PURGATIVES).

LEAD has no action itself upon the system, but its salts, when absorbed in any quantity, or for any length of time, have very important effects. When a lead salt comes in contact with a wound or with any mucous surface, it combines with the albuminous material of the discharge or secretion to form a whitish glaze, which affords a degree of protection to the surface. Further, the lead salt has an astringent action upon the blood-vessels, and therefore helps to stop bleeding or relieve the congestion of inflammation. If one of the soluble lead salts is taken internally, in large amount, it has an irritant action, and the acetate (sugar of lead), subacetate, and nitrate of lead are irritant poisons when taken into the stomach, although their action is comparatively feeble.

Uses: Externally, subacetate of lead is used in the form of Goulard's water, for application to painful areas, such as inflamed joints, bruises, sprains. (See GOULARD'S WATER.) In eczema this solution, sponged upon the affected area, often gives relief from itching. Lead lotion and lead and glycerin lotion are similarly used. Litharge, or lead monoxide, is used as a basis for many adhesive plasters, which are known as diachylon plasters. Lead with opium suppositories are used for the treatment of bleeding piles.

LEAD POISONING: Acute poisoning by lead acetate (sugar of lead) is an accident which sometimes, though rarely, happens to a child, and is treated, like cases of irritant poisoning generally, by administering diluents such as milk together with Epsom salts, which form an antidote, followed by emetics.

Chronic poisoning is apt to affect those who come in contact with lead or its salts, either in the production of these or in the course of their use. In Great Britain in 1978–1979 there were 24 cases of certified incapacity due to lead poisoning arising out of the victim's work but only one case in 1984. Thus lead-smelters, plumbers, file-makers, pottery workers who use lead in glaze, painters, dyers, above all, those who make white-lead, are liable to suffer. Another industrial lead health hazard is tetraethyl lead which is added to petrol as an 'anti-knocking' agent. The risk here is to workers cleaning petrol storage tanks. Whether it has any effect on the general population in this automobile-ridden age is still a moot point, but the lead content of petrol is being reduced. Lead-containing paint was a common cause of lead poisoning in children in the form of pica (qv) which manifests itself by the chewing of painted woodwork. Lead may also be introduced into system through food and water, in those who have nothing to do with the metal in their work. For example, drinking-water is sometimes contaminated by lead which it has dissolved off the pipes through which it passes. Cider, made in leaden presses, may so readily take up lead that 'Devonshire colic' was once a name given to lead-poisoning occurring in this part of the country, where cider forms a favourite beverage. The experts differ as to the critical level of lead in the blood. For many years it has been accepted that blood lead concentrations of over 80 micrograms per decilitre are likely to pose health risks, with clear evidence of the risk of mental and behavioural impairment above this level. Conversely the general view has been that blood lead levels of under 35 micrograms per decilitre will not normally produce a health hazard. The current view is that it would be a wise precaution to accept this lower level and to investigate any individual in whom the blood lead level exceeds 35 micrograms per decilitre.

Control over lead in food in England and Wales is exercised by the Lead in Food Regulations 1961 (revised in 1979). These Regulations lay down a limit of 1 mg per kg for most foods, with different levels for certain specified foods including canned meat and meat pastes, fish and fish pastes, for which a maximum of 5 p.p.m. is permitted. There are similar regulations for Scotland and Northern Ireland. Subsequent Regulations created a new category for foods specially prepared for infants and young children, and set a limit of 0·5 p.p.m. for this category. The upper allowable limit for lead in potable water is 0·1 mg per litre. Under an EEC directive the permitted quantity is 0·05 mg per litre. As regards drinking-water there is, in general, no danger, because the minerals in the water form, with the lead, insoluble compounds which are deposited in a thin coat upon the inside of the pipes. A greater danger exists in peaty or soft water, or in water contaminated by organic impurities, both of which give the water a high power of dissolving lead. Not only may the lead be introduced into the system through the skin of those who constantly handle lead-containing materials, and by way of the stomach, but in some of the most rapidly produced and serious cases – for example, among white-lead workers, and glazers of pottery – the lead is inhaled as dry dust. Lead is often similarly inhaled by men engaged in cutting up iron plates which have been fitted by the aid of red lead; this, being driven off by the heat of the blow-pipe employed, is apt to be inhaled.

Symptoms: Among the early symptoms of a chronic and insidious case are constipation, muscular weakness, and pallor of the skin. A blue line on the margin of the gums, due to deposit of lead sulphide in this locality, is also an important sign of the condition. Colic of a very painful nature, affecting the centre of the abdomen and lasting often for several days at a time, appears and forms one of the most prominent symptoms in almost every case. Lead has a specially damaging action upon the nervous system, causing an inflammatory process in the nerves, which results in tremors and paralysis, usually affecting the muscles on the back of the wrist first of all, and later those on the front and outer side of the leg, and causing wrist-drop and foot-drop. Convulsions, which may develop rapidly and may end in death, are also produced by poisoning of the nervous system, leading to a brain disorder known as lead encephalopathy. Occasionally, though fortunately rarely, affection of the optic nerve leads to blindness, which is either temporary or permanent. Owing to interference with the kidney functions, the urine becomes scanty, while a destructive action on the blood leads to anaemia.

Treatment: With regard to workers in lead and its salts, government regulations have been introduced which very effectively protect them. Among these preventive measures are included: personal cleanliness in washing the hands and changing the clothes before partaking of meals, the use of respirators by those who come in contact with white-lead dust, the provision of exhaust flues and electric fans beneath the tables at which pottery glazers work, and the drinking of at least a glass of milk daily. These and other measures confer a great degree of protection upon those engaging in these otherwise dangerous trades. Workers who begin to show symptoms of lead poisoning should at once undergo treatment. A frequent recurrence of symptoms shows a special liability to this form of poisoning, and indicates that the worker should seek some totally different employment. In the case of drinking-water the source of contamination must, of course, be removed. The drug which is of special use in treatment of lead-poisoning is sodium calcium-edetate, by which lead salts deposited in the tissues are dissolved, to be afterwards excreted from the body. Colic is treated by hot fomentations, magnesium sulphate, and belladonna, and a high calcium diet.

In acute cases of lead colic the intravenous administration of calcium gluconate or calcium chloride gives immediate relief.

LEBER'S DISEASE, or HEREDITARY OPTIC ATROPHY, is a hereditary disease in which blindness comes on at about the age of twenty.

LECITHIN is a very complex fat found in various tissues of the body, but particularly in the brain and nerves, of which it forms a large part. It is also found in large quantities in the yolk of an egg.

LEECHES are animals belonging to the class Vermes, provided with suckers and living a semi-parasitic life, their food being mainly derived from the blood of other animals. They abstract blood by means of a sucker surrounding the mouth, which is provided with several large sharp teeth. The medicinal leech, *Hirudo medicinalis*, was formerly employed for the abstraction of small quantities of blood in inflammatory and other conditions.

LEG: This term is generally applied to the whole lower extremity but, properly speaking, includes that part between the knee and ankle joints. The lower limb is attached to the pelvic bones by strong muscles, especially the gluteal and hamstring muscles behind and the abductor muscles on the inner side of the thigh. The head of the femur, or thigh bone, lies in a deep cup-shaped hollow, the acetabulum, on the outer side of the pelvis. The femur, which is the longest and strongest bone in the body, forms at its lower end the joint of the knee with the tibia. The knee-joint is protected in front by the patella or knee-cap. Along the outer side of the tibia lies the smaller fibula, which does not extend up to the knee but which, along with the tibia, forms the ankle joint. The two prominences on the ankle (*malleoli*) are formed by the tibia on the inner side and the fibula on the outer side. Seven tarsal bones comprise the hinder part of the foot, of which the talus takes the weight of the body from the tibia and fibula. There are five metatarsal bones in the front portion of the foot and each toe has three phalangeal bones, excepting the great toe which has two. The powerful quadriceps extensor muscle in front of the thigh is attached to the knee-cap, which in turn is attached to the front of the tibia by the patellar ligament. This muscle straightens the knee and keeps the body in an erect posture. Below the knee the muscles of the calf, attached to the heel through the tendo calcaneus, or tendon of Achilles, raise the heel off the ground in walking. In front of and to the outside of the leg lie the tibial and peroneal muscles, which bend the ankle upwards and raise the toes. In the sole of the foot are a number of small muscles which bend the toes downwards. The arch of the foot is a very important structure. (See FOOT.)

Most of the blood supply to the lower limb is carried by the femoral artery, which issues from the abdomen in the middle of the groin where its pulse can be felt. This passes down the inner side of the thigh to reach the middle of the back of the knee where it is known as the popliteal artery. Below the knee it divides into anterior and posterior tibial vessels. The former of these runs down the front of the leg and upper surface of the foot, and the latter, which is the larger, passes behind the inner ankle where its pulse can be felt about a finger's breadth behind the bony prominence. The blood returns from the leg partly by deep veins lying alongside the arteries, but to a large extent by the great saphenous vein, which can be seen or felt under the skin for most of the distance from the ankle up the inside of the leg and thigh to the inner side of the groin, where it joins the femoral vein.

The chief nerve in the lower limb is the sciatic nerve which runs down the middle of the back of the thigh deeply embedded in muscles. Above the knee it divides into two parts: the tibial and common peroneal nerves. The former of these runs down the back of the leg, deeply embedded in muscles, to the foot, and the latter passes round the upper end of the fibula on the outer side of the leg, where it can be felt and is liable to be damaged.

The arch of the foot is liable to give way, especially in debilitated or overworked people, thus producing flat foot. The ankle joint is liable to sprains which consist of tearing of the ligaments, especially on the inner side. The fibula is liable to be fractured near its lower end (a common accident in professional soccer players), either by twists of the foot or by a blow on the outer side of the leg. Fracture of the tibia is also a common accident and, as the tibia lies immediately beneath the skin, this fracture is in danger of becoming compound. The knee-joint, by reason of its great strength, is seldom dislocated, but the partial displacement of a cartilage in the knee is a common occurrence. Fracture of the femur is a serious accident, requiring a period of several months for complete union of the bone. The long and poorly supported vein on the inner side of the leg and thigh is very apt to become distended along with its branches, producing the condition known as varicose veins with resultant eczema and ulcer. The bursa in front of the knee-cap, in people who kneel a lot, readily becomes inflamed and thickened in the condition known as 'housemaid's knee'. (See also FOOT; FRACTURES; JOINTS; KNEE; LIMBS; VEINS.)

LEGIONNAIRE'S DISEASE is a form of pneumonia due to a bacterium known as *Legionella pneumophila*. The bacterium is widely distributed in nature and is commonly found in surface water and soil. Legionnellae are ubiquitous in water. Stationary water and sludge in water tanks provide favourable conditions for primary multiplication. Inhalation of water aerosols seems the most likely way that people acquire the disease. The organism is able to multiply at water outlets. Some rubber outlets in showers and taps are able to support the growth of legionnellae so that high concentrations of the organism are released when the tap is first used in the morning. In the presence of the disease the treatment of infected water systems is essential by cleaning, chlorination or heating or a combination of all three.

The pneumonia caused by legionnellae has no distinctive clinical or radiological features, so that the diagnosis is based on laboratory findings. This depends on the detection of antibodies by the indirect fluorescent antibody test. There is no evidence that the disease is transmitted directly from person to person. The predominant root of infection is by inhalation. The incubation period is two to ten days. The disease starts with aches and pains followed rapidly by a rise in temperature, shivering attacks, cough and shortness of breath. The X-ray tends to show patchy areas of consolidation in the lungs. The assessment of treatment is still hampered by the lack of proper clinical trials but it does seem that erythromycin and rifampicin are the most useful antibiotics. Rifampicin, however, should never be given alone because of the rapid development of drug resistance. In England in 1984 there were 151 cases reported to the Public Health Surveillance unit. Between 1985 and 1987 200 cases were reported each year.

LEGS, INEQUALITY OF: This may be due to one leg being longer or shorter than the other. Most usually it is due to one leg being abnormally short. This may be congenital in origin, or due to trauma resulting in damage to the epiphysis (qv), poliomyelitis (qv), or some infection such as osteomyelitis (qv) or septic arthritis (qv). If the shortening is only slight, this may be remedied by deepening the sole of one shoe. In more severe cases it may be treated by surgery. This is a complicated procedure which can only be carried out in special hospitals. It is also a lengthy procedure, requiring skilled physiotherapy as well as skilled surgery, but in carefully selected cases the results can be most satisfactory.

LEIOMYOMA is a tumour made up of unstriped or involuntary muscle fibres.

LEISHMANIASIS is a group of diseases due to infection with a number of parasites, of the genus known as Leishmania. The parasite is transmitted to man by the bite of certain sandflies. It is estimated that there are 400,000 new cases every year.

VISCERAL LEISHMANIASIS or KALA-AZAR, also known as DUM-DUM FEVER, occurs in tropical and sub-tropical Africa and Asia, the Mediterranean area and in tropical South America. It is caused by a parasite known as *Leishmania donovani*. The source of the infection, the type of sandfly that transmits it to man, and the common age of infection vary from one area to another. Thus, in the Mediterranean region it is predominantly a disease of infants, whereas in Africa it tends more to occur in adolescents and young adults. The onset may be sudden or gradual. In the well-established case there is enlargement of the spleen and of the liver, accompanied by fever and generalized glandular enlargement. The diagnosis is established by removing a piece of bone marrow, spleen or liver, and examining it for the presence of the causative parasite. Untreated the disease is usually fatal in at least 70 per cent of cases either in the acute stage or after two years or so.

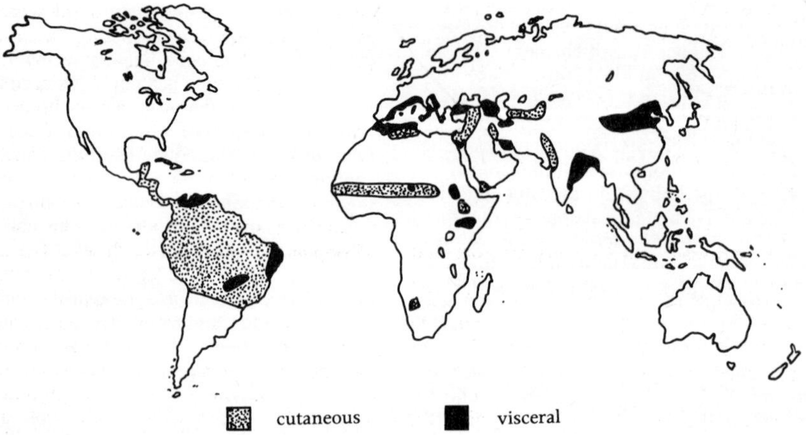

Distribution of cutaneous and visceral leishmaniasis.

Treatment: Sodium stibogluconate, a pentavalent antimonial compound, is the drug of choice. The response to treatment varies with the area in which the infection occurs. Thus, in India, the disease usually responds to one ten-day course of injections, whereas in the Mediterranean region two or three such courses may be needed. A high proportion of cases are cured in this way.

CUTANEOUS and MUCO-CUTANEOUS LEISHMANIASIS is the form of the disease in which the parasite involves predominantly the skin and mucous membranes, and sometimes also cartilage. It is caused by a variety of species of Leishmania, and is known by different names in different geographical areas. Thus, in South America it is known as espundia, whereas in Asia it is known variously as oriental sore, Delhi boil, Aleppo boil, Baghdad boil, Biskra boil (or button). In the Old World it tends to be restricted to the skin, producing a chronic ulcer, whereas in the New World it tends to be more diffuse, involving the nose and throat, and leading to widespread erosion of the nasal cartilage; it may well terminate in a fatal broncho-pneumonia.

Treatment is by sodium stibogluconate, but most of the cases in the Old World heal spontaneously, though slowly, and the affected area merely needs to be protected and kept clean.

LEMON is used in the form of the fresh peel, tincture, syrup, and oil. Its main value, however, is as a source of vitamin C (or ascorbic acid), the average content of ascorbic acid in the juice being 45 mg per 100 grams. (See also CITRIC ACID; and VITAMINS.)

LENS OF THE EYE (see EYE).

LENTIGO is another name for freckles (qv).

LEPROSY is a chronic disease which affects particularly the skin, mucous membranes, and nerves.

History: Some authorities say that leprosy originated in the upper reaches of the Nile. Others claim that it originated in the region of the Indus. Wherever it originated, its subsequent history is difficult to trace because of the confusion as to what the older writers meant by the term 'leprosy'. The term is used in the Authorized Version of The Bible, but experts differ as to whether this is the correct translation of the Hebrew word, *Tsaraath*. It was used for the true disease and for every disorder that was formerly supposed to be leprosy. In Europe, to which it was probably introduced by the troops of Alexander the Great returning to Greece from the Indian campaign of 327–326 BC, it reached its highest incidence between AD 1000 and AD, 1400 thereafter slowly declining. The last indigenous case in Great Britain died in 1798 – in the Shetland Islands. So far as the American continent is concerned, the available evidence suggests that it was introduced there originally by Columbus's soldiers, and much later by the slave trade from West Africa.

Causes: The causative organism of leprosy is the *Mycobacterium leprae* which was discovered by Hansen in 1872. It is a straight or slightly curved rod which closely resembles the *Mycobacterium tuberculosis* in its size and acid-fast staining reaction.

The total number of cases in the world has been conservatively estimated at between 10 and 11 million: 6·5 million in Asia (mainly in the Indian Subcontinent and the Far East); 3·5 million in Africa; and 350,000 in the Americas (mainly Central and South America). In Europe it is largely confined to countries bordering the Mediterranean, European Russia and European Turkey. It is estimated that there are 25,000 cases in Europe. It has reappeared in Britain as a result of the recent influx of immigrants from countries in which leprosy is endemic. In 1985, in England there were 304 registered cases of leprosy, 279 of which were known to be quiescent; 19 cases were notified during the year. Since the disease became notifiable in Britain in 1951 no case has been reported of the disease being acquired in this country. All have been cases in which the infection was acquired overseas. The incubation period, or latent period between the infection being acquired and the disease manifesting itself is considered to be between 3 and 5 years or even longer. Males are more commonly infected than females. It is uncommon below the age of 4 years, and no case has yet been reported before the age of 18 months. The variation of incidence among different races is due to contact rather than racial susceptibility, but the type of the disease varies in different races. Thus, the European and Mongol races appear to be more likely to acquire the serious lepromatous type of leprosy than the Indian and African races. There is some evidence that malnutrition may increase susceptibility to the disease. The disease is transmitted by contact with open cases of leprosy. The nasal secretion of such open cases is swarming with leprosy bacilli, and this is the likeliest source of infection for people in contact with open cases. The bacillus can also be present in the breast milk of infected mothers. Only a few of the people exposed to infection develop the disease, and those in contact with tuberculoid cases are much less likely to develop the disease than those in contact with lepromatous cases.

Symptoms: There are two distinct types of leprosy: tuberculoid and lepromatous. The differentiation is important because the former runs a relatively benign course and is often self-healing, whereas the latter is a steadily progressive form of the disease. The differentiation, however, is not always clear cut, and there is a group of 'indeterminate' or 'dimorphous' cases in which lesions similar to tuberculoid and lepromatous leprosy are seen in the same patient. The differentiation of those three types is a matter for the expert, and no attempt will be made here to go into the details of the different types.

Whatever form of leprosy may be present, the symptoms and signs can be divided into two main groups: those involving the skin and those arising from involvement of the nerves. The skin manifestations range from areas of whitening of the skin to massive nodules. The nerve manifestations range from localized swellings of the nerve to extensive areas of anaesthesia in the skin. The ultimate destruction of the nerves leads to the deformities which used to be such a marked feature of leprosy before adequate means of treatment became available. These included foot-drop, wrist-drop, claw-foot, extensive ulceration of the extremities leading to loss of the fingers and toes, and absorption of bone. The eyes may also be infected, leading to blindness, and ulcers may occur in the mouth and in the larynx. In the larynx they may cause hoarseness or even go on to the stage of producing complete blockage of it. These tragic cases of gross deformity, which in the past have made leprosy such a terrifying disease, should no longer occur. As Cochrane has pointed out: 'With the introduction of modern therapy the vast majority of cases, if treated adequately before extensive deformity has set in, should recover without any disability. Nevertheless, until adequate treatment and properly administered therapy are within the reach of all, the shadow of tragic deformity will remain, particularly where there is a failure to understand the importance of physiotherapy in preventing this'.

Treatment: For centuries chaulmoogra (hydnocarpus) oil was the great stand-by in the treatment of leprosy.

In 1941, the outlook was entirely changed by the discovery that a sulphone derivative was effective in the treatment. Widespread use of the sulphones has gone far to bringing leprosy under control. The most widely used sulphone is dapsone, which is given by mouth. Given over long periods of time, most cases of leprosy respond satisfactorily. Various other drugs have been introduced during recent years for the treatment of leprosy. The most promising are rifampicin, clofazimine, and ethionamide. Unfortunately the *Mycobacterium leprae* is developing resistance to dapsone when this is given alone. To reduce this risk to a minimum, it is necessary to give it along with some other anti-leprosy drug. At the moment the recommended combination is rifampicin, dapsone and clofazimine. Preliminary results suggest that BCG vaccine (qv) may be of value in the prevention of leprosy, but it is too early yet to assess the real significance of this observation. Hopes are also arising that it may be possible to produce an effective vaccine against the disease.

Chemotherapy, however, has not diminished the importance of physiotherapy in the treatment and prevention of deformity in leprosy. Equally important is the role of plastic and orthopaedic surgery in treating these deformities when they have reached a stage in which physiotherapy is of little use. Many patients with advanced leprosy, hitherto condemned to a life of chronic invalidism as a result of their deformities, are now being returned to the community as useful members who are able to use their hands and feet sufficiently to be able to earn a living and lead a reasonably active life.

The salient points about leprosy are summed up as follows in a *Memorandum on Leprosy* published by the Department of Health and Social Security.

(1) Leprosy is normally a curable disease.
(2) It is only slightly contagious and most people are, to some extent, naturally immune to the disease.
(3) If it is treated early enough, it can be arrested without deformity.
(4) Only a few people need to continue treatment for life.
(5) Leprosy is slow to develop and takes considerable time to treat.
(6) Patients with leprosy who are undergoing treatment for the disease can live at home, and continue normal family life and work.

LEPTAZOL is a synthetic organic drug introduced as a respiratory stimulant.

LEPTOMENINGITIS means inflammation of the inner and more delicate membranes of the brain or spinal cord.

LEPTOSPIRA is a group, or genus, of spiral micro-organisms, normally found in rodents and other small mammals in which they cause no harm. When transmitted to man by these animals, either directly or indirectly as through cows, they give rise to various forms of illness.

LEPTOSPIROSIS is the disease caused by infection with Leptospira. The three most common members of this group in the United Kingdom are *L. icterohaemorrhagiae*, *L. canicola*, and *L. hebiomadis*. It is an occupational hazard of farmers, sewage and abattoir workers, fish cutters and veterinary surgeons, but the infection can also be acquired from bathing in contaminated water. There were 72 cases, seven of them fatal, in the British Isles in 1981. Nine of them were due to immersion in polluted water. The figures for 1984 show a reduction in the incidence in sewage workers but a rise in the incidence in farmers. The disease varies in intensity from a mild influenza-like illness to a fatal form of jaundice due to severe liver disease. The kidneys are often involved and there may be meningitis. Penicillin or tetracycline are the usual treatment but unless they are given early in the disease their effect is limited.

SPIROCHAETOSIS ICTEROHAEMORRHAGICA, or WEIL'S DISEASE, is the term applied to infection with the *Leptospira icterohaemorrhagiae* which is transmitted to man by rats, these animals excreting the organism in their urine; hence the liability of sewer workers to the disease. The condition is characterized by fever, jaundice, enlarged liver, nephritis, and bleeding from mucous membranes. There were 39 cases in the British Isles in 1981.

LESION meant originally an injury, but is now applied generally to all disease changes in organs and tissues.

LETHARGY or LASSITUDE means a loss of energy. It is a common presenting complaint to both the general practitioner and hospital consultant. It may have a physical cause or a psychological cause. It may be the result of inadequate rest, environmental noise, boredom, insomnia or recent illness. It may be the result of drugs, the most common of which are beta-blockers and diuretics. The common psycho-social problems producing lethargy are depression and anxiety. If the patient with lethargy runs a fever the differential diagnosis is that of a PUO (Pyrexia of unknown origin). Many patients with fatigue can establish the onset of the symptom to a febrile illness even though they no longer run a fever. The lethargy that follows glandular fever and other viral infections is well recognized. Some of these patients have a true depressive illness and their presentation and response to treatment is little different to sufferers from any other depressive illness. Organic causes of lethargy include anaemia, malnutrition, hypothyroidism, uraemia, alcoholism and diabetes mellitus.

LETTUCE is a green vegetable consisting of leaves of *Lactucasativa.* It is a relatively rich source of vitamin A. The content of vitamin C is variable, ranging from 1 to 17 mg per 100 grams.

LEUCINE is one of the essential, or indispensable, amino-acids (qv). They are so called because they cannot be synthesized, or manufactured, in the body, and are therefore essential constituents of the diet.

LEUCO- (or LEUKO-) is a prefix meaning white.

LEUCOCYTE is the term applied to the white blood cells. Leucocytes differ from erythrocytes in that they contain no haemoglobin and are therefore colourless, and contain a well-formed nucleus. Most of them are larger than erythrocytes, being 8 to 15 micrometres in diameter, and there are many fewer in the blood – usually about 8000 per cubic millimetre of blood. There are three main classes of white cells: granulocytes, lymphocytes, and monocytes. *Granulocytes*, or polymorphonuclear leucocytes as they are sometimes termed, which normally constitute 70 per cent of the white blood cells, have a lobed nucleus and a granular cytoplasm. They are divided into three groups according to the staining reactions of these granules: neutrophils, which stain with neutral dyes and constitute 65 to 70 per cent of all the white blood cells; eosinophils, which stain with acid dyes (eg. eosin) and constitute 3 to 4 per cent of the total white blood cells; and basophils, which stain with basic dyes (eg. methylene blue) and constitute about 0·5 per cent of the total white blood cells. *Lymphocytes*, which constitute 25 to 30 per cent of the white blood cells, have a clear non-granular cytoplasm and a relatively large nucleus which is only slightly indented. They are divided into two groups: small lymphocytes which are slightly larger than erythrocytes (about 8 micrometres in diameter); large lymphocytes, which are about 12 micrometres in diameter. *Monocytes*, which constitute about 5 per cent of the white blood cells, are 10 to 15 micrometres in diameter and differ from lymphocytes in having a rather smaller nucleus which tends to be more indented and to be placed more eccentrically. Monocytes are motile phagocytic cells that circulate in the blood and migrate into the tissues where they develop into various forms of macrophages such as tissue macrophages and Kupffer cells. They remove micro-organisms from the body and identify and present antigenic material to lymphocytes. The cytoplasm is non-granular.

Site of origin: The granulocytes are formed in the red bone marrow. The lymphocytes are formed predominantly in lymphoid tissue. There is some controversy as to the site of origin of monocytes: some say they arise from lymphocytes, whilst others contend that they are derived from histiocytes: ie. the reticulo-endothelial system (qv).

Function: The leucocytes constitute one of the most important of the defence mechanisms against infection. This applies particularly to the neutrophil leucocytes. (See LEUCOCYTOSIS.)

(See also ABSCESS; BLOOD; INFLAMMATION; PHAGOCYTOSIS; WOUNDS.)

LEUCOCYTOSIS means a temporary condition in which the polymorphonuclear leucocytes in the blood are increased in number. It occurs in many different circumstances, and forms a valuable means of diagnosis in certain diseases. It may occur, however, as a normal reaction in certain conditions: eg. pregnancy, menstruation, and during muscular exercise. Apart from these conditions, leucocytosis is usually due to the presence of inflammatory processes. It is part of the body's defence mechanism against infection with micro-organisms, the purpose of the increase in the number of leucocytes being to help to destroy the invading bacteria. Thus, during many acute infective diseases, such as pneumonia, the number is greatly increased. In all suppurative conditions there is also a leucocytosis, and if it seems that an abscess is forming deep in the abdomen, or in some other site where it cannot be readily examined, as, for example, an abscess resulting from appendicitis, the examination of a drop of blood gives a valuable aid in the diagnosis, and may be sufficient, in the absence of other signs, to point out the urgent need of an operation. Typhoid fever constitutes the major exception to the statement that acute infective diseases show this increase of white corpuscles in the blood, and, accordingly, in the case of this disease, the presence of an increase is a specially reliable sign of abscess formation, or other severe complication.

Other infective conditions in which a leucocytosis does not occur include measles and influenza.

LEUCODERMA, or LEUCODERMIA, is a condition of the skin in which areas of it become white, as the result of various skin diseases.

LEUCOPENIA is a condition in which the white corpuscles of the blood are greatly reduced in numbers.

LEUCOPLAKIA is a chronic condition of the tongue in which, as the result of various forms of irritation, hard, smooth, whitish patches develop on its surface.

LEUCORRHOEA (see WHITES).

LEUCOTOMY (see PSYCHOSURGERY).

LEUKAEMIA, or LEUCOCYTHAEMIA, is a disease in which the number of white corpuscles in the blood is permanently increased. The disease is also characterized by great enlargement of the spleen, changes in the marrow of the bones, and by enlargement of the lymph glands all over the body. The condition may be either acute or chronic. According to the type of corpuscles chiefly present the acute form is called acute lymphoblastic leukaemia, or acute myeloblastic leukaemia. The names for the corresponding chronic forms of the disease are chronic lymphatic leukaemia, and chronic myeloid leukaemia. Acute lymphoblastic leukaemia is most common in the first five years of life, and rare after the age of 25. Acute myeloblastic leukaemia is most common in children and young adults, but may occur at any age. Chronic lymphatic leukaemia occurs at any age between 35 and 80, most commonly in the 60's, and is twice as common in men as in women. Chronic myeloid leukaemia is rare before the age of 25, and most common between 30 and 65. Men and women are equally affected.

Cause: The cause of the disease is unknown. In many ways it resembles a form of malignant disease characterized by uncontrolled overproduction of the white blood corpuscles.

Symptoms: In the acute cases the patient shows pallor, occasional purpuric rash, and enlargement of the lymphatic glands and spleen. The temperature is raised, and the condition may be mistaken for an acute infection. Such cases usually run a rapid course, lasting a few weeks or months. In the chronic type of the disease the onset is gradual, and the first symptoms which occasion discomfort are either swelling of the abdomen and shortness of breath, due to painless enlargement of the spleen, or the enlargement of glands in the neck, armpits and elsewhere, or the pallor, palpitation, and other symptoms of anaemia which often accompany the malady. Occasional haemorrhages from the nose, stomach, gums, or bowels may occur, and may be severe. Generally, there is a slight degree of fever. When the blood is examined microscopically, not only is there an enormous increase of the white corpuscles, which may be multiplied thirty- or sixty-fold, but various immature forms of corpuscles are found. In the lymphatic form of the disease the white corpuscles consist chiefly of corpuscles resembling in some measure the lymphocytes, which, in healthy blood, are present only in small numbers. In the myeloid form, myelocytes, or large immature corpuscles out of the bone-marrow, which are never present in healthy blood, appear in large numbers, and there may also be large numbers of immature, nucleated, red blood corpuscles.

Although there is still no cure, the outlook in both acute and chronic leukaemia has changed considerably for the better; particularly is this the case in the acute form of the disease. Thus, in the case of acute lymphoblastic leukaemia, which accounts for around 85 per cent of all childhood leukaemia, only 30 per cent of the cases seen at The Hospital for Sick Children, Great Ormond Street, London, in 1958–59 were alive after twelve months, and less than 10 per cent after two years. In 1966–67, however, 81 per cent survived for twelve months and 28 per cent were still alive three years later. In Britain as a whole the position today is that the chance of inducing a remission in children with acute lymphoblastic leukaemia is much better than 90 per cent, and in 50 per cent of cases the remission is maintained over a promisingly long period. The results in acute myeloblastic leukaemia are not nearly so satisfactory. In the case of chronic lymphatic leukaemia the average period from the time of diagnosis to death is around six years, although quite a number of cases, particularly the elderly, survive for ten years or more. In chronic myeloid leukaemia the average survival time is around three to four years, with 20 per cent surviving for more than five years.

Treatment: Unfortunately, there is no known cure for either the acute or the chronic forms of leukaemia but, as has been noted, promising results are being obtained in the control of the disease, especially by means of chemotherapy and bone-marrow transplantation. In the case of acute leukaemia the drugs now being used include mercaptopurine, methotrexate, cyclophosphamide, and vincristine. But cortisone and its derivatives sometimes produce dramatic temporary improvement. Blood transfusion plays an important part in controlling the condition during the period before the response to chemotherapy or hormone therapy can be expected. Chemotherapy has almost completely replaced radiotherapy in the treatment of chronic leukaemia. For the myeloid form busulphan is the most widely used drug, replaced by hydroxyurea, mercaptopurine, or one of the nitrogen mustard derivatives (qv) in the later stages of the disease. For the lymphatic form the drugs used are chlorambucil, cyclophosphamide, and the nitrogen mustard derivatives.

LEUKOTRIENES are a group of slow-reacting substances (SRSS) which have powerful smooth-muscle stimulating properties.

LEVALLORPHAN TARTRATE is an antidote to morphine. It is more potent and has a slightly longer action than nalorphine (qv). It is usually given intravenously. In opium poisoning the dose is 1 to 2 mg, repeated if necessary.

LEVAMISOLE is a drug that is proving of value in the treatment of ascariasis (qv). Its main advantage seems to be in mass treatment as one dose may prove effective. It is also being used in the treatment of a group of diseases of obscure origin including Crohn's disease (qv) and rheumatoid arthritis.

LEVODOPA is a drug that is being used in the treatment of Parkinsonism (qv).

LEVORPHANOL is a synthetic derivative of morphine. It is an effective analgesic but, like morphine, is a drug of addiction.

LIBIDO is the desire for sexual intercourse. Lack of desire or diminished libido may occur in any general medical illness as well as in endocrine diseases when there is a lack of production of the sex hormones. It is frequently associated with psychiatric diseases and may be the result of certain drugs. It must be distinguished from impotence where the desire for intercourse is normal but the performance is defective due to the inability to achieve or maintain an erection.

LICE (see INSECTS IN RELATION TO DISEASE; PEDICULOSIS).

LICHEN is a term applied to a group of chronic skin diseases characterized by thickening and hardening of the skin, with the formation of papules (qv). *Lichen simplex* develops as a result of persistent scratching. The cause of the itching is often obscure. The disease is more common in women than in men. In women it occurs most commonly in the nape of the neck. It also occurs on the back of the forearm, the inner part of the thigh, the back of the knee and around the ankle. The skin becomes thickened, and has been compared in appearance to that of morocco leather, but there are no papules. Treatment consists of that of the underlying condition if this can be recognized, and the application of corticosteroid cream and emollients. *Lichen planus* begins on the wrists and then spreads to the body and legs. The eruption is characteristic, consisting of purplish, shiny papules with thickening of the surrounding skin. The papules are often found as well in the mouth. The cause is obscure. In some it is apparently nervous or emotional in origin. In some it is due to drugs, including the organic arsenical drugs, gold, mepacrine, chloroquine, and para-aminosalicylic acid (PAS). It usually persists for some three months, but occasionally it may last for years. Treatment consists of the corticosteroids (qv) given by mouth and applied locally.

LICK ECZEMA is an irritating eruption round the mouth, which occurs in children who persistently suck their thumbs or lick their lips. It is due to the resulting constant soaking of the skin in saliva. The eruption disappears when the child is persuaded to give up the causative habit. If troublesome, it may be relieved by liberal applications of petroleum jelly.

LIDOFLAZINE (CLINIUM) (see CALCIUM ANTAGONISTS).

LIENTERIC DIARRHOEA is a mild form of diarrhoea in which the bowels move soon after every meal.

LIGAMENTS are strong bands of fibrous tissue which serve to bind together the bones entering into a joint. They are, in some cases, cord-like, in others flattened bands, whilst most joints are surrounded by a fibrous capsule or capsular ligament. (See JOINTS.)

LIGATURE means a cord or thread used to tie round arteries in order to stop the circulation through them, or to prevent escape of blood from their cut ends. Ligatures are generally made of catgut or silk, and are tied with a reef-knot.

LIGHT TREATMENT: The visible spectrum of white light, extending from red to violet, gives waves of different character. Beyond these, in the infra-red and ultra-violet regions, are numerous varieties of waves. Thus, in the infra-red region we have radiant heat and electric waves, which are used for practical purposes in high-frequency apparatus and radio and television; in the ultra-violet region are the chemically active rays used in heliotherapy, and then, much higher in the series, X-rays and gamma rays emitted by radioactive substances.

From the point of view of treatment, radiant energy is utilized in the following ways:

(1) *Sunlight treatment* or heliotherapy.

(2) *Radiant heat*, obtained by artificial means from incandescent or arc lamps, or by diathermy.

(3) *Ultra-violet radiation.*

(4) *X-rays; radium; radiotherapy;* and *isotopes.*

The first three are treated here. For the fourth see X-RAYS; RADIOTHERAPY.

SUNLIGHT TREATMENT, or HELIOTHERAPY: Sunlight is essential to the well-being of all living things. In the towns of Britain too much of the therapeutic efficiency of the solar rays is still filtered out by moisture, dust, and smoke. This has a specially harmful effect upon child life, and various disabling diseases, such as tuberculosis and rickets, are traceable in part to lack of sunlight. On the other hand, in the clear air of high mountains, especially over snow, which acts as a reflector, the ultra-violet rays are at a maximum.

This is why it is essential that everyone, and especially children, should get as much sunshine as possible – by abolishing atmospheric pollution and by going to the country or seaside for an annual holiday. Much of the benefit of sunshine is derived from its ultra-violet rays, and natural sunshine is preferable to ultra-violet rays produced by an ultra-violet lamp as it contains the complete spectrum of rays as well as those of light and heat.

ULTRA-VIOLET RADIATIONS assist the natural defensive powers of the body and enable them to combat disease. They produce an erythema of the skin and, acting upon 7-dehydrocholesterol in the skin convert it into vitamin D_3, the natural vitamin D present in skin, milk, and fish-liver oils. Calciferol, or vitamin D_2, generally used in preventive and therapeutic medicine, is obtained by ultra-violet irradiation of ergosterol.

Professor Finsen's discovery in 1893 that the rays in this part of the spectrum were bactericidal in their action induced him to try their local effect on lupus vulgaris (tuberculosis of the skin), in which disease he recorded very happy results. In addition to the original Finsen lamps, the mercury vapour lamp and especially the Tungsten arc-lamp, which gives a very high proportion of ultra-violet rays, are favourite forms. In the use of these lamps, the patient's eyes are protected by wearing coloured glass goggles. A few minutes' exposure at a time is usually sufficient.

Excellent results were obtained by ultra-violet radiation in the treatment of lupus and some other forms of tuberculosis before the introduction of the anti-tuberculosis drugs. It is of use in hastening the cure of septic skin diseases, such as ulcers. Exposure to ultra-violet light is one way of treating rickets, as it converts the 7-dehydrocholesterol of the skin into vitamin D_3. Ultra-violet light is bactericidal, and ultra-violet-light 'barriers' have been used in children's wards to prevent the spread of infection. Irradiation of the upper part of the atmosphere of schools has been used in an attempt to control the spread of common infections among school children.

INFRA-RED RADIATIONS employed in treatment are those with wave-lengths immediately below those of luminous rays. Infra-red rays are given out by bodies at a dull red or glowing temperature. The best source of these is sunshine, and they are also derived from incandescent light bulbs with tungsten filament, carbon arc lamps, and ordinary electric radiators at a red heat. These infra-red rays penetrate through the skin to a depth of 6 to 25 mm (¼ to 1 inch), and their action in moderate dosage is to dilate blood vessels and so produce an increased blood supply to the exposed part, and to exert a soothing action on its sensory nerves. They are useful therefore in rheumatic conditions, injury near the surface, to promote absorption and relieve pain, and in certain septic skin conditions such as boils and carbuncles. Apparatus is obtainable which supplies infra-red rays without luminous rays, but this has no advantage over sunshine or electric bulbs, which supply both infra-red and luminous rays, except in cases in which strong light is objectionable, as for example in treatment of conditions near the eyes. When deep penetration of heat is required, diathermy apparatus is used. (See DIATHERMY.)

LIGHTING: Daylight from a clear sky is the best illuminant, and in schools, offices and the like, the position of those working at desks should be arranged so that the light falls from behind, or from behind and to the left, and is not reflected straight up into the worker's eyes. Abundance of light, properly placed, is important, in order to avoid habitual strain of the eyes. The Illuminating Engineering Society Code (1973) recommends illuminance of 150 lux for casual reading, 300 lux for such activities as sewing and prolonged reading, and an increase of 50 to 100 per cent above these levels in old people's homes.

LIGHTNING INJURIES are not uncommon – it is estimated that lightning strikes somewhere on the earth an average of 100 times a second, but the majority of those struck by lightning recover. A direct hit, however, means instantaneous death, with the clothes torn off, and the victim may be hurled quite a long distance. Even the individual who recovers falls unconscious the moment he is struck. Those who are a little farther away experience tingling of the skin and their hair may stand on end.

Preventive measures indoors during a lightning storm consist of keeping away from the fireplace, the main electrical switch, the bathroom, the kitchen sink and the television aerial. It is perfectly safe to use the telephone. There is no point in drawing the curtains, pulling down the blinds, covering mirrors or taking off metal-frame spectacles. Out of doors, solitary trees, walls, wire fences and other metallic structures such as sheds, park seats and tent-poles, ponds and river banks should be avoided. So also should flat open spaces, such as golf courses, where an individual may form the highest point. To use a metal-tipped umbrella or a golf club is asking for trouble. There is no risk inside a motor car, but it is wise to avoid moors or hills and make for the nearest low ground. If the storm is really severe, the safest thing is to lie down in a ditch. In Britain, there are around 10 deaths a year from being struck by lightning.

Treatment of an individual struck by lightning consists of artificial respiration, which may need to be prolonged for several hours.

LIGNOCAINE is a local anaesthetic. It is also used in the treatment of certain disorders of cardiac rhythm known as ventricular arrhythmias which may be particularly dangerous following a coronary thrombosis (qv).

LIMBS are outgrowths from the sides of the body, which, in man as in all the higher animals, number four. The limbs of all the higher animals, though differing much in outward appearance, are constructed on a similar plan, modified to suit the requirements of the owner, the fore-limb, for example, developing in birds into a wing, in seals into a flipper. In all, however, the various muscles, bones, and blood-vessels, though differing in size and shape, correspond in arrangement. Also, between the upper and lower limb, a strict comparison is possible, and the bones, muscles, and main arteries of the arm, forearm, and hand have all representatives in the thigh, leg, and foot. (See ARM; LEG.)

The union of the lower limb with the body is, however, more intimate than that of the upper limb. For, whilst the shoulder-blade and collar-bone of the upper limb are separated from the organs of the chest by the ribs and their muscles, the haunch-bone is applied on each side directly to the spine and forms the side of the pelvis.

In structure, each limb consists of four segments, the shoulder, arm, forearm, and hand in the case of the upper limb, corresponding to the haunch, thigh, leg, and foot in the lower limb. Upon the surface, the limb is enveloped by skin which, over the hand, is specially rich in its supply of sensory nerves. Beneath the skin is a layer of loose cellular tissue containing an amount of fat which varies with the corpulence of the individual. Next comes a strong layer of fibrous tissue, known as fascia, which provides a complete investment for the limb, and supplies a separate sheath for each muscle. The chief bulk of the limb is made up by the muscles or flesh. Finally, in the centre of the limb lie the bones which give it rigidity; and in general the large arteries and nerves are embedded among the muscles close to the bones.

The diseases affecting the limbs are those of the skin, muscles, bones, etc., forming them. (For injuries of the limbs see FRACTURES; HAEMORRHAGE; JOINTS, DISEASES AND INJURIES OF; WOUNDS.)

LIME, CALX, QUICKLIME, or OXIDE OF CALCIUM, is a caustic, highly infusible solid which is prepared by calcining white marble, Iceland-spar, lime-stone shells or other forms of calcium carbonate ($CaCO_3$). Heating calcium carbonate drives off carbon dioxide, leaving lime or CaO. If water is sprinkled on it, the lime swells up, becomes hot, and breaks down into a white powder, known as calcium hydroxide or hydrated lime or slaked lime, the chemical formula of which is $Ca(OH)_2$. If a large quantity of water is added to this, a thick white liquid is formed, known as milk of lime, which used to be for whitewashing walls. If the milk of lime is filtered, a clear liquid, having an alkaline reaction, and known as lime-water, is obtained. This lime-water contains a small amount of slaked lime in solution: about 1 part in 700 of water. Chlorinated lime is prepared by passing chlorine gas over slaked lime, and is much used for bleaching and for disinfection. (See CHLORINATED LIME.) When slaked lime is exposed to the air for some time it gradually hardens, as in mortar and plaster, changing into carbonate of lime. Carbonate of lime exists extensively naturally, being used in medicine in the form of chalk.

Action: Quicklime has a caustic action upon parts of the body with which it is brought in contact. It is a fairly common accident for quicklime or slaked lime to get into the eye, upon the delicate surface of which it is destructive. (See EYE DISEASES AND INJURIES.) Internally, lime-water and chalk have a soothing and astringent action upon the bowels, although lime is absorbed only to a small extent into the blood.

Uses: Lime-water mixed with milk is administered to invalids and children in order to make the curd less hard and so render this food more easily digested, and also in order to exert a soothing action upon the stomach when there is a tendency to vomit. For this purpose two or three tablespoonfuls are generally added to a tumblerful of milk. As an astringent in diarrhoea, Aromatic Chalk with Opium Mixture, BPC, is used in doses of 10 to 20 millilitres for an adult, and 2 to 5 millilitres for a young child.

LIME-JUICE is a yellow liquid obtained by squeezing lime-fruit, *Citrus limetta*. In common with lemon-juice, it is a rich source of vitamin C (16·8 to 62·5 mg per 100 ml) and contains a large quantity of citric acid. It is used as a refreshing drink and as a preventive of, and remedy for, scurvy (qv). Lime-juice which has been boiled, or preserved for a prolonged period, loses its anti-scorbutic properties.

LIMP (see CHILDREN, PECULIARITIES OF).

LINCOMYCIN is an antibiotic derived from *Streptomyceslincolnensis*. It is active against a relatively limited number of bacteria, including staphylococci, streptococci, pneumococci and *B. anthracis*.

LINCTUS is a term applied to any thick syrupy medicine. Most of these are remedies for excessive coughing.

LINEA ALBA is the line of fibrous tissue stretching down the mid-line of the belly from the lower end of the sternum to the pubic bone. The linea alba gives attachment to the muscles of the belly wall.

LINEA NIGRA: During pregnancy the linea alba (qv) becomes pigmented and appears as a dark line down the middle of the belly, and is called the *linea nigra*.

LINEAR ACCELERATOR (see RADIOTHERAPY).

LINIMENTS, or EMBROCATIONS, are preparations intended for external application, generally with rubbing. Almost all are of an oily nature, and are highly poisonous, being dispensed therefore in green or blue bottles. Liniments should never be kept alongside medicines intended for internal use, because many fatalities occur through careless administration, a dose being poured out of the wrong bottle. Among the chief liniments are: aconite, belladonna, and camphor liniments, often mixed together in equal parts to form ABC liniment, which is used for neuralgia, rheumatism, and other painful conditions; iodine liniment, used to paint over enlarged glands, and swollen joints; methyl salicylate liniment, used to apply in various painful rheumatic conditions; white liniment, which contains turpentine, used especially for sprains, bruises, and rheumatic conditions; liniment of ammonia, popularly known as 'hartshorn and oil', used for the same purpose; and soap liniment, known also as 'opodeldoc', of like application.

LINSEED is used either as the seeds or in the form of linseed meal obtained by grinding the seeds of *Linum usitatissimum*, the common flax.
Uses: Externally, linseed meal is used in poultices (qv); for internal use, linseed tea is an old domestic remedy for the treatment of cough.

LINT was originally made of teased-out linen; now it consists of a loose cotton fabric, one side of which is fluffy, the other being smooth and applied next to the skin when the surface is broken. Marine lint consists of tow impregnated with tar, and is used where large quantities of some absorbent and deodorizing dressing are required. Cotton lint is impregnated with various substances, the most common being boracic lint. Lint containing perchloride of iron (15 per cent) is valuable as a styptic.

LIPAEMIA means the presence of an excessive amount of fat in the blood.

LIPASE is an enzyme widely distributed in plants, and present also in the liver and gastric and pancreatic juices, which breaks down fats to the constituent fatty acids and glycerol.

LIPID is a term which is used rather loosely. Strictly speaking, it means a substance which is insoluble in water but soluble in fat solvents such as alcohol and ether. The important lipids, so far as medicine is concerned, are the fats (or triglycerides), and the phospholipids which play an important part in the functioning of the membranes of the cells of the body.

LIPODYSTROPHY is a congenital maldistribution of fat tissue. Subcutaneous fat is totally absent from a portion of the body and hypertrophied in the remainder. Another form of lipodystrophy occurs at the site of insulin injections. These are much less frequently seen nowadays as the new synthetic preparations of insulin are pure and unlikely to cause this reaction which was not uncommon with the older preparations. Occasionally the converse occurs at the site of insulin injections where the lipogenic action of insulin stimulates the fat cells to hypertrophy. This can also be disfiguring and usually results from using the same site for injections too frequently.

LIPOMA is a tumour mainly composed of fat. Such tumours arise in almost any part of the body, developing in fibrous tissues, particularly in that beneath the skin. They are simple in nature, and seldom give any trouble beyond that connected with their size and position. (See TUMOURS.)

LIPOSOMES are essentially tiny oil droplets consisting of layers of fatty material known as phospholipid separated by aqueous compartments. Drugs can be incorporated into the liposomes, which are then injected into the bloodstream or into the muscles, or given by mouth. Using this method of giving drugs, it is possible to protect them from being broken down in the body before they reach the part of the body where their curative effect is required: for example, in the liver or in a tumour.

LIPPITUDO means a chronic condition of inflammation at the margins of the eyelids, which ultimately renders the person 'bleareyed'.

LIPS form a pair of curtains before the mouth, each composed of a layer of skin and of mucous membrane, between which lies a considerable amount of fat and of muscle fibres.

The diseases to which the lips are liable are not numerous. *Fissures*, coming on in cold weather, form a troublesome condition often difficult to get rid of. Such peeling and cracking of the vermilion of the lips is common in those exposed for long periods to wind and sunlight. Treatment consists of the application of aqueous cream BP. If the main cause is excessive exposure to sunlight, in which case the lower lip is mainly affected, the best application is mexenone cream BPC. Mexenone is also available as a proprietary lipstick (Uvistat). *Herpes*, in the form of what are known as 'cold sores', often develops on the lip as a result of a cold or other feverish condition, but quickly passes off. (See HERPES.) *Ulcers* may form on the inner surface of the lip, usually in consequence of bad teeth or of dyspepsia, while in infants ulceration on the lips may be a sign of inherited syphilis. *Boils* sometimes form on the upper lip; if large they produce a serious condition. (See BOILS.) Small *cysts* sometimes form on the inner surface of the lip, and are seen as little bluish swellings filled with mucus; they are of no importance. *Hare-lip* is a deformity sometimes present at birth. (See PALATE, MALFORMATIONS OF.) *Cancer* of the lip sometimes occurs, almost always in men, and usually on the lower lip. (See also MOUTH, DISEASES OF.)

LIQUOR (see SOLUTION).

LIQUORICE is the root of *Glycyrrhiza glabra*, a plant of southern Europe and Asia. It is a mild expectorant, but is mainly used to cover the taste of disagreeable and more powerful drugs. Solid and liquid extracts are made from it, but the most commonly used preparation is compound liquorice powder, which contains also senna and sulphur. (See also GLYCYRRHETINIC ACID.)

LISTERIOSIS is an infectious, contagious disease of animals which is sometimes transmitted to man, in whom it usually affects the central nervous system, causing meningitis and encephalitis. It sometimes occurs in new-born babies as a result of infection through the placenta from the mother. The causative microorganism is *Listeria monocytogenes*. The infection responds well to penicillin and other antibiotics. There were 32 cases of meningitis and 54 of septicaemia reported in 1984. In 1987, 200 cases were reported.

LITHAGOGUE is the term given to any agent which expels calculi from the body.

LITHIASIS is a general name applied to the formation of calculi and concretions in tissues or organs: eg. cholelithiasis means the formation of calculi in the gall-bladder.

LITHIUM CARBONATE is a drug widely used in the treatment of certain forms of mental illness. About one person in two thousand in Britain is said to be prescribed it. The major indication for its use is acute mania. It induces improvement or remission in over 70 per cent of such patients. In addition, it is effective in the treatment of manic-depressive patients, preventing both the manic and the depressive episodes. There is also evidence that it lessens aggression in prisoners who behave antisocially and in mentally retarded patients who mutilate themselves and have temper tantrums. It is not recommended for children. Because of its possible toxic effects it is a drug that must only be administered under medical supervision and with monitoring of the blood levels. Because of the risk of its damaging the unborn child, it should not be prescribed, unless absolutely necessary, during pregnancy, particularly in the first three months. Neither should mothers take it while breast feeding as it is excreted in the milk in high concentrations.

LITHOPAEDION is a foetus which has died while in the mother's body and has become calcified.

LITHOTOMY is the operation of cutting for stone in the bladder. The operation is of great historic interest, because more has probably been written about it in early times than about any other department of surgery, and because, for long, it formed almost the only operation in which the surgeon dared to attack diseases of the internal organs. It seems, from the fact that large numbers of people were cut for stone, and also from the fact that this operation remained, in France at least, in the hands of a special class of surgeons, referred to as lithotomists, that stone in the bladder must have been far commoner two or three centuries ago than it is today.

LITHOTRIPSY: Extracorporeal shock-wave lithotripsy (ESWL) causes disintegration of renal stones without contact and is therefore an attractive procedure both for patients with renal stones and for their surgeons. Urolithiasis of the upper urinary tract is a common condition in the United Kingdom causing considerable morbidity and requiring large and lengthy operations with an extensive convalescent period. Percutaneous renal surgery has changed this picture but it requires at least puncture of the kidney and possibly open nephrolithotomy for large branched calculi. Extracorporeal shock-wave lithotripsy causes disintegration of the stone without contact and is therefore a far more attractive procedure.

The generation of shock waves as a form of treatment for urinary calculi was first described in 1955 by the Russian engineer Yutkin. Shock waves generated outside the body can be accurately focused with a reflector whilst the patient is suspended in water to facilitate transmission of the waves. These are focused on the calculus. The resultant fine fragments are passed spontaneously in the urine with minimal, if any, discomfort. The procedure has been shown to be safe and effective and is most acceptable to patients. It is clearly a specialised urological procedure. There is an extremely brief convalescent period after discharge which affects large savings to the hospital, patient and community. A report of the first 50 patients treated for upper tract urinary calculi by ESWL has recently been published and the average stay for an in-patient was 3·7 days. All patients suffered minimal post-operative discomfort and nearly all resumed normal activity within one day after discharge.

LITHOTRITY, or LITHOLAPAXY, is the term applied to the operation in which a stone in the bladder is crushed by an instrument introduced along the urethra, and the fragments washed out through a catheter. It has now, to a great extent, replaced lithotomy, except in patients in whom a stone is very hard and very large, and in boys whose urethra is too small to admit the passage of a lithotrite. The lithotrite, or stone-crusher, consists of two blades, one of which fits into a groove in the other, so that, when the inner blade is screwed home, the lithotrite is little larger than and similar in shape to a catheter, and can be easily passed along the urethra. The instrument is made of tough steel and provided with a powerful screw, so that when fragments of stone are caught between the blades they are easily crushed.

LITMUS, which is prepared from several lichens, is a vegetable dye-substance, which on contact with alkaline fluids becomes blue, and on contact with acid fluids, red. Slips of paper, impregnated with litmus, form a valuable test for the acidity of the secretions and discharges.

LITTLE'S DISEASE is a form of cerebral palsy. (See CEREBRAL PALSY.)

LIVE-FLESH is a popular term applied to fine muscular tremors or twitchings seen especially in the eyelids and muscles of the hands. It is usually due simply to tiredness caused by overuse of the twitching muscles, but when persistent it may be a sign of some serious nervous disorder, such as progressive muscular atrophy.

LIVER: The liver is a solid organ of dark-brown colour and the largest gland in the body. It discharges several functions, acting both as an excreting organ and as an elaborator and storehouse of nourishment.

Form: The shape of the liver is generally described as that of a right-angled triangular prism, with the right angle rounded off. It has five surfaces, superior, anterior, right, posterior, and inferior, of which the anterior and posterior surfaces are triangular, with the base towards the right side and tapering off to the left. The surfaces are separated from one another by rounded margins, except in the case of the lower surface, which is divided from the right, front, and upper surfaces by a sharp edge. The organ is divided also into four lobes. The great bulk of it constitutes the right lobe; the left lobe is small and extends a little way into the left half of the abdomen, to end in a sharp left border, whilst the quadrate and caudate lobes are two small divisions upon the back and under surface. About the middle of the under surface, towards the back, is placed the porta hepatis, a transverse fissure, by which the hepatic artery and portal vein carry blood into the liver, and by which the right and left hepatic ducts emerge, carrying off the bile formed in the liver. The *gall-bladder* is attached to the under surface of the right lobe and projects from beneath the lower margin, where, if distended, it may be felt as a rounded swelling immediately beneath the end of the ninth rib. The connection of the gall-bladder – in which bile is stored –with the liver is rather complicated. The hepatic ducts emerge at the porta hepatis, one coming from the right and one from the left lobe. They immediately join to form the common hepatic duct, which is about 3 cm (1¼ inches) long, and joins the cystic duct, coming from the gall-bladder, at an acute angle. The hepatic and cystic ducts by their union form the bile duct, which is about 75 mm (3 inches) in length, and opens into the small intestine. Bile, which passes down from the liver by the hepatic duct, may either pass directly into the bile duct and so into the intestine, or it may pass upwards through the cystic duct into the gall-bladder, to be stored there, and later retraces its way through the cystic duct to the bile duct, and so to the intestine. The cystic duct and gall-bladder therefore together form a cul-de-sac in the bile passages.

Position: The liver occupies the right-hand upper portion of the abdominal cavity. Its upper surface is in contact with the diaphragm, which also separates its right surface from the right lower ribs. About four-fifths of the organ lies to the right of the middle line of the body. As it is of a rounded shape it fills up the dome of the diaphragm, the lower part of the right lung being hollowed out to receive the liver, from which it is separated only by the diaphragm and pleural membrane. The liver, in turn, rests upon various abdominal organs, the right kidney and suprarenal gland, the large intestine, the duodenum, and the stomach all making impressions upon it. In addition, the liver is swung from the walls of the abdomen by five ligaments, four of which consist of thickened parts of the peritoneal membrane lining the whole abdominal cavity, and reflected from the upper part of the liver to its walls. These are the coronary ligament, right and left triangular ligaments, falciform ligament, and a dense fibrous cord, the round ligament, or ligamentum teres.

Dimensions: The vertical thickness of the liver amounts, towards the right side, to over 12 cm (5 inches), and its extent from side to side is considerably more. Its weight is over 1·5 kg (50 ounces), varying with the size of the person, but making up about $\frac{1}{40}$ or thereabout of the whole body weight. In young children it is relatively larger, accounting, to a large extent, for their protuberant abdomen, and making up about $\frac{1}{18}$ of the weight of the whole body.

Vessels: The blood supply of the organ differs from that of any other part of the body, in that the blood collected from the stomach and bowels into the portal vein does not pass directly to the heart, but is distributed to the liver, in the substance of which the portal vein breaks up into capillary vessels. The effect of this is that some harmful substances, absorbed from the stomach and bowels, are abstracted from the blood-stream and destroyed, while various consituents of the food are stored up in the liver for gradual use. In addition, the liver receives a large hepatic artery from the coeliac axis, which also distributes branches to the stomach and pancreas, this blood supply serving to nourish the organ. After the blood has circulated through capillaries, it is collected together from both sources and emptied into the hepatic veins, which pass directly from the back surface of the liver into the inferior vena cava.

Minute structure: The liver is enveloped in a capsule of fibrous tissue, Glisson's capsule, from which strands run along the vessels, and, penetrating to the farthest recesses of the organ, bind its structure together. The hepatic artery, portal vein, and bile-duct divide and subdivide, the branches of each lying alongside corresponding divisions of the other two, till the finest divisions of artery, vein, and bile-duct, known as interlobular vessels, lie between the lobules, of which the whole gland is built up. These lobules, each about the size of a pin's head, form each in itself a complete secreting unit, and the liver is built up of many hundred thousands of such exactly similar lobules.

A lobule has the following structure: from the small vessels lying round its margin capillaries, or sinusoids, lined with stellate Kupffer cells (qv), are given off which run in towards the centre of the lobule, where they empty into a small central vein. These central veins from neighbouring lobules collect together, and ultimately the blood passes into the hepatic veins, and so leaves the liver. Between the capillaries, which radiate from the central vein to the edge

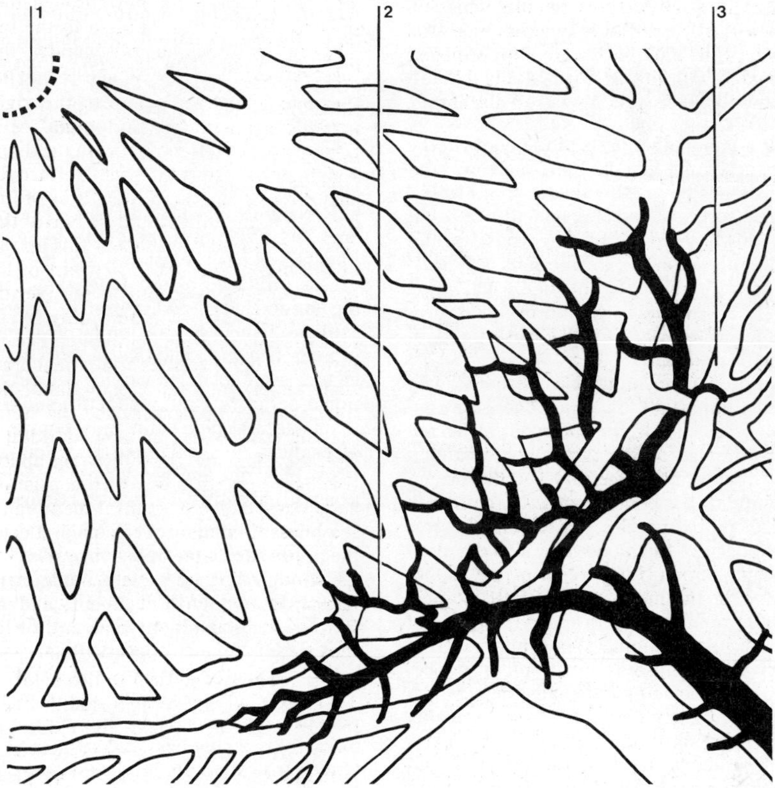

1 central vein connected by network of sinusoids with 2
2 interlobular bile-duct commencing in network of intercellular bile-canaliculi within the lobule
3 peripheral or interlobular veins

Diagram of liver lobule.

of the lobule, lie rows of large liver cells, these forming the distinctive tissue of the organ, upon which its activity depends. Between the rows of cells also lie fine bile capillaries, which collect the bile produced by the cells and discharge it into the bile-ducts lying along the margins of the lobules. The liver cells are among the largest cells in the body, and each contains one or two large, round nuclei. In the cells can often be seen droplets of fat or granules of glycogen, ie. animal starch.

Functions: The liver is a vast chemical factory. The heat produced by the chemical changes taking place in it forms an important contribution to the general warming of the body. The liver secretes bile, the chief constituents of which are the bile salts (sodium glycocholate and taurocholate), the bile pigments (bilirubin and biliverdin), cholesterol, and lecithin. The bile acids from which the salts are obtained are formed in the liver by the union of glycine and taurine with cholic acid. The bile salts are absorbed from the intestine and so find their way back to the liver again. The bile pigments are the iron-free and globin-free remnant of haemoglobin, being formed in the Kupffer cells of the liver. Bile pigments can, however, be formed in many other parts of the body: in the spleen, the lymph glands, bone-marrow, connective tissues (giving the colour to a bruise). Bile, then, serves to excrete pigment, the result of breakdown of old red blood corpuscles, and to aid the digestion of fat. Bile salts aid digestion of fat by emulsifying the fat, by activating pancreatic lipase, and by promoting fat absorption. Bile is necessary for the absorption of vitamins D and E.

In addition to forming bile the liver has a number of important functions. These are enumerated briefly: (1) In the embryo it forms red blood corpuscles, and in the adult stores vitamin B, a substance necessary for the proper functioning of the bone-marrow in the manufacture of red corpuscles. (2) It manufactures the fibrinogen of the blood, and also the albumin and globulin. (3) It stores iron and copper necessary for the manufacture of red corpuscles. (4) It produces heparin and, with the aid of vitamin K, prothrombin. (5) Its Kupffer cells in the liver blood-sinusoids are an important element in the reticulo-endothelial system, which breaks down red corpuscles, and probably manufactures antibodies. (6) It detoxicates noxious products made in the intestine and absorbed into the blood. (7) It stores carbohydrate in the form of glycogen, and maintains the two-way process: glucose $\rightleftarrows$ glycogen. (8) It forms vitamin A from carotene and stores the B vitamins. (9) It splits up amino-acids and manufactures urea and uric acids. (10) It plays an essential part in the storage and metabolism of fat.

LIVER DISEASES: The liver may be extensively diseased without any very urgent symptoms, unless the circulation through it is impeded, the outflow of bile checked, or neighbouring organs implicated. Jaundice, which is a symptom of several liver disorders, is dealt with elsewhere. Ascites, which may be caused by interference with the circulation through the portal vein of the liver, as well as by other causes, is also considered separately. The presence of gall-stones is a complication of some diseases connected with the liver, and is treated under GALL-BLADDER, DISEASES OF. For hydatid cyst of the liver see TAENIASIS.

INFLAMMATION OF THE LIVER, or HEPATITIS, may occur as part of a generalized infection or may be a localized condition. Infectious hepatitis, which is the result of infection with a virus, is one of the most common forms of hepatitis. (See HEPATITIS, ACUTE INFECTIVE.) There are many other viruses that can cause hepatitis, including that responsible for glandular fever (qv). Certain spirochaetes may also be the cause, particularly that responsible for leptospirosis (qv), as can many drugs. In tropical countries amoebic hepatitis, which often goes on to abscess formation, is an important complication of amoebic dysentery. (See ABSCESS, CHRONIC; DYSENTERY.) Other tropical conditions in which the liver is always involved include malaria and yellow fever. Hepatitis may also occur if there is obstruction of the bile duct, as by a gall-stone.

CIRRHOSIS OF THE LIVER: The cause of cirrhosis (qv) of the liver is still obscure. Experimentally it has been shown that the condition can be produced by a deficiency of certain of the amino-acids found in protein, but this only explains a small proportion of the cases found in man. It is probable that in most cases three factors are involved in varying degrees: a nutritional deficiency, a toxic factor, and an infective factor. Alcohol is the most common cause of cirrhosis in the United Kingdom and the USA. In Africa and many parts of Asia, infection with hepatitis B virus is a common cause.

Symptoms: In one form of cirrhosis the liver is much contracted (atrophic or coarse cirrhosis), its blood-vessels are pressed upon, and ascites results. In another form there is great enlargement of the organ (hypertrophic or biliary cirrhosis) and jaundice appears. In all cases there is loss of appetite and other signs of dyspepsia. There is a variable degree of anaemia. There may be a low-grade fever. In a certain number of cases, two characteristic signs may appear. One is so-called spider naevi (see NAEVUS). Each has a central red spot and may measure up to a centimetre in diameter. They rarely appear below the waist. The nose-bleeds which occur in around 20 per cent of cases may be due to naevi in the nose. The other is so-called liver palms, or reddening of the palms of the hands, most marked on the ball of the thumb and the outer edge of the hand.

Treatment: Nothing can be done to repair a cirrhosed organ, but the cause, if known, must be removed and further advance of the process thus prevented. In the case of the liver a high-protein, high-carbohydrate, low-fat diet is

given, supplemented by liver extract and vitamins B and K. The consumption of alcohol should be banned.
ABSCESS OF THE LIVER: When an abscess develops in the liver, it is usually a manifestation of amoebic dysentery, appearing sometimes late in the disease, even after the diarrhoea is cured. It may also follow upon inflammation of the liver due to other causes; and abscesses may form in this organ as in other sites in cases of blood-poisoning. The symptoms of abscess are much the same as in other types of inflammation, only they are more pronounced, and accompanied often by rigors, severe pain over the liver which may also be referred to the right shoulder, and by great enlargement of the liver. In the case of an amoebic abscess treatment consists of oral metronidazole. Aspiration of the contents of the abscess is now rarely necessary.
ACUTE YELLOW ATROPHY, or ACUTE HEPATIC NECROSIS as it is now known, is a destructive and often fatal disease of the liver which is very rare. It may be due to chemical poisons, such as carbon tetrachloride, chloroform, phosphorus and industrial solvents derived from benzene. It may also be the cause of death in cases of poisoning with fungi. Very occasionally it may be a complication of acute infectious hepatitis. It is also a rare complication of pregnancy. It sets in with a slight degree of jaundice, which cannot be distinguished from simple jaundice, and lasts several days. Then the jaundice suddenly deepens, there is pain in the region of the liver, convulsions and delirium appear, the heart grows very weak, and death ensues in a day or two. Crystals of leucine and tyrosine are found in the urine. The destruction of the liver as a secreting organ may be complete, but occasionally areas here and there only are affected, and recovery may then take place with restoration of the damaged areas after a prolonged illness.
CANCER OF THE LIVER is not uncommon, although it is rare for the disease to begin in the liver, the involvement of this organ being usually secondary to disease situated somewhere in the stomach or bowels. Cancer originating in the liver is more common in Asia and Africa. It usually arises in a fibrotic (or cirrhotic) liver and in carriers of the hepatitis B virus. There is great emaciation, which increases as the disease progresses. The liver is much enlarged, and its margin and surface are rough, being studded with hard cancer masses of varying size, which can often be felt through the abdominal wall. Pain may be present. Jaundice and oedema often appear. (See also TRANSPLANTATION.)

LIVER-FLUKE is the popular name of *Fasciola hepatica*, a parasite which infests sheep, and which is occasionally found in the bile-passages and liver of man. (See FASCIOLIASIS.)

LIVER PILLS (see CHOLAGOGUES).

LIVER SPOT is a popular term applied to brownish marks which appear on the skin, especially of the face. This is sometimes caused by the growth of a parasite (*Tinea versicolor*) in the surface layers of the epidermis. It also frequently accompanies pregnancy or the presence of abdominal tumours. It may also be due simply to some long-continued form of local irritation.

LOBE is the term applied to the larger divisions of various organs, such as to the four lobes of the liver, the three lobes of the right and the two lobes of the left lung, which are separated by fissures from one another, and to the lobes or superficial areas into which the brain is divided. The term lobar is applied to structures which are connected with lobes of organs, or to diseases which have a tendency to be limited by the boundaries of lobes, such as lobar pneumonia.

LOBECTOMY is the operation of cutting out a lobe of the lung in such diseases as abscess of the lung and bronchiectasis.

LOBELIA, or INDIAN TOBACCO, is a remedy used for asthma. It consists of the leaves and tops of *Lobelia inflata*, a common weed in the United States. In large doses, it causes vomiting and paralyses the heart's action, being a dangerous poison, but in moderate doses it relieves the spasm to which asthma is due. It is a constituent of many burning powders made for smoking by asthmatics, but it is more commonly used in the form of tincture of lobelia combined with other drugs.

LOBOTOMY is the cutting of a lobe.

LOBSTER CLAW (see CLEFT FOOT).

LOBSTER FOOT (see CLEFT FOOT).

LOBSTER HAND (see CLEFT HAND).

LOBULE is the term applied to a division of an organ smaller than a lobe: for example, the lobules of the lung are of the size of millet seeds, those of the liver slightly larger. Lobules form the smallest subdivisions or units of an organ, each lobule being similar to the others, of which there may be perhaps several hundred thousand in the organ.

LOCHIA is the discharge which takes place during the first week or two after child-birth. During the first four days it consists chiefly of blood; after the fifth day the colour should become paler, and after the first week the quantity should diminish and the appearance be creamy. There should at no time be any putrid odour, the presence of this being an indication of dangerous septic infection. The presence of blood after the second week indicates that the patient has been too active or that the natural absorptive changes are not duly taking place. (See PUERPERIUM.)

LOCKJAW is a prominent symptom of tetanus (qv) and is the popular name for this condition.

LOCOMOTOR ATAXIA (see TABES DORSALIS).

LOFEPRAMINE (GAMANIL) (see ANTIDEPRESSANTS).

LOGORRHOEA is the technical term for garrulousness, a feature which may be exaggerated in certain states of mental instability.

LOGWOOD (see HAEMATOXYLON).

LOIASIS is the disease caused by the filarial worm *Loa loa*, a thread-like worm which differs from *W. bancrofti* in that it is shorter and thicker, and it is found in the blood-stream during the day, not at night. It is transmitted by the mango fly, *Chrysops dimidiata*, but other flies of this genus can also transmit it. It is confined to West and Central Africa. The characteristic feature of the disease is the appearance of fugitive swellings which may arise anywhere in the body in the course of the worm's migration through the body. These are known as Calabar swellings. The worm is often found in the eye, hence the old name of the worm in Africa – the eye worm. Satisfactory results are being reported from the use of diethylcarbamazine in the treatment of this form of filariasis (qv).

LOIN is the name applied to the part of the back between the lower ribs and the pelvis. (For pain in the loins see BACKACHE; LUMBAGO.)

LONG-SIGHT (see REFRACTION).

LOPERAMIDE is a drug that is proving of value in the treatment of diarrhoea.

LOPRAZOLAM (DORMONOCT) (see BENZODIAZEPINES).

LORAZEPAM is a tranquillizer that is proving of value as a sedative for administration before operation. Its advantage, compared with other similar drugs, is that it stimulates, rather than depresses, breathing. It is used in the treatment of pre-eclampsia (qv) on the grounds that it has less of a depressant effect on the new-born child than other tranquillizers.

LORDOSIS means an unnatural curvature of the spine forwards. It occurs chiefly in the lumbar region, where the natural curve is forwards, as the result of muscular weakness, spinal disease, etc. (See SPINAL COLUMN.)

LORMETAZEPAM (LORAMET, NOCTAMID) (see BENZODIAZEPINES).

LOSS OF BLOOD (see HAEMORRHAGE).

LOTIONS are fluid preparations intended for bringing in contact with, or for washing, the external surface of the body. Lotions are generally of a watery or alcoholic composition, and many of them are known as 'liquors'. Those external applications which are of an oily nature, and intended to be rubbed into the surface, are known as liniments.

LOUSE (see INSECTS IN RELATION TO DISEASE).

LOZENGES, also known as TROCHES, or TROCHISCI, consist of small tablets containing drugs mixed with sugar, gum, glycerin-jelly, or fruit-paste. They are used in various affections of the mouth and throat, being sucked and slowly dissolved by the saliva, which brings the drugs they contain in contact with the affected surface. Some of the substances used in lozenges are benzalkonium, benzocaine, betamethasone, bismuth, formaldehyde, hydrocortisone, liquorice, penicillin.

LUES is the Latin word for a serious infectious disease, the term being especially applied to syphilis.

LUGOL'S SOLUTION is a compound solution of iodine and potassium iodide.

LUMBAGO is a term applied to a painful ailment affecting the muscles of the lower part of the back, generally regarded as of rheumatic origin. It is the cause of 60 per cent of sickness absence due to rheumatism and 15 per cent of total sickness absence from work. The incidence of backache among nurses is said to be greater than among manual workers in industry, and it is estimated that 20,000 nurses a year sustain back injury as a result of lifting and moving patients. (See also BACKACHE; PROLAPSED INTERVERTEBRAL DISC; RHEUMATISM.)

Cause: Lumbago seems to be brought on by exposure to cold and damp, and by other exciting causes of rheumatism. Sometimes it follows a strain of the muscles of the loins. The pain accompanying rheumatic manifestations in this region is believed to be due to an inflammatory condition in the connective tissues of the muscles, causing congestion of the blood-vessels and consequent pressure upon the endings of the sensory nerves. To this condition the term *fibrositis* is applied. Lumbago is specially apt to occur in the back muscles after they have been the seat of a strain or other injury leading probably to a tear in the muscle fibres, and the pain in such a case is largely produced by violent spasm of the surrounding muscle. A not uncommon cause is a prolapsed intervertebral disc (qv). In other cases lumbago occurs in gouty subjects and the attacks take the place of an ordinary attack of gout.

Symptoms: An attack of lumbago may occur alone, or be associated with rheumatism in other parts of the body at the time. It usually comes on as a seizure, often sudden, of pain in one or both sides of the small of the back, of a severe cutting or stabbing character, greatly aggravated on movement of the body, especially in attempting to rise from the recumbent posture, and also in the acts of drawing a deep breath, coughing, or sneezing. So intense may it be that it is apt to suggest the existence of inflammation in some of the neighbouring internal organs, such as the kidneys or bowels. The attack is in general short but occasionally it continues for a long time, not in such an acute form as at first, but rather as a feeling of soreness and stiffness on movement.

Prevention: Care should be exercised in performing any exertion involving bending of the back.

Treatment: The treatment includes that for rheumatic affections in general (see RHEUMATISM), and the application of local remedies of counter-irritant nature, such as hot fomentations with turpentine or laudanum applied by means of flannel to the part; or the rubbing in, if this can be borne, of liniments. The old and homely plan of counter-irritation by applying a heated iron to the part with a sheet of brown paper or blanket interposed is often beneficial in chronic cases. The hot-air bath, and various electrical applications, including faradization, static breeze, diathermy, and high-frequency currents, are also of value. Should there be localized areas of tenderness, the injection into these of procaine may give relief. During the acute stages, relief is obtained from the taking of analgesics such as aspirin. (See BATHS; ELECTRICITY IN MEDICINE.)

LUMBAR is a term used to denote structures in, or diseases affecting, the region of the loins, as, for example, the lumbar vertebrae, lumbar abscess.

LUMBAR PUNCTURE is a procedure for removing cerebrospinal fluid from the spinal canal in the lumbar region in order: (1) to diagnose disease of the nervous system; (2) to introduce medicaments: spinal anaesthetics, or drugs, or serum.

LUMBRICUS is a name sometimes applied to the roundworm or *Ascaris lumbricoides*. (See ASCARIASIS.)

LUNAR CAUSTIC is another name for nitrate of silver.

LUNATIC is a general term applied to people of disordered mind, because lunacy was supposed at one time to be largely influenced by the moon. (See MENTAL ILLNESS.)

LUNGS: The lungs form a pair of organs situated in the chest, and discharge the function of respiration. (See RESPIRATION.) Whilst this is their primary function, they also act as a filter for the blood. The air, which enters through the nose and passes down the throat, larynx, and windpipe in succession (see AIR PASSAGES), reaches the lungs by the right and left bronchial tubes, into which the windpipe divides within the chest, at the level of the second rib. The texture of the lungs is very highly elastic, so that when the chest is opened each lung collapses to about one-third of its natural bulk.

Form and position: Each lung is roughly conical in shape, with an apex projecting into the neck, and a base resting upon the diaphragm. The rounded outer surface of each is in contact with the ribs of its own side, while the heart, lying between the lungs, hollows out the inner surface of each to some extent. There is an anterior border, along which the outer and inner surfaces meet, and the borders of the two lungs touch one another for a short distance behind the middle of the breast-bone. The apex, which is blunt, extends 35 mm (1½inches) or more into the neck above the line of the collar-bone, being covered here by the muscles of the neck. The base is deeply hollowed, in correspondence with the domed shape of the diaphragm, which is pushed up by the liver on the right side, and by the stomach and spleen on the left. The right lung is split by two deep fissures into three lobes; the left has two lobes divided by a single fissure. The weight of the two lungs together is about 1·1 kg, the right being rather heavier than the left. The lungs of men are heavier than those of women. There is a tendency for lung mass to increase throughout life. Each lung is enveloped in a membrane, the pleura or pleural membrane, in such a way that one layer of the membrane is closely adherent to the lung, from which indeed it cannot be separated, while the other layer lines the inner surface of one half of the chest. These two layers form a closed cavity, the pleural cavity, which everywhere surrounds the lung except at the point where the bronchi and vessels enter it. This cavity is, in the natural state, a merely potential space, the two layers of pleural membrane being separated only by a thin layer of fluid, which enables them to glide with very little friction over one another as the lung expands and retracts in breathing; but, in certain states, fluid collects in the pleural cavity, so that several pints of fluid may be effused there, compressing the lung. In some circumstances air escapes into the pleural cavity, and the lung then collapses temporarily upon its root, but air in the pleural cavity is usually absorbed, and the lung comes to occupy its original volume.

Colour: In children, the colour of the lungs is rose-pink but, as life advances, they become more and more of a slaty hue, mottled with streaks and patches of dark grey and black, which are due to deposits in the lymph spaces of dust inhaled on the breath. Eskimos and others who live in an atmosphere free from dust retain the colour of childhood; on the other hand, the lungs of coal-miners become often of an almost uniform jet-black shade.

Changes at birth: Before birth, and in stillborn children, the lungs are of a yellowish colour, of solid gland-like appearance, and packed away in the back of the chest. Further, such lungs do not float in water, and their weight amounts to about 1/70 of the whole body-weight. Immediately upon birth a remarkable change takes place: the tissue of the lungs expands, like the petals of an opening flower; the colour changes to rose-red, and the weight is suddenly doubled from the inrush of blood; the consistency becomes spongy, as air is drawn into the lungs, and if the child should die after drawing a few breaths, any portion of the lung which may be cut off floats in water. These changes are of importance, from the medico-legal point of view, in determining whether a dead infant was born alive or not.

Connections with heart: Not only does the heart lie in contact with the two lungs, so that changes in the volume of the lungs cannot fail to have an effect upon the heart's action, but the heart is also connected by vessels with both lungs. The pulmonary artery passes from the right ventricle and divides into two branches, one of which runs straight outwards to each lung, entering its substance along with the bronchial tube at the hilum or root of the lung. From this point also emerge the pulmonary veins, which carry the blood purified in the lungs back to the left atrium.

Minute structure: Each main bronchial tube, entering the lung at the root, divides into branches, which subdivide again and again, to be distributed all through the substance of the lung, till the finest tubes, known as respiratory bronchioles, have a width of only 0·25 mm (1/100 inch). In structure, all these tubes consist of a mucous membrane surrounded by a fibrous sheath. The windpipe as well as the larger and medium bronchi have in the fibrous layer large pieces of cartilage, which in the windpipe and largest bronchial tubes form regular hoops, and in the medium-sized tubes are disposed as irregular plates. These pieces of cartilage have the function of preventing the tubes from closing or being compressed, and so obstructing the passage of air. The larger and medium bronchi are richly supplied with glands secreting mucus, which is poured out upon the surface of the membrane. This surface is composed of columnar epithelial cells, which are provided with cilia. These have a co-ordinated beating action which sweeps mucus and bacteria upwards towards the throat. The wall of the bronchial tubes is rich in fibres of elastic tissue, and immediately beneath the mucous membrane is a layer of circularly placed unstriped muscle fibres, which is specially well developed in the smaller bronchi. This muscular layer plays an important role in the removal of mucus by coughing; it is also of great importance in connection with the causation of asthma. (See ASTHMA.)

The smallest divisions of the bronchial tubes, or bronchioles, divide into a number of tortuous tubes known as alveolar ducts and these branch into expanded passages known as atria, each of which leads into a terminal air saccule. The walls of the alveolar ducts, atria and air saccules are covered with minute sacs, known as alveoli, of which there are around 300 million. Each alveolus consists of a delicate membrane composed of flattened, plate-like cells, strengthened by a wide network of elastic fibres, to which the great elasticity of the lung is due; and in these thin-walled air-cells the important function of the lungs is carried on.

The branches of the pulmonary artery accompany the bronchial tubes to the farthest recesses of the lung, dividing like the latter into finer and finer branches, and ending in a dense network of capillaries, which lies everywhere between the air-vesicles, the capillaries being so closely placed that they occupy a much greater area than the spaces between them. The air in the air-vesicles is separated therefore from the blood only by two delicate membranes: the wall of the air-vesicle and the capillary wall, through which an exchange of gases readily takes place. The blood from the capillaries is collected by the pulmonary veins, which also accompany the bronchi to the root of the lung.

Another and much smaller set of bronchial blood-vessels runs actually upon the walls of the bronchial tubes, and these serve the purpose of nourishing the lung tissue.

There is in the lung also an important system of lymph vessels, which start in spaces situated between the air-vesicles, under the pleural membrane and in the walls of the bronchial tubes. These vessels leave the lung along with the blood-vessels, and are connected with a chain of bronchial glands lying near the end of the windpipe.

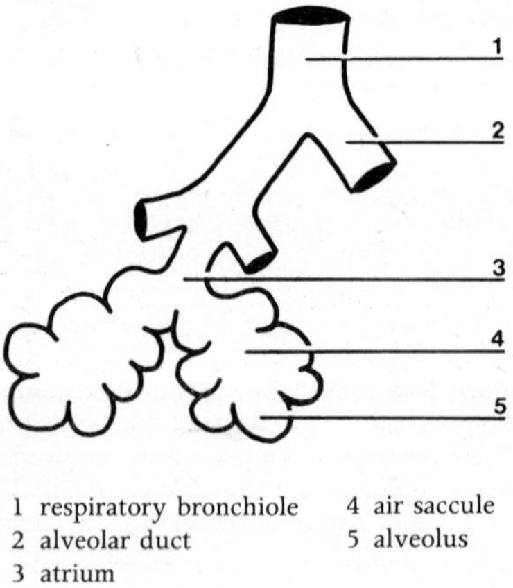

Diagram of the internal divisions of the air tubes.

LUNG DISEASES: The general symptoms and signs produced by disease of the lungs are mentioned under CHEST DISEASES and the chief affections to which these organs are liable are also treated under special headings. (See BRONCHIECTASIS; BRONCHITIS; CHEST, DEFORMITIES OF; CHILLS AND COLDS; EMPHYSEMA; EXPECTORATION; HAEMOPTYSIS; HAEMORRHAGE; PLEURISY; PNEUMONIA; OCCUPATIONAL DISEASES; PULMONARY EMBOLISM; TUBERCULOSIS.)

INFLAMMATION OF THE LUNGS is generally known as pneumonia when it is due to infection, as alveolitis when the inflammation is immunological and as pneumonitis when it is due to physical or chemical agents. (See PNEUMONIA.)

ABSCESS OF THE LUNG is a comparatively rare condition, and consists, like abscesses elsewhere, of a collection of pus in one or more areas of the lung. It may result from an acute pneumonia which does not clear up properly, or it may be due to a wound of the lung from without, or to the presence of foreign bodies, such as buttons, pins, or fragments of food, which have been sucked down the air passages. An abscess may also occur in the lung, as in other organs, during the course of blood poisoning (pyaemia), or may be produced by the bursting of an abscess into the lung after its formation in some neighbouring organ. The condition may be difficult to differentiate from cavity formation due to tuberculosis, although the failure to find tubercle bacilli in the expectoration, after repeated examination, is an important point against the latter condition.

An abscess in the lung may burst into one of the bronchial tubes, and, after the pus is spat up, healing and recovery may take place. Most cases respond to appropriate antibiotics and postural drainage (qv) but occasionally it may be necessary to resort to surgery and drain the abscess through the chest wall.

GANGRENE OF THE LUNG may also follow pneumonia in those of poor constitution or debilitated by serious illness. Just as in the case of gangrene of the limbs, a portion of lung dies and putrefies, giving rise to a most offensive smell, as the dead and broken-down lung tissue is spat up. The prospect of recovery is small, even when the portion of lung involved is very limited.

CONGESTION OF THE LUNGS is a term which is used in two quite different senses. The term is popularly used for acute inflammation of the lung in its early stages. When the patient recovers after a few days, the illness is often described as an attack of acute congestion.

In a strict medical sense, the term is used to mean quite a different condition of a more chronic nature: passive or mechanical congestion of the blood-vessels in the lungs due to some defect in the pumping action of the heart. Passive congestion arises under two sets of conditions. A very serious form, known as hypostatic congestion, arises when the heart is failing, towards the end of severe and long-continued fevers, such as typhoid fever; after severe surgical operations; and in old people who, for any reason, such as the occurrence of a broken leg, are confined for some weeks to bed. It occurs in the back parts of the lungs, as the feeble heart is unable to drive out the blood which gravitates into these dependent parts. Inflammation is very apt to arise in these congested parts, and hypostatic pneumonia often ends the life of old or feeble people confined to bed. The other form of passive congestion is due, not so much to weakness in the pumping action of the heart, as to some obstruction which hinders the escape of blood from the lungs into the left atrium of the heart. Narrowing of the opening which leads from the left atrium to the left ventricle (mitral stenosis) is the chief cause of this, and, although the condition is by no means so serious as the hypostatic form of congestion, it predisposes the people affected by this form of heart disease to sharp attacks of blood-spitting on exertion, to bronchitis, and to pneumonia. The treatment, in both cases, must be directed towards the heart.

OEDEMA OF THE LUNGS results when the left ventricle myocardium is unable to handle the blood delivered to it. There is an abrupt increase in the venous and capillary pressure in the pulmonary vessels followed by flooding of fluid into the interstitial spaces and alveoli. The commonest cause of acute pulmonary oedema is myocardial infarction which reduces the ability of the left ventricular myocardial muscle to handle the blood delivered to it. Pulmonary oedema may result from other causes of left ventricular failure such as hypertension or valvular disease of the mitral and aortic valves. The initial symptoms are cough with breathlessness and occasionally with wheezing. The patient becomes extremely short of breath with a sensation of imminent death. In a severe attack the patient is pale, sweating and cyanosed and obviously gasping for breath. Frequently frothy suputum is produced which may be blood stained.

COLLAPSE OF THE LUNG occurs under several conditions. The lungs are so resilient in consequence of the elastic fibres with which they are everywhere interspersed that, if air is admitted to the pleural cavities, the lungs immediately collapse to a third of their natural bulk. Accordingly, if one side of the chest is wounded and air is admitted (pneumothorax), the lung collapses, although, after the wound is healed, the air is absorbed from the pleural cavity and the lung quickly regains its size. Also, when fluid is effused into the pleural cavity the lung is compressed and collapses, and if the fluid is not absorbed or drawn off within some weeks, the collapse is apt to be permanent through the formation of adhesions round the lung. Again, if anything blocks a bronchial tube, the part of the lung to which it leads collapses, since these tubes do not communicate with one another. Thus, in children suffering from bronchitis or pneumonia areas of the lung may collapse through a plug of mucus sticking in a bronchus which the child is not sufficiently strong to free by coughing. A similar result is brought about by foreign bodies drawn into the air passages. It also occurs when the chest is opened on one side to drain away a collection of pus. The second lung, being healthy, is sufficient to overtake the needs of respiration, expanding as a rule somewhat in the process. The lungs of an infant at birth are collapsed in the sense that they have never been expanded, and any signs of expansion in the lungs of a dead infant form a sure token that he has been born alive. (See LUNGS.)

TUMOURS OF THE LUNG: Since the beginning of the twentieth century cancer of the lung has become increasingly frequent, particularly so in the last decade, and in 1984 was responsible for 35,739 deaths in England, compared with 10,360 deaths from carcinoma of the stomach and 13,409 deaths from carcinoma of the breast. It was the commonest form of cancer among cancer deaths in men, accounting for 39 per cent of all cancer deaths, and the second commonest among women (14 per cent), the commonest site for whom is the breast (20 per cent). Tumours may arise in the mediastinum or in connection with the pleura. Hydatid cysts are found from time to time in the lungs. (See TAENIASIS.)

WOUNDS OF THE LUNG are serious both by reason of the damage they may do to this organ and by admitting air into the pleural cavity, so that the lung collapses. The lung may be wounded by the end of a fractured rib, or by some sharp body pushed between the ribs, and it may also be torn as the result of disease: for example, a tuberculous and excavated lung may be perforated during a fit of coughing. If by any cause a free opening is made between the pleural cavity and air passages, immediate difficulty of breathing, due to collapse of the lung, ensues. Generally, however, the person recovers from the immediate symptoms, and, if the perforation is caused by an external wound, the wound may heal without leaving any permanent damage. Frequently, in such cases, blood is effused into the pleural cavity (haemothorax). This is gradually absorbed, leaving usually some thickening of the pleural membrane and adhesions between the lung and chest wall. Such a wound is liable, at the time of infliction, to become infected by organisms, and empyema (qv) may then result, with a tedious illness.

Wounds of the lung are chiefly dangerous on account of the risk of wounding large blood-vessels. Spitting of blood in any quantity after a wound of the chest has been received is a sign that the lung has been injured. A stab or bullet wound, which does not injure any large vessel, may traverse the lung without any serious consequences, but if one of the main veins or arteries is torn, death is likely to ensue.

LUPUS is a term used to designate a group of skin diseases of intractable character. There are two chief types of the disease: *Lupus vulgaris*, which is due to the *Mycobacterium tuberculosis*; and *Lupus erythematosus*, which is of unknown origin.

LUPUS VULGARIS begins most commonly before the age of 20, and, not infrequently, persists all through life, healing in one place to break out a short distance off. The nose, cheeks, brow, and sides of the neck are most commonly attacked, although the hands and the mucous membrane inside the nose and mouth are also common seats of the malady. The first sign of the disease is a small, soft nodule of yellowish transparent appearance, on this account often called an 'apple-jelly' nodule. No pain or itching accompanies the disease, but the skin gradually becomes thickened and discoloured, other nodules appear, and finally ulcers or small abscesses form. The disease progresses very slowly, but, after it has been in existence some years, the deformity produced may be very great. The nose may be partly or wholly eaten away; the lower eyelids, if attacked, become drawn down, showing the red inner surface. The condition is of little infective power.

Treatment: These horrors have now been removed by the excellent results obtained from the use of anti-tuberculous drugs. In certain cases it is still sometimes helpful to remove individual nodules by excision or by curettage, followed by the application of trichloracetic acid. The local application of intensive ultraviolet light is also sometimes of value.

LUPUS ERYTHEMATOSUS is a disease of unknown etiology. It occurs in two forms. The more common form, *discoid lupus erythematosus*, which is more common in women, involves only the skin and consists of rounded, red, and slightly raised patches, which are distributed most commonly on the nose and cheeks. These patches, by fusing together at their edges, sometimes give a characteristic butterfly-like appearance to the reddened nose and cheeks. There is no tendency to the formation of ulcers, as in lupus vulgaris, and deformity in consequence does not result, although the patches of red alternating with white and atrophied skin can render the complexion quite unsightly.

The second form, *systemic lupus erythematosus*, occurs predominantly in women in the proportion of nine women to one man. It is an auto-immune disease. There is some evidence that people who possess certain antigens (qv) are more vulnerable to it. It may be precipitated by a virus, exposure to sunlight, infection or the administration of sulphonamide drugs. Its manifestations vary considerably and include eruptions on the skin as in the discoid form, painful joints, involvement of the kidneys, alveolitis (qv), enlargement of the spleen, and fever. With adequate supervision the outlook is much better than was at one time thought to be the case, particularly if detected at an early stage. The disease usually responds dramatically to treatment with corticosteroids. Patients with systemic lupus erythematosus can obtain help and advice from the Lupus Society, c/o Arthritis Care, 5 Grosvenor Crescent, London SW1X 7ER (01–235 0902).

LUX is the unit of illumination. The abbreviation is lx.

LUXATION is another word for dislocation. (See DISLOCATIONS.)

LYCANTHROPY is the delusion entertained by an insane person that he or she is a wolf.

LYCOPODIUM is a fine, yellow powder, which consists of the spores of the club-moss, *Lycopodium clavatum*. It is used as a powder in which to roll pills, and is also a good dusting-powder for moist skin surfaces, such as the skin of infants.

LYING-IN (see LABOUR).

LYMPH is the fluid which circulates in the lymphatic vessels of the body. It is a colourless fluid, like blood plasma in composition, only rather more watery. It contains salts similar to those of blood plasma, and the same proteins, though in smaller amount: fibrinogen, serum albumin, and serum globulin. It also contains colourless lymph corpuscles, or lymphocytes as they are known, derived from the glands. In certain of the lymphatic vessels, the lymph contains, after meals, a great amount of fat in the form of a fine milky emulsion. These are the vessels which absorb fat from the food passing down the intestine, and convey it to the thoracic duct; they are called lacteals on account of the milky appearance of their contents. (See CHYLE.)

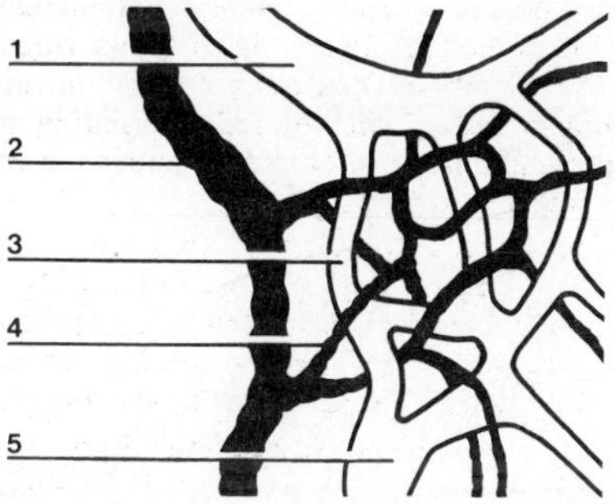

1 vein
2 lymphatic vessel
3 blood capilleries
4 lymph capilleries
5 small artery

Diagram showing the relation of the blood and lymph streams along the tissues.

The lymph is derived, in the first place, from the blood, the watery constituents of which exude through the walls of the capillaries into the tissues, conveying material for the nourishment of the tissues and absorbing waste products.

The various gaps and chinks in the tissues communicate with lymph capillaries, which have a structure similar to that of the capillaries of the blood-vessel system, being composed of delicate flat cells joined edge to edge. These unite to form fine vessels, resembling minute veins in structure, to which the name of lymphatics is applied. These ramify all through the body, passing here and there through lymphatic glands, and ultimately discharge their contents into the blood circulation once more, by opening into the jugular veins in the root of the neck. Other lymph vessels commence in great numbers as minute openings on the surface of the pleura and peritoneum, and act as drains for these otherwise closed cavities. When fluid is effused into these cavities, as in a pleural effusion, for example, its absorption takes place through the lymphatic vessels. The course of these vessels is described under GLANDS.

The circulation of the lymph is effected in some of the lower animals by lymph-hearts, which pump the lymph, just as the heart belonging to the blood-vessels keeps the blood in circulation. In man and most of the higher animals there is no heart for the lymph, which circulates partly by reason of the pressure at which it is driven through the walls of the blood capillaries, but mainly in consequence of incidental forces. The lymph capillaries and vessels are copiously provided with valves, which prevent any back flow of lymph, and every time these vessels are squeezed, as by the contraction of a muscle, or movement of a limb, the lymph moves on a little, leaving room for the exudation of fresh lymph. From this fact one can perceive the immense importance of regular exercise in maintaining the free circulation of lymph.

Lymph, like blood, possesses, in virtue of the fibrinogen which it contains, the power of clotting, forming, when it does so, a faintly yellow or colourless coagulum. This can be seen in the case of small wounds, after the blood has ceased to flow.

The term lymph is also applied to the serous fluid contained in the vesicles which develop as the result of vaccination, and used for the purpose of vaccinating other individuals. (See VACCINATION.)

The term lymph is also loosely applied to the layers and flakes of fibrin which are derived from the lymph and are found on the pleura and other serous membranes as the result of inflammation.

LYMPHADENITIS means inflammation of lymphatic glands. (See GLANDS, DISEASES OF.)

LYMPHADENOMA is another name for Hodgkin's disease (qv).

LYMPHANGIECTASIS means an abnormal dilatation of the lymph vessels, as in filariasis (qv).

LYMPHANGIOGRAPHY, or LYMPHOGRAPHY, is the procedure whereby the lymphatics (qv) and lymphatic glands can be rendered visible on X-ray films by means of the injection of radio-opaque substances.

LYMPHANGITIS means inflammation situated in the lymphatic vessels.

LYMPHATICS is the term applied to the vessels which convey the lymph (qv). (For an account of their arrangement, see GLANDS.)

LYMPHOCYTE is a variety of white blood corpuscle produced in the lymphoid tissues and lymphatic glands of the body. It contains a simple rounded nucleus surrounded by protoplasm generally described as non-granular. Two varieties of lymphocyte are described, small lymphocytes and large lymphocytes, and together they form over 20 per cent of the white corpuscles of the blood. They play an important part in the production of antibodies (qv), and in the rejection of transplanted organs such as the heart. (See TRANSPLANTATION.) This they do in two different ways. What are known as B lymphocytes produce antibodies, while T lymphocytes attack and destroy antigens (qv) directly. They are known as T lymphocytes because they are produced by the thymus gland. Their numbers are increased in tuberculosis and certain other diseases. Such an increase is known as lymphocytosis.

LYMPHOEDEMA means dropsical swelling of a part or organ due to obstruction to the lymph-vessels draining it.

LYMPHOGRANULOMA INGUINALE, LYMPHOGRANULOMA VENEREUM; PORADENITIS VENEREA; LYMPHOPATHIA VENEREUM, is a venereal disease in which the chief characteristic is enlargement of glands in the groin, the infecting agent being a virus. There were 17 cases in England in 1985.

LYMPHOKINES: Lymphokines are polypeptides that are produced by lymphocytes as part of their immune response to an antigen and their function is to communicate with other cells of the immune system. Some lymphokines stimulate B cells to differentiate into antibody-producing plasma cells; others stimulate T lymphocytes to proliferate and other lymphokines become interferons.

LYMPHOMA is a tumour of lymphoid tissue, one variety of which is found in children in Africa; sometimes called Burkitt's lymphoma after the surgeon who first described it. Because of its geographical distribution it is thought to be due to a virus which is transmitted by mosquitoes, but no virus has yet been definitely isolated from the tumour.

LYMPHOSARCOMA is a malignant growth of the lymphoid elements of the body, and is characterized by generalized enlargement of the lymphatic glands, spleen, and liver. The majority of cases –about 55 per cent – occur in the 60 to 70 age-group, but it may occur at any age. The prognosis is poor, 80 per cent of cases dying within six years. Treatment is by means of irradiation or chemotherapy.

LYSERGIC ACID, or LYSERGIC ACID DIETHYLAMIDE, popularly known as LSD, belongs to the ergonovine group of alkaloids. In minute doses it induces psychic states in which the individual becomes aware of repressed memories. Under the influence of the drug he feels he is watching himself and relives feelings from his childhood and infancy. It is proving of value in the treatment of certain anxiety states, but is a drug that must only be used under skilled supervision. (See DRUG ADDICTION.)

LYSIS means the gradual ending of a fever, and is opposed to crisis, which signifies the sudden ending of a fever. (See CRISIS.) It is also used to describe the process of dissolution of a blood-clot, or the loosening of adhesions.

LYSOFORM is a liquid soap containing formalin, which gives it a strong antiseptic power.

LYSOL is a brown, clear, oily fluid with antiseptic properties, made from coal-tar and containing 50 per cent cresol. When mixed with water it forms a clear soapy fluid. (See CRESOL.)

LYSOL POISONING: When lysol is swallowed there is a sense of burning about the mouth and throat. There are signs of corrosion around and in the mouth, with brown discoloration, and the characteristic smell of lysol is very evident in the breath. If the lysol is not speedily removed, unconsciousness and stupor gradually come on and death may occur within 24 hours. Septic pneumonia is also liable to supervene, and may produce death at a later period. **Treatment**: If the skin has been contaminated with the lysol, it must be washed with water, and any lysol-contaminated clothing must be taken off. Large quantities of tepid water and salt may be given at once to dilute the lysol if it has been swallowed, and produce vomiting.

LYSOZYME is a bactericidal substance present in tears.

LYSSA is another term for rabies or hydrophobia.

M

McBURNEY'S POINT is an area of small size on the front of the abdomen, at which the tenderness experienced in appendicitis is felt with special keenness. It is situated between the navel and the prominent anterior superior spine of the right iliac bone, about 50 mm (2 inches) from the latter.

MACERATION is the softening of a solid by soaking in fluid.

MACROCYTE is an unusually large red blood corpuscle especially characteristic of the blood in pernicious anaemia.

MACROGLOSSIA means an abnormally large tongue.

MACROPSIA: Condition in which objects appear larger than normal. It can be due to disease of the macula.

MACULES are spots or stained areas of brown or purplish-brown colour in the skin. They may be due to old haemorrhages, sunburn, disease of internal organs, pregnancy, skin diseases such as eczema and psoriasis, syphilis, and burns.

MADURA FOOT is the name given to a disease found in the Tropics in which the foot becomes swollen and its bones and other tissues riddled by sinuses. It is caused by the presence of a fungus.

MAGNESIUM is a light metallic element. Magnesium is one of the essential mineral elements of the body, without which it cannot function properly. The adult body contains around 25 grams, the greater part of which is in the bones. More than two-thirds of our daily supply come from cereals and vegetables. As most other foods also contain useful amounts, there is thus seldom any difficulty in maintaining an adequate amount in the body. It is an essential constituent of several vital enzymes (qv). Deficiency leads to muscular weakness and interferes with the efficient working of the heart. The salts of magnesium used as drugs are the hydroxide of magnesium, the oxide of magnesium, generally known as 'magnesia', and the carbonate of magnesium, all of which have an antacid action; also the sulphate of magnesium generally known as 'Epsom salts', which acts as a purgative.
Uses: Light and heavy carbonates of magnesia are used to correct hyperacidity of the stomach, as are the hydroxide and the light oxide. They are also used as feeble laxatives. Cream of magnesia, the official *British Pharmacopoeia* name of which is Magnesium Hydroxide Mixture, is a widely used, effective antacid. In large doses it is a useful safe laxative.

Magnesium sulphate is the most commonly used saline purge. (See EPSOM SALTS.)

MAGNETISM (see ELECTRICITY IN MEDICINE).

MAIDISM is another name for PELLAGRA (qv).

MALACIA is a term applied to softening of a part or tissue in disease: eg. osteomalacia or softening of the bones.

MALABSORPTION SYNDROME includes a multiplicity of diseases, all of which are characterized by faulty absorption from the intestine of essential foodstuffs, such as fat, vitamins and mineral salts. Among the conditions in this syndrome are coeliac disease (qv) and sprue (qv).

MALAISE means a vague feeling of feverishness, listlessness, and languor, which often precedes the onset of serious acute diseases, or accompanies passing derangements, such as dyspepsia, chills, and colds.

MALARIA, which derives its name from *mala aria* – the Italian for bad air – and also known as AGUE, PALUDISM, JUNGLE FEVER, MARSH FEVER, PERIODIC FEVER, is a disease caused by the presence of certain parasites in the blood. It consists at first of a series of febrile attacks, which may come on every day, every second day, or every third day; later it assumes a chronic form, in which a poor state of health known as chronic malaria or malarial cachexia is developed, and there is a tendency towards frequent relapses.
History: It has been known from the earliest times, having been recorded as far back as 1500 BC. Devastating malarial epidemics contributed significantly to the fall of the Roman Empire. Not only is it described by many of the medical writers of antiquity, but numerous references to it exist in general literature, such as the works of Horace. From these it appears that its connection with swampy ground was recognized even in ancient times.

The first important advance was made in 1640, when the Countess of Chinchon, wife of the Viceroy of Peru, brought home to Europe the bark by which the South American Indians had learned to treat the disease successfully. From this bark, named after her Cinchona bark (by Linnaeus who made a mistake in her name), and also known as Jesuit's bark, since the secret had been learned by priests from the Indians, quinine is derived. By this drug a means of treating the paroxysms of fever, as well as an aid in warding off the disease, was obtained. From the fact that quinine is an antiseptic it was assumed that the disease must be due to some poison circulating in the blood which the quinine could destroy.

In 1880 Laveran, a French military surgeon, discovered the presence of minute parasites in the corpuscles of blood drawn from malarious persons and examined them under the microscope. He described more than one form of the parasites, and subsequent observers demonstrated that the parasites go through a process of development, leading up to the production of spores, which are formed all through the blood of the affected person at one time, and from which a new set of parasites develops.

It had long been noticed, even by West African natives, that mosquitoes seem to flourish together with malaria, and several scientists endeavoured to establish a connection between the two. This was successfully proved by Manson in 1894, through bringing from Italy live mosquitoes which had been allowed to suck blood from malarious persons in that country, and allowing the insects to bite healthy people in London, who had no other possible connection with the disease. The experiment was successful, and those people who had offered themselves for the experiment proved conclusively that malaria is carried by mosquitoes. Others proved the converse of this proposition, and showed, by living for some months in a malarious district, such as the Roman Campagna, that infection does not take place if mosquitoes are kept off by gauze and other means.

From the examination of the blood in malarious people, Manson reasoned that the parasites go through a stage of their development in the bodies of the mosquitoes, passing, in the tissues of those insects, through a sexual stage, in which male and female forms unite in the production of masses of new parasites. The arduous work of demonstrating this was undertaken by Ross, then a military surgeon in India. The difficulty of this work is understood when one considers that the dissection of a great number of mosquitoes and their examination under the microscope were necessary before Ross was able in 1898 to confirm the truth of Manson's theory, by demonstrating the genus Anopheles as the insect in which the development of the malaria parasite takes place. Other observers confirmed his observations, and traced out in detail the changes which the parasites undergo while in the mosquito.

Causes: As shown by these discoveries, the presence of people infected by the malarial parasite and the access of the Anopheles mosquito to these and to healthy people form two of the conditions producing infection of fresh cases. But there are various factors which aid or retard the development of the parasite and of the mosquito. The disease is known all round the world, but is chiefly found in tropical climates, spreading here and there into temperate regions, where it occurs in summer and autumn, if the other conditions are suitable. The presence of swamps, pools of surface water, rank vegetation, and a poorly fed population are also important factors. Its chief seats are Africa, India, South East Asia and Central America. The estimated world incidence is 150 million. There is a growing incidence of it in the United Kingdom in people who have acquired the disease abroad. In 1986, 1,663 cases were reported in the United Kingdom.

The parasites of malaria are three in number, corresponding to the tertian fever, the quartan fever, and the malignant tertian malaria. The parasites are protozoa, belonging to the order *Sporozoa*, and to the genus *Plasmodium*. The specific names for benign tertian, quartan, and malignant malaria are, respectively, *Plasmodium vivax, P. malariae,* and *P. falciparum*. As has been stated, the malarial parasite passes one phase of its life-cycle in man and the other in the stomach and tissues of the mosquito (the sexual phase). After sexual union of male and female forms in the mosquito's stomach, the resulting offspring – the asexual sporozoites – eventually find their way into the mosquito's salivary gland. Once a mosquito has become infected it remains infective for life.

When the infected female mosquito bites a human being, these filamentous sporozoites are injected into the blood. They then find their way into the liver where they develop into what are known as schizonts. After a period ranging from six to sixteen days (depending on the species of plasmodium) these schizonts have reached maturity, and in the course of maturation each one has produced up to 40,000 merozoites. These merozoites are then released into the blood stream where they penetrate the red blood cells and form trophozoites or rings. These in turn enlarge, each to the capacity of the red corpuscle. The large trophozoite thus formed finally splits into numerous small parasites now called merozoites. These burst out of the red blood corpuscle into the blood stream and then attack other red corpuscles, the whole asexual cycle repeating itself once more. The paroxysm of malarial fever coincides with the bursting of the red blood corpuscles and the setting free of the merozoites into the bloodstream. Sexual forms – male and female gametocytes – also develop in the blood, but they undergo no further change until a mosquito bite sucks them into the mosquito's stomach.

Symptoms: For a day or two before the actual fever sets in, there may be headache, vague pains about the body and limbs, chilliness, and slight rises of temperature. When the parasites have multiplied up to the stage already mentioned, the attack suddenly comes on.

The acute malarial attack has, in general, three stages, although in occasional cases one of the stages may be excessively marked or may be wanting. These are the cold stage, the hot stage, and the sweating stage.

The cold stage begins with a feeling of chilliness even in the hottest weather. This increases till the person has to betake himself to bed and heap himself with clothes, face and nails being blue with cold, and the whole body shaken with shivering (rigors). Nevertheless, if the temperature is measured, it is found to be considerably raised. This stage lasts an hour or less.

The hot stage comes on as the temperature of the body rises, beginning with hot flushes, which lengthen till the body feels burning hot, the temperature rising to 40·5° to 41·1°C (105° or 106°F). There are also headache, dizziness, sickness, pain throughout the body, and sometimes even delirium. This stage may last several hours.

The sweating stage comes on after the fever reaches its height, as the temperature begins to fall. Profuse perspiration breaks out, the person begins to feel decidedly better, and the headache and pains at the same time pass off. Finally, after two or three hours the patient feels quite well, though much weakened, and remains so till the next attack begins.

If the parasite present is that of *quartan fever* there is an intermission of two days before the next attack: that is to say, if the first attack is on the 1st day of the month the succeeding ones are on the 4th, 7th, and so on. If the parasite is that of *tertian fever*, the attacks are on the 1st, 3rd, 5th, and so on; whilst in the severe *malignant tertian fever*, each attack may last considerably over a day, so that there may not be time for one to pass off completely before the next begins. The patient then is in a continued state of fever, known as *subtertian fever*. A person may get a double or treble infection of the malarial parasites, and then the fever may also occur every day. When the fever occurs every day, whatever the cause, it is sometimes called a *quotidian fever*.

As a rule people, after passing through an ague, feel completely recovered till the next attack is due, but now and then the attack may develop seriously. Thus hyperpyrexia (qv) may develop, the temperature continuing to rise till death occurs before the sweating stage sets in. Insensibility may set in and the person die owing to blockage of the small vessels in the brain by immense numbers of the parasites; this is known as cerebral malaria. Severe vomiting or diarrhoea may also endanger the patient's life, or he may become very collapsed during the sweating stage. One of the most dread complications is blackwater fever (qv).

If treatment is adopted between two attacks, the succeeding attack or the next after that is generally checked. Even when no treatment takes place, after a few weeks of the attacks these gradually get less and less marked and finally disappear. The parasites become so diminished that they are unable to cause fever, but they are not entirely destroyed in the blood, and so the affected person is subject after some weeks or months to a relapse, when the attacks of ague are repeated as in the first seizure. These rallies and relapses may go on for several years, especially if the person leads an exposed, laborious life, or is poorly nourished. Anything which depresses the vitality, such as a chill, is apt to lead to a fresh relapse. On the other hand, under efficient treatment complete recovery occurs.

If the disease becomes chronic, various symptoms set in. The person becomes very anaemic in consequence of the large number of blood corpuscles destroyed by the parasites in each paroxysm of fever. A feeble state of health, accompanied by bodily wasting and yellow discoloration of the skin, ensues, and the spleen and liver, particularly the former, become enlarged.

Treatment: This falls into two important sections, preventive and curative.

PREVENTIVE TREATMENT may be directed either against the parasites or against the mosquitoes which convey them. The drugs recommended by the Medical Committee of the Hospital for Tropical Diseases, London, for the prevention of malaria are: (a) Africa (except Kenya and Tanzania coastal areas), Arab States, Pakistan, India (except East India), Pacific Islands: proguanil 200 mg daily (first choice), or chloroquine 300 mg weekly. (b) Eastern India, Bangladesh, South East Asia, Central and South America, Papua New Guinea: Maloprim (pyrimethamine and dapsone) one tablet twice weekly, or Fansidar (pyrimethamine and sulfadoxine) one tablet weekly. Fansidar should not be taken by pregnant women or by those sensitive to sulphonamides. This geographical variation in the choice of recommended drugs is due to the increasing evidence of resistance to drugs being acquired by the causative organism, particularly *P. falciparum* to chloroquine in South Asia. Travellers should start taking antimalarial drugs one week before setting out and should continue taking them for at least four weeks after their return to the United Kingdom. Full details of which drugs to take and when, are given in two leaflets – *Notice to Travellers* published by the Department of Health and Social Security, and *Advice to Travellers* published by the Health Education Council – which are available from travel agencies, as well as in *Preservation of Personal Health in Warm Climates* published by the Ross Institute of Tropical Hygiene, Keppel Street, London WC1E 7HT.

It is still more important to attack the mosquitoes in their developing stage. The eggs are laid on or near pools of stagnant water in which the larvae and pupae swim just below the surface, breathing through a tube which projects above the surface of the water. These larvae may be destroyed by pouring on the surface of these pools some fluid through which the breathing-tube of the larva cannot be protruded. Crude petroleum and a special oil known as 'malariol' are used for this purpose, and when poured upon pools the oil spreads out instantly into a film which will remain intact for several days if not destroyed by rain or wind. Further, all small pools in gardens should be filled up, tubs, flowerpots, cisterns, and other collections of water emptied regularly at least once a week, and in public works, such as railways, it should be made illegal, as in Italy, to leave holes and ditches where water can collect. Anopheline breeding grounds can be sprayed with Paris green. Fish which feed on the larvae can be introduced into ponds and lakes.

Although these methods are still of value, they have largely been replaced or supplemented by the use of insecticides such as DDT, benzene hexachloride (BHC) and dieldrin which have proved most effective in destroying mosquitoes.

Wire-gauze screens to all the windows of a house, and muslin mosquito netting over the beds, form an efficient protection, and it should be remembered that not only should mosquitoes be kept away from healthy people by these means, but that it is even more important that the insects should not gain access to those suffering from the disease, by whose blood they become infected and made carriers of malaria to the healthy. The importance of suitable clothing, eg. long sleeves and long trousers, must also be borne in mind.

CURATIVE TREATMENT depends upon a wide range of drugs, including chloroquine, primaquine, pyrimethamine, and quinine. In cases in which the malaria organism has become resistant to these the World Health Organization recommends amodiaquine or sulfadoxine. (See also BLACKWATER FEVER.)

MALATHION is one of the less toxic organophosphorus insecticides (qv).

MALE FERN, or FILIX MAS, is a remedy once widely used for the expulsion of tapeworms.

MALFORMATION (see DEFORMITIES).

MALIGNANT is a term applied in several ways to serious disorders. Tumours are called malignant when they grow rapidly, tend to infiltrate surrounding healthy tissues, and to spread to distant parts of the body, leading eventually to death. (See CANCER, CARCINOMA AND SARCOMA.) The term is also applied to types of disease which are much more serious than the usual form, such as malignant hypertension, malignant smallpox. Malignant pustule is another name for anthrax (qv).

MALIGNANT FEVER, also known as MALIGNANT HYPERPYREXIA and MALIGNANT HYPERTHERMIA, is a rare, but dangerous, complication of general anaesthesia, commoner in children and adolescents than adults. The overall frequency is 1 in 15,000 anaesthetics in children and 1 in 50,000 in adults. It is characterized by a sudden rise in the temperature of the patient during anaesthesia. This may occur after a few minutes or several hours, and the temperature may rise as high as 44°C (112°F). It is associated with an abnormality of the muscles which tends to run in families. This may be detected by estimating the level of creatine phosphokinase in the blood, which is raised in those liable to develop this condition. The shorter the duration of the anaesthesia and the smaller the rise in temperature, the greater are the chances of recovery, which is one reason why a careful check is kept of the patient's temperature during general anaesthesia. In those liable to develop this complication, operations are carried out under regional or local anaesthesia whenever possible. (See ANAESTHESIA.)

MALIGNANT HYPERTENSION has nothing to do with cancer. It derives its name from the fact that, if untreated, it runs a rapidly fatal course. It is still undecided whether it is a disease entity in itself or is merely a terminal stage in certain cases of essential hypertension (qv). Its characteristic features are that it occurs in a younger age-group than essential hypertension, and that there is a very high diastolic blood-pressure, with papilloedema (qv) and kidney failure. This is the type of hypertension in which the antihypertensive drugs (see ESSENTIAL HYPERTENSION) have proved so successful. Indeed, the introduction of these drugs has revolutionized the outlook. At one time an invariably fatal disease within two years, many patients with this condition can now enjoy many years of comparatively good health.

MALINGERING is a term applied to the feigning of illness. In the great majority of cases a person who feigns illness has a certain amount of disability, but exaggerates the illness or discomfort for some ulterior motive.

MALLEOLUS is the term applied to either of the two bony prominences at the ankle. (See LEG.)

MALLET FINGER is due to sudden forced flexion of the terminal joint of a finger, resulting in rupture of the tendon. As a result the individual is unable to extend the terminal part of the finger which remains bent forward. The middle, ring and little fingers are most commonly involved. Treatment is by splinting the finger. The end result is satisfactory provided the victim has sufficient patience.

MALLET TOE is the condition in which it is not possible to extend the terminal part of the toe. It is usually due to muscular imbalance but may be due to congenital absence of the extensor muscle. A callosity (qv) often forms on it which may be painful. Should this be troublesome, treatment consists of removal of the terminal phalanx.

MALOPRIM is a combination of pyrimethamine (qv) and dapsone (qv) which is used for the prevention of malaria (qv). It has the advantage of only needing to be taken once weekly. It should not be taken by anyone hypersensitive to sulphonamides, and should not be used for the treatment of an acute attack.

MALT is a substance derived from barley by allowing a certain amount of growth to take place in the moistened grain, which is then dried and crushed. It contains a ferment named diastase, together with a large amount of maltsugar and dextrin, the latter constituents being still further developed from the starch of the barley by the action of the ferment, when the malt is allowed to digest in water at a temperature approaching 40°C (104°F). Similarly, the ferment will convert into sugar a large amount of the starch in flour mixed with malt, and so perform some of the functions of the saliva and pancreatic juice.

For these reasons malt is mixed with various proportions of flour to form some of the popular foods for children. It is also used in the form of malt extracts, 28 grams of which is equivalent to 80 Calories.

MALTA FEVER (see BRUCELLOSIS).

MAMMARY GLAND (see BREAST).

MAMMILLA is the Latin term for the nipple.

MAMMOGRAPHY is the special technique whereby X-rays can be taken that reveal the structure of the breast. It is an effective way of distinguishing benign from malignant tumours. It can detect tumours that are not palpable. In a multi-centre study in the USA, called The Breast Cancer Detection Demonstration Project, which involved nearly 300,000 women in the 40–49 age group, 35 per cent of the tumours were found by mammography alone, 13 per cent by physical examination and 50 per cent by both methods. Two recent Dutch studies published in 1984 have confirmed the benefits of breast screening with a reduction in mortality of 50 to 70 per cent in screened women. The optimum frequency of screening is debatable. The American College of Radiologists recommends a baseline mammogram at the age of 40 years with subsequent mammography at one to two year intervals up to the age of 50. Thereafter, annual mammography is recommended. As breast cancer is the commonest malignancy in Western women and is increasing in frequency, the importance of screening for this form of cancer is obvious.

MANDELIC ACID is a non-toxic keto-acid used in the treatment of infections of the urinary tract, especially those due to the *Escherichia coli* and the *Streptococcus faecalis* or *Enterococcus*. It is administered in doses of 3 grams several times daily. As it is only effective in an acid urine, ammonium chloride must be taken at the same time.

MANDIBLE is the bone of the lower jaw.

MANDL'S PAINT consists of iodine 1·25 grams, potassium iodide 2·5 grams, water 2·5 ml, oil of peppermint 0·4 ml, alcohol (90 per cent) 4 ml, glycerin to 100 ml. It is used as a throat paint in pharyngitis and tonsillitis. It should be well shaken before use.

MANGANESE is a metal, oxides of which are found abundantly in nature. Permanganate of potassium is a well-known disinfectant. (See PERMANGANATE OF POTASSIUM.)

MANIA is a form of mental disorder characterized by great excitement. (See MENTAL ILLNESS.)

MANIC-DEPRESSIVE INSANITY, or CYCLOTHYMIA, is a form of madness characterized by alternate attacks of mania and depression. (See MENTAL ILLNESS.)

MANIPULATION is the term applied to the forceful passive movement of joints. In skilled hands it is a most effective means of treatment of stiff joints or of pain in the back due to a prolapsed intervertebral disc (qv).

MANNITOL (OSMITROL) is an osmotic diuretic (qv) given intravenously. (See DIURETICS.)

MANOMETER is an instrument for measuring the pressure or tension of liquids or gases. (See BLOOD-PRESSURE.)

MANTOUX TEST, also known as MENDEL'S TEST, is a test for tuberculosis. It consists in injecting into the superficial layers of the skin (ie. intradermally) a very small quantity of old tuberculin. A positive reaction of the skin – swelling and redness – shows that the person so reacting has been infected with the *Mycobacterium tuberculosis*. But it does not mean that such a person is suffering from active tuberculosis. (See TUBERCULIN.)

MANUBRIUM is the uppermost part of the breast-bone.

MANZULLO'S TELLURITE TEST consists in applying to the throat of someone suspected of having diphtheria a 2 per cent potassium tellurite solution. If diphtheria bacilli are present the solution blackens. But some other germs also reduce the tellurite solution. As a negative test it has some use, because if no reduction occurs it is highly improbable that the patient has diphtheria.

MAPLE-SYRUP URINE DISEASE is a condition in which there is an association between mental defect and a disorder of amino-acid metabolism. It is so named because the urine has the odour of maple-syrup.

MAPROTILINE (LUDIOMIL) (see ANTIDEPRESSANTS).

MARASMUS means progressive wasting, especially in young children, when there is no ascertainable cause. It is generally associated with defective feeding. (See ATROPHY; INFANT FEEDING.)

MARBURG DISEASE, also known as GREEN MONKEY DISEASE and VERVET MONKEY DISEASE because the first recorded cases acquired their infection from monkeys of this genus, is a viral infection with a high mortality rate. The incubation period is 4 to 9 days. The onset is sudden with marked nausea and severe headache.

This is followed by rising temperature, diarrhoea, and vomiting. Towards the end of the first week a rash appears which persists for a week and is accompanied by internal bleeding. In those who recover convalescence is slow and prolonged. The world distribution of the causative virus is unknown, but apart from laboratory infections acquired through working with vervet monkeys, all the cases so far reported have occurred in Africa.

MARCH FRACTURE is a curious condition in which a fracture occurs of the second (rarely the third) metatarsal bone in the foot without any obvious cause. The usual story is that a pain suddenly developed in the foot while walking (hence the name) and that it has persisted ever since. The only treatment needed is immobilization of the foot and rest, and the fracture heals satisfactorily.

MARCH HAEMOGLOBINURIA is a complication of walking and running over long distances. It is due to damage to red blood cells in the blood-vessels of the sole of the feet. This results in haemoglobin (qv) being released into the bloodstream, which is then voided in the urine, the condition known as haemoglobinuria (qv). No treatment is required, but the complaint may be minimized by wearing shoes with resilient soles and, so far as possible, avoiding running on hard surfaces.

MARIHUANA is another term for CANNABIS INDICA, or hemp, or hashish. (See DRUG ADDICTION.)

MARRIAGE GUIDANCE (see RELATE NATIONAL MARRIAGE GUIDANCE).

MARROW means the softer substance enclosed in the interior of bones. It is of two kinds: *yellow marrow*, which occupies the large tubular space in the shaft of a long bone, such as a limb bone, and *red marrow*, which fills up the spaces in the interior of the ribs, sternum, and vertebral bodies, as well as the ends of the shafts of the long bones such as the femur and humerus. There is no essential difference between the two, although yellow marrow owes its colour to the large amount of fat contained in it, whilst red marrow is of a highly cellular structure. The marrow is the site of formation of red blood corpuscles, platelets, and granular white blood cells.

MARSH FEVER (see MALARIA).

MARSHMALLOW ROOT is the root of *Althaea officinalis*, which has long been credited as a domestic medicine, with a soothing influence upon mucous membranes, as well as exerting a diuretic action. It is used chiefly as an ingredient of lozenges for cases of sore throat.

MASSAGE, or RUBBING, is a method of treatment in which the operator uses his hands, or occasionally other appliances, to rub, knead, or press the skin and deeper tissues of the person under treatment. It is often combined with (*a*) passive movements, in which the masseur moves the limbs in various ways, the person treated making no effort; or (*b*) active movements, which are performed with the combined assistance of masseur and patient. Massage is also often combined with baths and gymnastics in order to strengthen various muscles. The beneficial effects of massage are exerted in different ways. Applied gently, it has a soothing action; applied more vigorously, certain methods have the effect of quickening the circulation of lymph and blood, and so leading to the rapid absorption of waste products in the muscles. Other forms of massage cause muscular contractions and so provide exercise for the muscles in cases in which movements of the whole body are not desired.

Varieties: STROKING, or *effleurage*, consists of gentle pressure with the hand moved in one direction. It soothes the nerves of the part treated and empties the main lymph-vessels and veins, thus increasing the circulation locally. It is carried out either with the flat of the hand or with the edges of thumb and first finger widely separated.

KNEADING, or *pétrissage*, is the most commonly employed form, and consists of squeezing, kneading, rolling, or rubbing movements coupled with a considerable amount of pressure, effected, it may be, with the fingers or knuckles, but generally with the pulp or the ball of the thumb. It has a still greater effect than stroking in moving on the lymph and blood circulation of deep-seated parts, and so leading to the absorption of inflammatory thickenings in and around joints, tendon-sheaths, and muscles. (See LYMPH.)

STABILE MOVEMENTS include such applications as the following. *Pressing* may be done with the finger-tips or with the knuckles; it is usually combined with rubbing. *Tapping* is done with the points of the fingers from the wrist, and, when applied gently, has a soothing effect. *Thrusting*, which consists in poking up the deeper parts with the points of the fingers, and *hacking*, in which the muscles are struck with the inner edge of the hand, the arms moving from the elbows, are employed to cause muscular contractions.

VIBRATORY MOVEMENTS are made either by tapping (as above) or by special pads, to which a very rapid oscillation is communicated from an electric motor. This form of massage has been used in order to exert a soothing influence, for example, in cases of headache.

PASSIVE MOVEMENTS are made chiefly for their effect upon the joints. The synovial fluid is increased if scanty, and tends to be absorbed if excessive, while adhesions, which limit the motions of the joint or render these painful, are broken down by passive movements of a more forcible type. This type of massage is the form chiefly employed in the treatment of stiff joints by bone-setters.

ACTIVE MOVEMENTS of a carefully regulated type, in which the person's will is concentrated upon the movement made, are specially useful for developing the muscles brought into play thereby. The amount of muscular force required is graduated and increased by the masseur resisting the movements with varying degrees of force.

Uses: Massage can only be employed to full advantage by fully trained masseurs (or masseuses). A complete list of members of the *Chartered Society of Physiotherapy* who are qualified to give massage can be obtained on application to the Secretary of the Society, 14 Bedford Row, London, WC1R 4ED (01-242 1941). The types of case in which massage is useful are extremely various. Neuralgia, sciatica, and muscular rheumatism are among the painful conditions in which some relief is generally obtained. In muscular wasting, and paralysis due to nerve conditions –such as lead-poisoning, peripheral neuritis, crutch palsy, Bell's paralysis, and poliomyelitis – the muscles affected may be kept in a state of good nutrition till the nerve weakness has disappeared, and so recovery may be materially hastened. In various other nervous conditions, such as hysteria, chorea, loss of sensation, and writer's cramp, massage often proves of great benefit. Several types of joint disease, such as chronic rheumatism and stiffness due to previous slight injuries, such as sprains, are specially amenable to treatment by passive movements combined with deep rubbing, but any such interference with joints which have been recently the seat of tuberculous disease is very dangerous, as by these means the disease may be more widely spread. In several general conditions such as corpulence and constipation associated with a flabby body, massage may be of use.

Massage may be combined with electrical applications. For example, high-frequency and static electricity may be used along with gentle massage to obtain a soothing effect. The interrupted galvanic, sinusoidal, and faradic currents are useful combined with more forcible massage to stimulate muscular contraction in various cases of paralysis. (See also CARDIAC MASSAGE.)

MASS HYSTERIA (see HYSTERIA).

MASS MINIATURE RADIOGRAPHY is a method of obtaining X-ray photographs of the chests of large numbers of people at about the rate of two per minute. It has been used on a large scale as a means of screening the population for pulmonary tuberculosis.

MASTALGIA is the term applied to pain in the breast.

MAST CELLS are round or oval cells found predominantly in the loose connective tissues. They contain histamine (qv) and heparin (qv), and carry immunoglobulin E, the antibody which plays a predominant part in allergic reactions. Although known to play a part in inflammatory reactions, allergy, and hypersensitivity, their precise function in health and disease is still not quite clear.

MASTECTOMY is the operation for removal of a breast. It is an operation that can cause considerable psychological disturbance. Those who find it difficult to adjust to the situation after the operation will obtain helpful advice from the Breast Care and Mastectomy Association of Great Britain, 26a Harrison Street, Kings Cross, London WC1H 8JG (01–837 0908).

MASTICATION is the act whereby, as a result of movements of the lower jaw, lips, tongue, and cheek, food is reduced to a condition in which it is ready to be acted on by the gastric juices in the process of digestion. Adequate mastication is an essential part of the digestive process. (See DIGESTION.)

MASTITIS is the term applied to inflammation of the breast. (See BREAST, DISEASES OF.)

MASTOID PROCESS is the large process of the temporal bone of the skull which can be felt immediately behind the ear. It contains numerous cavities, one of which, the mastoid antrum, communicates with the middle ear, and is liable to suppurate when the middle ear is diseased. (See EAR, DISEASES OF.)

MASTURBATION is the production of an orgasm, or at least a modicum of sexual pleasure, by self-manipulation of the penis or clitoris.

MAT BURN is a combination of a burn and an abrasion which occurs in wrestlers when the skin over the bony points is rubbed against the unyielding canvas mat. It is particularly liable to become infected. Treatment consists of thorough cleansing and the application of a dressing such as gauze and chlorhexidine covered by cotton-wool and firmly fixed by a bandage or elastoplast – depending on the extent of the injury.

MATCH-WORKERS' DISEASE (see PHOSPHORUS POISONING).

MATERIA MEDICA is that branch of medical study which deals with the sources, preparations, and uses of drugs.

MATERNITY and CHILD WELFARE: The high rate of infantile mortality which used to prevail in the larger towns drew attention to the great loss of infant life which was produced partly by ignorance on the part of the mothers and partly by poverty. A movement was accordingly begun early in the present century in some of the larger cities to provide trained women as health visitors for giving advice to working-class women on the proper methods of rearing their children. This was at first a voluntary effort conducted by philanthropic agencies, but it was soon taken up by local authorities throughout the country. The necessary information as to the existence of newly born infants was provided by the Notification of Births which was demanded by Acts passed in 1907 and 1915. Women health visitors were appointed to visit the homes of such newly born infants, and shortly afterwards INFANT CONSULTATION CENTRES and CLINICS were established by various local authorities and voluntary agencies.

At first the movement for child welfare was limited to infants from birth to 1 year of age, but shortly afterwards the necessity for supervising the health of children until they came under school discipline at 5 years was recognized. Still later it became evident that it was desirable to watch over the health of the expectant mother and to provide skilled attendance prior to and during confinement. This led, accordingly, to the establishment of MATERNITY AND CHILD WELFARE CENTRES and CLINICS by many local authorities. The schemes which have now been devised for combating infantile mortality are very wide. They include better housing, health visitors, consultation centres for mothers, infant milk depots, the provision of milk, vitamin preparations and iron tablets for expectant and nursing mothers, and hospital accommodation for expectant mothers before and during confinement. The provision of Child Welfare Centres to which parents may bring their infants at stated times produces valuable results, both by advice to the mothers and by keeping records of increase in weight and other important facts regarding the infants, and also by interesting and stimulating the mothers to greater efforts. The Centre also provides opportunities for giving instruction in health, cookery, sewing, etc., to the mothers, and for distributing food and clothing as may be necessary. Antenatal Clinics, which provide education and assistance for the expectant mother, form an important section of this work.

HEALTH VISITORS have been described as 'truly medico-social workers – playing a full part in both preventive medicine and social action'. Their duties cover maternity and child welfare, school nursing, health education, tuberculosis, venereal disease, infectious diseases, mental illness, welfare of the aged and the handicapped, family welfare services, and cooperation with general practitioners. Health visitors must pass the examination for the Health Visitor's Certificate. Candidates for this examination must be either: (*a*) Nurses who have undergone a three-years' course of training at a recognized general or children's hospital, who have obtained Part I of the Midwifes Certificate of the Central Midwives Board, and who have attended an approved whole-time course in public health work lasting for nine months; *or* (*b*) Women, not being trained nurses, who have undergone an approved course of training in public health work for two years together with six months' training in hospital, and who have obtained Part I of the Certificate of the Central Midwives Board.

ANTENATAL CLINICS are considered to be of great value, because the fatality among the unborn from stillbirth, abortion, etc., is higher than the mortality of infants during the first year of life; it is generally believed, further, that by the medical attention provided at such clinics many of these antenatal deaths could be prevented, and the number of infants born prematurely and of feeble constitution could be much reduced. Thus, it has been shown that the perinatal death rate (qv) is nearly five times higher in the children of mothers who are late in attending antenatal clinics than in the children of those who start attending early. Health visitors follow up cases seen at antenatal clinics and ensure that the medical instructions given at the clinic are carried out, and proper steps taken to prepare for the confinement.

Under the National Insurance Acts in Great Britain, a woman receives a maternity grant in respect of each child, and also a home confinement grant if the confinement takes place at home. A woman who ordinarily follows a gainful occupation is also given a maternity allowance for 18 weeks beginning about 11 weeks before her confinement provided that she abstains from work. Under the Employment Protection (Consolidation) Act 1978, a woman has the right to return to work after confinement provided (a) she has been continuously employed for not less than two years and has worked at least 16 hours a week; (b) she was employed until 11 weeks before the expected week of confinement. She is also entitled to maternity pay.

INFANT CONSULTATION CLINICS are conducted usually by local authorities, and, in cases where it is desirable, mothers are urged to bring infants to these clinics regularly. Many of the disabling illnesses of early childhood are thus prevented, and the attendance should continue as required during the first five years of the child's life.

DAY NURSERIES, or crèches, are provided in many places in connection with these clinics, at which children can be left when the mothers are out at work.

Most local authorities have schemes for supplying special foods or nutritious diet to mothers of children who after medical examination at the Clinic are found to require such assistance. SPECIAL TREATMENT CLINICS are also provided in many places for the examination and care of teeth, eyes, ears, nose, throat, and skin of children. Also there is at present a movement for the treatment of cases in which children are crippled as the result of early disease. Further, in connection with the clinics, many local authorities possess convalescent homes, or arrange with voluntary agencies for admission to their convalescent homes of children who are in need of special care and open-air regime. Indirectly connected with these clinics in many places there have also been established play centres and kindergartens for young children.

Under the National Health Service Act, 1946, all these services were unified under Local Health Authorities. A statutory duty was imposed upon Local Health Authorities to provide health centres, maternity and child welfare, domiciliary midwifery, health visiting, home nursing, vaccination and immunization, and ambulances. They were also empowered to provide home-help services, and care and after-care. Maternity and child welfare covers the care of expectant and nursing mothers and of children under 5 years of age who are not attending school. It includes antenatal clinics, postnatal clinics, child-welfare clinics, and a priority dental service for both expectant and nursing mothers and young children. Further reorganization of the National Health Service introduced in 1974 and 1982 aimed at a closer co-ordination of these services with the hospital service and the family doctor service.

MATTER (see PUS).

MATTOID is a term applied to a person who, though passing as sane, is eccentric or mentally unbalanced in some particular direction.

MAW-WORMS is another name for round-worms. (See ASCARIASIS.)

MAXILLA is the name applied to the upper jaw-bones, which bear the teeth.

MEASLES, also known as MORBILLI, is an acute infectious disease occurring mostly in children. The name, measles, comes from the teutonic root, *maes*, meaning a spot. Morbilli is a diminutive of morbus, a disease; it has also, rather fancifully, been suggested that, as it strictly means a 'little disease', it was applied to this disease as it primarily affected 'little ones'. It appears to have been known from an early period in the history of medicine, mention being made of it in the writings of Rhazes and others of the Arabian physicians in the tenth century. For long, however, its specific nature was not recognized, and it was held to be a variety of smallpox. Measles and scarlet fever were long confounded with each other; and in the account given by Sydenham of epidemics of measles in London in 1670 and 1674, it is evident that even that accurate observer had not as yet clearly perceived their pathological distinction, although it would seem to have been made a century earlier by Ingrassia, a physician of Palermo. The disease known as German measles, or rubella, is a much milder disease than measles. Measles is compulsorily notifiable in Britain.

Causes: Measles is a disease of the earlier years of childhood. Like most other infectious maladies, it is rare in infants under 6 months old on account of the antibodies that they have acquired from their mothers before birth. It is comparatively seldom met in adults, largely due to the fact that most have undergone an attack in early life, or have been repeatedly exposed to the infection of measles and so have probably acquired a certain amount of immunity, for, among communities where measles is not prevalent, the old suffer equally with the young, when infection is once introduced. Some countries enjoy long immunity from outbreaks of measles, but in such cases the disease, when introduced, spreads with great rapidity and virulence. Two classical examples of the last century were: the epidemic in the Faroe Islands in 1846, where, within six months after the arrival of a single case of measles, more than three-fourths of the entire population were attacked and many perished; and the similarly produced and still more destructive outbreak in Fiji in 1875, in which it was estimated that about one-fourth of the inhabitants were cut off by the disease within three months. In such cases it is generally held that epidemics arising on what may be termed a virgin soil are apt to possess a special severity.

In many lands, such as the United Kingdom and the United States, measles is rarely absent, especially from large towns, where sporadic cases are found in greater or less number at all seasons. But every two years, especially from December to February, epidemics arise and spread among the children who are not protected by a recent attack. In 1986 there were 82,061 cases in England and Wales. One attack of measles does not necessarily give complete immunity from future attacks, but second attacks are rare.

There are few diseases so infectious as measles, and its rapid spread in epidemics is no doubt due to the fact that infection is most potent in the earlier stages, even for several days, before its real nature has been shown by the appearance of the rash. Hence the difficulty of timely isolation and the readiness with which the disease is spread, which is mostly by infected droplets from the nose and throat coughed or sneezed into the air. (See INFECTION.) Another fact, which sometimes assists the spread of measles, is that the temperature often falls to normal on the second day and the child appears to be much better, so that he is again allowed to mix with his play-fellows, owing to the mistaken idea that he is suffering merely from a cold, till the rash appears on the fourth day and shows the real nature of the malady. The infecting agent is a virus.

Symptoms: After the infection has been received into the system, a period of incubation or latency precedes the development of the disease, during which scarcely any disturbance of the health is perceptible. This period appears to vary in duration, but it may be stated as generally lasting for from ten to fifteen days, when it is followed by the invasion of the symptoms specially characteristic of measles. These consist in the somewhat sudden onset of acute catarrh of the mucous membranes. Sneezing, accompanied with a watery discharge, sometimes bleeding from the nose, redness and watering of the eyes, cough of a short, frequent, and noisy character, with little or no expectoration, hoarseness of the voice, and occasionally sickness and diarrhoea, are the chief symptoms of this stage. There is well-marked febrile disturbance, the temperature being elevated to 37·7° to 39°C (100° to 102°F), and the pulse rapid, while headache, thirst, and restlessness are usually present to a greater or less degree. In some instances these initial symptoms are so slight that they almost escape notice, and the child is allowed to associate with others at a time when the contagion of the disease is most active. In rare cases, especially in young children, convulsions usher in, or occur in the course of, this stage of invasion which lasts as a rule for three or four days, the febrile symptoms, however, showing a characteristic tendency to pass away temporarily (remission) on the second and sometimes also on the third day. About the fourth day after the invasion, sometimes later, rarely earlier, the characteristic eruption appears on the skin, being first noticed on the brow, cheeks, chin, also behind the ears, and on the neck. It consists of small spots of a dusky red or crimson colour, slightly elevated above the surface, at first isolated, but tending to become grouped together into patches of irregular, occasionally crescentic, outline, with portions of skin free from the eruption intervening. The face acquires a swollen and bloated appearance, which, taken along with the catarrh of the nostrils and eyes, is almost characteristic, and renders the diagnosis at this stage a matter of no difficulty. Even before it appears on the skin, the rash is sometimes visible within the mouth, as bluish-white spots on the mucous membrane, known as Koplik spots. The eruption spreads downwards over the body and limbs, which are soon thickly studded with the red spots or patches. Sometimes these become confluent over a considerable surface, giving rise to a larger area of uniform redness.

The rash continues to come out for two or three days, and then begins to fade in the order in which it first showed itself: namely, from above downwards. By the end of about a week after its first appearance, scarcely any trace of the eruption remains beyond a faint staining of the skin. Occasionally during convalescence slight peeling of the epidermis takes place, but much less distinctly than is the case in scarlet fever. At the start of the eruptive stage, the fever, catarrh, and other constitutional disturbances, which were present from the beginning, become aggravated, the temperature often rising to 40·5°C (105°F) or more, and there are headache, thirst, furred tongue, and soreness of the throat, upon which red patches similar to those on the surface of the body may be observed. These symptoms usually decline as soon as the rash has attained its maximum, and often there occurs a sudden and extensive fall of temperature, indicating that the crisis of the disease has been reached. In favourable cases, convalescence proceeds rapidly, the patient feeling perfectly well even before the rash has faded from the skin.

Measles may, however, occur in a very severe or malignant form, in which the symptoms throughout are of urgent character, the rash but feebly developed and of dark-purple hue, while there is great prostration of strength, accompanied with intense catarrh of the respiratory or gastro-intestinal mucous membrane. Such cases, always of serious import, are happily rare, occurring mostly in circumstances of bad hygiene, both as regards the individual and his surroundings. On the other hand, cases of measles are often met of so mild a form throughout that the patient can scarcely be persuaded to submit to treatment.

Measles derives its chief importance from the risk of certain complications which are apt to arise during its course. The commonest of these are inflammatory affections of the respiratory organs. These are most liable to occur in very young and delicate children. It has been already stated that irritation of the respiratory passages is one of the symptoms characteristic of measles, but that this subsides with the decline of the eruption. Not infrequently, however, these symptoms, instead of abating, become aggravated, and bronchitis, bronchiolitis or pneumonia develop. By far the greater proportion of the mortality in measles is due to its complications, of which those just mentioned are the most common, but which also include infection of the ear (otitis media), infection of the eyes, diarrhoea, and encephalitis. A rare complication, except in grossly debilitated children, is a form of gangrene affecting the tissues of the mouth or cheeks and other parts of the body (CANCRUM ORIS), leading to disfigurement and even endangering life. (See also SUBACUTE SCLEROSING PANENCEPHALITIS.)

Treatment: The patient should be isolated, but quarantine of contacts is used much less than it used to be, though it is probably a wise precaution to keep infants away from the infected child. During an epidemic children under the age of 5 years should not be admitted to a nursery school, nursery class or infant school unless they are known to have had the disease or have been immunized against it. Child contacts of measles should be allowed to go to school provided they are sent home on the first suggestion of fever or malaise. Measles can be prevented or attenuated with gamma-globulin, and its use should be considered in young family contacts or older children suffering from some other disease. A vaccine is now available which gives a high degree of protection against the disease. It is usually given during the second year of life. Unfortunately the vaccination rate is only around 50 per cent, compared with, for example, The Netherlands where it is over 90 per cent. There is a comparably high rate in the USA, which has been followed by a decrease in the number of cases from 13,255 in 1978 to 2961 in 1980, compared with an average of nearly 100,000 in the United Kingdom with a population less than a quarter of that in the USA. The figure for 1986 in the UK was 82,061.

As regards special treatment, in an ordinary case of measles little is required beyond what is necessary in febrile conditions generally. Routine administration of sulphonamides or penicillin is not indicated, but the latter is indicated in: (*a*) children under 2 years of age; (*b*) children with previous middle-ear disease; (*c*) children suffering from some other disease; (*d*) children who are very ill. Confinement to bed so long as the temperature is raised; light, nourishing diet (eg. soups, milk puddings, glucose). The drug treatment of measles is mainly symptomatic. Linctus codeine is useful for the irritating cough. There is no need to darken the room as used to be the practice. If the patient resents the light, he can easily turn his face away from it.

The serious chest complications of measles are to be dealt with by those measures applicable for the relief of pneumonia or bronchitis. (See BRONCHITIS; PNEUMONIA.) Crusting of the eyes should be treated with bathing with warm water and weak saline compresses. Ear complications, if they come on, usually appear with a discharge as the child is getting better (see EAR, DISEASES OF). Diarrhoea is treated by the usual remedies, such as codeine phosphate or Loperamide. Mixtures of chalk and Kaolin are alternatives but fluid replacement is of prime importance in acute diarrhoea, especially in children. (See DIARRHOEA.)

Isolation can end seven days from the appearance of the rash if all discharges have dried up.

MEASURES (see WEIGHTS AND MEASURES).

MEAT (see PROTEIN).

MEATUS is a term applied to any passage or opening: eg. external auditory meatus, the passage from the surface to the drum of the ear.

MECHANOTHERAPY is the provision of active physical exercise by means of a mechanical contrivance which necessitates the expenditure of physical work before it can be moved or used. Examples of mechanotherapy are dumbbells, Indian clubs and parallel bars. One of the advantages of mechanotherapy, as opposed to other forms of physical exercise, is that it allows the amount of exercise performed to be accurately measured.

MECKEL'S DIVERTICULUM is a hollow process sometimes found attached to the small intestine. It is placed on the small intestine about 90 to 120 cm (3 or 4 feet) away from its junction with the large intestine, is several cms long, and ends blindly.

MECILLINAM (see ANTIBIOTIC).

MECONIUM is the brown, semi-fluid material which collects in the bowels of a child prior to birth, and which should be discharged either at the time of birth or shortly afterwards. It consists partly of bile secreted by the liver before birth, partly of debris from the mucous membrane of the intestines.

MEDAZEPAM (NOBRIUM) is a tranquilliser which is proving of value in the treatment of anxiety neurosis. (See BENZODIAZEPINES.)

MEDIAN TIBIAL SYNDROME (see SHIN SPLINTS).

MEDIASTINUM is the space in the chest which lies between the two lungs. It contains the heart and great vessels, the gullet, the lower part of the windpipe, the thoracic duct, the phrenic nerves, as well as numerous structures of less importance.

MEDULLA OBLONGATA is the hindmost part of the brain and is continued into the spinal cord. In it are situated several of the nerve-centres which are most essential to life, such as those governing breathing, the action of the heart, swallowing. (See BRAIN.)

MEFENAMIC ACID is a drug with pain-relieving, anti-inflammatory and antipyretic actions that is proving of value in the treatment of osteoarthrosis and rheumatoid arthritis.

MEFRUSIDE (BAYCARON) (see BENZOTHIADIAZINES).

MEGA- and MEGALO- are prefixes denoting largeness.

MEGALOMANIA is a delusion of grandeur or an insane belief in a person's own extreme greatness, goodness, or power.

MEGRIM is another name for migraine (qv).

MEIBOMIAN GLANDS: Numerous glands within the tarsal plates of the eyelids. Their secretions form part of the tears.

MEIOSIS or REDUCTION DIVISION is the form of cell division that only occurs in the gonads, that is the testis and the ovary, giving rise to the germ cells of the sperms and the ova. Two types of sperm cells are produced. One contains 22 autosomes and a Y sex chromosome and the other contains 22 autosomes and an X sex chromosome. All the ova, however, produced by normal meiosis have 22 autosomes and an X sex chromosome. Two divisions of the nucleus occur and only one division of the chromosomes, so that the number of chromosomes in

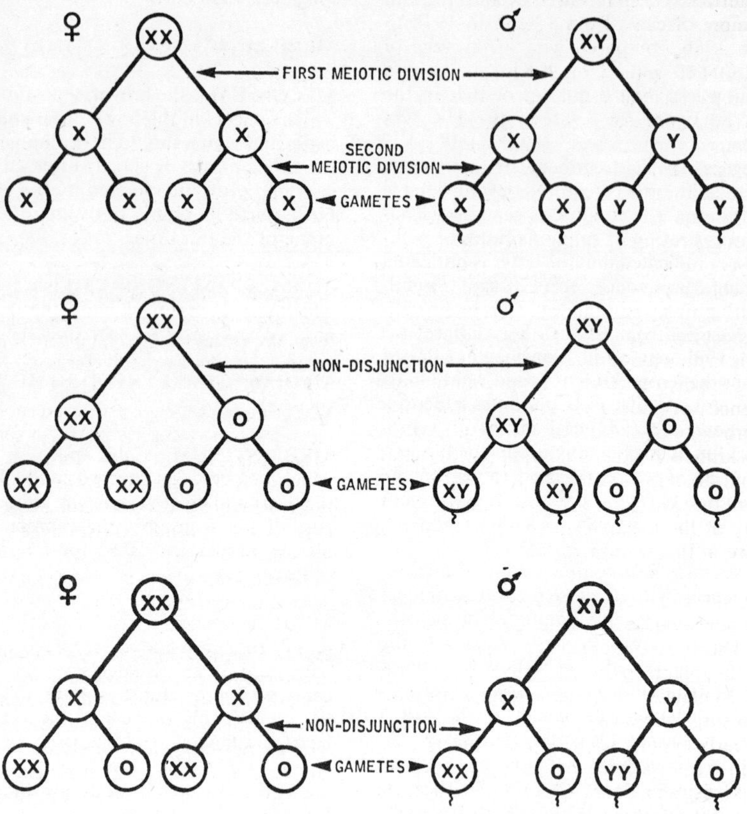

The formation of gametes. Top, normal meiosis. Centre, non-disjunction at first meiotic divison. Bottom, non-disjunction at second meiotic division.

the ova and sperms is half that of the somatic cells. Each chromosome pair divides so that the gametes receives only one member of each pair. The number of chromosomes is restored to full complement at fertilization so the the zygote has a complete set, each chromosome from the nucleus of the sperm pairing up with its corresponding partner from the ovum.

The first stage of meiosis involves the pairing of homologous chromosomes which join together and synapse lengthwise. The chromosomes then become doubled by splitting along their length and the chromatids so formed are held together by centromeres. As the homologous chromosomes, one of which has come from the mother and the other from the father, are lying together genetic interchange can take place between the chromatids and in this way new combinations of genes arise. All four chromatids are closely interwoven and recombination may take place between any maternal or any paternal chromatids. This process is known as crossing over or recombination. After this period of interchange homologous chromosomes move apart, one to each pole of the nucleus. The cell then divides and the nucleus of each new cell now contains 23 and not 46 chromosomes. The second meiotic division then occurs, the centromeres divide and the chromatids move apart to opposite poles of the nucleus so there are still 23 chromosomes in each of the daughter nuclei so formed. The cell divides again so that there are four gametes, each containing a half number (haploid) set of chromosomes. However, owing to the recombination or crossing over the genetic material is not identical with either parent or with other spermatozoa.

MELAENA means a condition of the stools in which dark, tarry masses are passed from the bowel. It is due to bleeding from the stomach or from the higher part of the bowel, the blood undergoing chemical changes under the action of the secretions, and being finally converted in large part into sulphide of iron.

MELANCHOLIA is a form of mental illness characterized by great mental and physical depression. (See MENTAL ILLNESS.)

MELANIN is the dark pigment found in the skin and hair, as well as the choroid coat of the eye. It is the amount of melanin which decides the colour of the skin and hair. In white skin it occurs as granules in cells known as melanocytes situated in the stratum basale of the skin (qv). On exposure to ultra-violet light these granules are released and pass into the superficial layers of the skin where they produce the brown colour known as sun-tan which protects the skin against the harmful effects of continued exposure to the ultra-violet rays of the sun. Genetic factors play an important role in determining the distribution of melanin in the skin and hence its colour. Thus in those with genetically brown or black skin, as well as sun-tanned white-skinned people, there is a widespread distribution of melanin in the more superficial layers of the skin. This is due more to increased activity of the melanocytes than to an actual increase in their number.

MELANOMA is a tumour arising from the cells that produce melanin (qv). A highly malignant form, known as malignant melanoma, arises from the pigmented cells of moles (qv) or naevi. Malignant melanoma, which responds well to surgical removal provided this is done at an early enough stage, is much more common in white people living in sunny climes such as Australia, South Africa and parts of the USA, but it can occur in the United Kingdom. The hazards of ultra-violet light in causing malignant melanoma cannot be ignored in the British Isles, particularly in those who holiday abroad. The incidence is steadily rising and, as one expert has pointed out, 'is likely to continue to rise so long as our society remains addicted to the sun'. He adds: 'Though ultra-violet light is not the sole cause of malignant melanoma, excessive exposure is an important factor... particularly in people whose skin has a tendency to go red whether or not it subsequently tans. The prophylactic use of sun-screening agents should be a routine for such people'. (See SUNBURN.)

MELORHEOSTOSIS is an abnormal condition of bone in which pathological hardening and denseness extend in a linear direction through one of the long bones of a limb, causing deformity and limitation of movement of the limb.

MELPHALAN (ALKERAN) is one of the alkylating agents (qv) which is proving of value in the treatment of certain forms of malignant disease. (See CYTOTOXIC DRUGS.)

MEMBRANES (see BRAIN; CROUP; DIPHTHERIA; LABOUR).

MEMORY (see FORGETFULNESS).

MENAPHTHONE is a synthetic vitamin K_1 preparation. (See VITAMINS.)

MENARCHE is the term applied to the beginning of the menstrual function. The average age at which it occurs in British girls is 12½ years. In London girls it is 13·1 years. There is considerable racial and geographical variation.

MENDELISM is the term applied to a law enunciated by G. J. Mendel that the offspring is not intermediate in type between its parents, but that the type of one or other parent is predominant. Characteristics are classed as either dominant or recessive. The offspring of the first generation tend to inherit the dominant characteristics, whilst the recessive characteristics remain latent and appear in some of the offspring of the second generation. If individuals possessing recessive characters unite, recessive characters then become dominant characters in succeeding generations. The law may be expressed by the following formula:

$$n(DD+2DR+RR),$$

in which DD represents dominant offspring, RR recessive offspring, and DR offspring with mixed characters.

MENIÈRE'S DISEASE, so called after the Frenchman, Prosper Menière, who first described it in 1861, is a disease characterized by tinnitus (qv), deafness and intermittent attacks of vertigo. It usually occurs in middle age, and is slightly more common in men than in women. The first manifestation is usually deafness on one side. Then, as a rule many months later, there is a sudden attack, without any warning, of intense vertigo. This often occurs during sleep, waking the patient up. It is soon followed by vomiting and sweating. The acute giddiness usually lasts for two to three hours but, after the attack, some unsteadiness persists for a few days. The time interval between attacks varies from a week to a few months. When they do recur, they tend to occur in clusters. The tinnitus, which tends to be high-pitched, comes on about the same time as the deafness. It is often described as being like rushing water or escaping steam. The deafness becomes gradually worse until it is complete. The condition is due to excessive fluid in the labyrinth of the ears (see EAR). The cause of this accumulation is not known, though it has been suggested that it might be a form of allergy, or might be due to spasm of the small blood-vessels.

Treatment consists of restricting the daily intake of fluid to 1·5 litres (2½ pints), and controlling the daily consumption of salt by not adding it to food at the table. A multiplicity of drugs has been recommended, including diuretics such as frusemide (qv), drugs to prevent vomiting such as dimenhydrinate (qv), and prochlorperazine (qv), and vasodilating drugs such as nicotinic acid (qv). If these all fail and the condition persists, then destruction of the labyrinth is carried out by operation or by ultrasound. An alternative is to cut the vestibular nerve; this has the advantage of preserving hearing, which the other surgical procedures do not do. (See TINNITUS.)

MENINGES are the membranes surrounding the brain and spinal cord. (See BRAIN.) The membranes include the dura mater, a tough, fibrous membrane closely applied to the inside of the skull; the arachnoid, a more delicate membrane, enveloping the brain but separated from its irregular surface by spaces containing fluid; and the pia mater, a delicate network of fibres containing blood-vessels and uniting the arachnoid to the brain. The two last are sometimes referred to as the pia-arachnoid. These membranes bear the blood-vessels which nourish the surface of the brain and the interior of the skull. Meningeal haemorrhage from these vessels forms one of the chief dangers arising from fracture of the skull.

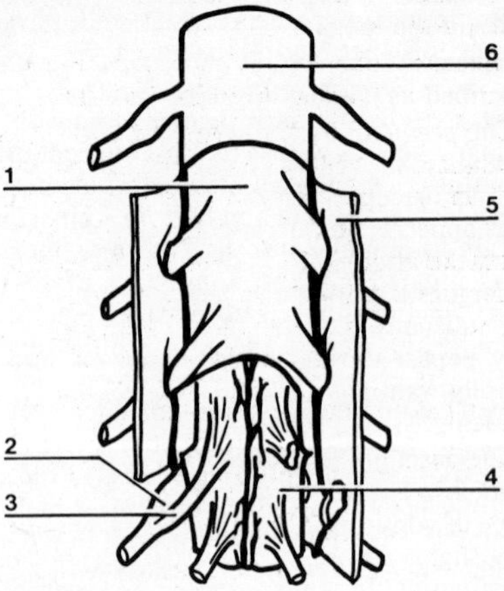

1 arachnoid
2 spinal ganglion
3 ventral nerve root
4 ligamentum denticulatum
5 dura mater, cut and turned backwards
6 dura mater

The membranes of the spinal cord.

MENINGISM is a condition with symptoms closely resembling those of meningitis, but due simply to a feverish state.

MENINGITIS is inflammation affecting the membranes of the brain (cerebral meningitis) or spinal cord (spinal meningitis), or both. Either the dura or the pia-arachnoid may be inflamed. In the former case the condition is known as pachymeningitis; in the latter, leptomeningitis. Pachymeningitis is the less common of the two, is often local and secondary to disease of the bone (eg. tuberculous or syphilitic), and may be cranial or spinal. Leptomeningitis is the more common, is usually extensive in distribution, greatly alters the composition of the cerebrospinal fluid, and may be primary or secondary to infection elsewhere in the body.

Meningitis may be classified according to the infecting organism as pneumococcal, pyogenic, tuberculous, syphilitic, meningococcal. The all-important evidence is gained by lumbar puncture and examination of the CEREBROSPINAL FLUID (qv). In meningitis the pressure of this fluid is increased, changes in its appearance and constituents occur, and the infecting agent can usually be isolated from it. In meningitis the protein and the number of cells increase and the glucose decreases. A decrease in the amount of chlorides of the cerebrospinal fluid is characteristic of tuberculous meningitis. Increase in the number of cells may make the normally clear cerebrospinal fluid opalescent, as in tuberculous meningitis, or turbid, as in pneumococcal and pyogenic meningitis. Clinically, the symptoms are due to irritation of the meninges and rise in the intracranial pressure: headache, vomiting, photophobia, rigidity of the neck, Kernig's sign (qv), convulsions, paralyses, coma.

In England, in 1986, there were 2172 cases of acute meningitis, 820 of which were due to the meningococcus. (See MENINGOCOCCAL MENINGITIS.)

PNEUMOCOCCAL MENINGITIS is usually secondary to infection with the pneumococcus elsewhere: for example, empyema or otitis media. This formerly fatal condition is now in many cases successfully treated by penicillin given intravenously.

PYOGENIC MENINGITIS is due to secondary infection with staphylococci, streptococci, *H. influenzae*, gonococci, or anthrax bacilli – especially the first two. The introduction of antibiotics has altered the previously fatal prognosis of these cases. Satisfactory results are obtained from the use of chloramphenicol in the treatment of meningitis due to *H. influenzae*.

TUBERCULOUS MENINGITIS is an inflammation of the membranes caused by the *Mycobacterium tuberculosis*. The disease is most common in children under the age of 10 years, but is by no means confined to that period of life, and may affect adults. The determining factor in the disease is exposure to infection with the bovine or the human *Mycobacterium tuberculosis*. All too often a grandparent with a chronic cough due to pulmonary tuberculosis is the unsuspected source of infection of the grandchild. In numerous cases associated factors are bad hygienic conditions, with insufficient or improper feeding, or some disease of childhood, particularly measles or whooping-cough. When it occurs in adults it is usually secondary to some chronic manifestation of tuberculosis in another part of the body, especially in the lungs.

Symptoms: Tuberculous meningitis is usually described as passing through three stages.

The *premonitory symptoms* are mostly such as relate to the general nutrition. The patient, if a child, becomes listless and easily fatigued, loses appetite, and is restless at night. There is headache after exertion, and the temper often undergoes a marked change, the child becoming unusually and irritable. These symptoms may persist during many weeks, or may be entirely wanting, the disease developing quite suddenly.

The onset of the *first stage*, or *stage of excitement*, is in most instances marked by the occurrence of vomiting, often severe, but sometimes only slight, and there is, in general, obstinate constipation. In some cases, the first symptoms are convulsions, which, however, may in this early stage subside, and remain absent, or reappear at a later period. Headache is one of the most constant of the earlier symptoms, and is generally intense and accompanied by sharper paroxysms, which cause the patient to scream with a peculiar and characteristic cry. There is great intolerance of light and sound and general nervous sensitiveness. The neck shows rigidity so that the head cannot be so readily bent forwards as usual, and similar rigidity in the lower limbs is almost invariably present. The latter symptom forms an important sign (Kernig's sign) of meningitis. If the knee is raised from the bed, stiffness and pain are experienced in the muscles behind the thigh when the attempt is made to straighten the leg at the knee-joint, whereas in the healthy child the whole lower limb can be readily flexed on the abdomen with the knee straight. Fever is present to a greater or less extent, the temperature ranging from 37·8° to 39·4°C (100° to 103°F); yet the pulse is not quickened in proportion, being on the contrary rather slow, but exhibiting a tendency to irregularity, and liable to become rapid on slight exertion. This slowness of the pulse is of great importance in distinguishing the disease from others which resemble it, and in which the heart beats more rapidly in proportion to the temperature. Symptoms of this character continue for a period varying from one to two weeks, when they are succeeded by the stage of depression.

In the *second stage*, or *stage of depression*, there is a marked change in the symptoms, which is apt to lead to the belief that a favourable turn has taken place. The patient becomes quieter and inclines to sleep, but on careful watching it will be found that this quietness is but a condition of apathy or partial stupor into which the child has sunk. The vomiting has now ceased, and there is less fever; the pulse is slower, and shows a still greater tendency to irregularity than before, while the breathing is of markedly unequal character, being rapid and shallow at one time, and long drawn out and sinking away at another. There is manifestly little suffering, although the peculiar cry may still be uttered, and the patient lies prostrate, occasionally rolling the head uneasily upon the pillow, or picking at the bedclothes or at his face with his fingers. He does not ask for food, but readily swallows what is offered. The eyes present important alterations, the pupils being dilated or unequal, and scarcely responding to light. There may be double vision, or partial or complete blindness. Squinting is common in this stage, and there may also be drooping of an eyelid, due to paralysis of the part, and one or more limbs may be likewise paralysed.

To this succeeds the *third stage*, or *stage of paralysis*, in which certain of the former symptoms recur, while others become intensified. There is generally a return of the fever, the temperature rising sometimes to a very high degree. The pulse becomes feeble, rapid, and exceedingly irregular, as is also the case with the breathing. Coma is profound, but the patient may still be got to swallow nourishment, though not so readily as before. Convulsions are apt to occur, while paralysis, more or less extensive, affects portions of the body or groups of muscles. The pupils are now widely dilated, and there is often complete blindness or deafness. In this condition the sufferer's strength undergoes rapid decline and the body becomes markedly emaciated. Death takes place suddenly in a fit, or, more generally, from exhaustion. Shortly before the fatal event it is not uncommon for the patient, who, it may be for some days previously, lay in a state of profound stupor, to wake up, ask for food, and talk to those around. But the hopes which may be thus raised are quickly dispelled by the setting in of the symptoms of rapid decline. The diagnosis is clinched by the finding of *Mycobacterium tuberculosis* in the cerebrospinal fluid.

The disease used to be invariably fatal, but the outlook has been entirely altered by the introduction of anti-tuberculous drugs. With modern treatment the mortality depends largely on the stage at which treatment is initiated. If this is in the early stages, 95 per cent recover, but if treatment is not started until later in the disease, only 60 per cent or fewer will recover.

Treatment: The drugs used in the treatment of tuberculous meningitis are streptomycin, isoniazid, rifampicin and ethambutol. The administration of streptomycin and isoniazid in this condition requires skilled medical and nursing supervision such as is available only in hospital. Every child (or adult) with tuberculous meningitis, or suspected tuberculous meningitis, therefore should be examined as early as possible by an experienced children's (or tuberculosis) specialist, in order that an expert opinion may be obtained.

SYPHILITIC MENINGITIS is usually a chronic inflammation (but sometimes producing acute symptoms) occurring in most cases within the first four years of infection. It may spread from the pia-arachnoid into the brain – a meningo-encephalitis – or it may attack the dura mater and the overlying bone. The pressure of the cerebrospinal fluid is raised; the fluid itself is clear and contains an increased number of lymphocytes. Headache is a common symptom. Paralysis of cranial nerves (resulting, for example, in a squint) can occur as a result of strangulation of the nerve in inflamed meninges at the base of the brain. Hydrocephalus may arise suddenly, with headache, vomiting, sleepiness, mental changes, and congestion of the optic discs as symptoms and signs, or syphilitic meningitis may come on acutely. The treatment is as for syphilis.

MENINGOCOCCAL MENINGITIS, also known as EPIDEMIC CEREBROSPINAL MENINGITIS, CEREBROSPINAL FEVER, SPOTTED FEVER, MALIGNANT PURPURIC FEVER, and POST-BASIC MENINGITIS, is a dangerous epidemic condition characterized by painful contractions of the muscles of the neck, retraction of the head, and mental symptoms. It was first distinctly recognized in the year 1837, when it prevailed as an epidemic, chiefly among troops in the south-west of France. In 1846 it appeared in Ireland, especially in the workhouses of Belfast and Dublin. Since that time it has appeared repeatedly both in Europe and America, notably in a severe epidemic in the large towns of Scotland in 1907–09, in a slighter form among the troops during the war of 1914–18, and a fair-sized epidemic in Great Britain in the winter of 1939–40. The disease is notifiable. Epidemics of it sweep across tropical Africa with great regularity.

Causes: When an outbreak takes place, it usually occurs about the months of February, March, and April, and affects a closed community such as a school, garrison, camp, or prison. The direct cause is an organism, the *Neisseria meningitidis* or *meningococcus*, which is found in the exudation round the nervous system, in the blood, and often in the nasal discharge. The organism is of four different types. It is believed that the infection takes place through the nose and that a large number of persons who do not contract the disease harbour the meningococcus in the nasal discharge and form sources of infection to more susceptible people, especially children, by coughing and sneezing – they are known as carriers. Factors favouring infection are a high carrier-rate, the virulence of the organism, a closed community (eg. a camp), nasopharyngeal catarrh, bad ventilation, insufficient space between beds, introduction of susceptible persons into a closed community, season of the year (winter and spring). Young children are much more susceptible than adults. The incubation period is 2 to 10 days (commonly 2 to 5).

Symptoms: The onset is usually sudden, sometimes startlingly so. As a rule, vomiting, headache, and shivering first appear, followed in a few hours by stiffness of the neck. In children, convulsions are common. In a case of very sudden onset, the patient, while going about as usual, may fall down suddenly in a convulsion, or he may go to bed perfectly well and be found unconscious on the following morning. If the patient is not unconscious, headache and pain with stiffness in the back of the neck continue, squinting is often seen, the tongue is furred and dry, and there is a rise of temperature: 37·8° to 40°C (100° to 104°F). The patient is irritable, the body tender to the touch, and the limbs stiff so that bending up of the lower limbs on the abdomen with the knee straight becomes impossible (Kernig's sign). The patient is often sleepless or delirious, and there is a great tendency for the symptoms to go and come. Purpuric spots, from which the disease takes its name of 'spotted fever', appear over the surface of the trunk during the first week of the disease in greater or less numbers in about one-quarter of the cases. Death occurs in a large number of the cases within a week of the onset, taking place very often suddenly from heart failure. After the first week, if life is prolonged, the disease usually abates gradually and in the course of some weeks the rigidity may have disappeared and the temperature may have become normal. On the other hand, the disease may pass into a chronic state with great wasting, and, if the patient is a young child, head retraction in these cases usually becomes very marked and the body is greatly bent backwards. The patient during the course of this chronic stage may become blind or deaf or may show marked mental deterioration. The child often falls a victim to some complication, such as broncho-pneumonia.

In those patients who die, it is common to find the surface of the brain and the spinal cord covered with thick pus and the blood-vessels markedly congested. If death has occurred at a very early period, nothing more may be visible than very intense congestion of the membranes on the surface of the brain. The interior of the brain shows more than the usual amount of fluid.

The prognosis in this disease has been revolutionized by the introduction of the sulphonamides and penicillin. Formerly the mortality rate in epidemics was 70 to 80 per cent, whilst in fulminating cases it might even be 100 per cent. Today, with efficient treatment it has fallen to 7 to 10 per cent. The main factors governing the prognosis are: (1) The age of the patient: the disease is particularly dangerous in infants and old people. (2) The type of onset: a fulminating onset carries a bad prognosis. (3) The stage of the disease at which treatment is begun: the earlier the better.

Treatment: The patient must be isolated and, whenever possible, should be treated in hospital. Treatment consists essentially of the administration of full doses of penicillin injections intravenously. The patient is confined to bed and given a light nutritious diet. For insomnia sedatives are usually required, whilst the pains in the joints and limbs are usually best relieved by warm baths. The headache usually responds to a combination of aspirin, paracetamol, and codeine but, if particularly severe, lumbar puncture may be necessary.

Quarantine of contacts is useless, but there is some evidence that, in the event of an outbreak in a semi-closed community (eg. a residential school or a military camp) the administration of sulphadiazine to all contacts may be of value. A vaccine is now available which is proving of value in the control of epidemics in Africa, but the duration of its action is still not certain.

MENINGOCELE is a protusion of the meninges of the brain through a defect in the skull. (See SPINA BIFIDA.)

MENINGOCOCCUS (see NEISSERIA).

MENINGOENCEPHALITIS is the term applied to infection of the membranes, or meninges, of the brain and the underlying brain matter. In practically all cases of meningitis (qv) there is some involvement of the underlying brain. It is when this involvement is considerable that the term, meningoencephalitis, is used. One form that has attracted attention in recent years is that caused by amoebae (qv), particularly that known as *Naegleria fowleri*, in which the infection is acquired through bathing in contaminated water. Effective chlorination of swimming baths kills this micro-organism.

MENINGOMYELOCELE is a protrusion of the meninges of the spinal cord through a defect in the spine. (See SPINA BIFIDA.)

MENISCUS is the term applied to a crescentic fibro-cartilage in a joint, such as the cartilages in the knee-joint.

MENOPAUSE is the term applied to the cessation of menstruation at the end of reproductive life. Usually it occurs between the ages of 45 and 50, although it may occur before the age of 30 or after the age of 50. It can be a psychologically disturbing experience which is quite often accompanied by physical manifestations. These include hot flushes, tiredness, irritability, lack of concentration, palpitations, aching joints and vaginal irritation. There may also be loss of libido. Most women can and do live happy, active lives through the menopause, the length of which varies considerably. The chauvinists would say that it was a natural event and it is those women that can accept it as such who are least likely to suffer from its manifestations. This is not true. The loss of oestrogen which occurs at the menopause causes atrophy of the genital tract. Vasomotor instability in the form of hot flushes, sweats and palpitations occur and can be very debilitating. The urinary urge, loss of libido and depression are not uncommon manifestations and are remediable with treatment.

One of the major problems of the menopause which does not give rise to symptoms until many years later is the osteoporosis which follows the cessation of menstruation. Osteoporosis is a metabolic bone disease characterised by a reduction in the total amount of bone but without any abnormality in the actual bone present. After the menopause 1 per cent of the bone is lost per annum to the end of life. This accounts for the frequency of fractures of the femur in elderly women as a result of osetoporosis but it can be prevented by hormone-replacement therapy. Oestrogens are more effective than tranquillisers or sedatives in relieving the short-term symptoms such as hot flushes, sweats and vaginal dryness. Atrophic vaginitis and vulvitis also usually respond to treatment with oestrogens. Oestrogen therapy reduces the demineralisation of bone which normally occurs after the menopause and if it is started early and continued for years it may prevent the development of osteoporosis. Oestrogen is far more effective than calcium supplements and has been shown to greatly reduce fractures affecting the spine, wrists and legs after the age of 50. Cyclical therapy is necessary to avoid abnormal bleeding in women who have reached the menopause. If oestrogens are given alone there is a slightly increased risk of endometrial hyperplasia which may proceed to endometrial cancer. This can be prevented by the administration of oestrogen-progestogen combinations. There is good evidence that a combination of oestrogen and a progestogen avoids the endometrial hyperstimulation produced by the oestrogen alone and relieves most of the symptoms of vasomotor instability of the menopause and prevents the bone loss associated with the menopause. It has been suggested there was a relationship between oestrogen treatment and breast tumours. However a study by the Boston collaborative drug surveillance program showed that there was no evidence of any association between oestrogen therapy and either benign or malignant breast tumours. There is good evidence that before the age of 50 men are a greater risk of developing myocardial infarction but in the post-menopausal women the risks are the same. It has thus been suggested that the secretion of oestrogens protects against cardiovascular disease in the reproductive years. Nevertheless there is no evidence that the administration of oestrogens in the menopause increases the risk of developing atherosclerotic vascular disease, breast cancer, thrombo-embolic disorders or hypertension.

MENORRHAGIA means an over-abundance of the menstrual discharge.

MENSTRUATION is a periodic change occurring in human beings and the higher apes, and consists chiefly in a flow of blood from the cavity of the womb, and associated with various slight constitutional disturbances. It begins between the ages of 12 and 15, as a rule, although its onset may be delayed till as late as 20, or it may begin as early as 10 or 11. Along with its first appearance the body develops the secondary sex characteristics of the sex: eg.

enlargement of the breasts, characteristic hair distribution. The duration of each menstrual period varies in different persons from two to eight days. It recurs in the great majority of cases with regularity, most commonly at intervals of twenty-eight days or thirty days, less often with intervals of twenty-one or twenty-seven days, ceasing only during pregnancy and lactation, till the age of 45 or 50 arrives, when it stops altogether, as a rule ceasing early if it has begun early, and vice versa. The final stoppage is known as the menopause (qv) or the climacteric (qv).

Menstruation depends upon a functioning ovary and this upon a healthy pituitary gland. The regular rhythm may depend upon a centre in the hypothalamus, which is in close connection with the pituitary. After menstruation the denuded uterine endometrium is regenerated under the influence of the follicular hormone, oestradiol. The epithelium of the endometrium proliferates, and about a fortnight after the beginning of menstruation great development of the endometrial glands takes place under the influence of progesterone, the hormone secreted by the corpus luteum. These changes are made for the reception of the fertilized ovum. In the absence of fertilization the uterine endometrium breaks down in the subsequent menstrual discharge.

Disorders of menstruation: In the majority of healthy women, menstruation proceeds regularly for thirty years or more, with the exceptions connected with childbirth. In many persons, as the result either of general or local conditions, the process may be absent or excessive, or may be attended with great discomfort or pain. The term *amenorrhoea* is applied to cases in which menstruation is absent, *menorrhagia* and *metrorrhagia* to cases in which it is excessive, the former if the excess occurs at the regular periods, the latter if it is irregular, whilst *dysmenorrhoea* is the name given to cases in which the process is attended by pain.

AMENORRHOEA: If menstruation has never occurred the amenorrhoea is termed *primary*. If it ceases after having once become established it is known as *secondary amenorrhoea*. The only value of these terms is that some patients with either chromosome abnormalities or malformations of the genital tract fall into the primary category. Otherwise the age of onset of symptoms is more important.

The causes of amenorrhoea are numerous and treatment requires dealing with the primary cause. The commonest cause is pregnancy. Hypothalamic disorders such as psychological stress or anorexia nervosa cause amenorrhoea. Poor nutrition or loss of weight by dieting may cause amenorrhoea and any serious underlying disease such as tuberculosis or malaria may also result in the cessation of periods. The excess secretion of prolactin, whether this is the result of a micro-adenoma of the pituitary gland or whether it is drug induced, will cause amenorrhoea and possibly galactorrhoea as well. Malfunction of the pituitary gland will result in a failure to produce the gonadotrophic hormones with consequent amenorrhoea. Excessive production of cortisol, as in Cushing's syndrome, or of androgens, as in the adreno-genital syndrome or the polycystic ovary syndrome, will result in amenorrhoea. Amenorrhoea occasionally follows use of the oral contraceptive pill and may be associated with both hypothyroidism and obesity. It is thus important to take a careful history with emphasis on psychological factors, weight fluctuations and the use of drugs that may stimulate the release of prolactin and it is also important to look for evidence of virilisation. A gynaecological examination is necessary in primary amenorrhoea to exclude malformations of the genital tract. Estimations of the gonadotrophic hormone levels will reveal whether the amenorrhoea is primary ovarian failure or secondary to pituitary disease.

In view of the frequent psychosomatic origins of amenorrhoea, reassurance of the patient is of great importance, in particular with reference to marriage and the ability to conceive. When weight loss is the cause of amenorrhoea, restoration of body weight alone can result in spontaneous menstruation. Patients with raised concentration of serum gonadotrophin hormones have primary ovarian failure. It is not amenable to treatment. Cyclical oestrogen/progestogen therapy will usually establish withdrawal bleeding. If the amenorrhoea is due to mild pituitary failure menstruation may return after treatment with clomiphene. Clomiphene is a non-steroidal agent which competes for oestrogen receptors in the hypothalamus. The patients who are most likely to respond to clomiphene are those who have some evidence of endogenous oestrogen and gonadotrophin production.

MENORRHAGIA: Excessive menstruation may be due to the same general conditions which produce amenorrhoea, the same diseases, such as glomerulonephritis or tuberculosis, causing stoppage or excess in different women. Thus, in some people an excessive loss is brought about by these conditions, and the effects of the general disease are much increased by the loss of blood. In heart disease, the womb may share in the general internal congestion, and the menses in consequence are increased. In some people, menstruation at its first appearance is excessive; whilst this is so often the case as to be almost the general rule at the time when the menstrual periods are about to stop, ie. at the menopause, when they also tend to become irregular. But it is most often a local condition that produces menorrhagia: in this case, as a rule, not only is the periodic loss increased but there is bleeding at irregular times (metrorrhagia). Polypus, fibroid, and other tumours, displacements of the womb, and some inflammation consequent upon childbirth or miscarriage, are the most common causes of this type. In the treatment, rest and various internal remedies which check haemorrhage, together with careful attention to the general health between the periods, are essential. (See UTERUS, DISEASES OF.)

DYSMENORRHOEA may vary from mere discomfort to agonizing colic, accompanied by prostration and vomiting. Anaemia is sometimes a cause of painful menstruation as well as of stoppage of this function. Chills and exhaustion may produce pain for a single period in women whose periods are usually painless.

Inflammation of various internal organs, eg. of the womb itself, the ovaries, or the Fallopian tubes, is one of the commonest causes of dysmenorrhoea which comes on for the first time late in life, especially when the trouble follows the birth of a child. In this case the pain exists more or less at all times, but is aggravated at the periods. It is relieved by various local means directed towards checking the inflammation present.

Many cases of dysmenorrhoea appear with the beginning of menstrual life, and accompany every period. It has been estimated that 5 to 10 per cent of girls in their late teens or early twenties are severely incapacitated by dysmenorrhoea for several hours each month. In some of these it is of an obstructive type, due to spasm of the neck of the womb, in consequence of which a severe uterine colic is set up. In many cases, the spasm appears to be one manifestation of a nervous temperament. In other cases the pain appears to be due to difficulty in the separation of the surface layer of mucous membrane, which comes away in healthy menstruation in fragments with the blood. In these cases, the lining of the uterus, after great difficulty, is finally expelled in the form of a complete membranous cast of the interior, and the pain then abates, In other cases, the spasm may be due in part to defective development of the womb, producing either narrowness of its mouth or causing it to be bent upon itself, and occasionally these cases are benefited, or cured by an operation designed to stretch the neck of the womb, or otherwise relieve the defect. Yet a further cause for this pain, it has been suggested, is an excessive production of prostaglandins (qv). In not a few –indeed some would say the majority – there is a large psychological factor. This may be the sole cause, or it may be an ancillary cause exacerbating the pain, or discomfort, induced by some physical cause. Whatever the psychological factor –whether due to inadequate sex instruction, fear, mental, domestic, or work disharmony – the sooner it is discovered and dealt with, the more likely is the dysmenorrhoea to come under control. For the temporary relief of dysmenorrhoea, rest in bed, or, at all events, in the recumbent position, a hot water bottle to the lower part of the abdomen, and aspirin orally, are the remedies which prove most useful.

MENTAL HANDICAP is also referred to as intellectual handicap or learning difficulties. Terms such as mental deficiency, mental retardation, mental subnormality, and still more outdated words such as imbecility, feeblemindedness and idiocy, are often now regarded as pejorative and offensive to the people they label, as indeed may be the term mental handicap itself.

A person with a mental handicap has been defined as 'an individual who, by reason of developmental intellectual impairment, needs additional services to live a normal life, or as normal a life as possible.' The World Health Organization International Classification of Diseases defines mental retardation as a condition of arrested or incomplete development of mind which is especially characterized by subnormality of intelligence and social functioning. The American Association on mental deficiency defines mental retardation as significantly subaverage intellectual functioning existing concurrently with deficits in adaptive behaviour and manifest during the developmental period. The 1983 Mental Health Act uses the term 'mental impairment' to describe that small minority of mentally handicapped people who also show 'abnormally aggressive or seriously irresponsible conduct'.

The degree of mental handicap is often further subdivided on IQ grounds into profound (under 20), severe (20–35), moderate (35–49), and mild (50–70). The profound, severe and moderate groups are often grouped together as major mental handicap. However it must be emphasized that IQ testing is not a precise science, that due account must be taken of the individual's linguistic, social and cultural background, and that individuals who function normally in society cannot be said to be handicapped.

Occurrence: Estimates vary as to how common mental handicap is, depending on the definitions used and the age of the populations being examined. In general it seems that the incidence (of new cases within a particular period of time) of mental handicap is decreasing in the UK but that, because people with a mental handicap now live longer, the prevalence is increasing. IQ tests are commonly statistically designed to ensure that about 2.5 per cent of the population tested scores below IQ 70. Not all these people will have significant impairment of adaptive function or need special services. For school age children it is generally agreed that major mental handicap occurs in about 0·4 per cent of the population. In countries with a high infant mortality the percentage may well be lower because children with handicaps are more vulnerable.

Causation: All degrees of handicap result from a complex interaction between genetic make-up and past and present and environmental features. The greater the degree of impairment the more likely it is to have an organic basis, ie. to be caused by maldevelopment of, or damage to the brain. For major mental handicap it is possible to identify a medical cause for the handicap in about three quarters of those affected. There is less but increasing evidence for an organic component in mild mental handicap.

Forty per cent of major mental handicap is caused by chromosome abnormalities, mainly trisomy 21 (Down's syndrome). Other genetic defects account for a further 15 per cent. Another 10 per cent occur within pregnancy or the perinatal period and 10 per cent of mental handicap occurs after birth as a result of accidents, child abuse, infections and brain tumours. The cause in the remaining quarter is unknown. Prenatal diagnosis is now available for many of the conditions causing major mental handicap.

Medical complications: Since major mental handicap is usually caused by maldevelopment of, or damage to the brain, and sometimes other body systems, it is not surprising that people with such handicaps are also more liable to physical ill health and handicap. Down's syndrome may involve malformation of the heart and intestines, and people with the syndrome are more liable to develop other illnesses subsequently. Some people with major mental handicap are paralysed or have other motor disorders. Sensory handicaps are also more common and must be identified to prevent secondary handicap resulting from them. About one third of people with major mental handicap have epileptic fits. People with a mental handicap will in the first place use normal primary care services, but may need referral on to specialist medical services.

Psychological and psychiatric needs: The lives many mentally handicapped people lead, their learning difficulties and the presence of brain damage, all predispose to the development of disturbed behaviour. This may require a change of environment or a range of psychiatric and psychological interventions, from behaviour therapy to psychotropic drugs. This may be provided by mental-illness services or specialist mental-handicap services.

Residential needs: It is now recognized that people with a mental handicap neither wish nor need to live in hospitals, though obviously they may need to be admitted when acutely ill. Most live at home, usually with family members but occasionally alone. People with mental handicap may want to leave home or their families may want them to do so. They will need a variety of accommodation: both staffed and unstaffed houses, group homes and hostels with appropriate specialist support.

Education: People who learn slowly obviously have special educational needs. These may be met by special schools or, increasingly, by special provision within mainstream education. The 1981 Education Act requires local authorities to provide for children with special educational needs which are defined in the Warnock report, including special means of access, equipment or resources, modification of the environment or specialist teaching techniques, the provision of a specialized or modified curriculum, and attention to the social and emotional climate in which education takes place. Each child's special needs must be assessed, and a decision made as to where these can best be met. Parents must be involved in drawing up the statement of special needs under the 1981 act.

People with a mental handicap are entitled to remain at school until the age of 19 and further education may be available to them. Many can find employment on the open market, but for others specialist help or sheltered employment may be needed.

Parents or other relatives of mentally subnormal children can obtain helpful advice from The Mental Health Foundation, 8 Hallam Street, London W1N 6DH (01-580 0145); The Royal Society for Mentally Handicapped Children & Adults, 123 Golden Lane, London EC1Y ORT (01-253 9433); or the Scottish Society for the Mentally Handicapped, 13 Elmbank Street, Glasgow G2 4QA (041-226-4541).

MENTAL ILLNESS: Problems of feeling, thinking and behaving may be regarded as a mental illness if they become excessive for the particular individual in relation to the difficulties experienced.

Mental illness exists in many forms which may overlap with one another. Help and treatment may be sought by the sufferer, or less commonly may be imposed against his or her will. So long as symptoms of mental disorder do not result in behaviour which is markedly opposed to prevailing social custom, society does not interfere with the person in a restrictive way. When people's conduct becomes a risk to their own health and safety, or that of others, they can be compulsorily admitted to a psychiatric unit under the Mental Health Act 1983 (U.K.). Approximately 10 per cent of psychiatric admissions in England and Wales are compulsory. A large number of people with socially maladapted personalities may be found in the prison population.

The medical approach, which regards mental disorder as a disease to be treated on the same lines as other diseases, is generally regarded as having begun with the publication of Pinel's *Traité médico-philosophique sur l'aliénation mentale ou la manie* in 1801. A great amount of attention was paid during the next fifty years to the study of mental diseases, and during this period a large number of asylums for the humane treatment of mentally disordered people were founded. The emphasis now, however, is more on care in the community.

The question of legal responsibility may arise in various civil or criminal matters, including the ability to make a valid will. (In order to be 'of sound disposing mind', individuals should know the nature and extent of their property, know the persons having a claim on it as possible beneficiaries and the relative strengths of their claims and be able to express themselves on this question clearly and without ambiguity.) The development of mental illness subject to detention under the Mental Health Act 1983 does not excuse the patient from the fulfilment of a contract, provided he was not eligible to be detained at the time when the contract was entered into.

When a crime is committed, the question of responsibility is often very difficult to decide. The general principle accepted is that, if the accused person suffers from a delusion, but is not insane in other matters, he is held responsible for his offence, unless he has acted in such a way as would have been permissible if the facts about which his delusion exists had been true. In other words, in order to establish a defence on the ground of insanity, it must be proved that 'at the time of committing the act the party accused was labouring under such a defect of reason, from disease of the mind, as not to know the nature and quality of the act he was doing or, if he did know it, that he did not know he was doing it, or that he did not know he was doing what was wrong'. The principle is also recognized that, if the mind is so diseased or so defective that there is complete absence of the power of self-control, so that the person acts under an ungovernable impulse, then he is not held responsible. This inability to exercise self-control does not, however, exonerate a person in whom the loss of self-control is due to his own fault, as, for example, when he is intoxicated.

Causes: Mental illness, like normal mental functioning, is complex and a single causal explanation is not often sufficient on its own. Any one causative agent may increase the risk of mental illness but by no means make it inevitable. It may be helpful to think in terms of the predisposing causes and the precipitating causes, and sometimes the perpetuating causes.

(1) PREDISPOSING CAUSES: It is often difficult to distinguish between the roles of genetic inheritance and family upbringing among the more distant predisposing causes. Modern research suggests that, for some illnesses, genetic loading significantly increases the risk but may not be a sufficient cause on its own. Even an identical twin, with exactly the same genetic constitution, has only a substantial risk, rather than a complete certainty, of developing the same illness.

Birth trauma is another physical cause increasing the risk of mental illness, as is the presence of any sort of physical illness.

Socio-cultural factors, such as family size, class or ethnic background may predispose to some illnesses. The individual's psychology and personality, shaped on the basis of inherited features by upbringing, are often relevant in their mental resilience to different types of stresses. Loss of a parent in childhood has been shown in some subjects slightly to increase the risk of depression many years later. Some researchers argue that the characteristic pattern of thinking, or cognitive approach, may make some individuals vulnerable to anxiety or depression.

(2) PRECIPITATING CAUSES: Physical disorders may again be relevant. A depressive episode following influenza is well known, as is emotional disequilibrium following childbirth, even if this more often takes the form of 'the blues', or more rarely a depressive illness. A post-puerperal psychosis is rare. Acute confusional states, especially in the elderly, may have an infective or metabolic origin. Diseases of the *endocrine glands*, particularly myxoedema and thyrotoxicosis but also abnormalities of adrenal function, can cause mental symptoms. Medication related to these, as well as other medication, can be a factor.

Legal but non-therapeutic drugs like alcohol are often implicated, partly because people take them as a way of modifying their response to stress and particularly if there are withdrawal reactions after dependence has occurred. Opiates, such as heroin, cause marked withdrawal reactions which are not regarded as a mental illness. Other drugs, such as amphetamines, cocaine and, rarely, cannabis, can precipitate a psychotic reaction.

There has been much study of social precipitants of mental illness, known technically as life events. Although it is sometimes unclear whether the illness has caused the event (such as loss of job) or vice versa and, although they only increase the risk of illness rather than determine it, the association is well established. Among the most stressful events are bereavement, divorce or separation and moving house.

(3) PERPETUATING CAUSES may include any of the above factors but the victim may have suffered additional social dislocation as a result of the illness itself, for example, through the loss of job or eviction. Psychologically, patients may experience real or imagined stigma and their self-confidence may have been impaired by the 'breakdown'.

Symptoms of mental disorder: EARLY SYMPTOMS: Mental illness rarely develops suddenly and indications of vulnerability to an approaching mental breakdown may be gathered from some early prodromal symptoms. These are often non-specific symptoms of anxiety or depression including insomnia, mental and physical tension and other bodily symptoms of anxiety such as rapid pulse, sweating and gastrointestinal upset, as well as difficulty concentrating.

GENERAL SYMPTOMS of mental illness may be classed as psychotic and non-psychotic. *Psychotic symptoms*, such as delusions or hallucinations, imply that the patient has lost touch with reality to some degree. A *delusion* is a fixed false belief, held with unshakeable conviction, not in conformity with the information available to the patient or with the social and cultural background of his or her peers. There are many types of delusions. In delusions of reference, for example, patients think people in the street or on the television are referring to them. In paranoid delusions, others, human or supernatural, are intent on harming the person, although there is no basis in reality. Delusions of grandeur or of having remarkable attributes are typically associated with mania. Delusions of guilt, hypochondriacal or 'nihilistic' delusions (that part of the patient's body is being or has been destroyed) are characteristic of the psychotic extremes of depression. Other delusions are religious or jealous. In some delusions people, places or situations may be misidentified or misinterpreted. There may be delusions that feelings, actions, willpower or thoughts are being interfered with or controlled.

Hallucinations are false perceptions of the senses, which occur in the absence of external stimuli. They are not misinterpretations or distortions of actually existing stimuli ('*illusions*'). Patients complain that they hear voices speaking to them when there is no one there. *Pseudo-hallucinations* are experienced within the mind and are not truly psychotic but true. *Auditory hallucinations* are heard through the ears. These voices may be well known to them or unknown. They may be persecutory, condemnatory or imperative with direct instructions. They may comment on the patient's actions or several voices may argue. Hallucinations of sight are suggestive of some organic disorder. Hallucinations of smell may imply pathology in the temporal lobe of the brain.

Obsessions are included among the neurotic symptoms. Although an obsessional trait such as over-tidiness is quite common, obsessions are relatively rare. They are the persistent intrusion of unwelcome thoughts, feeling or impulses, despite the fact that the sufferer tries to resist them. They are often repugnant or bizarre, violent, sexual or blasphemous in nature. A 'compulsion' is technically an act which is similarly bizarre but which the individual is compelled to perform, despite resisting. Nevertheless obsessions and compulsions are clearly recognized as part of the subject's own mind and are not delusions.

Phobias are more common than obsessions. The fear is disproportionate to the situation; it cannot be reasoned away or controlled voluntarily. It may cause intense subjective and bodily symptoms of anxiety and the subject characteristically avoids the feared situation. Some fears, of spiders or the dark, are common in childhood. A list of recognized objects of phobia runs well into three figures but is now considered most usefully under three main headings: (a) *agoraphobia*, includes fear of congested places or leaving the house. It does not mean fear of open spaces and psychiatrists do not use the term claustrophobia separately to indicate a fear of closed spaces. Crowded shops, lifts, buses and underground trains are typical feared situations. (b) animal or other *specific phobias*, eg. of spiders, birds or snakes. (c) *social phobias* of meeting and being exposed to scrutiny by others, going beyond natural shyness, often with feelings of intense anxiety or panic and usually resulting in relative social isolation.

Derealization and depersonalization are rare but normal experiences. Respectively, subjects have a sudden intense feeling that their surroundings are somehow unreal, as if part of a video or stage set, or that they themselves are unreal or even out of their own body. These may be due to a dissociative mechanism in a situation which the subject would otherwise find very stressful and should not be regarded as psychotic phenomena.

Suicide may be the result of profound mental depression but is also more common with schizophrenia. It is associated with men, older years and concurrent painful physical disease. The number of deaths due to suicide in England and Wales is approximately 4,000 a year.

Attempted suicide is roughly ten times more common and ranges from a failed serious attempt, to a cry for help or an overdose of tablets to ensure a prolonged sleep. The assessment of someone who has attempted suicide should exclude any serious psychiatric illness and evaluate all the evidence about how determined the attempt was.

MANIA: The term, mania, should strictly be reserved for cases in which there are hallucinations or delusions. Hypomania is less florid and includes all the other symptoms, most typically, elevation of mood. Patients are in a state of over-activity, loquacious, garrulous, often clever in repartee; they flit from one subject to another; the mind never rests and sleeplessness is common. In the more pronounced form there may be pressure leading to incoherence of speech, intense restlessness and distractability. Social, sexual and financial disinhibition may be of concern. Patients may seem to be unaware of fatigue, either of mind or body, and wear themselves out, with very occasionally a fatal result. The illness characteristically occurs in episodes, lasting several weeks or months. When episodes of both depression and hypomania have occurred, the illness is termed manic-depressive disorder.

DEPRESSION is characterized by feelings of misery that are excessive in relation to the circumstances. In milder forms the depression is not very great and may exist only as a symptom on its own, rather than as a cluster of associated symptoms constituting a syndrome or medical illness. Patients may be able to pull themselves together in the presence of strangers and when it is necessary. Sometimes, especially after a severely depressed state has lasted for some time, patients are retarded in their movements, sit staring straight in front of them and are persuaded with difficulty to take food. In severe agitated depression, patients show restlessness and agitation, wringing their hands, swaying their body, weeping, or showing inability for the slightest concentration upon any one subject. Depressive delusions may be present, and patients think they have wronged themselves and their family, that they are responsible for the illness or misfortune of other people, that they are going to be burned, tortured or otherwise maltreated and, in such people, the impulse to suicide may be very strong. Along with the mental symptoms, physical signs are often present, including disordered digestion with constipation. Recovery is usual but a person of depressive personality is liable to subsequent episodes.

PARANOIA is a condition in which there are delusions in the absence of hallucinations, which gradually form into a system that can be complex. Used more loosely, the term applies to abnormal suspiciousness that one is a victim of persecution by others.

SCHIZOPHRENIA is the collective name given to a group of conditions characterized during an acute episode by positive symptoms such as hallucinations (typically taking the form of voices talking to or about the afflicted person), strange experiences (for example, that mental or bodily functions are being interfered with by some outside force such as radio waves or telepathy) and inability to think clearly. Such symptoms may lead to bizarre speech and behaviour. Acute episodes usually respond to treatment with medication, the phenothiazines being the class of drugs most commonly used.

In about 25 per cent of cases the condition clears up completely after one or a few such attacks. Unfortunately, many conditions become chronic and a 'negative' type of syndrome becomes prominent. This is characterized by slowness, lack of energy and social withdrawal. About 25 per cent of those with schizophrenia become severely disabled. The rest, about half, are subject to occasional relapses (particularly if medication is discontinued) and to a moderate degree of disability. About one in a hundred individuals develops schizophrenia at some time during their lives, a proportion that seems to vary by, at most, a factor of 10 between extremes in different parts of the world. The causes are not known but a genetic factor is present in a proportion of cases, indicating a possible biochemical vulnerability.

In recent years there has been an intensive search for a biochemical basis for schizophrenia: a theory apparently supported by the response of the condition to certain potent tranquillizing drugs.

Undue environmental stress can precipitate a relapse. A degree of support may therefore be necessary, although not so great as to discourage the individual from becoming as independent as possible.

Apart from the people who are themselves afflicted by schizophrenia, those chiefly involved are the relatives and close friends. A voluntary organization, the National Schizophrenia Fellowship, has been formed to promote the welfare of sufferers and families. There are branches in most parts of the UK. Enquiries should be addressed to the General Secretary, NSF, 78 Victoria Road, Surbiton, Surrey KT6 4NS (01–390 3651).

ALCOHOLIC PSYCHOSIS: Alcoholism and drug habits are also sometimes regarded as mental disorders and alcohol, in turn, can produce organic changes in the nervous system which lead to chronic mental illness.

CONFUSIONAL STATES: This type of mental disorder usually is due to organic factors, such as infections, metabolic disturbances or poisons such as alcohol. The patient has difficulty in understanding simple questions. Hallucinations are common and patients may see faces in the air or insects crawling on the bedclothes and mistake persons near them for old friends or enemies. Commonly too, patients have no idea where they are. They may also be disorientated with regard to time. Memory is often disordered and restlessness is frequent. Recovery usually depends on the treatment of the underlying condition.

DEMENTIA is a condition of general impairment of most mental faculties. It usually starts gradually with impairment of short-term memory. Approximately 5 per cent of those over 65 in England and Wales have mild and a further 5 per cent severe dementia. The two commonest varieties are due to impairment of blood circulation and Alzheimer's disease. The Alzheimer's Disease Society address is 158/160 Balham High Road, London SW12 9BN, (01–675 6557).

Treatment: *Depression* is the commonest psychiatric disorder encountered both in general practice and in hospital medicine. A relatively mild depression responds to supportive psychotherapy, whilst a psychotic depression with delusions and hallucinations will require admission to hospital and possible electro-convulsive therapy. Depressive illness has a spontaneous remission rate of about 50 per cent within several months and, if anti-depressant drugs are given, the recovery rate increases to over 70 per cent. The advantage of drugs treatment is that recovery is made more rapidly and the patient's suffering is therefore curtailed and the risk of suicide reduced. Tricyclic antidepressant drugs act, apparently, by promoting the transmission of impulses between nerves by noradrenaline or serotonin. Depressed patients with agitation or anxiety respond best to a sedative tricyclic antidepressant such as amitriptyline or dothiepin. Retarded, apathetic patients are best treated with a less sedative antidepressant, such as imipramine. The side-effects of the tricyclic antidepressants (particularly amitriptyline) are due to atropine-like effects which lead to a dry mouth, constipation, pupillary dilatation and blurring of close vision. The monoamine oxidase inhibitors are best reserved for those neurotic or atypical cases, where the depression is accompanied by a great deal of anxiety and phobic behaviour. The monoamine oxidase inhibitors are associated with severe side-effects if the patient eats cheese or any substance that contains tyramine or catecholamines. Electro-convulsive therapy may also facilitate the transmission of nerve impulses. It is now given under brief general anaesthetic with a muscle relaxant. It is an effective treatment in severe depressive illness and the response is at least as good and probably more rapid than the response to tricyclic antidepressants.

People with *hypomania* require admission to hospital. The most useful drugs are the phenothiazines, such as chlorpromazine and the butyrophenones such as haloperidol, which act by blocking central dopamine receptors. Lithium carbonate has anti-manic properties but as it has little effect for seven to ten days it is generally reserved for prophylaxis of recurrent manic depressive disorder.

In the treatment of anxiety states, patients must be given an opportunity to ventilate their worries and be counselled on stress management and relaxation. Since many patients with anxiety states are often concerned that the commonly associated physical symptoms indicate an underlying organic disorder, they should be reassured (see PSYCHOSOMATIC DISEASES). If an acute stress cannot be managed in this way, long-acting benzodiazepines may be indicated (see BENZODIAZEPINES). Short-acting benzodiazepines are more suitable for elderly patients or patients with renal or hepatic impairment. These drugs should in general be prescribed only for a few weeks at most, as patients often become tolerant to their effects and dependent on them. In patients who experience a rapid pulse or tremor, beta-blockers (see ADRENERGIC RECEPTORS) are useful and do not cause dependence.

The treatment of *schizophrenia* usually requires admission to a psychiatric unit for clarification of the diagnosis. The treatment is both pharmacological and psycho-social. The drugs most commonly used for the treatment of schizophrenia are neuroleptics including the phenothiazines, such as chlorpromazine, and the butyrophenones, such as haloperidol. The efficacy of neuroleptics in acute schizophrenia is demonstrated by the fact that 75 per cent of patients given phenothiazines are substantially better after four weeks compared to 25 per cent given a placebo. Psycho-social treatment is also important. During the acute phase the schizophrenic patient needs support, reassurance and simple counselling. Schizophrenic individuals are vulnerable to social pressures that most people can take in their stride. Despite the introduction of drug treatment, schizophrenic patients still occupy about one-sixth of all hospital beds in England and Wales. Drug treatment needs to be prolonged as 50 per cent of patients will relapse when drugs are discontinued. As a high proportion of psychiatric outpatients fail to comply with oral medication, long-acting depot-neuroleptics are commonly used, such as fluphenazine and flupenthixol. Patients may experience side-effects with the neuroleptics. These take the form of abnormal muscle movements or rigidity, as well as restlessness in the legs and increased salivation. Some of them can be controlled with other medication and recede with time.

After treament has been established and florid symptoms are controlled, the patient is encouraged to resume activities by degrees. If living at home is not desirable, a hostel or group home may be indicated.

Like the 1959 Mental Health Act, the 1983 Act continues the principles (1) that as much treatment as possible, both in hospital and outside, should be given on a voluntary and informal basis; (2) that the care of people with mental illness should be shifted as far as possible from the institutions to care within the community. Psychiatric units attached to or in district general hospitals are now regarded as the norm and there is a widespread move to close large separate mental hospitals.

The 1983 Act strengthened the checks and protected the civil liberties of the 10 per cent of in-patients who are admitted to psychiatric hospitals involuntarily.

Under the Act, mental disorder is defined as mental illness, arrested or incomplete development of mind, psychopathic disorder, or any other disability of mind.

Under Section 2 it provides for the compulsory admission of a patient to hospital for a maximum of 28 days on the grounds: (a) that he is suffering from mental disorder of a nature or degree which warrants his detention for assessment (or for assessment followed by medical treatment); and (b) that he ought to be so detained in the interests of his own health or safety or with a view to the protection of other persons.

Under Section 3 compulsory admission to hospital for treatment is for a maximum of six months, subject to renewal.

Patients detained in hospital must be informed of their rights and may apply to a Mental Health Tribunal to be released. Medical staff and hospital managers also have the power to discharge a patient from the compulsory provisions at any time.

Other sections of the Act permit involuntary detention for shorter periods of time under certain conditions and provide for guardianship in the community, although this last provision has been little used.

Persons coming before the courts who are mentally disordered may be detained in hospital or received into guardianship if the court considers it a suitable course. In certain circumstances higher courts may also make restriction orders, in which case the patient may not be discharged without the consent of the Home Secretary. Persons detained in prison or approved school who are found to be mentally disordered may be transferred to hospital by the Home Secretary.

Institutions, known as Special Hospitals, exist for mentally disordered people who, in the opinion of the minister, require treatment under conditions of special security on account of their dangerous, violent, or criminal tendencies.

The Mental Health Act Commission has been set up to provide special safeguards for detained patients. It gives second opinions in certain matters affecting the treatment of patients, will visit detained patients, investigate complaints, review the use of legal powers and advise staff on good practice. Some treatments are not permitted without the patient's consent and an independent second opinion; some may be given without consent but only if the second opinion agrees, whilst others can be given for up to three months without consent or a second opinion.

The checks on and safeguards of civil liberties of detained patients in the 1983 Act are detailed. Further information can be obtained from the Mental Health Commission, Hepburn House, Marsham Street, London SW1P 4HW, telephone 01-211 8061 and from MIND, The National Association for Mental Health, 22 Harley Street, London W1N 2ED, telephone 01-637 0741. MIND also acts as a campaigning and advice organization on all aspects of mental health.

MENTHOL is a white crystalline substance deposited from oil of peppermint when it is cooled. It comes principally from Japan, being derived from several species of *Mentha*. It dissolves freely in alcohol, ether, chloroform, and olive oil, and also to a slight extent in water, to which it gives a strong odour and taste of peppermint. Mixed with a little oil of peppermint, it can be moulded into cones, sticks, or pencils. When menthol is rubbed up with thymol, carbolic acid, chloral, or camphor, the two solids form a clear oily liquid which can be painted on the skin, exerting the effects of both drugs.
Action: Applied to the skin, menthol has weak antiseptic properties, and it acts upon the sensory nerves, causing first a hot, tingling sensation, followed quickly by a cool, numb feeling. When applied to inflamed mucous membranes, such as those of the nose and throat, menthol relieves irritability, diminishes congestion, and checks excessive secretion. Menthol has the merit of being non-poisonous.
Uses: In neuralgia, cones and sticks of menthol are used to rub over the affected part. In toothache, cotton-wool dipped in one of the oily fluids named above and placed in the cavity of the carious tooth quickly relieves the pain. In many itchy conditions of the skin a strong solution of menthol in olive oil (1 part in 10) relieves the sense of irritation at once. Menthol plaster is useful in gout, rheumatism, and neuralgia, and so are mixtures with chloral or camphor painted over the painful parts. For inflamed conditions of the nose and throat, the oily compounds of menthol are diluted with parolene and sprayed on the part affected, or in the case of the throat various lozenges and pastilles containing menthol are sucked. In bronchitis menthol crystals in hot water, from which the vapour is inhaled, give much relief.

MEPACRINE HYDROCHLORIDE is a synthetic acridine product used in the treatment of malaria. It came to the fore during the 1939–1945 War, when supplies of quinine were short, and proved of great value both as a prophylactic and in the treatment of malaria. It is also used in the treatment of infestation with tapeworms. (See MALARIA; TAENIASIS.)

MEPROBAMATE is one of the tranquillizer drugs. It is mainly used for the relief of states of tension, mild anxiety states and persistent insomnia.

MEPYRAMINE MALEATE is one of the antihistamine drugs (qv).

MERALGIA PARAESTHETICA is a condition characterized by pain and paraesthesia (qv) on the front and outer aspect of the thigh. It is more common in men than in women, and the victims are usually middle-aged, overweight and out of condition. It is due to compression of the lateral cutaneous nerve of the thigh. It is exacerbated by an uncomfortable driving position when motoring long distances. Reduction in weight, improvement in general fitness and correction of faulty posture usually bring relief. If these fail, surgical decompression of the nerve may bring relief.

MERCAPTAMINE is a drug that is proving of value in the treatment of paracetamol poisoning.

MERCAPTOPURINE (PURI-NETHOL) is one of a group of drugs known as antimetabolites which are proving of value in the treatment of certain forms of malignant disease, especially acute leukaemia. It is believed that they act by depriving rapidly dividing malignant cells of factors essential for their metabolism. Hence the generic name for the group of drugs – antimetabolites. It is also proving of value in the treatment of Crohn's disease (qv). (See CYTOTOXIC DRUGS.)

MERCUROCHROME is an organic salt of mercury with weak antiseptic action, which is sometimes used as an antiseptic to wash out the bladder when infected.

MERCURY, also known as QUICKSILVER or HYDRARGYRUM, is a heavy fluid metal which, with its salts, has been used in medicine for many centuries.
Action: The salts of mercury fall into two groups: the mercuric salts, which are very soluble and powerful in action; and the mercurous salts, which are less soluble and act more slowly and mildly. The mercuric salts are all highly poisonous both to man and to bacterial life, so that they are strongly antiseptic. In strong solutions, several act as caustics, and in weaker solutions they are irritants. Taken internally, the first effect of the mercuric, and to a less degree of the mercurous salts, is by their irritating action to set up copious purging. They are also credited with the power of increasing the flow of bile, and for this reason blue pill, which contains mercury, and mercurous chloride, ie. calomel, were at one time much used as purgatives.
Uses: Externally the mercuric salts are used as disinfectants and antiseptics. Ammoniated mercury ointment, or white precipitate ointment, is used in the treatment of impetigo. The yellow oxide of mercury ointment is used for an

application to the eyelids when a mild antiseptic ointment is required. Internally, mercurial salts were widely used at one time as purges, particularly calomel, the dosage of which is 30 to 200 mg for an adult, and blue pill 250 to 500 mg. They are best taken at night, and followed by a saline draught in the morning. They are seldom used nowadays.

A complex organic salt of mercury (mersalyl) is used as a diuretic in the treatment of oedema but it has largely been replaced by the oral benzothiadiazine and loop diuretics.

MERCURY POISONING is of two kinds: (1) acute mercury poisoning, due to swallowing one of the soluble mercury salts, such as perchloride of mercury or one of the organic mercury compounds used as fungicides; and (2) chronic mercury poisoning, produced either by continuing repeated medicinal doses of mercurials for too long a time, or by handling the metal or inhaling its fumes, as happens sometimes among mirror and barometer makers and dental technicians.

ACUTE POISONING. **Symptoms**: There is burning pain, first in the mouth, then in the stomach, followed by diarrhoea and vomiting. The lips and mouth are generally burned white, and a metallic taste is left in the mouth. This may be followed by shock, and the person may die in a few hours. If death does not take place at an early stage, the kidneys are liable to remain seriously damaged by the drug.

Treatment: The stomach should be washed out as quickly as possible with sodium bicarbonate. Some albuminous preparation, such as egg white or milk, should then be given, as, with corrosive sublimate, this forms an insoluble and harmless compound. Dimercaprol (BAL) (qv) or penicillamine (qv) should also be given. If signs of shock appear, the patient is treated accordingly. (See SHOCK.)

CHRONIC POISONING. **Symptoms**: When too much mercury is being taken into the system in small doses, the first signs are an excessive discharge of saliva into the mouth, and tenderness about the teeth when the mouth is tightly shut. Next, the odour of the breath becomes bad, the gums tender, spongy, and ready to bleed at the slightest touch, and the tongue swollen. Finally, the teeth become loose and drop out, the jaw-bone may become diseased, the person becomes generally weak and bloodless, and may indeed die. People who work with metallic mercury may develop these symptoms to some extent, and in addition they become affected by trembling and palsy in various parts of the body. Such trembling induced by mercury in the felt hat industry was known as 'hatters' shakes'. A form of psychic disturbance known as erethism often develops. This is characterized by self-consciousness, shyness, indecision, timidity, lack of concentration, depression and irritability. It is this condition that was responsible for the phrase 'mad as a hatter'.

Treatment consists in stopping the mercury if it is being administered as medicine, and change of employment if the symptoms are due to work. If the condition is sufficiently severe, a course of injections of dimercaprol (qv) or penicillamine (qv) is given.

MERYCISM is another name for rumination, in which the contents of a meal are returned to the mouth some time after they have been swallowed and are once again chewed.

MESCALINE is derived from the Mexican peyote cactus, *Anhaloniumlewinii*. It is probably the most powerful of all the hallucinogens and has been used for many centuries by Indian tribes in Mexico as an intoxicant to produce ecstatic states for religious celebrations. (See DRUG ADDICTION.)

MESENCEPHALON is the mid-brain connecting the cerebral hemispheres with the pons and cerebellum.

MESENTERY is the double layer of peritoneal membrane which supports the small intestine. It is of a fan shape, and its shorter edge is attached to the back wall of the abdomen for a distance of about 15 cm (6 inches), while the small intestine lies within its longer edge, for a length of over 6 metres (20 feet). The terms mesocolon, mesorectum, etc., are applied to similar folds of peritoneum that support parts of the colon, rectum, etc.

MESMERISM (see HYPNOTISM).

MESOCOLON is the double fold of peritoneum by which the large intestine is suspended from the back wall of the abdomen.

MESTEROLONE (PRO-VIRON) is a synthetic androgen (qv) which is being used in the treatment of hypogonadism (qv). (See ANDROGENS.)

METABOLISM means tissue change and includes all the physical and chemical processes by which the living body is maintained, and also those by which the energy is made available for various forms of work. The constructive, chemical and physical, processes by which food materials are adapted for the use of the body are collectively known as anabolism. The destructive processes by which energy is produced with the breaking down of tissues into waste products is known as catabolism. *Basal metabolism* is the term applied to the energy changes necessary for essential processes such as the beating of the heart, respiration, and maintenance of body warmth. This can be estimated, when a person is placed in a state of complete rest, by measuring the amounts of oxygen and carbon dioxide exchanged during breathing under certain standard conditions. (See CALORIE.)

METACARPAL bones are the five long bones which occupy the hand between the carpal bones at the wrist and the phalanges of the fingers. The large rounded 'knuckles' at the root of the fingers are formed by the heads of these bones. (See HAND.)

METAPHYSIS is the extremity of a long bone where it joins the epiphysis (qv).

METAPLASIA is the term applied to a change of one kind of tissue into another.

METASTASIS and METASTATIC are terms applied to the process by which malignant disease spreads to distant parts of the body, and also to the secondary tumours resulting from this process. For example, a cancer of the breast may produce metastatic growths in the glands of the armpit, cancer of the stomach may be followed by metastases in the liver.

METATARSAL bones are the five bones in the foot which correspond to the metacarpal bones in the hand, lying between the tarsal bones, at the ankle, and the toes. (See FOOT.)

METATARSALGIA is pain affecting the metatarsal region of the foot. It is common in adolescents associated with flat-foot (qv). In adults it may be a manifestation of rheumatoid arthritis. *Morton's metatarsalgia* is a form associated usually with the nerve to the second toe cleft often induced by the compression of tight shoes.

METATARSUS is the group name of the five metatarsal bones in the foot (qv). *Metatarsus varus* is the condition characterized by deviation of the forefoot towards the other foot. It is a common condition in new-born babes and almost always corrects itself spontaneously. Only in the rare cases in which it is due to some deformity of the bones or muscles of the foot is any treatment required.

METEORISM means the distension of the abdomen by gas produced in the intestines. (See FLATULENCE.)

METFORMIN is a biguanide (qv) which lowers the blood sugar. This it does by increasing cellular uptake of glucose. It is active when taken by mouth and is proving of value in the treatment of certain cases of diabetes mellitus.

METHADONE, or PHYSEPTONE, is an analgesic with morphine-like properties. It has much less hypnotic action than morphine, and is used as a linctus for the alleviation of troublesome cough. It has some of the addiction-forming properties of morphine.

METHAEMOGLOBIN is a derivative of haemoglobin in which the iron has been oxidised from ferrous to ferric form. It does not combine with oxygen and therefore plays no part in oxygen transport. Normal concentration of methaemoglobin in red blood cells is less than one per cent of the total haemoglobin. When a large concentration of the haemoglobin is in the form of methaemoglobin the patient will suffer from hypoxia and will be cyanosed. Most cases of methaemoglobinaemia are due to chemical agents.

METHAEMOGLOBINAEMIA is a condition due to the presence in the blood of methaemoglobin (qv). It is characterized by cyanosis (qv) which turns the skin and lips a blue colour, shortness of breath, headache, fatigue and sickness. There are two main forms: a *hereditary* form and a *toxic* form. The latter is caused by certain drugs, including acetanilide, phenacetin, the sulphonamides and benzocaine. The treatment of the toxic form is the withdrawal of the causative drug. In the more severe cases the administration of methylene blue or ascorbic acid may also be needed, and these are the drugs used in the hereditary form.

In recent years attention has been drawn to a form known as *infantile methaemoglobinaemia* in bottle-fed babies under the age of 6 months. This is due to the presence of excess nitrate in the drinking water. Nitrate pollution of water has been increasing due to the purification of sewage effluent to a high standard before its discharge to water-courses, and to changes in agricultural policy leading to better drainage of land and increased use of artificial fertilizers. As a result, especially where rainfall is low and the land low-lying, as in eastern and south-east England, underground supplies of water contain more than 50 mg of nitrate per litre, which is the level recommended by the World Health Organization, and may even exceed the maximum acceptable level of 100 mg per litre. High nitrate concentrations may also occur in surface waters after heavy rain. The cause of the methaemoglobinaemia is nitrite into which the nitrate is converted either in the baby's bottle or in his gut. Few serious cases have been recorded in Britain, and most of those which have occurred have been due to water from private sources.

Arrangements are now in force whereby Water Authorities inform the appropriate Health Authority if water with a nitrate content of 50 mg per litre has to be supplied, and alternative low-nitrate water is made available, sometimes in the form of bottled water, by Local Authorities for infants below the age of 6 months. The EEC has recommended an even more stringent criterion: that water used for baby feeds should not contain more than 25 mg of nitrate per litre.

METHALLENOESTRILL (VALLESTRIL) (see OESTROGENS).

METHICILLIN (see PENICILLIN, ANTIBIOTIC).

METHOHEXITONE is an ultra-short-acting barbiturate which is proving of value as a short-acting anaesthetic – particularly in dentistry.

METHOTREXATE (EMTEXATE) is an antimetabolite (qv) which is proving of value in the treatment of choriocarcinoma (qv). (See CYTOTOXIC DRUGS.)

METHOTRIMEPRAZINE (NOZINAN, VERACTIL) (see ANTI-PSYCHOTIC DRUGS).

METHYCLOTHIAZIDE (ENDURON) (see BENZOTHIADIAZINES).

METHYL is an organic radical whose chemical formula is CH_3, and which forms the centre of a wide group of substances known as the methyl group. For example, methyl alcohol is obtained as a by-product in the manufacture of beet-sugar, or by distillation of wood; methyl salicylate is the active constituent in oil of wintergreen; methyl hydride is better known as marsh gas.

Methyl alcohol, or wood spirit, is distilled from wood and is thus a cheap form of alcohol. It has actions similar to, but much more toxic than, those of ethyl alcohol. It has a specially pronounced action on the nervous system, and in large doses is apt to cause neuritis, especially of the optic nerves, leading to blindness, partial or complete.

METHYLCELLULOSE is a colloid (qv) which absorbs water to swell to about 25 times its original volume. It is used in the treatment of constipation and also in the management of obesity. The rationale for its use in obesity is that by swelling up in the stomach it reduces the appetite.

METHYLDOPA is one of the drugs introduced for the treatment of high blood-pressure. It is the drug most commonly used to control high blood-pressure in pregnancy.

METHYLENE BLUE is another name for methylthionin chloride (qv).

METHYLPREDNISOLONE is a preparation with an action comparable to that of prednisolone (qv), but effective at a somewhat lower dose.

METHYLTESTOSTERONE (VIRORMONE) is a derivative of the testicular hormone, testosterone (qv), which is active when taken by mouth. (See ANDROGENS.)

METHYLTHIONIN CHLORIDE, or METHYLENE BLUE, is a dark powder forming a deep-blue solution, used for various tests. It is also used in the treatment of methaemoglobinaemia (qv).

METHYSERGIDE is a drug that is being used in the prevention of attacks of migraine (qv). Its precise value is still not clear, and it has to be used with care because of the toxic effects it sometimes produces, such as nausea, drowsiness and retroperitoneal fibrosis.

METOCLOPRAMIDE is a drug that is proving of value in the treatment of vomiting. It is said to restore normal co-ordination and tone to the upper digestive tract. It is proving of value in the early treatment, and prevention, of migraine (qv).

METOLAZONE (METENIX) (see BENZOTHIADIAZINES).

METOPROLOL (BETALOC, LOPRESSOR) is a beta-adrenergic receptor blocking agent. (See ADRENERGIC RECEPTORS.)

METRE is the basic unit of length in the modern version of the metric system, known as the International System of Units (SI). (See WEIGHTS AND MEASURES.) It is equivalent to 39·37 inches.

METRITIS means inflammation of the womb.

METRONIDAZOLE is a drug, administered by mouth, which is proving of value in the treatment of various diseases including balantidiasis (qv), giardiasis (qv), amoebic dysentery (see DYSENTERY) and trichomonal vaginitis. (See TRICHOMONAS VAGINALIS.) It is also active against Gram-negative anaerobic micro-organisms.

METROPATHIA HAEMORRHAGICA, or ESSENTIAL UTERINE HAEMORRHAGE, is a diseased state characterized by haemorrhage from the uterus, cysts in the ovaries, and thickening of the uterine mucosa.

METRORRHAGIA means bleeding from the womb otherwise than at the proper period. It is usually due to a uterine lesion. (See MENSTRUATION.)

METYRAPONE is a drug that is used in the treatment of Cushing's syndrome (qv).

MEXENONE is a substance that has the property of absorbing ultra-violet light over a wide range, and is therefore used in the prevention of sunburn. It has the practical advantage of not being readily removed from the skin by washing or sweating, and thereby provides long protection.

MEZLOCILLIN (see ANTIBIOTIC).

MIANSERIN (BOLVIDON, NORVAL) (see ANTIDEPRESSANTS).

MICONAZOLE is a drug that is proving of value in the treatment of the group of diseases known as the mycoses (qv).

MICROANGIOPATHY means disease of the capillaries (qv).

MICROBE (see BACTERIA).

MICROBIOLOGY is the branch of biology concerned with the study of micro-organisms. (See BACTERIOLOGY.)

MICROCEPHALY is abnormal smallness of the head. (See MENTAL SUBNORMALITY.)

MICROCYTE means a small red blood corpuscle.

MICROGRAM is the 1/1000th part of a milligram. The abbreviation for it is μg.

MICROMETRE, or MICRON, is the 1/1000th part of a millimetre. The abbreviation for it is μm.

MICRO-ORGANISM (see BACTERIA).

MICROPSIA: Condition in which objects appear smaller than normal. It can be due to disease of the macula.

MICROSPORON is the genus of fungi which includes the fungi responsible for ringworm of the scalp. (See RINGWORM.)

MICROSURGERY is surgery performed with the use of an operating microscope. It is used routinely in certain operations on the eye, the ear and the larynx. In recent years it has been used, with increasing success, in attempts to reunite severed legs and arms. Under the operating microscope, surgical sutures invisible to the naked eye are used to reunite blood vessels 0·5 millimetre in diameter. The severed limb will survive for up to eight hours at room temperature, longer if cooled – as by ice in the ambulance taking the patient to hospital. Success depends primarily on restoration of the circulation to the limb. Once this has been achieved, attention is later turned to restoring the continuity of the nerves.

MICROWAVES are non-ionizing electro-magnetic radiations in the frequency range of 30-300,000 megahertz. They are emitted from electronic devices, such as heaters, some domestic ovens, television receivers, radar units and diathermy units. There is no scientific evidence to justify the claims that they are harmful to man or produce any harmful effect in the genes (qv). The only known necessary precaution is the protection of the eyes in those using them in industry, as there is some evidence that prolonged exposure to them in this may induce cataract. (See also DIATHERMY.)

MICTURITION means the act of passing water.

MIDGES (see BITES AND STINGS).

MIDWIFERY (see LABOUR).

MIGRAINE, or HEMICRANIA as it is sometimes known from the Greek word for half a skull, is a common condition characterized by recurring intense headaches. It is much commoner in women than men. There are said to be six million victims of it in Britain. It has been defined as 'episodic headache accompanied by visual or gastro-intestinal disturbances, or both, attacks lasting hours with total freedom between episodes'.

It usually begins at puberty and often tends to stop in middle age: eg. in women attacks often cease after menopause. It often disappears during pregnancy. In susceptible individuals attacks may be provoked by a wide variety of causes including:

Anxiety, emotion, depression, shock, and excitement

Physical and mental fatigue

Prolonged focusing on television or cinema screen

Noise, especially loud and high-pitched sounds

Certain foods: eg. chocolate, cheese, citrus fruits, pastry

Alcohol

Prolonged lack of food

Irregular meals

Menstruation and the pre-menstrual period

Indeed, it has been said that anything that can provoke a headache in the ordinary individual can precipitate an attack in a migrainous subject. It seems as if there is an inherited predispostion that triggers a mechanism whereby in the migrainous subject the headache and the associated sickness persist for hours, a whole day or even longer.

The precise cause is not known, but the generally accepted view is that in susceptible individuals one or other of these causes produces spasm or constriction of the blood-vessels of the brain. This in turn is followed by dilatation of these blood-vessels which also become more permeable and so allow fluid to pass out into the surrounding tissues. This combination of dilatation and outpouring of fluid is held to be responsible for the headache.

The typical attack is very characteristic. It consists of an intense headache, usually situated over one or other eye. The headache is usually preceded by a feeling of sickness and blurring of sight. In 15 to 20 per cent of cases this disturbance of sight takes the form of bright lights: the so-called aura of migraine. The majority of attacks are accompanied by vomiting. The duration of the headache varies, but in the more severe cases the victim is usually confined to bed for twenty-four hours.

Treatment consists, in the first place, of trying to avoid any precipitating factor. Patients must find out which drug, or drugs, give them most relief, and they must always carry these about with them wherever they go. This is because it is a not uncommon experience to be aware of an attack coming on and to find that there is a critical quarter of an hour or so during which the tablets are effective. If not taken within this period, they may be ineffective and the unfortunate victim finds himself prostrate with headache and vomiting. In addition he should immediately lie down, and at this stage a few hours' rest may prevent the development of a full attack. When an attack is fully developed, rest in bed in a quiet, darkened room is essential; any loud noise or bright light intensifies the headache or sickness. The less food that is taken during an attack the better, provided the individual drinks as much fluid as he wants. Group therapy, in which groups of around ten migrainous subjects learn how to relax, is often of help in more severe cases, whilst in others the injection of a local anaesthetic into tender spots in the scalp reduces the number of attacks. Drug treatment is not very satisfactory. Perhaps the most effective remedy for the condition is ergotamine tartrate which causes the dilated blood vessels to contract, but this must only be taken under medical supervision. In many cases metoclopramide, followed ten minutes later by three tablets of either aspirin or paracetamol, provides a most effective form of treatment if taken early in an attack. In milder attacks, aspirin, with or without codeine and paracetamol, may be of value.

Migraine Clinics: There are four migraine clinics in London:

The City of London Migraine Clinic, 22 Charterhouse Square, EC1M 6DX (01-251 3322).

Charing Cross Hospital, (Fulham) Fulham Palace Road, W6 8RF (01-748 2040).

King's College Hospital, Denmark Hill, SE5 (01-274 6222).

The National Hospital for Nervous Diseases, Queen Square, WC1N 3BG (01-837 3611).

There are eight in the provinces:

The Birmingham and Midland Eye Hospital, Church Street, Birmingham, B3 2NS (021-236 4911).

Royal Surrey County Hospital, Egerton Road, Park Barn, Guildford GU2 5XX.

Hull Royal Infirmary, Anlaby Road, Hull HU3 2JZ (0482 28541).

Radcliffe Infirmary, Oxford OX2 6HE (0865 249891).

Regional Neurological Centre, Newcastle General Hospital, Newcastle-upon-Tyne, NE4 6BE.

Neurological Department, Royal Devon & Exeter Hospital (Wonford), Barrack Road, Exeter, EX2 5DW.

Department of Neurology, Royal Preston Hospital, Sharoe Green Lane, Preston PR2 4HT (0772 716565).

Paediatric Department, John Radcliffe Hospital, Oxford (children only).

There are two in Scotland:

Neurological Unit, Northern General Hospital, Ferry Road, Edinburgh EH5 2DQ (031-332 2525).

Southern General Hospital, 1345, Govan Road, Glasgow G51 4TF.

Patients must first obtain a covering letter from their general practitioner before requesting an appointment for consultation. All correspondence should be addressed to The Secretary, The Migraine Clinic.

People with migraine and their relatives can obtain help and guidance from the British Migraine Association, 178A High Road, Byfleet, Weybridge, Surrey KT14 7ED (09323 52468).

MILIA: These are small keratin cysts appearing as white papules on the cheek and eyelids.

MILIARIA is the name applied to the group of diseases of the skin caused by disturbances of perspiration. The best known is MILIARIA RUBRA, or PRICKLY HEAT (qv).

MILIARY is a term, expressing size, applied to various disease products which are about the size of millet seeds: eg. miliary aneurysms, miliary tuberculosis.

MILIUM is the term applied to a small, whitish nodule in the skin, especially of the face. (See ACNE.)

MILK is the natural food of all animals belonging to the class of mammalia for a considerable period following their birth. It is practically the only form of animal food in which protein, fat, carbohydrate, and salt are all represented in sufficient amount, and it therefore contains all the constituents of a standard diet. Milk is important in human nutrition because it contains first-class animal protein of high biological value, because it is exceptionally rich in calcium, and because it is a good source of vitamin A, thiamine and riboflavine. It also contains a variable amount of ascorbic acid (vitamin C) and of vitamin D, the amount of the latter being higher during the summer months than during the winter months. Raw milk yields 67 Calories per 100 millilitres, in which are present (in grams) 87·6 of water, 3·3 of protein, 3·6 of fat, 4·7 of carbohydrate, and 0·12 of calcium. Heat has no effect on the vitamin A or D content of milk, or on the riboflavine content, but it causes a considerable reduction in the vitamin C and thiamine content.

The milk of different cows varies, especially in the amount of fat and of the fat-soluble vitamins A and D, but the mixed milk of a herd should reach a certain standard. It should contain over 12 per cent of solids. Half a litre (about one pint) of milk provides approximately 400 Calories of energy value. The percentage of cream by volume should be not less than 10 per cent. The amount of cream contained in milk can readily be discovered by allowing the milk to stand overnight in a cylindrical graduated vessel, when the cream rises to the top, and its volume can be measured off.

The ready digestibility of milk, especially when mixed with lime water, or when 125 to

	Human Milk	Cow's Milk
Vitamin A (summer)	450 μg	45 μg
Vitamin A (winter)		30 μg
Vitamin D (summer)	0·03 μg	0·04 μg
Vitamin D (winter)		0·01 μg
Thiamine	17 μg	40 μg
Riboflavine	30 μg	150 μg
Nicotine acid	170 μg	80 μg
Vitamin C	3·5 mg	2 mg
Calcium	25 to 35 mg	120 mg

Vitamin and calcium content of human and cow's milk (per 100 millilitres).

200 mg of citrate of soda have been added for 30 ml of milk in order to soften the curd, makes it a specially suitable food for children, invalids, and people suffering from fever; its blandness and the completeness with which it is absorbed and assimilated adapt it admirably for the general staple of nourishment in many disease; and its high nutritive value compared with its cost renders it a valuable article of diet for the healthy. As a complete diet, for an adult doing hard work, about 5 litres (9 pints) of milk would be required daily; but for a person confined to bed and restricted in the matter of food, 1 · 5 litres (3 pints) daily afford sufficient nourishment for two or three weeks.

Preparation of milk: Milk may be prepared for food in various ways. *Boiling* destroys the bacteria, especially any *Mycobacteriatuberculosis* which the milk may contain. It also partly destroys vitamin C and thiamine, as does *pasteurization. Curdling* of milk is effected by adding rennet, which carries out the initial stage of digestion and thus renders milk more suitable for people who could not otherwise tolerate it. *Souring* of milk is practised in many countries before milk is considered suitable for food; it is carried out by adding certain organisms such as the lactic acid bacillus, the Bulgarian bacillus, and setting the milk in a warm place for several hours. (See LACTIC ACID BACILLI.) *Sterilization*, which prevents fermentation and decomposition, is usually carried out by raising the milk to boiling temperature (100°C) for fifteen minutes and then hermetically sealing it. *Condensed, unsweetened milk* – usually known as *evaporated milk* – is concentrated *in vacuo* at low temperature; the milk is then placed in tins, which are sealed, and is sterilized by heat at a temperature of 105°C. This destroys 60 per cent of the vitamin C and 30 to 50 per cent of the thiamine. *Sweetened condensed milk* is not exposed to such a high temperature. The sugar, which prevents the growth of micro-organisms, is added before the condensing, and finally reaches a concentration of about 40 per cent. In a good, well-prepared, sweetened condensed milk, only 15 per cent of vitamin C and 5 to 10 per cent of thiamine may be lost. The sweetened form is apt to lead in children to flatulence and diarrhoea. *Dried milk* is prepared by evaporating all the fluid so that the milk is reduced to the form of powder. In *spray-drying* a very fine spray of milk is forced into a heated chamber, where drying is almost instantaneous. Milk powder thus prepared is nearly completely soluble in water. During the drying process about 20 per cent of the vitamin C and 10 per cent of the thiamine are lost. There is about a 5 per cent decrease in the biological value of the milk proteins (casein, lactalbumin, lactoglobulin). The calcium is unaffected. *Roller-dried milk* is prepared by spreading a thin film of milk over steam-heated revolving metal cylinders; the powder is removed by a stationary scraper. Roller-dried milk is less soluble in water than spray-dried milk; in its preparation the loss of vitamin C and thiamine is higher and there is slightly greater deterioration of protein. *Peptonized milk* is prepared by treating fresh milk with peptonizing powder, and although the milk is rendered less palatable by this means, it is easily digested and is readily tolerated in weak conditions of the stomach and intestines. (See PEPTONIZED FOODS.) *Humanized milk* is cow's milk treated to render it closely similar to human milk.

Grades of milk: In England and Wales the grades of milk that are now officially recognized are:

1. *Untreated milk.*

2. *Heat-treated milk*, which is divided into three categories: pasteurized, sterilized, and ultra heat-treated.

Pasteurized milk is milk that has been treated in one of two ways. One is the 'Holder Process', in which the milk is retained at a temperature of not less than 63°C and not more than 65 · 5°C for at least half an hour and then immediately cooled to a temperature of not more than 10°C. The other is the 'High Temperature Short Time Process', in which the milk is retained at a temperature of not less than 71 · 7°C for at least fifteen seconds and then immediately cooled to a temperature of not more than 10°C. Pasteurization will not make satisfactory milk that was unsatisfactory in the first instance but, provided satisfactory milk is used in the first instance, it does provide a safe milk of good keeping qualities without affecting its nutritive value to any appreciable extent. *Sterilized milk* is milk that has been filtered or clarified, homogenized and then heated to, and maintained at, a temperature of at least 100°C for such a period as to ensure that it complies with the turbidity test as described in the appropriate regulations. It is heat treated in bottles and after treatment the bottles are sealed with an airtight seal and labelled 'Sterilized Milk'. It is a perfectly safe milk though there is some decrease in the nutritive value. *Ultra heat-*

treated milk is milk which has been retained at a temperature of at least 132°C for not less than one second. It is required to satisfy the bacteriology colony count test as laid down in the appropriate regulations. It keeps much better than pasteurized milk: packed in sterile cartons it will keep for several weeks without refrigeration.

In Scotland the grades of milk are:

1. *Untreated milk*, which is known as *Premium* or *Standard milk*.
2. *Heat-treated milk*, which, as in England and Wales, is available as *Pasteurized, Sterilized*, or *Ultra heat-treated milk*.

MILK, DISEASES DUE TO: Milk has a remarkable power of absorbing gases and vapours to which it is exposed, so that it readily becomes tainted. Milk is also liable to be infected by dirt, or from water, or from the hands of milkers suffering from disease, and in these circumstances epidemics of enteric fever, scarlet fever, diphtheria and food poisoning are traceable to the milk supply. Between 1970 and 1979, in Scotland, where 10 per cent of all milk retailed was neither pasteurized nor heat treated in any way, there were 29 outbreaks of salmonella food poisoning, with a mean of 84 people per attack and an attack rate of 47·6 per 100,000 population. In England and Wales, where only 3 per cent of milk was not pasteurized or heat treated in some way, the attack rate in the same period for milk-borne salmonella food poisoning was only 1·9 per 100,000, with a mean of 14 people per attack. On the other hand in England and Wales between 1951 and 1980, there were 233 outbreaks of communicable disease attributed to milk or dairy products. These involved 9411 patients, four of whom died. Milk may also transmit *Brucella abortus*, the causative organism of undulant fever. Diarrhoea in children is often due to milk containing large quantities of bacteria. Tuberculosis may be communicated by the milk from disease affecting the cow itself. Efficient protection against these diseases is obtained by boiling or pasteurizing the household supply of milk. Although the sale of untreated milk is being phased out, in England and Wales regulations made in 1980 permit the continued sale of farm-bottled untreated milk. In Scotland, however, legislation phased out untreated milk in 1983. (See also LACTOSE INTOLERANCE.)

MILK TEETH are the temporary teeth of children. (For the time of their appearance, see TEETH.)

MILLILITRE is the 1000th part of 1 litre. It is practically the equivalent of a cubic centimetre ($1\ cm^3 = 0\cdot999973$ ml). Ml is the usual abbreviation.

MINOCYCLINE is a long-acting tetracycline (qv) which is proving of value in the treatment of carriers of meningococci, or *Neisseria meningitidis* (see MENINGITIS), and in some cases of chronic bronchitis.

MIOSIS: Condition of constriction of the pupil.

MISCARRIAGE (see ABORTION).

MITHRAMYCIN (MITHRACIN) (see CYTOTOXIC DRUGS).

MITHRIDATISM is a term applied to immunity against the effects of poisons produced by administration of gradually increasing doses of the poison itself. The process is named after Mithridates, King of Pontus, who rendered himself immune against poisoning by this means.

MITOCHONDRIA are the rod-like bodies in the cells of the body which contain the enzymes (qv) necessary for the activity of the cell. They have been described as the 'power plant of the cell'. (See CELLS.)

MITOSIS is the process of cell division for somatic cells and for the ovum after fertilization. Each chromosome becomes doubled by splitting lengthwise and forming two chromatids which remain held together by the centromere. These chromatids are exact copies of the original chromosomes and contain duplicates of all the genes they bear. When cell division takes place the pull of the spindle splits the centromere and each double chromatid separates, one passing to one pole of the nucleus and the other to the opposite pole. The nucleus and the cell itself then also divide, forming two new daughter cells containing precisely the same 23 pairs of chromosomes and carrying exactly the same complement of genes as did the mother cell.

MITRAL STENOSIS is the narrowing of the opening between the left atrium and left ventricle of the heart as a result of rigidity of, and adhesion between, the cusps of the mitral valve. It is due, almost invariably, to the infection of rheumatic fever.

MITRAL VALVE, so called from its resemblance to a bishop's mitre, is the valve which guards the opening between the atrium and ventricle on the left side of the heart. (See HEART.)

MOGIGRAPHIA is a term sometimes applied to writer's cramp. (See CRAMP.)

MOLAR TEETH are the last three teeth on each side of the jaw. (See TEETH.)

MOLE is a term used in two quite different senses. In the first place, a mole on the skin is a darkly pigmented spot, usually raised above the surrounding surface, rough, and covered with hair. These moles are of developmental origin, and malignant growths may spring from some of them late in life. Secondly the term hydatidiform mole is applied to cases in which, following upon conception, a degenerative mass forms in the womb, the embryo dying in the process; whilst the term carneous mole, is applied to an ovum that has died in the early months of pregnancy.

MOLLUSCUM CONTAGIOSUM a disease in which small papules, seldom larger than peas, develop on the surface of the skin. It is due to a virus and is highly contagious, being most commonly conveyed from individual to individual in swimming pools and Turkish baths. They may disappear spontaneously. Treatment is by freezing the nodules with liquid nitrogen. Alternatively, each nodule may be spiked with a sharpened orange stick which has been dipped in pure phenol, or in 10 per cent podophyllin in industrial methylated spirit.

MOLYBDENUM is a metallic element that occurs in all animal tissue. There is some evidence that deficiency of it plays a part in the causation of dental caries, and that a high intake of it, like fluorine, may protect against caries. There is also some evidence linking deficiency of molybdenum with cancer of the oesophagus (gullet).

MONGOLIAN BLUE SPOTS are irregularly shaped areas of bluish-black pigmentation found occasionally on the buttocks, lower back or upper arms in new-born infants of African, Chinese and Japanese parentage and sometimes in the babies of black-haired Europeans. They measure from one to several centimetres in diameter, and usually disappear in a few months. They are commonly mistaken for bruises.

MONGOLISM (see DOWN'S SYNDROME).

MONILIASIS is the infection caused by monilia, the genus of fungi now known as *Candida albicans*. The infection may occur in the mouth, where it is known as thrush (qv), lungs, intestine, vagina, skin, or nails.

MONKEYPOX is a smallpox-like disease, due to a virus which occurs in monkeys kept in captivity. Since 1970, when first reported, 48 human cases have been recorded. Most of these have been in Zaïre, and all have been in the equatorial rain-forest of West and Central Africa (Zaïre, Liberia, Sierra Leone, Nigeria, Ivory Coast and Cameroon). The case-fatality rate to date has been 17 per cent. It does not appear to be highly infectious and it is not at the moment considered to be a great risk to human beings.

MONKSHOOD (see ACONITE).

MONOAMINE OXIDASE INHIBITORS are drugs that destroy, or prevent the action of, monoamine oxidase (MAO). Monoamines, which include noradrenaline (qv) and tyramine, play an important part in the metabolism of the brain, and there is some evidence that excitement is due to an accumulation of monoamines in the brain. MAO is a naturally occurring enzyme (qv) which is concerned in the breakdown of monoamines.

An excessive accumulation of monoamines can induce a dangerous reaction characterized by high blood-pressure, palpitations, sweating and a feeling of suffocation. Hence the care with which MAO inhibitor drugs are administered. What is equally important, however, is that in no circumstances should a patient receiving any MAO inhibitor drug eat cheese, yeast preparations such as Marmite, tinned fish, or high game. The reason for this ban is that all these foodstuffs contain large amounts of tyramine which increases the amount of certain monoamines such as noradrenaline in the body.

There are also certain drugs, such as amphetamine and pethidine, which must not be taken by a patient who is receiving an MAO inhibitor drug.

MONOMANIA is a form of partial insanity, in which the affected person has a delusion upon one subject, though he can converse rationally and is a responsible individual upon other matters.

MONOPLEGIA means paralysis of a single limb or part. (See PARALYSIS.)

MONOSACCHARIDE is a sugar having six carbon atoms in the molecule, such as glucose, galactose, and laevulose.

MOOREN'S ULCER: A particular form of peripheral corneal ulceration (see EYE, DISEASE AND INJURIES OF).

MORBID means diseased.

MORBIFIC means disease-producing. For example, the *Vibriocholerae* may be called the morbific agent in cholera.

MORBILLI is another name for measles.

MORBILLIVIRUSES are the group of viruses which include those responsible for measles, canine distemper and rinderpest.

MORBUS, the Latin word for disease, is used in such terms as morbus cordis (heart disease), morbus coxae (hip-joint disease).

MORON is the term applied to a feeble-minded person whose defect is relatively slight and whose mental age is somewhere between 8 and 12 years.

MORPHOEA is a form of circumscribed scleroderma. (See SCLERODERMA.)

MORPHINE, or MORPHIA, is the name of the chief alkaloid upon which the action of opium depends. (See OPIUM; DRUG ADDICTION.)

MORTALITY (see DEATH, CAUSES OF; DEATH RATE; INFANT MORTALITY).

MORTIFICATION is another name for gangrene. (See GANGRENE.)

MOSAICISM: If non-dysjunction occurs after the formation of a zygote, that is during a mitotic cell division and not a meiotic cell division, some of the cells will have one chromosome consitution and others another. The term mosaicism describes a condition in which a substantial minority of cells differ from the majority in their chromosome content. How substantial this minority is will depend on how early during cleavage the zygote undergoes non-dysjunction.

MOSQUITOES. (See ANOPHELES; BITES AND STINGS.)

MOTILIN is a hormone (qv) formed in the duodenum (qv) and the jejunum (qv) which plays a part in controlling the movements of the stomach and the gut.

MOTOR NEURON DISEASE. (See PARALYSIS.)

MOUNTAIN-SICKNESS is the name given to the group of symptoms which appear when people reach great heights, either in climbing mountains or in aeroplanes. Some people suffer at lower altitudes than others, but prolonged residence at a high level does not seem to prevent mountain-sickness when the person climbs higher. Those who live habitually at a high altitude develop an increased proportion of red corpuscles in the blood and thus obtain a greater amount of oxygen from the rarefied air, and lose the tendency to mountain-sickness. Exhaustion, want of food, exposure to cold and a too rapid ascent bring it on sooner, but every one seems to begin to suffer when a height over about 4900 metres (16,000 feet) is reached. Shortage of oxygen is the main cause. Weakness, difficulty of breathing, palpitation of the heart, giddiness, sickness, vomiting and finally unconsciousness are the main symptoms, but these rapidly pass off, causing no permanent damage, when the person again reaches a lower lever. Acetazolamide (qv) is said to be useful as a prophylactic.

MOUTH is the start of the alimentary canal. It is bounded anteriorly by the lips and posteriorly by the fauces which is the narrow passage between the tonsils. Immediately behind the lips are the teeth, embedded in the jaw, and behind the lower teeth is the tongue. The upper part of the mouth is the palate. The anterior or hard palate is firm and immovable as it consists of bone covered by mucosa, while the posterior part is soft and mobile. The soft palate moves during swallowing and speech. The salivary glands discharge their saliva into the mouth through small ducts. Two of these ducts are large and can be easily seen; the parotid duct opens into the cheek opposite the upper second molar tooth and the submandibular gland duct can be seen under the tongue in the midline.

Food in the mouth is prepared for digestion by being broken up by the teeth and mixed with saliva prior to being projected into the stomach via the oesophagus.

MOUTH, DISEASES OF: The mucous membrane of the mouth can indicate the health of the individual and internal organs, eg. pallor or pigmentation may indicate anaemia, jaundice or Addison's disease. The musculature of the tongue can also act as a guide to the health of other muscles and of the nervous system in generalized disease.

CONDITIONS OF THE TONGUE: At rest the tongue touches all the lower teeth and is slightly arched from side to side. It has a smooth surface with a groove in the middle and an even but definite edge. It is under voluntary control and the tip can be moved in all directions.

Ankyloglossia or tongue-tie is found when the frenum or band connecting the lower surface of the tongue to the floor of the mouth is so short or tight that the tongue cannot be protruded. This is said to interfere with speech but, if it does, it is only to a small degree. The restricted movement makes it difficult to remove food from round the teeth which may encourage decay.

Gross enlargement of the tongue can make speech indistinct or make swallowing and even breathing difficult. This is known as macroglossia and may be such that the tongue is constantly protruded from the mouth. The cause may be congenital as in severe cases of Down's Syndrome or it may occur as a result of acromegaly or be due to abnormal deposits as in amyloid disease.

In general debility the tongue may appear flabby, large and pale with the edge indented by the teeth.

A marked tremor of the tongue when protruded may be seen in various nervous diseases but is common in excessive indulgence in alcohol and cannot be concealed.

After a stroke involving the motor nerve centre the control of one side of the tongue musculature will be lost. This will result in the protruded tongue pointing to the side of the body which is paralysed. The sense of taste on one side of the tongue may also be lost in some diseases of the brain and facial nerve.

The presence of fur on the tongue may be obvious and distressing. This is due to thickening of the superficial layers of the tongue which may appear like hairs which trap food debris and become discoloured. Furring is common in the presence of fever, mouth breathing and smoking. Debility and loss of appetite will prevent the normal cleaning movements of the tongue and result in a build-up of debris between elongated papillae. A prominent brown fur with a yellow edge on a red mucous membrane is commonly seen in typhoid fever. In scarlet fever the description *strawberry tongue* is used when the surface of the tongue is covered with a white fur through which red spots of mucosal papillae project. Constipation and bowel obstruction are associated with a thick white or brownish fissured fur. Gastritis particularly when related to alcohol excess is associated with a thin white fur which wears off as the day progresses. Stomach cancers and ulcers are not particularly associated with furring of the tongue. Inflammatory lesions of the throat such as tonsillitis may accompany a thick moist fur on the tongue.

In some conditions the tongue may appear dry, red and raw. An inflamed *beefy tongue* is characteristic of pellagra, a disease caused by deficiency of nicotinic acid in the diet. A magenta-coloured tongue may be seen when there is a lack of riboflavin.

THRUSH is characterized by the presence of white patches on the mucous membrane which bleeds if the patch is gently removed. It is caused by the growth of a parasitic mould known as Candida Albicans. Thrush is frequently found under the upper denture of elderly people who wear their dentures day and night and whose oral hygiene is poor. A more florid form is seen in feeble babies and in adults with a chronic severe illness. A less obvious form may be found in some patients after they have been taking antibiotics. Antifungal agents usually suppress the growth of Candida. Candidal infiltration of the mucosa is often found in cancerous lesions.

LEUKOPLAKIA literally means a white patch. In the mouth it is often due to an area of thickened cells from the horny layer of the epithelium. It appears as a white patch of varying density and is often grooved by dense fissures. There are many causes, most of them of minor importance. If, however, it is associated with spirits, smoking, syphilis, chronic sepsis or trauma from a sharp tooth, then cancer must be excluded.

A bright red bare area of tongue surrounded by a definite whitish yellow margin is known as *geographical tongue*. The areas may change position from week to week and there may be a slight burning sensation. Apart from an association with digestive disorders, it is of no great importance.

Ulcers of the tongue are similar to those elsewhere in the mouth. The most common are aphthous ulcers which are small red and painful and last for about ten days. They are associated with stress, mild trauma, and occasionally with folic acid and vitamin B deficiency. Ulcers of the tongue are sometimes found in patients with chronic bowel disease.

STOMATITIS (inflammation of the mouth) arises from the same causes as inflammation elsewhere, but among the main causes are the cutting of teeth in children, sharp or broken teeth, excess alcohol, tobacco smoking and general ill-health. The mucous membrane becomes red, swollen and tender and ulcers may appear. The avoidance of spicy foods and other irritants make the patient more comfortable until the condition resolves. Treatment consists mainly of preventing secondary infection supervening before the stomatitis has resolved. Antiseptic mouthwashes are usually sufficient.

Gingivitis (see TEETH, DISEASES OF) is inflammation of the gum where it touches the tooth. It is caused by poor oral hygiene and is often associated with the production of calculus or tartar on the teeth. If it is neglected it will proceed to periodontal disease.

ULCERS OF THE MOUTH: These are usually small and arise from a variety of causes. *Aphthous ulcers* are the most common. They are round with a bright red margin and uncomfortable as they tend to occur near a sharp tooth or on a mobile part of the mucosa where they are easily stretched open or torn. They last about ten days and usually heal without scarring. They may be associated with stress or dyspepsia. There is no ideal treatment.

Herpetic ulcers are similar but usually there are many ulcers and the patient appears feverish and lethargic. It is more common in children and may arise from mothers who have cold sores on their lip.

Undernourished children may develop an ulcer in the cheek which causes pain, an increased flow of saliva and a foetid breath. This rarely progresses to a condition known as cancrum oris in which much of the cheek may be destroyed.

In whooping cough the underside of the tongue may be frequently forced against the lower teeth as it is protruded during the coughing bouts and this will cause an ulcer under the tongue. Larger ulcers may be tuberculous, syphilitic or cancerous in origin.

ALVEOLAR ABSCESS, DENTAL ABSCESS or GUMBOIL. This is an abscess caused by an infected tooth. It may present as a large swelling or cause trismus (inability to open the mouth). Treatment is drainage of the pus, extraction of the tooth or antibiotics.

CALCULUS (a) *Salivary*: A calculus or stone may develop in one of the major salivary gland ducts. This may result in a blockage which will cause the gland to swell and be painful. It usually swells before a meal and then slowly subsides. The stone may be passed but often has to be removed in a minor operation. If the gland behind the calculus becomes infected, then an abscess forms and, if this persists, the removal of the gland may be indicated. (b) *Dental*, also called TARTAR: This is a hard substance which adheres to the teeth. Some people produce more than others. It is a mixture of calcified material and bacteria and often starts as the soft debris found on teeth which have not been well cleaned and is called plaque. If not removed, it will gradually destroy the periodontal membrane and result in the loss of the tooth.

RANULA: This is a cystlike swelling found in the floor of the mouth. It is often caused by mild trauma to the salivary glands with the result that saliva collects in the cyst instead of discharging into the mouth. Careful surgical removal is required as cysts can become quite large.

MUCOCOELE or MUCOUS CYST: This is a collection of saliva in the lip following mild trauma. It is similar to a ranula but does not become so large. Treatment is surgical removal.

MUMPS is an acute infective disorder of the major salivary glands. It causes painful enlargement of the glands which lasts for about two weeks.

TUMOURS occur in all parts of the mouth. They may be benign or malignant. Benign tumours are common and may follow mild trauma or are an exaggerated response to irritation. Polyps are found in the cheeks and on the tongue and become a nuisance as they may be bitten frequently. They are easily excised.

A *mucocoele* (qv) is found mainly in the lower lip.

An *epulis* is a lump on the gum. One form is seen during pregnancy and may bleed easily but disappears spontaneously at the end of the gestation. Another form is more persistent and may recur after excision and removal of the associated teeth. An *exostosis* or bone outgrowth is often found in the mid-line of the palate and on the inside of the mandible. This only requires removal if it becomes unduly large or pointed and easily ulcerated.

Malignant tumours within the mouth are often large before they are noticed, whereas those on the lips are usually seen early and are more easily treated. The cancer may arise from any of the tissues found in the mouth including epithelium, bone, salivary tissue and tooth-forming tissue remnants. In England and Wales in 1984 there were 2,093 new cases of malignant disease in the mouth and major salivary glands. Nearly 600 of these were in the tongue.

Cancer of the mouth is less common below the age of 40 years and more common in men. It is often associated with chronic irritation from a broken tooth or ill-fitting denture. It is also more common in those who smoke and those who chew betel leaves. Leukoplakia (qv) may be a precursor of cancer. Spread of the cancer is by way of the lymph nodes in the neck. Early treatment by surgery or radiotherapy will often give a five-year cure, except for the posterior of the tongue where the prognosis is very poor. Although surgery may be extensive and potentially mutilating, recent advances in repairing defects and grafting tissues from elsewhere have made treatment more acceptable to the patient.

MUCILAGE is prepared from acacia or tragacanth gum, and is used as an ingredient of mixtures containing solid particles in order to keep the latter from settling, and also as a demulcent. (See DEMULCENTS.)

MUCOCELE is an abnormally dilated cavity in the body due to the accumulation of mucus; such a 'cyst' may therefore form wherever there is mucous membrane.

MUCOCUTANEOUS LYMPH NODE SYNDROME is a disease that has been reported from Japan, Korea, Hawaii, Greece and the USA, but not yet from Britain. The cause is not known. It occurs in young children, usually under the age of 5 years. It is characterized by fever, a generalized rash which becomes bright red on the hands and feet, and enlargement of the glands in the neck. Recovery usually occurs in two to four weeks. Complications sometimes occur in the form of meningitis, arthritis, jaundice, or myocarditis. The mortality rate is 1 to 2 per cent. There is no specific treatment.

MUCOLYTIC is the term used to describe the property of destroying, or lessening the tenacity of, mucus. It is most commonly used to describe drugs which have this property and are therefore used in the treatment of bronchitis (qv). The inhalation of steam, for example, has a mucolytic action.

MUCOMEMBRANOUS COLIC is a disorder in which constipation, abdominal pain, and the passage of mucus or casts of mucus in the stools occur in highly strung or neurotic people, especially women. The spasm of the colon causing these symptoms may be allergic in origin.

MUCOUS MEMBRANE is the general name given to the membrane which lines many of the hollow organs of the body. These membranes vary widely in structure in different sites, but all have the common character of being lubricated by mucus, derived in some cases from isolated cells on the surface of the membrane, but more generally from definite glands placed beneath the membrane, and opening here and there through it by ducts. The air passages, the alimentary canal and the ducts of glands which open into it, and also the urinary passages, are all lined by mucous membrane.

In structure a mucous membrane consists of a basis of fibrous tissue resembling the true skin, though looser and lighter in texture, in which the blood-vessels, nerves, and mucous glands lie. This is covered on its surface by a layer of epithelium resembling the epithelium covering the skin, although the cells are in all cases of a more soft and succulent nature than those on the outer surface of the body.

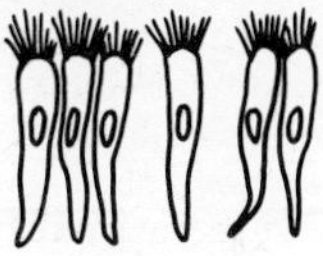

Ciliated epithelial cells from the air passages.

It is in the character and properties of these cells that the various mucous membranes chiefly differ. In the air passages they are – almost everywhere except over the vocal cords –of a pillar-like shape and provided with thread-like processes, being known as ciliated cells. On the vocal cords the cells, which are exposed to constant friction, resemble those of the skin. In the alimentary system generally they are of a simple pillar-like or columnar type placed side by side, though in the mouth and gullet, where the food causes much friction, the surface, like that of the vocal cords, closely resembles the epidermis of the skin.

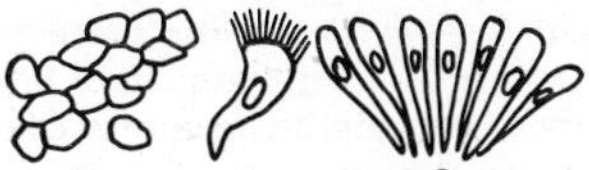

1 surface view of the ends of a group of cells
2 columnar cell from the mucous membrane of the small intestine
3 side view of a group of cells

Columnar epithelium.

Lying close beneath the epithelium there is, in most mucous membranes, a thin layer of involuntary muscle fibres, and to this, coupled with the extremely loose attachment of mucous membranes to the organs which they line, is due the great pliability and elasticity of these membranes.

MUCOUS PATCH is the name given to the syphilitic eruption as it affects mucous membranes. These patches are seen especially about the lips, mouth, and throat, and consist of slightly raised areas, reddish at the edge, and covered by a velvety whitish layer. They are very infectious. (See SYPHILIS.)

MUCOVISCIDOSIS (see FIBROCYSTIC DISEASE OF THE PANCREAS).

MUCUS is the general name for the slimy secretion derived from mucous membranes. It is mainly composed of a substance called mucin, which varies according to the particular mucous membrane from which it is derived, and it contains other substances, such as cells cast off from the surface of the membrane, ferments, and dust particles. From whatever source derived, mucin has the following characters: it is viscid, clear, and tenacious; when dissolved in water it can be precipitated by addition of acetic acid; and when not in solution already, it is dissolved by weak alkalis, such as lime-water.

Under normal conditions the surface of a mucous membrane is lubricated by only a small quantity of mucus; the appearance of large quantities is a sign of inflammation.

MULLERIAN DUCTS: The Mullerian and the Wolffian ducts are separate sets of primordia that transiently co-exist in embryos of both sexes. In female embryos the Mullerian ducts grow and fuse in the midline producing the Fallopian tubes, the uterus and the upper third of the vagina whereas the Wolffian ducts regress. In the male the Wolffian ducts give rise to the vas deferens, the seminal vesicles and the epididymis and the Mullerian ducts disappear. This phase of development requires a functioning testis from which an inducer substance diffuses locally over the primordia to bring about the suppression of the Mullerian duct and the development of the Wolffian duct. In the absence of this substance development proceeds along female lines regardless of the genetic sex.

MULTIGRAVIDA is a pregnant woman who has had more than one pregnancy.

MULTIPARA is a woman who has borne several children.

MULTIPLE BIRTHS: Twins occur about once in eighty pregnancies, triplets once in 6000, quadruplets about once in 500,000. Quintuplets are exceedingly rare. Such is the natural state of affairs. In recent years, however, the position has been altered by the introduction of the so-called fertility drugs, such as clomiphene (qv), and human menopausal gonadotrophin which, through the medium of the pituitary gland, stimulate the production of ova. Their wide use in the treatment of infertility has resulted in an increase in the number of multiple births, a recognized hazard of giving too large a dose. So far as fraternal, or binovular, twins are concerned, multiple pregnancy may be an inherited tendency; it certainly occurs more often in certain families, but this may be partly due to chance. A woman who has already given birth to twins is ten times more likely to have another multiple pregnancy than one who has not previously had twins. In 1974, a Swedish mother, who had not had any fertility drugs, gave birth to her third lot of twin girls. Both she and her husband were twins themselves. The statistical chance of a third pair of twins is 1 in 512,000. Identical twins do not run in families.

Twins may be binovular or uniovular. *Binovular*, or *fraternal, twins* are the result of the mother releasing two ova within a few days of each other and both being fertilized by separate spermatozoa. They both develop separately in the mother's womb and are no more alike than is usual with members of the same family. They are three times as common as *uniovular*, or *identical, twins*, who are developed from a single ovum fertilized by a single spermatozoon, but which has split early in development. This is why they are usually so remarkably alike in looks and mental characteristics. Unlike binovular twins, who may be of the same or different sex, they are always of the same sex.

The relative proportion of twins of each type varies in different races. Identical twins have much the same frequency all over the world: around 3 per 1000 maternities. Fraternal twins are rare in Mongolian races: less than 3 per 1000 maternities. In Whites they occur two or three times as often as identical twins: between 7 (Spain and Portugal) and 10 (Czechoslovakia and Greece) per 1000 maternities. They are more common in Negroes, reaching 30 per 1000 maternities in certain West African populations. (See also SIAMESE TWINS.)

In England and Wales 353 triplets were born in the four-year period, 1971–1975. This gives an incidence of 1 in 9824 births, and a ratio of triplets to twins of 1 : 96. Of the 1059 triplets, 541 were girls. The sexes were identical in 150 sets: 77 all girls and 73 all boys. The peak age for mothers having triplets was 35–39 years. The stillbirth rate for triplets was 41·5 per 1000 live births and stillbirths, compared with 30·6 for twins and 9·4 for all births.

'False twins' are not uncommon, when 'twin' children have been fathered by different men.

Parents of twins can obtain advice and help from the Twins and Multiple Births Association, Hon. Secretary, 41 Fortuna Way, Aylesby Park, Grimsby, South Humberside DN37 9SJ.

MULTIPLE SCLEROSIS is a disease of the brain and spinal cord, which, though slow in its onset, in time may produce marked symptoms, such as paralysis and tremors, and may ultimately render people suffering from it confirmed invalids. It consists of hardened patches, from the size of a pin-head to that of a pea or larger, scattered here and there irregularly through the brain and cord, each patch being made up of a mass of the connective tissue (neuroglia), which should be present only in sufficient amount to bind the nerve-cells and fibres together. In the earliest stage, the insulating sheaths of the nerve-fibres in the hardened patches break up, are absorbed, and leave the nerve-fibres bare, the connective tissue being later formed between these.

Cause: Although this is one of the most common diseases of the central nervous system in Europe – there are around 50,000 affected individuals in Britain alone – the cause is still not known. The disease comes on in young people (onset being rare after the age of 40), apparently without previous illness. It is more common in first and second children than in those later in birth order, and in small rather than big families. There may be a hereditary factor, but this is by no means proven. If such exists it is of an obscure nature and linked more to a defect in the individual's reaction to infection than to any precise defect in the nervous system. The actual changes in the nervous system appear to be due to the action of some substance which dissolves or breaks up the fatty matter of the nerve-sheaths.

Symptoms: These depend greatly upon the part of the brain and cord affected by the sclerotic patches. Temporary paralysis of a limb, or of an eye muscle, causing double vision, and tremors upon exertion, first in the affected parts, and later in all parts of the body, are early symptoms. Stiffness of the lower limbs causing the toes to catch on small irregularities in the ground and trip the person in walking, is often an annoying symptom and one of the first to be noticed. Great activity is shown in the reflex movements obtained by striking the tendons and by stroking the soles of the feet. The latter reflex shows a characteristic sign (Babinski sign) in which the great toe bends upwards and the other toes spread apart as the sole is stroked, instead of the toes collectively bending downwards as in the normal person. Tremor of the eye movements (nystagmus) is usually found. Trembling handwriting, interference with the functions of the bladder, giddiness, and a peculiar 'staccato' or 'scanning' speech are common symptoms at a later stage. Numbness and tingling in the extremities occur commonly, particularly in the early stages of the disease. As the disease progresses, the paralyses, which were transitory at first, now become confirmed, often with great rigidity in the limbs. Many cases progress very slowly and show little or no tendency to shortening of the duration of life.

People with multiple sclerosis, and their relatives, can obtain help and guidance from the Multiple Sclerosis Society of Great Britain and Northern Ireland, 25 Effie Road, London SW6 1EE (01-736 6267). Another helpful organization is Action for Research into Multiple Sclerosis, 4A Chapel Hill, Stansted, Essex CM24 8AG (0279 815553), which provides a 24-hour telephone counselling service (01–222 3123) for those with the disease and their families. Those with sexual or marital problems arising out of the illness can obtain information from SPOD (Association to Aid the Sexual and Personal Relationships of People with a Disability), 286 Camden Road, London N7 0BJ (01–602 8851/2).

Treatment is unsatisfactory, because the most that can be done is to lead a life as free from strain as possible, to check the progress of the disease. It is important to keep the nerves and muscles functioning, and therefore the patient should remain at work as long as he or she is capable of doing it, and in any case should regularly exercise the lower limbs by walking and the upper limbs by carrying out movements requiring co-ordination, such as knitting or embroidery. Corticosteriods seem to be as effective a means as any of slowing up the progress of the disease, but they can only be used under skilled medical supervision.

MUMPS, also known as EPIDEMIC PAROTITIS, is an infectious disease characterized by inflammatory swelling of the parotid and other salivary glands, often occurring as an epidemic, and affecting mostly young people. Its name comes from the old verb, 'mump', meaning to mope or assume a disconsolate appearance –an apt description of the victim of the disease at its height.

Causes: Mumps is due to infection with a virus and is highly infectious from person to person. It is predominantly a disease of childhood and early adult life, but it can occur at any age. Epidemics usually occur in the winter and spring. It is infectious for two or three days before the swelling of the glands appears. A vaccine is now available that gives a high degree of protection against the disease.

Symptoms: There is a long incubation period of two to three weeks after infection before the glands begin to swell. The first signs are fatigue, slight feverishness, and sore throat, which may precede the swelling by a day or two. The gland first affected is generally the parotid, situated in front of and below the ear. Along with the swelling there is often some face-ache and considerable rise of temperature to 38·3° or even 40°C (101° or 104°F). The swelling usually spreads to the submaxillary and sublingual glands lying beneath the jaw, and to the glands on the side opposite that first affected. There is hardly ever any redness or tendency to suppuration in the swollen parts, although interference with the acts of chewing and swallowing may occasion a good deal of trouble, and the swelling is tender to touch. After continuing four or five days, the swelling abates, the temperature having generally already fallen. In 15 to 30 per cent of males, inflammation of the testicles (orchitis) develops. This usually occurs during the second week of the illness, but may not occur until two or three weeks later. It may result in partial atrophy of the testicles, but practically never in infertility. In a much smaller proportion of females with mumps, inflammation of the ovaries or breasts may occur. Inflammation of the pancreas, accompanied by tenderness in the upper part of the abdomen and digestive disturbances, sometimes occurs. Meningitis is also an occasional complication. The various complications are found much more often when the disease affects adults than when it occurs in childhood.

Treatment: The patient must be confined to bed for at least a week or ten days, and kept in isolation for 14 days from the onset of the disease or 7 days from the subsidence of all swelling. Soft food, and the protection of the inflamed parts by a strip of flannel or by cotton-wool and a handkerchief are all the treatment usually required. If there is much face-ache, it is relieved by warm fomentations or aspirin.

MURIATIC ACID is an old name for hydrochloric acid.

MURMUR is the uneven, rustling sound heard by auscultation over the heart and various blood-vessels in abnormal conditons. For example, murmurs heard when the stethoscope is applied over the heart are highly characteristic of valvular disease of this organ.

MUSCAE VOLITANTES ('FLYING FLIES'): Spots before the eyes due to small opacities in the vitreous humour casting shadows on the retina. In themselves vitreous floaters are harmless but anyone with 'spots before the eyes' of sudden onset should seek specialist advice.

MUSCARINE is the poisonous principle found in some toadstools. (See FUNGUS-POISONING.)

MUSCLE, popularly known as FLESH, is the tissue by which, because of its power of contraction, movements are made in the higher animals. Muscular tissue is divided, according to its function, into two main groups, *voluntary muscle* and *involuntarymuscle*, of which the former is under control of the will, whilst the latter discharges its functions independently. The term *striped muscle* is often given to voluntary muscle, because under the microscope all the voluntary muscles show a striped appearance, whilst involuntary muscle is, in the main, unstriped or plain. There are exceptions to the latter statement, for the heart muscle, which is involuntary, is partially striped, while certain muscles of the throat, and two small muscles inside the ear, not controllable by will-power, are also striped.

Structure of muscle: VOLUNTARY MUSCLE is disposed in a regular method over the body, being mainly attached to the skeleton, and hence often called skeletal muscle. There are certain definite muscles, and these vary as to shape only slightly in different persons, although in one person particular muscles may be developed to a much greater bulk than in others. Each muscle is enclosed in a sheath of fibrous tissue, known as fascia or epimysium, and, from this, partitions of fibrous tissue, known as perimysium, run into the substance of the muscle, dividing it up into small bundles. Each of these bundles, if carefully examined, will be found to consist in turn of a collection of fibres, which form the units of the muscle. Each fibre is about 50 micrometres in thickness and ranges in length from a few millimetres to 300 millimetres. If the fibre is cut across and examined under a high-powered microscope, it is seen to be further divided into fibrils. Each fibre is enclosed in an elastic sheath of its own, which allows it to lengthen and shorten, and is known as the sarcolemma. Within the sarcolemma lie numerous nuclei belonging to the muscle fibre, which was originally developed from a simple cell. To the sarcolemma, at either end, is attached a minute bundle of connective-tissue fibres which unites the muscle fibre to its neighbours, or to one of the connective tissue partitions in the muscle, and by means of these connections the fibre produces its effect upon contracting. The sarcolemma is pierced by a nerve fibre, which breaks up upon the surface of the muscle fibre into a complicated end-plate, and by this means each muscle fibre is brought under the guidance of the central nervous system, and the discharge of energy which produces muscular contraction is controlled. When the muscle fibre within the sarcolemma is examined by a high magnifying power, it is found to show alternate light and dark transverse stripes, with a fine dotted line, called Dobie's line or Krause's membrane, across the middle of each light stripe. These appearances are due to the fact that the fibre is composed of segments made up partly of fibrous connective material, partly of semi-fluid contractile tissue, in which visible changes take place as the fibre contracts.

Between the muscle fibres, which have, on account of their relative length and width, a pillar-like shape, run many capillary blood-vessels. They are so placed that the contractions of the muscle fibres empty them at once of blood, and thus the active muscle is ensured a specially good blood supply. None of these vessels, however, pierces the sarcolemma surrounding the fibres, so that the blood does not come into direct contact with the muscular tissue, whose nourishment is carried on by the lymph that exudes from the blood-vessels. The lymph circulation is also automatically varied, as required, by the muscular contractions. Between the muscle fibres, and enveloped in a sheath of connective tissue, lie here and there special structures known as muscle-spindles. Each of these contains thin muscle fibres, numerous nuclei, and the endings of sensory nerves. They appear to be the sensory organs of the muscles. (See TOUCH.)

INVOLUNTARY MUSCLE includes, as already stated, the heart muscle and unstriped muscle. The heart muscle stands in structure between striped and unstriped muscle. Each fibre is short, has a nucleus in its centre, communicates with its neighbours by short branches, shows a faintly striped appearance near its exterior, and is devoid of sarcolemma.

Plain or unstriped muscle is found in the following positions: the inner and middle coats of the stomach and intestines; the ureters and urinary bladder; the windpipe and bronchial tubes; the ducts of glands; the gall-bladder; the uterus and Fallopian tubes; the middle coat of the blood- and lymph-vessels; the iris and ciliary muscle of the eye; the dartos muscle of the scrotum; and in association with the various glands and hairs in the skin. The fibres are very much smaller than those of striped muscle, although they vary greatly in size. Each is pointed at the ends, has one or more oval nuclei in the centre, and a delicate sheath of sarcolemma enveloping it. The fibres are grouped in bundles, much as are the striped fibres, but they adhere to one another by cement material, not by the tendon bundles found in voluntary muscle.

Development of muscle: All the muscles of the developing individual arise from the central layer (mesoderm) of the embryo, each fibre taking origin from a single cell. Later on in life, muscles have the power both of increasing in size, as the result of use, for example, in athletes, and also of healing, after parts of them have been destroyed by injury. This takes place partly by the growth and splitting of the original fibres to form new fibres, and partly from reserve cells, known as sarcoplasts, which lie in every muscle between the muscle fibres. An example of the great extent to which unstriped muscle can develop, to meet the demands made upon its power, is given by the womb, whose muscular wall develops so much during pregnancy that the organ increases from the weight of 30 to 40 grams (1 to 1½ ounces) to a weight of around 1 kilogram (2 pounds), decreasing again to its former small size in the course of a month after child-birth.

Physiology of contraction: A muscle is an elaborate chemico-physical system for producing heat and mechanical work. The total energy liberated by a contracting muscle can be exactly measured. From 25 to 30 per cent of the total energy expended is used in mechanical work. The heat of contracting muscle makes an important contribution to the maintenance of the heat of the body. (See also MYOGLOBIN.)

The energy of muscular contraction is derived from a complicated series of chemical reactions. Complex substances are broken down and built up again, supplying each other with energy for this purpose. The first reaction is the breakdown of adenyl-pyrophosphate into phosphoric acid and adenylic acid (derived from nucleic acid); this supplies the immediate energy for contraction. Next phosphocreatine breaks down into creatine and phosphoric acid, giving energy for the resynthesis of adenyl-pyrophosphate. Creatine is a normal nitrogenous constituent of muscle. Then glycogen through the intermediary stage of sugar bound to phosphate breaks down into lactic acid to supply energy for the resynthesis of phosphocreatine. Finally part of the lactic acid is oxidized to supply energy for building up the rest of the lactic acid into glycogen again. If there is not enough oxygen, lactic acid accumulates and fatigue results.

There are some points to be noticed in this version of muscular activity. First, muscle contraction and relaxation take place in the absence of oxygen – the anaerobic phase. Secondly, oxygen comes into the picture in the phase of recovery, and by oxidizing some of the lactic acid winds up the contractile mechanism once more. Thirdly, the energy of contraction does not come directly from the breakdown of glycogen.

All of the chemical changes are mediated by the action of several enzymes.

Involuntary muscle has several peculiarities of contraction. In the heart *rhythmicality* is an important feature, one beat appearing to be, in a sense, the cause of the next beat. *Tonus* is a character of all muscle, but particularly of unstriped muscle in some localities, as in the walls of arteries. Muscles are not held either slack or taut, but in a slightly stretched condition, so that when occasion arises they are ready for instant action, while the arteries owe their elasticity and strength mainly to this fact. The involuntary muscle, forming the middle coat of the bowels, gland-ducts, and other tubes, contracts in the so-called *vermicular movement*, or peristalsis, which means that a ring of contraction passes slowly along the tube, at a rate of about 25 mm (1 inch) per second, the muscle relaxing as the ring of contraction passes on.

Fatigue of muscle comes on when a muscle is made to act for some time. It is due, not to wearing out of the muscle's power, but to the accumulation of waste products, especially sarcolactic acid, produced by the muscle's activity. These substances affect the end plates of the nerve controlling the muscle, and so prevent destructive over-action of the muscle. As they are rapidly swept away by the blood, the muscle, after a rest, particularly if the rest is accompanied by massage or by gentle contractions to quicken the circulation, recovers rapidly from the fatigue. After great muscular activity over the whole body, a more lasting fatigue is produced by the accumulation of these products, and by their action upon the central nervous system, this being recovered from after a prolonged rest, during which the waste substances are excreted by the lungs, kidneys, and other excretory organs.

Another factor that comes into play is the accumulation of fluid in the muscles on unaccustomed exercise. Active tissues swell because of the increased blood flow through them. This results in an increased amount outside the blood-vessels but within the tissues themselves. Normally the body can cope with this state of affairs but on occasion, as when an under-trained individual undertakes excessive exercise, the accumulation of fluid in the muscles may be so great that the body cannot absorb it quickly enough, and the muscles swell and become tense and painful. This is the cause of the muscle stiffness which follows unaccustomed exercise. In those areas of the body where the space available for muscles is restricted, this increase of fluid may cause trouble and produce what is known as the compression syndrome. The classical example of this is the *anterior tibial syndrome*, in which the muscles on the front and outer aspect of the shin, lying within a tight fascial envelope, as they do, become tense and painful, and there may be actual damage to the muscles as a result of interference with their blood supply. (See MUSCLES, DISEASES OF.)

Rigor mortis is a condition which comes on in the muscles after death, and to which the general stiffening of the dead body is due. It consists in a state of permanent, wasteful contraction, beginning in the muscles of the neck and lower jaw at a period which varies from ten minutes to seven hours after death, and spreading gradually over the whole body. It comes on quickest after death from exhaustion, or from some weakening disease; and, occasionally, after violent injuries causing death, it comes on instantaneously, so that the posture of the body is fixed in the attitude in which death occurs. The rigidity lasts usually from sixteen to twenty-four hours, but its duration is extremely variable, being longer, as a rule, when its onset has been slow. (See DEATH, SIGNS OF.)

Muscular system, popularly known as 'the flesh', comprises all the voluntary muscles, and amounts in an average man of 70 kg (154 pounds) to about 35 kg (77 pounds), or half of the whole body weight. The total number of the voluntary muscles, each of which is named, amounts to around 620, including the muscles of both sides. Each muscle constitutes a separate organ, controlled by a special nerve or nerves, which connect it with the spinal cord and brain, where, however, actions and combined movements are represented rather than individual muscles. (See BRAIN.) The fleshy part of the muscle is known as its belly, and there is usually at either end a tendon, by which the muscle is inserted into bone or other structure, upon which it acts. One end is more fixed than the other, as a rule, the rigid end being known as the origin of the muscle, the more mobile end as its insertion.

UPPER LIMB: *Between the trunk and limb* run the following muscles: the trapezius, latissimus dorsi, large and small rhomboids, and levator of the angle of the scapula, behind; and the large and small pectoral, the subclavius, and serratus anterior muscles in front. *In the shoulder region* lie the deltoid, supraspinatus, infraspinatus, large and small teres, and the subscapular muscles. *In the upper arm* the coracobrachialis, biceps, and brachialis occupy the front, while the triceps fills up the back of the arm. *In the forearm* the muscles in front that bend the wrist and fingers, or turn the hand palm downwards, are the pronator teres, the radial flexor of the wrist, the long palmar, the ulnar flexor of the wrist, the superficial and deep flexors of the fingers, the long flexor of the thumb, and the pronator quadratus; while the muscles on the back of the forearm that extend the fingers and bend the wrist backwards, or turn the hand palm upwards, are the supinator, longer and shorter radial extensors of the wrist,

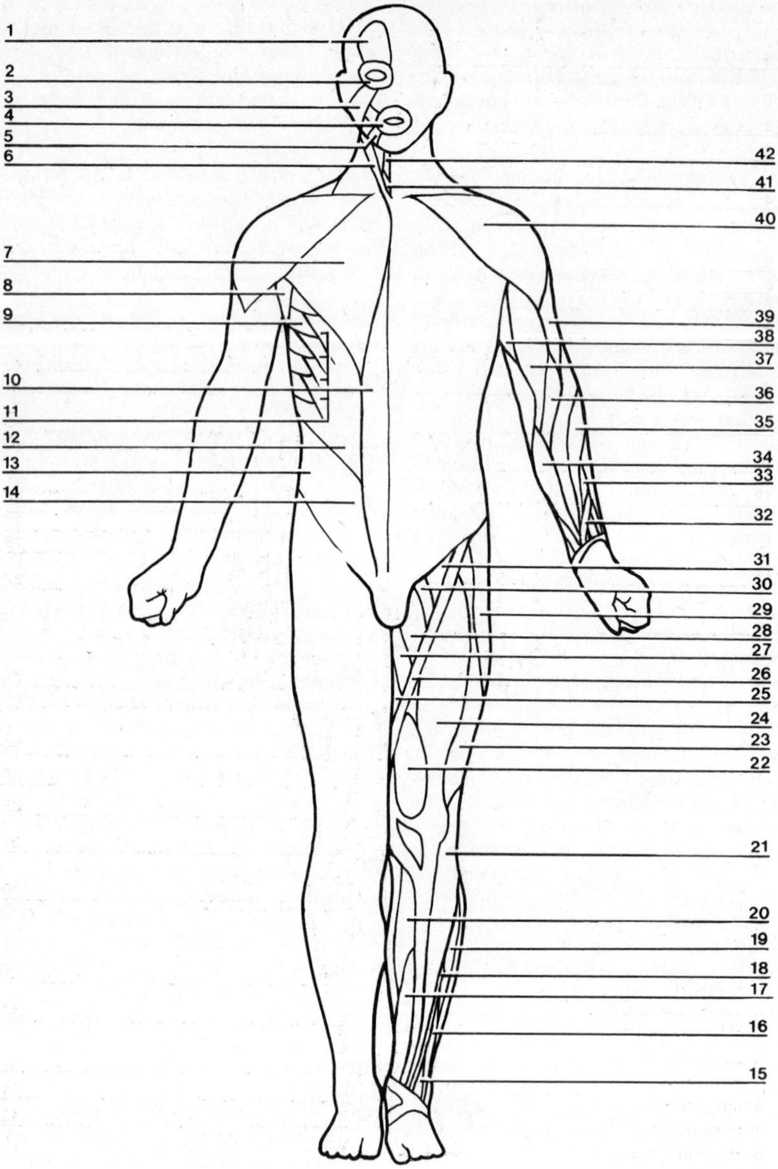

1 frontalis	15 extensor hallucis longus	29 tensor fasciae latae
2 orbicularis oculi	16 peroneus brevis	30 iliopsoas
3 masseter	17 soleus	31 iliacus
4 orbicularis oris	18 extensor digitorum longus	32 abductor pollicis longus
5 depressor anguli oris	19 peroneus longus	33 extensor carpi radialis brevis
6 sternocleidomastoid	20 gastrocnemius	34 flexor carpi radialis
7 pectoralis major	21 anterior tibial	35 extensor carpi radialis longus
8 latissimus dorsi	22 vastus medialis	36 brachialis
9 serratus anterior	23 vastus lateralis	37 biceps brachii
10 rectus abdominis	24 rectus femoris	38 coracobrachialis
11 external intercostals	25 gracilis	39 triceps brachii
12 sheath of rectus abdominis	26 sartorius	40 deltoid
13 external oblique	27 adductor longus	41 sternothyroid
14 internal oblique	28 pectineus	42 sternohyroid

Muscles on the front of the body.

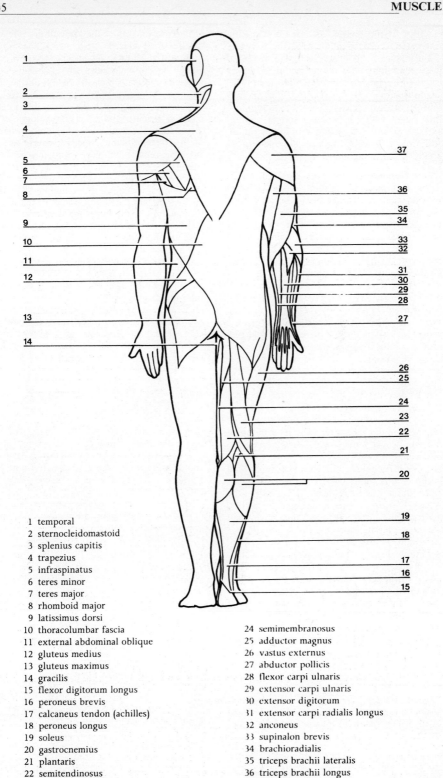

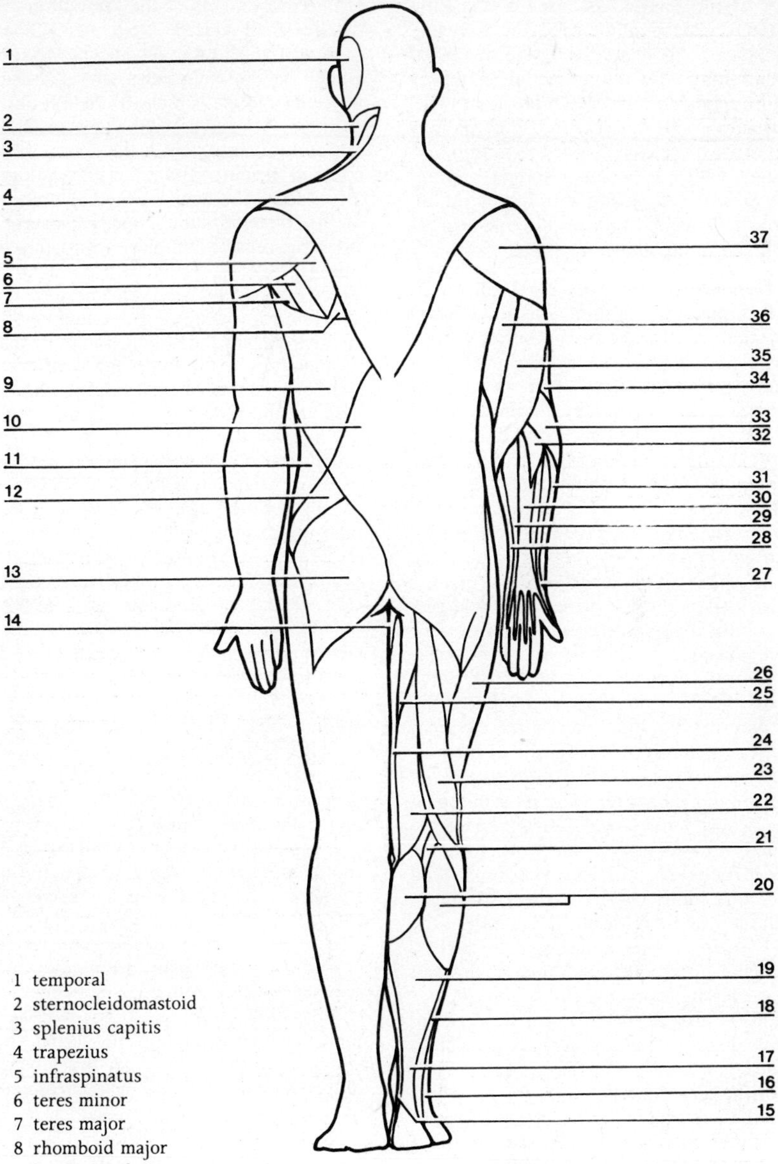

1 temporal
2 sternocleidomastoid
3 splenius capitis
4 trapezius
5 infraspinatus
6 teres minor
7 teres major
8 rhomboid major
9 latissimus dorsi
10 thoracolumbar fascia
11 external abdominal oblique
12 gluteus medius
13 gluteus maximus
14 gracilis
15 flexor digitorum longus
16 peroneus brevis
17 calcaneus tendon (achilles)
18 peroneus longus
19 soleus
20 gastrocnemius
21 plantaris
22 semitendinosus
23 biceps femoris (short head),(long head)
24 semimembranosus
25 adductor magnus
26 vastus externus
27 abductor pollicis
28 flexor carpi ulnaris
29 extensor carpi ulnaris
30 extensor digitorum
31 extensor carpi radialis longus
32 anconeus
33 supinalon brevis
34 brachioradialis
35 triceps brachii lateralis
36 triceps brachii longus
37 deltoid

Muscles on the back of the body.

extensor of the fingers, extensor of the little finger, ulnar extensor of the wrist, the extensors of the metacarpal bone, of the first joint, and of the second joint of the thumb, and the extensor of the forefinger. *In the palm of the hand* there are four lumbrical muscles, the short palmar muscle, three muscles each for the thumb and little finger, which respectively abduct, oppose, and flex these digits, an adductor of the thumb, and, in the spaces between the metacarpal bones, seven interosseous muscles.

LOWER LIMB: *Muscles of the hip* are the iliacus in front, and, behind, the three gluteus muscles forming the prominence of the buttock, with the pyriform, external and internal obturator, two gemelli, and quadratus femoris muscles under cover of the largest gluteal muscle, while to the outer side lies the tensor of the sheath of the thigh. *On the back of the thigh* lie the biceps, semitendinosus, and semimembranosus muscles, whose tendons, standing out prominently behind the knee, are known collectively as the ham-strings. *In front of the thigh* are placed the sartorius, which is the longest, and the quadriceps extensor of the leg, which is the largest muscle of the body. *Onthe inner side of the thigh* lie the gracilis and pectineus muscles, with the long, the short, and the large adductors. *On the front of the leg* are placed the tibialis anterior, the long extensor of the great toe, the long extensor of the toes, and the peroneus tertius muscles. *On the outer side of the leg* are two muscles, the long and short peroneal muscles, whose tendons pass down behind the outer ankle to the foot. *On the back of the leg* are two groups of muscles. The superficial group of three muscles, consisting of the gastrocnemius, a double-bellied muscle, the soleus, which is flat and projects slightly beneath the gastrocnemius, and the small plantaris muscle, forms the calf of the leg, and ends in the tendo calcaneus, or Achilles tendon, behind the heel. The deep group lies close upon the bones, and consists of the popliteus, long flexor of the toes, long flexor of the great toe, and tibialis posterior muscles, the tendons of the last three passing down behind the inner ankle. *In the foot* there is one muscle, the short extensor of the toes, upon the 'dorsum' or upper surface; while in the sole of the foot are four layers of small muscles, comprising the short flexor of the toes, and abductors of the great and little toes; the accessory flexor of the toes, and four lumbrical muscles; the short flexor of the great toe, oblique and transverse adductors of the great toe, and short flexor of the little toe; and in the fourth layer seven interosseous muscles, as in the hand.

FACE AND HEAD: Attached to the auricle of the ear are three weak muscles which raise, draw back, and flatten the auricle. The eyelids, nose, and lips are provided with numerous flattened muscles, which dilate and draw together these openings, and which form the means of varying facial expression.

The movements of the eye-ball are effected by six small muscles. (See EYE.) The movements of the lower jaw in chewing are controlled by four muscles on each side: the masseter muscle, which can be felt on the hinder part of the cheek as the jaws are closed; the temporal muscle, felt in the region of the temple; and the outer and inner pterygoid muscles, attached to the deep surface of the jaw-bone. Within the mouth the tongue consists of certain intrinsic muscle bundles, together with four muscles on each side, which connect it with the lower jaw, hyoid bone, and base of the skull. The floor of the mouth is formed by four muscles, which pass from the hyoid bone in front of the neck up to the lower jaw and base of the skull. The throat or pharynx, which is open in front to the nose, the mouth, and the larynx, one beneath the other, is closed behind by three broad, flat muscles, the superior, middle, and inferior constrictors of the pharynx, and is swung from the base of the skull by the stylopharyngeus muscle on either side. The soft palate, which separates the hinder part of the cavities of nose and mouth from one another, consists of five muscles on each side covered by mucous membrane. The larynx is controlled by eleven small muscles, which open or close its opening, and render the vocal cords more or less tense in the production of the voice.

FRONT OF NECK: The most prominent feature of the neck is the thick sternocleidomastoid muscle, which on each side runs from behind the ear downwards and forwards to the breast-bone and collar-bone. Partly under cover of these and protecting the front of the larynx are four small muscles on each side: the sternohyoid, sternothyroid, thyrohyoid, and omohyoid muscles. Deep in the neck, behind, and to either side of the windpipe, gullet, and large blood-vessels, lie the anterior, middle, and posterior scalene muscles, which pass from the spinal column to the upper two ribs. Lying close upon the spine are three rectus muscles on each side, which bend the head upon the spine, and the long muscle of the neck, which bends the spine in this region.

BACK OF THE NECK AND TRUNK: The muscles in this region form a very complicated system, most arising from the spines or transverse processes of several vertebrae or from a number of ribs, and running upwards to be attached to another series of vertebrae or ribs some distance above, whilst the upper muscles of the set are attached to the hinder portion of the skull. These muscles form a couple of strong columns running the whole length of the back from the loins to the head, with a groove between in which the line of vertebral spines can be felt. The upper and lower serrated muscles of the back are muscles of respiration passing from ribs to spine, and, together with the splenius muscle in the neck, form a superficial layer. Beneath them the erector spinae, the great muscle which supports the back, runs the whole distance from the sacrum to the skull, obtaining at numerous points attachments to the spines and transverse processes of the vertebrae and to the neighbouring portions of the ribs. This muscle, along with those about to be mentioned, is of great power, having, even in moderately strong persons, a lifting power of 90 to 180 kg (200 to 400 pounds). Covered by the erector is the transversospinalis group of muscles, in which all the muscles ascend with an inward inclination; a series of short muscles connecting succeeding vertebrae with one another; and four small muscles passing from the uppermost two vertebrae to the skull. These last-named muscles incline and rotate the trunk and head from side to side.

CHEST: The diaphragm is the chief muscle of this part of the body. (See DIAPHRAGM.) Next in importance come the outer and inner intercostal muscles, which form a double layer of oblique fibres filling up the gaps between the ribs, the fibres of the two muscles running in different directions. There are also levators of the ribs, which pass each from a vertebra to the rib beneath it, and subcostal muscles which are of feeble development. All these muscles share in the act of inspiration.

ABDOMEN: The sides and front of the abdomen, unprotected by any bone beneath the level of the ribs, are enclosed by thick muscular layers strengthened by sheets of fibrous tissue. On the sides of the abdomen are three muscles: the external oblique, consisting of fibres which run downwards and forwards from the lower eight ribs; the internal oblique, under cover of the first, consisting of fibres which run upwards and forwards from the haunch-bone, and fibrous layers in its neighbourhood; and thirdly, the transversalis muscle, the fibres of which run horizontally forward from the lower six ribs, the lumbar vertebrae, and the haunch-bone. The fibres of all three muscles end along a curved line, the semilunar line, which is plainly visible upon the surface of the abdomen, running with a curve from its upper to its lower end, and distant, at the level of the navel, some 10 or 12·5 cm (4 or 5 inches) from the middle line. From the curved line a sheet of dense fibrous tissue runs inwards, those of the two sides meeting down the middle line of the body. Embedded in this fibrous sheet is a strong muscle upon each side, the rectus abdominis, which is 7·5 or 10 cm (3 or 4 inches) broad, almost 25 mm (1 inch) thick in muscular persons, and runs vertically from the front of the pelvis up to the lower part of the chest. It is a muscle of great strength, and is divided into four or five sections, by tendinous intervals, which run across the muscle, and which, in well-developed persons, form distinct transverse depressions on the front of the abdomen. The quadratus lumborum is still another muscle situated, behind, in the gap between the last rib and the haunch-bone. Other small muscles close the lower opening of the pelvis, and are associated with the functions of the bowel and genital organs.

MUSCLE CRAMP is a sudden painful involuntary maximal contraction of a muscle or muscle group. It may last up to 10 minutes and occurs in individuals with no neurological or muscle disease. Cramps usually occur in bed at night when the individual is at rest. Night cramps are especially common in the elderly, during pregnancy and in cases of diabetes or peripheral vascular disease. They can be caused by sodium loss from excessive sweating, vomiting or diarrhoea. It may also be due to hypokalaemia as a result of treatment with diuretics. Drugs such as the beta-adrenergic stimulants may be responsible. Sometimes an attack can be thwarted by actively contracting the opposing muscle. The most common cramp is in the calf or foot, so the foot should be dorsiflexed at the ankle and the leg straightened. When the cramp is in the calf muscles, getting out of bed and standing up will stretch the calf muscles and ease the attack. When attacks of cramp occur frequently at night, treatment with quinine bisulphate is beneficial.

MUSCLE RELAXANTS are drugs which cause relaxation of muscles. The most effective of them, such as tubocurarine (qv), gallamine and pancuronium, act by antagonizing the action of acetylcholine (qv). Acetylcholine is the natural transmitter of nerve impulses to muscle. When an impulse passes down a motor nerve to voluntary muscle it causes release of acetylcholine at the nerve endings, which in turn causes contraction of the muscle. This it does by action on specific receptors in the muscle. The group of drugs which includes tubocurarine combine with these receptors and so prevent acetylcholine from performing its natural functions. This results in relaxation, or paralysis of the muscle. Other drugs, such as suxamethonium, act principally by reducing the excitability of muscle. Others again, such as some of the tranquillizers (qv), act through the brain; these, however, cannot be used as muscle relaxants because of their overpowering sedative action. The main use of muscle relaxants is in anaesthesia to produce adequate relaxation of muscles. They are also used to control convulsions, as in status epilepticus, tetanus, electric convulsion therapy, and poisoning with convulsant drugs such as strychnine.

MUSCLES, DISEASES OF: The muscles are singularly free from liability to diseases which commonly affect other tissues, this being the result, probably, of their activity, good blood supply, and the changes constantly taking place in them. Wasting of muscles sometimes occurs as a symptom of disease in other organs: for example, damage to the nervous system, as in poliomyelitis or in the disease known as progressive muscular atrophy. (See PARALYSIS.)

INFLAMMATION (MYOSITIS) of various types may occur. As the result of injury, an abscess may develop (see ABSCESS), although wounds affecting muscle generally heal well. Tuberculous inflammation in muscles is almost unknown. A growth due to syphilis, known as a gumma, sometimes forms a hard, almost painless swelling in a muscle. Rheumatism is a type of chronic inflammation (see RHEUMATISM) to which muscles are very liable. The most common form of myositis is the result of immunological damage as a result of auto-immune disease. Because it affects many muscles it is called polymyositis.

MYOSITIS OSSIFICANS, or deposition of bone in muscles, may be congenital or acquired. The congenital form, which is rare, first manifests itself as painful swellings in the muscles. These gradually harden and extend until the child is encased in a rigid sheet – the 'stone man' who used to be one of the unfortunate 'freaks' in circus side-shows. There are usually associated congenital abnormalities of the toes and fingers. The condition is fatal sooner or later. There is no effective treatment, though in some cases diphosphonates seem to delay the onset of calcification.

The acquired form arises as a sequel of a direct blow on muscle, most commonly on the front of the thigh. The condition should be suspected whenever there is severe pain and swelling following a direct blow over muscle. The diagnosis is confirmed by hardening of the swelling. Even when the condition is only suspected it is essential to avoid immobilization of the patient, and to avoid massage. Treatment consists of short-wave diathermy (see DIATHERMY) with gentle active movements. Recovery is usually complete, though slow surgical removal of residual calcified areas may be necessary.

RUPTURE of a muscle may occur, without any external wound, as the result of a spasmodic effort. It may tear the muscle right across, as sometimes happens to the feeble plantaris muscle in running and leaping, or part of the muscle may be driven through its fibrous envelope, forming a hernia of the muscle. The severe pain experienced in many cases of lumbago is due to tearing of one of the muscles in the back. These conditions give rise to considerable pain, but are relieved by rest and massage. Partial muscle tears, such as occur in sport, require more energetic treatment. In the early stages this consists of the application of cold (see COLD, USES OF), firm compression, elevation of the affected limb and rest. After forty-eight hours gradual mobilization is started, with active exercises and short-wave diathermy (see DIATHERMY) or ultrasonics (qv).

COMPRESSION SYNDROME is the tense painful state of muscles induced by excessive accumulation of interstitial fluid (qv) in them, following unusual exercise. It is particularly likely to occur in those parts of the body where the space available for muscles is restricted, as on the front and outer aspect of the shin, where the muscles lie within a tight fascial membrane. Here the syndrome is known as the *anterior tibial syndrome*. Prevention consists of always keeping fit and in training for the amount of exercise to be undertaken. Equally important is what is known in sporting circles as 'warming down': ie, at the end of training or a game, exercise should be gradually tailed off. Treatment consists of elevation of the affected limb, compression of it by compression bandages, with ample exercise of the limb within the bandage, and massage. In more severe cases diuretics (qv) may be given. Occasionally surgical decompression may be necessary.

MYASTHENIA (see MYASTHENIA GRAVIS) is muscle weakness due to a defect of neuro-muscular conduction.

PAIN, quite apart from any inflammation or injury, may be experienced on exertion. This type of pain, known as myalgia, occurs especially in weakly persons, and is then relieved by rest and physiotherapy. It is also one of the common forms of rheumatism. In young children, pains of an aching character are often experienced in the muscles, especially of the legs and back, and are known as growing pains (qv). These come on especially after exertion and are relieved by resting.

PARASITES sometimes lodge in the muscles, the most common being *Trichinella spiralis*, producing the disease known as trichinosis (qv).

TUMOURS are occasionally met with, the most common being fibroid, fatty, and sarcomatous growths.

MYOPATHY is a term applied to an acquired or developmental defect in certain muscles. (See MYOPATHY.)

MUSCULAR DYSTROPHY (see MYOPATHY).

MUSHROOM POISONING (see FUNGUS-POISONING).

MUSHROOM-WORKER'S LUNG is a form of lung disease that occurs in mushroom workers as a result of their being hypersensitive to mushrooms. (See ALVEOLITIS.)

MUSTARD, or MUSTARD FLOUR as it is technically known, is a yellowish powder, consisting of the dried, ripe seeds of *Brassica nigra* and *Brassica alba* mixed together. The former contains an active principle called sinigrin, the latter contains sialbin, while both contain a quantity of a ferment named myrosin, which in the presence of water converts the two active principles into the volatile oil to which the action of mustard is due. This oil is extremely irritating to skin and mucous surfaces with which it is brought in contact.

Uses: Externally mustard is used made into a paste with water and spread upon brown or cartridge paper, or made up (2 per cent) with linseed into a poultice, for its irritant action upon the skin, in cases of rheumatism, inflamed joints, neuralgia, and for application to the chest and abdomen when organs in these cavities are inflamed. These applications should not, as a rule, last longer than twenty minutes. Liniment of mustard is used for similar purposes. In a hot or cold bath one or two tablespoonfuls of mustard have an invigorating effect. Added to hot water it makes a refreshing foot-bath. (For Mustard Pack, see WET PACK.) The effect of mustard, if too pronounced, may be relieved by applying olive oil.

Internally, mustard is used in small quantities as a stimulant to digestion, and in large quantities as an emetic, a tablespoonful (10 grams) of mustard flour being stirred up in a tumblerful (200 ml) of cold water for the latter purpose.

MUSTINE is the *British Pharmacopoeia* name for the *bis* form of nitrogen mustard. The nitrogen mustards have an action comparable to that of ionizing radiation and inhibit cell division. Mustine is used in the treatment of chronic leukaemia and Hodgkin's disease. (See CYTOTOXIC DRUGS.)

MUTISM (see VOICE AND SPEECH).

MYALGIA means pain in a muscle. (See BORNHOLM DISEASE; LUMBAGO; RHEUMATISM.)

MYALGIC ENCEPHALOMYELITIS is a disorder which occurs in epidemics in closed communities such as schools and hospitals. It is presumed to be of viral origin. By definition there must be evidence of encephalomyelitis at the start of the illness. This usually takes the form of a febrile illness with meningism and sometimes double vision, urinary retention and sensory changes. It is characterized by headaches, diffuse muscle aches, variably enlarged lymph nodes and physical exhaustion with mood disturbance. It may persist over long periods. Although there is no mortality, there is considerable morbidity in that over 50 per cent of individuals are not working six months after. The condition has been variously named epidemic neuromyasthenia, Royal Free disease, Icelandic disease and epidemic myalgic encephalomyelitis. A much more common condition characterized by extreme fatigue and emotional disturbance without any evidence of encephalomyelitis follows acute viral illnesses and this is better referred to as the post-viral fatigue syndrome. As there is no evidence of encephalomyelitis this disorder should not be called myalgic encephalitis. (See POST-VIRAL FATIGUE SYNDROME.)

MYASTHENIA GRAVIS is a serious disorder in which the chief symptoms are muscular weakness and a special tendency for fatigue to come on rapidly when efforts are made. The prevalence is around 1 in 30,000. Two-thirds of the patients are women, in whom it develops in early adult life. In men it tends to develop later in life.

It is a classical example of an auto-immune disease (see AUTO-IMMUNITY). The body develops antibodies which interfere with the working of the nerve endings in muscle that are acted on by acetylcholine (qv). It is acetylcholine that transmits the nerve impulses to muscles. If this transmission cannot be effected, as in myasthenia gravis, then the muscles are unable to contract. Not only the voluntary muscles, but those connected with the acts of swallowing, breathing, and the like, become progressively weaker, though there is no very marked wasting. Rest and avoidance of undue exertion, so as carefully to husband the strength, are necessary, and regular doses of neostigmine bromide, or pyridostigmine at intervals enable the muscles to be used and in some cases have a curative effect. These drugs act by inhibiting the action of cholinesterase. This is an enzyme (qv) produced in the body which destroys any excess of acetylcholine. In this way they increase the amount of available acetylcholine which compensates for the deleterious effect of antibodies on the nerve endings.

The dose of anticholinesterase that gives the maximum therapeutic response must be established. This may not restore muscle strength to normal and patients often have to live with some degree of disability. If the dose of drugs is increased above the maximum response level, in the forlorn hope of improving physical activity, the opposite effect will be produced, with progressive muscle weakness, possibly ending in what is called a cholinergic crisis. Anticholinergic drugs have no affect on the underlying disease, they merely increase the concentration of acetylcholine at receptor level.

The thymus gland plays the major part in the cause of myasthenia gravis, possibly by being the source of the original acetylcholine receptors to which the antibodies are being formed. At all events, thymectomy, or removal of the thymus, is increasingly important in the management of patients with myathenia gravis. The incidence of remission following thymectomy increases with the number of years after the operation. Complete remission or substantial improvement can be expected in 80 per cent of patients.

The other important aspect in the management of patients with myasthenia gravis is immunosuppression. Drugs are now available that suppress antibody production and so reduce the concentration of antibodies to the acetylcholine receptor. The problem is that they not only suppress abnormal antibody production, but also suppress normal antibody production. The main groups of immunosuppressive drugs used in myasthenia gravis are the corticosteroids and azathioprine. Improvement following steroids may take several weeks to become manifest and an initial deterioration is often found during the first week or ten days of treatment. Azathioprine is also effective in producing clinical improvement and reducing the antibodies to acetylcholine receptors. These affects occur more slowly than with steroids and the mean time for an azathioprine remission is nine months.

The British Association of Myasthenics has been established to relieve and comfort those who suffer from myasthenia gravis, to bring myasthenics together into a meaningful association where they may be offered help and understanding, and to provide the opportunity where myasthenics also help each other to overcome many of their common problems and disabilities. The BAM also encourages families and friends to accompany myasthenics in order that they too may learn more about the symptoms and effects of the disorder, and so offer the real help and understanding that is required. The British Association of Myasthenics was created and is supported by myasthenics, their families and friends. Its address is Keynes House, 77 Nottingham Road, Derby DE1 3QS (0332–290219).

MYCOPLASMA is a genus of micro-organisms which differ from bacteria in that they lack a rigid cell wall. They are responsible for widespread epidemics in cattle and poultry. For a long time the only member of the genus known to cause disease in man was *Mycoplasma pneumoniae* which is responsible for the form of pneumonia known as primary atypical pneumonia (see PNEUMONIA). Another, *Mycoplasma genitalium*, has now been isolated which is responsible for certain cases of non-gonococcal urethritis. (See NON-SPECIFIC GENITAL INFECTION.)

MYCOSIS is the general term applied to diseases due to the growth of fungi in the body. Among some of the simplest and commonest mycoses are ringworm, favus, and thrush. The Madura foot of India, actinomycosis, and occasional cases of pneumonia and suppurative ear disease are also due to the growth of moulds in the bodily tissues. Other forms of mycosis include aspergillosis (qv), candidiasis (qv), cryptococcosis (qv) and histoplasmosis (qv).

MYCOSIS FUNGOIDES is a rare neoplastic condition of the reticulo-endothelial system, characterized in its later stages by multiple tumours of the skin. The course is prolonged and almost invariably ends fatally.

MYDRIASIS: Condition of dilatation of the pupil.

MYELIN is a white fat-like substance forming a sheath round medullated or myelinated nerve-fibres in the nerves and in the central nervous system.

MYELITIS is inflammation of the spinal cord.

MYELOCYTE is the name given to one of the cells of bone-marrow from which the granular white corpuscles of the blood are produced. They are found in the blood in certain forms of leukaemia.

MYELOGRAPHY is the injection of a radio-opaque substance into the central canal of the spinal cord in order to assist in the diagnosis of diseases of the spinal cord or spine.

MYELOMA is a tumour made up of bone-marrow cells and generally occurring in the marrow of more than one bone at the same time.

MYELOMALACIA is morbid softening of the spinal cord as a result of injury, pressure, inflammation, or arterial disease.

MYELOMATOSIS is a malignant process involving the bone marrow. It runs an invariably fatal course.

MYIASIS is a term applied to any disease caused by maggots or flies.

MYOCARDIAL INFARCTION (see CORONARY THROMBOSIS).

MYOCARDITIS means inflammation of the muscular wall of the heart.

MYOCARDIUM is the muscular substance of the heart.

MYOCLONUS is a brief, twitching muscular contraction which may involve only a single muscle or many muscles. It may be too slight to cause movement of the affected limb, or so violent as to throw the victim to the floor. The cause is not known, but in some cases may be a form of epilepsy. A single myoclonic jerk in the upper limbs occasionally occurs in petit mal. (See EPILEPSY.) The myoclonic jerks which many people experience in falling asleep are a perfectly normal phenomenon.

MYOGLOBIN is the protein which gives muscle (qv) its red colour. It has the property of combining loosely and reversibly with oxygen. This means that it is the vehicle whereby muscle extracts oxygen from the haemoglobin in the blood circulating through it, and then releases the oxygen for use by the muscle.

MYOMA is the term applied to a tumour, almost invariably of a simple nature, which consists mainly of muscle fibres. These muscle tumours often occur in the uterus.

MYOMETRIUM is the muscular coat of the uterus (qv).

MYOPATHY, also known as MUSCULAR DYSTROPHY or IDIOPATHIC MUSCULAR ATROPHY, is a condition in which wasting takes place in certain muscles, with or without previous increase in bulk of these muscles, and apparently without any affection of the nervous system. The cause of the condition is still obscure, although the disease appears to run in families, being transmitted, like some other hereditary diseases, by the mother. Generally the disease appears in early childhood. The changes which are found after death show that a simple wasting away of the muscle fibres takes place, and that these are in some cases to a great extent replaced by fatty and fibrous tissue.

Symptoms: There are three chief types of myopathy. The commonest, known as pseudo-hypertrophic muscular dystrophy, affects particularly the upper part of the lower limbs of children. The muscles of the buttocks, thighs and calves seem excessively well developed, but nevertheless the child is clumsy, weak on his legs, and has difficulty in picking himself up when he falls. In another form of the disease, which begins a little later, as a rule about the age of 14, the muscles of the upper arm are first affected, and those of the spine and lower limbs become weak later on. In a third type, which begins about this age, the muscles of the face, along with certain of the shoulder and upper arm muscles, show the first signs of wasting. All the forms have this in common: that the affected muscles grow weaker till their power to contract is quite lost. In the first form, the patients seldom reach the age of 20, falling victims to some disease which, to ordinary people, would not be serious. In the other forms the wasting, after progressing to a certain extent, often remains stationary for the rest of life. Myopathy may also be acquired when it is the result of disease such as thyrotoxicosis, osteomalacia or Cushing's disease, and the myopathy resolves when the primary disease is treated.

Treatment: The general health must be well maintained. Massage, electricity and exercise short of fatigue are of the utmost importance, and above all, care must be taken that these invalids are not exposed unduly, as they succumb easily to chest affections.

The education and management of these unfortunate children raise many difficulties. Much help in dealing with these problems can be obtained from the Muscular Dystrophy Group of Great Britain, 35 Macaulay Road, London, SW4 0QP (01–720 8055, Fax 01–498 0670).

MYOPIA (see REFRACTION).

MYOSITIS means inflammation of a muscle. (See MUSCLES, DISEASES OF.)

MYOSITIS OSSIFICANS (see MUSCLE).

MYOTONIA is a condition in which the muscles, though possessed of normal power, contract only very slowly. The stiffness disappears as the muscles are used.

MYRINGOTOMY is the operation of cutting the drum of the ear in cases of acute inflammation of the middle ear.

MYRRH is a gum-resin obtained from *Commiphora molmol*, an Arabian myrtle tree. It stimulates the function of mucous membranes with which it is brought in contact or by which it is excreted. Tincture of myrrh is used for a gargle in sore throat, as a tooth-wash when the gums are inflamed, and as an ingredient of cough mixtures.

MYXOEDEMA is a disease due to underactivity of the thyroid gland. The thyroid gland secretes two hormones – thyroxine and triodothyronine – and these hormones are responsible for the metabolic activity of the body. Hypothyroidism may result from developmental abnormalities of the gland or a deficiency of the enzymes necessary for the synthesis of the hormones. It may be a feature of endemic goitre and cretinism, but the most common cause of hypothyroidism is the autoimmune destruction of the thyroid known as chronic thyroiditis. It may also occur as a result of radio-iodine treatment of thyroid overactivity and is occasionally secondary to pituitary disease in which inadequate TSH production occurs. It is a common disorder, occurring in fourteen per one thousand females and one per one thousand males. Most patients present between the age of thirty and sixty years. The term myxoedema was introduced in 1878 to describe the swelling of the skin and sub-cutaneous tissues that characterised severe forms of hypothyroidism.

Symptoms: As thyroid hormones are responsible for the metabolic rate of the body hypothyroidism usually presents with a general slowing-up. This affects both physical and mental activities. The intellectual functions become slow, the speech deliberate and the formation of ideas and the answers to questions takes longer than in healthy people. Physical energy is reduced and patients frequently complain of lethargy and generalized muscle aches and pains. Patients become intolerant of the cold and the skin becomes dry and swollen. The larynx also becomes swollen and gives rise to a hoarseness of the voice. Most patients gain weight and develop constipation. The skin becomes dry and yellow due to the presence of increased carotine. Hair becomes thinned and brittle and even baldness may develop. Swelling of the soft tissues may give rise to a carpal tunnel syndrome and middle-ear deafness. The diagnosis is confirmed by measuring the levels of thyroid hormones in the blood which are low and of the pituitary TSH which is raised in primary hypothyroidism.

Treatment consists of the administration of thyroxine. Although triodothyronine is the metabolically active hormone, thyroxine is converted to triodothyronine by the tissues of the body. Treatment should be started cautiously with a small dose of not more than 0·05 mg of thyroxine and this can be slowly increased to 0·2 mg daily, the equivalent of the maximum output of the thyroid gland. If too large a dose is given initially palpitations and tachycardia are likely to result and in the elderly heart failure may be precipitated.

MYXOMA is a tumour consisting of very imperfect connective tissue, and containing a peculiar mucus-like juice.

MYXOVIRUSES include the influenza viruses A, B and C; the para-influenza viruses, types 1 to 3; and respiratory syncytial virus which is an important cause of respiratory disease in the early years of life.

N

NAEVUS is the term applied to a mass of dilated blood-vessels. They most commonly occur as birthmarks. These structures may take the form of the large port-wine stain often seen on the face, for which little can be done, or they may occur as swellings of a more restricted nature, usually of a red or bluish colour. Many naevi tend to decrease in size as the child advances in years; if not, the blemish can often be removed by excision of the piece of skin that is involved, or by electrolysis. There is a form known as spider naevi which occur in cirrhosis of the liver. (See LIVER, DISEASES OF.)

NADOLOL (CORGARD) (see ADRENERGIC DRUGS).

NAFCILLIN (see ANTIBIOTIC).

NAIL-BITING is a common practice in schoolchildren, most of whom gradually give it up as they approach adolescence. Too much significance should therefore not be attached to it. In itself it does no harm, and punishment or restraining devices do nothing but harm. It is a manifestation of tension or insecurity, the cause of which should be removed.

NAILS (see SKIN).

NAILS, DISEASES OF: The nails are subject to relatively few diseases. On the other hand, any interference with the natural appearance of the finger-nails is very unsightly, whilst the sensitive matrix of both finger- and toe-nails is extremely tender when diseased.

INFLAMMATION of the nails and of the bed in which they rest occurs in various skin diseases: eg. psoriasis, eczema, fungus infections (see RINGWORM). The nails then become rough, thickened, irregular, discoloured, and split readily into layers. Most acute febrile diseases are accompanied by irregularities in growth of the nails, producing a transverse furrow in the nail, as it grows onwards, and these furrows on the nails serve to date a severe illness fairly accurately, the furrow gradually approaching the free margin of the nail and disappearing in about six months' time.

Brittle nails tend to be troublesome in the elderly. To reduce this brittleness, nails should be kept trimmed and as short as possible. A hand cream, consisting of equal parts of salicylic acid ointment and glycerin of starch, should be applied all over the finger tips and nails on going to bed every night. In some instances the brittleness may be due to, or associated with, poor local circulation to the finger. This may be ameliorated by taking a small dose (250 mg) of inositol nicotinate daily during the cold weather.

Spoon-shaped or concave nails (KOILONYCHIA) are often associated with iron deficiency, especially in middle-aged women, and become normal when this is treated.

ABSCESS may occur at the root of the nail (see WHITLOW) or underneath it near its edge. As a rule, these abscesses are caused by a minute poisoned wound, such as that due to a splinter of wood. The condition is generally very painful, but is relieved by opening, so as to allow free exit for the pus, the nail being snipped up with a pair of scissors if necessary. The nail in these cases is often cast off.

INJURY to the nail by a blow is often followed by an extravasation of blood beneath it, the nail first turning black, and then often being shed. In all these cases in which the nail is shed, a new nail generally appears quickly, and replaces the old one in six months, unless the matrix has been very seriously diseased or injured. While the new nail is growing, the point of the finger merely requires the protection of a finger-stall.

INGROWING NAIL is a troublesome condition affecting only the nails of the toes. It is due to a variety of causes, chief among which are the pressure of badly fitting shoes, cutting away of the corners in paring the nails, and want of attention to the nails, whereby scarf-skin and dirt collect beneath the nail, and by inflammatory changes causing ulceration of the skin at the sides. The condition commonly occurs in old, bedridden people, mainly for the last-named reason. The treatment is simple, though sometimes tedious. It consists in the wearing of well-made footwear, cutting of the nails square across without paring away the corners and the packing two or three times daily of a shred of boric lint between the corner of the nail and the skin which it is chafing. These measures are generally sufficient after a little time, but sometimes the nail is so much thickened that the edges cannot be raised up to admit the threads of lint. In this case the centre of the nail may be softened by dabbing on caustic potash, and then the nail is easily thinned down by scraping with a sharp knife till it becomes pliable. When the skin at the side of the nail bleeds very readily, this is remedied by touching with bluestone or with nitrate of silver. In severe cases a minor surgical operation may be required. Anyone having trouble with ingrowing toe-nails, especially elderly people, should consult a chiropodist.

NALIDIXIC ACID is a drug, active against Gram-negative micro-organisms, which is proving useful in the treatment of infections of the urinary tract.

NALORPHINE HYDROBROMIDE reduces or abolishes most of the actions of morphine and similarly acting narcotics, such as pethidine. It is used as an antidote in the treatment of overdosage with these drugs.

NALOXONE is the most efficient drug in the treatment of morphine poisoning. It blocks the effects of most opiates. Administration by mouth is unreliable but, when given intravenously, it acts within two or three minutes.

NANDROLONE DECANOATE (DECA-DURABOLIN) (see ANABOLIC STEROIDS).

NANDROLONE PHENYLPROPIONATE (DURABOLIN) (see ANABOLIC STEROIDS).

NANOMETRE is a millionth of a millimetre. The approved abbreviation is nm.

NAPPY RASH is the eruption which tends to occur on the buttocks of infants, due to too infrequent changing of soiled nappies or inadequate laundering of nappies. There is some evidence that it is more common in bottle-fed, than in breast-fed, babies. It has become much less common since the advent of disposable nappies.

Prevention consists of four main measures. (i) When the baby is bathed, particular attention must be paid to the creases and folds of the skin which must be carefully washed, then equally carefully dried and sprinkled with a bland baby powder. (ii) Nappies must not be washed in strong soaps or detergent solutions. After washing they must be carefully rinsed out in several changes of clean water. (iii) Soiled nappies must be changed frequently. (iv) Waterproof pants should be reserved for special social occasions, and not used all and every day.

Should the skin become inflamed, washing it with a 1 per cent solution of sodium sulphate, followed by careful drying and the application of calamine lotion, is often useful. An alternative application which has stood the test of time is zinc and castor oil ointment.

NAPRAPATHY is a system of healing which attributes disease to disorder in the ligaments and connective tissues.

NAPROXEN (NAPROSYN) (see NON-STEROIDAL ANTI-INFLAMMATORY DRUGS).

NARCISSISM is an abnormal mental state characterized by excessive admiration of self.

NARCOLEPSY is a condition in which uncontrollable episodes of sleep occur two or three times a day. It starts at any age and persists for life. The attacks, which usually last for 10 to 15 minutes, come on at times normally conducive to sleep, such as after a meal, or sitting in a bus, but they may occur when walking in the street. In due course, usually after some years, they are associated with cataplectic attacks when for a few seconds there is sudden muscular weakness affecting the whole body. These attacks are commonly brought on by amusement with laughter. In others they may be induced by anger or by a sense of triumph. In the first of these groups the affected individual soon learns to sit down when jokes are going around. The attacks of narcolepsy seem to be reduced in number if the individual takes a 15-minute nap after meals. Affected people should carry 5 mg tablets of dexamphetamine about with them and take one or two to tide them over special occasions when an attack could be embarrassing. Some doctors recommend the regular taking of dexamphetamine, but this is deprecated by others in view of the possible adverse effect of such continued treatment on the mental state. The cataplectic attacks are controlled by imipramine or clomipramine.

Familial narcolepsy is well recognised and recently a near 100 per cent association between narcolepsy and the histocompatability antigen HLA-DR2 has been discovered. This has given rise to the notion that narcolepsy is an immune-related disease. The Narcolepsy Association (United Kingdom) has recently been founded to help patients with this strange disorder. The address is c/o Dorothy Pownall, 6 Derwent Close, Holmes Chapel, Crewe, Cheshire CW4 7JY.

NARCOSIS is a condition of profound insensibility, resembling sleep so far that the unconscious person can still be roused slightly by great efforts, or at all events is not entirely indifferent to sensory stimuli. It is most commonly produced by drugs, such as opium, but may also be due to poisons formed within the body, as in uraemia.

NARCOTICS (see HYPNOTICS).

NARES is the Latin word for the nostrils.

NASOPHARYNX is the upper part of the throat, lying behind the nasal cavity. (See NOSE.)

NATAMYCIN is an antibiotic isolated from *Streptomyces natalensis* which is proving of value in the treatment of moniliasis (qv).

NATIONAL HEALTH SERVICE: The current structure of the National Health Service was established by The Health Services Act 1980 and was introduced in 1982. The Secretary for State for Social Services is responsible for the N.H.S. in England while in Scotland and Wales the Secretary for State for the appropriate province is responsible. The country is divided into 14 regions, each with a Regional Health Authority. In England there are 192 District

Health Authorities (D.H.A.s) which are responsible for the provision of hospital and community health services in their districts. In addition there are a small number of Special Health Authorities and Boards of Governors directly accountable to The Secretary of State for the services provided by highly specialised hospitals and post graduate teaching hospitals. Family Practitioner Committees (F.P.C.s) are responsible for the services provided by General Practitioners, Dentists and Opticians. The populations served by District Health Authorities vary from 100,000 to more than 800,000 and the financial resources given to them are dependent on the population they serve. Smaller District Health Authorities receive money in the order of £20,000,000 per annum whilst larger District Health Authorities have annual resources in excess of £100,000,000. Currently Family Practitioner services are independent contractors and not subject to cash limits, though the government has stated its intention to supervise these services. Community Health Councils exist for each District Health Authority. They do not provide services but act as the consumer's watchdog. They are financed by a cash limit fixed by the Regional Health Authority.

In 1985 the government decided to implement the recommendations of the Griffiths' report on the management of the National Health Service. This report has identified a number of weaknesses in the management of Health Authorities and made some recommendations for overcoming these failings. The most important of these decisions was to introduce a general management function into the National Health Service. This would allocate personal responsibility for drawing together planning, implementation and control of performance to a single person at each level of the service. These individuals would be called General Managers. They were to be appointed at three main management levels of the Health Service: (i) The 14 Regional Health Authorites, which are the bodies responsible for strategic planning, some with budgets of more than one billion pounds; (ii) the 192 District Health Authorities with responsibility for planning and delivering services at local level, with budgets of about £50,000,000, and (iii) perhaps the most important, the 700 or so Units, that is the hospitals, clinics and health centres in which patients are treated.

A Health Service Supervisory Board and an N.H.S. Management Board have been established. The Health Services Supervisory Board (H.S.S.B.) is chaired by the Secretary of State and includes the Minister of Health, the Permanent Secretary and the Chief Medical Officer. It deals with the objectives and resource allocation and performance of the National Health Service. The N.H.S. Management Board is responsible for all the existing N.H.S. management responsibilities in the Department of Health and Social Security. The Chairman is drawn from outside the National Health Service and acts as the right-hand man to the Secretary of State and the Accounting Officer for N.H.S. expenditure.

The introduction of general management is a positive attempt to improve facilities provided by the National Health Service and time will tell how successful this has been.

NATIONAL LISTENING LIBRARY is a charity which produces recorded books for handicapped people who cannot read, with the exception of the blind who have their own separate organization, the Royal National Institute for the Blind. Otherwise it caters for all those who are deprived of the ability to read through any form of disability, including arthritis. Its catalogue includes over 700 titles, ranging from thrillers to theology, as well as children's books. Its address, from which full details can be obtained, is: National Listening Library (Talking Books for the Handicapped and Mental Patients), 12 Lant Street, London SE1 1QR (01–407 9417). (See also CALIBRE.)

NAUSEA means a feeling that vomiting is about to take place. (See VOMITING.)

NAVEL, or UMBILICUS, is the scar on the abdomen marking the point where the umbilical cord joined the body in embryonic life. (See AFTER-BIRTH.)

NEAR SIGHT (see REFRACTION).

NEBULA is the term applied to a slight opacity on the cornea producing a haze in the field of vision, and also to any oily preparation to be sprayed from a nebulizer, an apparatus for splitting up a fluid into fine droplets.

NEBULIZERS: A nebulizer makes an aerosol by blowing air or oxygen through a solution of a drug. Many inhaled drugs such as salbutamol, ipratropium and beclomethasone can be given in this way. It has the advantage over a medihaler in that no special effort is required to co-ordinate breathing and a nebulizer allows a much greater concentration of the drug to be delivered compared with that of a medihaler. The use of higher doses of bronchodilator drugs made possible by the nebulizer means that the risk of unwanted side-effects is also increased.

NECATOR AMERICANUS is a hookworm, closely resembling but smaller than the *Ancylostoma duodenale*. (See ANCYLOSTOMIASIS.)

NECK is that portion of the body which extends from the upper limit of the chest to the base of the skull. Its main function is to support the head. Through its front part run the passages for the air and the food. The great bulk of the neck is composed of seven cervical vertebrae with the muscles attached thereto, in front and behind. (See MUSCLES.) Within the canal formed by the rings of these vertebrae lies the cervical part of the spinal cord, from which proceed the nerves that control the movements of the neck and arms.

In front of the spinal column lies the pharynx, or throat-cavity, extending from the base of the skull above down to the lower edge of the sixth vertebra, where the gullet continues it directly downwards, while the larynx opens out of it in front. The larynx is close to the surface of the front of the neck, and the thyroid cartilage can be readily seen and felt beneath the skin. (See LARYNX.) The larynx is continued downwards by the windpipe, and just beneath the larynx the isthmus of the thyroid gland can be felt crossing the windpipe and connecting the two lobes of the gland which lie one on either side of the larynx. The strong sternocleidomastoid muscle is prominent on each side of the neck, running from the mastoid process of the skull down to the breast-bone and inner end of the clavicle; under cover of it lies a fibrous sheath containing the carotid artery, internal jugular vein and vagus nerve. The sternocleidomastoid muscle divides each side of the neck into two triangular areas, in which lie important nerves and branches of these blood-vessels, as well as chains of lymphatic glands. Several large superficial veins run down the neck, and are of importance, because in wounds of the neck they may give rise to much bleeding. The chief of these are the external jugular vein, running straight downwards from the angle of the jaw, and the anterior jugular vein, running downwards from beneath the chin, not far from the middle line. At the root of the neck the apex of each lung projects a short distance from the chest into the neck.

NECROPSY is a post-mortem examination which produces almost no disfigurement. The brain is examined by an opening across the scalp, afterwards hidden by the hair, and the contents of chest and abdomen are inspected through an opening down the middle line in front. If necessary minute pieces of organs are removed for microscopic examination. It is a social duty of the deceased person's relatives to permit or request a post-mortem examination in cases in which the disease was a matter of uncertainty.

NECROSIS means death of a limited portion of tissue, the term being most commonly applied to bones when, as the result of disease or injury, a fragment dies and separates. (See BONE, DISEASES OF.)

NEEDLING is an operation performed by means of a needle, especially in the discission or tearing of a cataract so as to allow the fluid in the anterior chamber of the eye to dissolve it.

NEGATIVISM means a morbid tendency in a person to do the opposite of what he is desired or directed to do. It is specially characteristic of schizophrenia, but is not uncommon in non-psychotic persons.

NEISSERIA is a group, or genus, of rounded bacteria that occur in pairs and are therefore known as diplococci (see BACTERIOLOGY). They are named after Albert Neisser, the German physician who discovered the gonococcus, the causative organism of gonorrhoea (qv), which is now known as *Neisseria gonorrhoea*. The group also includes the causative organism of cerebrospinal meningitis (see MENINGITIS): *Neisseria meningitidis*.

NEMATODE is a roundworm. (See ASCARIASIS.)

NEOMYCIN is an antibiotic derived from *Streptomyces fradiae*. It has a wide antibacterial spectrum, being effective against the majority of Gram-negative bacilli. Its use is limited by the fact that it is liable to cause deafness and kidney damage. For this reason it is never given by injections. Its main use is for application to the skin, either in solution or as an ointment, for the treatment of infection of the skin. It is also given by mouth for the treatment of certain forms of enteritis due to *E. coli*.

NEONATAL means pertaining to the first month of life.

NEONATAL MORTALITY is the mortality of infants under one month of age. In England and Wales this has fallen markedly in recent decades: from 28·28 per 1000 related live births in 1939 to 5·6 in 1984 and 4·1 in 1986. This improvement can be attributed to various factors: better antenatal supervision of expectant mothers; care to ensure that expectant mothers receive adequate nourishing food; improvements in the management of the complications of pregnancy and of labour. Nearly three-quarters of neonatal deaths occur during the first week of life. For this reason, increasing emphasis is being laid on this initial period of life. Between 1960 and 1979, in England, the number of deaths in the first week fell from 9772 to 4208, representing a fall in the rate per 1000 live births from 13·2 to 6·7. The chief causes of deaths in this period are immaturity of the infant, birth injuries, congenital abnormalities and asphyxia. After the first week the commonest cause is infection.

NEOPLASM, which means literally a 'new formation', is another word for tumour.

NEPENTHE is a solution of opium in alcohol and water given in the same dose as laudanum.

NEPHRECTOMY is the operation for removal of the kidney. (See KIDNEY, DISEASES OF.)

NEPHRITIS means inflammation of the kidneys. (See GLOMERULONEPHRITIS.)

NEPHROLITHIASIS is the term applied to a condition in which calculi are present in the kidney.

NEPHROPEXY is the fixation of a floating kidney in its original position.

NEPHROPTOSIS means the condition in which a kidney is movable or 'floating'. (See KIDNEY, DISEASES OF.)

NEPHRORRHAPHY is the operation by which a movable kidney is fastened by stitches in its proper place.

NEPHROSTOMY is the operation of making an opening into the kidney to drain it.

NEPHROTIC SYNDROME is one of proteinuria, hypo-albuminaemia and gross oedema. The primary cause is the leak of albumin through the glomerulus. When this exceeds the liver's ability to synthesise albumin the plasma level falls and oedema results. The nephrotic syndrome is commonly the result of primary renal glomerular disease (see GLOMERULO NEPHRITIS). It may also be a result of metabolic diseases such as diabetic glomerular sclerosis and amyloidosis. It may be the result of systemic auto-immune diseases such as systemic lupus erythematosis and polyarteritis. It may complicate malignant diseases such as myelomatosis, Hodgkin's disease and lymphocytic leukaemia. It is sometimes caused by nephrotoxins such as gold or mercury and certain drugs, and it may be the result of certain infections such as malaria and Crohn's disease.

NEPHROTOMY means the operation of cutting into the kidney, in search of calculi or for other reasons.

NERVES: The nervous system consists in part of cells and in part of fibres, each of which is a long process extending from a nerve-cell. The brain and spinal cord are often spoken of together as the central nervous system; the nerves which proceed from them, forty-three on each side, are named the cerebrospinal, or peripheral nerves; whilst the third great division, situated in the neck, thorax and abdomen, and intimately connected with the cerebrospinal nerves (though in its action largely independent of the brain and cord) is known as the autonomic nervous system. The last-named consists of ganglia containing nerve-cells, which are profusely connected by plexuses of nerve-fibres.

The nerve-cells originate, or receive, impulses and impressions of various sorts, which are conveyed from them to muscles, blood-vessels, and elsewhere, by efferent nerves, or received by them through afferent nerves coming from the skin, organs of sense, joints, etc. The autonomic system is concerned mainly with the movements and other functions of the internal organs, secreting glands and blood-vessels, the activities of which proceed independently of the will.

Structure: (1) NERVE-FIBRES: The nerves vary much in size. The sciatic nerve, deeply buried in the muscles on the back of the thigh, is the largest nerve in the body, being as thick as a pencil or more; other nerves reach about the size of goose-quills, and from these there are all gradations, down to the minute single fibres distributed to muscle-fibres or to skin. A nerve, such as the sciatic, possesses a strong, outer fibrous sheath, called the epineurium, within which lie bundles of nerve-fibres, divided from one another by partitions of fibrous tissue, in which run blood-vessels that nourish the nerve. Each of these bundles is surrounded by its own sheath, known as the perineurium, and within the bundle fine partitions of fibrous tissue, known as endoneurium, divide up the bundle into groups of fibres. The blood-vessels and lymphatics of the nerves divide into fine branches, which run in these sheaths and partitions of fibrous tissue. The finest subdivisions of the nerves are the fibres, and these are of two kinds: medullated and non-medullated fibres. The *medullated fibres* vary in thickness from 2 to 15 micrometres, some nerves containing a greater proportion of the small fibres than others. Under the microscope, all have the appearance of tubes, this being due to the fact that each has an outer membranous sheath, the neurilemma, within which is a clear white material, the medullary (or myelin) sheath, in the centre of which runs the axis-cylinder or nerve-fibre proper. The neurilemma is a strong but thin sheath with nuclei at regular intervals on its inner surface. The medullary sheath is composed of fatty material containing lecithin and cholesterin, and to it the white colour of the nerves is mainly due. It is divided at regular intervals by short gaps, situated about 1 mm apart, known as the nodes of Ranvier, but across these gaps the neurilemma and axis-cylinder are continuous. This medullary, or myelin, sheath is regarded as fulfilling a purpose similar to the insulating material upon electric wires and preventing nerve impulses from passing beyond the nerve-fibre by which they are conveyed. The axis-cylinder, or axon, is the conducting part of the nerve, for whilst the neurilemma is absent from the fibre in its course through the brain and spinal cord, and the medullary sheath is absent from non-medullated nerves, the axis-cylinder never fails. It has a striped appearance, seeming to consist of a number of fibrils which, however, cannot be separated from one another. The *non-medullated fibres* are very much thinner than the average of medullated fibres, from which they differ only in the fact of not possessing a medullary sheath, and of being therefore greyish in colour.

(2) NERVE-CELLS, from one of which springs each nerve-fibre, are found in the grey matter of the brain and spinal cord. In the brain alone it is calculated there are some 600,000,000 of these cells. They also exist in the ganglia of the sympathetic system, in connection with some of the nerves of special sense, and on the posterior roots of the spinal nerves. The shape of these nerve-cells varies. The most common

appearance is that of a large clear cell, containing an oval nucleus, and running out at various points into long processes, which, as a rule, branch again and again, after the manner of a tree, these dendritic processes, as they are called, meeting with similar processes from neighbouring cells. The ends of the branching processes from one cell meet the ends of similar processes from another cell, the points of apposition being known as *synapses.* The state of closure or openness of these synapses is believed to be of great importance in quickening or blocking nerve impulses. The body of the cell has a mottled appearance, owing to its containing many bodies, known as Nissl's granules, which appear to be of the nature of food material, destined to be used up when the cell is stimulated to work till reduced to a state of fatigue.

In the cerebrum, the cells are distinctly pyramidal in shape, and one of the processes of each cell is much longer than the rest, forming indeed a nerve-fibre, which may run a long distance down the spinal cord. Other cells are bipolar, ie. they possess just two processes, and others are unipolar, ie. they possess only one process, which, a short distance from the cell, divides in a T-shaped manner, as, for example, the cells in the ganglia upon the posterior roots of the spinal nerves. Other cells are found in the grey matter of the brain, which are known as neuroglia cells. These are provided with innumerable processes that form a supporting feltwork for the nerve-cells and nerve-fibres, and act merely as connective tissue cells.

(3) NERVE-ENDINGS: Each nerve-fibre proceeds from a nerve-cell to end in a definite organ, to or from which it carries a special form of nerve impulse. The manner in which the fibre ends in the organ to which it proceeds varies in different cases. The simplest mode of ending is that of the non-medullated fibres which proceed to the involuntary muscle-fibres, as, for example, those of the intestine. These fibres form a complex network between the layers of muscle, from which fine fibres pass between the muscle-fibres. In the heart the nerves end in a similar manner. In voluntary muscles the arrangement is more complicated. Each nerve-fibre splits up into numerous branches, which go to neighbouring muscle-fibres. Each branch pierces the membrane surrounding its muscle-fibre, and ends by spreading out into a plate composed of granular material and numerous nuclei. The endings of sensory nerves in the skin have a special arrangement. Most of these end, not in the epidermis, which is devoid of sensation, but in the projections of the corium beneath it, where each nerve-fibre enters a small rounded bulb. Some of these bulbs found beneath the skin of the fingers are known as Pacinian corpuscles: around 2·5 mm long and half that in width. These consist of a large number of thin coats enclosing the swollen end of a nerve-fibre. Other much smaller bodies, around 0·08 mm long, known as touch-corpuscles, are found close beneath the epidermis all over the skin, and consist of a framework of connective tissue in which the nerve-fibre winds round and round. Similar bodies are found on the front of the eye. In other cases the nerves appear to end abruptly in cells in the deepest layer of the epidermis.

Development and repair: The whole nervous system is developed from the ectoderm or outer layer of the embryo, the brain and spinal cord arising from an infolding of the surface along the back to form a tube, and all the nerves being

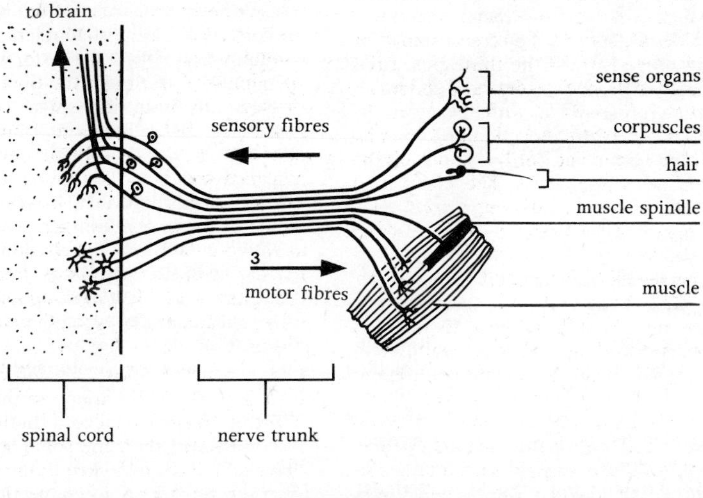

Diagram showing nervous connections between the central nervous system and muscle and skin.

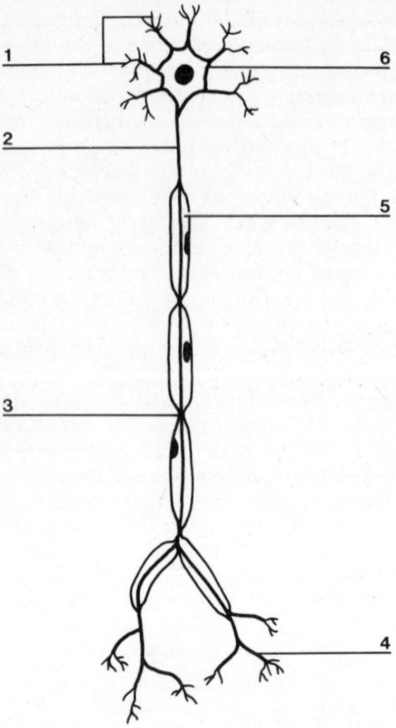

1 dendrites
2 axon
3 node of Ranvier
4 bare axons
5 myelin sheath
6 cell body

Diagram of a nerve.

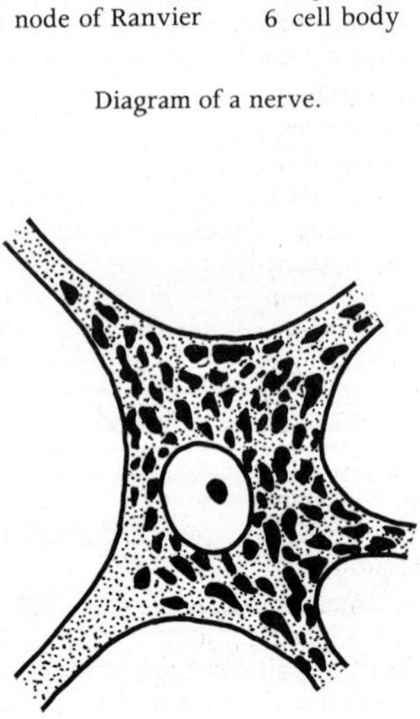

A nerve cell, showing Nissl's granules.

formed directly or indirectly as out-growths from this tube, which increase in length till they reach the muscle, skin or other structure for which they are destined. Each nerve-fibre, as already stated, is the process of a nerve-cell, and, if a nerve is cut, that portion of its fibres which is separated from the cells immediately starts to degenerate, the medullary sheath and axis-cylinder, as a rule, breaking up. Within a few days or weeks, however, a bundle of small new fibres grows out from the cut end of each fibre in that portion which has not been cut off from connection with the nerve-cells, and these grow through the scar and down the sheath of the degenerated portion till they reach the organs to which the nerve originally proceeded. Thus the nerve is restored. This process is quickened when the cut ends have been carefully brought together, and indeed there are reasons for believing that, sometimes when this is done, no degeneration takes place, but the nerve heals and again transmits impulses at once.

Functions of nerves: The greater part of the bodily activity originates in the nerve-cells, food material being used up in the process. As a result of this activity, impulses are sent down the nerves, which act simply as transmitters. The impulse which passes from a nerve-cell along a nerve-fibre to a muscle may be compared to the electric spark which explodes a mine, since the nerve impulse causes sudden chemical changes in the muscles as the latter contract. (See MUSCLES.) Similarly, the impulse which passes from a sensory ending in the skin along a nerve-fibre to affect nerve-cells in the spinal cord and brain, where it is perceived as a sensation, may be compared to the electric current which passes along a telephone cable to affect the receiver. Nevertheless, it must be understood that the impulse passing along a nerve is a form of motion quite different from electricity: travelling at the slow rate of about 30 metres (100 feet) per second, and probably more nearly resembling the motion of air-particles which produces sound. (See NERVOUS IMPULSE.)

The important fact that the anterior root of each spinal nerve is motor in function was discovered in 1811 by Sir Charles Bell. This was confirmed by Magendie in 1822, and the discovery also made that the posterior roots are sensory in function. They therefore concluded that the anterior roots consist of motor fibres to muscles, the posterior roots of sensory fibres from the skin. The terms, efferent and afferent, are applied to these roots more correctly because, in addition to motor fibres, fibres through which blood-vessels are contracted and relaxed, and fibres which control secreting glands leave the cord in the anterior roots, while, in addition to sensory fibres, fibres which bring in impulses from muscles, joints and other organs, and inform the sense of locality as well as the sense of feeling, also enter the cord by the posterior roots.

Sensation is popularly supposed to be derived through five senses: smell, sight, hearing, taste and touch. In addition to these, impulses are brought by special nerve-fibres and converted in the brain into sensations which furnish a sense of movement and locality, a sense of pain, and a sense of heat and cold. (See TOUCH.)

The connection between the sensory and motor systems of nerves is important. The simplest form of nerve action is that known a

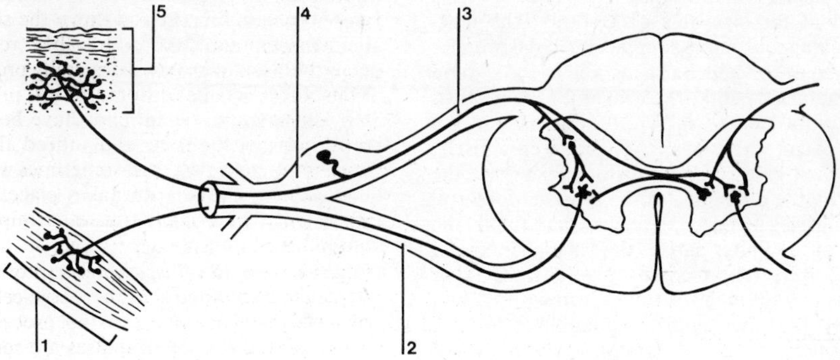

1 muscle
2 ventral root
3 dorsal root
4 dorsal root ganglion
5 skin

Diagram of a reflex arc.

automatic action. In this a part of the nervous system, controlling, for example, the lungs, goes on rhythmically, making discharges from its motor cells sufficient to keep the muscles of respiration in regular action, influenced only by occasional sensory impressions and chemical changes from various sources, which increase or diminish its activity according to the needs of the body.

In *reflex action* the parts engaged are a sensory ending, say in the skin; a sensory nerve leading from it to the spinal cord, where it ends by splitting up into processes near the nerve-cells; a nerve-cell which is stimulated by the sensory impulse, and which immediately sends a motor impulse down its nerve; and a muscle which contracts as the result. A simple example of reflex action is given by the drawing away of the hand when it is pricked with a pin, before and independently of the conscious perception of pain.

Voluntary acts are more complicated than reflex ones. The same mechanism is involved, but, in addition, the controlling power of the brain is brought into play. This exerts first of all an inhibitory or blocking effect, which prevents immediate reflex action, and then the impulse, passing up to the cerebral hemispheres, sets up activity in a series of cells there, the complexity of these processes depending upon the intellectual processes involved. Finally, the inhibition is removed and an impulse passes down to motor cells in the spinal cord, and a muscle or set of muscles is brought into play through the motor nerves.

The *trophic function* of nerves is another most important part of their activity, for it appears as if the constant passage of nerve impulses down the nerves of any part were important for its nutrition. Thus, if sensory nerves are diseased or injured, ulceration of the skin, bed sores and other changes are liable to occur, while muscles waste and disappear if their motor nerves are permanently destroyed.

Nervous system: The brain and its twelve pairs of cranial nerves are treated under BRAIN; the spinal cord and the origin of its thirty-one pairs of nerves are treated under SPINAL CORD.

Each of these spinal nerves arises by two roots, the posterior root being larger than the anterior, and being furnished with a ganglion. Just before they emerge from the side of the spinal canal, the two roots unite to form a single nerve, their fibres mix, and then the nerve separates into two divisions.

One division immediately turns backwards to supply the skin and muscles of the back (posterior division), the other runs forwards (anterior division).

These anterior divisions supply the skin on the front and sides of the body and on the limbs, as well as all the muscles of the trunk and limbs, excepting those on the back. They do not run straight to these parts, but form a series of plexuses in which the nerve-fibres from different levels of the cord to the limbs are given off. The upper four cervical nerves unite to produce the *cervical plexus.* From this the muscles and skin of the neck are mainly supplied, and the phrenic nerve, which runs down through the lower part of the neck and the chest to innervate the diaphragm, is given off. The *brachial plexus* is formed by the union of the lower four cervical and first dorsal nerves, and, in addition to nerves which proceed to some of the muscles in the shoulder region, and others to the skin about the shoulder and inner side of the arm, it gives off the following large nerves that proceed down the arm: the musculocutaneous nerve, the median nerve, the ulnar nerve, and the radial nerve, each of which is about the size of a goose-quill. The musculocutaneous nerve supplies the large muscles in front of the upper arm, as well as the skin on the radial side of the forearm as far as the wrist. The radial nerve winds round the back of the upper arm, where it supplies the triceps muscle, and then gives branches which innervate the skin on the outer side of the arm and forearm, the muscles behind the forearm, and finally the skin on the outer part of the back of the hand and fingers. The median nerve and the ulnar nerve run through the upper arm without giving off branches, and it is possible to feel the ulnar nerve as a cord running between the two marked bony prominences behind the elbow. The median nerve supplies most of the muscles in front of the forearm, a few of the small muscles in the hand and the skin of the palm and front of the thumb, index finger, middle finger and half of the ring finger. The ulnar nerve supplies two muscles in the forearm, most of the small muscles in the hand and the skin down the inner side of the forearm and palm and the skin in front of the little finger and half the ring finger.

The *thoracic* or *dorsal nerves*, with the exception of the first, do not form a plexus, but each runs round the chest along the lower margin of the rib to which it corresponds, whilst the lower six extend on to the abdomen. In this course they supply both the skin and muscle of the trunk.

The *lumbar plexus* is formed by the upper four lumbar nerves, and its branches are distributed to the lower part of the abdomen, and front and inner side of the thigh.

The *sacral plexus* is formed by parts of the fourth and fifth lumbar nerves, and the upper three and part of the fourth sacral nerves. It gives branches directly to the muscles and skin about the hip and fork, and supplies the skin down the back of the thigh, but the main bulk of the plexus is collected into the sciatic nerve. This, the largest nerve in the body, is buried in the muscles on the back of the thigh, which it supplies. It continues down to the back of the knee, and there divides into two branches, the internal popliteal (tibial) nerve and the external (common) popliteal nerve, which between them supply all the muscles below the knee and the greater part of the skin covering the leg and the foot.

The *sympathetic system* is joined by a pair of small branches given off from each spinal nerve, close to the spine. This system consists of two great parts. There is, first, a pair of cords running down on the side and front of the spine, and containing on each side three ganglia in the neck, and beneath this a ganglion opposite each vertebra. From these two ganglionated cords numerous branches are given off, and these unite in the second place to form plexuses connected with various internal organs, and provided with numerous large and irregularly placed ganglia. The chief of these plexuses are the cardiac plexus, the solar or epigastric plexus, the diaphragmatic, suprarenal, renal, spermatic, or ovarian, aortic, hypogastric and pelvic plexuses, the name in each case indicating the organ upon which, or the part of the abdomen within which, the plexus is placed.

NERVE INJURIES are produced by several causes. Continued or repeated severe pressure

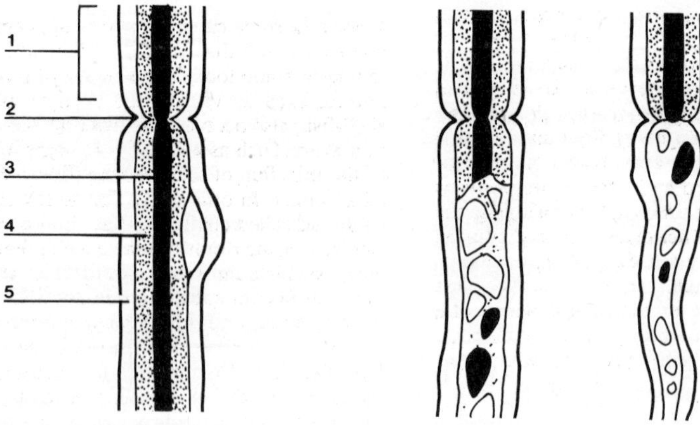

1 Schwann cell
2 node of Ranvier
3 axon
4 myelin
5 neurilemma

Diagram of (left) a healthy nerve, (centre) degenerating nerve cell after two days, (right) and after a week.

may be enough to damage a nerve seriously, as in the case of a badly made crutch pressing into the armpit and causing drop-wrist. Bruising due to a blow which drives a superficially placed nerve against a bone may inflict severe damage upon a nerve such as the radial nerve behind the upper arm. A wound may sever nerves, along with other structures; this accident is specially liable to occur to the ulnar nerve in front of the wrist, owing to falls upon broken glass, and to various nerves in the armpit when the humerus is fractured near its upper end.

Symptoms: When a sensory nerve is injured, sensation is immediately more or less impaired in the part supplied by the nerve. When the nerve in question is a motor one the muscles governed through it are instantly paralysed. In the latter case, the portion of nerve beyond the injury degenerates and the muscles gradually waste, and lose their power of contraction in response to electrical applications. Finally, deformities result and the joints become fixed. This is particularly noticeable when the ulnar nerve is injured, the hand and fingers taking up a claw-like position. The skin may also become cold, glossy and even ulcerate, owing to the loss of its nerve supply.

Treatment: The nerve, if wounded, should be carefully stitched with the ends touching one another, and, if injured by other causes, should be carefully protected from a repetition of the injury. In some cases recovery takes place within a few days, but usually, if the nerve is completely severed or seriously injured, the muscles supplied by it do not regain their power for several weeks at least. The reason for this is that the part cut off from connection with the brain and cord degenerates rapidly, and the new nerve has to grow all the way down the sheath of the old one. (See NERVES.) An operation designed to unite a damaged nerve and relieve paralysis may sometimes be successfully performed even some weeks or months after the wound has closed. When the ends of the damaged nerve are so shortened that they cannot be got to meet, a portion of a sensory nerve or of a nerve from an animal is sometimes inserted and carefully stitched between the divided ends. Nerve anastomosis is also sometimes practised by bringing the ends of the divided nerve up to a neighbouring nerve and carefully stitching them within its sheath. For example, the facial nerve when injured at the side of the face is sometimes anastomosed with the healthy hypoglossal nerve, and the facial paralysis which has resulted is thus relieved. Massage and galvanism of the muscles will keep them from wasting till the nerve is ready to take up its functions again. The power of the muscles to react again to faradic electricity is a most important sign, as showing that repair of the nerve is taking place. (See ELECTRICITY IN MEDICINE.)

NERVOUS DEBILITY (see NEURASTHENIA).

NERVOUS DISEASES: This class of disease is one of the most difficult to diagnose. The brain and spinal cord being enclosed in the skull and spine, beyond the reach of direct examination, and the nerves being almost everywhere deeply buried in the tissues, the nature of nervous diseases must be made out from the disturbances of organs governed by the affected nerves.

The following conditions are discussed under their individual headings: APHASIA; APOPLEXY; BRAIN DISEASE; CATALEPSY; CHOREA; CRAMP; EPILEPSY; FORGETFULNESS; HYSTERIA; LOCOMOTOR ATAXIA; MENTAL SUBNORMALITY; MENTAL ILLNESS; MULTIPLE SCLEROSIS; NERVE INJURIES; NEURALGIA; NEURITIS; PARALYSIS; PYSCHOSOMATIC DISEASE; SPINAL CORD, DISEASES OF.

NERVOUS IMPULSE: The effects of nervous activity are now believed in all cases to be transmitted chemically, by the formation at nerve-endings of chemical substances. When, for example, a nerve to a muscle is stimulated, there appears at the junction of nerve-ending and muscle the chemical substance, acetylcholine. Acetylcholine also appears at endings of the parasympathetic nerves and transmits the effect of the parasympathetic impulse. When an impulse passes down a sympathetic nerve, the effect of it is transmitted at the nerve-ending by the chemical liberated there: adrenaline or an adrenaline-like substance.

NETTLE-RASH, or URTICARIA, is a disorder of the skin characterized by an eruption resembling the effect produced by the sting of a nettle, namely, raised red or red-and-white patches, occurring in parts or over the whole of the surface of the body, and attended with great itching and irritation. It may be acute or chronic.

Causes: In some cases the attack appears to be connected with digestive derangements, or the taking of some foods particularly of a protein nature, such as various kinds of meat, fish, shell-fish, also occasionally from the use of certain drugs, such as penicillin. In some it is due to the injection of sera, or may follow the bite of an insect. In others it is due to exposure to cold – so-called cold urticaria – and occasionally may be the result of effort. There remains a considerable number of cases in which it is difficult to incriminate any one specific causal factor. The general consensus of opinion is that urticaria is an allergic reaction on the part of the affected individual to some substance to which he or she is hypersensitive. In other words, it comes into the same category as asthma and hay fever. In all three conditions the individual is allergic to some factor or factors, but the allergic response varies: in asthma it is the bronchioles of the lungs that are involved; in hay fever it is the mucous membrane of the nasopharynx, sinuses and eyes; whilst in urticaria it is the skin that gives the allergic response.

Symptoms: In severe cases there is at first considerable feverishness and constitutional disturbance, together with sickness and faintness, which either precede or accompany the appearance of the rash. The eruption may appear on any part of the body, but is most common on the face and trunk. In the former position it causes swelling and disfigurement while it lasts, and is apt to excite alarm in those unacquainted with its nature. The attack may pass off in a few hours, or may last for several days, the eruption continuing to come out in successive patches. The lesions are accompanied by severe itching. Occasionally a similar process takes place in the throat, and there is then considerable danger from blockage of the larynx. (See also ALLERGY.)

Treatment: The treatment of urticaria has been revolutionized by the introduction of the antihistamine drugs. There is now a large number of these, and it is necessary to find which particular preparation suits a particular individual. In addition, it is necessary to discover, if possible, the causative factor and to remove it. For instance, if an attack always follows the taking of a certain article of diet, this should be carefully noted and avoided in future.

NEURALGIA, literally *nerve pain*, is a term which is often employed both technically and popularly in a somewhat loose manner, to describe pains the origin of which is not clearly traceable. In its strict sense it means the existence of pain in some portion of, or throughout the whole of, the distribution of a sensory nerve, without any distinctly recognizable structural change in the nerve or nerve-centres. This strict definition, if adhered to, however, would not be applicable to a large number of cases of nerve pain; for in many instances the pain is connected with pressure on, or inflammation of, the nerve. Hence the word is generally used to indicate pain affecting a particular nerve or its branches, whatever be the cause.

Symptoms: Although the pain is generally localized, it may spread beyond the area where it first occurs. It is usually of paroxysmal character, and often periodic: that is to say, it occurs at a certain time of the day or night. It varies in intensity, being often of the most agonizing character, and again less severe and more of a tingling kind. Various forms of perverted nerve function may be found along with or following neuralgia. Thus there may be over-sensitiveness of the skin, loss of feeling, paralysis or alterations of nutrition, such as wasting of muscles, whitening of the hair. Attacks of neuralgia are apt to recur, particularly when the general health is low, and some people unhappily continue to suffer from occasional attacks during the greater part of their lifetime.

Varieties: The nature of the disease is best described under the names of the forms in which it most commonly occurs. These are trigeminal neuralgia (qv) or tic douloureux; intercostal neuralgia; and sciatica (qv). Other forms, affecting other nerves, are of much less frequent occurrence.

INTERCOSTAL NEURALGIA is pain affecting the nerves which emerge from the spinal cord and run along the spaces between the ribs to the front of the body. This form of neuralgia affects the left side more than the right, is more common in women than in men, and occurs generally in enfeebled states of health. It might be mistaken for pleurisy or some inflammatory affection of the lungs; but the absence of any chest symptoms, its occurrence independently of the acts of respiration, and other considerations establish the distinction. The specially painful points are chiefly where the nerve issues from the spinal canal, and at the extremities towards the front of the body, where it breaks up into filaments which ramify in the skin. This form of neuralgia is occasionally the precursor of an attack of shingles (*herpes zoster*) as well as a result of it. (See HERPES.)

Treatment: With all forms of neuralgia it is of the first importance to ascertain, if possible, whether any constitutional condition is associated with the symptom.

Naturally also one looks for, and as speedily as possible removes, any source of local irritation, such as a decayed tooth, and also any such reflex source as uterine or intestinal disorder.

During the time an acute attack lasts, various local applications give relief, the most useful being, perhaps, hot fomentations applied over the painful part. Bathing with water as hot as can be borne is also beneficial in many cases. Rubbing or painting with anodyne liniments, such as a mixture of the liniments of aconite, belladonna and chloroform (ABC Liniment), or a mixture, in equal parts, of chloral, camphor and menthol, rubbed up together and painted over the part, is soothing, especially perhaps for those cases in which the pain begins as soon as the sufferer gets warm in bed at night. Ointment of aconitine is also recommended by some to be rubbed on the painful spot. Hypodermic injections of morphine, although they give temporary relief, are not to be recommended because of the great danger that their use will become a habit. In the case of purely sensory nerves, like the fifth nerve, injection of pure alcohol into the nerve has a deadening effect and often gives relief for a long time.

Internally, during an acute attack, many remedies are given. Those which are most generally useful, and which may be safely used without any tendency to bring about habitual use, are aspirin, paracetamol and codeine.

Local measures in the chronic state include the application of blisters or counter-irritation by touching the skin with the button-cautery. The blister is made of an oblong shape, with its length corresponding to the line of the nerve, and the spots at which the cautery is applied generally also follow the affected nerve. The use of galvanic electricity is often beneficial in both the acute and the chronic stage. (See ELECTRICITY IN MEDICINE.) Diathermy is also employed with soothing effect. (See DIATHERMY.) Massage, though it increases the pain in the acute state, may be of great benefit in chronic cases due to some inflammatory process in the nerve.

Some cases resist all forms of medicinal treatment, and for these surgical procedures are sometimes tried, such as division and removal of a portion of the nerve, or injection of absolute alcohol into the nerve.

NEURALGIA TRIGEMINAL: This form of neuralgia affects the sensory nerve which supplies most of the face. Usually two out of the three main branches are involved. It is a severe pain often initiated by light pressure on the skin. It is generally diagnosed after excluding all other likely causes of facial pain. Treatment may be with the long-term use of the analgesic carbamezepine or partial or complete destruction of the appropriate branch of the nerve. The nerve may be destroyed by freezing, coagulating or injection of an alcohol round it. If untreated or suppressed the pain may be present for many months, then disappear, only to recur a year or so later.

NEURASTHENIA means a condition of nervous exhaustion in which, although the patient suffers from no definite disease, he becomes incapable of sustained exertion. It was never a very well-defined entity, and the term has now been largely given up. The condition which it represented is now recognized to be a form of neurosis (qv) or psychosomatic disease (qv).

NEURECTOMY is an operation in which part of a nerve is excised: for example, for the relief of neuralgia.

NEURILEMMA is the thin membranous covering which surrounds every nerve-fibre. (See NERVES.)

NEURITIS means inflammation affecting a nerve or nerves which may be localized to one part of the body, as, for instance, in sciatica, or which may be general, being then known as multiple neuritis, or polyneuritis. Owing to the fact that the most peripheral parts of the nerves are usually at fault in the latter condition, ie. the fine subdivisions in the substance of the muscles, it is also known as peripheral neuritis.

Causes: In cases of LOCALIZED NEURITIS the fibrous sheath of the nerve is usually at fault, the actual nerve-fibres being only secondarily affected. This condition may be due to inflammation spreading into the nerve from surrounding tissues, to cold or to long-continued irritation by pressure on the nerve, and the symptoms produced vary according to the function of the nerve, in the case of sensory nerves being usually neuralgic pain (see NEURALGIA), in the case of motor nerves more or less paralysis in the muscles to which the nerves pass.

In POLYNEURITIS, which is always due to some general or constitutional cause, the nerve-fibres themselves in the small nerves degenerate and break down. Hence the very protracted nature of this malady, since, if recovery takes place, it must be brought about by the growth of new nerve-fibres from the healthy part of the nerve, down the sheath of the nerve, to the muscle. The cause of this degeneration may be said, in general terms, to be some poison either taken into or produced in the body, and circulating in the blood. By far the commonest of these poisons is alcohol, and the disease especially affects women who are quiet, steady tipplers. The condition also arises in men, though more rarely, but the abuse of alcohol in this sex tends more to produce delirium tremens, from which women are almost exempt. Next in importance comes lead, wrist-drop and other features of neuritis being among the most prominent symptoms of lead-poisoning. (See LEAD-POISONING.) Arsenic is occasionally responsible for neuritis, particularly when the effect of arsenic is combined with over-indulgence in alcohol, as in an epidemic of neuritis, due to beer contaminated with arsenic, in the Midlands of England about the year 1900. Bisulphide of carbon, naphtha and other solvents of rubber are apt to produce the disease when inhaled in large quantity by the workmen in rubber factories. Those who suffer from diabetes mellitus are prone to neuritis, the condition sometimes being the result of deficiency of thiamine in the diet. This deficiency probably also accounts for some cases of alcoholic neuritis. The disease known as beri-beri (qv) is a form of neuritis which persists in certain localities of the world, in consequence of thiamine deficiency.

Symptoms: The chief symptom of a LOCALIZED NEURITIS, whether pain or paralysis, varies according to the functions of the nerve. In cases following diphtheria, or other infective disease, the neuritis of an outlying nerve often shows, as its most prominent and annoying feature, a paralysis of a group of muscles in the arm or leg, leading to weakness of the part concerned. This may cause inability for some months to grasp objects with the hand, to lift the foot in walking and similar troublesome symptoms. These, however, usually pass off completely in time. The area of skin associated with the affected nerve is, in addition, often much changed, becoming glossy, or developing an ulcer or, especially about the face and trunk, breaking out in shingles. (See HERPES.) A case of neuritis of this type may come on very quickly, developing fully in a few days.

POLYNEURITIS, as a rule, takes longer to show itself. In most cases it begins with vague pains and tingling in the limbs; weakness and wasting of the muscles in the feet and legs, in the hand and arms, or in other parts, following later. Wrist-drop, the peculiar steppage gait in which the person lifts his feet as if he were constantly stepping over small obstacles, squinting, loss of voice, difficulty of breathing, enfeeblement of the heart's action appear according to the muscles whose nerves are affected. The knee-jerks and other deep reflexes are generally lost in all forms of neuritis, if severe in character. A peculiar feature of alcoholic neuritis is the wandering delirium from which the patient often suffers, her imagination conjuring up the most vivid delusions as to journeys she is making, and the mind being quite confused, especially in matters regarding time and place.

The course of the disease is usually very slow, and particularly is this the case when a poison, as in the case of alcohol or lead, has been taken into the system over a long period. Months, or even a year or two, may elapse before health is restored. The ultimate hope of recovery is, however, good. Except in the case of beri-beri, which is fatal unless treated, and in those cases of poisoning by alcohol, or of diphtheria, in which the mechanism of the heart or that of respiration becomes affected, the mortality is low.

Treatment: For the treatment of LOCALIZED NEURITIS see under NEURALGIA.

The first essential in the treatment of POLYNEURITIS is to discover and remove the cause by which the nerves are being poisoned. This applies particularly to alcoholism, lead poisoning and neuritis due to manufacture of rubber. In the case of alcoholism there is always the moral difficulty of preventing the patient from obtaining fresh supplies of stimulants, so that treatment must be carried out in a hospital or nursing-home. Rest in bed is the next essential to prevent over-fatigue of the weakened nerves and muscles. In the early stages the muscles are too tender to permit much handling, but, later on, massage helps to prevent wasting of muscles, and the deformities which arise through fixation of the joints in one position. These deformities must be prevented as far as possible during the earlier stages by frequently changing the position of the patient's limbs as he lies in bed. Electrical treatment may also help as recovery advances. Much benefit is sometimes gained from injections of thiamine or administration of foods containing it, such as Bemax or Marmite.

NEURODERMATOSES, sometimes grouped under the name of NEURODERMATITIS, are disorders of the skin in which stress is one of the important factors, if not the most important cause. In some conditions, such as pruritus (see ITCHING) and rosacea (qv) this is the principal cause. In others, such as atopic eczema (see ECZEMA) and lichen simplex (see LICHEN), it is a secondary, but nonetheless often important, factor, any mental or emotional stress or strain bringing on an exacerbation, or flaring up, of the skin condition. In others again, such as *dermatitis artefacta* the emotional, or mental, instability may be the sole cause, the individual deliberately damaging his or her skin, without divulging the cause. The extreme form of this manifestation of mental illness is parasitophobia, in which the individual has a morbid terror of parasites and is quite convinced that he or she is infested with some parasite which is causing the itching which in turn has been scratched until the skin has broken down.

NEUROGLIA is the name applied to a fine web of tissue and branching cells which supports the nerve fibres and cells of the nervous system. (See NERVES.)

NEUROLEPTIC is an anti-psychotic drug: ie. a drug used in the treatment of a psychosis (qv).

NEUROLOGY is the branch of medical practice and science which deals with the nervous system and its diseases.

NEUROMA means a tumour connected with a nerve, such tumours being generally composed of fibrous tissue, and of a painful nature.

NEUROMYASTHENIA is a disease, which often occurs in epidemics, and which is characterized by headache, stiffness of the neck and back, muscular weakness and pain, fever and often diarrhoea. When it occurs in epidemics it is known as epidemic neuromyasthenia, Icelandic disease or Royal Free disease. This last name results from an outbreak among the nurses at the Royal Free Hospital, London. The epidemic form is most common among women. The cause is not known but has been attributed to a virus or to hysteria (qv).

NEURON is a single unit of the nervous system, consisting of a nerve cell with its various processes and the nerve fibre or fibres to which it gives origin. As applied to the motor part of the nervous system, two neurons are specially recognized: the *upper neuron*, which includes a cell on the surface of the brain and a fibre extending down into the spinal cord; the *lowerneuron*, which consists of a cell in the grey matter of the cord with a nerve fibre extending outwards to end in a fibre of the muscle with which it is connected. The former has a controlling influence over the latter, whilst the latter is more directly concerned with the changes that result in the contraction of the muscle fibre and with nutritional influences over it. (See NERVES.)

NEUROSIS is a general term applied to mental or emotional disturbance in which, as opposed to psychosis, there is no serious disturbance in the perception or understanding of external reality. However, the boundaries between neurosis and psychosis are not always clearly defined. Neuroses are usually classified into anxiety neuroses, depressive neuroses, phobias, hysteria and obsessional neuroses.

ANXIETY NEUROSIS, or ANXIETY STATE, constitutes the commonest form of neurosis. Fortunately it is also almost the most responsive to treatment. It is more likely in people of anxious personality. Once the neurosis develops, they are in a state of persistent anxiety and worry, 'tensed up', always feeling fatigue and unable to sleep at night. In addition, there are often physical complaints, eg. palpitations or headache. OBSESSIONAL NEUROSES are much less common and constitute only about 5 per cent of all neuroses. Like other neuroses, they usually develop in early adult life. (See MENTAL ILLNESS.)

NEUROSURGERY is surgery performed on some part of the nervous system, whether brain, spinal cord or nerves.

NEUROTIC is a general term of indefinite meaning applied to a person of nervous temperament, whose actions are largely determined by emotions or instincts rather than by reason.

NEUROTRANSMITTER is a substance which transmits the action of a nerve to a cell. It is now recognized that this is how nerves work. If there should be a lack or deficiency of the appropriate neurotransmitter, then the nerve cannot carry out its action. A classical example of this is dopamine (qv), lack of which is responsible for the condition known as Parkinsonism (qv). Other neurotransmitters include acetylcholine (qv) which is the neurotransmitter for the parasympathetic system (qv) and noradrenaline which is the neurotransmitter for the sympathetic nervous system.

NEUTRON is one of the particles that enter into the structure of the atomic nucleus. (See ISOTOPE.)

NEUTROPENIA denotes a reduction in the number of neutrophil leucocytes per cubic millimetre of circulating blood to a figure below that found in health. There is still some disagreement over the precise limits of normality, but a count of less than 2500 per c.mm would be generally accepted as constituting neutropenia. Several infective diseases are characterized by neutropenia, including typhoid fever, influenza and measles. It may also be induced by certain drugs, including chloramphenicol, phenylbutazone, the sulphonamides and chlorpromazine.

N.H.S. MANAGEMENT BOARD (see NATIONAL HEALTH SERVICE).

NICLOSAMIDE is the drug of choice in the treatment of tapeworm infestation. It is also known as YOMESAN.

NICOFURANOSE (BRADILAN) (see HYPERLIPIDAEMIA).

NICOTINAMIDE, the amide of nicotinic acid, is sometimes used instead of nicotinic acid (qv).

NICOTINE is the active principle in tobacco. (See TOBACCO.)

NICOTINIC ACID, or NIACIN, is a member of the vitamin B complex. It is essential for human nutrition, the normal daily requirement for an adult being about 15 to 20 mg. A deficiency of nicotinic acid is one of the factors in the etiology of pellagra (qv), and either nicotine acid or nicotinamide is used in the treatment of this condition. (See HYPERLIPIDAEMIA.)

NIFEDIPINE (ADALAT) is a drug that is being used in the treatment of angina pectoris (qv). It is said to reduce the requirements of the heart muscle for oxygen. It is also proving of value in the treatment of high blood-pressure. It is one of the calcium antagonists (qv). (See CALCIUM ANTAGONISTS.)

NIGHT BLINDNESS (see BLINDNESS).

NIGHTMARE (see SLEEP).

NIGHT SWEATS consist in copious perspiration occurring in bed at night and found in conditions such as tuberculosis, brucellosis and lymphomas.

NIKETHAMIDE is a drug which stimulates the respiratory centre.

NIPPLES, DISEASES OF (see BREAST, DISEASES OF).

NIRIDAZOLE is a drug which is proving of value in the treatment of schistosomiasis (qv) and guinea-worm infections (see DRACONTIASIS).

NITRAZEPAM (MOGADON) is a tranquillizer introduced as a hypnotic. (See TRANQUILLIZERS, BENZODIAZEPINES.)

NITRE, also known as SALTPETRE, NITRATE OF POTASSIUM and, in the form of sticks, as SAL PRUNELLE, is a crystalline substance of a sharp saline taste, found in India, Persia and other places. It is very irritating to the stomach and is not now used internally, but was of use for inhalation in the treatment of asthma, since the nitrate in burning gives off nitrites.

NITRIC ACID is one of the strongest of the mineral acids, and is a clear, heavy liquid, becoming brownish with age. It is kept in dark, stoppered bottles, and immediately the stopper is removed from the bottle, irritating white fumes are given off.

Action: In its pure state, nitric acid acts as a powerful caustic upon the tissues of the body, which it turns a bright yellow colour. In weaker solution it is, like all acids, an antiseptic, but is very irritating. Internally, in small doses it has a stimulating action upon the gastric mucous membrane.

Uses: Nitric acid is one of the most effective caustics for warts, and is also used as a powerful antiseptic and caustic for destroying foul ulcers which threaten to spread, leaving clean ulcers in their place. It is applied to warts drop by drop with a glass rod, and its action can be checked by applying similarly a few drops of solution of common salt.

NITRITES are salts which have a powerful effect in paralysing the action of involuntary muscle, and they therefore dilate the blood-vessels, and check spasm of all sorts. The most commonly used nitrites are nitrite of amyl, of ethyl, and of sodium. Erythrol tetranitrate and nitroglycerin have a similar action. (See GLYCERYL TRINITRATE.)

NITROFURANTOIN is a synthetic nitrofuran derivative which has a wide range of antibacterial activity and is effective against many Gram-positive and Gram-negative micro-organisms. It is used mainly in the treatment of infections of the urinary tract.

NITROGEN MUSTARDS are nitrogen analogues of mustard gas. They are among the most important alkylating agents (qv) used in the treatment of various forms of malignant disease. They include mustine, trimustine, uramustine, busulphan, chlorambucil and melphalan.

NITROHYDROCHLORIC ACID, or AQUA REGIA, so called because of its power to dissolve gold, is a yellow liquid prepared by adding 1 part of nitric acid to 4 parts of hydrochloric acid. It is a caustic in its pure state, but is only used for internal administration in a diluted form. It is used in the treatment of dyspepsia associated with a low gastric acidity.

NITROUS OXIDE GAS, also known as LAUGHING GAS, is, at ordinary pressures, a gas devoid of odour but of a slightly sweetish taste. Its use in medicine is to produce insensibility to pain, which it does very quickly, and with a great degree of safety, though the effect is of very short duration, not extending beyond two or three minutes. Its use is therefore applicable only for short operations, such as extraction of a tooth, unless it is repeatedly administered in association with oxygen. (See ANAESTHETICS.)

NOCTURIA denotes excess passing of urine during the night. Among its many causes are glomerulonephritis (qv) and enlargement of the prostate. (See also URINE, EXCESS OF.)

NOCTURNAL ENURESIS is the involuntary passing of urine during sleep. It is a condition predominantly of childhood. In a small minority of cases it is due to some organic cause such as infection of the genito-urinary tract, but in the vast majority of cases it is due to inadequate or improper training of the child or psychological ill health. Traditionally it is said to be associated with threadworms, but there is little, if any, evidence to support this tradition.

Before deciding that a child is suffering from nocturnal enuresis, it is necessary to remember that the age at which a child achieves full control of bladder function varies considerably. Such control is usually achieved in the second year, but more commonly in the third year of life, and there are some children who do not normally achieve such control until the fourth, or even fifth, year.

It is a difficult condition to cure in the absence of an organic cause. If there should be an organic cause, treatment consists of its eradication. In the absence of such a cause, treatment consists essentially of reassurance and firm but kindly and understanding training. In quite a number of cases the use of a buzzer alarm which wakens the child should he start passing water is helpful provided that it is backed up by psychological support from the parents and the family doctor.

NODE: The term node is widely used in medicine. For instance, the smaller lymphatic glands (qv) are often termed lymph nodes. It is also applied to a collection of nerve cells forming a subsidiary nerve centre found in various places in the sympathetic nervous system, such as the sinuatrial node and the atrio-ventricular node which control the beating of the heart.

NOISE (see DEAFNESS).

NOMA is another name for cancrum oris. (See CANCRUM.)

NOMIFENSINE (MERITAL) (see ANTIDEPRESSANTS).

NON-SPECIFIC GENITAL INFECTION, or NON-SPECIFIC URETHRITIS, is an inflammatory condition of the urethra (qv) due to infection with certain types of micro-organism. The most common is *Chlamydia trachomatis*. Others include *Ureaplasmaurealyticum* and *Mycoplasma genitalium*. In England it is the commonest sexually transmitted disease: 134,079 cases were reported in 1983. It produces pelvic inflammatory disease in women, which often results in sterility, the risk of ectopic pregnancy (see ECTOPIC), and recurrent pelvic pain. Most cases respond well to tetracycline (qv). Abstinence from sexual intercourse should be observed during treatment and until cure is complete. Children born to infected mothers may have their eyes infected during birth, producing the condition known as ophthalmia neonatorum (qv). This is treated by the application to the eye of chlortetracycline eye ointment. The lungs of such a child may also be infected, resulting in pneumonia. The eye may also be infected in adults with the disease or those who are in contact with infected sexual partners.

NON-STEROIDAL ANTI-INFLAMMATORY DRUGS act by inhibiting the formation of prostaglandins which are mediators of inflammation. They act both as analgesics to relieve pain and as inhibitors of inflammation. Aspirin is a classic example of such a compound. Newer compounds have been synthesized with the aim of producing fewer and less severe side-effects. They are sometimes preferred to aspirin for the treatment of conditions such as rheumatoid arthritis, osteoarthritis, sprains, strains and sports injuries. Their main side-effects are gastro-intestinal. Gastric ulcers and gastric haemorrhage may result. This is because prostaglandins are necessary for the production of the mucous protective coat in the stomach and when the production of prostaglandin is inhibited the protection of the stomach is compromised. They should therefore be used with caution in patients with dyspepsia and gastric ulceration. The various non-steroidal anti-inflammatory drugs differ little from each other in efficacy though there is considerable variation in patient response. Naproxen (Naprosyn) is one of the first choices in this group of drugs as it combines good efficacy with a low incidence of side effects and administration is only required twice daily. Other drugs in this series include diflunisal (Dolobid), sulindac (Clinoril) fenoprofen (Fenopron), flurbiprofen (Froben), ibuprofen (Brufen), ketoprofen (Orudis), azapropazone (Rheumox), feprazone (Methrazone), piroxicam (Feldene), diclofenac (Voltarol), fenbufen (Lederfen), fenclofenac (Flenac), indoprofen (Flosint), tiaprofenic acid (Surgam) and tolmetin (Tolectin).

NORADRENALINE is a precursor of adrenaline (qv) in the medulla of the suprarenal glands. It is also present in the brain. Its main function is to mediate the transmission of impulses in the sympathetic nervous system (qv). It also has a transmitter function in the brain.

NORETHANDROLONE (NILEVAR) (see ANABOLIC STEROIDS).

NORETHISTERONE is a synthetic preparation that has the action of progesterone (qv), but is active when given by mouth.

NORETHYNODREL is a synthetic substance which has a progesterone-like action. (See PROGESTERONE.) Originally, and still, used for the treatment of various menstrual disorders, these progestogens, as they are known, have also the property of inhibiting ovulation. It is this property that led to their use as oral contraceptives. (See CONTRACEPTION.)

NORMAL is a term used in several different senses. Generally speaking, it is applied to anything which agrees with the regular and established type. In chemistry the term is applied to solutions of acids or bases of such strength that each litre contains the number of grams corresponding to the molecular weight of the substance in question. In physiology the term normal is applied to solutions of such strength that, when mixed with a body fluid, they are isotonic and cause no disturbance: eg. normal saline solution. (See ISOTONIC.)

NORMOBLAST is the term applied to the precursor of a red blood corpuscle which still contains the remnant of a nucleus.

NORTRIPTYLINE (ALLEGRON, AVENTYL) is an antidepressant drug which is also a sedative. (See ANTIDEPRESSANTS.)

NORWEGIAN SCABIES is the name given in Scotland to the severe form of scabies (qv) in which the skin becomes greatly thickened and fissures develop.

NOSE: The nose has three main functions. It is the natural pathway whereby air enters the body in the course of respiration (qv). In the nose the incoming air is warmed, moistened and filtered before passing on into the lungs. It has also a protective function. Irritation of it by dust or the like induces sneezing (qv) which expels the irritant from the nose and so prevents it getting into the lungs. It is also the organ of smell (qv).

The *external nose* is formed partly of bone and partly of cartilage, covered by skin. In its upper part, the two nasal bones, one on each side, project downwards from the frontal bone for about 25 mm (1 inch), and, supported by a process of the upper jaw-bone, form the hard bridge of the nose between the eyes. The ending of the bony part can be seen or felt on most noses, and, beneath this, two cartilages on each side, the lateral cartilages and the cartilages of the aperture give shape, firmness, and pliability to the lower two-thirds of the nose. The gap between the cartilages of the aperture can be distinctly felt on the point of the nose. The spaces between the cartilages are filled up and the cartilages firmly bound to the bones and to one another by fibrous tissue. When the nose is injured, some of the cartilages are apt to be dislocated, thus altering the shape of this organ. However, most injuries resulting in deformity of the nose are due to injuries to the bones of the nose.

In its *interior*, the nose is completely divided into two narrow cavities, one on each side, by a septum or partition running from front to back. This septum is a thin plate composed partly of bone, partly of cartilage, consisting in about its hinder two-thirds of the central plate of the ethmoid bone and of the vomer bone, and in about its anterior third of a four-sided plate of cartilage, which along one edge touches the nasal bones, the lateral cartilages, and the cartilages of the aperture. On both surfaces this septum is covered by the general mucous membrane that lines the nose.

The cavities on either side of the septum, known as the *nasal fossae*, are extremely narrow, being at their widest point less that 6 mm (¼ inch) in breadth, though in height they correspond to the length of the nose, and run directly backwards about 5 cm (2 inches). At its upper end each cavity is separated from the interior of the skull by a thin plate of bone containing many minute apertures for the passage of the filaments of the olfactory nerve. The front part of each cavity consists of the space enclosed by the cartilages of the nose, is lined by skin, which is furnished with stiff hairs or vibrisae that grow downwards and protect the entrance, and is known as the vestibule. Farther back the outer surface of each cavity is rendered very complicated, and the space in the cavity greatly filled up, by three projections known as the nasal conchae or turbinates. These bones form ridges which run from before backwards with an inclination downwards, and, in section, each ridge is curled over so that its edge looks downwards. There are therefore three passages (meatus) running from before backwards, each under cover of a corresponding nasal turbinate. As each of these bones, in common with the whole of the cavity, is covered with very vascular and thick mucous membrane, the air in its passage through the nose is by this arrangement brought in contact with a large surface of mucous membrane, and thus is considerably warmed before it enters the broncial tubes and lungs. In addition, this mucous membrane, which is covered with cilia (qv), secretes more that 500 millilitres of sticky mucus every 24 hours. This traps dust particles and the like, which are then moved on by the cilia and usually swallowed unnoticed. It is the excessive production of this mucus, in response to irritations or infection, that is known as nasal catarrh (qv). The front portion of the inferior and of the middle nasal concha can be seen as two red projections by looking up the nostril with a bright light, when the nostril is slightly opened by a speculum. The superior meatus beneath the superior nasal concha is a narrow passage, and, upon this bone and passage as well as upon the corresponding part of the septum, the nerves of smell end in the mucous membrane. The wider and longer middle meatus and inferior meatus are the passages through which the air mainly passes out and in during respiration.

Certain *sinuses* lie concealed in the bones of the skull, into which air enters freely by apertures connecting them with the nose. These cavities occupy spaces in the frontal bone over the eyebrow (frontal sinus), in the upper jawbone, filling in the angle between the eye and the nose (maxillary sinus or antrum of Highmore), in the sphenoid bone (sphenoidal sinus), and in the lateral part of the ethmoid bone (ethmoidal sinus). The function of the sinuses is, as yet, unknown. The most capacious is the maxillary sinus, which is a cubical cavity, often over 12 mm (½inch) in measurement each way. The frontal sinus, maxillary sinus, and ethmoidal sinus open by small apertures about the centre of the middle meatus, the sphenoidal sinus above this. Into the front part of the inferior meatus opens the nasal duct, which carries the tears off from the eye. (See EYE.) The latter fact explains the frequent blowing of the nose which becomes necessary when a person is weeping. On a level with the inferior meatus, but situated in the part of the throat into which the nose opens, is placed the orifice of the Eustachian, or auditory, tube leading to the middle ear. (See EAR.)

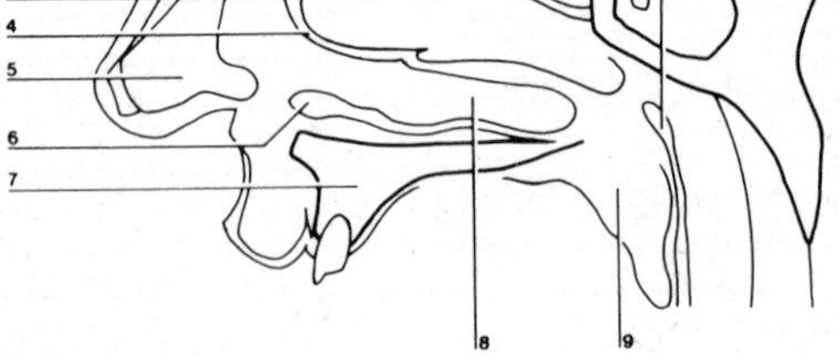

1 frontal sinus
2 atrium of middle meatus
3 middle nasal concha
4 middle meatus
5 vestibule
6 inferior meatus
7 maxilla
8 inferior nasal concha
9 soft palate
10 sphenoidal sinus
11 auditory tube
12 sphenoethmoidal recess and higher nasal concha
13 superior nasal concha
14 superior meatus

The lateral wall of the right half of the nasal cavity.

NOSE, DISEASES OF: The nose, so far as the skin-covering is concerned, is subject to the same diseases as the skin of other parts. Redness of the skin of this part may, on account of its disfiguring character, be very annoying. It may be due to poor circulation in cold weather, partaking of the nature of a chilblain (see CHILBLAINS); occasionally it is due to acne rosacea. Among the skin diseases, acne (qv), lupus (qv), and erysipelas (qv) are specially prone to affect this site.

ACUTE INFLAMMATION of the nose is generally a viral infection affecting the mucous membrane of the nose and paranasal sinuses and is commonly known as a cold in the head. (See CHILLS AND COLDS.) It may be due, though less commonly, to the inhalation of irritating gases. Boils occasionally develop just within the entrance to the nose, in connection with the hairs there, and in this locality give rise to great pain and considerable danger. (See BOILS.) Diphtheria used to be a form of severe rhinitis but this is now extremely rare. Hay fever is a distressing form of acute rhinitis. (See HAY FEVER.)

MALFORMATIONS OF THE NOSE are of various kinds. The external nose varies much in shape in different races, even in different families, and it is possible for persons who desire for aesthetic reasons to alter the character of their noses to undergo some form of surgery. This is known as rhinoplasty. As to the interior of the nose, the two cavities are practically never of equal size, the septum almost always bulging to one or other side, so that the passage of air is slightly freer on one side than on the other. When this bulging is so marked that the septum touches the nasal conchae on one side, or when, owing to injury or other cause, spurs and crests have developed on the septum, considerable irritation may arise, and this may form the starting-point for chronic inflammation of the nose, hay fever or asthma. These imperfections, though they often exist without the least ill-effect, and are only discovered accidentally, are readily removed by the specialist if necessary, such operations being attended by but little pain. A more common abnormality is that in which the nose becomes obstructed as the result of nasal polyps, adenoids and other causes and in consequence the person breathes through the mouth.

ADENOIDS means an overgrowth of the glandular tissue which is naturally found in small amount on the back of the upper part of the throat, into which the nose opens.

Causes: This glandular tissue is similar in structure to the tonsils and lymphatic glands, and in children may be large enough to obstruct the posterior openings of the nose into the nasopharynx. This obstruction therefore leads to nasal obstruction and may also obstruct the Eustachian tubes.

Symptoms: Generally this overgrowth subsides as the child reaches puberty but the continued enlarged state of the adenoids for a prolonged period of time may produce serious problems for the child's health. This constant obstruction often leads to the typical appearance of the child suffering from enlarged adenoids. The mouth is kept constantly open since breathing proceeds through it and, as a result, the child snores at night. The point of the nose is often pinched and the nostrils narrow, and the bridge of the nose is often flattened. The palate is highly arched and the front teeth often prominent. This condition varies in its severity in that there may be minimal symptoms or there may be significant obstruction with excessive mouth breathing, snoring at night and periods in the night where the child actually stops breathing for short spells. This leads to episodes of hypoxia and may have associated cardiovascular implications. Although the parents often think that the child is sleeping well and is in a deep sleep because of the excessive snoring, the sleep pattern is in fact grossly disturbed and the children are often irritable the next day, they may be somnolent, and performance at school may be affected. The association between enlarged adenoids and Eustachian-tube dysfunction remains controversial, but a substantial number of children with enlarged adenoids do have secretory otitis media (glue ear). Children with a problem of enlarged adenoids and some or all of these symptoms should seek specialist opinion.

Treatment: If symptoms are severe with the complications mentioned above, operation is usually necessary. The operation is called adenoidectomy and may or may not be associated with tonsillectomy if enlarged tonsils are also contributing to the obstruction of the upper airway.

POLYPI: Nasal polyps are growths of soft, jelly-like character, with more or less of a stalk, usually arising from the ethmoid and maxillary sinuses, but they may also grow from the middle nasal turbinate. They arise from chronic inflammation associated with allergic rhinitis, chronic sinusitis, asthma and aspirin abuse. This chronic inflammation leads to oedema or swelling of the mucous membrane of the nose and paranasal sinuses which becomes so extensive as to produce polypi.

Treatment: When polyps become extremely large they can cause erosion of the nasal bones and should therefore generally be removed. Limited success has been reported using inhaled steroids in the nose, in that the polyps may regress, but this is, as yet, unproved and generally polyps are treated by surgical removal. Removal may be performed under local anaesthetic but is more commonly performed under general anaesthesia. Malignant tumours are occasionally found growing in the nose but are very rare. When they do occur, they are hard in texture and are unlike the soft nasal polyps mentioned above.

BLEEDING FROM THE NOSE, or EPISTAXIS (see HAEMORRHAGE).

FOREIGN BODIES At first the foreign body may set up no reaction and produce no symptoms but, in time, there will be obstruction of the affected nostril, with a foul-smelling discharge, which is often bloody from that side. The foreign body may remain in the nose for years until symptoms are noticed, but the presence of a unilateral foul-smelling bloody discharge should always alert one to the possible presence of a foreign body.

Treatment: Foreign bodies require removal. This may be done by the general practitioner but, if any difficulty is encountered in removing the foreign body, specialist referral should be sought. It may be possible to remove the foreign body with the patient awake but, in some cases, a general anaesthetic may be necessary.

LOSS OF SENSE OF SMELL, or ANOSMIA may be temporary or permanent. Temporary anosmia is caused by conditions of the nose which are reversible, whereas permanent anosmia is caused by conditions which destroy the olefactory nerves. Temporary conditions are those such as the common cold, or other inflammatory conditions of the nasal mucosa or the presence of nasal polyps. Permanent anosmia may follow and influenzal neuritis or it may also follow injuries to the brain and fractures of the skull involving the olfactory nerves.

SINUSITIS is of fairly frequent occurrence and most commonly follows an upper-respiratory-tract infection involving the nose and paranasal sinuses. The maxillary sinus is the sinus most commonly prone to sinus infection, followed by the ethmoid sinuses, then the frontal sinuses and, finally, the cells of the sphenoid sinus. Maxillary sinusitis may also arise from dental infection if the roots of the upper teeth penetrate into the floor of that sinus.

Symptoms: When suppuration occurs in the *frontal sinuses*, severe headache is apt to result as well as discharge from the nose. When suppuration takes place in the *sphenoidal sinuses*, there is constant purulent discharge either from the nose or into the throat, and there may be a state of general debility, or inflammatory changes may be set up in the eye or its optic nerve, which lie in close relation to these sinuses. The effects of a collection of pus in the *maxillary sinus*, or antrum, may be very slight; intermittent pain of a neuralgic character often felt above one eye, tooth-ache and slight swelling of one cheek may be the only signs for a long time. Generally, however, attention is called to the nose by a slight intermittent discharge of matter from one nostril, especially when the head is laid upon the opposite side.

Treatment: Sinusitis is generally treated by the administration of antibiotics and decongestants. Topical decongestants are of more benefit than systemic decongestants, as these help to open the sinus openings and facilitate drainage of the affected sinus. In more severe cases, it may be necessary to drain the sinus through an opening made between the sinus and the nose. This is done by an ear, nose and throat surgeon and may be performed under local or general anaesthesia. At this procedure pus is aspirated from the affected sinus and the sinus then washed out with warm water. Should the infection in the maxillary sinus be of dental origin, the offending tooth should be dealt with. In severe cases of frontal sinusitis, associated with orbital complications, a frontal sinus trephine is performed. This is done under general anaesthetic and involves making an incision above the eye. Drainage of the sphenoid sinus is also performed under general anaesthetic.

NOSOLOGY is the term applied to scientific classification of diseases.

NOSOPHOBE is a person who has a morbid fear of contracting a certain disease.

NOSTALGIA means a form of melancholy or aggravated home-sickness occurring in persons who have left their home.

NOTIFIABLE DISEASES are diseases, usually of an infectious nature, which are required by law to be made known to a health officer or local authority. (See INFECTION.) Certain occupational diseases (qv) are also notifiable.

Notifiable Diseases as at 1 October 1988

Under the Public Health (Control of Disease) Act 1984:
Cholera
Plague
Relapsing fever
Smallpox
Typhus

Under the Public Health (Infectious Diseases) Regulations 1988:
Acute encephalitis
Acute poliomyelitis
Anthrax
Diphtheria
Dysentery (amoebic or bacillary)
Leprosy
Leptospirosis
Malaria
Measles
Meningitis
Meningiococcal septicaemia (without meningitis)
Mumps
Ophthalmia neonatorum
Paratyphoid fever
Rabies
Rubella
Scarlet fever
Tetanus
Tuberculosis
Typhoid fever
Viral haemorrhagic fever
Viral hepatitis
Whooping cough
Yellow fever

NOVOBIOCIN is an antibiotic derived from cultures of *Streptomyces spheroides* or *Streptomyces niveus.* It is particularly active against staphylococci, and has proved especially useful in the treatment of staphylococcal infections which have not responded to treatment with other antibiotics, or in which the causative micro-organism is resistant to such antibiotics.

NUCHA is the Latin name for the back of the neck.

NUCLEAR MAGNETIC RESONANCE is a new method of scanning the body which is promising to be more reliable than X-rays in detecting abnormalities in the soft tissues of the body. It is based on the fact that certain types of atomic nuclei, including those in living tissue, give off an identifiable signal when placed in a strong magnetic field and energized by radio waves. These signals reveal the dispersion of body fluids and fats, and thereby are of value in detecting, for example, intra-abdominal tumours, as in the liver. It is also proving of value in pin-pointing diseases in the brain and spinal cord, such as multiple sclerosis. One of its practical advantages, compared with X-rays, is that it does no harm to the tissues of the body, as X-rays can do unless used with discrimination. (See X-RAYS.)

NUCLEAR MEDICINE is that branch of medicine that is concerned with the use of radioactive material in the diagnosis, investigation and treatment of disease.

NUCLEIC ACID is a substance constructed out of units known as nucleotides which consist of a purine or pyrimidine base linked to a pentose sugar which in turn is esterified with phosphoric acid. Two types of nucleic acid occur in nature: deoxyribonucleic acid (DNA) and ribonucleic acid (RNA). (See DNA; RNA.)

NUCLEUS means the central body in a cell, which controls the activities of the latter. (See CELL.)

NUCLEUS PULPOSUS is the inner core of an intervertebral disc. (See SPINAL COLUMN.)

NULLIPARA is the term applied to a woman who has never borne a child.

NUMBNESS (see TOUCH).

NUMMULAR SPUTUM is expectoration which when spat into water flattens out into a shape like coins. (See EXPECTORATION.)

NURSING as a profession requires an elaborate training, although people are often called upon to nurse relatives and friends without any previous experience of the subject.

Professional nursing falls into four divisions: (*a*) *Hospital nursing*, which forms a training for all the other kinds of nursing. (*b*) *Private nursing*, ie. nursing of a single patient, to whom the nurse's undivided attention is given, at home. (*c*) *District nursing*, which is the most arduous, and requires the greatest skill in the nurse. In this type of nursing, patients are visited at home, and not only a long and varied training but great self-reliance are required. (*d*) *Midwifery nursing*, which includes the care of mother and child for about a month after the latter is born. Full details about openings in nursing, details of training and of training schools can be obtained from the Royal College of Nursing, 20 Cavendish Square, London W1M 0AB (01-409 3333). The Nurses, Midwives and Health Visitors Act 1979 provides for the establishment of a United Kingdom Central Council and four National Boards for nursing, midwifery and health visiting. The Central Council, supported by the Boards, will eventually assume sole responsibility for registration and the setting and maintaining of standards of education and of conduct of nurses, midwives and health visitors throughout the United Kingdom. There is to be a handover period before the Act comes into force.

NURSING-BOTTLE MOUTH is the state of rampant caries of the teeth induced in children who are allowed to suck a bottle when put to bed at night or in their prams during the day. While the caries is more likely to occur if the 'comforter bottle', as it is popularly known, contains a sweetened drink, as it all too often does, it may also occur if the contents are milk. The reason for this is that with the child lying down the drink, whatever it is, is not swallowed promptly but tends to remain in the mouth and thus damage the teeth. This bottle-induced caries is most likely to occur in children who are allowed to engage in this pernicious habit after they have been weaned on to an ordinary diet. In no circumstances should a 'comforter bottle' be used. The same applies to the so-called comforter or dummy. By itself it is not as dangerous as the comforter bottle but, if sweetened, it is truly 'accursed' and should never be used by any parent who has any respect for her (or his) children. (See also TEETH, DISEASES OF.)

NUTS, which consist to the extent of one-half or more of vegetable fat, form a highly concentrated form of nourishment, and if suitably prepared, for example, by roasting to render them more digestible, become of higher nourishing value than cheese, and may to a considerable extent act as substitutes for meat.

NUX VOMICA is the seed of *Strychnos nux-vomica*, an East Indian tree. It has an intensely bitter taste. The medicinal properties of the plant are almost entirely due to two alkaloids, strychnine and brucine, which it contains. (See STRYCHNINE.)

NYCTALOPIA: Technical term for night blindness.

NYSTAGMUS (see EYE, DISEASE AND INJURY OF).

NYSTATIN is an antibiotic isolated from *Streptomyces noursei*. It was the first antibiotic to be isolated which was active against fungus diseases, and is proving particularly useful in the treatment of moniliasis (qv).

O

OBESITY is a condition of the body characterized by over-accumulation of fat under the skin and around certain of the internal organs.

Causes: Various causes are assigned for the production of obesity. Thus, in some instances it may be due to disturbances of some of the endocrine glands, such as the thyroid, pituitary and sex glands. In some families there appears to be a hereditary predisposition to an obese habit of body, upon which precautions in living seem to have little effect. But, beyond this, it is unquestionable that certain habits favour the occurrence of corpulence.

An inactive or sedentary life is a well-recognized predisposing cause. The more immediate exciting causes are overfeeding and the large use of fluids of any kind, but especially alcohol. Fat people are not always great eaters, although many of them are; while again, leanness and inordinate appetite are not infrequently associated. Still, it may be stated generally that indulgence in food beyond what is requisite to repair daily waste goes towards the increase of fat. This is more especially the case when the non-nitrogenous (the fatty, sugary and starchy) elements of the food are in excess. It is generally held that the fat of the body is mainly, if not entirely, formed from these foods, while nitrogenous foods (proteins) increase oxidation and lead to tissue waste. Alcohol, when taken to a considerable extent, also tends to the formation of fat, partly because many drinks, eg. beer, contain much sugar, and partly no doubt because a portion of the body heat is derived from the alcohol and a corresponding amount of the starchy and sugary food spared and converted into fat.

Women are more prone to become corpulent than men, and appear to take on this condition more readily after having borne a child, and after the cessation of menstruation.

In young people excessive weight is sometimes associated with defective action of some of the endocrine glands, especially the pituitary and thyroid glands. In slighter cases of such defect the gland usually gains its full development as life advances, and the corpulence passes off when adult age is reached.

Defective muscular exertion has been mentioned as a cause of obesity, but it is sometimes observed that stout men, when they begin to take active exercise, become fatter still, the reason being that the appetite is sharpened and still more food is taken.

It is rare for obesity to have an established endocrine basis, although most patients insists that their problem is metabolic. However, formal studies of food intake support the view that obese subjects do not eat more than lean subjects and this applies to adults, adolescents and children. Obesity tends to be familial and the normal-weight children of obese patients tend to eat less calories than their lean counterparts. Apart from physical exercise there are three components of energy expenditure: (1) the basal metabolic rate; (2) non-shivering thermogenesis; (3) luxus comsumption (post-prandial thermogenesis). The basal metabolic rate is concerned with the synthetic activities of the body such as protein synthesis, the mechanical working of the body such as the pumping of the heart, and the osmotic processes of the body that keep the sodium out of cells and the potassium within the cells. The basal metabolic rate accounts for 60 per cent of daily energy expenditure. Non-shivering thermogenesis is the means of producing heat by the release of chemical energy through processes which do not involve muscular contraction, ie. shivering. Obese individuals have a reduced drive for non-shivering thermogenesis and when exposed to cold their body temperature falls more than with lean individuals. The term luxux consumption was introduced over 80 years ago by Neumann to describe the dissipation of excess heat on over-feeding. He maintained his weight constant over a three-year period despite increasing his daily energy intake from 1766 kcal/day to 2403 kcal/day. The excess energy was dissipated by increasing heat production. It appears that obese subjects have a lower luxus consumption than lean ones and therefore gain weight more easily when over-eating. There is also little doubt that physical exercise enhances diet-induced thermogenesis and probably non-shivering thermogenesis as well.

Symptoms: Health cannot be long maintained with excessive obesity, for the increase in bulk of the body, rendering exercise more difficult, leads to relaxation and defective nutrition of muscle, while the accumulations of fat in the chest and abdomen occasion embarrassment to the functions of the various organs in these cavities. In general, the mental activity of the highly corpulent becomes impaired, although there have always been notable exceptions to this rule.

The corpulent are at least as liable as the spare to be attacked by acute diseases, and they succumb much more readily to them than do the latter. Diabetes mellitus, gall-stones, gout, arterial disease, high blood-pressure and varicose veins are all more common in the obese individual. Various skin conditions, such as eczema, and particularly a chafed and painful condition of the skin at folds where two surfaces meet (see CHAFING), are also troublesome. It is therefore not surprising that the corpulent have a poor expectation of life. Life insurance statistics show that an increase of 11 kg (25 pounds) above standard weight reduces the life expectancy of a man of 45 by 25 per cent. This means that he is likely to die at 60, whereas he might have expected to live until 80 if he had not been obese.

Treatment: When the obesity is due to myxoedema (qv), excellent results are obtained from the administration of thyroxine, but this form of treatment should not be used for the treatment of obesity except under careful medical supervision.

Of far greater importance than any drugs is the question of the regulation diet, exercise and sleep. Rapid loss of weight is apt to be attended with serious impairment of health, and, generally speaking, it is not advisable to aim at losing weight at a greater rate than about 1·4 or 1·8 kg (3 or 4 pounds) in each week.

Various Continental spas have elaborate courses of treatment, in which rigid rules are laid down. Since a person submits himself more easily to, and obeys more implicitly, the rules in these places than he would do at home, such a 'cure' is attended with special benefit.

Unless the individual is grossly overweight it is inadvisable to reduce weight too rapidly. Provided the diet is carefully adhered to, it is seldom necessary to give a diet containing less than 1000 to 1200 Cal. Fats and carbohydrates must be reduced as much as possible. This means that sugar, sweets, jams, tinned fruit, potatoes and fried food must be banned. It is advisable to exclude all alcohol, but if the individual is so used to these that complete abstinence would be a real hardship, then a little dry wine may be allowed. Beer, sweet wines, spirits and aerated waters must not be taken. Items which can be partaken of freely include green vegetables (salad dressings must be made with vinegar or lemon juice, *not* olive oil), coffee (without milk), tea and clear soups. Saccharine, of course, can be used freely for sweetening purposes.

Exercise should be abundant, and clothing should be light when an attempt is made to reduce corpulence, but care must be taken that the food is not at the same time increased to satisfy the sharpened appetite, or the effect of exercise is defeated. Sleep is a matter of importance. The person should go to bed early, and should limit the duration of rest to seven or at most eight hours, while the habit of sleeping during the day should be broken off.

In the grossly obese individual who fails to respond to any other form of treatment, a reduction in weight may be obtained by an operation in which a large section of the small intestine is by-passed, thereby reducing the amount of food that is absorbed into the body. A similar operation is being used to by-pass the stomach. The results, however, are far from impressive, and the procedure is not without its hazards to life and health. Surgical treatment is always the last resort and should not be used in patients who have not consistently dieted for a minimum of five years. Other less drastic measures being used are dental splintage, which is safe but not very effective, and inserting balloons in the stomach to reduce its capacity.

In no circumstances should so-called 'slimming drugs' be taken except under medical supervision. Such appetite suppressant drugs do not replace dietary control. They are merely supplementary and for use in individuals who are grossly overweight, and whose weight is not responding to a controlled diet.

OBSESSION in medicine means the sudden domination of the mind by an idea or emotion, leading to impulsive acts which are beyond the control of the will, the power of judgment being for a time lost. (See MENTAL ILLNESS.)

OBSTETRICS means the art of midwifery. (See LABOUR.)

OBSTRUCTION OF THE BOWELS (see INTESTINE, DISEASES OF).

OCCIPUT is the lower and hinder part of the head where it merges into the neck.

OCCUPATIONAL DISEASES: The increasing complexity of industrial and manufacturing processes, and the large proportion of the population of the country who are employed in industry, render occupational or industrial diseases of increasing importance. Whenever a new process is introduced into industry every care should be taken to ensure that it will involve no hazards to those employed in it. Even so, it is not always possible to foresee all possible risks, and therefore the management and the industrial medical officer must always be on the look-out so as to be able to detect any such hazard at the earliest possible stage before irreparable harm is done to the health of men or women handling the process. In many cases freedom from the hazards to health inherent in industrial or manufacturing processes is, in part at least, dependent upon the active cooperation of workers and involves such simple procedures as the wearing of respirators, careful washing of the hands before eating, the application of barrier creams to the hands and arms, and the like. The obtaining of such cooperation is one of the main aims of efficient industrial management at the present day. The magnitude of the problem involved can be gathered from the fact that it is estimated that there are about 2000 diseases which can be attributed to an individual's occupation. It says much therefore for the efficiency of the precautionary measures, and the care and skill with which they are employed, that there are so relatively few industrial diseases in any given year in such a highly industrialized country as Great Britain.

The Health and Safety Commission is charged with taking appropriate steps to secure the health, safety and welfare of people at work, to protect the public generally against risks to health and safety arising out of the work situation, and to give general direction to the Health and Safety Executive which is its main operative arm. The Health and Safety Executive includes six executives: Alkali and Clear Air; Factories; Mines and Quarries; Nuclear Installations; Explosives; and Agriculture. It also includes the Employment Medical Advisory Service under the direction of the Director of Medical Services. This is an organization of doctors and nurses who give advice about occupational health and examine suspected health hazards at work.

Although many industrial diseases entitle the victims to compensation, only a few are compulsorily notifiable. The following are the diseases which, if contracted in a factory, must be notified by the medical practitioner to the Chief Inspector of Factories: poisoning by lead, phosphorus, manganese, arsenic, mercury, carbon bisulphide, and aniline; chronic benzene poisoning, toxic jaundice, anthrax, epitheliomatous ulceration, chrome ulceration, compressed air illness, byssinosis, asbestosis, nasal adenocarcinoma, and toxic anaemia.

Lead is used widely throughout industry, and the following are some of the occupations in which it constitutes a hazard to health unless adequate precautions are taken: smelting, plumbing and soldering, shipbreaking, printing, pottery industry, painting. In the case of pottery and printing the risk has been almost entirely eliminated by the use of modern methods. The lead salts used in industry which are most dangerous to health are the oxide, the carbonate, and the chromate. The lead usually enters the body by the inhalation of dust or fumes. One of the practical difficulties in detecting and preventing lead poisoning is that it is often insidious in onset. (See LEAD POISONING.)

Phosphorus has practically been eliminated as a cause of industrial poisoning in Great Britain. The first cases to be reported in this country since 1919 occurred during the 1939–45 War – one in 1941 and 1944. Yellow and white phosphorus are the dangerous forms. The red phosphorus used in the making of safety matches is relatively harmless. The match industry, in the days when white phosphorus was used for this purpose, was the classical source of phosphorus poisoning. The phosphorus gained admission through abrasions in the gums and caused destruction of the jaw, the condition known as phossy jaw. Luminous paints are another potential source of danger, principally when used to paint luminous watch dials. (See PHOSPHORUS POISONING.)

Manganese is not a common cause of industrial disease, but it is important because the results are so serious. It affects the brain and causes a condition very like post-encephalitic Parkinsonism (qv) and leaves the victim a permanent invalid. The dioxide is the dangerous salt, and the risk occurs in the handling of manganese ore, or in the handling of manganese dioxide itself, from exposure to the dust.

Arsenic is encountered in industry in the smelting and refining of ores, the subliming of white arsenic, and the manufacture of sheep dip and Paris green. White arsenic is used as a preservative of furs, hides, and skins, whilst Paris green is used as an insecticide for fruit trees. Poisoning from arsenic in industry usually results from inhalation of, or contact with, the dust of arsenic compounds, and results in eczema and neuritis. Occasionally it takes a more serious and acute form, when it results from the inhalation of arseniuretted hydrogen. (See ARSENIC; NEURITIS.)

Mercury constitutes an industrial hazard in three forms: (i) exposure to the dust or vapour of metallic mercury; (ii) contact with mercury fulminate; (iii) exposure to organic mercury compounds. The industries or processes in which exposure to mercury may occur include: mercury mining and the separation of the metal from the ore; the manufacture of barometers, thermometers, and certain types of electric bulbs; water gilding; the felt-hat industry; dental technicians. Mercury fulminate is used in the making of explosives, and is particularly liable to attack the skin. Organic mercury compounds are mainly used in the manufacture of seed dressings and fungicides, and in the pharmaceutical industry. (See MERCURY POISONING.)

Carbon bisulphide, for long used in the cold curing of rubber and as a solvent for rubber, oil, and fats, has in more recent years been used in large amounts in the manufacture of certain forms of artificial silk. One of its dangers is that it vaporizes at ordinary temperatures, and the breathing of 1150 parts per million parts of air for 30 to 60 minutes is dangerous. Its main

Cause	*Occupation*	*Disease*
Coal dust	Coal mining	Coal-workers' pneumoconiosis
Silica	Gold mining Iron and steel industries (metal casting) Metal grinding Stone dressing Pottery	Silicosis
Asbestos	Asbestos mining Manufacture of fireproof and insulating materials	Asbestosis
Iron oxide	Arc welding	Siderosis
Tin dioxide	Tin ore mining	Stannosis
Beryllium	Aircraft and atomic energy industries	Berylliosis
Cotton, flax or hemp dust	Textile industries	Byssinosis
Fungal spores from mouldy hay, straw or grain, bagasse, mushroom compost	Agriculture and related industries	Farmer's lung Metalworker's lung Bagassosis Mushroom worker's lung

Some occupational lung diseases. Davidson and Macleod.

effect is upon the nervous system: neuritis, anxiety, depression, and impairment of memory.

Aniline is used in a wide variety of industrial processes: dyeing, painting, varnishing, rubber processing, and the manufacture of dyes, explosives, pharmaceutical products, and photographic chemicals. Absorption takes place mainly through the skin but may also occur through the lungs. The chief early manifestation of poisoning is a greyish-blue colour of the skin followed by shortness of breath. In chronic cases anaemia develops.

Benzene, a coal-tar derivative, is used on a large scale: the distillation of coal tar, the blending of motor fuels, and in the chemical industry. It is also used as a solvent in the rubber, aeroplane, linoleum, and celluloid industries and in the manufacture of paints, varnishes, glue, and artificial fertilizer. The main manifestation of chronic benzene poisoning is anaemia due to a toxic effect of the benzene upon the bone marrow. Benzene is absorbed by inhalation.

Cadmium may cause disease in two different ways. Its fumes, encountered in melting cadmium or cadmium alloy, or from the use of cadmium electrodes, and the manufacture of ceramics, may cause an influenza-like illness, with shortness of breath, cough, irritation of the throat and sickness. Cadmium oxide dust produces diarrhoea, pneumonitis (qv) and proteinuria (qv). There may be a long period between exposure to cadmium and the first signs of poisoning by it. There is some evidence that there may be an increased incidence of cancer of the prostate and the lung in workmen occupationally exposed to cadmium. (See CADMIUM.)

Nitrobenzene is used in the manufacture of aniline dyes and explosives, and is a constituent of shoe and floor polish. It is also used as a perfume in cheap soaps. The main route of absorption is through the skin. It acts upon the nervous system, causing headache, giddiness, and numbness in the limbs, and upon the blood, causing anaemia and cyanosis.

Dinitrobenzene, which is used in the manufacture of dyes and explosives, is absorbed through the skin. Its principal toxic effect is upon the blood, resulting in cyanosis, which manifests itself by a blue discoloration of the skin. It also causes anaemia.

Trinitrotoluene, better known as TNT, is used in the making of explosives. It is mainly absorbed through the skin, and causes dermatitis, jaundice, and anaemia.

Chrome, used in chromium plating, attacks the skin, causing dermatitis. It also attacks the septum of the nose, leading to chrome ulceration and perforation of the septum. It is the cartilaginous part of the septum and not the bone which is attacked.

Toxic jaundice may be caused by trinitrotoluene, tetrachloroethane, arseniuretted hydrogen, carbon tetrachloride, and certain benzene derivatives.

Epitheliomatous ulceration, a form of cancer, may arise among workers with tar, pitch, bitumen, or mineral oil. The best known form is mule-spinner's cancer.

Anthrax may occur among workers in wool, hides, and hair infected with the anthrax bacillus. The infection may be acquired through the skin, where it causes the so-called malignant pustule, or through the lungs by breathing in the bacillus, when pulmonary anthrax results. Its incidence among people handling infected wool gave rise to the name woolsorters' disease. (See ANTHRAX.)

Brucellosis is the disease caused by *Brucella abortus*, the micro-organism responsible for contagious abortion in cattle. It is a disease therefore to which farm workers, veterinary surgeons and abattoir workers are particularly susceptible. (See BRUCELLOSIS.)

Occupational asthma is asthma which develops after a period of symptomless exposure to a sensitizing agent encountered at work. Workers who suffer from occupational asthma are able to claim industrial injuries benefits provided this is due to one of the following groups of agents: platinum salts, isocyanates, epoxy resin curing agents, colophony fumes, proteolytic enzymes (eg biological washing powders), animals and insects in laboratories, dusts arising from milling or handling flour (eg baker's asthma), from harvesting, drying, transporting and storing grains. (See ASTHMA.)

Viral hepatitis is an inflammatory disease of the liver caused by a virus. Industrial injuries benefits are now payable to employees whose work brings them into close and frequent contact with human blood, human blood products or patients with viral hepatitis. The majority of people affected will be employed in the health sector, particularly doctors, nurses, laboratory technicians and similar groups of workers. (See HEPATITIS.)

Polymer fume fever is an influenza-like illness that occurs in people who work with polytetrafluoroethylene (Teflon). (See POLYMER FUME FEVER.)

Pneumoconioses: This is a group of diseases of the lungs due to the inhalation of dust. The most important dust in this connection is silica. The resulting disease is known as silicosis (qv). Other diseases in this category are asbestosis (qv), bagassosis (qv), berylliosis (qv), byssinosis (qv), siderosis (qv), stannosis (qv), and farmer's lung (qv).

Asbestosis is a form of pneumoconiosis, but its main hazard is the risk of cancer of the lung or pleura, or sometimes of the ovary. It is caused by the inhalation of asbestos dust, either in the mining or quarrying of it, or in one of the many industries in which it is used: eg. as an insulating material, in the making of paper, cardboard and brake linings. (See ASBESTOSIS.)

Byssinosis is another form of pneumoconiosis, caused by the inhalation of dust in textile factories. (See BYSSINOSIS.)

Kaolinosis is a form of pneumoconiosis caused by the inhalation of clay dust.

Nasal adenocarcinorna is a form of cancer of the nose, and sometimes of the associated air sinuses, that sometimes develops in workers making wooden furniture.

Vinyl chloride, which is used to make polyvinyl chloride, one of the most widely used plastics today, is known to cause a rare form of cancer of the liver (angiosarcoma), and it may possibly cause cancer elsewhere in the body. There is a long period between first exposure to vinyl chloride and the diagnosis of cancer: 12 to 29 years in one series of cases. It can also cause a non-malignant disease of the liver (non-cirrhotic portal cirrhosis) and an unusual finger condition (acro-osteolysis).

Tungsten carbide, which is used in metal machining and metal working, may cause a disease characterized by cough, shortness of breath and tightness of the chest. (See HARD METAL DISEASE.)

Dermatitis is now one of the most important industrial diseases. It may be caused by a wide variety of agents, including alkalis, oil, petrol, paraffin, French polish, various chemicals. Its importance lies in the fact that, with reasonable care, it can often be avoided, or, if it be detected early, it responds well to treatment. On the other hand, if allowed to persist for any length of time, it may become resistant to all but one form of treatment: ie. change of occupation to one in which the individual will not come into contact with the offending substance. Preventive measures ensure adequate washing facilities and their full use by all workpeople exposed to risk; maximum cleanliness at work, which reduces the risk of the individual coming into contact with the offending substance; the wearing of protective clothing; the use of barrier creams where this is possible. (See DERMATITIS.)

Cramps and paralyses: Cramps may occur in individuals whose work involves repeated use of the same groups of muscles. Perhaps the best known example of this is *writer's cramp*. Another example is *twister's cramp* which occurs in the cotton and woollen industries among those whose job is the twisting of cotton or woollen yarns. Although in a somewhat different category, reference may also be made here to the painful condition which develops in the arms of those handling *powerful pneumatic tools*. It is liable to be accompanied by insomnia and tremors. No effective treatment is known.

Miner's nystagmus is a distressing condition, characterized by persistent uncontrollable movements of the eye, which occurs in coalminers. It is now generally accepted that the main cause is inadequate illumination; the introduction of adequate lighting into mines has gone far towards reducing its incidence. (See NYSTAGMUS.)

Compressed air illness, formerly known as caisson disease, occurs in divers and in those who work in caissons. It is due to the affected individuals being decompressed, or returned to atmospheric pressure, too quickly. Divers and caisson workers work under high pressures, and if this pressure is reduced too quickly, bubbles of nitrogen are released in the body which cause pain in various areas – usually muscles or joints. These painful areas are known as bends. Adherence to official decompression tables should prevent such accidents, but when they do occur, the treatment consists of recompression until the pain goes, followed by slow decompression.

Radiation-induced diseases include heat cataract in workers with frequent or prolonged exposure to rays from molten or red-hot metal. They also include a disease characterized by inflammation, ulceration or malignant disease of the skin or subcutaneous tissues or of the bones, a blood disorder, or cataract, due to electro-magnetic radiations (other than radiant heat), or to ionising particles.

OCCUPATIONAL THERAPY is the treatment of physical and psychiatric conditions through specific selected activities in order to help people reach their maximum level of function and independence in all aspects of daily life.

Occupational therapists work from hospital and community bases. They do much more than keep patients occupied with diverting hobbies. The arts and crafts still have a place in modern therapy techniques but these now also include household chores, industrial work, communication techniques, social activities, sports and educational programmes. An Occupational Therapy Department may have facilities for woodwork, metalwork, printing, gardening, cooking, art and drama. Occupational therapists will use any combination of activities to strengthen muscles, increase movement and restore co-ordination and balance. With mentally ill people similar activies are used. They help provide order, comfort and support and aim to build up self-confidence. Occupational therapists plan courses of treatment which are individually tailored to the needs of the patient. The aim is to help the patient practise all the activites involved in daily life. The therapists are part of a team including doctors, nurses, social workers, home helps, housing officers, physiotherapists, speech therapists and psychologists. Occupational therapists are mainly employed by the National Health Service and by Local Authority Social Services and they work in hospitals, special centres and in the handicapped person's own home. State Registration is essential for employment as an occupational therapists. There are 15 occupational therapy schools in the United Kingdom where the course leading to the diploma of the College of Occupational Therapists can be followed. The course lasts three academic years. (See REHABILITATION; REMPLOY.)

OCHRONOSIS is a rare condition in which the ligaments and cartilages of the body, and sometimes the conjunctiva, become stained by dark brown or black pigment. This may occur in chronic carbolic poisoning, or in a congenital disorder of metabolism in which the individual is unable to break down completely the tyrosine of the protein molecule, the intermediate product, homogentisic acid, appearing in the urine – this being known as alkaptonuria.

OEDEMA means an abnormal accumulation of fluid beneath the skin, or in one or more of the cavities of the body.

Causes: Oedema is not a disease, although this is a popular idea, supported by the fact that at one time many deaths were recorded as due to 'dropsy' without a further statement of the cause. Oedema may be due to one of three conditions: (1) weakening of the walls of the capillary vessels, by injury of the part in which oedema occurs, by ill-health of the body generally, by poverty of the blood circulating through and nourishing the vessels, or by poisonous materials in the blood; (2) obstruction to the blood-flow through the veins; (3) a watery condition of the blood allowing fluid to escape through the capillary walls. Oedema may also result from obstruction to the flow of lymph in the lymph channels.

Heart disease, which produces increased pressure in the veins, and also an impaired circulation of the blood, in consequence of the defective pumping action of the heart, and *glomerulonephritis* in which the kidneys fail in their functions of excreting poisonous substances and a certain amount of water from the blood, are the main causes of general oedema. In heart disease the oedema is more marked after exertion; in kidney disease it is found chiefly after resting. Thus one of the chief characters of oedema due to glomerulonephritis is that it appears in the morning, affects loose tissues like the skin beneath the eyes, and passes off as the day advances. Oedema due to heart disease, on the other hand, tends to appear towards evening, affects dependent parts like the feet, and diminishes during the night.

In *hunger oedema* due to diminution of the amount of protein in the blood as a result of starvation, the oedema is generalized, but in the earlier stages is most marked in the feet and legs, especially after exertion. The swelling which sometimes follows snake bites, beestings or the eating of poisonous shell-fish, and constitutes an extreme and rapidly ensuing form of *nettle-rash*, is a special variety of oedema. *White-leg*, which may appear after some acute disease like typhoid fever or pneumonia, or after the birth of a child, due to a thrombosis or plugging of the main vein in the affected limb, is one of the localized forms of oedema. A similar condition may be caused by a *tumour* pressing upon a large vein of the arm or leg. Oedema in the legs may be due to varicose veins. *Cirrhosis*, tumours, and other diseases of the liver may, by interference with the circulation through it, cause oedema, first of the abdomen and later of the lower limbs.

Treatment: There is no general treatment which will meet every case. The particular cause has, in each case, to be removed. Oedema due to heart or kidney disease yields as the disease producing it is alleviated. In cases of localized oedema, elevation of the oedematous part is of great importance, and the person should adopt the recumbent position. In the case of heart disease, digitalis, which improves the action of the heart, and benzothiadiazine diuretics form the chief means employed. In acute kidney disease the treatment of the oedema consists in the routine treatment of glomerulonephritis. In oedema due to liver conditions, occasional purges with blue-pill or calomel may help the condition. When the oedema will not yield to drugs, some of the fluid may have to be drawn off (see ASPIRATION); when this is done partially, the kidneys are sometimes enabled to cope with the remainder of the fluid.

OEDEMA OF THE LUNGS results when the left ventricle myocardium is unable to handle the blood delivered to it. There is an abrupt increase in the venous and capillary pressure in the pulmonary vessels followed by flooding of fluid into the interstitial spaces and alveoli. The commonest cause of acute pulmonary oedema is myocardial infarction which reduces the ability of the left ventricular myocardial muscle to handle the blood delivered to it. Pulmonary oedema may result from other causes of left ventricular failure such as hypertension or valvular disease of the mitral and aortic valves. The initial symptoms are cough with breathlessness and occasionally with wheezing. The patient becomes extremely short of breath with a sensation of imminent death. In a severe attack the patient is pale, sweating and cyanosed and obviously gasping for breath. Frequently frothy sputum is produced which may be blood stained.

OESOPHAGOSCOPE is an instrument constructed on the principle of the telescope, which is passed down the oesophagus and enables the observer to see the state of the oesophagus. (See FIBROSCOPE.)

OESOPHAGUS, or GULLET, is the tube which conveys the food and drink from the throat down to the stomach. It begins above at the level of the sixth cervical vertebra, and, lying close against the left side and front of the spinal column, passes downward through the neck and chest to pierce the diaphragm, and then opens into the stomach. It consists of three coats: a strong outer coat of muscle fibres in two layers, the outer running lengthwise, the inner being circular; inside this a loose connective tissue coat containing blood-vessels, glands, and nerves; and finally a strong mucous membrane lined by epithelium, which closely resembles that of the mouth and skin.

OESOPHAGUS, DISEASES OF: The oesophagus, or gullet, may be the seat of catarrhal or inflammatory conditions causing discomfort in swallowing, but the more important ailments are those which arise from local injuries, such as the swallowing of scalding or corrosive substances. This may cause ulceration followed by the formation of a scar which narrows the passage and produces the symptoms of *stricture* of the oesophagus: namely, pain and difficulty in swallowing, with regurgitation of the food. In all cases of organic stricture the food does not necessarily return at once, but seems as if it has passed into the stomach. In reality, however, it has passed into the dilated or pouched portion of the gullet, which is almost always present immediately above the seat of stricture, where it remains until, from its amount, it regurgitates back into the mouth, when it can be seen, by the absence of any evidence of digestion, that it has never been in the stomach. The severity of the case will necessarily depend upon the amount of narrowing and consequent mechanical obstruction, but in some instances this has occurred to such an extent as practically to close the canal. Cases of oesophageal stricture of this kind may sometimes be dilated by the use of suitable instruments.

A still more serious and frequent cause of oesophageal stricture is that due to *cancer*, which may occur at any part, but is most common at the lower end, in the vicinity of the entrance into the stomach. The chief symptoms of this condition are increasing difficulty in the passage downwards of the food, steady decline in strength, together with enlargement of the glands in the neck. The diagnosis is rendered the more certain by the absence of any cause, such as local injury, for the formation of a stricture, and by the age (as a rule at or beyond middle life). Traditionally it is said to be much more common in men than women, but of the 3572 fatal cases in England in 1980, 1518 were in women, compared with 2054 in men. In many cases treatment can only be palliative, but recent advances in surgery are producing promising results. In some cases treatment with irradiation produces relief, if not cure. In those in whom neither operation nor radiation can be performed life may be prolonged and freedom from pain obtained by fluid food which is either swallowed or passed down a tube. The operation of gastrostomy, by which an opening is made through the front of the abdomen, allows food to be directly introduced into the stomach.

Strictures of the oesophagus may also be produced by the pressure of tumours or aneurysms within the cavity of the chest but external to the gullet.

An important cause of difficulty in swallowing is the condition known as *cardiospasm* or *achalasia of the cardia*. The latter is the more accurate description as the condition is due to failure of the cardiac sphincter (the sphincter at the lower end of the oesophagus) to relax when food is swallowed. The cause is not known. The condition occurs usually in young adults, who complain of food sticking behind the breastbone. This results in vomiting and, of course, loss of weight. Treatment consists of passing special bougies down the oesophagus to dilate the sphincter. As this may need to be done before every meal for several months, the patient learns to pass the bougie himself. Such treatment, though prolonged, is usually successful.

Finally, difficulty in swallowing sometimes occurs in certain serious nervous diseases from paralysis affecting the nerves supplying the muscular coats of the pharynx, which thus loses its propulsive power (*bulbar paralysis*). When such complications occur, they usually denote an advanced stage of the brain disease with which they are connected, and a speedily fatal termination.

Foreign bodies which lodge in the respiratory part of the throat, ie. at the entrance to, or in the cavity of, the larynx, set up immediate symptoms of choking. (See CHOKING.) Those which lodge in the gullet, on the contrary, do not usually set up any immediately serious symptoms, although their presence causes considerable discomfort. Such bodies are divided, for practical purposes, into two classes. One class includes smooth bodies like coins or fruit stones, which may be pushed down into the stomach or pulled up into the mouth by means of a bougie or a special instrument known as a coin-catcher, or, better still, by forceps passed down under the direct guidance of the oesophagoscope. The other, and more dangerous, class comprises bodies which are too large to be pushed down into the stomach and safely passed by the bowels, or too rough to be pulled back into the mouth, such as large pieces of bone, or large plates of artificial teeth. In cases in which it is impossible to dislodge a foreign body up or down, it becomes necessary to perform an operation in order to remove the body from the gullet directly through the side of the neck.

OESTRADIOL is the name given to the oestrogenic hormone secreted by the ovarian follicle. Oestradiol is responsible for the development of the female sexual characteristics, of the breasts, and of part of the changes that take place in the uterus before menstruation.

OESTRADIOL VACERATE (PROGYNOVA) (see OESTROGEN).

OESTRIOL (OVESTIN) (see OESTROGEN).

OESTROGEN is the term applied to any substance that will induce oestrus or 'heat'. In human medicine it is applied to the substances, natural or synthetic, that induce the changes in the uterus that precede ovulation. They are also responsible for the development of the secondary sex characteristics in women: that is the physical changes that take place in a girl at puberty, such as enlargement of the breasts, appearance of pubic and axillary hair and the deposition of fat on the thighs and hips. They are used in the management of disturbances of the menopause, and also in the treatment of cancer of the prostate and certain cases of cancer of the breast.

The oestrogenic hormones of the ovary are oestradiol and oestrone and they are interconvertible. The natural oestrogens, like the hormones of the testis and the adrenal cortex, are steroids. They are rapidly metabolized in the body and excreted in the urine as inactive conjugates. The rapid degradation of natural oestrogens limits their use as therapeutic agents. Chemical substitution of the steroid molecule, as in ethinyl oestradiol, or the use of a non-steroidal synthetic oestrogen such as stilboestrol, greatly reduces the rate of degradation and enhances the therapeutic action. A further development has been the use of compounds which are not actually oestrogenic themselves, but which are slowly metabolized to oestrogenic substances, or substances such as chlorotrianisene, which are taken up in the body fat and then slowly released into the circulation. There is in fact little to choose between the various synthetic oestrogens. Preparations such as equine oestrogens or chlorotrianisene have little therapeutic advantage and are considerably more expensive. Ethinyl oestradiol is the most potent oral oestrogen, being twenty times more active than stilboestrol.

The following oestrogens are in therapeutic use: chlorotrianisene (Trace), cyclofenil (Ondonid), cyproterone (Androcure), dinoestrol (Armo-noestrol), equine oestrogens (Premarin), ethinyl oestradiol (Lynoral), hexoestrol, methallenoestril (Vallestril), oestradiol valerate (Progynova), oestriol (Ovestin), oestrone, piperazine oestrone sulphate (Harmogen), quinestradol (Pentovis), stilboestrol (Pabestrol), stilboestrol diphosphate (Honvan), quinestrol (Estrovis).

OESTRONE (see OESTROGEN).

OFFICIAL is a term applied to drugs and preparations which are authorized by pharmacopoeias and other recognized lists.

OFFICINAL is a term applied to drugs and preparations which are regularly kept in stock for sale in chemists' shops.

OILS are divided into *fixed oils* and *volatile* or *essential oils*. FIXED OILS are of the nature of liquid fats composed of a fatty acid and glycerin: for example olive oil, which consists of a mixture of glycerin compounds of oleic acid and palmitic acid. Other examples of fixed oils are almond oil, linseed oil, and cod-liver oil. Fixed oils are used as foods, and in large quantities as mild aperients. Some fixed oils have important special properties by virtue of active principles that they contain: for example castor oil, which acts as a purgative. Fixed oils are obtained from the fruits or seeds of plants or from animal tissues by pressure, or by boiling with water and skimming off the melted oil. Fats are fixed oils which are solid at ordinary temperatures and are extracted by combination of heat and pressure. An example of an animal fat is lard, and of a vegetable fat, cocoa butter. Fixed oils can be dissolved in ether and chloroform.

VOLATILE or ESSENTIAL OILS resemble fixed oils in being soluble in ether or chloroform and in being lighter than water. Examples of these are the oils of dill, anise, cajuput, caraway, cloves, cinnamon, eucalyptus, juniper, lavender, lemon, peppermint, rosemary, rue, mustard, and turpentine. The volatile oils have some actions in common by being in small doses antispasmodics and analgesics, and by possessing a mild antiseptic and disinfectant action. Most of them are prepared by distillation. Their composition varies considerably, some being of the nature of alcohols, others ketones, others allied to carbolic acid. Volatile oils can be dissolved to a small extent in water, to which they communicate their scent and other properties, and these aquae or waters are used in treating colic and other spasmodic conditions, usually in doses of one or two tablespoonfuls. Volatile oils are also readily soluble in spirit containing 90 per cent alcohol, and these spirits usually contain about 10 per cent of the volatile oil and are given in doses of from 5 to 30 drops.

For oils of the petroleum series, see PARAFFIN.

OINTMENTS are semi-solid mixtures of medicinal substances with lard, benzoated lard, paraffin or yellow soft paraffin, and wool-fat (lanolin), intended for external application. They are used for three main purposes: (i) as emollients, that is to soften the skin; (ii) as a protective preparation to be applied to the skin; (iii) as a means for the local application of medicaments to be absorbed through the skin.

Other substances occasionally used to form the body of an ointment are almond oil, beeswax, camphor, glycerin, oleic acid, spermaceti, and prepared suet.

Among the most useful ointments are the following: *Simple Ointment* BP, which contains 5 per cent each of wool fat, hard paraffin, and cetostearyl acid in white or yellow soft paraffin, and is used for application to chafed surfaces. *Cold Cream*, made of beeswax, spermaceti, almond oil, rose water, and attar of rose, is used for a similar purpose. *Zinc and Castor Oil Ointment* BP, which contains 7·5 per cent zinc oxide and 50 per cent w/w castor oil has a well-earned reputation for the prevention and treatment of napkin rash. *Mercuric Oxide Eye Ointment* BPC, or yellow oxide of mercury eye ointment as it is sometimes known, is used for treating inflammation about the eye.

OLD AGE (see AGE, NATURAL CHANGES IN).

OLEANDOMYCIN is an antibiotic derived from *Streptomycesantibioticus.* It is active against many Gram-positive micro-organisms and some Gram-negative micro-organisms.

OLEIC ACID is the commonest of naturally occurring fatty acids, being present in most fats and oils in the form of triglyceride. It is used in the preparation of ointments, but not eye ointments.

OLFACTORY NERVE, the nerve of smell, is the first cranial nerve.

OLIGAEMIA means a diminution of the quantity of blood in the circulation.

OLIGOMENORRHOEA is infrequent menstruation.

OLIGURIA means an abnormally low excretion of urine, such as occurs in acute nephritis.

OLIVE OIL is the oil obtained by pressure from the fruit of *Oleaeuropaea*. It is practically a pure fat.

OMENTUM is a long fold of peritoneal membrane, generally loaded with more or less fat, which hangs down within the abdominal cavity in front of the bowels. It is formed by the layers of peritoneum that cover the front and back surfaces of the stomach in their passage from the lower margin of this organ to cover the back and front surfaces of the large intestine. Instead of passing straight from one organ to the other, these layers dip down and form a sort of fourfold apron. It is to the increasing deposit of fat in this structure that the prominence of the abdomen is largely due in people of middle age who are large eaters. This omentum is known as the greater omentum, to distinguish it from two smaller peritoneal folds, one of which passes between the liver and stomach (the hepatogastric omentum), and the other between the liver and duodenum (the hepatoduodenal omentum). Together they are known as the lesser omentum.

OMPHALOCELE is another name for exomphalos – a hernia of abdominal organs through the umbilicus.

OMPHALUS is another name for the navel or umbilicus.

ONCHOCERCIASIS is infestation with the filarial worm, *Onchocercavolvulus*. It is found in many parts of tropical Africa south of the Sahara, in Central and South America, and in the Yemen and Saudi Arabia. It is estimated that there are more than 20 million victims of it. It is transmitted by gnats of the genus *Simulium*. After a period of nine to eighteen months, the young filarial worms, injected into the body by the bite of an infected *Simulium*, mature, mate and start producing young microfilariae. The females live for up to fifteen years and during this period each may produce several thousand microfilariae a day. It is these microfilariae, which have a life-span of up to two years, that produce the characteristic features of the disease: an itching rash of the skin and the appearance of nodules in different parts of the body. There may also be involvement of the eyes and the worm may invade the optic nerve and so cause blindness; hence the name of African river blindness. Treatment consists of diethylcarbamazine and suramin. An international campaign is now under way in an attempt to destroy *Simulium* in the affected zones. Meanwhile the only means of prevention is to avoid so far as possible being bitten by the gnat. One means of achieving this is by wearing long trousers, shoes and socks.

ONCOGENE is a specific segment of DNA (qv) which confers the property of malignancy.

ONCOLOGY is that part of medical science which is concerned with the management of malignant disease such as cancer.

ONYCHIA means an inflammation affecting the nails. (See NAILS, DISEASES OF.)

ONYCHOGRYPHOSIS is a distortion of the nail in which it is much thickened, overgrown and twisted on itself. This usually affects a toenail and is the result of chronic irritation and inflammation.

ONYCHOLYSIS means separation of the nail from the nail-bed.

OOPHORECTOMY is a term applied to removal, by operation, of an ovary. When the ovary is removed for the presence of a cyst, the term ovariotomy is usually employed.

OOPHORITIS is another name for ovaritis or inflammation of an ovary.

OOPHORON is another name for the ovary.

OPHTHALMIA means inflammation of the eye, the term being used sometimes instead of conjunctivitis. (See CONJUNCTIVITIS under EYE DISEASES AND INJURIES.)

OPHTHALMOPLEGIA means paralysis of the muscles of the eye. Internal ophthalmoplegia refers to paralysis of the iris and ciliary body, external ophthalmoplegia refers to paralysis of one or all of the muscles that move the eyes.

OPHTHALMOSCOPE: An instrument for examining the interior of the eye. There are different types of ophthalmoscope, all have a light source to illuminate the inside of the eye and a magnifying lens to make examination easier.

OPIATE is a preparation of opium (qv).

OPIPRAMOL is a drug with antidepressant properties.

OPISTHOTONOS is the name given to a position assumed by the body during one of the convulsive seizures of tetanus. The muscles of the back, by their spasmodic contraction, arch the body in such a way that the person for a time may rest upon the bed only by his heels and head.

OPIUM is the dried juice of the unripe seed-capsules of the white Indian poppy, *Papaver somniferum*. It is cultivated mainly in India, but it is also produced in Iran, China, and the Asiatic provinces of Turkey. Opium possesses its medicinal properties only when produced under favourable conditions of soil and climate, and the juice of other species of poppies grown in temperate climates is almost useless. The juice is obtained by scarifying the seed-capsules of the poppies before they are ripe, and next day collecting the gummy sap which has exuded from the cuts. This is dried with great care, kneaded, and carefully tested. Good opium should contain about 10 per cent of morphine, to which its action is chiefly due. It is a brown, resinous-looking substance, or brown powder, with characteristic smell and bitter taste. The action of opium depends upon the twenty to twenty-five alkaloids it contains. Of these, the chief is morphine, the amount of which varies from around 9 to 17 per cent. Other alkaloids include codeine, narcotine, thebaine, papaverine, and naceine, and as the action of these differs considerably, the effect of the opium naturally varies according to the proportion of each that it contains. Turkish opium, which is purest in morphine, is generally regarded as the best, the use of Indian opium, which contains a large proportion of narcotine, being more apt to cause sickness. Opium, which is exported from the country of its production in balls or cakes, is often adulterated with sugar, vegetable extracts, gum, molasses, and even stones concealed in the middle of the cakes, and it is therefore very carefully tested before sale.

The importation into Britain of opium is very carefully regulated under the *Dangerous Drugs Acts*. Similar regulations govern the sale and distribution of any preparation of morphine or diamorphine (heroin) stronger than 1 part in 500.

The preparations of opium are numerous. Powdered opium (containing 10 per cent morphine) is used in doses ranging from 30 to 200 mg. Among the other solid preparations are ipecacuanha and opium powder, better known as Dover's powder (containing 10 per cent opium), in doses of 300 to 600 mg; aromatic chalk with opium powder (containing 0·25 per cent morphine), used for the treatment of diarrhoea, in doses of 500 mg to 5 grams. Of the liquid preparations, the tincture of opium, also known as laudanum (containing 1 per cent morphine), is the most used, in doses of 0·3 to 2 ml; the camphorated tincture of opium, also known as paregoric (containing 0·05 per cent morphine), is given in doses of 2 to 10 ml. (See PAREGORIC.) A preparation of opium known as nepenthe is particularly useful in children, the dose being 0·06 ml for each year of age.

The alkaloids, morphine and codeine, are administered in various forms. Morphine hydrochloride and morphine sulphate are

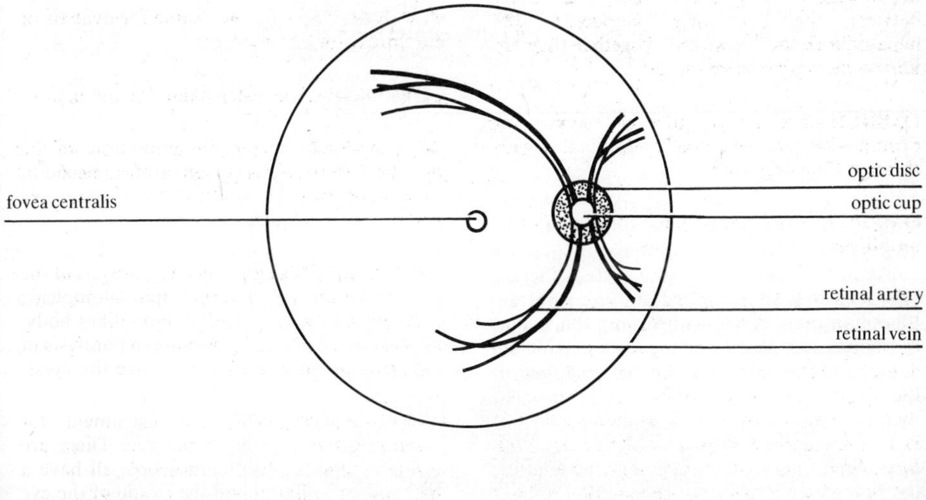

View through an ophthalmoscope of the fundus of the right eye.

given in doses from 7·5 to 20 mg; codeine phosphate in doses from 10 to 60 mg. Morphine hydrochloride solution (containing 1 per cent of morphine) is used like laudanum, in doses from 0·5 to 2 ml. A suppository of morphine (containing 15 mg of morphine), is used for painful conditions of the lower bowel.

Action: The action of opium varies considerably, according to the source of the drug and the preparation used; it varies even more according to the age, race, and temperament of the individual. The unstable nervous system of children is profoundly affected by even the smallest doses, and the death of an infant has been caused by a few drops of laudanum, so that the drug is unsuited for use, except with great care, during childhood.

In small doses, opium produces a state of gentle excitement, the person finding his imagination more vivid, his thoughts more brilliant, and his power of expression greater than usual. This stage lasts for some hours, and is succeeded by languor. In larger, ie. medicinal, doses this stage of excitement is short and is followed by deep sleep, from which the person can still be aroused as from natural sleep. When very large, ie. poisonous, doses are taken, sleep comes on quickly, and passes into coma and death. The habitual use of opium obtains for it a great degree of tolerance, so that opium users require to take large quantities daily before experiencing its pleasurable effects. The need for opium also confers tolerance, so that people suffering great pain may take, with apparently little effect beyond dulling the pain, quantities which at another time would be dangerous.

It checks all secretions, except the sweat, and slows the processes of tissue change, this action being sometimes useful, sometimes a hindrance to its employment.

Uses: Internally, its great use is to relieve severe pain, such as that of renal colic or cancer; for this purpose morphine is often given with atropine, which aids the effect in diminishing any spasm present, and at the same time is an antidote to the poisonous qualities of morphine. In conditions in which there is constant, irritating, useless cough, some preparation of opium or morphine may be used as an ingredient in cough mixtures to relieve this. In cases of pelvic pain, whether arising in the bowel, bladder, womb, or ovaries, morphine may be used in the form of suppositories to afford relief. Apart from the relief of pain, the main use of opium is in the treatment of left ventricular failure as it causes dilatation of the venous system, thereby reducing the load on the heart. All preparations of opium must be prescribed with the utmost discrimination, in view of the marked tendency to habit-formation. (See DRUG ADDICTION.)

OPIUM POISONING: Perhaps there is no drug in which the amount that can produce serious consequences varies so much as in the case of opium. Two drops of laudanum have been recorded as fatal to an infant, whereas addicts of the drug have been known to drink it like wine, with only a stimulating effect.

Symptoms: When a poisonous dose of any of the preparations of the drug has been taken, sleep rapidly comes on, becomes deeper and deeper, and passes gradually into a state of complete insensibility, usually within half-an-hour, although the effect may be postponed for several hours, particularly when the drug is taken along with alcoholic liquor. Convulsions sometimes occur, especially in children, and vomiting may take place before sleep becomes deep, or as the person is recovering. The breathing is slow, quiet, and shallow; and these characteristics become more and more marked as death approaches,the person dying, indeed, as the result of paralysis of the respiratory centre in the brain. The lips and face become livid and covered with cold sweat, and the pupils are much contracted. As a rule, death occurs in from seven to eighteen hours after the dose has been taken.

Treatment: An emetic should be given as soon as possible (see EMETICS), and after this has acted, a cup of strong coffee should be swallowed. Even after an emetic has acted, and certainly if it fails to act, the stomach should be washed out with water containing potassium permanganate, which destroys the alkaloids of the opium. As an antidote, full doses of naloxone, levallorphan or nalorphine should be given. Should none of these be immediately available, injections of caffeine sodium benzoate, amphetamine, or nikethamide may be given.

It is important to keep the patient awake; and for this purpose he must be walked up and down the room if possible, or one may tap him on the forehead with the finger-nails, flick him with wet towels, or apply other painful stimuli. From time to time strong coffee, and other stimulants may be given internally. If, in spite of all these measures, he becomes unconscious and the breathing begins to fail, artificial respiration must be performed. Generally speaking, by twelve hours after taking the poison the patient is either dead or is showing signs of recovery.

OPODELDOC is an old name for soap liniment.

OPSONINS are substances present in the serum of the blood which act upon bacteria, so as to prepare them for destruction by the white corpuscles of the blood.

OPTIC NERVE (see EYE).

ORANGE is an excellent source of vitamin C: 100 millilitres of orange juice contain 50 mg of ascorbic acid (ie. vitamin C). It is also used as a flavouring agent in the form of infusion, tincture and syrup of the peel. Fresh orange is also employed, often mixed with glucose, in feverish conditions for the action of the citric acid it contains. (See CITRIC ACID.)

ORBIT (see EYE).

ORCHIDECTOMY is the operation for the removal of the testicles (one or both).

ORCHIDOPEXY: When testes do not descend into the scrotum normally in young children (cryptorchidism) an operation is necessary to bring the testes in to the scrotum. This is called surgical orchidopexy.

ORCHITIS means inflammation of the testicle. (See TESTICLE, DISEASES OF.)

ORCIPRENALINE is an adrenaline-like drug that is proving of value in the relief of the bronchial spasm in asthma. It is given either by mouth or by inhalation. It is being replaced by the more selective beta-2 adrenoreceptor stimulants.

ORF is a widespread viral infection of sheep and goats which is sometimes transmitted to man, in whom it manifests itself as a skin eruption, usually on the hands, fingers, forearms and face.

ORGANIC DISEASE is a term used in contradistinction to the word functional, to indicate that some structural change is responsible for the faulty action of an organ or other part of the body.

ORGANIC SUBSTANCES are those which are obtained from animal or vegetable bodies, or which resemble in chemical composition those derived from this source. Organic chemistry has come to mean the chemistry of the carbon compounds.

ORGANO-PHOSPHORUS INSECTICIDES are a group of insecticides which act by inhibiting the action of cholinesterase. (See ACETYLCHOLINE.) For this reason they are also toxic to man and must therefore be handled with great care. The most widely used are parathion (qv) and malathion (qv).

Some of them are of value in agriculture because, when applied to plants, they are absorbed, and distributed to all parts of the plant, where they may kill sucking insects such as aphids.

ORIENTAL SORE, also known as DELHI BOIL and as ALEPPO EVIL, is a disease of tropical climates in which an ulcer begins in a small pimple, spreads, and then heals very slowly; leaving an unsightly scar. (See LEISHMANIASIS.)

ORNITHOSIS is an infection of birds with the micro-organism known as *Chlamydia psittaci*, which is transmissible to man.

ORPHENADRINE is a drug used in the treatment of Parkinsonism (qv).

ORTHODONTICS is the branch of dentistry concerned with the prevention and treatment of dental irregularities and malocclusion.

ORTHOPAEDICS: Originally the general measures, surgical and mechanical, which can be used for the correction or prevention of deformities in children. Now, that branch of medical science dealing with skeletal deformity, congenital or acquired.

ORTHOPNOEA is a form of difficulty in breathing so severe that the patient cannot bear to lie down, but must sit or stand up. As a rule, it occurs only in serious affections of the heart or lungs.

ORTHOPTIC TREATMENT involves the examination and treatment by exercises of squints and their sequelae.

OSGOOD-SCHLATTER'S DISEASE is the form of osteochondrosis (qv) involving the tibial tubercle – the growing point of the tibia (qv). It occurs around puberty, mainly in boys, and first manifests itself by a painful swelling over the tibial tubercle at the upper end of the tibia. The pain is worst during and after exercise. A limp with increasing limitation of movement of the knee joint develops. Treatment consists of immobilization of the knee joint in plaster of Paris for six to eight weeks, with gradual return to activity over the next few months. Thereafter progressive return to sport may be allowed, but intense activity must be banned for many months.

OSMOSIS means the passage of fluids through a membrane, which separates them, so as to become mixed with one another. Osmotic pressure is a term applied to the strength of the tendency which a fluid shows to do this, and depends largely upon the amount of solid which it holds in solution.

OSSIFICATION means the formation of bone. In early life, centres appear in the bones previously represented by cartilage or fibrous tissue, and from these the formation of true bone and deposit of lime salts proceed. When a fracture occurs, the bone mends by ossification of the clot which forms between the fragments. (See FRACTURES.) In old age an unnatural process of ossification often takes place in parts which should remain cartilaginous, eg. in the cartilages of the larynx and of the ribs, making these parts unusually brittle.

OSTEITIS means inflammation in the substance of a bone. *Traumatic osteitis* is a condition particularly common in footballers, in which the victim complains of pain in the groin following exercise, particularly if this has involved much hip rotation. Examination reveals difficulty in spreading the legs and marked tenderness over the symphysis pubis. It responds well to rest and the administration of anti-inflammatory drugs such as indomethacin.

OSTEITIS DEFORMANS (see PAGET'S DISEASE OF BONE).

OSTEITIS FIBROSA is a pathological rather than a clinical entity. The term refers to the replacement of bone by a highly cellular and vascular connective tissue. It is the result of osteoclastic and osteoblastic activity and is due to excessive parathyroid activity. It is thus seen in a proportion of patients with primary hyperparathyroidism and in patients with uraemic osteodystrophy; that is, the secondary hyperparathyroidism that occurs in patients with chronic renal disease.

OSTEOARTHROSIS, or OSTEOARTHRITIS, is a term applied to a chronic degeneration of the bones composing a joint, and leading to deformity. (See RHEUMATISM.)

OSTEOCHONDRITIS is inflammation of both bone and cartilage. It is a not uncommon cause of backache in young people, particularly gymnasts.

OSTEOCHONDROSIS includes a group of diseases involving degeneration of the centre of ossification (see BONE) in the growing bones of children and adolescents. They include Kohler's disease (qv), Osgood-Schlatter's disease (qv), and Perthes' disease (qv).

OSTEOGENESIS IMPERFECTA is a hereditary disease due to an inherited abnormality of collagen (qv). It is characterized by extreme fragility of the skeleton, resulting in fractures and deformities. It may be accompanied by blue sclera (the outermost, normally white coat of the eyeball), transparent teeth, hypermobility (excessive range of movement) of the joints, deafness, and dwarfism (shortness of stature). The cause is not known, though there is some evidence that it may be associated with collagen formation (see COLLAGEN). Parents of affected children can obtain help and advice from the Brittle Bone Society, Unit 4, Block 20, Carlunie Road, Dunsinane Estate, Dundee DD2 3QT (0382–817771).

OSTEOMALACIA is the adult form of rickets. It is due to inadequate mineralisation of osteoid tissue caused by a deficiency of vitamin D. This deficiency may arise because of inadequate intake or it may be due to impaired absorption such as occurs in intestinal malabsorption. It may also be due to renal disease as the kidney is responsible for the hydroxylation of cholecalciferol, which has virtually no metabolic action, to dihydroxy-cholecalciferol, the metabolically active form of the vitamin. (See VITAMIN D.)

OSTEOMYELITIS means inflammation in the marrow of a bone. (See BONE, DISEASES OF.)

OSTEOPATHY is the name applied to a system of healing in which diseases are treated by manipulating bones and other parts with the idea of thereby restoring functions in the bodily mechanism that have become deranged.

OSTEOPHYTES are bony spurs or projections. They occur most commonly at the margins of points involved in osteoarthrosis (qv).

OSTEOPOROSIS is a reduced mass of normal bone. It is due to excessive resorption of bone rather than decreased bone synthesis. The quality of the bone that is present is normal, it is just the quantity that is deficient. It is a feature of ageing so that osteoporosis is common in the elderly. After the menopause women lose one per cent of their bone each year so that post-menopausal osteoporosis is a common disorder unless hormone replacement therapy is given. Osteoporosis is also a feature of Cushing's syndrome and of patients who have been on long-term treatment with corticosteroids. Information and advice about the disease can be obtained from the National Osteoporosis Society, PO Box 10, Radstock, Bath BA3 3YB (0761–32472).

OSTEOSARCOMA is the most common, and most malignant, tumour of bone. It occurs predominantly in older children and young adults. The commonest site for it is at the ends of the long bones of the body: ie. the femur, tibia and humerus. Treatment is by amputation of the limb followed by radiotherapy and chemotherapy. The 5-year survival rate is only 20 per cent.

OSTEOTOMY is the operation of cutting of a bone.

OS TRIGONUM is a small accessory bone behind the ankle joint which is present in about 7 per cent of the population. It may be damaged by energetic springing from the toes in ballet, jumping or fast bowling.

OTITIS means inflammation of the ear. (See EAR, DISEASES OF.)

OTOLOGY is that branch of medical science which is concerned with disorders and diseases of the organ of hearing, one practising this branch being called an OTOLOGIST.

OTOMYCOSIS (see EAR, DISEASES OF).

OTORRHOEA means discharge from the ear. (See EAR, DISEASES OF.)

OTOSCLEROSIS is a condition in which abnormal bone is deposited around the foot-plate of the stapes resulting in fixation of that bone and causing a progressive conductive hearing loss due to immobility of the ossicular chain. There is an hereditary pattern to the disease and its onset is usually in the third decade. It tends to be slightly commoner in women and is often accelerated in pregnancy. Treatment involves supplying a hearing aid or performing an operation known as stapedectomy. Rarely the deposition of abnormal bone may affect the inner ear as well.

OUABAIN, or Strophanthin-G, is a glycoside first obtained from the African tree, *Acokanthera ouabaio*: it was used as an arrow poison in West Africa. It is now obtained from the African tree *Strophanthus gratus*. It is a cardiac stimulant, having a similar action to that of digitalis.

OVARIES are the glands in which are produced, in the female sex, the ova, capable, if fertilized, of developing into new individuals. They are situated, one on each side, in the cavity of the pelvis, corresponding on the surface of the body approximately to the centre of the groin. Each is shaped something like an almond, is about 3 cm long, 1·5 cm wide, and 1 cm in thickness, and is whitish in colour. It is attached to the broad ligament running from the womb to the side of the pelvis, by one edge along which blood-vessels and nerves enter. One end is connected to the expanded end of the Fallopian tube, as well as by a ligament to the side of the pelvis, and the other end to a ligament to the side of the womb. The ovary therefore lies to a considerable extent free in the pelvis.

The chief bulk of the ovary is made up of connective tissue, which differs from ordinary fibrous tissue in being composed of spindle-shaped cells. On the surface is a layer of columnar cells, and beneath this a dense connective tissue layer, the tunica albuginea. Beneath the tunica albuginea the structure appears to the naked eye to be of a granular character, this appearance being due to the presence of a layer of follicles, estimated at around 2,000,000 in number in each ovary at birth. By puberty they are reduced to around 40,000 in each ovary, a mere 400 of which will be shed at ovulation during the child-bearing period. Each follicle contains one (seldom more) ovum, each of these ova being capable of developing into a new individual. Every follicle consists essentially of a hollow ball of cells, embedded in which is a single large cell, the ovum. Each ovary contains follicles in all stages of maturity, from the rudimentary ones described above to several which are greatly increased in size to 35 micrometres in diameter through multiplication of the cells surrounding the ovum and the formation among them of a cavity distended with fluid. One at least of these follicles comes to maturity, when it is known as a Graafian follicle, about half-way between two menstrual periods, distends till it reaches the surface of the ovary, and finally bursts allowing the escape of the contained ovum, measuring 110 micrometres in diameter, which finds its way down the corresponding Fallopian tube into the womb. This process is know as ovulation. (See MENSTRUATION.)

For ovarian secretions, see Ovaries under ENDOCRINE GLANDS, and also OESTRADIOL; OESTROGEN; PROGESTERONE.

OVARIES, DISEASES OF: When diseased, the ovaries can be responsible for much ill-health. INFLAMMATION OF THE OVARY (OVARITIS) seldom, if ever, occurs alone and is usually associated with inflammation of the Fallopian tubes (ie. salpingitis) and of the pelvic peritoneum. It may be acute or chronic. The acute form is due to gonorrhoea, infection during the puerperium or following abortion, or infection from the alimentary tract: eg. the appendix. If the acute form is not successfully overcome, it is liable to become chronic with exacerbations. In the chronic stage adhesions form which bind down and displace the ovaries, the Fallopian tubes, and the uterus. Bladder function is also liable to be interfered with. In all cases of infection of the ovaries and Fallopian tubes the possibility of this being due to tuberculosis must be considered, particularly in young patients.

Symptoms: In the acute form these may be mild or severe, consisting of pain in the lower part of the abdomen, usually during or just after menstruation, prolongation of menstruation, and fever. There may also be pain on passing water, sickness and vomiting. In severe cases with high temperature there may be rigors. In chronic cases there may be backache, usually worse after a day's work, fatigue, excessive or painful menstruation, pain on passing water, sterility and debility. In more severe cases there may be a discharge from the vagina (ie. leucorrhoea) and anaemia. Sometimes an abscess develops in the ovary or in the Fallopian tubes, and in these cases the general health is more likely to suffer because of toxic absorption.

Treatment: In the acute cases this consists of rest in bed and the administration of an antibiotic. Hot fomentations are useful to relieve pain. Hot douches to the vagina are not used as much as they were at one time, as they are sometimes liable to increase the pain. The diet should be light and nourishing. Care is necessary to ensure regular emptying of the bowels, but violent purgatives must not be used for this purpose. The majority of cases respond to such treatment. Operation is only indicated when there are signs of general peritonitis, or when there is no evidence of the condition responding to medical treatment in two to three weeks. The treatment of chronic cases is similar, but here hot douches to the vagina twice daily are also of value. Operation is required for chronic cases if the general health is affected, if there are acute exacerbations, or if there is much persistent local pain and menorrhagia.

OVARIAN TUMOURS may be of several kinds. Solid tumours, either simple or malignant, are relatively rare, though cancer of the ovary causes the death of more than 3000 women in Britain every year. Far commoner are the cystic forms, which often reach a huge size. The largest ever reported weighed 148 kg (328 pounds). These cysts are of several types, sometimes consisting of a distended condition of the Graafian follicles, at other times being simple cysts filled with a complex papillary growth, again being dermoid tumours and containing fat, hair, teeth, and other structures associated with the skin, and yet again arising from the distension of some part of the parovarium, a rudimentary structure attached to the ovary.

The fluid in these cysts is sometimes of a greenish-grey or brown colour and viscid, ropy consistence, at other times clearer and thinner, and, in the case of dermoid tumours, usually of a greasy nature.

Symptoms: These cystic tumours generally remain painless till the weight and distension caused by their increasing size give trouble. They arise often in young women without any apparent cause. If they are not removed, some, which stand on the verge of being malignant tumours, increase rapidly in size, and all lead to great discomfort and loss of health, and finally shorten life.

Treatment: The one method of treatment adopted now consists in *oophorectomy* ie. removal of the affected ovary. This operation should be performed early in the course of the disease, because, as the tumour grows, it contracts adhesions to surrounding organs, and these are the source both of most distressing symptoms and of the chief difficulty and danger in a later operation. Most cases operated upon at an early stage recover well, the operation being one of the safest major operations in surgery.

OVARIOTOMY or OOPHORECTOMY is the operation of removal of an ovary or an ovarian tumour.

OVERLAYING OF INFANTS is the term applied to the process whereby an infant sleeping in the same bed as an adult is suffocated as a result of the adult lying on top of the infant. In most cases the adult is under the influence of alcohol.

OVUM is the single cell derived from the female, out of which a future individual arises, after its union with the spermatozoon derived from the male. It is about 35 micrometres in diameter. (See FOETUS; OVARIES.)

OXALIC ACID is not used in medicine, but it is of importance because it is an irritant poison, and has a domestic use for cleaning purposes: eg. removing ink stains and iron mould, and cleaning leather. Oxalic acid, or binoxalate of potassium (salt of sorrel), is occasionally taken by mistake for Epsom salts or for cream of tartar. This substance is also important, because oxalate of lime is found in urinary sediment, and sometimes composes urinary calculi. (See BLADDER, DISEASES OF.) Oxalate of lime in the urine is derived partly from articles of food, like rhubarb, that contain it, and is partly produced within the body as the result of tissue change.

When poisoning is the result of taking oxalic acid or binoxalate of potassium, chalk or whiting well diluted with water should be given, and, if vomiting is not already present, an emetic; afterwards the irritation resulting in the stomach and bowels is to be soothed by demulcents. The antidote to oxalic acid is Calcium Gluconate Injection BP.

OXACILLIN (see ANTIBIOTIC).

OXPRENOLOL (APSOLOX, LARACOR, TRASICOR) (see ADRENERGIC RECEPTORS).

OXYCEPHALY, or STEEPLE HEAD, describes a deformity of the skull in which the forehead is high and the top of the head pointed. There is also poor vision and the eyes bulge.

OXYGEN is a colourless gas, devoid of smell, slightly heavier than common air. It was discovered by Joseph Priestley in 1772. It forms rather more than one-fifth by volume of the atmosphere. It may be obtained by the fractional distillation of liquid air, or by the electrolysis of water. It is stored at high pressure (up to 120 atmospheres) in steel cylinders, from which it is obtained at any desired rate by turning a stop-cock.

Action: Oxygen is necessary to life, and the process of respiration (see RESPIRATION) has, as one of its main objects, the supply of oxygen to the blood (see also HAEMOGLOBIN). Applied to the unbroken skin, oxygen has little effect, but when brought in contact with a wound or ulcer, it increases the circulation and acts as a stimulant.

The condition of oxygen want, or anoxia, may be produced by various conditions, such as damage to the lung by tumours, or defects of the circulation, eg. valvular disease of the heart, in which the circulation is so slow that the tissues do not receive their proper amount of oxygen, and in cases of anaemia and poisoning where the blood is not capable of carrying its normal amount of oxygen. In these states, and above all in cases of anaemia and valvular disease, when the pulse is quick and feeble, when the patient's lips and ears are blue, and when the breathing is rapid and shallow, the administration of oxygen gives great relief.

Uses: In severe cases of anoxia the rate at which oxygen may require to be delivered to the patient is between 4 and 6 litres per minute. A tube is attached to the head of the cylinder, which passes through the tubes of a wash-bottle and is continued to either a mask, which fits over the patient's nose and mouth, or to a catheter which is passed into one of the nostrils and fixed in position at the side of the face by a strip of sticking plaster. The use of the latter is unaccompanied by any sense of oppression to the patient.

Great advances have been made in recent years in the development of both oxygen masks and tents. The advantage of the latter is that the patient is breathing all the time in an atmosphere saturated with oxygen.

A recent development in oxygen therapy is what is known as *hyperbaric oxygen*. This is the use of oxygen at high pressures, such as 3 atmospheres. Originally introduced as an adjunct to radiotherapy in the treatment of cancer, it is now being used in the treatment of carbon monoxide poisoning, *Clostridium welchii* infections (qv) and coronary thrombosis. The most convenient method of administering hyperbaric oxygen is in a special pressure chamber.

Substances which contain oxygen and are capable of giving it off, such as permanganate of potassium, and peroxide of hydrogen, have a powerful effect as disinfectants either by destroying organisms or oxidizing noxious products of their growth. Such substances are therefore used in the treatment of ulcers and various skin diseases and as antiseptics.

OXYMETHOLONE (ANAPOLON) (see ANABOLIC STEROIDS).

OXYPERTINE is an anti-psychotic drug related to the phenothiazines.

OXYTETRACYCLINE is an antibiotic derived from a soil organism, *Streptomyces rimosus*. Its range of antibacterial activity is comparable to that of tetracycline (qv).

OXYTOCIC means hastening parturition or stimulating uterine contraction, or a drug or procedure that has this effect.

OXYTOCIN is the extract isolated from the pituitary posterior lobe which stimulates the uterine muscle to contract. It can also be synthesized. (See PITUITARY BODY.)

OXYURIS is another name for the threadworm.

OZAENA is a chronic disease of the nose of an inflammatory nature, combined with atrophy of the mucous membrane and the formation of extremely foul-smelling crusts in the interior of the nose. (See NOSE, DISEASES OF.)

OZONE is a specially active form of oxygen in which three volumes of the gas are condensed into the space ordinarily occupied by two. It has a characteristic smell, which may be noticed in the neighbourhood of dynamos, as ozone is produced by the passage through the air of electric sparks. It exists free in small quantities in the air of pine-clad mountains and of the seaside, where the invigorating properties of the fresh air may be partly due to its presence. It has also a powerful deodorant action.

P

PACEMAKER (see CARDIAC PACEMAKER).

PACHYDERMIA means hypertrophy or thickening of the skin. PACHYDERMIA LARYNGIS is a name applied to thickening of the vocal cords due to chronic inflammation or irritation.

PACHYMENINGITIS means inflammation of the dura mater of the brain and spinal cord. (See MENINGITIS.)

PACINIAN CORPUSCLES, or lamellated corpuscles, are minute bulbs at the ends of the nerves scattered through the skin and subcutaneous tissue, and forming one of the end-organs for sensation.

PACKS (see WET PACK).

PAEDIATRICS means the branch of medicine dealing with diseases of children.

PAGET'S DISEASE OF BONE, or OSTEITIS DEFORMANS, is a chronic disease in which the bones – especially those of the skull, limbs, and spine – gradually become thick and also soft, causing them to bend. It is said to be the commonest bone disease in the world, and it is estimated that some 600,000 people in England may suffer from it. It seldom occurs under the age of 40. Pain is its most unpleasant manifestation. The cause is not known, and there is no known cure, but satisfactory results are being obtained from the use of calcitonin (qv) and a group of drugs known as diphosphonates (eg. etidronate). Those with the disease can obtain help and advice from The National Association for the Relief of Paget's Disease, 413 Middleton Road, Middleton, Manchester M24 4OZ (061-643 1998).

PAIN is a necessary part of conscious existence, all our sensations being accompanied by more or less feeling of pleasure or pain. In the former case we seek the repetition of the sensations; in the latter case we instinctively avoid them, unless, by an act of will, we avoid the sense of pleasure or bear that of pain for some ulterior motive. The ability to perceive pain constitutes a special sense which the body has evolved, or with which it has been furnished, in order that it may preserve itself, by avoiding conditions that produce damage.

Pain is of various types. The most important is that caused by injury of the skin, as by a prick, burn, or pinch. This sense is quite distinct from that of touch. There are special nerve-fibres for the conduction of painful impressions, running up the spinal cord near its central canal, while the fibres conveying the impressions for touch run up in the posterior part of the cord. This is proved by the destruction of the sense of pain in the disease known as syringomyelia (which affects the central part of the cord), notwithstanding the fact that the slightest touch can still be felt in the parts of the body incapable of feeling pain. It is probable that these nerves of pain have special endings in the skin, since pain does not appear to be felt uniformly, but, like the other senses, at special spots thickly scattered over the surface. And it is also likely that there is a special centre in the brain for the reception of painful impressions.

Internal parts are much less sensitive than the skin, and diseases in them usually give rise to quite a different sensation. Indeed these parts, not being liable to damage by external objects, are not endowed with the power of feeling pain due to sudden injury, so that the bowel, when brought out through the skin, may be cut with scissors or knife, though the individual, unless he sees it, is quite unaware of what is taking place; tendon, muscle, and bone are also very insensitive, so that the two former may be cut or scraped without more than a slightly sickening sensation, or the ends of a broken bone rubbed together without causing severe pain.

Nevertheless inflammatory changes in these deep-seated structures, and disturbances in their functions, are capable of influencing the brain so as to produce the severest type of pain. This inflammation, particularly when seated in dense structures which cannot expand so as to prevent the congested blood-vessels of the part from pressing upon its nerves, is accompanied by throbbing pain, and, in bone particularly, this is apt to be of a boring, excruciating character. The gnawing pain of a tumour invading surrounding tissues is of a similar nature, and any source of irritation on the course of a nerve is apt to produce the severe pain of neuralgia. Over-action of a weak part or muscle leads to continued pain of an aching character, due probably to an irritating deposit of the chemical products of muscular activity, or may produce spasm, as in the stitch of the side caused by unwontedly violent exercise. Of a similar nature is the colic or griping pain, caused by irritation of the bowels, bile-ducts, and ureters, which in its severest forms may properly be designated agony. (See COLIC.) The burning pain of certain forms of dyspepsia is due to the action of an excessively acid gastric juice, and, like burns of the skin, is apparently due to irritation of the sensitive nerve-endings at points where the surface of the mucous membrane has become eroded.

Ordinary sensations of all sorts become painful when they are excessive, and thus liable to damage the organ in question: eg. bright light, loud sound.

Painful sensations depend much also upon the state of the nervous system, varying according to the power of the nerves to conduct, and of the brain to receive, impressions. Some people are notoriously better at bearing pain than others, and the healthy and strong are less affected by trivial injuries than those whose nervous system is in a state of ready irritability through chronic ill-health. People with strong will-power can undoubtedly inhibit painful impressions, like those from a surgical operation, just as they can control irregular movements. Thus by a mental effort not only do such people bear pain better, but they actually feel less pain. Similarly the mind that is dominated by an idea unconsciously inhibits painful impressions, so that they gain no entrance for the time, as in the case of soldiers wounded in the heat of battle.

On the other hand, pain may be of a purely functional character, and a person with a highly strung or disordered nervous system may suffer pain without any external cause, the mind misinterpreting or exaggerating sensations which by the healthy person would not be noticed. (See HYSTERIA.)

These facts are well known to those faith-healers and others who attempt to cure by a direct mental impression, and who by this means often succeed in alleviating pain, although only in special cases, such as the functional pains just mentioned, are they successful in curing the disease to which the pain is due, and of which it is the warning.

Pain in a certain part is not necessarily due to disease in the same part. In the case of injury to the skin covering the body, the mind, as the result of experience, very accurately refers the painful impressions down the nerves which bring them, to the parts from which they come. But when impressions come to the central nervous system from organs or parts of the body not usually liable to injury or disease, the mind is apt to refer the pain to some other part which is more commonly the seat of pain, and whose nerve-fibres enter the same part of the brain or spinal cord as do those coming from the part which is really affected. For example, in the early stages of hip-joint disease, the pain is more often felt down the inner side of the thigh and knee than in the deep-seated hip-joint, since branches from the same nerves (obturator and femoral) supply the hip-joint and the skin of this particular area. For the same reason, the pain of spinal disease, due to pressure upon the large nerve roots close to the point where they enter the cord, is often referred, not to this unfamiliar seat of pain, but to the sides and front of the body where these nerves end in the skin. In this connection it may be stated that pain felt equally on both sides of the body is almost always due to some affection of the central nervous system.

In the case of the internal organs whose nervous control is derived from the sympathetic nervous system (in the case of the heart, lungs, stomach, and bowels partly also from the tenth cranial, or vagus, nerve), through which they often obtain complicated and very distant connections with the brain and cord, pain is often referred, in what seems at first sight to be a bizarre manner, to distant points. *Referred pain* is often, in the case of the heart, stomach, liver, and bowels, felt on the surface situated over these organs, and the skin may be so tender that gentle pressure or even the slightest touch cannot be borne. Heart conditions are liable also to cause pain running down the inner side of the left, and in some cases of the right, arm to the elbow. In dyspepsia, due to irritation of the stomach, the pain is often referred to the pit of the stomach or middle of the back. In conditions affecting the liver there may be pain in the region of the right shoulder. Affections of the lower end of the bowel commonly cause pain down the back of the thighs, especially of the left thigh, to the knee. Pain due to disorders of the womb is felt internally much less often than in the lowest part of the back and the thighs; and, when the ovaries or Fallopian tubes also are affected, the pain may have a wide distribution, including the small of the back, the groin, and the front of the thigh, or it is occasionally referred to the hip or knee-joint, so that the case may for a time be mistaken for disease in one of these joints.

Treatment of pain: There are three general principles by which the relief of pain may be attempted. (1) The most natural way is to remove the cause of pain, such as a decayed tooth, ulcer, abscess, or inflammatory condition of some internal organ, or to soothe the nerves of the affected part by warmth or some other means. (2) The nerves which convey impressions from the affected region may be treated so that their conducting power is lessened or stopped, as, for example, by administration of sedatives, use of electricity, local anaesthetics, or by chordotomy (qv) (see NEURALGIA). (3) The part of the brain which receives the impressions of pain may be dulled by drugs, or the influence of these impressions may be inhibited by powerful mental impressions, as, for example in hypnotism, faith-healing. (See also ANAESTHETICS; ANALGESICS; ANODYNES; TRANSCUTANEOUS ELECTRICAL NERVE STIMULATION; and under the headings of the various diseases that give rise to pain.)

PAINS (see LABOUR).

PAINTER'S COLIC (see COLIC; LEAD POISONING).

PALATE is the partition between the cavity of the mouth, below, and that of the nose, above. It consists of the *hard palate* towards the front, which is composed of a bony plate covered below by the mucous membrane of the mouth, above by that of the nose; and of the *soft palate* farther back, in which a muscular layer, composed of nine small muscles, is similarly covered. The hard palate extends a little farther back than the wisdom teeth, and is formed by the maxillary and palate bones. The soft palate is concave towards the mouth and convex towards the nose, and it ends behind in a free border, at the centre of which is the prolongation known as the uvula. When food or air is passing through the mouth, as in the acts of swallowing, coughing, or vomiting, the soft palate is drawn upwards so as to touch the back wall of the throat and shut off the cavity of the nose. Movements of the soft palate, by changing the shape of the mouth and nose cavities, are important in the production of speech.

PALATE, MALFORMATIONS OF: The palate is subject to certain alterations, as the result of defective development. The hard palate may be much more arched than usual: this is sometimes due to the failure to breathe through the nose, caused by the presence of adenoid vegetations in the throat. (See NOSE, DISEASES OF.)

In early embryonic life (see FOETUS) there are certain clefts in the region of the throat and face, the nose being formed by the junction of one process which grows down from between the eyes (fronto-nasal process) and two which grow in, one from either side (maxillary processes). The fronto-nasal process produces the external nose, the septum of the nose, the central part of the upper lip, and that part of the upper jaw which carries the two front teeth. The maxillary processes form the remainder of the upper jaw and the palate on each side. These three should unite completely prior to birth, but if they fail to do so, a Y-shaped gap is left. This gap runs from the back of the palate forward to a point a little distance behind the front teeth, from which point a limb of the gap runs forwards to each nostril and through the upper lip. A complete state of *cleft palate* may occur; or there may be only a partial gap in the soft palate, the parts having closed in front; or again, there may be closure behind and only a notch be left in the lip or a single cleft in the edge of the upper jaw. The notch of the lip is known as *hare-lip*, from a fanciful resemblance to the hare, which has a notch in the centre of its lip.

The incidence of cleft lip (hare-lip) and cleft palate seems to be increasing and one child in approximately 700 normal births has some degree of cleft lip and palate. The increase is probably due to more of these babies surviving, as a result of improved surgical techniques, and getting married and having children. As a rough guide, it can be said that if a child is born with a cleft, and there is no family history as far back as the parents' grandparents, the chances of another malformed child is about the same as in the general population. When one parent is affected, the risk is around 1 in 80 but, when a mother with a cleft palate produces a daughter with a cleft palate, the risk to a second daughter is as high as 1 in 7.

Cleft-palate and hare-lip should, if possible, be rectified by operation, because both are a serious drawback to feeding in early life, while later, hare-lip is a great disfigurement, and cleft-palate gives to the voice a peculiar twang. When there is merely a slight degree of hare-lip, it is usual to operate a few weeks or even some days after birth, although, when the notch is very large, it may be necessary to wait till the child is several months old. The closure of a large cleft in the palate, which is a more formidable operation, is usually deferred till the child has gained some strength, and the most suitable time is generally held to be between eighteen months and two and a half years of age, because the fault must be remedied before the child has learned to speak. The operations performed vary greatly in details, but all consist in paring the edges of the gap and drawing the soft parts together across it.

Until a hare-lip has been remedied, it is often necessary to feed the child with a spoon, as he cannot suck. When a cleft palate is too wide for operation, its effects can be diminished in later life by wearing an artificial palate.

Parents of such children can obtain help and advice from the Cleft Lip and Palate Association, 1 Eastwood Gardens, Kenton, Newcastle-upon-Tyne NE3 3DQ (091–2859396), or the Dental Department, Hospital for Sick Children, Great Ormond Street, London WC1.

PALINDROMIC RHEUMATISM is a form of rheumatism in adults characterized by multiple, afebrile attacks of acute arthritis, and inflammation of the surrounding tissues, with pain, swelling, redness, and disability of one or more small or large joints, the attacks coming on suddenly, lasting a few hours to a few days then disappearing completely, to recur at irregular intervals.

PALLAESTHESIA means sensibility to the vibrations of a tuning-fork applied to the neighbourhood of a bone. Loss of this sense is an early feature of certain nervous diseases, such as tabes dorsalis.

PALLIATIVE is a term applied to the treatment of incurable diseases, in which the aim is to mitigate the sufferings of the patient, not to effect a cure.

PALPATION means the method of examining the surface of the body and the size, shape, and movements of the internal organs, by laying the flat of the hand upon the skin.

PALPITATION is a condition in which the heart beats forcibly or irregularly, and the person becomes conscious of its action.

Causes: As a rule we are quite unconscious of the beating of the heart, but when the nervous system is unduly excited its action may become unpleasantly palpable. A disorder of the rhythm of the heart (arrhythmia) may cause the heart to beat rapidly and give rise to palpitations. Sudden emotions, such as fright, and occasionally dyspepsia, may bring it on. A common cause consists in over-use of tobacco, tea, coffee, or alcohol. Sometimes it may appear in cases of organic heart disease.

Symptoms: There may simply be a fluttering of the heart and a feeling of weakness, which is often expressively described as 'gone-ness', or the heart may be felt pounding and the arteries throbbing, causing great distress to the affected person. In some cases the subject of palpitation is conscious of the heart missing beats.

Treatment: Mental quietness is the great requisite to still the overaction, and all sources of excitement must be avoided. The person should understand that, however unpleasant the condition may be, there is no danger from it, and that serious disease is not usually the cause. Moderate exercise is a good thing. If the person is a heavy smoker, this is probably the cause, and tobacco should be given up. Similarly tea, coffee, and alcohol should be partaken of sparingly, and any food likely to cause flatulent dyspepsia should be avoided. In the cases due to organic disease, the condition causing palpitation must be treated. The beta adrenoreceptor antagonists are the most useful drugs in controlling the palpitations of anxiety and those due to some cardiac arrhythmias.

PALSY is another name for paralysis. (See PARALYSIS.)

PALUDRINE (see PROGUANIL).

PAN- is a prefix meaning all or completely.

PANACEA is a term applied to a remedy for all diseases, or more usually to a remedy which benefits many different diseases.

PANARITIUM is a term applied to a whitlow which remains chronic and destroys part of the finger.

PANCARDITIS means inflammation of the pericardium, myocardium, and endocardium at the same time.

PANCREAS, or SWEETBREAD, is a long secreting gland situated in the back of the abdomen, at the level of the first and second lumbar vertebrae. It lies behind the lower part of the stomach, an expanded portion, called the head of the pancreas, occupying the bend formed by the duodenum or first part of the small intestine, whilst a long portion known as the body extends to the left, ending in the tail, which rests against the spleen. A duct runs through the whole gland from left to right, joined by many small branches in its course, and, leaving the head of the gland, unites with the bile duct from the liver to open into the side of the small intestine about 7·5 to 10 cm (3 or 4 inches) below the outlet of the stomach.

Minute structure: The gland resembles one of the salivary glands, being composed of tubes of columnar cells bound together by loose connective tissue. These cells are arranged with one end abutting on a central lumen into which the secretion of the cells passes, and each group of tubes ends in a small duct, which unites with other small ducts to join the main pancreatic duct running to the intestine. The cells present an outer, clear zone, and an inner zone filled with granules of the materials secreted by the activity of the cell. Blood-vessels and nerves in large numbers run in the connective tissue of the gland.

Scattered through the pancreas are collections of cells known as the islets of Langerhans, of which there are around a million in a normal individual. These do not communicate with the duct of the gland, and the internal secretion of the pancreas –insulin – is formed by these cells and absorbed directly into the blood.

Functions: The most obvious function of the pancreas is the formation of the pancreatic juice, which is poured into the small intestine after the partially digested food has left the stomach. This is the most important of the digestive juices, is alkaline in reaction, and contains, in addition to various salts, four enzymes. These enzymes are: trypsin and chymotrypsin, which digest proteins; amylase, which converts starchy foods into the disaccharide maltose; lipase, which breaks up fats. For the action of these see DIGESTION.

Inadequate production of insulin by the islets of Langerhans leads to the condition known as diabetes mellitus (qv). In addition to insulin, another hormone is produced by the pancreas. This is glucagon which has the opposite effect to insulin and raises the blood sugar by promoting the breakdown of liver glycogen.

PANCREAS, DISEASES OF: Abscesses, cysts, calculi, and tumours may occur in the pancreas as in other organs, but are not very common. The most important disease of the pancreas, though again, fortunately, not very common, is acute pancreatitis. This is sudden in onset, accompanied by acute pain, and causes severe shock and collapse. It carries a mortality rate of around 20 per cent, even when treated adequately and early. Chronic pancreatitis is a much more indeterminate disease, commonly associated with disease of the gall-bladder, particularly gall-stones, and chronic alcoholism. Pancreatitis may occur as a complication of mumps. Cancer of the pancreas is on the increase: from 3070 deaths in England and Wales in 1962 to 4414 cases in 1970. In 1984 it was responsible for 6037 deaths in England. There is an established association with heavy cigarette smoking, and it is twice as common in patients with diabetes mellitus as compared with the general population. Reference has already been made to the association between the islets of Langerhans and diabetes mellitus (qv).

PANCREATIN contains three ferments: trypsin, lipase, and amylase. Thereby it hydrolyses fats to glyceryl and fatty acids, changes protein to proteoses and derived substances, and converts starch into dextrins and sugars (see DIGESTION). It is given by mouth for the relief of pancreatic deficiency in conditions such as pancreatitis (qv) and fibrocystic disease of the pancreas (qv). It is also used for the preparation of predigested, or so-called peptonized, foods. For peptonizing milk, pancreatin is added to tepid water to which milk previously heated to 38°C is added. The mixture is stirred and maintained at 38°C for 15 minutes, and then raised to boiling point. It is then transferred to a cool place. It should be used within 24 hours. Various farinaceous foods may be similarly predigested.

PANDEMIC is an epidemic which affects a vast area, such as a country or a continent.

PANHYSTERECTOMY is an operation by which the uterus is completely removed.

PANNICULITIS means inflammation of the subcutaneous fat, and may occur anywhere on the body surface.

PANNUS: Blood vessels growing into the cornea beneath its epithelium. Seen in trachoma and to a lesser extent in patients who are long-term soft contact lens wearers.

PANTOTHENIC ACID, which has now been prepared synthetically, is part of the vitamin B complex. It is known as the chick anti-dermatitis factor because if it is absent from the chick's diet the bird develops dermatitis, and degeneration of nerve-fibres in the spinal cord also occurs. In rats lack of pantothenic acid produces greying of the hair, but there is no evidence that in man greying is due to lack of this vitamin. Indeed, little is known about the significance of pantothenic acid in man, except that it is one of the essential constituents of the diet. The daily requirement is probably around 10 milligrams. It is widely distributed in foodstuffs, both animal and vegetable. Yeast, liver, and egg-yolk are particularly rich sources.

PAPAIN, PAPYAOTIN, and PAPOID are names given to a ferment, or mixture of ferments, obtained from the juice of the pawpaw, the unripe fruit of *Carica papaya*, which has an action similar to that of the ferments of the gastric and pancreatic juices. It is accordingly sometimes used to peptonize foods for invalids, as it does not give them the same bitter taste that pepsin gives. It is widely used as a meat tenderiser.

PAPAVERETUM consists of the hydrochlorides of alkaloids of opium (qv). It has the pain-relieving and narcotic effects of morphine (qv), but fewer side-effects. It is largely used in association with anaesthesia.

PAPILLA means a small projection, such as those with which the corium of the skin is covered, and which project into the epidermis and make its union with the corium more intimate; or those covering the tongue and projecting from its surface.

PAPILLITIS is the term applied to inflammation of any papilla, but especially of the prominence formed by the end of the optic nerve in the retina, also known as optic neuritis.

PAPILLOEDEMA: Swelling of the optic disc specifically due to raised intra-cranial pressure.

PAPILLOMA means a tumour composed of papillae growing from the surface of skin or mucous membrane. These tumours may be either simple or malignant in nature. Such a tumour is found occasionally in the bladder, and the chief symptom of its presence is the painless presence of blood in the urine.

PAPOVAVIRUS is a group of viruses, one of which is responsible for warts (qv).

PAPULE means a pimple.

PARA- is a prefix meaning near, aside from, or beyond.

PARA-AMINO SALICYLIC ACID was one of the early antituberculous antibiotics. It tended to cause a lot of dyspepsia and has been replaced by newer antituberculous drugs with less side-effects. The first-line drugs for tuberculosis are now rifampicin, isoniazid, and ethambutol.

PARACENTESIS is the puncture by hollow needle or trocar and cannula of any body cavity (eg. abdominal, pleural, pericardial), for tapping or aspirating fluid pathologically accumulated. (See ASPIRATION.)

PARACETAMOL has antipyretic and analgesic actions similar to those of aspirin. The dose is 500 to 1000 milligrams.

PARACETAMOL POISONING: Paracetamol is one of the safest of drugs when taken in correct dosage. When an overdose is taken, however, it is a very dangerous one because of the toxic effect on the liver. This is why cases of poisoning with it must be taken to hospital as quickly as possible. In the early stages there is only sickness and vomiting without any loss of consciousness. Once in hospital, treatment consists of washing out the stomach, and the administration of drugs, such as cysteamine and acetylcysteine, to protect the liver.

PARACUSIS means any perversion of the sense of hearing.

PARAESTHESIA is a term applied to unusual feelings, apart from mere increase, or loss, of sensation, experienced by a patient without any external cause: for example, hot flushes, numbness, tingling, itching. Various paraesthesiae form a common symptom in some nervous diseases.

PARAFFIN is the general name used to designate a series of saturated hydrocarbon bodies, discovered by Reichenbach in 1830 and first produced as a commercial product by Young in 1850. The higher members of the series, paraffin-waxes, are solid at ordinary temperatures, some being hard, others soft. Lower in the scale comes petroleum, which is liquid at ordinary temperatures. Naphtha, petroleum spirit, and hydramyl are lower members of the series which are very volatile, and lowest comes methane, better known as marsh-gas, which is a gaseous body.
Uses: In the form of the *British Pharmacopoeia* preparation, liquid paraffin, it is used in the treatment of constipation.

Externally, the hard and soft paraffins are used in various consistencies, being very useful as ointments and lubricants as they are apparently harmless.

PARAFORMALDEHYDE is used as a source of formaldehyde. For disinfecting rooms it is prepared in the form of tablets which are vaporized on an electric hotplate. It is also used as lozenges. These should be allowed to dissolve slowly in the mouth. To keep catheters and other surgical instruments aseptic, it is enclosed with them in airtight containers.

PARAGANGLIOMA is the term used to describe two types of tumour. One known as a CHROMAFFINOMA or PHAEOCHROMOCYTOMA, is a tumour containing chromaffin cells (qv), most often found in the medulla of the suprarenal gland, where chromaffin cells are normal constituents. An important sign of these tumours is paroxysmal high blood-pressure. The other, also known as a CHEMODECTOMA, occurs in the carotid body (qv) and the comparable aortic body. It is usually quite small and is more common in women than men.

PARAGONIMIASIS is the condition caused by *paragonimus*, a genus of trematode or fluke, the most common being *Paragonimus westermani*, which is most often found in the Far East, but is also found in India, South America and parts of Africa. The disease is also known as endemic haemoptysis, as the presenting feature is haemoptysis, or the coughing up of blood, due to the worm settling in the lungs. The infection is acquired by eating inadequately cooked crayfish or crab. Bithionol is the drug most commonly used in treatment. Chloroquine is also used.

PARAGRAPHIA is misplacement of words, or of letters in words, or wrong spelling, or use of wrong words in writing as a result of a lesion in the speech region of the brain.

PARAINFLUENZA VIRUSES are divided into four types, all of which cause infection of the respiratory system. Infection with type 3 begins in May, reaches a maximum in July or August and returns to baseline level in October. Types 1 and 2 are predominantly winter viruses. In 1981, 455 cases of parainfluenza type 3 infection were reported. Children aged 1 to 11 months were the most commonly affected age-group. The manifestations include croup (qv), fever, a rash, and occasionally convulsions. It is of interest that the virus was isolated from the upper respiratory tract of three children, aged 7 weeks, 2 months and 4 months, with a diagnosis of cot death (qv).

PARALDEHYDE is a clear, colourless liquid with a penetrating ethereal odour, and a burning taste followed by a cool sensation in the mouth. Although in small quantities it may cause excitement, in larger doses it is a soporific, with little depressing effect, and productive of quiet, refreshing sleep.

Uses: It is given when a powerful hypnotic action is required, and is particularly useful in inducing sleep in mentally unstable patients. Its unpleasant taste restricts its use, but has the compensatory advantage that it usually prevents the patient receiving paraldehyde from becoming an addict. It is sometimes given per rectum as a general anaesthetic.

PARALYSIS, or PALSY, means loss of muscular power due to interference with the nervous system. When muscular power is weakened as the result of some affection of the nervous system, but not entirely lost in the parts concerned, the term *paresis* is often used instead of paralysis. Various terms are used to designate paralysis distributed in different ways. Thus *hemiplegia* is the term applied to paralysis affecting one side of the face, with the corresponding arm and leg, as the result of disease on one side of the brain; *diplegia* means a condition of more or less total paralysis, in which both sides are affected in this manner; *monoplegia* is the term applied to paralysis of a single limb; and *paraplegia* signifies paralysis of both sides of the body below a given level, usually from about the level of the waist; *quadriplegia* is paralysis of all four limbs.

Certain descriptive terms are used in popular language in connection with the word paralysis; thus *creeping paralysis* is a vague term applied most often to tabes dorsalis *shaking paralysis* is the popular name for paralysis agitans or Parkinsonism, and *wasting paralysis* commonly means progressive muscular atrophy.

Paralysis should be regarded rather as a symptom than as a disease by itself, and it is generally connected with well-marked disorder of some portion of the nervous system. According to the locality and extent of the nervous system affected, so will be the form and completeness of the paralysis.

Reference can here be made only to the more common types of paralysis, and that merely in general terms.

1. PARALYSIS DUE TO BRAIN DISEASE: Of this, by far the most common form is palsy affecting one side of the body, or **Hemiplegia**. It usually arises from disease of the hemisphere of the brain opposite to the side of the body affected, such disease being in the form of haemorrhage into the brain substance (*cerebral haemorrhage*), or the plugging up of blood-vessels by a locally formed clot (*cerebral thrombosis*) or by a clot dislodged from some other part of the body (*cerebral embolism*), and conse-

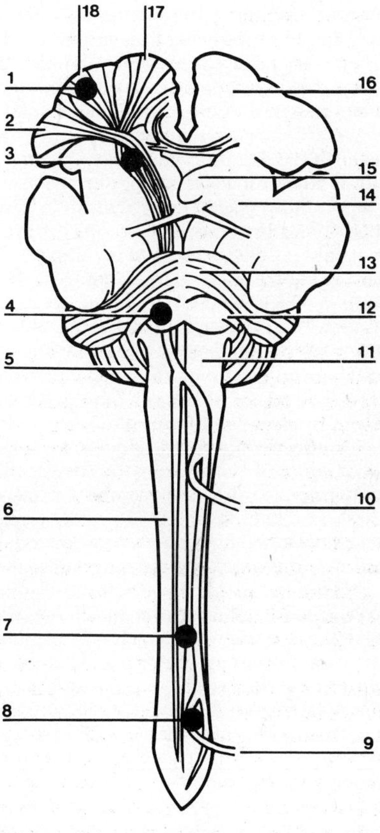

Brain and spinal cord, showing motor paths and positions of injuries causing various forms of paralysis. 1 position of haemorrhage causing paralysis of left arm; 2 face; 3 position of haemorrhage causing complete paralysis of left side; 4 position of haemorrhage followed by paralysis of left arm and leg with right side of face (crossed paralysis); 5 cerebellum; 6 spinal cord; 7 position of disorder causing paralysis of both lower limbs (paraplegia); 8 position of the disease responsible for poliomyelitis in the left leg; 9 to leg; 10 to arm; 11 medulla oblongata; 12 seventh nerve (facial); 13 pons; 14 lentiform nucleus; 15 thalamus; 16 cerebral hemisphere; 17 leg; 18 arm.

quent arrest of blood supply to an area of the brain; or again, it may result from an injury, or be due to a tumour in the tissues of the brain. The character of the seizure and the amount of paralysis vary according to the situation of the disease or injury, its extent, and its sudden or gradual occurrence. The attack may come on as a stroke (see STROKE), in which the patient becomes suddenly unconscious, and loses completely the power of motion of one side of the body, or a like result may arise more gradually and without loss of consciousness. In either type of complete hemiplegia, the paralysis affects on one side the muscles of the face, tongue, body, and limbs. Speech is indistinct and thick, and the tongue, when protruded, points towards the paralysed side owing to the unopposed action of its muscles on the unaffected side. The muscles of the face implicated are chiefly those about the mouth. The paralysed side hangs loose, and the corner of the mouth is depressed, but the muscles closing the eye are, as a rule, unimpaired, in consequence of the fact that movements like that of shutting the eyes, which are performed usually on both sides together, are controlled from either side of the brain. As a result the eye on the paralysed side can be shut, unlike what occurs in another form of facial paralysis (Bell's palsy), in which the fault lies in the nerve. The muscles of respiration on the affected side are seldom more than slightly weakened for deep breathing, but those of the arm and leg are completely powerless. Sensation may at first be impaired (anaesthesia), but as a rule returns soon, unless the portion of the brain involved be that which is connected with this function. Rigidity of the paralysed members is usually present as a later symptom. In many cases of even complete hemiplegia, improvement takes place after the lapse of weeks or months, and is in general indicated by a return of motor power, first in the face, next in the leg, while that of the arm follows after a longer or shorter interval, and is rarely complete. Such recovery of movement is, however, only partial in a large proportion of cases and the side remains weakened. In such instances the gait of the patient is characteristic. In walking, he leans to the sound side and swings round the affected limb from the hip, the foot scraping the ground as it is raised and advanced. The paralysed parts retain their contractility when stimulated by electric currents, but they are apt to suffer in their nutrition from disuse and to assume an attitude of rigidity unless treatment is carefully carried out.

In many instances the hemiplegia is only partial, and instead of the symptoms of complete paralysis just described, there exist in varied combination only certain of them, their association depending on the extent and locality of the damage to the brain. Thus there may be impairment of speech and some amount of facial paralysis, while the arm and leg may be unaffected, or the paralysis may be present in one or both extremities of one side while the other symptoms are absent. Further, the paralysis may be incomplete throughout, and the whole of the side be weak, but not entirely deprived of motor power. To partial paralysis of this latter description the term PARESIS is applied.

Besides hemiplegia, various other forms of paralysis may arise from cerebral disease. Thus occasionally there is CROSSED PARALYSIS, one side of the face and the opposite side of the body being affected simultaneously. Or again, as is often observed in the case of tumours of the brain, the paralysis may be limited to the distribution of one or more of the cranial nerves, and may produce a combination of symptoms (such as squinting, drooping of the eyelid, and impairment or loss of vision) which may enable the seat of the disease to be accurately localized. The condition of DIPLEGIA, in which both sides are affected, sometimes occurs in infants, and is due generally to some inflammation of the brain occurring soon after birth.

Trembling palsy, PARALYSIS AGITANS; PARKINSONISM or SHAKING PARALYSIS (see PARKINSONISM).

Cerebral palsy (see CEREBRAL PALSY).

Functional paralysis includes other forms of paralysis which, being of cerebral origin, should be mentioned here, although they are not connected with any discoverable disease of the brain. These forms of paralysis are amenable to psychological treatment, the cause of the paralysis often being traceable to some deep-seated mental conflict having its origin in childhood. (See HYSTERIA.)

2. PARALYSIS DUE TO DISEASE OF THE SPINAL CORD: Of paralysis from this cause, there are numerous varieties, depending on the nature, the site, and the extent of the disease. Frequently defects in muscular action, due to disease in the spinal cord, are not of a paralytic nature, and these must be carefully distinguished. For example, in disease of the posterior part of the cord, involving the sensory paths, the condition of *ataxia* is produced, and the patient, though sufficiently strong, cannot control his movements, as he is unconscious of the directions in which his limbs move till he sees the movements made. Or again, in disease of the lateral parts of the cord, involving the controlling motor paths from the brain, the condition of *spasticity* results, and when muscles contract they do so excessively, so that freedom of movement is impossible.

Paraplegia, paralysis of both lower extremities, including usually the lower portion of the trunk, and occasionally also the upper portion – indeed, all the parts below the seat of the disease in the spinal cord – is a form of paralysis which is a common result of injuries or disease of the vertebral column; also of inflammation affecting the spinal cord (myelitis), as well as of haemorrhage or tumours involving its substance. When it is due to disease, this is generally situated in the lower portion of the cord. The symptoms necessarily vary in relation to the locality and the extent of the disease in the cord. Thus, if in the affected area the posterior part of the cord, including the posterior nerve roots, suffer, the function of sensation in the parts below is impaired because the cord is unable to transmit the sensory impressions from the surface of the body to the brain, and the condition of ataxia affects the power of motion. If, on the other hand, the anterior portion of the cord and the anterior nerve roots be affected, the motor impulses from the brain cannot be conveyed to the muscles below the seat of the injury or disease, and consequently their power of movement is abolished. Whilst, if the lateral portions of the cord be affected, a condition of spastic paralysis is set up. In many forms of this complaint, particularly in the case of injuries, the whole thickness of the cord is involved (transverse myelitis), and both sensory and motor functions are lost below the level at which the cord is affected. Further, the functions of the bladder and bowels are apt to suffer, and either spasm, or more often paralysis, of these organs is the result. The nutrition of the paralysed parts tends to become affected, and bed sores and wasting of the muscles are common. Occasionally, more especially in cases of injury, recovery takes place, but in general this is incomplete, the power of walking being more or less impaired. When the paralysis is due to pressure caused by a diseased or injured spine, an operation designed to relieve this pressure is often completely successful, and entire power is restored, even after the paralysis has lasted for several months. On the other hand, the patient may linger on for years bedridden, and at last succumb to bed sores or to a septic affection of the paralysed bladder spreading up to the kidneys. Advances in recent years, however, have gone a long way towards ameliorating the lot of the paraplegic patient and allowing him or her to lead a reasonably active life at home and in the community. Patients and their relatives can obtain help and advice from the Spinal Injuries Association, Newpoint House, 76 St James's Lane, London N10 3DF (01-444 2121) and the Scottish Spinal Cord Injuries Association, Unit 22, 100 Elderpark Street, Glasgow G51 3TR (041-440 0960).

Infantile paralysis (see POLIOMYELITIS).

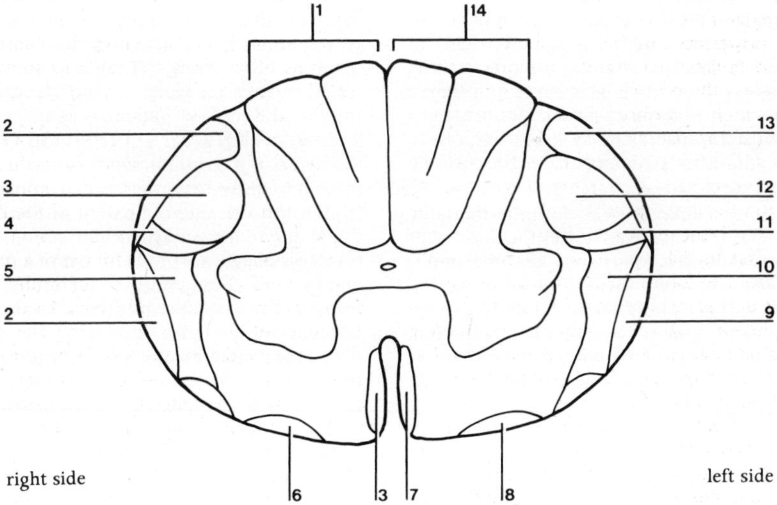

1 conscious muscle sense, direct touch
2 unconscious muscle sense
3 voluntary control of striated muscle
4 involuntary control of striated muscle
5 pain, heat and cold
6 crossed touch
7 ventral corticospinal tract (pyramidal)
8 ventral spinothalmic tract
9 ventral spinocerebellar tract
10 lateral spinothalmic tract
11 rubrospinal tract (extrapyramidal)
12 lateral corticospinal tract (pyramidal)
13 dorsal spinocerebellar tract
14 posterior columns

Diagram of a cross-section of spinal cord. Nerve tracts are shown on the right and their function on the left.

Motor neuron disease is a disease usually occurring in middle life. Pathologically it is characterized by degeneration: (*a*) of the anterior horn cells of the grey matter of the spinal cord, with corresponding degeneration of the peripheral motor nerves and wasting of the muscles innervated by them; (*b*) of the nerve cells in the bulb of the brain from which the motor cranial nerves arise: hypoglossal, facial, trigeminal, oculomotor, accessory, glossopharyngeal, vagus; (*c*) in some cases the large motor neurones of the cerebral cortex that give rise to the cortico-spinal tract. There is diffuse atrophy of the white matter of the spinal cord, excepting the posterior, sensory columns. The cause of the degeneration is not known. Approximately one person in 50,000 develops it each year, and it is estimated that there are around 5000 victims of it in the United Kingdom.

From this it can be seen that spastic paralysis and profound wasting of muscle may be combined, as in amyotrophic lateral sclerosis (qv); that a purely spastic paralysis may occur when the degenerative process affects principally the motor cells of the cerebral cortex; that a wasting of groups of muscles will occur when predominantly the anterior horn cells of the spine are involved as in progressive muscular atrophy; and that the clinical picture will be that of a bulbar paralysis when the motor nuclei of cranial nerves degenerate.

Amyotrophic lateral sclerosis is the most common form of the disease. It usually begins in middle age. The first manifestation is wasting of one hand. It is insidious in onset and it may be many months before the wasting spreads to other muscles, accompanied by fibrillation, or fasciculation (fine twitching of the fibres of the wasting muscles).

The other palmar muscles suffer in the same way, and as the disease advances the muscles of the arm, shoulders, and trunk become implicated if they have not themselves been the first to be attacked. The malady tends to spread symmetrically, involving the corresponding parts of both sides of the body in succession. It is slow in its progress, but, although it may occasionally undergo arrest, it tends to advance and involve more and more of the muscles of the body, until the sufferer is reduced to a condition of extreme helplessness. Should some other ailment not be the cause of death, the fatal result may be due to the disease extending so as to involve the muscles of respiration.

Progressive muscular atrophy is similar in its general manifestations. Indeed the modern tendency is not to differentiate between the two, but to refer to them both as simply motor neurone disease. Differences between the two include the fact that in progressive muscular atrophy there may be a long delay – in some cases a matter of years – before the initial wasting of the hand muscles begins to spread to other parts of the body. In some cases, however, it is rapid and widespread, finally involving the neck muscles to such an extent that the head droops and flops passively as the patient sits up or lies down.

Bulbar paralysis may occur as a form of motor neuron disease, or as a complication of other diseases, including rabies, diphtheria, and polyneuritis. The muscles of facial expression, of mastication, of articulation, and of swallowing suffer progressive loss of power.

Treatment: All forms of motor neuron disease run an inexorable course to a fatal termination. There is no treatment in the strict sense of the term, but much can be done to make the lot of the victim more comfortable. How this can be done is admirably summarized by the following guidelines provided by a nurse, whose doctor-husband died of the disease.

'To those caring for a patient I would suggest the following guidelines:

Care and prevention of the 'choke'

(a) Avoid excessively hot, salt, or sweet foods.
(b) Always have a cup of water at the ready.
(c) Check position and posture frequently – particularly head and neck.
(d) Reassure patient and other people present.

Care and prevention of the 'fall'

(a) Provide a rubber-tipped walking stick.
(b) Fix hand supports in appropriate places around the home, particularly in the bathroom and lavatory.
(c) Train the patient to fall correctly to avoid breaking bones (a physiotherapist can help with this).
(d) After a fall always allow the patient time to collect himself, then help him up by using graduated heights – books, stools, chairs.
(e) Always be on hand to guide limbs in the position desired by patient – as in getting in and out of the bath.

Provision of maximum comfort

(a) Allow maximum chest expansion.
(b) Ensure adjacence of bell or alarmbuzzer and telephone to attract attention.
(c) Use specially adapted knife, fork and spoon, and geriatric plate. Food should be chopped up as patient feels necessary. (I believe some need to have it 'Moulied'.)
(d) Ensure maintenance of 'fresh air' without draughts.
(e) Ensure exact positioning of pillows, and pads and sheepskins, to obtain maximum comfort.
(f) Provide arm rests to ensure that the patient can support chin in hands to ease dyspnoea.' (*British Medical Journal*, vol. 284, 1982.)

Much help can also be obtained from the Motor Neuron Disease Association, 61 Derngate, Northampton NN1 1UE (0604-25050 or 22269).

Progressive muscular dystrophy, MYOPATHY, or PSEUDOHYPERTROPHIC MUSCULAR DYSTROPHY, is one of the muscular dystrophies. (See MYOPATHY.)

3. PERIPHERAL PARALYSIS, or local paralysis of individual nerves, is of frequent occurrence. Only the most common and important examples of this condition will be briefly referred to.

Facial paralysis and BELL'S PALSY are the terms applied to paralysis involving the muscles of expression supplied by the seventh cranial nerve. It is unilateral. The cause is not known, but it sometimes follows exposure of one side of the head to a draught of cold air, which sets up inflammation of the nerve. It may also be due to injury or disease either affecting the nerve near the surface or deeper in the bony canals through which it passes, or in the brain itself, involving the nerve at its origin. The paralysis is manifested by a marked change in the expression of the face, the patient being unable to move the muscles of one side in such acts as laughing, and whistling, or to close the eye on that side. The mouth is drawn to the sound side, while, although the muscles of mastication are not involved, the food in eating tends to lodge between the jaw and cheek on the palsied side. Occasionally, when the nerve is injured as it passes through the skull, the sense of taste is impaired. In the ordinary cases of this disease, such as those due to exposure, recovery usually takes place in about six weeks, the improvement being first shown in the power of closing the eye, which is soon followed by the disappearance of the other signs. Recovery may be speeded up by the administration of prednisolone (qv), especially if this is given at an early stage of the disease. It is more effective in younger patients (under the age of 45) than older ones. When the paralysis proceeds from wounding of the nerve, disease of the temporal bone, or from tumours in the brain, it is more apt to be permanent, and is in many cases of serious import.

Lead palsy is a common form of local paralysis. It is due to the poisonous action of lead upon the system, and, like the other symptoms of lead poisoning, affects chiefly workers in that metal. (See LEAD POISONING.)

A form of peripheral paralysis, resembling this often results from chronic alcoholism. Other poisons also act similarly, as, for example, arsenic. (See NEURITIS.) Injury to a nerve may cause paralysis in the muscles which it should supply, and this may follow on wounds, severe bruises, or even long-continued pressure, as in crutch-palsy. (See DROP-WRIST; NERVE INJURIES.) The paralysis occurring after diphtheria, another example of the peripheral variety, has been already mentioned, and similar paralyses, for example of the foot, follow sometimes on other infectious diseases. (See DIPHTHERIA; DROP-FOOT.)

Treatment: It is impossible in a brief notice like the present to enter at any length into the treatment of the different varieties of paralysis. Generally speaking, the treatment consists of measures which aim at supporting the patient's strength and maintaining his health while the nervous system is slowly restoring itself so far as may be. The conditions of the disease in any particular case can only be understood and appreciated by the medical expert, under whose direction alone treatment can be advantageously carried out.

An important point in the treatment is that, since paralysed muscles tend to undergo degenerative changes, their action should be maintained as long as possible. With the view of improving the circulation in the muscles, and also in order to prevent stiffening of the joints, massage is very useful. In order to exercise the muscles, the faradic current or, failing it, the interrupted galvanic current, may be applied daily.

In the case of paraplegia there is a necessity for highly skilled nursing, since not only the patient's comfort but his life depends upon careful management, directed towards preventing bed sores (see BED SORES), and inflammation of the bladder (see CATHETERS) in cases in which the act of urination is interfered with. A similar remark applies to bulbar palsy, in which special care is necessary in feeding the patient, owing to his difficulty in swallowing.

In all forms of paralysis, particularly the more severe cases, such as paraplegia, cheerfulness is an essential ingredient of treatment combined with reassurance. In few afflictions does the will to survive and live as full a life as possible play a more important role in obtaining the optimum return to normality.

PARAMETRITIS means inflammation in the cellular tissue at the side of the womb.

PARAMNESIA is a derangement of the memory in which words are used without a comprehension of their meaning; it is also applied to illusions of memory in which a person in good faith imagines and describes experiences which never occurred to him.

PARAMYOCLONUS is the name applied to an affection in which paroxysmal jerking contractions of the muscles of the limbs take place; it is sometimes due to organic disease of the nervous system, sometimes hysterical.

PARANOIA is a form of mental illness characterized by fixed delusions, usually of persecution. Many sufferers are able to go about freely and carry out activities with which their delusions do not interfere. In loose English usage, 'paranoia' means 'subject to any sorts of feelings of persecution'. (See MENTAL ILLNESS.)

PARAPHASIA is misplacement of words, or use of wrong words, in speech as a result of a lesion in the speech region of the brain.

PARAPHRENIA is a form of paranoia (qv). (See also MENTAL ILLNESS.)

PARAPLEGIA means paralysis of the lower limbs, accompanied generally by paralysis of bladder and rectum. (See PARALYSIS.)

PARAQUAT is a contact herbicide widely used in agriculture and horticulture. A mouthful is enough to kill. Its major misuse has resulted in its being decanted from the professional pack into soft drink bottles and kept in the domestic kitchen. The resultant potential for accidental and probably fatal ingestion is obvious. It is involved in around 40 cases of suicide every year. The eyes and skin must be carefully protected so as not to come into contact with it. So widespread is its use that nineteen medical centres have been set up throughout the country to provide treatment in cases of poisoning with it. Details of these can be obtained from the National Poisons Information Service centres in London (Tel: 01-407 7600), Edinburgh (031-229 2477) and Cardiff (0222 492233).

PARASITICIDE is a general term applied to agents or substances destructive to parasites.

PARASUICIDE is non-fatal self-poisoning or self-injury, or attempted suicide. It is most common in the 12–15 age-group. The intention is not as a rule to commit suicide, but a cry for help to resolve an acute domestic upset.

PARASYMPATHETIC NERVOUS SYSTEM is that part of the autonomic nervous system which is connected with the brain and spinal cord through certain nerve centres in the mid-brain, medulla, and lower end of the cord. The nerves from these centres are carried in the 3rd, 7th, 9th, and 10th cranial nerves and the 2nd, 3rd, and 4th sacral nerves. The action of the parasympathetic system is usually antagonistic to that of the sympathetic system. Thus it inhibits the action of the heart and augments the action of the intestine, whereas the sympathetic augments the action of the heart and inhibits that of the intestine.

PARATHION is one of the organophosphorus insecticides (qv). It is highly toxic to man and must therefore be handled with the utmost care.

PARATHYROID is the name applied to four small glands, about 5 mm in diameter, which lie to the side of and behind the thyroid gland. These glands regulate the metabolism of calcium and of phosphorus. If for any reason there is a deficiency of the secretion of the parathyroid glands, the amount of calcium in the blood falls too low and the amount of phosphorus increases. The result is the condition known as tetany (qv), in which there is great restlessness and spasm of muscles. The condition is checked by the injection of calcium gluconate – which causes an increase in the amount of calcium in the blood. The commonest cause of this condition, or hypoparathyroidism as it is known, is accidental injury to or removal of the glands during the operation of thyroidectomy for the treatment of thyrotoxicosis (qv). This is one of the hazards of thyroidectomy in view of the very close relationship of the parathyroid glands to the thyroid gland. If there is over-production of the parathyroids there will be an increase of calcium in the blood. This extra calcium is drawn from the bones, in which, as a consequence, thin cysts form and greatly weaken the bones, these breaking easily as a result. This cystic disease of bone is known as OSTEITIS FIBROSA CYSTICA (qv). Tumours of the parathyroid glands result in this overactivity of the parathyroid hormone, and the resulting increase in the amount of calcium in the blood leads to the formation of stones in the kidneys. The only available treatment is surgical removal of the tumour. This state of increased activity of the parathyroid glands, or hyperparathyroidism, is always considered as a possible cause in dealing with a case of stones in the kidneys. (See KIDNEYS, DISEASES OF.)

PARATYPHOID FEVER (see ENTERIC FEVERS).

PAREGORIC, or CAMPHORATED OPIUM TINCTURE, is a preparation of opium much used for cough mixtures. It contains 5 per cent of tincture of opium, together with oil of anise, benzoic acid and camphor. The dose is 2 to 10 ml. Scotch paregoric, or ammoniated opium tincture, contains 10 per cent of tincture of opium, together with dilute ammonia solution, oil of anise and benzoic acid. The dose is 2 to 4 ml.

PARENCHYMA is a term meaning originally all the soft tissues of internal organs except the muscular flesh, though now reserved for the secreting cells of the glandular organs.

PARENTERAL is the word applied to the administration of drugs by any route other than by the mouth or by the bowel.

PARENTERAL NUTRITION: In severely ill patients, especially those who have had major surgery or with sepsis, burns, acute pancreatitis and renal failure, the body's reserves of protein become exhausted. This results in weight loss, reduction of muscle mass, a fall in the serum albumin and lymphocyte count and an impairment of cellular immunity. Severely ill patients are unable to take adequate food by mouth to repair the body protein loss so that enteral or parenteral nutrition is required. Enteral feeding is through the gastro-intestinal tract with the aid of a naso-gastric tube. Parenteral nutrition involves the provision of carbohydrate, fat and proteins by intravenous administration. Intitally the carbohydrate glucose was the sole energy substrate used, but it soon became appreciated that regimes supplying an equal proportion of carbohydrate and fat were preferable in the vast majority of cases. Over the last decade a multitude of nitrogen solutions have been developed for the purpose of intravenous nutrition. As with enteral nutrition there are few indications for the administrations of pure amino acids. All patients requiring intravenous nutrition will require, in addition, a supply of vitamins and essential minerals.

Methods of vascular access have improved remarkably over recent years. The preferred route for the infusion of hyperosmolar solutions is via a central venous catheter. If parenteral nutrition is required for more than two weeks it is advisable to use a long-term type catheter such as the Broviac, Hickman or extra corporeal type, which is made of silastic material and is inserted via a long subcutaneous tunnel, which not only helps to fix the catheter but minimises the risk of ascending infection.

Dextrose is considered the best source of carbohydrate and may be used as a 20 per cent or 50 per cent solution. Amino acids should be in the laevo form and should contain the correct proportion of essential and non-essential amino acids. Preparations such as Vamin glucose 9, Synthamin 9 (low nitrogen solution), Synthamin 14 and 17 (high nitrogen solutions) are available with or without electrolytes. Intralipid is the safest fat emulsion and is used either as 10 per cent or 20 per cent solution.

The main hazards of intravenous feeding are blood-borne infections made possible by continued direct access to the circulation, and biochemical abnormalities related to the composition of the solutions infused. The continuous use of hypertonic solutions of glucose can cause hyperglycaemia and glycosuria and the resultant polyuria may lead to dehydration. Treatment with insulin is needed when hyperosmolality occurs, and in addition the water and sodium deficits will require to be corrected.

PARESIS means a state of partial paralysis. (See PARALYSIS.)

PARIETAL is the term applied to anything pertaining to the wall of a cavity: eg. parietal pleura, the part of the pleural membrane which lines the wall of the chest.

PARKINSONISM, or PARKINSON'S DISEASE, so called after the London general practitioner who first described the condition in 1817, is also known as PARALYSIS AGITANS. It is a progressive disease of insidious onset which comes on in the second half of life, and is due to degenerative changes in the ganglia at the base of the cerebrum. This results in a deficiency of a neurotransmitter known as dopamine (qv), and it is this deficiency of dopamine which is responsible for most cases. In some, however, deficiency of neurotransmitters other than dopamine may be the cause. It is much commoner in men than in women. In some cases the disease is a sequel to encephalitis lethargica. The disease first manifests itself by increasing rigidity of the muscles. In the face this results in a loss of the natural play of expression and produces a mask-like expression. The voice is also affected by the rigidity of the muscles of the larynx, tongue and lips, loses its tone and inflexion and develops into a monotone. Later the limbs become rigid, and this is typified by the peculiar running gait. The patient always seems to be tottering and taking short steps as if running after himself. Later a coarse tremor develops in the muscles, best typified in the rolling movements of the fingers as if a cigarette were always being rolled. The tremor is exaggerated by excitement and self-consciousness and ceases during sleep. In the hands and arms it may interfere grossly with eating and dressing.

Treatment: There is now an increasing number of drugs that keep the condition under control. None is curative, and the effort to find the most suitable one for any given individual is usually a matter of trial and error, the successful outcome of which depends largely upon understanding cooperation between family doctor and patient. The most promising one at the moment is levodopa which is a precursor of dopamine. Its introduction has revolutionized the outlook in this disease. Unfortunately it has considerable side-effects, which means that it must only be administered under skilled medical supervision. Current opinion is that it produces spectacular improvement in one-fifth of patients, moderate improvement in two-fifths, modest improvement in one-fifth, and no improvement in one-fifth. A recently introduced drug proving of value in supplementing the benefit of levodopa is selegiline.

Patients with the disease and their relatives, seeking advice and help, are recommended to get in touch with the Parkinson's Disease Society of the UK, 36 Portland Place, London W1N 3DG (01–255 2432).

PAROMOMYCIN is an antibiotic derived from a sub-species of *Streptomyces rimosus*, which is proving of value in the treatment of certain cases of both bacillary and amoebic dysentery.

PARONYCHIA is the term applied to inflammation near the nail. In the *acute* form it is usually due to infection with *Staphylococcus aureus*, and is most often seen in nurses and others handling septic material. It usually starts at one corner of the nail-fold and then spreads to the other side and deeply under the base of the nail. There is local pain and tenderness, with swelling of the nail-fold. Treatment in mild cases consists of applying an adhesive dressing and giving penicillin. In more severe cases the swelling has to be opened. A new nail grows in two or three months, displacing the old one in front of it. *Chronic paronychia* occurs usually in women who have their hands much in water. In men it occurs in fishmongers and chefs. It may affect one or more fingers. Treatment consists of keeping the finger dry and giving a suitable antibiotic. (See WHITLOW.)

PAROSMIA means a perverted sense of smell; everything usually smells unpleasant to the affected individual. The most common cause is some septic condition of the nasal passages, but it may occasionally be due to a lesion in the brain involving the centre responsible for the sense of smell.

PAROTID GLAND is one of the salivary glands (qv). It is situated just in front of the ear, and its duct runs forwards across the cheek to open into the interior of the mouth on a little projection opposite the second last tooth of the upper row. The parotid gland is generally the first of the salivary glands to become enlarged in mumps.

PAROTITIS means inflammation of the parotid gland. Epidemic parotitis is another name for mumps (qv).

PAROVARIUM is a rudimentary structure situated near the ovary, in which tumours sometimes arise.

PARSLEY is the leaves and fruit of *Apium petroselinum*. It has a stimulant and diuretic action. It should not be confused with *fool's parsley*, or lesser hemlock, *Aethusa cynapium*, which is highly poisonous.

PARTHENOGENESIS is non-sexual reproduction. In other words, development of the ovum into an individual without fertilization by a spermatozoon. It is a rare spontaneous event. In *The Lancet* in 1955 it was reported that a woman had had a daughter where parthenogenesis could not be disproved. It has been produced in animals experimentally. There is, however, no certain record of the birth of a parthenogenetic animal. The most that has been achieved is that parthogenetic mice and rabbit embryos have developed normally to about halfway through pregnancy but have then died and been aborted.

PARTOGRAM is a method of recording the degree of dilatation, or opening, of the cervix (or neck) of the uterus in labour, which is of value in assessing how labour is progressing.

PARTURITION (see LABOUR).

PARULIS is another name for gumboil or abscess of the gum.

PARVOVIRUSES (from *parvus*, Latin for small) is a group of viruses responsible for outbreaks of winter vomiting disease (qv).

P.A.S. is a commonly used abbreviation for para-aminosalicylic acid (qv).

PASTEURELLA is a group of bacilli. They are essentially animal parasites that under certain conditions are transmitted to man. They include the micro-organism responsible for plague and tularaemia.

PASTEURIZATION is a method of sterilizing milk. In many parts of the world pasteurization has done away with milk-borne infections, of which the most serious is bovine tuberculosis, affecting the glands, bones, and joints of children. Other infections conveyed by milk are scarlet fever, diphtheria, enteric fever (typhoid and paratyphoid), undulant fever (brucellosis), and food poisoning (eg. from salmonellae or the toxins of the staphylococcus). The case therefore is very clear for the compulsory pasteurization of all milk. Yet 10 per cent of all milk retailed in Scotland is neither pasteurized nor heat treated in any way. The comparable figure for England and Wales is 3 per cent.

HIGH-TEMPERATURE SHORT-TIME (HTST) PASTEURIZATION consists in heating the milk at a temperature not less than 71·7°C (161°F) for at least fifteen seconds, followed by immediate cooling to a temperature of not more than 10°C (50°F).

LOW-TEMPERATURE PASTEURIZATION, or 'HOLDER' PROCESS, consists in maintaining the milk for at least half-an-hour at a temperature between 63° to 65°C (145°F and 150°F), followed by immediate cooling to a temperature of not more that 10°C (50°F). This has the effect of considerably reducing the number of bacteria contained in the milk and of preventing the diseases conveyed by milk referred to above. This procedure is sufficient for the sale of milk as 'pasteurized milk' in England. (See MILK.)

PATELLA, also known as the knee-pan or knee-cap, is a flat bone shaped somewhat like an oyster-shell, lying in the tendon of the extensor muscle of the thigh, and protecting the knee-joint in front. (See BONES; KNEE; FRACTURES.)

PATHOGENIC means disease-producing, and is a term, for example, applied to bacteria, capable of causing disease.

PATHOGNOMONIC is a term applied to signs or symptoms which are specially characteristic of certain diseases, and on the presence or absence of which the diagnosis depends. Thus the discovery of the *Mycobacterium tuberculosis* in the expectoration is said to be pathognomonic of pulmonary tuberculosis.

PATHOLOGY is the science which deals with the causes of, and changes produced in the body by, disease.

PAUL-BUNNELL TEST is a test for glandular fever (qv) which is based upon the fact that patients with glandular fever develop antibodies which agglutinate sheep red blood cells.

PECTIN is a polysaccharide substance allied to starch, contained in fruits and plants, and forming the basis of vegetable jelly. It has been used as a transfusion fluid in place of blood in cases of haemorrhage and shock.

PECTORAL means anything pertaining to the chest, or a remedy used in treating chest troubles.

PECTORILOQUY means the resonance of the voice, when spoken or whispered words can be clearly heard through the stethoscope. It is a sign of consolidation, or of a cavity, in the lung.

PEDICULOSIS is infestation with lice.

Pediculi, or lice, are of three species, which vary in shape and size as well as in the area of the body they infest.

PEDICULUS HUMANUS var. CAPITIS (*Pediculus capitis*), or the head louse, is similar in practically all respects to the body louse, except that it occurs in the head and not on the trunk of the body. It is more common in girls and women than boys and men. The eggs, commonly known as nits and visible as little white specks, are usually laid in the hairs of the back of the head; behind the ears is also a favourite site. On infested heads the hairs are often matted together by the exudate which results from irritation and scratching. The glands behind the ears and in the back of the neck are often enlarged.

PEDICULUS HUMANUS var. CORPORIS (*Pediculus vestimenti*), or the body louse, is found on the underclothing on the trunk and upper arms, rather than on the skin. The female louse, which has a life of almost a month, lays seven to ten eggs a day. The eggs hatch out in 7 to 10 days and become mature in another week. Without food the adult dies in nine days and the newly hatched louse in two days. The eggs are viable for much longer (up to a month) and are usually found in the more inaccessible parts of the clothing: eg. the seams.

PEDICULUS PUBIS, popularly known as the crab louse, is broader and shorter. It is found predominantly on the short hairs of the pubic region, to which it adheres very tenaciously. It may also infest the eye-lashes, beard, and leg and under-arm hairs. It causes intense itching. So far as is known, it does not carry any disease. It is most commonly transmitted from one person to another by sexual contact. Live lice have been found on lavatory seats, and the eggs may be spread from a lousy person by attachment of their infected hairs to towels and clothing.

(For further details, see INSECTS IN RELATION TO DISEASE.)

PELLAGRA is a nutritional disorder, showing a number of nervous, digestive, and skin symptoms.

Causes: It occurs in those parts of the world where the inhabitants live on a diet of maize without adequate first-class protein in the form of milk and meat. It is due to deficiency of the nicotinic acid component of the vitamin B complex, in association with deficiency of protein. For long the puzzling feature was that it occurred predominantly in maize-eating areas of the world, yet maize has as much nicotinic acid as wheat but the disease did not occur in wheat-eating areas. The explanation is that the nicotinic acid in maize is in a bound form that the consumer cannot utilize. Further, maize is deficient in the amino-acid, tryptophan, from which the human body can make nicotinic acid.

Symptoms: Pellagra is known as the disease of the three D's: dermatitis, diarrhoea and dementia. The course of pellagra lasts many years, with digestive disturbances including loss of appetite and diarrhoea or constipation, headache, and irritability of temper. The skin manifestations consist at first of redness resembling severe sunburn on the parts of the body exposed to the sun, such as the hands, forearms, chest, neck, and face. The irritation usually lasts about a fortnight, is followed by desquamation, and the skin remains rough, thickened, and permanently brownish in colour. This brownish and roughened appearance on the hands is the most prominent feature of the disease, and from this the disease takes its name. Tremors, sleepiness, and weakness of the legs also appear. For several years the disease may recur in this manner every spring, the attacks gradually becoming more severe, the patient slowly growing emaciated and in some cases completely paralytic or demented.

Treatment: The disease is prevented or cured by adding to the diet foods such as fresh meat, eggs, milk, liver, and yeast extracts, and nicotinic acid, as well as by improvement of the general conditions of life.

PELOTHERAPY is the therapeutic use of mud or peat. It is prescribed either as general or local baths or in the form of a pack.

PELVIS is that divison of the skeleton which is made up of the haunch-bones, one on each side, and the sacrum and coccyx behind. It connects the lower limbs with the spine. Each haunch-bone is composed of three originally separate bones, in the adult pelvis firmly fused together: the ilium; the ischium, with a rounded part below, the tuberosity, upon which the body rests in sitting; and the pubis in front. The expanded parts of the iliac bones incompletely surround the lower part of the abdomen, known as the false pelvis, and are separated by a distinct line, known as the brim or inlet, from the true pelvis beneath. The true pelvis, as its name implies, is basin-shaped; though in the dried state it has a wide outlet beneath, yet in the living body this is well closed and rounded off by ligaments and muscles so as to leave small openings only for the urinary and genital passages and for the rectum. This soft floor of the pelvis is composed mainly of two muscles, the levators of the anus, whilst the deep notch, between the haunch-bone and sacrum behind, is closed in by a pair of strong sacro-sciatic ligaments.

The pelvis varies considerably in the two sexes. In the female it is shallower and the ilia are more widely separated, giving great breadth to the hips of the woman; the inlet is more circular and the outlet larger; whilst the angle beneath the pubic bones (subpubic angle), which is an acute angle in the male, is obtuse in the female. All these points are of importance in connection with child-bearing.

The contents of the pelvis are the urinary bladder and rectum in both sexes; in addition the male has the seminal vesicles and the prostate gland surrounding the neck of the bladder, whilst the female has the womb, ovaries, and their appendages.

In addition to these sex differences, there are differences in the pelvis of different races, those of certain races, such as the Negro race, being, generally speaking, longer from before back and from above down than those of Caucasians: the so-called anthropoid pelvis.

PEMPHIGUS is an autoimmune skin condition characterized by the appearance of large blebs. *Pemphigus neonatorum* is really a form of impetigo in which Bullae (or large blisters) occur. (The term Pemphigus Neonatorum is misleading and should be abandoned.) It is liable to occur in nurseries and maternity hospitals and is highly infectious. Strict isolation of cases is essential and the prognosis is satisfactory provided active treatment is started at an early stage. In addition to the local treatment recommended for impetigo in older children and adults, an antibiotic or sulphonamide should be given provided the staphylococcus responsible or the condition is sensitive to it. Unfortunately *Staphylococcus aureus*, especially that which occurs in hospital, is so often resistant to penicillin that this antibiotic is of no avail, and some other has to be used. *Pemphigus vulgaris*, which occurs in the middle-aged, particularly Jews, is a comparatively rare condition. The skin eruption is accompanied by marked constitutional disturbances and, until the introduction of the corticosteroids (qv) it was almost invariably fatal, though it still carries a mortality rate of 30–50 per cent. With large doses of corticosteroids, however, the condition can usually be kept under control. The local application of zinc cream or calamine lotion is soothing. *Pemphigus foliaceus*, in which practically the whole of the skin may be involved, is not marked by such constitutional disturbances. Treatment is as for pemphigus vulgaris. *Pemphigoid* is the form of the disease as it occurs in old age. It responds well to corticosteroids. It may occur as a complication of Penicillamine or Gold therapy and usually clears on withdrawal of the offending drug.

PENICILLAMINE is a metabolite of penicillin which is a chelating agent (qv). It is sometimes used in Rheumatoid arthritis that has not responded to the first-line remedies and it is particularly useful when the disease is complicated by vasculitis. Penicillamine is also used as an antidote to poisoning by heavy metals, particularly copper and lead, as it is able to bind these metals and so remove their toxic effects. Because of its ability to bind copper it is also used in Wilson's disease where there is a deficiency in the copper-binding protein so that copper is able to become deposited in he brain and liver, damaging these tissues.

PENICILLIN is the name given by Sir Alexander Fleming, in 1929, to an antibacterial substance produced by the mould *Penicillium notatum*. This mould was first described in 1911 in Scandinavia, where it was discovered in decaying hyssop. The story of penicillin is one of the most dramatic in the history of medicine, and its introduction into medicine initiated a new era in therapeutics comparable only to the introduction of anaesthesia by Morton and Simpson and of antiseptics by Pasteur and Lister. The two names that will always be primarily associated with penicillin are those of Sir Alexander Fleming, of St Mary's Hospital, London, who discovered its anti-bacterial action, and Lord Florey, of Oxford, who did so much to develop its practical use during the 1939–45 War. The two great advantages of penicillin are that it is active against a large range of bacteria and that, even in large doses, it is non-toxic. Among the organisms against which it is active are: staphylococcus, streptococcus, pneumococcus, meningococcus, gonococcus, and the organisms responsible for syphilis, and for gas gangrene.

Penicillin has been synthesized in the laboratory, but it is such a complex and unstable substance that there is no reason to believe that it will be possible to synthesize it on a commercial scale – at least not for a long time to come. This means that the main method of obtaining penicillin is by the laborious technique of cultivating the penicillin mould, *Penicillium chrysogenum*. Partial synthesis of penicillin, however, has been achieved by the isolation of the penicillin nucleus – 6-aminopenicillanic acid. This can still only be obtained by culture of the penicillin mould but, now that the nucleus can be isolated, it has proved possible to add side-chains to it and so produce a large number of different –semi-synthetic as they are known – penicillins.

Various forms of penicillin are now available. *Benzylpenicillin* is available as the sodium or potassium salt. It is given intramuscularly, and is the form that is used when a rapid action is required. It can also be given by mouth but, as the proportion absorbed varies greatly, it is unreliable in action when given in this way. *Procaine penicillin* is a relatively insoluble form of penicillin. A single daily intramuscular injection of 600,000 units will maintain a bacteriostatic level in the blood for twenty-four hours. *Benzathine penicillin* is a relatively insoluble derivative of penicillin which is often given by mouth. When given intramuscularly it gives low but very prolonged blood levels of penicillin. *Phenoxymethyl penicillin* is given by mouth but is absorbed inconstantly.

Phenethicillin is the first of the new penicillins obtained by adding a side chain to the penicillin nucleus. It is effective when taken by mouth and produces a blood concentration of penicillin which is twice as great as that following a comparable dose of phenoxymethylpenicillin. *Ampicillin* is another of the new penicillins derived by semi-synthesis from the penicillin nucleus. It, too, is active when taken by mouth, but its special feature is that it is active against Gram-negative micro-organisms such as *E. coli* and the salmonellae. *Cloxacillin* is yet another of the semi-synthesized penicillins. It has a relatively weak antibacterial action, but has the advantage of being active against penicillin-resistant staphylococci. *Propicillin* is alpha-phenoxypropyl penicillin, which is active when taken by mouth, and against penicillin-resistant staphylococci. *Phenbenicillin* is potassium phenoxybenzylpenicillin and is active when taken by mouth.

Methicillin is another of the new penicillins derived from the penicillin nucleus. It is active against penicillin-resistant staphylococci but has to be given by injection as it is destroyed by the acid secretion of the stomach. *Carbenicillin*, yet another of the new semi-synthetic penicillins, must be given by injection, which may be painful. Its main use is in dealing with infections due to *Pseudomonas pyocanea*. It is the only penicillin active against this micro-organism. *Carfecillin* is another semi-synthetic penicillin. It is given by mouth and in the body is converted into carbenicillin, to which it owes its antibiotic properties. It is proving of particular value in the treatment of infection of the urinary tract such as cystitis and pyelonephritis. *Flucloxacillin*, also a semi-synthetic penicillin, is active against penicillin-resistant staphylococci and has the practical advantage of being active when taken by mouth. *Amoxycillin* and *talampicillin* are orally administered semi-synthetic penicillins with the same range of action as ampicillin but less likely to cause side-effects. *Mezlocillin*, another semi-synthetic penicillin, is comparable to ampicillin in its range of action, but is particularly active against *H. influenzae*, gonococci, and *Proteus* micro-organisms. *Mecillinam* is yet another in this series, though of slightly different chemical origin. It is proving of value in the treatment of infections with salmonellae (see SALMONELLA INFECTIONS), including typhoid fever, and with *E. coli* (see ESCHERICHIA). It is given by injection. There is a derivative, *Pivmecillinam*, which can be taken by mouth.

PENIS is the organ down which, in the male, passes the urethra, the tube by which the contents of the urinary bladder and those of the seminal vesicles escape.

PENNYROYAL is a popular name for several plants such as *Menthapulegium* (European pennyroyal) and *Hedeoma pulegioides* (American pennyroyal). These plants contain a volatile oil which is used for rubbing into the skin to prevent the bites of midges and mosquitoes and to allay the itching caused by them.

PENTAMIDINE is a drug that is used in the prevention and treatment of African trypansomiasis, and in the treatment of leishmaniasis.

PENTAZOCINE is a pain-relieving drug with similar actions and uses to those of morphine, but much less likely to lead to addiction. It is given, usually by injection, for the relief of moderate to severe pain, especially postoperative pain, and to relieve the pain of myocardial infarction, or coronary thrombosis.

PEPPER is the unripe fruit of *Piper nigrum*, a vine of the East Indies, and possesses an active principle, piperine. It is used externally as a counter-irritant and internally as a stimulant to digestion.

PEPPERMINT is the leaves and tops of *Mentha piperita*. It has an aromatic odour, due to the presence of an oil from which is obtained menthol, a camphor-like substance. (See MENTHOL.) Peppermint water is a useful remedy for flatulence and colic in infants. Oil of peppermint is used like the other volatile oils.

PEPSIN is the name given to a ferment found in the gastric juice which digests proteins by converting them into peptides and amino-acids. Pepsin is used in medicine in cases of weak digestion either to digest food before it is taken or more frequently to administer after meals. It is a light yellowish-brown or white powder prepared from the fresh mucous membrane of the stomach of pigs, sheep, or calves. (For the predigestion of food, see PEPTONIZED FOODS.)

PEPTIC ULCER is the term commonly applied to ulcers in the stomach and duodenum. (See DUODENAL ULCER; STOMACH, DISEASES OF.)

PEPTIDE is a compound formed by the union of two or more amino-acids.

PEPTONIZED FOODS are foods which have been predigested by pancreatin (qv) and thereby rendered more digestible.

PERCUSSION is an aid to diagnosis practised by striking the body with the fingers, in such a way as to make it give out a note. It was introduced in 1761 by Leopold Auenbrugger (1722–1809) of Vienna, the son of an innkeeper, who derived the idea from the habit of his father tapping casks of wine to ascertain how much wine they contained. According to the degree of dullness or resonance of the note, an opinion can be formed as to the state of consolidation of air-containing organs, the presence of abnormal cavities in organs, and the dimensions of solid and air-containing organs, which happen to lie next to one another. Still more valuable evidence is given by auscultation (qv).

PERCUTANEOUS is a term applied to any method of administering remedies by passing them through the skin, as by rubbing in an ointment or carrying in drugs on the galvanic current.

PERFORATION is one of the serious dangers attaching to any ulcerated condition of the stomach or bowels. When a perforation from one of these hollow organs takes place into the peritoneal cavity, many bacteria, are poured into this cavity and there set up peritonitis. (See PERITONITIS.) The immediate signs that a perforation has taken place are usually a state of collapse, and increase of pain over the abdomen, together with, in some cases, the evidence of free fluid and gas in the peritoneal cavity.

PERHEXILINE is a drug used in the treatment of severe cases of angina pectoris (qv).

PERI- is a prefix meaning around.

PERIARTERITIS NODOSA (see POLYARTERITIS NODOSA).

PERICARDITIS means inflammation of the pericardium. (See HEART DISEASES.)

PERICARDIUM is the smooth membrane that surrounds the heart. (See HEART.)

PERICYAZINE (NEULACTIL) (see ANTIPSYCHOTIC DRUGS).

PERIMETRITIS means a localized inflammation of the peritoneum surrounding the womb.

PERINATAL MORTALITY consists of deaths of the foetus after the 28th week of pregnancy and deaths of the new-born child during the first week of life. Today, more individuals die within a few hours of birth than during the following forty years. It is therefore not surprising that the perinatal mortality rate, which is the number of such deaths per 1000 total births, has come to be looked upon as a valuable indicator of the quality of care provided for the mother and her new-born baby. In 1984, the perinatal mortality rate was 10·0 in England, compared with 32·5 in 1960. This is still much higher than in several other countries. Thus, in 1977, the perinatal mortality rate was 10·1 in Sweden, 10·6 in Denmark and 11·2 in Switzerland. In Northern Ireland it was 21·1. Overall, in 1977, the latest year for which comparable figures are available the perinatal mortality rate for England and Wales was the 19th lowest of the 32 countries which provided statistics.

The causes of perinatal mortality include intrapartum anoxia (that is, difficulty in the birth of the baby, resulting in lack of oxygen), congenital abnormalities of the baby, antepartum anoxia (that is, conditions in the terminal stages of pregnancy preventing the foetus getting sufficient oxygen), and injuries to the brain of the baby during birth.

In 1984 perinatal deaths in England and Wales numbered 6,464 (which number includes still births). The deaths during the first weeks of life numbered 2,821. The commonest cause of perinatal death was some complication of placenta, cord or membranes. The next most common was congenital abnormality. Intra-uterine hypoxia and birth asphyxia comprised the third most common cause.

PERINEUM, or FORK, or CROTCH, is the region situated between the opening of the bowel behind and of the genital organs in front. In women it is apt to be lacerated in the act of childbirth.

PERIOD (see MENSTRUATION).

PERIODIC PARALYSIS is a condition characterized by the onset of weakness of the voluntary muscles. It usually occurs in young adults. As a rule the onset is in the morning on awakening. The weakness usually lasts for several hours. Attacks may also be brought on by a heavy meal or severe cold. It is a familial condition of obscure origin. There is one form, probably the most common, which is apparently due to a low level of potassium in the blood and is relieved by the taking of potassium chloride – 10 grams in water. There are other forms, however, in which the blood potassium may be raised or normal.

PERIODONTAL MEMBRANE (see TEETH).

PERIOSTEUM is the membrane surrounding a bone. The periosteum carries blood-vessels and nerves for the nutrition and development of the bone. When it is irritated, an increased deposit of bone takes place beneath it; if it is destroyed, the bone may cease to grow and a portion may die and separate as a sequestrum. (See BONE.)

PERIOSTITIS means inflammation on the surface of a bone affecting the periosteum. (See BONE, DISEASES OF.)

PERIPHERAL NEURITIS means inflammation of the nerves in the outlying parts of the body. (See NEURITIS.)

PERISTALSIS is the worm-like movement by which the stomach and bowels propel their contents. It consists of alternate waves of relaxation and contraction in successive parts of the tube. When any obstruction to the movement of the contents exists, these contractions become more forcible and are liable to be accompanied by the severe form of pain known as colic.

PERITONEOSCOPY is viewing of the peritoneal cavity through a tube fitted with mirrors and light. The instrument (resembling a CYSTOSCOPE (qv)) is entered just below the umbilicus. The peritoneal cavity is then inflated with air. This simple operation may obviate a more drastic one: for example, if peritoneoscopy shows deposits of cancer in the peritoneum or the liver. Colour photographs of the liver have been taken through the peritoneoscope.

PERITONEUM is the membrane lining the abdominal cavity, and forming a covering for the organs contained in it. That part lining the walls of the abdomen is called the parietal peritoneum, and that part covering the viscera is known as the visceral peritoneum. The two are continuous with one another at the back of the abdomen, and form a closed sac. One may understand its relation to the organs by conceiving them to have been pressed against the outside of this sac from behind, and each to have become wrapped up in the hinder part of the sac without being forced through to its interior, while the front wall of the sac remains quite smooth. The folds of peritoneum passing from one organ to another are thus very complicated, and receive special names in various parts. (See MESENTERY; OMENTUM.)

Although the peritoneum is said to form a closed sac, there is an exception in the female, the Fallopian tube on each side having an opening into the cavity at its end large enough to admit a bristle. There is, however, no large outlet for drainage of fluid, so that a small amount is always present to lubricate the membrane, while a large amount collects in conditions that are associated with dropsy. From this arises one great reason for the danger of inflammation affecting this membrane, since there is no escape from it for the pus and other products of inflammation, which accumulate and increase the state of irritation.

In structure the peritoneum consists of a dense, though thin and elastic, fibrous membrane covered, on its inner side, by a smooth glistening layer of plate-like epithelial cells. Here and there between the cells are minute openings (stomas), each of which communicates with a lymphatic vessel, so that the fluid in the cavity is constantly draining off into the general lymphatic circulation.

PERITONITIS means inflammation of the peritoneum or membrane investing the abdominal and pelvic cavities and their contained viscera. It may exist in an acute or a chronic form, and may be either localized in one part or generally diffused. Inflammation of this membrane varies much as regards its causes, severity, and danger, according as it is acute or chronic.

ACUTE PERITONITIS: **Causes**: As a rule it arises in consequence of the entrance of micro-organisms into the peritoneal cavity, which gain entrance through wounds from the exterior or pass out of some of the abdominal organs. The great danger which follows upon stabs and other penetrating wounds of the abdomen originates from the risk of peritonitis. On the other hand, the danger may come from within, and all conditions which lead to perforation of the stomach, bowels, bile-ducts, bladder, and other hollow organs may produce it. Thus gastric ulcer, typhoid fever, gall-stones, rupture of the bladder, strangulated hernia, and obstructions of the bowels may end in peritonitis. Again, abscesses and cysts developed in connection with various organs may burst and so produce it, appendicitis, abscesses of the ovary and Fallopian tubes being specially dangerous. Peritonitis may also arise within a few days after delivery.

The changes which take place in the peritoneum are similar to those undergone by other serous membranes when inflamed: (1) congestion; (2) exudation of fibrin in greater or less abundance, at first greyish in colour and soft, thereafter yellow and becoming tough in consistence, causing the folds of intestine to adhere together, and so tending to limit the spread of the inflammation; (3) effusion of fluid, either clear, turbid, bloody, or purulent; (4) absorption, more or less complete, of the fluid and fibrin, or, in cases which proceed to a serious issue, the formation of grey or greenish-grey pus. Occasionally shreds or bands of unabsorbed fibrin remain, and become converted into fibrous tissue, thus producing adhesions which constitute a subsequent danger of strangulation of the bowel, although this risk follows more often upon recovery from the chronic form.

In some cases the peritonitis becomes *localized* by adhesions between neighbouring organs due to the deposit of fibrin upon their surface. This process takes place with great rapidity, and it makes a great deal of difference to the result of the disease whether it be thus shut in to one part of the abdomen or whether it spreads so rapidly, or is of so virulent a type, as quickly to become *general*.

The bacteria causing peritonitis are numerous, but among the most common are the *Escherichia coli*, which is always present in the intestine; streptococci, which produce the most virulent form of inflammation; and the gonococcus.

Symptoms: The symptoms usually begin by a rigor, together with vomiting and pain in the abdomen of a peculiarly severe and sickening character, accompanied with extreme tenderness, so that the slightest pressure causes intense aggravation of the pain. The patient lies on the back with the knees drawn up, and the hands often rest upon the head, and it will be noticed that the breathing is rapid and shallow and performed by movements of the chest only, the abdominal muscles remaining rigid, unlike what takes place in healthy respiration. The abdomen becomes swollen by flatulent distension of the intestines, which increases the patient's distress. There is usually constipation. The skin is hot, and the temperature rises to 40° to 40·5°C (104° or 105°F), although there may be no perspiration; the pulse is small in volume; the urine is scanty and high coloured, and passed with pain. The patient's aspect is one of anxiety and suffering. These symptoms and signs may subside in a day or two, but if they do not, the case is apt to go on rapidly to a fatal termination. In such an event, the pain and tenderness subside, the abdomen becomes more distended, hiccup and vomiting of brown or blood-coloured matter occurs, the temperature falls, the face becomes pinched, cold, and clammy, the pulse exceedingly rapid and feeble, and death takes place from collapse, the patient's mental faculties generally remaining clear till the close. When the peritonitis is due to perforation, as may happen in the case of a gastric ulcer, or the ulcers of typhoid fever, the above-mentioned manifestations and the fatal collapse may all take place in from twelve to twenty-four hours. But usually the disease lasts four or five days, and the patient sometimes survives as long as a week. The puerperal form of this disease, which comes on within a day or two after parturition, is always very serious.

Treatment: The patient should lie recumbent on the back, with a pillow beneath the knees, so as to bend up the thighs, and a cage over the abdomen to support the weight of the bed-clothes. Externally, either an ice-bag or hot laudanum fomentations give relief, though sooner or later morphine or pethidine is necessary to give relief from the pain. The patient must be given ample fluid, but this must not be given by mouth or in the form of enemas. It must be given parenterally – preferably intravenously but, if facilities for this are not available, it can be given subcutaneously. The fluid may be normal saline (see ISOTONIC) or one-fifth normal saline with 4·2 per cent dextrose. If it is to be given intravenously, plasma or blood is given. Once vomiting occurs, it is usual in hospital to pass a tube through the nose into the stomach (a naso-gastric tube) and keep the stomach clear by aspirating the stomach contents through this tube.

The introduction of antibiotics has resulted in a great improvement in the outlook for this serious condition.

The question of operation arises in every case of peritonitis. In cases due to perforation of the stomach or intestine which are discovered early, operation is always advisable, because there is a good prospect of freeing the abdomen from the septic material which has entered it, and, if no operation is performed, the patient will almost certainly die. In cases in which peritonitis has become localized the question of when to operate is often a difficult one and can only be answered by an experienced doctor or surgeon. The operation consists in making an opening into the abdomen, carefully cleansing the outer surface of the bowels, and attending to the original cause of the peritonitis, whether it be a perforation, obstruction, abscess, or appendicitis, after which it is usual to insert drainage tubes.

CHRONIC PERITONITIS: **Causes**: In the great majority of cases this is tuberculous in origin and secondary to tuberculous disease of bones, joints, glands, or bowels. There is also a localized form of chronic peritonitis, which is non-tuberculous. This latter form is due to long-continued inflammation in an abdominal organ or to ulceration which threatens to perforate. This type of peritonitis is advantageous, because it produces great thickening and adhesions over the part in question, thus lessening the risk of perforation or of infection of the general peritoneal cavity: eg. in appendicitis.

Symptoms: The chief symptoms of tuberculous peritonitis are abdominal pain and distension, along with disturbance of the functions of the bowels, there being either constipation or diarrhoea, or each alternately. Along with these local manifestations, there exist the usual phenomena of tuberculous disease: fever, with emaciation and loss of strength. The abdominal pain may, however, be so slight as only to reach a feeling of uncomfortable weight and fullness.

The simple localized form is characterized mainly by recurring attacks of sharp pain, and sometimes the thickening of the peritoneum is so great as to resemble and be mistaken for a tumour.

Treatment: The same rules, as to diet and a healthy life, that pertain to the treatment of pulmonary tuberculosis, apply to tuberculous peritonitis (see TUBERCULOSIS). In addition, the patient is treated with an anti-tuberculous chemotherapy.

PERITONSILLAR ABSCESS is the term applied to a collection of pus or an abscess which occurs complicating an attack of tonsillitis. The collection of pus forms between the tonsil and the superior constrictor muscle of the pharynx. This condition is also known as quinsy. The treatment of this condition involves drainage of the abscess and the administration of appropriate antibiotics.

PERLECHE (see CHEILOSIS).

PERMANGANATE OF POTASSIUM is a crystalline substance of brilliant purple hue. Permanganate of sodium is red, and is the chief ingredient in Condy's disinfectant fluid, having an action similar to that of the potassium salt. Potassium permanganate dissolved in water is brilliant purple and has a powerful oxidizing action, in exerting which it disintegrates alkaloidal poisons, foul and decomposing organic bodies, and kills low forms of life, such as bacteria. It is therefore a powerful antiseptic. It is non-volatile, and therefore has not the penetrating power of carbolic acid, and in exerting its oxidizing power it is itself reduced, so that it gradually loses strength.

Uses: Permanganate of potassium is a cheap disinfectant, and is conveniently kept in a saturated solution (1 part of potassium permanganate to 20 parts of water). If this is diluted with water twenty-five times (1 in 500), that is, to a crimson tint, or in the proportion of about a tablespoonful of the strong solution to a tumblerful of water, it forms an excellent lotion for washing ulcers and suppurating wounds, and, diluted to a pale pink colour, makes a good gargle for an ulcerated throat. In the latter strength, it may be poured down drains, when it both purifies them and destroys the smell proceeding from them. If the hands become brown after its use, this discoloration may be removed by oxalic acid. As an antidote to poisoning by opium, strychnine, colchicum, oxalic acid, and toadstools (muscarine), potassium permanganate is most valuable if administered at once; 200 or 250 mg may be given well diluted in water. A pale pink solution of potassium permanganate is also a test for the purity of drinking-water; a drop or two allowed to fall into a glass of water should tinge the latter pink, but, if the pink colour disappear, it indicates the presence of organic impurities.

PERNICIOUS ANAEMIA is an auto-immune disease in which the sensitised lymphocytes destroy the parietal cells of the stomach. These cells normally produce intrinsic factor which is the carrier protein for vitamin B12 that permits its absorption in the terminal ileum. Without intrinsic factor, vitamin B12 can not be absorbed and this gives rise to a macrocytic anaemia. The skin and mucosa become pale and the tongue smooth and atrophic. A peripheral neuropathy is often present and this is commonly manifest by paraesthesiae and numbness, and even ataxia. The more severe neurological complication of sub-acute combined degeneration of the cord is fortunately more rare. The anaemia gets its name from the fact that before the discovery of vitamin B12 it was uniformly fatal. Now a monthly injection of vitamin B12 is all that is required to keep the patient healthy.

PERONEAL is the name given to structures, such as the muscles, and nerves, on the outer or fibular side of the leg.

PERPHENAZINE (FENTAZINE) (see ANTI-PSYCHOTIC DRUGS).

PERSEVERATION is the senseless repetition of words or deeds by a person with a disordered mind.

PERSPIRATION, or SWEAT, is an excretion from the skin, produced by microscopic sweat-glands, of which there are around 2·5 million, scattered over the surface. There are two different types of sweat-glands, known as eccrine and apocrine. Perspiration takes place constantly by evaporation from the openings of the sweat-glands, and this insensible perspiration amounts in twenty-four hours to considerably over a litre. Under certain circumstances, as when the skin is heated or the person exerts himself, drops of sensible perspiration appear on the skin; to these the term sweat is generally confined, and the amount of sweat secreted may become very large: up to 3 litres an hour for short periods of time.

Eccrine sweat is a faintly acid, watery fluid containing less than 2 per cent of solids, made up mainly of salts and to a slight extent of fatty material, and including 0·3 per cent of urea (about the same concentration as in the blood), the substance which the kidneys excrete in large amount. When the action of the kidneys is defective, for example in glomerulonephritis, urea and other substances, which the kidneys normally excrete, pass out in increased amounts through the skin. This action of the skin is so marked that in a case of uraemia crystals of urea may be deposited on the surface as the sweat evaporates.

The *eccrine sweat-glands* in man are situated in greatest numbers on the soles of the feet and palms of the hands, and with a magnifying glass their minute openings or pores can be seen in rows occupying the summit of each ridge in the skin. Perspiration is most abundant in these regions, though it also occurs all over the body.

The chief object of perspiration is to regulate the amount of heat lost from the surface of the body and so maintain an even body temperature. Accordingly muscular activity, which sets free a great deal of heat, is the chief cause of sweating, and external heat is another. The process is regulated by nerves, some of which are the nerves controlling the size of the blood-vessels (vasomotor), and therefore the amount of blood in a part, whilst other nerves proceed to the sweat-glands (secretory) and directly influence secretion. These belong to the sympathetic nervous system (qv).

The *apocrine sweat-glands* are found in the armpits, the eyelids, around the anus in association with the external genitalia and in the areola and nipple of the breast. (The glands that produce wax in the ear are modified apocrine glands.) They are developed in close association with hairs and their ducts often open into hair follicles. They do not start functioning until puberty. The flow of apocrine sweat is evoked by emotional stimuli such as fear, anger, or sexual excitement. It is the decomposition of apocrine sweat in the armpits by the bacteria of the skin that produces the characteristic smell of armpit sweat.

Abnormalities of perspiration: LESSENED sweating under certain conditions may occur, as in the early stages of fever, in diabetes, and in some forms of glomerulonephritis. Certain persons are peculiar in the fact of being unable to sweat copiously after muscular exertion, or when exposed to heat, and such persons are often seriously affected by exposure to a hot sun or to the heat of an engine-room. (See HEAT-STROKE.) EXCESSIVE sweating or HYPERIDROSIS, may take place in any feverish condition, tending to be particularly marked in rheumatic fever, and, above all, in advanced pulmonary tuberculosis, where the night sweats are often copious enough to drench the patient's night-clothes and bedding. Such copious night-sweats also occur in certain cases of undulant fever. In a slighter degree, weak people of feeble muscular power are apt to perspire very freely on exertion or when exposed to heat. It may also be due to hyperthyroidism, obesity, diabetes mellitus, or an anxiety state. There is also a form of hyperidrosis, which may be localized or generalized, due to some disturbance of the nervous control of the sweat-glands. The troublesome form of excessive sweating in the armpits tends to run in families. Rare in children and the aged, it is usually induced or exacerbated by emotional stress.

OFFENSIVE perspiration, or BROMIDROSIS, is not uncommon. But it is sweating of the feet or armpits that is most offensive of all, this condition being often due to decomposition of the skin secretions by bacteria.

Treatment: LESSENED perspiration is treated when necessary by various drugs known as diaphoretics (see DIAPHORETICS), and by hot-air baths (see BATHS).

EXCESSIVE sweating occurring in febrile diseases, eg. pulmonary tuberculosis, is diminished by treatment of the condition responsible for the fever. In conditions such as pulmonary tuberculosis, in which the sweating is liable to be prolonged and is particularly irritating to the patient, sponging the skin with vinegar in water may be helpful. In other cases the administration of extract of belladonna by mouth may help.

Hyperidrosis, in which the perspiration is often offensive, is best treated by frequent baths. Regular shaving of the axillary, or armpit, hair is also helpful. The feet, armpits, and other sources of perspiration should be washed daily with hexachlorophane, coal-tar, or other mildly antiseptic soap, carefully dried, and thereafter dusted with talcum powder or bathed with hydrogen peroxide. Socks must be frequently changed. Shoes should be worn in preference to boots, so as to allow freer access of air to the feet, and for the same reason it is a good plan not to wear rubber soles. Sandals should be worn in hot weather. Sweating may also be considerably checked, if it is very copious, by rubbing the feet and armpits with liniment of belladonna or with spirit. Another useful plan in the case of excessive sweating of the feet is to soak the soles (not the entire foot) in 3 per cent formalin solution for five to ten minutes every night. There is also available a wide range of antiperspirant preparations, the active ingredient of which is often an aluminium salt. One of the most effective of these aluminium salts, is 25 per cent aluminium chloride hexahydrate in absolute alcohol, but this must only be used under medical supervision. A deodorant in powder form which has stood the test of time consists of: zinc peroxide 20 per cent; zinc stearate 10 per cent; boric acid 10 per cent; talc 60 per cent. In severe cases of localized excessive sweating, treatment by X-rays may be necessary and may give satisfactory results. Alternatively, in cases of excessive sweating in the armpits, which fails to respond to any other form of treatment, removal, by surgery or cryosurgery (qv), of a small area of skin (4 × 2·5 cm) at the dome of the armpit, where 70 to 80 per cent of the sweat-glands are present, may bring the condition under control.

PERTHES' DISEASE is an affection of the hip in children, due to fragmentation of the epiphysis (or spongy extremity) of the head of the femur. It occurs in the age-group, 4 to 10 years, with a peak between 6 and 8. It is ten times more common in boys than girls, and is bilateral in 10 per cent of cases. The initial manifestation is a lurching gait with a limp, accompanied by pain. Treatment consists of bed rest and traction of the affected limb so long as there is pain and spasm. The child is then allowed up and about with a walking calliper splint (qv) until the condition has healed. Spontaneous recovery occurs in about two years.

PERTUSSIS is another name for whooping-cough. (See WHOOPING-COUGH.)

PERUVIAN BARK is another name for cinchona bark, from which quinine is derived.

PES CAVUS is the technical name for claw-foot (qv).

PES PLANUS is the technical name for flat-foot (qv).

PESSARIES are either instruments designed to support a displaced womb, or solid bodies suitably shaped for insertion into the vagina, which are made of oil of theobromine or a glycerin basis and are used for applying local treatment to the vagina.

PEST is an old name for plague (qv).

PESTICIDES may be defined as any substance or mixture of substances intended for preventing or controlling any unwanted species of plants and animals, and includes any substances intended for use as plant growth regulators, defoliants or dessicants. The main groups of pesticides are: *herbicides* to control weeds; *insecticides* to control insects; *fungicides* to control or prevent fungal disease.

PETECHIAE are small spots on the skin, of red or purple colour, resembling flea-bites. They are small haemorrhages in the skin, as in purpura.

PETHIDINE HYDROCHLORIDE is a synthetic analgesic and antispasmodic drug, which is used in the treatment of painful and spasmodic conditions in place of morphine and atropine. It was at first thought that the drug would have an advantage over morphine in not encouraging addiction, but this has not proved to be the case.

PETIT MAL means the lesser type of epileptic seizure. (See EPILEPSY.)

PETRI DISHES are shallow, circular glass dishes, usually 10 cm in diameter, which are used in bacteriology laboratories for the growth of micro-organisms.

PETROLATUM is the United States National Formulary name for yellow soft paraffin B.P. (See PARAFFIN.)

PEYER'S PATCHES are conglomerations of lymphoid nodules in the ileum, or lower part of the small intestine. They play an important part in the defence of the body against bacterial invasion, as in typhoid fever.

PHAGEDAENA means a process of ulceration of so severe a type that pieces of skin become gangrenous and slough off. It is due either to great weakness on the part of the person attacked, or to excessive virulence of the bacteria concerned.

PHAGOCYTOSIS is a process by which the attacks of bacteria upon the living body are repelled and the bacteria destroyed through the activity of the white corpuscles of the blood.

The first observations upon this point were made by Metchnikoff in the case of the Daphnia or water-flea. This little animal, which exists in large numbers in pools of stagnant water, may often be observed to devour the large spores of a species of fungus. Metchnikoff observed that these spores, perforating the intestine of the Daphnia, found their way into its body cavity and there multiplied. They were, however, attacked at once by the white corpuscles circulating in the creature's vessels, which surrounded and took into their substance these spores, apparently in time digesting them, so that they broke down and disappeared. In some cases, however, he found that the spores developed quickly, the white corpuscles appeared to be sluggish in attacking them, and the creature died.

Similar observations have been made in the case of other bacteria in higher animals. The processes which precede phagocytosis – the slowing of the blood-stream in the part, collection of the white corpuscles on the walls of the vessels, their passage out of the vessels into the tissues (diapedesis), and their approach to the bacteria – are described under ABSCESS and INFLAMMATION. When bacteria are very virulent they seem to repel the white corpuscles instead of attracting them, and no phagocytosis takes place, but the bacteria develop unimpeded. (See OPSONINS.)

PHALANX is the name given to any one of the small bones of the fingers and toes. The phalanges are fourteen in number in each hand and foot, the thumb and great toe possessing only two each, whilst each of the other fingers and toes has three.

PHANTASY, or FANTASY, is the term applied to an imaginary appearance or day dream.

PHANTOM LIMB: Following the amputation of a limb it is usual for the patient to experience sensations as if the limb were still present. This condition is referred to as a phantom limb. In the vast majority of cases the sensation passes off in time.

PHARMACOLOGY is the part of medical science dealing with knowledge of the action of drugs.

PHARMACOPOEIA is an official publication dealing with the recognized drugs and giving their doses, preparations, sources, and tests. Most countries have a pharmacopoeia of their own. That for Great Britain and Ireland is prepared by the British Pharmacopoeia Commission under the direction of the Medicines Commission. Many hospitals and medical schools have a small pharmacopoeia of their own, giving the prescriptions most commonly dispensed in that particular hospital or school. The British National Formulary (qv) is a useful pocket book for those concerned with the prescribing or dispensing of medicines.

PHARMACY is the term applied to the art of preparing and compounding medicines, or to a place where this is carried out.

PHARYNGITIS is an inflammatory condition affecting the wall of the pharynx or throat proper. It is most commonly due to a viral upper respiratory tract infection. It may be confined to the pharynx or may also involve the rest of the upper respiratory tract, ie. the nose and the larynx. On examination the mucous membrane is red and glazed with enlarged lymph-follicles scattered over it. It produces considerable irritation, tickling in the throat and discomfort which may last longer if not treated. If a viral cause is suspected, then only symptomatic treatment is instituted, consisting of analgesia and various gargles. This may include the sucking of medicated pastilles or lozenges. If a bacterial cause is suspected, an antibiotic should be prescribed and in both conditions irritants, such as smoking and highly spiced foods should be avoided.

PHARYNX is another name for the throat. The term throat is popularly applied to the region about the front of the neck generally, but in its strict sense it means the irregular cavity into which the nose and mouth open above, from which the larynx and gullet open below, and in which the channel for the air and that for the food cross one another. It extends from the base of the skull down to the 6th cervical vertebra, separated from the upper six vertebrae only by some loose fibrous tissue, and is about 12·5 cm (5 inches) long.

It is completely closed behind by a layer of muscles, and by mucous membrane, but in front it opens into the nose, mouth, and larynx in succession from above down. In its upper part, the Eustachian tubes open one on either side, and between them on the back wall grows a mass of glandular tissue known as the third tonsil, which, if enlarged, produces the condition known as adenoids. (See NOSE, DISEASES OF.) The muscles which close in the sides and back of the pharynx are three in number on each side, and spring, one from the jawbone, the second from the hyoid bone, the third from the side of the larynx, each of these constrictors spreading out like a fan on the back of the pharynx. Two other small muscles run downwards on each side.

PHENACETIN is a white crystalline coal-tar product, at one time much used in fevers, influenza, headaches, and neuralgias of all kinds, on account of its power of reducing temperature and of deadening pain. As its regular use is not without danger, particularly to the kidneys, it is gradually being discarded, and in Britain is only now available on a doctor's prescription.

PHENAZOCINE is a powerful pain-reliever, or analgesic, which is said to be more potent, but less habit-forming, than morphine.

PHENAZONE, also known as ANTIPYRIN, is an antipyretic and analgesic.

PHENBENICILLIN (see PENICILLIN).

PHENCYCLIDINE (see DRUG ADDICTION).

PHENELZINE (NARDIL) is one of the widely used antidepressant drugs which are classified as monoamine oxidase inhibitors (qv). (See ANTIDEPRESSANTS.)

PHENETHICILLIN (see PENICILLIN, ANTIBIOTIC).

PHENINDIONE is a synthetic anticoagulant (qv) which is effective by mouth, and is used for the same purpose as heparin. It is slower in action than heparin, the full anticoagulant effect not being obtained until 36 to 48 hours after the initial dose.

PHENOBARBITONE is the *British Pharmacopoeia* name for one of the most widely used of all the barbiturate group of drugs. It is given in doses of 30 to 125 mg. Phenobarbitone Sodium is a soluble preparation which can be given by injection.

PHENOL is another name for carbolic acid (qv).

PHENOLPHTHALEIN is a substance much used as an indicator of reaction in urine, and gastric juice, for example, being colourless in acid media, brilliant red with alkalis, and varying in tint according to the acid concentration. It is also given internally in 60 to 300 mg doses as an aperient.

PHENOTHIAZINES are the group of major tranquillizers which are proving of value in the treatment of the psychoses (qv). They include chlorpromazine, prochlorperazine and thioridazine.

PHENOXYBENZAMINE is an alpha-adrenoceptor blocking drug (see ADRENERGIC RECEPTORS) that is proving of value in the treatment of some cases of enlargement of the prostate. (See PROSTATE.)

PHENOXYMETHYLPENICILLIN (see PENICILLIN).

PHENSUXIMIDE is a succinamide derivative used in the treatment of *petit mal* and the psychomotor type of epilepsy.

PHENYLKETONURIA is one of the less common, but very severe, forms of mental deficiency. The incidence in populations of European origin is around 1 in 15,000 births. It is due to the inability of the baby to metabolize the amino-acid, phenylalamine. Its outstanding interest lies in the fact that, if it is diagnosed soon after birth – and this can be done by a simple urine test or by a test carried out on a drop of blood – and the infant is then given a diet low in phenylalamine, the chances are that the infant will grow up mentally normal. Parents of children with phenylketonuria can obtain help and information from the National Society for Phenylketonuria and Allied Disorders (NSPKU), Worth Cottage, Lower Scholes, Pickels Hill, Keighley, West Yorkshire BD22 0RR (0535 44865).

PHENYTOIN SODIUM is one of the most effective drugs for the treatment of epilepsy. One of its advantages is that it does not make the patient feel particularly sleepy. Its use is not without risk and it must therefore be used only under medical supervision.

PHEROMONES are chemicals produced and emitted by an individual which produce changes in the social or sexual behaviour when perceived by other individuals of the same species. The precise role of these odours, for it is by their smell that they are recognized, in man is still not clear, but there is growing evidence of the part they play in the animal kingdom. Thus if a strange male rat is put into a group of female rats, this may cause death of the foetus, and this is attributed to the pheromones emitted by the male rat.

PHIMOSIS is a condition of great narrowing at the edge of the foreskin, for which the operation of circumcision (qv) may be necessary.

PHLEBITIS means inflammation of a vein. (See VEINS, DISEASES OF.)

PHLEBOGRAPHY is the study of the veins, particularly by means of X-rays after the veins have been injected with a radio-opaque substance.

PHLEBOLITH is the term applied to a small stone formed in a vein as a result of calcification of a thrombus.

PHLEBOTOMY is an old name for the operation of blood-letting by opening a vein. (See BLOOD-LETTING.)

PHLEGM is a popular name for mucus, particularly that secreted in the air passages. (See BRONCHITIS; EXPECTORANTS; MUCUS.)

PHLEGMASIA DOLENS is another name for white leg (qv).

PHLYCTENULE: A hypersensitivity reaction of the conjunctiva. At the turn of the century the commonest cause was tuberculosis. Nowadays it is most commonly due to hypersensitivity to *staphylococci*.

PHOBIA is an irrational fear of particular objects or situations. A well-known American medical dictionary lists 206 'examples' of phobias, ranging, alphabetically, from air to writing. Included in the list are phobophobia (fear of phobias) and triskaidekaphobia (fear of thirteen at table). It is a form of obsession, and not uncommonly one of the features of the anxiety state. (See MENTAL ILLNESS.) Those who suffer from what can be a most distressing condition can obtain help and advice from the Phobics Society, 4 Cheltenham Road, Chorlton-cum-Hardy, Manchester M21 1QN (061–881 1937).

PHOCOMELIA: This is a great reduction in the size of the proximal parts of the limbs. In extreme cases the hands and feet may spring directly from the trunk.

PHOLCODINE is the 3-(2-morpholinoethyl) ester of morphine. As it resembles codeine in suppressing cough, it is used for the relief of unproductive coughs.

PHONOCARDIOGRAPH is an instrument for the graphic recording of heart sounds and murmurs.

PHOSPHATES are salts of phosphoric acid, and, as this substance is contained in many articles of food as well as in bone, the nuclei of cells, and the nervous system, phosphates are constantly excreted in the urine. The continued use of an excess of food containing alkalis, such as green vegetables, and still more the presence in the urine of bacteria which lead to its decomposition, produce the necessary change from the natural mild acidity to alkalinity, and lead to the deposit of phosphates and to their collection into stones.

PHOSPHATURIA means the presence in the urine of a large amount of phosphates.

PHOSPHORIC ACID, either as the dilute acid or in the form of phosphates, forms a constituent of many so-called 'tonics'. Phosphate of lime is used in cases of debility and especially of bone disease. Sodium phosphate and effervescent sodium phosphate are much used as mild aperients, and acid sodium phosphate is used in cases of cystitis.

PHOSPHORUS BURNS: If particles of phosphorus settle on or become embedded in the skin, the resulting burn should be treated with a 2 per cent sodium bicarbonate solution, followed by application of a 1 per cent solution of copper sulphate. Fats and oils should not be employed.

PHOSPHORUS POISONING is now rare, and is produced only by the yellow, soluble form of phosphorus. Red phosphorus, from which safety matches are made, is harmless or nearly so. The main cause of acute phosphorus poisoning at the present moment is the swallowing of a rat poison containing phosphorus. When taken internally phosphorus acts first as an irritant poison, and, being thereafter absorbed, produces profound degenerative changes in the liver and other abdominal organs. There is also a chronic form of phosphorus poisoning, usually due to exposure to phosphorus fumes in chemical works. This consists of profound debility, and the occurrence of disease in the lower jaw-bone (phossy jaw), which necroses and comes away in large fragments, over a period of months or years. It is now believed by some authorities that this disease in the bone is due partly to infection occurring in the jaw as a result of toxic effects produced by the phosphorus.

Symptoms: When a child, for example, has taken a large dose he speedily suffers from pain, vomiting, colic, diarrhoea, and perhaps convulsions, and may die in a few hours. There is often a smell of garlic in the breath. Or partial recovery may take place, and the sufferer survive for several days, later developing jaundice and blood-stained urine.

Treatment: As phosphorus is absorbed slowly, washing out the stomach may succeed in removing the poison up to two hours after it has been swallowed. Copper sulphate, a 1 in 1000 solution, in water, may be given every ten minutes until vomiting occurs. Gastric lavage with a 1 in 5000 solution of potassium permanganate or with hydrogen peroxide solution may be tried instead. After emesis and gastric lavage 56 or 112 ml of liquid paraffin and a big dose of a saline purge should be given. No oils, fats, or milk should be taken so long as any phosphorus remains in the gastro-intestinal tract, for phosphorus is soluble in fats. If damage to the liver is threatened then treatment with sodium bicarbonate, glucose and insulin is indicated.

Chronic poisoning is prevented in chemical works dealing with phosphorus, by free ventilation, cleanliness, and periodic examination of the teeth of the match-workers.

PHOTOCOAGULATION: Coagulation of the tissues of the retina by laser for treatment of diseases of the retina such as diabetic retinopathy (see RETINA, DISEASES OF).

PHOTODERMATOSIS, or PHOTODERMATITIS, is the term applied to an eruption on areas of the skin exposed to sunlight, caused by sensitivity to sunlight. (See POLYMORPHIC LIGHT ERUPTION.) In some cases the sensitivity is caused by certain drugs, cosmetics or chemicals.

PHOTOPHOBIA: Sensitivity to light. It can occur in disorders of the eye, or in meningitis.

PHOTOPSIA: This is a description of the flashing lights which are a not uncommon aura preceding an attack of migraine.

PHOTOTHERAPY is treatment by means of light rays, the source of which is usually fluorescent light strips. Its main use is in the treatment of jaundice in the newborn infant. It is the blue section of the visual spectrum that is most effective in this respect. (See JAUNDICE.)

PHRENIC NERVE is the nerve which chiefly supplies the diaphragm. It springs from the 3rd, 4th, and 5th cervical spinal nerves, and has a long course down the neck, and through the chest to the diaphragm.

PHRENOLOGY is an old term applied to the study of the mind and character of individuals from the shape of the head. As the shape of the head has been shown to depend chiefly upon accidental characteristics, such as the size of the air spaces in the bones, and not upon development of special areas in the contained brain, this branch of science is now generally discredited.

PHTHALYLSULPHATHIAZOLE is a sulphonamide drug similar to succinylsulphathiazole (qv). Because of its poor absorption from the gut it is used as an intestinal antiseptic.

PHTHIRIASIS means the condition of eczema, matted hair, dirt, and enlarged glands caused by the crab louse (*Pediculus pubis*). (See PEDICULOSIS.)

PHTHISIS means wasting, and is the general term applied to that progressive enfeeblement and loss of weight that arise from tuberculous disease of all kinds, but especially from the disease as it affects the lungs.

PHYSIOLOGY is the branch of medical science that deals with the healthy functions of different organs, and the changes that the whole body undergoes in the course of its activities.

PHYSIOTHERAPY is the form of treatment involving the use of physical measures, such as exercise, heat and massage in the treatment of disease. An alternative name is PHYSICAL MEDICINE.

PHYSOSTIGMINE, or ESERINE, is an alkaloid obtained from Calabar bean, the seed of *Physostigma venenosum*, a climbing plant of West Africa. Calabar bean is known also as the ordeal bean, because preparations derived from it were at one time used by the natives of West Africa to decide the guilt or innocence of accused persons, the guilty being supposed to succumb to its action, while the innocent escaped. Its action depends on the presence of two alkaloids, the one known as physostigmine or eserine, the other as calabarine, the former of these being much the more important.

Action: Physostigmine produces the same effect as stimulation of the parasympathetic nervous system (qv): ie. it constricts the pupil, stimulates the gut, increases the secretion of saliva, stimulates the bladder, and increases the irritability of voluntary muscle. In poisonous doses it brings on a general paralysis.

Uses: It is used in medicine in the form of physostigmine salicylate. Its main use is to contract the pupil and thereby reduce the pressure inside the eyeball. For this purpose it is used as eye-drops or as lamellae. It is also given by subcutaneous injection to stimulate the gut when this is paralysed or atonic. It is the specific antidote (qv) to atropine and is therefore used in the treatment of atropine poisoning (qv).

PHYTOMENADIONE is the *British Pharmacopoeia* name for vitamin K. (See VITAMIN.)

PIA MATER is the membrane closely investing the brain and spinal cord, in which run blood-vessels for the nourishment of these organs. (See BRAIN; SPINAL CORD.)

PICA (Latin for magpie) is a term which means an abnormal craving for unusual foods. It is not uncommon in pregnancy. Among the unusual substances for which pregnant women have developed a craving are soap, clay pipes, bed linen, charcoal, ashes – and almost every imaginable foodstuff taken in excess. In primitive races it is taken to mean that it indicates the growing foetus requires such food. It is also not uncommon in children. (See APPETITE; LEAD POISONING.)

PICORNAVIRUSES derive their name from pico (small) and RNA (because they contain ribonuleic acid). They are a group of viruses which includes the enteroviruses (qv) and the rhinoviruses (qv).

PICRIC ACID, or TRINITROPHENOL, is used for preparing explosives, and so is employed in medicine only in solution. As it coagulates albumin, it produces a soothing pellicle over any raw surface with which it is brought into contact. It has antiseptic properties, but is rapidly going out of use because of its toxic effects.

PIGEON BREAST (see CHEST DEFORMITIES).

PIGEON-BREEDER'S LUNG, or BIRD FANCIER'S LUNG as it is sometimes known, is a form of extrinsic allergic alveolitis resulting from sensitization to pigeons. In pigeon fanciers skin tests have revealed sensitization to pigeons' droppings, eggs, protein and serum, even though there has been no evidence of any illness. (See ALVEOLITIS.)

PIGMENT is the term applied to the colouring matter of various secretions, blood, etc.; also to any medicinal preparation of thick consistence intended for painting on the skin or mucous membranes.

PILES, or HAEMORRHOIDS, consist of a varicose and often inflamed condition of the veins about the lower end of the bowel, known as the haemorrhoidal veins.

Varieties: It is usual to divide haemorrhoids into external piles, internal piles, and mixed piles. To understand this division, it is important to remember that at the margin of the anus the skin joins the mucous membrane of the bowel in a sharp line, and that the bowel is kept closed by two circular muscles, the external sphincter and internal sphincter. The external sphincter is a weak muscle situated immediately beneath the skin, while the internal sphincter is a stronger circular band, extending up the bowel for about 2½ cm. External piles are found outside the bowel, and are covered by skin, being brown or dusky purple in colour; internal piles are within the opening, covered by mucous membrane, and are bright red or cherry-coloured. Mixed piles are those situated just on the margin, and covered half by skin, half by mucous membrane. Even internal piles do not extend past the position of the internal sphincter muscle.

Causes: There is always a tendency for the veins in this situation to become distended, partly because they are unprovided with valves, partly because they form the lowest part of the portal system and are very apt to become overfilled when there is the least interference with the circulation through the portal vein, and partly because the muscular arrangements for keeping the rectum closed interfere with the circulation through the haemorrhoidal veins. Probably most people of middle life are troubled by this condition to some extent, especially men of sedentary habits who indulge in overeating and are troubled by constipation, as well as women who have borne many children. Habitual constipation is perhaps the principal cause of the presence of piles, and sitting on a cold stone or damp seat, or even a general chill, may suffice from time to time to irritate them and bring on what is popularly known as an 'attack of piles'.

It must be remembered, however, that in a certain number of cases piles are merely a symptom of disease higher up on the portal system, causing interference with the circulation. They often come on during pregnancy, passing off when this condition has terminated. They are common in heart disease, liver complaints, such as cirrhosis or congestion, and any disease affecting the bowels.

Symptoms: EXTERNAL PILES may be present for years and give no trouble whatever, beyond occasioning pain of a cutting or burning character now and then when a very costive motion is passed. When, in consequence of a chill or other cause, they become inflamed, they are very painful and tender from chafing against the thighs and clothing in walking, and from pressure upon the chair on which the person sits. The pile, or piles, in these circumstances become enlarged and red, and give off a thin blood-stained discharge. They may become so badly inflamed as to suppurate, and this sometimes results in a natural cure, or they may cure by filling with blood-clot and shrivelling up into hard little knots. Such an 'attack of piles' lasts generally a week or two, and then subsides.

INTERNAL PILES may be slight, and may give no sign of their presence beyond occasional bleeding, which may vary from a mere streak, when the bowels are opened, to a discharge of several ounces of dark blood. They are apt to produce a constant discharge of mucus tinged with blood which soils the linen, but unless very severe are not, as a rule, painful. These discharges of blood may, when copious and frequent, cause anaemia and become a serious menace to the health, though they are never fatal. When internal piles are large they may come down with the movement of the bowels, and may then become inflamed and painful from time to time, just like external piles.

Treatment: Constipation must, in the first place, be corrected. While the use of violent and irritating purgatives should be avoided, care must be taken, by regulation of the diet and other means, to secure soft motions. (See CONSTIPATION.) The diet should include plenty of fruit and vegetables, and should in all cases be of a simple nature. Alcoholic beverages tend to produce and perpetuate piles, and should therefore in bad cases be entirely abandoned. Regular exercise is necessary in order to carry off the blood to the limbs and so relieve the portal circulation.

Locally, great care must be taken not to irritate the piles, and when they are inflamed they should be washed with water and cotton-wool every time the bowels move. Bleeding and the tendency to inflammation may be controlled by applying a sponge full of very hot water, or by smearing on cocaine or adrenaline ointment after the motion. In the case of internal piles which come down at stool it is very important that they should be returned within the bowel each time by gentle steady pressure with the fingers. If they are down and inflamed, a hot bath followed by a cocaine and morphine suppository gives relief.

Often these means suffice to keep the piles from causing trouble or to cure them completely, but occasionally surgical treatment is necessary. The external piles are simply removed. Internal piles require, according to their size and position, to be ligatured, destroyed by clamp and cautery, or, when they extend all round the bowel, to be removed *en masse* along with the last inch of mucous membrane lining the bowel. In many cases, however, the most satisfactory treatment of internal piles consists of injecting them with a 5 per cent solution of phenol in arachis oil, to which 0·5 per cent of menthol has been added, or some other comparable solution. Alternative non-surgical methods of treatment that are now being advocated are ligation of the piles with rubber bands, cryosurgery (qv), and manual dilatation of the anus.

PILLS are small round masses containing active drugs held together by syrup, gum, glycerin, or adhesive vegetable extracts. They are sometimes without coating, being merely rolled in French chalk, but often they are covered with sugar, gelatin, or gilt. Some pills, designed to act upon the bowels only, are coated with keratin, salol or other substances which are insoluble in the gastric juice.

PILOCARPINE is an alkaloid derived from the leaves of *Pilocarpus microphyllus* (jaborandi). It produces the same effects as stimulation of the parasympathetic nervous system: ie. it has exactly the opposite effect to atropine (qv), but cannot be used in the treatment of atropine poisoning as it does not antagonize the action of poisonous doses of atropine on the brain. Its main use today is in the form of eye-drops to decrease the pressure inside the eyeball in glaucoma (qv).

PIMENTO, or ALLSPICE, is the dried fruit of *Pimenta officinalis*, a Central American shrub, from which oil of pimento, a volatile oil, is obtained. It is used in the form of aqua pimentae, or water of allspice, in doses of a tablespoonful or more in cases of colic, and to make up various medicines.

PIMPLES, technically known as papules, are small, raised, and inflamed areas on the skin. On the face the most common cause is acne (qv). Boils (qv) start as hard pimples. The eruption of smallpox and that of chickenpox begin also with pimples. (See also SKIN DISEASES.)

PINDOLOL (VISKEN) (see ADRENERGIC RECEPTORS).

PINE OIL is a nearly colourless oil with aromatic odour, distilled from the fresh needles of *Pinus silvestris*, the Scotch fir. Its action is similar to that of turpentine, and it is mainly used as an inhalation, prepared by adding a few drops to hot water.

PINEAL BODY is a small reddish structure, 10 mm in length and shaped somewhat like a pine cone (hence its name), situated on the upper part of the mid-brain. Many theories have been expounded as to its function, but there is increasing evidence that, in some animals at least, it is affected by light and plays a part in hibernation and in controlling sexual activity and the colour of the skin. This it seems to do by means of a substance it produces known as melantonin. There is also growing evidence that it may play a part in controlling the circadian rhythms (qv) of the body..

PINK DISEASE (see ERYTHROEDEMA).

PINK EYE: An obsolete term used to describe a highly infectious, usually viral infection of the conjunctiva.

PINS AND NEEDLES is a form of paraesthesia (qv), or disturbed sensation, such as may occur, for example, in neuritis (qv) or polyneuritis (qv).

PINT is a measure of quantity containing 16 fluid ounces (wine measure) or 20 fluid ounces (Imperial measure). The metric equivalent is 568 millilitres. (See WEIGHTS AND MEASURES.)

PIPERACILLIN (see ANTIBIOTIC).

PIPERAZINE is a drug used for the treatment of threadworms and ascariasis. (See ASCARIASIS; ENTEROBIASIS.)

PIPERAZINE OESTRONE SULPHATE (HARMOGEN) (see OESTROGENS).

PIPOTHIAZINE (PIPORTIL) (see ANTIPSYCHOTIC DRUGS).

PIRETANIDE (ARELIX) (see DIURETICS).

PIROXICAM (FELDENE) (see NON-STEROIDAL ANTI-INFLAMMATORY DRUGS).

PITHIATISM is a group of disorders in which the patient is subject to cure by persuasion or suggestion, the term being used as an equivalent for hysteria. (See HYSTERIA.)

PITUITARY BODY, also known as the PITUITARY GLAND and the HYPOPHYSIS, is an ovoid structure, weighing around 0·5 gram in the adult, attached to the base of the brain, and lying in the depression in the base of the skull known as the sella turcica on account of its resemblance to a Turkish saddle. It consists of an anterior and a posterior section divided by a clear line of cleavage. For long these two parts were known, respectively, as the anterior and the posterior lobes of the pituitary body, and the part of the gland that connected it to the brain was known as the stalk or infundibulum. This, however, was too simple a classification to be accurate, as was realized once information concerning the multifarious functions of the gland began to accumulate. It was therefore decided to divide it up according to its origin. The reason for this is that the pituitary has a double origin. The anterior part is derived in the embryo from the ectoderm (see FOETUS) of the primitive mouth, and this part of the gland is now known as the adenohypophysis. The posterior part is derived from the brain and is now known as the neurohypophysis. The gland is connected to the hypothalamus (qv) of the brain by a stalk known as the hypophyseal or pituitary stalk. The confusing thing about this new 'classification' of the pituitary is that it involves a certain amount of overlapping with the old classification. Thus, the adenohypophysis is made up of the anterior lobe which, in turn, is subdivided into a pars distalis and a pars tuberalis, and the pars intermedia of the posterior lobe. The neurohypophysis is also made up of three parts: the infundibular process (or neural lobe) of the posterior lobe, the nervous part of the stalk known as the infundibular or neural stalk, and the median eminence of the tuber cinereum.

The pars distalis, which accounts for the greater part of the gland, is composed of masses of cells which fall into three main groups: (1) chromophobe cells which do not stain and constitute about 50 per cent of the total; (2) acidophil cells which stain with acid dyes and constitute about 35 per cent of the total; and (3) basophil cells which stain with basic stains and constitute about 15 per cent of the total. The pars intermedia consists only of a few cells, whilst the pars tuberalis contains non-granular cells. The neurohypophysis is composed of nerve fibres and brown granular cells known as pituicytes.

The pituitary gland is the most important ductless, or endocrine, gland in the body. (See ENDOCRINE GLANDS.) It has been described as the master gland of the endocrine system, or the conductor of the endocrine orchestra. This over-all control it exerts through the media of a series of hormones which it produces. The adenohypophysis is the major producer of these, and those it produces will be dealt with first. Those which function through the media of other endocrine glands are known as trophic hormones and have therefore been given names ending with 'trophic' or 'trophin'. The thyrotrophic hormone, or thyroid stimulating hormone (abbreviated to TSH) as it is also known, exerts a powerful influence over the activity of the thyroid gland. The adrenocorticotrophic hormone, also known as corticotrophin (ACTH), stimulates the cortex of the adrenal glands. The growth, or somatotrophic, hormone, also known as somatotrophin (SMH), controls the growth of the body. There are also two gonadotrophic hormones which play a vital part in the control of the gonads: these are the follicle stimulating hormone (FSH), and the luteinizing hormone (LH) which is also known as the interstitial cell stimulating hormone (ICSH). (See GONADOTROPHINS.) The lactogenic hormone, also known as prolactin, mammotrophin and luteotrophin, induces lactation. The neurohypophysis produces two hormones. One is oxytocin which is widely used because of its stimulating effect on contraction of the uterus. The other is vasopressin, or the antidiuretic hormone (ADH), which acts on the renal tubules and the collecting tubules (see KIDNEYS) to increase the amount of water that they normally absorb.

Gigantism is the result of the over-activity of, or tumour formation of, the acidophil cells in the adenohypophysis which produce the growth hormone. If this over-activity occurs after growth has ceased a condition known as acromegaly (qv) arises, in which there is gross over-growth of the ears, nose, jaws, and hands and feet. Dwarfism may be due to lack of the growth hormone. Diabetes insipidus (qv), a condition characterized by the passing of a large volume of urine every day, is due to lack of the antidiuretic hormone. Enhanced productuion of ACTH by the basophil cells of the pituitary leads to Cushing's syndrom (qv). Excessive production of prolactin by micro or macro adenomas leads to hyperprolactinaemia and consequent amenorrhoea and galatorrhoea. Some chromophobe adenomas do not produce any hormone but cause effects by damaging the pituitary cells and inhibiting their hormone production. The most sensitive cells to extrinsic pressure are the gonadotrophin-producing cells and the growth-hormone producing cells, so that if the tumour occurs in childhood growth-hormone will be suppressed and growth will cease. Gonadotrophin hormone suppression will prevent the development of puberty and if the tumour occurs after puberty will result in amenorrhoea in the female and lack of libido in both sexes. The thyroid-stimulating hormone cells are the next to suffer and the pressure effects on these cells will result in hypothyroidism. Fortunately the ACTH producing cells are the most resistant to extrinsic pressure and this is teleologically sound as ACTH is the one pituitary hormone that is essential to life. However, these cells do suffer damage from intracellar tumours, and adrenocortical insufficienty is not uncommon.

PITYRIASIS ALBA is a form of chronic eczema which occurs mainly in children. It is characterized by rounded, scaly, white patches, usually on the face, but also sometimes on the upper arms and back. It is a self-limiting condition, but may drag on for several years. A bland cream controls the scaling if this is troublesome.

PITYRIASIS ROSEA is a skin eruption of unknown origin that occurs in young people. It starts characteristically with an oval, slightly red and scaly area – known as the herald patch – between the shoulder blades or on the lower abdomen. Three or four days later the eruption spreads all over the trunk. It consists of pink papules (qv) and oval brownish macules (qv), which tend to itch considerably. It usually lasts about six weeks, and does not usually recur. No specific treatment is called for. Hot baths should be avoided as they tend to accentuate the itching. If this itching is unpleasant, it can be relieved with calamine lotion or antihistamine tablets.

PIVAMPICILLIN (see ANTIBIOTIC).

PIVMECILLINAM is a derivative of the antibiotic, mecillinam. It differs from the latter in being active when taken by mouth. (See PENICILLIN, ANTIBIOTIC.)

PIX is another name for tar.

PLACEBO: No treatments of specific value are found in all the pages of Hippocrates. Nevertheless the placebo response occurred with sufficient frequency to enable the physician to command respect. The therapeutic opportunities are now very different. However, man himself has not changed. He still wants and expects to take medicine when he is ill and is still just as subject to persuasion and suggestion. Despite the scientific advances of this century the physician is still the most important therapeutic agent.

Placebo is the Latin for "I will please". Traditionally, placebos were used to pacify without actually benefitting the patient. They were inactive substances formerly given to please or gratify the patient but now only used in controlled studies to determine the efficacy of drugs. We now realise that pharmacologically inert compounds can relieve symptoms and we call this the placebo effect. The reassurance that is associated with placebo administration is accompanied by measurable changes in body function which are affected through autonomic pathways and humoral mechanisms. Alterations in blood pressure and pulse frequency are especially common. Placebos have the ability to relieve a variety of symptoms in a consistent proportion of the population. On average, one third of patients with symptoms such as pain or cough will respond to placebo medications and an even higher proportion of patients with psychological symptoms such as anxiety or insomnia is relieved. Current scientific jargon defines the placebo as any therapy or component of therapy that is deliberately or unknowingly used for its non-specific psychological or psycho-biological effect and that is without specific activity for the condition being treated.

PLACENTA is the technical name for the afterbirth. (See AFTERBIRTH.)

PLACENTA PRAEVIA (see LABOUR).

PLACENTOGRAPHY is the procedure of rendering the placenta, or afterbirth (qv), visible by means of X-rays. This can be done either by using what is known as soft-tissue radiography, or by injecting a radio-opaque substance into the blood-stream or into the amniotic cavity. (See AMNION.) The procedure is not without danger to both mother and foetus, and must therefore only be carried out under expert supervision but it is sometimes of value in assessing the cause of antepartum haemorrhage. The placenta and foetus can now be visualised by the non-invasive and safe method of ultrasound (qv).

PLAGIOCEPHALY is a congenital abnormality of the skull characterized by flattening of the forehead on one side and bossing or bulging on the other side. This results in the two orbits (qv) not being level. A minor form is common in infancy and tends to improve with time.

PLAGUE, or BUBONIC PLAGUE, is an infectious epidemic disease common to man and many of the lower animals. Its main characters are fever, swelling of the lymphatic glands, a rapid course, and a very high mortality, which has made it a much-dreaded scourge. In the Middle Ages it was known as the BLACK DEATH, which again and again ravaged Europe, though for the past century it has been almost confined to warm climates. The ancients referred to a disease which they called 'pestis', a term which possibly included several severe epidemic maladies; but, according to Hirsch, there is a recognizable description of an epidemic of what we know as plague infesting Libya, Egypt, and Syria between the second and third centuries BC. The first occurrence of the disease in Europe was the plague of Justinian, which swept through the Roman Empire in AD 542, devastating cities and country as it spread. Subsequently it periodically invaded Europe from the east, and spread westward, though with lessening severity in successive epidemics. The last occasion on which England was seriously invaded was at the time of the Great Plague in 1664–65, when 70,000 people died in London out of the total population of 460,000. In Glasgow a small outbreak occurred in 1900, which was quickly supressed. The disease had not invaded America till 1899-1900, when it broke out in Brazil, the Argentine Republic, San Francisco, and Mexico. At the present day 1000 to 6000 cases occur annually, with 100 to 200 deaths.

Causes: The disease is probably always present (endemic) in certain localities, such as in the south-west of China, among the hill people of India, and in East Africa. From these areas it spreads outwards at intervals, sometimes creeping from village to village, at other times being disseminated widely along trade-routes.

The bacillus (*Yersinia pestis*) which is the immediate cause was discovered independently by Kitasato and Yersin in 1894. (See BACTERIOLOGY.) It is found in the enlarged lymphatic glands, and the sputum in pneumonic cases, as well as in the blood of septicaemic cases.

Plague occurs first as an epizoötic (qv) in rats: especially in the black rat, *Rattus rattus*. The infection is then conveyed to man by the rat flea, especially *Xenopsylla cheopis*. The plague bacilli multiply in the gastro-intestinal tract of the flea, which may remain infectious for as long as six weeks. In pneumonic plague the bacillus may pass from man to man as a droplet infection.

The rat is not the only rodent which serves as a reservoir for *Yersinia pestis*. In the Caucasus, Siberia, and Manchuria the marmot is an important reservoir, whilst in Argentina it has been found in wild guinea-pigs. In the USA between the Rocky Mountains and the west coast plague is widespread among ground squirrels, wood rats, and prairie dogs. Between 1900 and 1951 rodent plague had spread through fifteen of the western states of the USA. This carries with it the risk of starting plague in any city with a large rat population. In South Africa, too, plague is prevalent in rodents, and human cases have cropped up from time to time. In England the last outbreak was in Suffolk in 1910.

Symptoms: After infection, an incubation period, varying from two to six days for bubonic plague, and three to four days for pneumonic plague, elapses, and then the disease sets in suddenly with fever, headache, great lassitude, and aching of the limbs. The temperature soon rises to 39·5°C (103°F) or more, the skin is hot and dry, the tongue furred, while thirst, prostration, and a feeling of utter weakness assail the sufferer. His features become drawn, his eyes sunken, and he sinks into a state of stupor or passes sometimes into wild delirium. There is often also sickness and vomiting.

In over two-thirds of all cases there are swollen glands, known as buboes, from which the malady has received the name of *bubonic plague*. These are situated most commonly in the groins, less often in the armpits, and give sometimes the first sign that the person has contracted the plague. There are also haemorrhages under the skin in many cases, which sometimes produce black gangrenous patches that lead to large ulcers, and hence the old name of black death. In favourable cases the fever abates at about the end of a week, the strength gradually returns, and the buboes soften, burst, and discharge foul-smelling pus.

There is a rapidly fatal form, associated with great weakness, in which the bacteria enter the blood, and the person dies on the second or third day, sometimes even in a few hours, before the buboes have time to form (*septicaemic plague*).

In other cases the lungs especially become affected, and pneumonia comes on, with death on the fourth or fifth day. This is said to be both the most infectious and the most fatal form of the disease (*pneumonic plague*).

In all epidemics, especially at the beginning and end of the epidemic, mild cases occur, in which the persons continue to go about, the buboes being almost the only sign of the malady. The matter from the buboes of such slight cases is, nevertheless, infectious, and these cases are therefore specially dangerous to other people.

The death-rate in untreated cases varies in different epidemics from 25 to 50 per cent. Untreated septicaemic plague and pneumonic plague is usually fatal, but modern treatment has reduced the fatality considerably, even in pneumonic plague.

Treatment: Preventive treatment is all-important in this disease. Plague is one of the six internationally quarantineable diseases, the others being cholera, louse-borne relapsing fever, smallpox, louse-borne typhus, and yellow fever. Contacts of plague are quarantined for six days. The strictest quarantine is apt to be ineffective, and measures directed against the spread of plague are essential. This includes the disinfestation of all contacts with insecticide powder, such as 5 to 10 per cent DDT powder. Clothes, skins, any soft merchandise which have been in contact with the plague-stricken preserve the bacilli, and consequently their infectiousness, for several months. Such articles must therefore be either destroyed or disinfected with DDT. Houses or huts in which plague has occurrred should either be carefully disinfected with DDT or, if valueless, burned to the ground. The inhabitants of a plague-infected village or district are not allowed to migrate, carrying infection with them, to other localities, but all who have been in contact with a plague-stricken person should be isolated as contacts or suspects in special houses or camps and dusted with DDT.

In time of plague, or when plague is approaching, a war of extermination should be waged against rats and other rodents which are responsible for spreading the disease, and the bodies should also be carefully examined. Various devices are adopted against the rats on ships. Thus the ships are generally moored a little way distant from the quay, the hawsers are rendered 'rat-proof' by slipping hollow metal cones round them, and sulphurous acid gas or hydrocyanic acid is pumped into the holds under closed hatches to kill vermin which may be among the merchandise.

Personal protection is gained by good feeding, and by living in bright, well-ventilated rooms or out of doors. The wearing of high boots and special clothing impervious to fleas is important for those who go into the neighbourhood of plague cases. The use of antiseptics for the hands and of disinfectant mouth-washes is important for those nursing the plague-stricken, and special precautions must be taken to seal up any small wounds on the hands, and so guard against inoculation.

Vaccination affords partial protection for six months, and is used in the control of local outbreaks of plague. The administration of the sulphonamides, sulphadiazine, sulphamerizine, or sulphadiamine, is recommended for the protection of those who have been exposed, particularly to pneumonic plague.

In the treatment of the disease the best results are obtained from streptomycin or one of the broad-spectrum antibiotics.

PLANTAR DERMATOSIS is a condition usually affecting children, characterized by cracks, or fissures, in the skin of the soles of the feet. The skin also assumes a glazed appearance. It is usually relieved by the regular rubbing in of paraffin ointment BPC, or one of its proprietary equivalents.

PLANTAR FASCIITIS (See FASCIITIS.)

PLAQUE is a coating of the teeth which forms as a result of neglect. It consists of food debris and bacteria and later calcium salts will be deposited in it to form calculus. It is therefore associated with both caries and periodontal disease.

PLASMA is the name applied to the fluid portion of the blood composed of serum and fibrinogen, the material which produces clotting. When the plasma is clotted, the thinner fluid separating from the clot is the serum.

PLASMA EXCHANGE involves the removal of the circulating plasma (qv) from the patient. It is done by removing blood from a patient and returning the red cells with a plasma expander. The plasma exchange is carried out through an in-dwelling cannula in the femoral vein and the red cells and plasma are separated by a hemonetics separator. Usually a sequence of three or four sessions is undertaken, at each of which two to three litres of plasma are removed. The lost plasma can either be replaced by human serum albumin or a plasma expander.

In auto-immune disorders the disease is due to damage wrought by circulating antibodies or sensitised lymphocytes. If the disease is due to circulating humoral antibodies, removal of these antibodies from the body should theoretically relieve the disorder. This is the principle on which plasma exchange was used in the management of auto-immune diseases due to circulating antibodies. Such disorders include Goodpasture's syndrome, systemic lupus erythematosis and myasthenis gravis. One of the problems in the use of plasma exchange in the treatment of such diseases is that the body responds to the removal of antibody from the circulation by enhanced production of that antibody by the immune system. It is therefore necessary to suppress this homeostatic response with cytotoxic drugs such as azathioprine. Nevertheless remissions can be achieved in auto-immune diseases due to circulating antibodies by the process of plasma exchange.

PLASMA TRANSFUSION is sometimes used instead of blood transfusion. Plasma, the fluid part of blood from which the cells have been separated, may be dried and in powder form kept almost indefinitely; when wanted it is reconstituted by adding sterile distilled water. In powder form it can be transported easily and over long distances. Transfusion of plasma is especially useful in the treatment of shock. One advantage of plasma transfusion is that it is not necessary to carry out testing of blood groups before using it. (See TRANSFUSION OF BLOOD.)

PLASMODIUM is the general term applied to minute protoplasmic cells, and particularly to those which cause malaria and allied diseases. (See MALARIA.)

PLASMON is a flour-like food consisting of the protein materials of milk.

PLASTER OF PARIS is a form of calcium sulphate, which, after soaking in water, sets firmly. For this reason it is widely used as a form of splinting in the treatment of fractures. It is used for this purpose in the form of bandages which consist of bleached cotton cloth impregnated with the plaster and suitably adhesive. Its great advantage, compared with an ordinary splint, is that it can be moulded to the shape of the limb. This technique was originally introduced by a Dutchman in 1852. A predecessor of it, which seemed to serve its purpose well, was a bandage stiffened by soaking in egg white and flour – a method still in use in parts of Africa.

PLASTERS (see ADHESIVE PLASTERS).

PLASTIC SURGERY is that branch of surgery which is concerned with the reformation and restoration of parts of the body which are damaged, lost, or deformed.

PLASTRON is the term applied to the skeleton on the front of the chest consisting of the breast bone and attached rib cartilages.

PLATELETS: Blood platelets, or thrombocytes, are small spherical bodies in the blood, which play an important part in the process of blood coagulation. Normally, there are around 300,000 per cubic millimetre of blood.

PLATING is a term used in connection with bacteriological investigation to mean the cultivation of bacteria on flat plates containing nutrient material. The term is also applied in surgery to the method of securing union of fractured bones by screwing to the sides of the fragments narrow metal plates, which hold them firmly together while union is taking place.

PLEOPTICS: A method of treatment of specific forms of squint.

PLETHORA means a condition of fullness of the blood-vessels in a particular part or in the whole body. The term is applied to a condition in which the volume of the blood is increased above normal; there may or may not be an increase in the total number of red blood corpuscles.

PLETHYSMOGRAPH is an apparatus for estimating changes in the size of any part placed in the apparatus; in this way changes in the volume of blood in a part can be measured.

PLEURA, or PLEURAL MEMBRANE, is the name of the membrane which, on either side of the chest, forms a covering for one lung. The two pleurae are distinct, though they touch one another for a short distance behind the breastbone. (See LUNGS.)

PLEURISY, or PLEURITIS, means inflammation of the pleura or serous membrane investing the lung and lining the inner surface of the ribs. It is a common condition, and may be either acute or chronic, the latter being usually tuberculous in origin.

The changes which take place are as follows. (1) Inflammatory congestion and infiltration of the pleura, which may spread to the tissues of the lung on the one hand, and to those of the chest wall on the other. (2) Exudation of fibrin on the pleural surfaces. This exudation consists mainly of coagulated fibrin along with epithelial cells and red and white blood corpuscles. Its presence causes roughening of the two pleural surfaces by material which may later break up or may become organized by the development of new blood-vessels and formation of fibrous tissue. This, by forming permanent adhesions, may obliterate the pleural sac throughout a greater or less space, and interfere with the free play of the lungs. (3) Effusion of fluid into the pleural cavity. This fluid may vary in its characters. Most commonly it is clear or slightly turbid, of yellowish-green colour, sero-fibrinous, and containing flocculi of fibrin. The amount may vary from an almost inappreciable quantity to 4–6 litres. When large in quantity, it may fill the pleural sac to distension, bulge out the thoracic wall externally, and compress completely the lung, which may in such cases have all its air displaced and be reduced to a mere fraction of its natural bulk lying squeezed up upon its own root. Other organs, such as the heart and liver, may in consequence of the presence of the fluid be shifted away from their normal position. In favourable cases the fluid is absorbed more or less completely and the pleural surfaces may unite by adhesions; or, all traces of inflammatory products having disappeared, the pleura may be restored to its normal condition. When the fluid is not speedily absorbed, it may remain long in the cavity and compress the lung to such a degree as to render it incapable of re-expansion as the effusion passes slowly away. The consequence is that the chest wall falls in, the ribs become approximated, the shoulder is lowered, the spine becomes curved and internal organs permanently displaced, while the affected side scarcely moves in respiration. Sometimes the unabsorbed fluid becomes purulent, and an *empyema* is the result. In such a case the pus may point as an abscess upon the chest or abdominal wall, or, on the other hand, burst into the lung and be discharged by the mouth, if it is not evacuated by surgical means.

Many cases of pleurisy are associated with only a little effusion, the inflammation consisting chiefly in exudation of fibrin. To this form the term *dry pleurisy* is applied. Further, pleurisy may be limited to a very small area, or, on the contrary, may affect, throughout a greater or less extent, the pleural surfaces of both lungs.

Causes: Pleurisy is often associated with other forms of inflammatory disease within the chest, more particularly pneumonia, bronchiectasis, and tuberculosis, and also occasionally accompanies pericarditis. It may also be due to carcinoma of the lung, or be secondary to abdominal infections such as subphrenic abscess. Further, wounds or injuries of the thoracic walls are apt to set up pleurisy. The connection of pleurisy with tuberculosis is important. Sometimes it happens that an attack of pleurisy, which apparently has passed off, returns and is eventually followed by tuberculosis, it may be after several years.

Symptoms: The symptoms of pleurisy vary, being generally well marked, but sometimes obscure.

DRY PLEURISY: In the case of dry pleurisy, which is, on the whole, the milder form, the chief symptom is a sharp pain in the side, felt especially on breathing. Fever may or may not be present. There is a slight, dry cough, which the individual does his best to suppress because of the pain which it causes. The breathing is quicker than normal and shallow. Should a deep breath be taken, it ends with a characteristic catch, due to the pain which it causes. If much pain is present, the body leans somewhat to the affected side, to relax the tension on the intercostal muscles and their covering, which are even tender to touch. On listening to the chest with the stethoscope the physician recognizes sooner or later friction, a superficial rough rubbing sound, occurring only with respiration and ceasing when the breath is held. It is due to the coming together during respiration of the two pleural surfaces which are roughened by the exuded fibrin. The patient may himself be aware of this rubbing sensation, and its vibration or fremitus may be felt by the hand laid upon the thoracic wall during breathing.

This form of pleurisy may be limited or may extend over the greater part of one or both sides. It is a frequent complication of pulmonary tuberculosis. In general it disappears in a short time, and complete recovery takes place; or, on the other hand, extensive adhesions may form between the surfaces of the pleura covering the ribs and the lung, preventing uniform expansion of the lung in respiration, and leading to emphysema. Although not of itself attended with danger, dry pleurisy must always be treated as a serious condition, as it may be accompanied by disease in the underlying lung.

PLEURISY WITH EFFUSION is usually more severe than dry pleurisy, and, although it may in some cases develop insidiously, it is in general ushered in sharply by shivering and fever, like other acute inflammatory diseases. Pain is felt in the side or breast, of a severe cutting or stabbing character. The pain is greatest at the outset, and tends to abate as the effusion takes place. A dry cough is almost always present, which is particularly distressing, owing to the increased pain the effort excites. The breathing is painful and difficult, tending to become shorter and shallower as the disease advances, and the lung on the affected side becomes compressed. The patient at first lies most easily on the sound side, but as the effusion increases he finds his most comfortable position on his back or on the affected side.

In most instances the termination is favourable, the acute symptoms subsiding, and the fluid (if not drawn off) gradually or rapidly becoming absorbed, sometimes after re-accumulation. On the other hand, it may remain long without undergoing much change, and thus a condition of *chronic pleurisy* becomes established. Such cases are to be viewed with suspicion, particularly in those who are predisposed to tuberculosis, of which it is sometimes the precursor.

In some cases the pleurisy is on the undersurface of the lung. This condition, known as *diaphragmatic pleurisy*, gives few signs on examination and is liable, when the symptoms are severe, to be mistaken for some acute inflammation of the abdomen.

The chief dangers in pleurisy are the occurrence of a large and rapid effusion, particularly if both sides be affected, causing much embarrassment to the breathing, and tendency to collapse; the formation of an *empyema* (often marked by recurring fever); severe collateral congestion of the other lung; imperfect recovery, and the supervention of tuberculosis.

Acute pleurisy is often merely an accompaniment of the severer condition of lobar pneumonia, the disease really being a *pleuro-pneumonia*.

Treatment: The treatment varies greatly with the form and severity of the attack. If it is tuberculous in origin, a full course of chemotherapy is given as for pulmonary tuberculosis. (See TUBERCULOSIS.) Should it be associated with an underlying infection of the lung, such as pneumonia, the appropriate antibiotics are given.

So far as the treatment of the pleurisy itself is concerned, in the early inflammatory stage, one of the chief symptoms calling for treatment is the pain, which may be soothed by opiates in the form of morphine or Dover's powder, along with the application to the chest of heat in the form of hot poultices, fomentations or a hot water bottle. Instead of these, an ice-bag may be applied to the side, and this has the effect of almost immediately soothing the acute pain.

In the case of pleurisy with effusion, in addition to these measures, aspiration of the fluid may be required. (See ASPIRATION.) The operation is all the more necessary if the accumulated fluid is interfering with the function of other organs, such as the heart, or is attended with marked embarrassment of the breathing. The chest is punctured in the lateral or posterior regions, and most physicians prefer to draw off not more than 850 ml or thereabout at one time and to repeat the operation if necessary. In general, the operation is unattended with danger, although not entirely exempt from such risks as sudden fainting. In many instances, not only is the removal of distressing symptoms speedy and complete, but the lung is relieved from pressure in time to enable it to resume its normal expansion. When there is any evidence that the fluid is purulent, the operation should be performed early. In such cases it is sometimes necessary to establish for a time a drainage of the pleural cavity by introducing a drainage tube through an opening in the lower part of the side, a portion of a rib being usually removed to admit the tube. The pleural cavity is then irrigated through the opening at regular intervals, and treated exactly as any other large abscess cavity. (See EMPYEMA.)

The convalescence from pleurisy requires care, and the expansion of the lung may be assisted by suitable breathing exercises.

After an attack of pleurisy, and particularly after a second attack, the person should submit himself from time to time to medical examination, in order to make sure that tuberculosis does not develop in the lung. He will thus be enabled, if this serious disease should show itself, to start its treatment at an early stage, when a cure may be expected.

PLEURODYNIA means a painful condition of the chest-wall. It may be due to rheumatism of the intercostal muscles or to neuralgia of the intercostal nerves, or, when of the sharp nature popularly known as a 'stitch in the side', to cramp.

PLEURO-PNEUMONIA means a combination of pleurisy with pneumonia. Acute pneumonia is practically always accompanied by a certain amount of pleurisy, to which the pain experienced in pneumonia is mainly due. The epidemic disease known as pleuro-pneumonia which is so fatal to horned cattle, does not affect man.

PLEXUS is a network of nerves or vessels: eg. the brachial and sacral plexuses of nerves and the choroid plexus of veins within the brain.

PLUMBISM is another name for lead poisoning. (See LEAD POISONING.)

PLUMMER-VINSON SYNDROME is a syndrome associated with certain cases of hypochromic anaemia. It consists of hyochromic anaemia, and difficulty in swallowing due to an oesophageal web. It is found practically only in women. (See ANAEMIA.)

PNEUMOCONIOSIS is the general name applied to a chronic form of inflammation of the lungs which is liable to affect workmen who constantly inhale irritating particles at work. It has been defined by the Industrial Injuries Advisory Council as: 'Permanent alteration of lung structure due to the inhalation of mineral dust and the tissue reactions of the lung to its presence but does not include bronchitis and emphysema'. Some of the trades liable to suffer are those of stone-masons, potters, steel-grinders, ganister workers, colour-grinders, coal-miners, millers, and workers in cotton, flax, or wool mills. In 1979, there were 797 fresh cases of pneumoconiosis in Great Britain, 538 of these in coalworkers and 125 in asbestos workers. (See OCCUPATIONAL DISEASES; TUBERCULOSIS.)

PNEUMONECTOMY is the operation of removing an entire lung in such diseases as bronchiectasis, tuberculosis, and cancer of the lung.

PNEUMONIA: Inflammation of the lung may be caused by allergic reactions, when the term *alveolitis* is used, or by chemical or physical agents, when the term *pneumonitis* is used. The classicial division of pneumonia into lobar and bronchial pneumonia is no longer relevant. The aetiology and management of pneumonia depends on whether it occurs in a healthy person or in a person who has some underlying chronic disease that has lowered his local bronchial defences or his general resistance to infection. In the latter case a multitude of organisms may be responsible, many of which have no special affinity for the lungs. Conditions predisposing to the lowering of local or general resistance are chronic bronchitis, diabetes mellitus, malnutrition, alcoholism, and in those patients in whom the immune mechanism is suppressed either by a disease such as leukaemia or by the treatment with immunosuppressive drugs which is always necessary after an organ transplant.

When pneumonia arises in a previously healthy person the three most common organisms are the streptococcus pneumoniae, a virus or mycoplasma pneumoniae. Staphlylococcus aureus is an important cause of pneumonia following an attack of influenza. Rarer causes of pneumonia in a previously healthy person include psittacosis, which is caused by a chlamydia, Q fever caused by a rickettsia, and legionnaire's disease which is caused by a bacterium. Organisms responsible for pneumonia in patients with pre-existing disease include Strep. pneumoniae, Staphlylococcus aureus, Haemophilus influenziae, Stre. pyogenes, Klebsiella and Gram Negative bacilli such as Pseudomomas aeruginosa, Escherichia coli and Proteus.

Immunosuppressive drugs predispose to what are called opportunist infections of the lung, which are infections by organisms that rarely cause pneumonia in ordinary circumstances. These include bacteria such as Nocardia, Cytomegalo virus, fungi and protozoa (Pneumocystic carinii).

Symptoms: The common symptoms with which pneumonia presents are cough, fever, especially when accompanied by rigors, pleuritic pain, dyspnoea or cyanosis. The elderly or infirm may have no fever. The sputum is usually purulent in patients with chronic bronchitis and watery and rusty in those with an overwhelming infection. In other cases sputum may be difficult to obtain during the early stages of the disease and this is partly because coughing is suppressed by pleuritic pain. It is however important to obtain a specimen of sputum so that the nature of the pneumonia can be ascertained by culturing the organism responsible.

Certain physical signs are usually present. Diminished movement of the affected side is noticeable, the healthy side of the chest performing most of the respiratory function. On percussion over the affected area a dull note is obtained which becomes particularly marked if fluid has collected in the pleural cavity. On auscultation over the affected area the breathing is usually harsh and high-pitched (bronchial breathing) but it sometimes shows no deviation from normal, especially in cases in which the deeper parts of the lung only are affected. Accompanying the breathing in the early stages of the disease crackling sounds may be heard.

It is advisable to obtain a specimen of sputum and to do a blood culture before antibiotics are given.

Treatment: The treatment of pneumonia requires eradication of the infection, correcting hypoxia, relieving cough and pleuritic pain, and dealing with any complications that may arise. If the patient is drowsy, cyanosed or confused hospital admission is indicated. Treatment of the infection with antibiotics should start at the earliest possible moment. The choice of antibiotic is based on the clinical judgement of the type of pneumonia with any microbiological support that is available. Microscopic examination of the sputum with the relevant stains will provide a clue to the nature of the prevailing organism but the results of culture may take 24 to 48 hours. Pus cells in the sputum and a leucocytosis suggest that the infection is bacterial rather than viral in origin. Pneumonia in a previously healthy person, particularly if there are rigors and herpes labialis and if there are pus cells and diplococci in the sputum, means that pneumonia is almost certainly due to Strep. pneumoniae and the antibiotic of choice is benzlypenicillin. If the clinical symptoms and signs suggest that the pneumonia is due to a virus, mycoplasma or other non-bacterial infection, then a broad spectrum antibiotic such as erythromycin or tetracycline or ampicillin is indicated. Pneumonia complicating chronic bronchitis should be treated with a broad spectrum antibiotic such as ampicillin or co-trimoxazole. Acute fulminating pneumonia accompanied by signs of respiratory or circulatory failure is probably staphylococcal in origin and this requires urgent intravenous treatment with flucloxacillin and either gentamicin or tobramicin. The optimum duration of antibiotic treatment depends on the response of the patient and the nature of the infection. Good nursing is also important. Pain and difficulty in breathing may be relieved by the application of hot-water bottles and by the administration of analgesics. Cough may be relieved by expectorants. Excessive fever may be controlled by sponging with tepid water. As regards feeding, the digestive powers are much reduced in such an acute infection and the patient should be fed with milk, soups and other light forms of nourishment. Oxygen is important for the hypoxic patient. However if the patient has chronic obstructive airways disease oxygen is the drive to respiration and if oxygen is given in too great a concentration respiration will be suppressed and the patient will die of hypercapnia and acidosis. Oxygen is therefore administered in a concentration of 28 per cent usually through a Venturi mask.

PNEUMONITIS is an inflammation of the lung due to chemical or physical agents. When the inflammation of the lung is due to infections it is called pneumonia and when it is caused by allergic reactions it is known as alveolitis.

PNEUMOPERITONEUM means a collection of air in the peritoneal cavity. Air introduced into the peritoneal cavity collects under the diaphragm which is thus raised and collapses the lungs. This procedure was sometimes carried out in the treatment of pulmonary tuberculosis in the pre-antibiotic days as an alternative to artificial pneumothorax.

PNEUMOTHORAX means a collection of air in the pleural cavity, into which it has gained entrance by a lesion in the lung or a wound in the chest wall. When air enters the chest the lung immediately collapses towards the centre of the chest, but, air being absorbed from the pleural cavity, the lung expands again in a short time. (See LUNG DISEASES.)

Artificial pneumothorax was an operation often performed in the pre-antibiotic days by which in a case of pulmonary tuberculosis air was run into the pleural cavity to cause collapse of one lung, which rests it and allows cavities in it to heal.

POCKET, DENTAL is a pathological space which develops between the root of a tooth and its socket when the periodontal membrane is destroyed.

PODAGRA is another name for gout affecting the foot. (See GOUT.)

PODOPHYLLIN is a resin derived from the root of *Podophyllumpeltatum*, a plant of the United States and Canada, or from *Podophyllum emodi*, a plant which grows in the Himalayas. It has a purgative action but is seldom used for this purpose now. It is also used as a local application in the treatment of venereal warts.

POIKILOCYTOSIS: This is a term used to describe the variation seen in the shape of red blood cells in some bone marrow disorders.

POISON IVY (*Rhus* (or *Toxicodendron*) *toxicodendron*), POISON OAK (*Rhus* (or *Toxicodendron*) *radicans*) and POISON SUMAC (*Rhus* (or *Toxicodendron*) *vernix*) are plants which grow widely in North America. In Britain, poison ivy and, less often, poison sumac, are grown in gardens for their attractive autumn tints. They contain a poisonous principle, urushiol, which induces a severe dermatitis in half the people who come in contact with the plant, and many severe effects, including kidney trouble, in 10 per cent. Treatment of the dermatitis consists of immediately washing the skin with soap and water to remove all the poison. This is followed by the application of wet dressings such as 1 per cent aluminium acetate, or 1 in 10,000 potassium permanganate. The accompanying itch is relieved by rubbing the crushed leaves of the common plantain on the affected part.

POISONS: It is difficult to give a concise definition of the word, poison, because substances which are injurious by their mechanical action, such as steel filings or powdered glass, cannot be classed as such; nor is boiling water a poison; nor can a substance be regarded as a poison if it owes its effect to some bodily peculiarity: as, for example, a draught of cold water taken by an overheated person. The following definition is, however, given by Guy: 'A poison is any substance or matter (solid, liquid, or gaseous) which, when applied to the body outwardly, or in any way introduced into it, can destroy life by its own inherent qualities, without acting mechanically, and irrespective of temperature'. Even this definition is not quite satisfactory because many substances are poisonous in large quantities, harmless in smaller amounts: eg. saltpetre, tartaric acid, Epsom salts. Further, a substance originally poisonous in a certain dosage may be tolerated in increasingly large doses as the individual continues to take it over a period of time, as in the case of arsenic and opium. (See OPIUM.) Again, different people and animals vary widely in susceptibility to poisons. Many herbivorous animals, like the cow, feed upon the deadly nightshade with impunity, and pigeons are almost entirely unaffected by opium.

Over the last two decades 4000 to 5000 deaths a year have been recorded from poisoning in Britain, but the total number of poisonings, fatal and non-fatal, now runs around 130,000 a year. The majority of these are self-poisonings.

Poisoning is a common accident in childhood, but the outcome is seldom fatal. In the twenty years, 1958–77, 598 deaths were registered in British children under the age of 10 years as due to accidental poisoning. Drugs were responsible for 484 of these deaths. Salicylates, mainly aspirin, were the cause in 23 per cent of these drug-induced deaths. Non-medicinal products were responsible for 111 deaths, with lead responsible for a third of these. There were only three deaths from poisonous plants and in one of these the role of the plant in causing death was doubtful. The plants involved were hemlock (qv) and *Amanitaphalloides* (see FUNGUS-POISONING.) It is of interest that this century no case of a death in a child from laburnum poisoning has been reported, and only one case in an adult.

Varieties: Many substances which are poisonous are valuable remedies when used in small quantities or properly applied externally. Others are common household substances or garden plants, and many have important uses in the arts. Under the heading of poisons must be included bacteria and the harmful substances which their growth produces, such as the poisons found in decomposing meat. (See BACTERIOLOGY; FOOD POISONING, and other headings.) The injuries inflicted by insects, snakes, and other animals which introduce some poison into the body are considered under BITES AND STINGS.

Leaving these out of account, we may classify poisons either according to their source or to their mode of action. Classified according to their source they are: *animal*, like cantharides; *vegetable*, like deadly nightshade; *mineral*, like sulphuric acid or perchloride of mercury; and *aerial*, like carbon monoxide gas. By this classification, however, substances with the most diverse actions are included in each group. A more practical arrangement is made, according to the mode of action, into:

Corrosives, which burn and destroy the parts with which they come in contact.

Irritants, which have generally an irritant action upon the stomach and bowels.

Narcotics, which affect the brain and spinal cord, causing a stuporous state.

Narcotico-irritants, which produce first of all an irritative effect upon the stomach or upon the nervous system, and finally act as narcotics.

The two last-mentioned groups are by some authorities placed together as *narcotics*.

(1) CORROSIVES go so far as to corrode, ulcerate, or even perforate the organs with which they come in contact. The chief corrosives are the strong mineral acids, like sulphuric, nitric, hydrochloric; the alkalis, like caustic soda or potash, their carbonates, and ammonia; and certain strong salts, like corrosive sublimate.

(2) IRRITANTS include vegetable acids and some acid salts, such as tartaric acid, white arsenic (arsenious acid), yellow arsenic (orpiment), acetate of lead (sugar of lead), sulphate of copper (blue vitriol), subacetate of copper (verdigris), arsenite of copper (Scheele's green), tartarated antimony (tartar emetic), chloride of antimony (butter of antimony), chloride of zinc (Burnett's disinfectant), nitrate of silver (lunar caustic), bichromate of potassium, sulphate of iron (green vitriol or copperas); also the leaves, roots, berries, or resins of many plants taken in large amount, such as colocynth, savin, gamboge, aloes, croton oil, elaterium.

(3) NARCOTICS include a large range of substances ranging from the age-old opium to the modern synthetic drugs. Few poisons have a purely narcotic action, most producing also sickness, delirium, or other signs of irritation. Among the narcotics are opium and its preparations, prussic acid (hydrocyanic acid), cyanide of potassium, alcohol, ether, chloral, chloroform. Most poisonous gases also belong to this group, the chief among them being carbon dioxide, carbon monoxide, water gas, sulphuretted hydrogen, sulphide of ammonium, and other sewer gases. The amount of these which is necessary in the air in order to produce serious symptoms, or even to cause death if breathed for long, is very small. (See ASPHYXIA.)

(4) NARCOTICO-IRRITANTS form a large group in which the individual substances cause varied symptoms of irritation, such as delirium and excitement, convulsions, or sickness and vomiting. The group includes carbolic acid, oxalic acid, binoxalate of potash (salt of sorrel), nux vomica, strychnine, meadow saffron (*Colchicum autumnale*), white hellebore (*Veratrum album*), foxglove (*Digitalis purpurea*), monkshood (*Aconitum napellus*), henbane (*Hyoscyamus niger*), deadly nightshade (*Atropa belladonna*), black or garden nightshade (*Solanum nigrum*), woody nightshade or bittersweet (*Solanum dulcamara*), potato tops and seeds (*Solanum tuberosum*), tobacco (*Nicotiana tabacum*), Indian tobacco (*Lobelia inflata*), thorn apple (*Datura stramonium*), spotted hemlock (*Conium maculatum*), water hemlock or cowbane (*Cicuta virosa*), hemlock-water dropwort (*Oenanthe crocata*), five-leaved water hemlock (*Phellandrium aquaticum*), fool's parsley (*Aethusa cynapium*), yew leaves and berries (*Taxusbaccata*), laburnum seeds and

bark (*Cytisus laburnum*), and many species of poisonous fungi. (See FUNGUS POISONING.)

Symptoms: The symptoms of poisoning, which come on soon after a meal, or at least after some substance has been swallowed, are of great importance, because the treatment varies according to the type of poison taken, as shown by the symptoms.

CORROSIVE POISONS produce immediate pain and swelling of the lips, mouth, and throat, which also show signs of discoloration, depending on the poison taken. If the dose is large, there may be speedy collapse and death.

IRRITANT POISONS produce vomiting, purging, and abdominal pain. In the case of the milder irritants, the results may be deferred for a few hours, particularly when a full meal has been taken along with the poison. Later, in very serious cases, collapse and insensibility come on.

NARCOTICS produce giddiness, headache, interference with sight, stupor, preceded occasionally by convulsions, followed by deepening insensibility ending in coma and death. No pain is produced by these. (For the means by which narcotic poisoning is distinguished from apoplexy, or alcoholic intoxication, see OPIUM.)

NARCOTICO-IRRITANTS produce at first the symptoms of the irritant poisons: vomiting, abdominal pain, and in many cases purging. Later, delirium or convulsions appear, ending in stupor and death.

Further details as to the symptoms and treatment connected with the more important poisons will be found under the headings of these poisons.

Poison	*Treatment*
Acids: Hydrochloric, Nitric, Sulphuric	Give lime-water, magnesia, chalk, whitening, or bicarbonate of soda in water, oil, or barely water; then albumin water.
Aconite	Lay patient down; give stimulants; wash out stomach with permanganate of potassium; give injection of atropine.
Alcohol	Wash out stomach; give stimulants.
Alkalis: Caustic soda, Caustic potash, Ammonia	Give vinegar in water, lemon juice, or dilute hydrochloric acid then linseed or olive oil.
Arsenic	Wash out stomach; give Glauber's salt; then magnesia or hydrated oxide of iron, prepared by mixing solution of perchloride of iron with solution of ammonia in equal parts, straining through a handkerchief, and stirring up the precipitate in water; then albumin water or barley water; give dimercaprol; give laudanum if much colic
Belladonna and atropine	Give emetic; wash out stomach with permanganate of potassium; neostigmine as antidote; artificial respiration.
Camphor	Give emetic, then a stimulant.
Carbolic acid, Cresol, Lyson, etc.	Give magnesium sulphate or Glauber's salt, then albumin water or milk; wash out stomach.
Chloral	Give emetic; wash out stomach with potassium permanganate; give stimulants; artificial respiration.
Cocaine	Give stimulants; wash out stomach; artificial respiration.
Corrosive sublimate (mercuric chloride)	Give albumin water or milk; wash out stomach with sodium bicarbonate; give dimercaprol.
Digitalis (Foxglove)	Give emetics; wash out stomach with permanganate of potassium.
Ether	Wash out stomach; cold douches.
Iodine	Give flour or other form of starch in water; wash out stomach.
Laudanum: Morphine, Opium, etc.	Give emetic; wash out stomach with permanganate of potassium; give strong coffee; keep patient awake; artificial respiration.
Lead acetate (sugar of lead)	Give magnesium sulphate or Glauber's salt; wash out stomach; then give albumin water or barley water.
Lysol	(See CARBOLIC ACID above).
Mushrooms: Fungi	Wash out stomach with water containing charcoal; hourly aspiration of duodenum; hypodermic injection of atropine.
Oxalic acid and binoxalate of potassium (salt of sorrel)	Give magnesia, chalk, or whitening (*not* bicarbonate or carbonate of soda); wash out stomach; give albumin water or milk.
Phosphorus (matches, etc.)	Give sulphate of copper as emetic; wash out stomach with potassium permanganate; give albumin water; avoid oils.
Silver nitrate (lunar caustic)	Give salt in water; wash out stomach; give albumin water or milk.
Strychnine	Wash out stomach with permanganate of potassium; give chloral.
Turpentine	Give emetics, then magnesium sulphate and albumin water or milk.
Zinc chloride	Wash out stomach; then give albumin water or milk.

Treatment: The first essential in the first-aid treatment of a case of poisoning is to arrange for the casualty to be seen by a medical practitioner, or removed to hospital as quickly as possible. If he is conscious he should be asked what poison he has taken, as he may lose consciousness any moment. If he is unconscious, or even semi-conscious, no attempt should be made to give him anything by mouth, as this may cause choking or asphyxia. He should be placed in what is known as the recovery position (illustration 344), which ensures that an open airway is maintained. This is done as follows:

(1) Kneel beside him.

(2) Turn him gently on his side by grasping the clothing at the hip.

(3) Draw up the upper arm until it makes a right angle with the body and then bend the elbow.

(4) Draw up the upper leg till the thigh makes a right angle with the body and then bend the knee.

(5) Draw out the under arm very gently backwards to extend behind his back.

(6) Bend the undermost knee slightly.

When a CORROSIVE POISON has been taken, first of all administer the chemical antidote to the poison, if there is one; and thereafter soothing substances should be given to allay the irritation in the mouth, throat, and stomach. The following corrosive poisons have such chemical antidotes. When acids have been taken, give a dilute alkali, such as lime-water, magnesia, chalk, whitening, or even plaster scraped from the walls and mixed with water. When caustic alkalis have been taken, give weak acids, such as copious draughts of vinegar in water or lemon juice in water. When corrosive sublimate is the poison, white of egg in water or milk combines with it to form a harmless substance.

After the poison has been neutralized, milk, white of egg in water, or other bland fluid may be given to mitigate the irritation it has caused.

In the case of the IRRITANT POISONS, draughts of water or milk to dilute the poison, together with an emetic consisting of a tablespoonful of mustard in water, or of 1·2 grams of sulphate of zinc in water, should be given as soon as possible. Still better is it to wash out the stomach with the stomach tube at the earliest possible moment.

The following irritant poisons have chemical antidotes, which may be given before the stomach is emptied. When oxalic acid or salt of sorrel has been taken, give chalk or magnesia, which forms in the stomach the harmless oxalate of lime. If lunar caustic has been swallowed, common salt in water neutralizes it by forming the inert chloride of silver. When sugar of lead has been swallowed, Epsom salts is an efficient antidote, producing the insoluble sulphate of lead in the stomach. Carbolic acid also has Epsom salts as an antidote. Arsenic is neutralized by a solution of hydrated peroxide of iron, when this is obtainable.

In the case of NARCOTIC AND NARCOTICO-IRRITANT poisons, an emetic administered at once is beneficial, and it is the usual practice for a medical man to wash out the stomach with a weak solution of permanganate of potassium, when he sees the case. Permanganate of potassium has the power of destroying many of these vegetable poisons which are of an alkaloidal nature. Many of these poisons, whose deadliness depends upon active principles, can be neutralized to some extent by other drugs.

WHEN THE POISON IS UNKNOWN, but the fact of poisoning suspected, the safest course is to administer tepid water containing common salt (sodium chloride) (see EMETICS), in order to expel the contents of the stomach, thereafter administering a drink of milk. The drink of salty water must not be repeated as too much salt may be harmful. Above all things it is necessary to keep all vomited matter and the remains of food that the poisoned person has been taking till the arrival of a medical man.

A National Poisons Information Service has been set up to give advice, preferably to doctors, on the diagnosis and treatment of cases of poisoning. It has centres in London (Tel. 01-407 7600), Edinburgh (031-229 2477) and Cardiff (0222 492233). (See also SELF-POISONING.)

POLDINE, or POLDINE METHYLSULPHATE, is a synthetic drug, with an atropine-like action (see ATROPINE), which is used in the treatment of gastric and duodenal ulcers.

POLICEMAN'S HEEL is a painful condition of the heel, most commonly found in those who stand and walk a lot, such as policemen (hence its name), waiters and maids. Obesity is a common associated condition. Most of the patients are over the age of 40. The cause is controversial. Some consider it to be a form of fasciitis (qv). In some cases it is associated with spurs of bone on the calcaneus; in others with rheumatoid arthritis. It is usually unilateral. If both heels are involved, it is more likely to be part of some generalized condition such as rheumatoid arthritis. One of its characteristics is that the pain tends to be worse after rest – especially with the first few steps in the morning. Most cases get better with rest and protection from direct pressure on the heel, as by a sorbo-rubber or plastic foam pad. In more severe cases the local injection of a corticosteroid may be beneficial.

POLIOMYELITIS, or INFANTILE PARALYSIS, is an infectious disease involving the spinal cord and the brain.

Cause: The first epidemic of poliomyelitis to be recorded occurred in Sweden in 1881. The disease then became of increasing importance, particularly in Scandinavia, USA and Australia, but with the successful introduction of poliomyelitis vaccination it rapidly became a relatively rare disease. In Great Britain the disease has been notifiable since 1912. Although sporadic cases may occur at any time, there is a definite seasonal incidence, epidemics tending to occur in the late summer and early autumn in the northern hemisphere and in March and

April in the southern hemisphere. In the tropics infection continues throughout the year. In 1979 there were six cases of paralytic poliomyelitis in England. Two of these were fathers of children recently vaccinated with oral poliovaccine. Three were adult nationals of the United Kingdom who contracted the disease in the Middle East. None had been vaccinated and one died. The sixth victim was a child from the Middle East who had the disease when she came to this country. In 1984 not a single case of poliomyelitis was reported in the UK.

The infecting organism is a virus, of which there are three types. Infection occurs from ingestion of the virus by mouth. The virus then passes to the lower alimentary tract and is excreted in the stools. It has been shown that the viruses are excreted by 90 per cent of paralytic cases, particularly children, and they are also excreted in the stools by healthy contacts of cases. It is in this way that the disease is spread: through contamination of the hands and then contamination of the mouth from such contaminated hands. Children are the most susceptible members of families, but during recent years there has been a definite tendency to severe paralytic cases occurring among young adults. One attack usually produces permanent immunity; second attacks are rare.

Pathology: The sites of selection for the virus are the motor cells in the anterior horn of the spinal cord, and there is a tendency for this to be more marked in the lumbar part of the cord. The cranial nerves and certain nuclei in the brain are also involved in some cases.

Symptoms: The incubation period is 3 to 21 days, commonly 7 to 12 days. The onset may be either sudden or gradual. In the case of the latter the child may merely be 'off colour' for a day or two and complain of aches or pains in the limbs; there may be only a slight rise in temperature. This may gradually pass into the stage of weakness, and then paralysis, of the limbs. In other cases, after a few days' vague illness, the paralysis of the limbs may come on quite suddenly, usually with a sharp rise in temperature. In cases of sudden onset, the victim complains of headache and aches and pains, and the temperature rises to 39·5°C (103°F) or higher. In other cases, particularly in children, the limbs may be found to be paralysed when the child wakens in the morning, although he was apparently quite well when he went to bed the previous evening.

The site and the distribution of the paralysis depend upon the extent to which the spinal cord and brain are involved. The most serious cases are those in which the diaphragm and the muscles of respiration (the intercostal muscles) are involved, as this prevents the patient breathing, and he may die in a very short space of time unless he is placed on a respirator. When the cranial nerves and brain are involved, there may be nystagmus (qv), hoarseness, and difficulty in swallowing. Convulsions may occur in young children. The cerebrospinal fluid contains an excess of cells in the first and second weeks and an increased amount of protein in the third week.

Prophylaxis: A high degree of protection is given by poliomyelitis vaccine. This is now given by mouth, and its use has practically banished the disease. Of the 6 cases in England in 1979, none had been immunized. The vaccine is given in childhood, but a booster dose should be given to adults, particularly young adults, when they are going to a country of high poliomyelitis incidence, which in practice means any country outside Europe and North America. It is also recommended that unvaccinated parents of a child being given oral vaccine should be given the vaccine at the same time.

In the presence of an epidemic the following measures should be taken. Children should not be allowed to go into crowded buildings such as cinemas. Public swimming baths should be avoided. Children, especially younger ones, should not be allowed to get overtired, particularly in hot weather. Particular care should be taken to protect food from flies and to ensure that the highest standards of cleanliness are observed in the handling of food. No operations for the removal of tonsils or adenoids should be performed. Immunization against diphtheria and whooping-cough and measles vaccination should, if at all possible, be postponed until the epidemic is over.

Treatment: The patient must be put to bed on the first sign of the disease, and the affected limbs completely rested. This is the one definite practical fact that has resulted from all the careful investigation of the disease during recent years: that the earlier the disease is detected, and therefore the earlier the patient is put to bed and the affected parts rested, the better the ultimate result. Splints may be necessary at this stage to give adequate rest to the affected muscles. Later, careful physiotherapy is necessary. If the breathing is affected, it may be necessary to put the patient on a respirator. To ensure the best possible results, after-treatment may need to be continued for two or three years. In cases in which severe paralysis and wasting of limbs persist, surgical treatment may be necessary to reduce the resulting disability to a minimum.

POLIOSIS means premature greying of the hair. It is also the term applied to whitening of the hair in segments, such as a forelock.

POLITZER'S BAG is a rubber bag with nozzle intended for inflation of the middle ears by blowing air up one nostril while the other is closed, and so clearing a blocked Eustachian tube. (See EAR, DISEASES OF.)

POLLEN consists of microspores formed in flowering plants and conifers. Between 4 and 7 million tons of it are said to be shed annually throughout the world. From ancient days it has had the reputation of being a specific against old age, and recent reports from Russia claim that bee-keepers live longer because they eat pollen. It contains protein, vitamins A, B, C, D and K, small amounts of minerals including calcium, copper, iron, magnesium, manganese, phosphorus, potassium, and sulphur, as well as several enzymes. It has a bitter taste, which is traditionally disguised by honey – the ambrosia of the Bible, the Koran and the Talmud. Sufferers from hay fever should not eat it during the hay-fever season as it may induce allergic reactions.

POLLEX is a Latin term for thumb.

POLYARTERITIS NODOSA, or PERIARTERITIS NODOSA as it is sometimes known, is a disease of unknown origin, in which prolonged fever and obscure symptoms referable to any system of the body are associated with local areas of inflammation along the arteries, giving rise to nodules in their walls. Recovery occurs in about 50 per cent of cases.

POLYCHROMASIA and POLYCHROMATOPHILIA are terms applied to an abnormal reaction of the red blood corpuscles in severe anaemia, whereby they have a bluish tinge instead of the normal red colour in a blood film stained by the usual method. It is a sign that the cell is not fully developed.

POLYCYSTIC OVARY SYNDROME: In 1935 Stein and Leventhan described seven hirsute and infertile women with amenorrhoea or oligomenorrhoea in whom bilateral cystic ovarian enlargement was found at laparotomy and thereby gave their names to a polycystic ovarian disorder. Since then, however, the protean manner of clinical presentation and the variability of biochemical changes in patients with this condition have lead some people to doubt the existence of a disease entity. Enlarged cystic ovaries may occur in the absence of the classical clinical characteristics originally described. Polycystic ovaries may be found in those who have conceived and are not hirsute, and they may be seen in infertile women who menstruate regularly and even in some patients with menorrhagia. On the other hand, the clinical features of oligomenorrhoea, hirsutism and infertility may occur in the absence of bilateral ovarian enlargement and cystic change may be found in normal sized or small ovaries.

Polycystic ovaries may have several causes. Whether large or small ovaries result may be determined by the duration and severity of the particular cause. Sclerocystic ovarian change would therefore be a better description, but the term polycystic is now firmly established by common usage. The choice of treatment is determined by the clinical presentation and the main complaint. If hirsutism is the main problem and there is evidence of androgen suppression after dexamethasone then corticosteroid treatment should be tried. The anti-androgen, cyproterone acetate, has recently been introduced and is probably more effective. If, however, fertility is the prime consideration then clomiphene should be given and wedge ressection of the ovaries considered if pregnancy does not result after three courses of the drug.

POLYCYTHAEMIA is an excess in the number of red corpuscles in the blood.

POLYDACTYLY means the presence of extra, or supernumerary, fingers or toes.

POLYDIPSIA means excessive thirst, which is a symptom of diabetes mellitus and some other diseases.

POLYGRAPH is an instrument for making simultaneous tracings of the pulse in two different parts of the circulation.

POLYMER FUME FEVER occurs in people who work with polytetrafluoroethylene (PTFE, Teflon). The fever is caused by degradation products, including hydrofluoric acid, which are produced at temperatures of 170°C and upwards. The likeliest source of these injurious products is cigarette smoking. Even the tiniest particles of PTFE on a burning cigarette will yield sufficient of these degradation products to cause fume fever.

The illness consists of an influenza-like illness, which lasts for a few hours.

POLYMORPH is a name applied to certain white corpuscles of the blood which have a nucleus of irregular and varied shape. These form between 70 and 75 per cent of all the white corpuscles. (See BLOOD.)

POLYMORPHIC LIGHT ERUPTION is a photodermatosis (qv) which occurs predominantly in females, appearing first as a rule in adolescence or early adult life. The eruption, which consists of a mixture of erythema (qv), papules (qv) and vesicles (qv), occurs on those parts of the body exposed to the sun, mainly the back of the hands, the forearms, the front of the neck, the cheeks and the nose. There are usually several attacks a year, depending on the amount of sunlight. The attacks start in the spring and continue until the winter. Apart from the fact that the rash is provoked by sunlight, the precise cause is not known. Treatment consists of avoiding sunlight, wearing protective clothing, and using sunscreening preparations. (See SUNBURN.)

POLYMYALGIA RHEUMATICA is a form of rheumatism characterized by gross early morning stiffness, which tends to ease off during the day, and pain in the shoulders and sometimes round the hips. It affects women more than men, and is rare under the age of 60. The cause is still obscure. It responds well to prednisolone, but treatment may need to be long continued. On the other hand the condition is not progressive and does not lead to crippling.

POLYMYXIN is the name applied to the group of antibiotics derived from various species of *Bacillus polymyxa.* Polymyxin B is the one available commercially, and is the antibiotic of choice in the treatment of infections due to *Ps. pyocyanea.*

POLYNEURITIS means an inflammatory condition of nerves in various parts of the body. (See NEURITIS.)

POLYPHARMACY is a term applied to the administration of too many drugs in one prescription.

POLYPOSIS means the presence of a crop, or large number, of polypi. The most important form of polyposis is that known as *familial polyposis coli*. This is a hereditary disease characterized by the presence of large numbers of polypoid tumours in the large bowel. Every child born to an affected parent stands a fifty-fifty chance of developing the disease. Its importance is that sooner or later one or more of these tumours undergoes cancerous change. If the affected gut is removed surgically before this occurs, and preferably before the age of 20, the results are excellent.

POLYPUS is a general name applied to tumours which are attached by a stalk to the surface from which they spring. The term refers only to the shape of the growth and has nothing to do with its structure or nature. Most polypi are of a simple nature, though malignant polypi are also found. The usual structure of a polypus is that of a fine fibrous core covered with epithelium resembling that of the surrounding surface. The sites in which polypi are most usually found are the interior of the nose, the outer meatus of the ear, and the interior of the womb, bladder, or bowels (see POLYPOSIS).

Their removal is generally easy, as they are simply twisted off, or cut off, by some form of snare or ligature. Those which are situated in the interior of the bladder or bowels, and whose presence is usually recognized by the presence of blood in the urine or stools, require a more serious operation to reach the organ into which they project.

POLYTHELIA is the condition in which extra or supernumerary nipples appear along a line between the armpit and the groin.

POLYTHIAZIDE (NEPHRIL) (see BENZOTHIADIAZINES).

POLYURIA means the passage of an amount of urine considerably in excess of the 1500 ml or thereabout which is the usual daily quantity. It is a symptom of diabetes mellitus, diabetes insipidus, chronic renal failure and psychogenic polydipsia.

POMPHOLYX is a form of eczema characterized by the appearance of deeply set vesicles (qv) on the palms and soles, fingers and toes. When it occurs on the fingers and hands it is known as CHEIROPOMPHOLYX. On the toes and feet it is known as PODOPOMPHOLYX.

PONS VAROLII is the bridge of the brain, mainly composed of strands of white nerve-fibres which unite various parts of the brain. (See BRAIN.)

POPLITEAL SPACE, or HAM, is the name given to the region behind the knee. The muscles attached to the bones immediately above and below the knee bound a diamond-shaped space through which pass the main artery and vein of the limb (known in this part of their course as the popliteal artery and vein), the tibial and common peroneal nerves (which continue the sciatic nerve from the thigh down to the leg), the external saphenous vein, as well as several small nerves and lymphatic vessels. The muscles, which bound the upper angle of the space and which are attached to the leg bones by strong prominent tendons, are known as the hamstrings. The lower angle of the space lies between the two heads of the gastrocnemius muscle, which makes up the main bulk of the calf of the leg.

POPPY as used in medicine is of two species: *Papaver somniferum,* the white opium-poppy (see OPIUM), and *Papaver rhoeas,* the red corn-poppy. The corn-poppy is chiefly used as a colouring agent, the syrup made from it having a brilliant crimson colour.

PORENCEPHALY, or PORENCEPHALIA, is a term applied to the presence of cysts in the surface of the brain due to an arrest of development or to birth haemorrhage. The condition is generally associated with serious mental defect.

POROPLASTIC is a thick kind of felt which is easily moulded into splints when softened by hot water and used for surgical purposes.

PORPHYRIA is a condition, or rather a series of conditions, characterized by an excessive production and excretion of porphyrins. Porphyrins are constituents of various blood and respiratory pigments found throughout the animal kingdom, including human beings. They are also found in plants and micro-organisms.

In porphyria there is some disturbance of their metabolism and this results in a variegated picture which includes discoloration of the urine due to excessive excretion of porphyrins, skin rashes due to sensitization of the skin to light, various forms of indigestion and mental disturbances.

PORT-A-CATH: The Port-a-cath system consists of a silicon catheter connected to a staileess steel chamber in which there is a silicon injection port. The catheter is inserted into a central vein and connected by a sub-cutaneous tunnel to the portal which is implanted sub-cutaneously on the chest wall. Its purpose is to provide a central venous access while avoiding repeated cannulation with its inevitable risk of sepsis.

PORRIGO is a general term applied to diseases of the skin covering the head, such as ringworm.

PORTAL VEIN is the vein which carries to the liver blood that has been circulating in many of the abdominal organs. It is peculiar among the veins of the body in that it ends by breaking up into a capillary network instead of carrying the blood directly to the heart, a peculiarity which it shares only with certain small vessels in the kidneys. The portal system begins below in the haemorrhoidal plexus of veins round the lower end of the rectum, and from this point, along the whole length of the intestines, the blood is collected into an inferior mesenteric vein upon the left, and a superior mesenteric vein upon the right side. The inferior mesenteric vein empties into the splenic vein, and the latter, uniting with the superior mesenteric vein immediately above the pancreas, forms the portal vein. The portal vein is joined by veins from the stomach and gall-bladder, and finally divides into two branches which sink into the right and left lobes of the liver. (For their further course, see LIVER.)

The organs from which the portal vein collects the blood are the large and small intestines, the stomach, spleen, pancreas, and gall-bladder.

POSSETTING is the technical term used to describe the quite common habit of healthy babies to regurgitate, or bring up, small amounts of the meal they have just taken.

POST- is a prefix signifying after or behind.

POST-MORTEM EXAMINATION (see NECROPSY).

POST-PARTUM is the term applied to anything happening immediately after child-birth: for example, post-partum haemorrhage.

POST-VIRAL FATIGUE SYNDROME is a disorder which may be epidemic or sporadic. It follows a virus infection and is characterized by physical exhaustion. The fatigue may be disabling and even incapacitating but recovery is the rule, although remission may take several months. It is more common in young people. Fatigue and lethargy are the characteristic symptoms. Physical exercise frequently aggravates the condition. Physical examination does not reveal any evidence of disease and the standard haematological and biochemical investigations are normal. Recent evidence has suggested that enteroviruses are causally related to the post-viral fatigue syndrome and the virus is usually Coxsackie B. However, other viruses such as influenza, varicella, rubella and Epstein-Barr may also precipitate the same syndrome. Although in some patients the disorder has a non-organic basis, it seems probable, in view of recent studies, that in the majority it is an organic illness of undetermined aetiology. Evidence of early intracellular acidosis of muscle during exercise has recently been demonstrated. Recent studies have also demonstrated persistence of the virus in individuals with the syndrome and there is some evidence of a correlation between the clinical improvement and the disappearance of the viral antigen from the circulation. Viral infections have long been known to be frequently followed by severe depression. This is particularly common following the Epstein-Barr viral infection of glandular fever. Mood disturbances hinder recovery from physical illness so that both the mind and the body need care and attention. This is particularly important as there is scant objective evidence of reduced muscle strength and fatigue ability when these are measured by electrical stimulation of muscle so that the fatigue is almost certainly central in origin rather than a sign of muscle weakness. However, recovery is the rule, although the symptoms may persist for many months.

POSTURAL DRAINAGE is the process whereby the drainage of secretions from dilated bronchi of the lungs is facilitated. The patient lies on an inclined plane head downwards and is encouraged to cough up as much secretion from the lungs as possible. The precise position depends on which part of the lungs is affected. It may need to be carried out for up to three hours daily in divided periods. It is of particular value in bronchiectasis (qv) and lung abscess.

POTASH, or POTASSA, is the popular name for potassium carbonate. Hydrated oxide of potassium is usually known as caustic potash, and its solution as potash solution.

POTASSIUM is a metal which, on account of its great affinity for other substances, is not found in a pure state in nature. Its salts are used to a great extent in medicine but, as their action depends in general not on their metallic radicle but upon the acid with which it is combined, their uses vary greatly and are described elsewhere. All salts of potassium have a depressing effect on the heart's action by virtue of the potassium ion.

POTASSIUM ASCORBATE EYE-DROPS were originally introduced for the treatment of glaucoma. They are now largely used in helping to prevent ulceration and perforation of the cornea (qv) following acid and alkali burns of the eye.

POTASSIUM CHLORATE, in addition to the general actions exerted by potassium salts, has a soothing action upon inflamed mucous membranes, and is used for a gargle in sore throat of every description.

POTT'S DISEASE is a name often applied to the angular curvature of the spine which results from tuberculous disease. (See SPINAL DISEASES.) The disease is named after Percivall Pott, an English surgeon (1714–88), who first described the condition.

POTT'S FRACTURE is a term applied to a variety of fractures around the ankle, accompanied by a varying degree of dislocation of the ankle. In all cases the fibula is fractured. Named after Percivall Pott, who suffered from this fracture and was the first to describe it (see FRACTURES), it is often mistaken for a simple sprain of the ankle.

POULTICES (see also FOMENTATION) are soft moist applications to the surface of the body, generally used hot. They soften the parts with which they come in contact, soothe irritated nerve-endings, relax spasmodically contracted muscle-fibres, and, after being applied for some time, dilate the vessels of the part they cover and increase the circulation through it. These applications are consequently used in all stages of inflammation to soothe pain and promote resolution, or in the late stages, when pus is forming, to aid the rapid formation of an abscess. (See ABSCESS.)

POUPART'S LIGAMENT, also known as the inguinal ligament, is the strong ligament lying in the boundary between the anterior abdominal wall and the front of the thigh.

POWDERS form a method in which drugs are prescribed, powerful drugs being made up with inert substances like sugar, gum, or ginger in order to give them sufficient bulk. The best known powders are Dover's powder (ipecacuanha and opium powder), containing opium; Gregory's powder (compound rhubarb powder); and Seidlitz powder (compound effervescent powder). Powders have largely been replaced by tablets.

PRAZEPAM (CENTRAX) (see BENZODIAZEPINES).

PRAZIQUANTEL is a drug that is proving of value in the treatment of schistosomiasis (qv).

PRE- is a prefix meaning before.

PRECORDIAL REGION is the area on the centre and towards the left side of the chest, lying in front of the heart.

PREDNISOLONE is a derivative of cortisone, which is five or six times as active as cortisone and has less of the salt- and water-retaining properties of cortisone. It is given by mouth.

PREDNISONE is the official name for deltadehydrocortisone, and has the same action as prednisolone.

PRE-ECLAMPSIA is a complication of pregnancy characterized by oedema, high blood-pressure and the presence of albumin in the urine. It is so called because, unless adequately treated in time, it may be a prelude to the onset of eclampsia (qv).

PREFRONTAL LOBOTOMY (see PSYCHOSURGERY).

PREGNANCY: This state is a natural one although it sets up great changes, not only in the womb, but throughout the whole body. Most of these changes subside quickly after delivery is accomplished, and though a few minor alterations persist throughout life, the mother returns to her normal state within about one month after the child is born.

Duration of pregnancy: It is generally accepted that pregnancy lasts about 280 days from the first day of the last menstrual period. In exceptional cases there may be considerable variation, but it is generally agreed that the shortest duration of a normal pregnancy is 240 days and the longest duration 313 days. The cause of these variations is not understood. The longest period of gestation that has ever been admitted in the Law Courts in Great Britain is 349 days, whilst the shortest that has been accepted is 174 days. On the other hand, a case was reported in 1971 of a mother giving birth to a child in a Sussex hospital after what was claimed to be a pregnancy of 381 days. For the purpose of calculating the probable date of confinement, it is usual to take the first day of the last period that occurred, to allow seven days for the duration of this and then to add 273 days for the duration of gestation, making in all 280 days from the beginning of the last menstruation. The actual date can be estimated roughly by adding seven days and then counting forwards nine calendar months; for example, supposing the last menstrual period began on 3rd October, adding seven days makes the 10th October, and nine months forwards from this gives the date of probable confinement as the 10th of July. It is usual to say that this day is the middle of the week in which the confinement may be expected.

Signs of pregnancy: (*a*) The stoppage of the menstrual flow is the sign which first attracts attention. This symptom may, however, be due to many other causes (see MENSTRUATION), but if it occurs quite suddenly it may usually be counted upon as an important sign. It is a popular mistake to suppose that pregnancy cannot occur in a woman while she is suckling a previous child, for this does occur even while the menses are in abeyance. (*b*) Swelling of the breasts is another important sign, appearing even in the second or third month of pregnancy. A thin fluid, known as colostrum, can, even at this early stage, be pressed from the nipples. At the same time the veins on the breasts become enlarged and visible, and the pigmented ring round the nipple (areola) becomes much darker than before, as well as showing small nodules (Montgomery's tubercles) round its edge. (*c*) Sickness in the morning immediately on rising is also a common sign, occurring in about two-thirds of all women. When the sickness is marked, however, it is a valuable sign, because it appears early in the course of pregnancy, during the second month, and lasts usually about a couple of months. (*d*) Quickening, or the fluttering sensation felt by the mother in consequence of the child's rapid movements, is a very important sign, though it does not usually occur till some time during the fifth month of pregnancy or even later. It is the first sign of life felt by the mother, though it is a popular error to suppose that the child only then begins to live. (*e*) Enlargement of the abdomen is a pronounced sign, though for the first three months the enlargement is not apparent. It must not be forgotten, however, that enlargement may be due to other causes, such as tumours, and even constipation or increasing development of fat. It is not an uncommmon mistake for an elderly childless woman to delude herself with the hope that she is about to bear a child, when the abdomen is enlarging simply for the last-named reason. This condition is known as pseudocyesis or false pregnancy. (*f*) The only absolutely certain sign of pregnancy is obtained when the medical attendant hears the beating of the foetal heart by auscultation over the lower part of the abdomen. The heart-sounds are rapid, much resembling the ticking of a watch, and are heard, in general, from the middle of the fifth month onwards. (*g*) There are various minor signs which are sometimes present, sometimes absent, some of which are noticeable by the mother, others appreciable only by the medical attendant. Such are the occurrence of varicose veins, mucous discharge from the vagina, changes in the neck of the womb.

Hygiene of pregnancy: It is unnecessary for a healthy woman to make any great change in her ordinary mode of life during pregnancy. Her diet must be good, but should be simple and moderate. Alcoholic liquors and smoking should preferably be abandoned during pregnancy. Because of the possible risk to the unborn child, no drugs should be taken during early pregnancy except on medical advice. A pregnant woman should drink at least half a litre (one pint) of milk a day, on account, amongst other things, of the calcium it contains. Cheese should also be taken for its calcium. (The foetus in the uterus needs calcium for its bones.) Iron-containing foods are also important for the development of the foetus's red blood corpuscles. Iron is present in such foods as eggs, green leafy vegetables, and in liver and meat. Vitamins are also of great importance to the pregnant woman, and these are present in such foods as eggs, milk, cheese, butter, wholemeal bread, brown bread, fresh vegetables, and fruit (especially oranges, lemons, currants, potatoes, and tomatoes), and fat fish, such as herring and salmon; in the winter months compound vitamin tablets may well be taken in addition. Constipation should be avoided by a suitable diet containing vegetables, fruit, and the like, or by mild aperients. The skin should be kept in good condition by regular bathing. Moderate exercise should be taken every day and late hours avoided. The dress should be loose and comfortable. It is inadvisable for sexual intercourse to take place during the last month of pregnancy. During pregnancy a healthy woman gains an average of 12·5 kg (28 pounds), but this varies considerably.

Special ailments: The misfortune which specially attaches to pregnancy is miscarriage (qv) but this is not likely to occur in healthy persons. Digestive disturbances are common. Thus the natural morning sickness may become very troublesome, or even dangerous, and require special treatment. Constipation or diarrhoea may be troublesome, but either of them is treated much as under ordinary circumstances. Varicose veins in the legs, piles, swelling of the feet, and cramps in the legs are all liable to be caused in the later months by pressure of the increasing womb upon the large vessels and nerves within the pelvis. These, however, are not serious signs, and must simply be tolerated till after the child is born, when they quickly improve. Varicose veins, if very severe, should be supported by elastic stockings or by bandaging the legs, and cramps may be relieved by the usual means. (See CRAMP.) Irritability of the bladder, showing itself by frequency of making water, is also a temporary inconvenience, similarly due to pressure.

More serious symptoms occasionally arise, such as those of kidney disease, various nervous disorders, and especially the condition known as eclampsia, in which convulsions occur. A sudden gain in weight in late pregnancy may indicate the onset of pre-eclampsia (qv).

It is because of the possibility of such ailments, whether mild or serious, occurring during pregnancy that every pregnant mother should be seen by her doctor, or attend an antenatal clinic, at regular intervals throughout pregnancy.

PREGNANCY TESTS: There are several tests for pregnancy in its early stages.

The Hogben test: This test is based upon the observation that the injection of pregnancy urine promotes ovulation in the female South African clawed toad (*Xenopus laevis*). It gives a result within twenty-four hours.

The Haemagglutination Inhibition test: This, and the subsequent tests to be mentioned, are

known as immunological tests, as opposed to that already mentioned which is known as a biological test. They are based upon the effect of the urine from a pregnant woman upon the interaction of red-blood cells, which have been sensitized to human gonadotrophin (qv), and anti-gonadotrophin serum. They have the great practical advantage of being performed in a test-tube or even on a slide, and therefore not requiring animals. Because of their ease and speed of performance (a result can be obtained in two hours), these tests are being used on an increased scale.
The *Latex test* and the *Gravindex test* are modifications of the haemagglutination test.

PREGNANDIOL is the excretion product of the hormone, PROGESTERONE (qv), manufactured by the corpus luteum of the ovary. Pregnandiol is excreted in the urine during the second half of the menstrual period, and its excretion rises steadily throughout pregnancy.

PREMATURE BIRTH (see ABORTION; BIRTH; FOETUS) is one that takes place before the end of the normal period of gestation. In practice, however, it is defined as a birth that takes place when the baby weighs less than 2·5 kilograms (5½ pounds). In the vast majority of cases the aim of management is to prolong the pregnancy and so improve the outlook for the unborn child. This consists essentially of rest in bed and sedation, but there are now several drugs, such as ritodrine (qv), that are used to suppress the activity of the uterus and so help to suppress premature labour.

PREMENSTRUAL SYNDROME has been defined as 'any combination of emotional or physical features which occur cyclically in a woman before menstruation and which regress or disappear during menstruation'. It is characterized by mood changes, discomfort, swelling and tenderness in the breasts, swelling of the legs, a bloated feeling in the abdomen, headache, fatigue and constipation. The mood changes range from irritability and mild depression to outbursts of violence. It may last for three up to 14 days. How common it is is not known, as only the more severe cases are seen by doctors, but it has been estimated that 1 in 10 of all menstruating women suffer from it severely enough to require treatment. The cause is not known, but it is probably due to some upset of the hormonal balance of the body. In view of the multiplicity of causes that have been put forward, it is not surprising that there is an equal multiplicity of treatments. Among these one of the most widely used is progesterone (qv). Others include pyridoxine (qv), danazol (qv), and gamma linolenic acid available in the form of oil of evening primrose. Whatever drug may be prescribed, psychological treatment is equally essential and, in many cases, is all that is required.

Although no-one denies that the syndrome is a real entity, and one which causes much suffering to a not inconsiderable number of unfortunate women, it is a diagnosis which is often abused, as exemplified by the fact that at the Premenstrual Syndrome Clinic at University College Hospital, London, the diagnosis of premenstrual syndrome is confirmed in only half of the women claiming to suffer from it. As a leading woman doctor with long experience in dealing with the condition has written: 'Premenstrual syndrome has been trivialized by the media, and feminine interests will best be served by our ability to distinguish the few genuine sufferers from the many malingerers whose claims can never be substantiated'.

PRENYLAMINE is a drug that is proving of value in the treatment of angina pectoris (qv).

PREPUCE is the free fold of skin that overlaps the glans penis.

PRESBYACUSIS is the deafness that comes on with increasing years. It is caused by increasing loss of elasticity in the hearing mechanism, combined with the slowing down of the mental processes that accompanies old age. It is characterized by particular difficulty in hearing high notes such as the telephone and the voices of women and children. Hearing in a background of noise, is also early affected. Modern, miniaturized, transistor 'within-the-ear' hearing aids are now available that are proving helpful in making life more bearable for the elderly in this respect. (See also DEAFNESS; HEARING AIDS.)

PRESBYOPIA (see ACCOMMODATION AND REFRACTION).

PRESCRIPTION means the written direction given by the doctor to the chemist for the compounding of medicine suitable to a patient's case.

At the present day the official recommendation is to prescribe in terms of milligrams and grams rather than grains and ounces, millilitres rather than minims, and in the *British Pharmacopoeia* and *British National Formulary* dosages are given in terms of the metric system only. Further, in the *British Pharmacopoeia* names of drugs are given in English, and not in Latin. (See also DOSAGE; DRUGS.)

Restrictions on prescribing and dispensing at public expense came into effect in the United Kingdom on 1st April, 1985. The restrictions are intended to reduce the enormous expenditure on pharmaceutical remedies. The aim was to exclude more expensive proprietary preparations when equivalent non-proprietary remedies were available at much less expense. The following groups of drugs were involved:

Antacids.
Laxatives.
Analgesics – used for mild or moderate pain.
Cough and cold remedies.

Bitters and tonics, vitamins.

Benzodiazepine tranquillisers and sedatives.

Medicines should be prescribed only when they are essential. This is particularly important in patients who are pregnant, where the risk to both patient and foetus must be considered –there are many drugs for which there is not sufficient evidence to be quite certain that they are harmless to the foetus. The most dangerous time is the first trimester of pregnancy.

Non-proprietary titles should normally be prescribed as this will enable the pharmacist to dispense any of the proprietary equivalents that he has in stock and thus avoid delay to the patient and expense to the Health Service. The pharmacist is not allowed to dispense a controlled drug unless the specific requirements of the "Mis-use of Drugs Regulations" of 1973 are met. The *British National Formulary* gives classified notes on drugs and preparations used in the treatment of diseases and their recommended doses. It is intended for the guidance of medical practitioners, pharmacists, nurses and other workers who have the necessary training and experience to interpret the information it provides. It is intended as a reference book for the pocket and should be supplemented by a study of more detailed publications when required. The councils of the British Medical Association and the Pharmaceutical Society have agreed that the name of the preparation should appear on the label of the bottle unless the prescriber indicates otherwise.

PRESENTATION means the appearance in labour of some particular part of the child's body at the mouth of the womb. This is a head presentation in 96 per cent of cases, but in a certain number the breech (or buttocks) may present, or the face, or foot, or even a part of the trunk in cases of cross-birth.

PRESSOR is the term applied to anything that increases the activity of a function: for example, a pressor nerve or pressor drug.

PRESSURE SORES (see BED SORES).

PRICKLY HEAT, or MILIARA RUBRA, is a troublesome skin condition affecting Europeans in tropical climates. It consists in the appearance of numbers of minute vesicles, produced by blocking of the outlet of the sweat or sebaceous glands in the skin, and accompanied by intolerable itching.

Causes: Nearly every European suffers from prickly heat during the early years of residence in the tropics, when the hot season comes round. It is due probably to the cells on the surface of the skin becoming sodden by the constant perspiration, and so swelling and blocking the outlets of the minute gland-ducts. Anything that leads to perspiration, such as hot drinks, hot soup, close rooms, or warm clothing, aggravates the condition.

Symptoms: The surface is covered by minute vesicles which cause extreme itching and pricking. The scratching which this entails often leads to the formation of boils and pustules, but the condition is not in itself a dangerous one. The extreme discomfort, and the loss of sleep arising from it, may, however, be a serious matter for invalids.

Treatment: The most important point is to avoid, so far as possible, all causes of excessive perspiration, such as warm drinks and rough underclothing. Curtailing the intake of salt and maintaining an adequate intake of fluid are also said to be helpful. Common soap should not be used in the bath, and each time after bathing, the skin should be dusted with an astringent and antiseptic dusting powder, such as one composed of boric acid, zinc oxide, and starch in equal parts. Equally effective is the use of an emollient cream or bath oil. If nothing else is immediately available, the application of olive oil is often helpful.

As a preventive, rubbing the body over after the bath with the juice of a lemon has been recommended. Calamine lotion (either alone or incorporating some menthol crystals) or carbolic acid lotion relieves the itching temporarily.

PRIMIDONE is a drug used for the treatment of epilepsy.

PRIMIPARA is the term applied to a woman who has given birth, or is giving birth, to her first child.

PRO- is a prefix meaning forwards.

PROBE is a slender, flexible instrument usually made of metal designed for introduction into a wound or cavity either to explore its depth and direction, to discover the presence of foreign bodies, or to introduce medicinal substances.

PROBENECID is a benzoic acid derivative. It interferes with the excretion by the kidney of certain compounds, including penicillin and para-aminosalicylic acid, and was originally introduced into medicine for this reason, as a means of increasing and maintaining the concentration of penicillin in the body. It has also proved of value in the treatment of chronic gout.

PROBUCOL (LURSELLE) (see HYPERLIPIDAEMIA).

PROCAINAMIDE is a derivative of procaine, which has been introduced for the treatment of certain cardiac arrythmias.

PROCAINE, or PROCAINE HYDROCHLORIDE, is a synthetic substance having a similar action to the natural alkaloid, cocaine. It is a powerful local anaesthetic with transitory effect. Procaine possesses the anaesthetic properties of cocaine, but has an advantage over the latter in being very much less poisonous, so that it can be administered in larger doses, and also in producing no tendency to contract a habit for its use.

PROCAINE PENICILLIN (see PENICILLIN).

PROCARBAZINE is a drug that is proving useful in the treatment of various forms of tumour, especially Hodgkin's disease (qv). It acts by interfering with the process of mitosis (qv), whereby the cells of the body, or tumours, reproduce themselves.

PROCHLORPERAZINE (STEMETIL, VERTIGON) is an anti-psychotic drug. It is also an effective drug for the prevention or treatment of vomiting, and has therefore been used in the treatment of Menière's disease (qv). (See ANTI-PSYCHOTIC DRUGS.)

PROCIDENTIA is another term for prolapse (qv).

PROCTALGIA is neuralgic pain in the anus or rectum. The term is usually reserved for rectal pain without local disease in the rectum to account for it.

Proctalgia fugax is a condition characterized by cramp-like pains in the rectum which may be excruciatingly painful. They are more common in men than women. They occur during the night, last up to fifteen minutes and may be accompanied by a feeling of faintness. The cause is not known. The taking of food or drink may bring relief, as may pressure on the perineum (eg. by sitting astride the edge of the bath). A finger in the rectum may also bring relief. The sucking of a 1 mg tablet of glyceryl trinitrate is said by some to bring prompt relief. The attacks are said to cease after the age of 50.

PROCTITIS means inflammation situated about the rectum or anus.

PRODROMATA is a term applied to the earliest symptoms of a disease, or those which give warning of its presence.

PROFLAVINE is a valuable antiseptic. It is an acridine derivative. Like all the acridine derivatives it is effective against both Gram-positive and Gram-negative bacteria and is not inactivated by body fluids or pus. It is also non-toxic and non-irritating.

PROGERIA is premature old age.

PROGESTOGEN is a preparation with an action like that of progesterone (qv).

PROGESTERONE is the hormone of the corpus luteum (qv). After the escape of the ovum from the ruptured follicle, the corpus luteum secretes progesterone, which stimulates the growth and secretion of the endometrial glands of the uterus during the fourteen days before menstruation. In the event of pregnancy, the secretion of progesterone continues until parturition. (See also ETHISTERONE; NORETHISTERONE; NORETHYNODREL; PREGNANDIOL; CONTRACEPTION; MENSTRUATION.)

PROGLOTTIS is a segment of a tapeworm.

PROGNOSIS is the term applied to a forecast as to the probable result of an illness or disease, particularly with regard to the prospect of recovery.

PROGRESSIVE MUSCULAR ATROPHY (see PARALYSIS).

PROGUANIL HYDROCHLORIDE is a synthetic antimalarial drug which has proved of value both in the treatment and the prevention of malaria, particularly the form known as malignant tertian malaria.

PROLACTIN is the pituitary hormone which initiates lactation. The development of the breasts during pregnancy is ascribed to the action of oestrogens (qv). Prolactin starts them secreting. If lactation does not occur or fails, it may be started by injection of prolactin.

The secretion of prolactin is normally kept under tonic inhibition by the secretion of a prolactin inhibitory hormone. This is formed in the hypothalamus and secreted into the portal capillaries of the pituitary stalk to reach the anterior pituitary cells. The prolactin inhibitory hormone has now been identified as the catecholamine dopamine. Drugs that deplete the brain stores of dopamine or antagonise dopamine at receptor level will cause hyperprolactinaemia and hence the secretion of milk from the breast and amenorrhoea. Methyldopa and reserpine deplete brain stores of dopamine and the phenothiazines act as dopamine antagonists at receptor level. Other causes of excess secretion of prolactin are pituitary tumours, which may be minute and are then called microadenomas, or may actually enlarge the pituitary fossa and are then call macroadenomas. The commonest cause of hyperprolactinaemia is a pituitary tumour. The patient may present with infertility, because patients with hyperprolactinaemia do not ovulate, or the patient may present with amenorrhea and even galactorrhoea.

Bromocriptine is a dopamine agonist. Treatment with bromocriptine will therefore control hyperprolactinaemia and restore normal menstruation and ovulation and suppress galactorrhoea. If the cause of hyperprolactinaemia is a macroadenoma, surgical treatment should be considered.

PROLAPSE means slipping down of some organ or structure. The term is applied chiefly to downward displacements of the rectum and womb. When the lower end of the bowel prolapses each time the bowels move – as may occur in children – it should be carefully sponged with cold water, replaced, and, if necessary, retained in place by a soft pad and bandage attached to a waist-belt, or by strapping the buttocks together with plaster. The condition tends to pass off as the child grows older. Prolapse which affects the womb may, in the earlier stages, cause protrusion of a fold of the bowel or bladder through the vagina, and in the later stages the womb itself may protrude to the exterior. The condition, which affects elderly women, is mainly due to injuries caused by childbirth. It may often be remedied by wearing a suitably shaped pessary, or by an operation designed to unite the torn parts.

PROLAPSED INTERVERTEBRAL DISC: The spinal column (qv) is built up of a series of bones, known as vertebrae, placed one upon the other. Between these vertebrae lies a series of thick discs of fibro-cartilage known as intervertebral discs. Each disc consists of an outer portion known as the annulus fibrosus, and an inner core known as the nucleus pulposus. The function of these discs is to give flexibility and resiliency to the spinal column and to act as buffers against undue jarring. In other words, they are most efficient shock absorbers. They may, however, prolapse, or protrude, between the two adjacent vertebrae. If this should happen they press on the neighbouring spinal nerve and cause pain. As the most common sites of protrusion, or prolapse, are between the last two lumbar vertebrae and between the last lumbar vertebra and the sacrum, this means that the pain occurs in the back, causing lumbago (qv) or down the course of the sciatic nerve causing sciatica (qv). The prolapse is most likely to occur in middle age, which suggests that it may be associated with degeneration of the disc involved, but it can occur in early adult life as well. It usually occurs when the individual is performing some form of exercise which involves bending, as in gardening. The onset of pain may be acute and sudden, or gradual and more chronic in intensity.

Treatment varies, depending, amongst other things, on the severity of the condition. In the acute phase rest in bed is essential. Later, exercise and physiotherapy are helpful, and in some cases manipulation of the spine brings relief by allowing the herniated, or prolapsed, disc to slip back into position. The injection of a local anaesthetic into the spine (epidural anaesthesia) is yet another measure that often helps the more chronic cases. The ultimate form of treatment is an operation to remove the prolapsed disc, but this is a procedure that is not now performed nearly as often as it once was. An alternative form of treatment is the injection into the disc of chymopapain, an enzyme (qv) obtained from the paw-paw, which dissolves the disc.

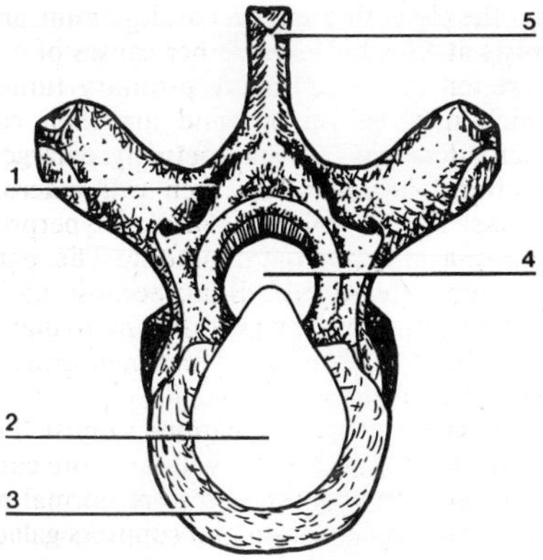

1 lamina
2 prolapsed disc
3 intervertebral disc
4 spinal cord
5 spinous process

Diagram of prolapsed intervertebral disc.

PROMAZINE (SPARINE, DOLMATIL) (see ANTI-PSYCHOTIC DRUGS).

PROMETHAZINE HYDROCHLORIDE is a widely used antihistamine drug with a prolonged action and a pronounced sedative effect. (See ANTIHISTAMINE DRUGS.)

PROMETHAZINE THEOCLATE, or AVOMINE, is a drug that is widely used in the alleviation or prevention of sea-sickness.

PRONATION is the movement whereby the bones of the forearm are crossed and the palm of the hand faces downwards.

PROPANTHELINE, or PROPANTHELINE BROMIDE, is a substance with an anti-cholinergic, or atropine-like action, which is used in the treatment of conditions such as duodenal ulcer and spastic colon.

PROPHYLAXIS means treatment or action adopted with the view of warding off disease.

PROPICILLIN (see PENICILLIN, ANTIBIOTIC).

PROPRANOLOL (ANGILOL, APSOLOL, BEDRANOL, BERKOLOL, INDERAL, SLOPROLOL) is a drug that is used in the treatment of angina pectoris, myocardial infarction, certain abnormal rhythms of the heart, and high blood-pressure. It is also proving of value in preventing attacks of migraine, and in certain anxiety states, particularly those associated with unpleasant bodily sensations, such as palpitations. It is a beta-adrenoceptor-blocking drug. (See ADRENERGIC RECEPTORS.)

PROPTOSIS: A condition in which the eye protrudes from the orbit. Some causes include thyroid disorders, tumours within the orbit, inflammation or infection of the orbit. Proptosis due to endocrine abnormality, eg. thyroid problems, is known as *exophthalmos*.

PROSTACYCLIN is a prostaglandin (qv) produced by the endothelial lining of the blood vessels. It inhibits the aggregation of platelets (qv), and thereby reduces the likelihood of the blood clotting. It is also a strong vasodilator.

PROSTAGLANDINS, so called because they were first discovered in the semen and thought to arise in the prostate gland, are a group of recently discovered substances with a wide range of activity. The richest known source is semen, but they are also present in many other parts of the body. Their precise mode of action is not yet clear, but they are potent stimulators of muscle contraction and they are also potent vasodilators (qv). They cause contraction of the womb and have been used to induce labour. They are also being used as a means of inducing therapeutic abortions. They play an important part in the production of pain, and it is now known that aspirin relieves pain by virtue of the fact that it prevents, or antagonizes, the formation of certain prostaglandins. In addition, they play some, though as yet incompletely defined, part in producing inflammatory changes. (See INFLAMMATION, NON-STEROIDAL ANTI-INFLAMMATORY DRUGS.)

Thus prostaglandins have potent biological effects but their instability and rapid metabolism make them short acting. They are produced but not stored by most living cells and act locally. The two most important prostaglandins are prostacycline and thromboxane. Prostacycline is a vaso-dilator and an inhibitor of platelet aggregation and may cause relaxation of the myometrium. Thromboxanes have the opposite effects and cause vaso-constriction and platelet aggregation. The non-steroidal anti-inflammatory drugs act by blocking an enzyme called cyclo-oxygenase which converts arachidonic acid to the precursors of the various prostaglandins. Despite their potent pharmacological properties, the role of prostaglandins in current therapeutics is limited and controversial. They have been used most successfully as an inhibitor of platelet aggregation in extra-corporeal haemoperfusion systems. The problems with the prostacyclines is that they have to be given intravenously as they are inactive by mouth, and continuous infusion is required because the drug is rapidly eliminated with a half-life of minutes. Side-effects tend to be severe because the drug is usually given at the highest dose the patient can tolerate. The hope for the future lies in the exploitation of the novel compound to generate stable orally active prostacycline analogues which will inhibit platelet aggregation and hence thrombotic events, and yet have minimal effects on the heart and blood vessels.

PROSTATE GLAND is a structure which lies at the neck of the bladder in men and surrounds that part of the urethra lying within the pelvis. This gland is of importance, especially because in late life it is apt to increase in size and change in shape in such a way as to obstruct the exit of urine from the bladder. Accordingly, great difficulty occurs in urinating. In some cases relief can be obtained, for a time at least, by the administration of phenoxybenzamine. In the large majority of cases, however, in which enlargement of the prostate produces such obstruction, removal by means of operation is now recommended. At the present day this operation, if performed by experienced surgeons, carries a relatively low mortality rate – 0·75 to 1 per cent – even though it is often carried out on old men who are far from fit. It has been estimated that one in every ten men will undergo this operation. The prostate is also one of the common sites of cancer in men, for which treatment takes various forms, including removal of the gland by operation, orchidectomy (qv), radiotherapy (qv), and administration of stilboestrol (qv).

PROSTATISM is the condition induced by benign enlargement of the prostate gland (qv).

PROSTHESIS is an artificial replacement, such as an artificial limb or eye, or a denture. (See ARTIFICIAL LIMBS.)

DENTAL PROSTHESIS is any artificial replacement of a tooth. There are three main types, a crown, a bridge and a denture. A crown is the replacement of the part of a tooth which sticks through the gum. It is fixed to the remaining part of the tooth and may be made of metal, porcelain, plastic or a combination of these. A bridge is the replacement of two or three missing teeth and is usually fixed in place. The replacement teeth are held in position by being joined to one or more crowns on the adjacent teeth. A denture is a removable prosthesis used to replace some or all the teeth. The teeth are made of plastic or porcelain and the base may be of plastic or metal. All these prostheses are individually made by skilled technicians and are matched to the patient's own teeth for size, shape and colour. Removable teeth may be held more firmly by means of implants (qv).

PROTAMINES are a class of proteins found in combination with nuclei and in the heads of fish spermatozoa. They have two main uses in medicine. When combined with insulin they produce a compound which exerts a slower and more prolonged anti-diabetic action. (See INSULIN.) They also act as an antidote to heparin (qv).

PROTEIN is the term applied to members of a group of non-crystallizable nitrogenous substances widely distributed in the animal and vegetable kingdoms and forming the characteristic materials of their tissues and fluids. They are essentially combinations of amino-acids.

They mostly dissolve in water and are coagulated by heat and various chemical substances. Typical examples of protein substances are white of egg and gelatin.

Proteins constitute an essential part of the diet as a source of energy and for the replacement of protein lost in the wear and tear of daily life. Their essential constituent from this point of view is the nitrogen they contain. To be absorbed, or digested, proteins have to be broken down into their constituent amino-acids. The adult human body can maintain nitrogenous equilibrium on a mixture of eight amino-acids, which are therefore known as the essential amino-acids. They are isoleucine, leucine, lysine, methionine, phenylalanine, threonine, tryptophan and valine. In addition, infants require histidine. It is because some of these essential amino-acids, particularly lysine, are lacking in cereals and pulses that these cannot alone constitute an adequate diet. Generally speaking, the major source of protein is animal food, although some vegetables, notably the pulses, contain protein. The use of a certain amount of nitrogenous food is necessary to the system, as from this source alone can the body derive all the building material it requires to repair daily waste. (See DIET.) Even carbohydrate foods contain a certain amount of protein, but if all the necessary protein were to be obtained from these it would incur the waste of much starch, or its formation into fat in the bodily tissues. Hence the main value of a mixed diet.

Meat in structure consists of long cylinders of semi-fluid, protein material enclosed in thin, fibrous tubes, and known as muscle fibres. (See MUSCLE.) These are bound together by fibrous tissue, enclosing more or less fat in its meshes. The protein material consists mainly of myosin, which clots when the muscle dies, and contains also albumin and haemoglobin. In addition, there are several chemical substances which can be extracted by steeping the meat in hot water, and which are therefore known as extractives. To these the flavour of meat is due, and the varying taste of different meats is to be explained by slight chemical differences in the extractives present. The feeding and habits of animals have much to do with these differences, and explain the variety in taste between the flesh of wild and tame rabbits, and of grouse and poultry. The shape of the muscle fibres has much to do with the digestibility of meat, short or fine fibres, as in poultry, being the most quickly dissolved. The fatness of meat, or rather the extent to which the fat is interspersed between the meat fibres, is of more importance in connection with digestibility and explains why pork, duck, and goose have a reputation for being indigestible. Sweetbreads and tripe, being held together by loose connective tissue, are, on the other hand, quickly digested, and therefore suitable for invalids. Liver and kidney, which contain much nuclein, a substance closely allied to uric acid, are bad for gout.

Jellies contain little but gelatin, obtained from the fibrous tissue of meat and sinews, and when made with a large quantity of water, ie. weak in gelatin, they are easily digested. Gelatin is of little or no use as building material, and the main value of jellies is to add bulk and variety to the invalid diet.

Soup consists of a small quantity of gelatin, fat, salts and extractives in hot water. To make soup or beef-tea from meat does not remove the nutritious materials, although it extracts all the flavour and hardens the meat. Clear soup contains practically no nourishment, although it is stimulating to the digestion by reason of the extractives it contains. Thick soup is nutritious only by reason of the vegetables and gelatin added to it. The same is true of the extract of meat introduced by Baron Liebig in 1865, and of its many more recent imitations. Each pint of beef-tea made from this extract represents the salts and extractives in about half a pound of lean meat, although it contains little or none of the nutritive materials. Its use is valuable, because it appears to play a part in helping on the processes of nutrition. It is useful therefore in fevers and in feeble conditions, when little food is needed, or when the digestive powers are weak. Beef-juice, obtained by chopping meat up finely, mixing with a little water and squeezing out cold, is quite another article, and contains a larger proportion of the nutritive materials as well as extractives.

Fish is an excellent source of protein, and, in the case of fatty fish, such as herring and mackerel, has the additional advantage of containing vitamins A and D. Haddock and whiting are among the most digestible fish, some of which, like cod, have a coarse fibre, and others, like salmon, are very fat. Herring is one of the most palatable forms of nitrogenous food, and two herrings contain as much animal protein as need enter into the daily dietary of an ordinary working man.

Milk is practically the only form of animal food in which protein, fat, carbohydrate and salt are all represented in sufficient amount. It contains 2 to 3 per cent of casein, from which cheese, an almost purely protein and fatty food, is made; a small quantity of milk-albumin; 4 per cent of fat in the form of a fine emulsion, which gradually rises to the surface as cream; and 4 to 5 per cent of milk-sugar, to the decomposition of which souring of milk is due. (See DIET; INFANT FEEDING; MILK.)

Eggs, each of which contains the material necessary to form a chicken, present the building material for the formation of bone and muscle in an easily convertible form, and are therefore an excellent food for convalescents, and for children. They do not contain any carbohydrate material, and therefore, to form a good article of general diet, should be mixed with rice, flour or other cereals, as is done in the shape of puddings. The digestibility is increased when an egg is beaten up with milk or water, and still more when the eggs are lightly boiled. One egg corresponds in nutritive value to about half a tumblerful of good milk, or to about 30 grams of meat.

Pulses, of which the chief are peas, beans and lentils, have been called the 'poor man's beef'. This, however, is misleading because, though they are cheap, they are not so digestible, contain little first-class protein, and are far from being so completely absorbed as meat unless carefully cooked, while in some people the gases formed by their decomposition in the bowels give rise to great flatulence. They are also poor in fat, hence the habit of eating them combined with fat foods, as pork and beans, duckling and peas, and butter with beans. Nevertheless, the pulses form a valuable form of food.

The necessity for protein and the reason for its combination with other foods is described under the article on DIET.

PROTEINURIA is the condition in which proteins are found in the urine. It is usually referred to as ALBUMINURIA (qv), but this is not strictly correct, as both of the two blood proteins – albumin and globulin – may be found in the urine.

PROTOPLASM is the viscid, translucent, glue-like material containing fine granules and composed mainly of proteins, which makes up the essential material of plant and animal cells and has the properties of life.

PROTRIPTYLINE (CONCORDIN) is an antidepressant drug. (See ANTIDEPRESSANTS.)

PROXIMAL is a term of comparison applied to structures which are nearer the centre of the body or the median line as opposed to more distal, or distant, structures.

PRURIGO is the name of a chronic skin disease in which small papules (qv) develop in the skin, accompanied by intense itching. The condition may either be permanent or may come and go.

PRURITUS is another name for itching (qv).

PRUSSIC ACID POISONING: Prussic, or hydrocyanic, acid is a very deadly poison with a sweet smell and pleasant taste, paralysing every part of the nervous system with which it comes in contact. In its dilute state it was once widely used as a remedy for irritable conditions of internal mucous membranes, such as that of the stomach, and for irritable skin diseases, being used in small doses to check vomiting or cough, and applied in lotions to relieve itching. It exerts this curative action by numbing the sensory nerves with which it is brought in contact. At the present day it is seldom used for therapeutic purposes.

As a poison it acts with great rapidity, and, since potassium cyanide is much used in the processes of electroplating and photography, and is almost as deadly in its effects as the acid, those using the cyanide should be acquainted with the treatment which may save life in a case of poisoning.

Symptoms: After a large dose, the poison is very rapidly diffused through the body, and only a few minutes or seconds elapse before the symptoms appear. These are slowness of breathing, slowness and irregularity of the heart's action, and blueness of the face and lips. In a few minutes, insensibility with gradual stoppage of breathing and of the heart's action comes on, preceded in some cases by convulsions.

The suddenness and character of the symptoms and the sweet smell of prussic acid on the breath make the cause evident.

Treatment: This is based upon the administration of nitrites, which convert cyanide in the blood into the harmless cyanmethaemoglobin. Amyl nitrite is given by inhalation for 30 seconds every two minutes and also, if the victim can still swallow, 0·5 gram of sodium nitrite in 10 millilitres of water, by mouth. Artificial respiration (see DROWNING, RECOVERY FROM) is started immediately, preferably by the Holger-Nielsn method (*not* by the mouth-to-mouth method), and oxygen is administered. Injections of sodium nitrite and sodium thiosulphate are then given, as well as analeptics. An 'Ampin' Cyanide Emergency Kit is available which allows these injections to be given quickly. The victim must be watched carefully for forty-eight hours. Another antidote that is proving of value is cobalt edetate.

PSEUDOCYESIS means spurious or false pregnancy, a condition characterized by enlargement of the abdomen, and even enlargement of the breasts and early morning sickness, the unfortunate woman being quite convinced that she is pregnant.

PSEUDOHYPERTROPHIC MUSCULAR DYSTROPHY, or PSEUDOHYPERTROPHIC PARALYSIS, is a condition in which certain muscles enlarge owing to a fatty and fibrous degeneration, giving a false appearance of increased strength. (See MUSCLES, DISEASES OF.)

PSEUDOXANTHOMA ELASTICUM: This is a hereditary disorder of elastic tissue. Degenerating elastic tissue in the skin produces lesions in the skin which look like soft yellow papules. Elastic tissue in the eye and blood vessels is also involved, giving rise to visual impairment, raised blood pressure and haemorrhages.

PSITTACOSIS is a contagious infection of parrots sometimes communicated to man and caused by a micro-organism known as *Chlamydia psittaci*. In 1979 five cases were reported in England attributable to an ill parrot in a consignment of parrots from Brazil which spent a few days in transit in an animal quarantine station at an airport before being shipped abroad. Four out of six persons in contact with the parrots in the quarantine station developed the disease, as did a man who had taken part in unloading the birds and driving them to the quarantine station. In 1980, there were 43 cases in which the source of infection were 'psittacine and other exotic birds'. The number of laboratory reports received at the Communicable Disease Surveillance Centre at Colingdale for Chlamydia B were 362 in 1983 and 410 in 1984.

PSOAS is a powerful muscle which arises from the front of the vertebral column in the lumbar region, and passes down, round the pelvis and through the groin, to be attached to the inner side of the thigh-bone not far from its upper end. The act of sitting up from a recumbent posture, or that of bending the thigh on the abdomen, is mainly accomplished by the contraction of this muscle. Disease of the spine in the lumbar region is apt to produce an abscess which lies within the sheath of this muscle and makes its way down to the front of the thigh, where it threatens to burst. Such an abscess is known as a psoas abscess. (See ABSCESS, CHRONIC.)

PSORIASIS is a disease of the skin in which raised, rough, reddened areas appear, covered with fine silvery scales. This eruption consists of a chronic inflammatory process in the corium, the papillae of which become considerably lengthened and more vascular than usual, together with changes in the epidermis which cause a defect in the horny formation that naturally takes place on the surface and results in an increased production of epidermal cells. The nails are also involved in about 50 per cent of cases. (See SKIN.)

Causes: The condition generally appears for the first time around adolescence or early adult life and, it has been estimated, affects around 2 per cent of the population in Britain. It is often a family disease. A child with one affected parent has a 25 per cent chance of developing the disease. The risk rises to 60 per cent if both parents are affected. If parents without the disease have a child with psoriasis the risk for a subsequent child is 17 per cent. It may be associated with arthritis and rarely gout. In some persons, psoriasis appears repeatedly at a particular season of the year, especially in the spring and autumn, but it is not infectious. Depressing influences seem to have something to do with its appearance, and people who are liable to it are troubled by its reappearance at any time when the general health is below par.

Symptoms: The eruption almost always appears first round the back of the elbows and front of the knees. It begins as small pimples, each covered with a white cap of scales, which enlarge in breadth till they form patches 5 to 7·5 cm (2 or 3 inches) wide. At the same time, patches appear on other parts of the body, trunk, back, limbs, scalp and in the more extensive disease the face is also affected. The disease is divided into several varieties according to the size, shape, and distribution of these patches.

Treatment: It is essential first of all to attend to the general health. A sympathetic approach to the patient is very important and an adequate explanation of the nature of the condition, the treatments available and what can be expected of these often helps to alleviate many an anxiety. It is important also for the individual to be well motivated, as the success of therapy depends to a great extent on his or her willingness to apply what are often messy creams several times a day for long periods. There is no cure for the condition and the best that can be hoped for is that it can be kept under control. Tar and dithranol are among the chief and most successful external applications. Satisfying results can also be obtained from the use of creams or ointments containing one or other of the corticosteroid preparations. Natural sunlight, or ultra-violet light, alone or in combination with tar preparations, produces a marked improvement in many cases. The latest form of treatment is that known as PUVA (qv). More recently, synthetic vitamin A is being used to treat one type of psoriasis, while cyclosporin (a drug used to prevent rejection in patients who have received a kidney transplant) is used in severe resistant cases. Patients with psoriasis can obtain help and advice by contacting the Psoriasis Association, 7 Milton Street, Northampton NN2 7JG (0604-711129).

PSYCHEDELIC DRUGS are drugs, such as lysergic acid diethylamide (LSD), that expand consciousness and perception. (See DRUG ADDICTION.)

PSYCHIATRY is that branch of medical science which treats mental disorder and disease.

PSYCHO-ANALYSIS is the term applied to the theories and practice of the school of psychology originating with Freud. It depends upon the theory that states of disordered mental health have been produced by a repression of painful memories or of conflicting instincts. By such repression these hurtful memories or instincts are kept constantly in a subconscious condition. As a result, the individual's mental power is needlessly occupied and diverted from the proper objects with which it should be concerned and he finds difficulty in concentrating his attention upon and adapting himself to the practical realities of everyday life.

Psycho-analysis aims at discovering these repressed memories which are responsible for the diversion of mental power and of which the affected person usually is only dimly aware or quite unaware. The fundamental method of psycho-analytical treatment is the free expression of thoughts, ideas and fantasies on the part of the patient. To facilitate this, in classical analysis, he or she lies on a couch to relax mind and body, and the analyst may sit so as to observe the patient but not to be observed by him. The analyst's task is to adopt a neutral attitude to the patient, to encourage the free association of ideas and to explain where explanation is necessary for the continuance of free association. The analyst will receive by way of transference good and bad fantasies of the patient and represent for him or her from time to time objects of love and hate, especially members of the patient's family. In the course of analysis the patient will re-explore his early emotional attitudes and tensions.

There is much that is speculative in the theories of psycho-analysis by the standards of orthodox experimental science but, at the same time, its fundamental conceptions have been widely adopted and developed by other schools of psychology to their enrichment. The new approaches to the study of the mind in health and disease opened up by the concepts of Freud have changed the attitude of the lay and the medical public to the problems of the neurotic, the morbidly anxious, the fearful and to the mental and emotional development of the child.

PSYCHOLOGY is the branch of science that deals with the mind and its methods of working.

PSYCHONEUROSIS is a general term applied to various functional disorders of the nervous system. (See NEUROSIS.)

PSYCHOPATHIC: Psychopathic disorder is defined by the Mental Health Act 1983 as a persistent disorder or disability of mind (whether or not including significant impairment of intelligence) which results in abnormally aggressive or seriously irresponsible conduct. The cardinal features are as follows: (1) Absence of normal feelings for other people such as love, affection, sympathy and condolence. (2) A tendency to anti-social impulsive acts with no forethought of the consequences. (3) A failure to learn by experience and to be deterred from crime by punishment. (4) Absence of any other form of mental disorder that would explain the unusual behaviour. The corresponding American terminology is 'anti-social personality disorder'.

PSYCHOSIS is a term applied to serious disorder of the mind, amounting to insanity.

PSYCHOSOMATIC DISEASES are illnesses resulting from the effects of excessive or repressed emotions upon bodily function or structure. They affect vast numbers of patients who are not out of their minds and yet do not have any organic disease to account for their illness. Functional symptoms must not be regarded as invented or imagined or as a mysterious state affecting an inferior personality. In psychosomatic disease the will may be strong and the mind normal, yet the emotions require treatment. Disorders precipitated by emotional factors may be psychotic, psychoneurotic or psychosomatic. In psychotic and psychoneurotic illnesses the symptoms are predoninantly psychological, whilst in psychosomatic disorders the symptoms may be entirely somatic. The concept of emotional disturbances contributing to bodily disease is not new. It was over 2400 years ago that Socrates stressed that "as you ought not to attempt to cure the eyes without the head, or the head without the body, so you should not treat body without mind". The rapid advances of scientific medicine have encouraged a preoccupation with the measurable and a neglect of the intangible. It has been estimated that one third of medical outpatients have psychiatric illness. In another third symptoms are largely dependent on an emotional factor even though organic disease is present. In gynaecological clinics emotional tensions are even more commonly encountered and exceed physical disease as a cause of illness. Over one quarter of all absence from work due to sickness is a result of an illness having an emotional basis.

The three major problems that lead to psychosomatic disorder are marital relationships; occupation, which includes the frustrations, disappointments and feelings of unfulfilment provoked by the patient's work; and finally, social relationships – the feelings which prevail between friends, neighbours and relations.

The many somatic symptoms due to anxiety result from enhanced activity of the sympathetic nervous system. Pain may be a manifestation of psychosomatic disease. Psychogenic fators may produce muscle tension and and cause a pain that is organic. The tension headache is due to the increased tone of the muscles of the neck and scalp.

The visceral reactions of emotional stimuli are of two types:

(1) Sympathetic. This is the part of the autonomic nervous system concerned with emergency situations in the external environment, the so-called preparation for fight or flight. The sympathetic nervous system which adjusts the body to such stresses inhibits the metabolic processes of the body and increases the heart rate and blood pressure, and mobilizes carbohydrate reserves. Its effects are mediated through the hormones adrenaline and noradrenaline.

(2) Parasympathetic. This is concerned with the conservation and anabolic processes of the body. Hence there is stimulation of gastrointestinal and bronchial secretions, a storing of sugar in the liver, and protective reflexes such as contraction of the pupil and spasm of the bronchiolar muscles as a protection against irritant substances. Parasympathetic effects are mediated through the secretion of acetylcholine. As a result of excess acetylcholine there is a feeling of warmth and flushing due to vasodilatation, and sweating due to cholinergic stimulation of the sweat glands. This is associated with nausea, vomiting and abdominal colic due to increased peristalsis and contraction of the intestines and the stomach. Thus, when emotional impulses are repressed, two possibilities arise. The patient may be in a constant state of preparedness for action and if this is never executed the sympathetic over-activity persists

with a chronic increase in muscle tension, tachycardia and raised blood pressure, and these may give rise to symptoms. An alternative reaction is emotional withdrawal from action into a dependent state of para-sympathetic overactivity. This would include diarrhoea, gastric acid hypersecretion, oesophageal spasm and other parasympathetic effects on the gastro-intestinal tract. Since the autonomic nervous system innovates practically every portion of the body, a somatic manifestation of emotional tension may be related to any area. Autonomic nervous overactivity may be manifest in the various systems as follows:

(1) Central nervous system. Headache. Often described as a pressure on the head. Dizziness, feelings of faintness, nervousness, tremors, sleeplessness and physical exhaustion.

(2) Cardiovascular system. Tachycardia, arrhythmia and precordial pains.

(3) Respiratory symptoms. Sighing respirations and a feeling of an inability to breathe deeply. Vasomotor rhinitis, chronic sore throat and asthma.

(4) Gastro-intestinal system. Anorexia, nausea, vomiting, indigestion, wind, heartburn, diarrhoea, constipation and sensations of a lump in the throat.

(5) Skin. Itching, sweating, parasthesiae and neuro-dermatitis.

Direct observations on the human colon through fistulae and colostomy openings and on the gastric mucosa through gastrostomy have shown that fear, anxiety and pain can cause an increase in peristalsis with reddening and swelling of the mucous membrane, whilst depression causes reduced motility and pallor of the mucosa. Psychosomatic symptoms may be the result of disorders of secretory functions, such as salivation, dry mouth, hyperchlorhydria, functional hyperinsulinism and mucous colitis, or alternatively they may be due to disorders of motor function such as oesophageal spasm, gastric hypermotility, spastic colon, constipation and diarrhoea. The skin plays an important part in the regulation of body temperature by sweating and its functions are controlled by the autonomic nervous system.

Vasoconstriction, vasodilatation, pilomotor activity and sweating are the four common physiological processes of the skin and are all largely controlled by the autonomic nervous system. Emotional sweating is most evident on the palms and soles and in the axilla. The influence of emotion on respiratory function is well recognized by the everyday expression, "it took my breath away". The autonomic innervation of the respiratory tract, which includes the nasal mucosa, consists of sympathetic and para-sympathetic nerves. Para-sympathetic nerves exert a constrictor effect on the smooth muscle of the respiratory tract and the sympathetic nerves have a relaxing influence. If para-sympathetic stimulation is excessive, mucous cells oversecrete and vasodilatation of blood vessels occurs. This produces swelling of the bronchial mucosa and congestion of airways.

Functional illness has its own characteristics and the diagnosis is not established by the mere exclusion of organic disease. It is suggested by the existence of emotional disturbance as a precipitating factor, by the presence of certain characteristic symptoms, by a family history of a similar disorder and by a phasic course characterized by remissions and relapses. It must always be remembered that organic disease may cause anxiety and may provide the stressful factor needed to precipitate psychosomatic disease.

PSYCHOSURGERY was introduced in 1936 by Egas Moniz, Professor of Medicine in Lisbon University, for the surgical treatment of certain psychoses. For his work in this field he shared the Nobel prize in 1949. The original operation, known as leucotomy, consisted of cutting white fibres in the frontal lobe of the brain. It was accompanied by certain hazards such as persistent epilepsy and undesirable changes in personality. Pre-frontal leucotomy is now regarded as obsolete. Modern stereotactic surgery may be indicated in certain intractable psychiatric illnesses in which the patient is chronically incapacitated, especially where there is a high suicide risk. Patients are only considered for psychosurgery when they have failed to respond to routine therapies. One contra-indication is marked histrionic or anti-social personality. The conditions in which a favourable response has been obtained are intractable and chronic obsessional neuroses, anxiety states and severe chronic depression.

Psychosurgery is now rare in Britain. The Mental Health Act 1983 requires not only consent by the patient, confirmed by an independent doctor, and two other representatives of the Mental Health Act Commission, but that the Commission's appointed medical representative must also advise on the likelihood of the treatment alleviating or preventing a deterioration in the patient's condition.

PSYCHOTHERAPY is the term applied to any form of treatment which operates through the mind. Almost every type of disease or injury has a mental aspect, even if this relates only to the pain or discomfort that it causes. In some diseases and with some temperaments, the mental factor is much more pronounced than in others; for such cases psychotherapy is particularly important. The chief methods employed are the following:

Suggestion is a commonly employed method, used in almost every department of medicine. It may consist, in its simplest form, merely of emphasizing that the patient's health is better, so that this idea becomes fixed in the patient's mind. A suggestion of efficacy may be conveyed by the physical properties of a medicine or by the appearance of some apparatus used in treatment. Again, suggestion may be conveyed

emotionally, as in religious healing. In occasional cases a therapeutic suggestion may be made to the patient in a hypnotic state.
Persuasion is a method of treatment in which appeal is made to a patient's reasoning faculties.
Analysis consists in the elucidation of the half-conscious or subconscious repressed memories or instincts that are responsible for some cases of mental disorder or personal conflicts.
Group therapy is a method whereby patients are treated in small groups and encouraged to participate actively in the discussion which ensues amongst themselves and the participating therapists. A modification of group therapy is *drama* therapy. Large group therapy also exists.
Education and employment may be important factors in rehabilitative psychotherapy.
Supportive therapy consists of sympathetically reviewing the patient's situation with him or her and encouraging the patient to identify and solve problems.
Short-term supportive psychotherapy is aimed at stabilizing and strengthening the psychological defence mechanisms of those patients who are confronted by a crisis which threatens to overwhelm their ability to cope, or who are struggling with the aftermath of major life events.
Long-term supportive psychotherapy is needed for patients with personality disorders or recurrent psychotic states, where the aim of treatment is to prevent deterioration and help the patient to achieve an optimal adaptation, making the most of his psychological assets. Such patients may find more profound and unstructured forms of therapy distressing.
Behavioural therapy and **cognitive therapy**, often carried out by psychologists, attempt to clarify with the patient specific features of behaviour or mental outlook respectively and identify step-by-step methods the patient can use for controlling the disorder. Behaviour therapy is commonly used for agoraphobia and other phobias, and cognitive therapy has been used for depression and anxiety.

PTERYGIUM: A degenerative disorder of the conjunctiva which grows over the cornea medially and laterally. The overgrowths look like wings. They are commonly seen in people who live in areas of bright sunlight, particularly when reflected from deserts or snowfields. Treatment involves excision of the overgrowth.

PTOSIS (see EYE, DISEASE AND INJURIES OF).

PTYALIN is the name of the enzyme contained in the saliva, by which starchy materials are changed into sugar, and so prepared for absorption. It is identical with the amylase of pancreatic juice. (See DIGESTION; PANCREAS.)

PTYALISM is a condition characterized by excessive production of saliva.

PUBERTY means the change that takes place when childhood passes into manhood or womanhood. This change is generally a very definite one, taking place at about the age of fourteen years, although it is modified by race, climate, and bodily health, so that it may appear a year or two earlier or several years later. At this time the sexual functions attain their full development, the contour of the body changes from a childish to a more rounded womanly, or sturdy manly form, and great changes take place in the mode of thought and feeling. In girls it is marked by the onset of menstruation and development of the breasts. Development of the breasts is usually the first sign of puberty to appear, and may occur from 9 years onwards. Most girls show signs of breast development by the age of 13. The time from the beginning of breast development to the onset of menstruation is usually around two years but may range from six months to five years. The first sign of puberty in boys is an increase in testicular size between the age of 10 and 14. The larynx enlarges in boys, so that the voice after going through a period of 'breaking', finally assumes the deep manly pitch. Hair appears on the pubis and later in the armpits in both boys and girls, whilst in the former it also begins to grow on the upper lip, and skin eruptions are not uncommon on the face. (See ACNE.)

The period is one of transition from a physical and mental point of view. Puberty is not to be regarded as a physiological 'coming of age', for full development is not attained till between twenty and thirty years of age. (See also MENARCHE; MENSTRUATION.)

PUBIS is the bone that forms the front part of the pelvis. The pubic bones of opposite sides meet in the symphysis and protect the bladder from the front.

PUBLIC HEALTH (see SANITATION; also DISINFECTION; INFECTION; SEWAGE AND SEWAGE DISPOSAL; VENTILATION; WATER SUPPLY).

PUERPERAL FEVER, or CHILD-BED FEVER, used to be the great dread of those attending women in child-birth.
Causes: This fever is of various types and grades of severity. After the birth of a child, the mother is specially liable, for several reasons, to contract any infectious disease to which she may be exposed. In the first place, she is weakened by the strain through which she has passed, and often by the loss of a considerable quantity of blood. In the second place, the injuries incidental to child-birth produce raw surfaces in the genital tract, from which absorption occurs with great facility. The organism most commonly involved is the *Streptococcus haemolyticus* (qv).
Symptoms: The symptoms vary according to the form that the infection takes, and most commonly appear on the second or third day after labour, the first three days being regarded as the critical period in recovery. Thus the organisms may, in the mildest form, develop

on the raw or wounded surface, to which they gain access without entering the system. In such a case, there are general discomfort and feverishness, rise of temperature, and quickening of the pulse.

When the organisms gain access to the surrounding lymphatic vessels and veins, inflammation in the cellular tissue of the pelvis results, and may be followed by abscesses, peritonitis, either localized or general (see PERITONITIS), or, later on, by the condition known as white leg, caused by blocking of the veins in one lower limb. In these conditions, which are less common, the symptoms are more severe. There are considerable fever, shivering, prostration, and quickening of the pulse as early signs, together with pain in the lower part of the abdomen, followed later on by the symptoms belonging to peritonitis, white leg, or other condition set up by the inflammation. The condition may be recovered from in a week or two, or long-continued ill-health may result, or the patient may speedily succumb.

If the organisms gain access to the general circulation, the serious condition known as septicaemia results (see BLOOD-POISONING), and is accompanied by high fever, great prostration, delirium, and increasing feebleness of the heart's action.

Treatment: The prevention of the condition is of the greatest importance. For this reason, care in the choice of a lying-in room, great care to shield the patient from every risk of infection, and above all, scrupulous cleanliness on the part of all the attendants, are necessary. (See also LABOUR.)

Treatment resolves itself into careful nursing, blood transfusion if haemoglobin falls below 6 g/dl, and administration of penicillin or the appropriate antibiotic.

PUERPERIUM is the period which elapses after the birth of a child until the mother is again restored to her ordinary health. It is generally regarded as lasting for a month. One of the main changes that occur is the enormous decrease in size that takes place in the muscular wall of the womb. (See MUSCLE.) There are often afterpains during the first day in women who have borne several children, less often after a first child. (See AFTERPAINS.) The discharge is blood-stained for the first two or three days, then clearer till the end of the first week, after which it becomes thicker and less in quantity, finally disappearing altogether, if the case goes well, at the end of two or three weeks. The breasts, which have already enlarged before the birth of the child, secrete milk more copiously, and there should be a plentiful supply on the third day of the puerperium.

Management: It is now realized that prolonged rest in bed is not necessary for the mother after a normal birth. Indeed, it may be harmful. The mother should start practising exercises to help to ensure that the stretched abdominal muscles regain their normal tone. There is no need for any restriction of diet, but care must be taken to ensure an adequate intake of fluid, including at least 580 ml (a pint) of milk a day. The bowels are generally sluggish and it is usual to take an aperient on the second or third day.

Milk, as already stated, appears copiously on the third day, but this is preceded by a secretion from the breast, known as colostrum, which is of value to the new-born child. The child should therefore be put to the breasts within six to eight hours of being born, in order to obtain the small amount of fluid they are secreting, and also because suckling stimulates both the breasts and the natural changes taking place during this period. Suckling is beneficial for both child and mother.

PULEX IRRITANS is the common human flea. It is between 2 and 4 mm in length. Of more importance is *Xenopsylla cheopis*, the rat-flea which transmits plague. Both are destroyed by DDT: 5 per cent solution in kerosene for buildings and furniture: 10 per cent powder for clothing. For pet animals DDT should be used as a powder and not as a solution. (See BITES AND STINGS.)

PULMONARY DISEASES (see LUNG DISEASES).

PULMONARY EMBOLISM is the condition in which an embolus (see EMBOLISM), or clot, is lodged in the lungs. The source of the clot is usually the veins of the lower abdomen or legs in which clot formation has occurred as a result of the occurrence of thrombophlebitis. (See VEINS, DISEASES OF.) Thrombophlebitis, with or without pulmonary embolism, is a not uncommon complication of surgical operations, especially in older patients. This is one reason why nowadays such patients are got up out of bed as quickly as possible, or, alternatively, are encouraged to move and exercise their legs regularly in bed. The severity of a pulmonary embolism, which is characterized by the sudden onset of pain in the chest, with or without the coughing up of blood, and a varying degree of shock, depends upon the size of the clot. If large enough it may prove immediately fatal. In other cases immediate operation may be needed to remove the clot, whilst in less severe cases anticoagulant treatment, in the form of heparin (qv), is given to prevent extension of the clot.

PULP (see TEETH).

PULSATION, or throbbing, is an appearance seen or felt naturally below the fourth and fifth ribs on the left side, where the heart lies, and also at every point where an artery lies close beneath the surface. In other situations, it may be a sign of aneurysm. In nervous people, particularly if thin, great pulsation can often be seen and felt in the upper part of the abdomen, due to the throbbing of the normal abdominal aorta.

PULSE: If the tip of one finger is laid gently on the front of the forearm, about 2·5 cm (one inch) above the furrows that mark the wrist, and about 1 cm (half an inch) from the outer edge, the pulsations of the radial artery can be felt. This is known as *the pulse*, but a pulse can be felt wherever an artery of large or medium size lies near the surface.

The cause of the pulsation lies in the fact that, at each heart-beat, 80 to 90 millilitres of blood are driven into the aorta, and a fluid wave, distending the vessels as it passes, is in consequence transmitted along the arteries all over the body. This pulsation gets less and less marked as the arteries grow smaller, and is finally lost in the minute capillaries, where a steady pressure is maintained. For this reason, the blood in the veins flows steadily on without any pulsation. Immediately after the wave has passed, the artery, by virtue of its great elasticity, regains its former size. In this wave the physician has a valuable means of studying both the state of the artery as regards elasticity and the heart's action.

The pulse rate is usually about 70 per minute, but it may vary in health from 50 to 100, and is quicker in childhood and slower in old age than in middle life; it increases in all feverish states.

Further, the character of the vessel wall is of great importance. In childhood and youth the vessel wall is so thin that, when sufficient pressure is made to expel the blood from it, the artery can no longer be felt. In old age, however, and in some degenerative diseases, the vessel wall becomes so thick that it may be felt like a piece of whipcord rolling beneath the finger. The extent to which this change has taken place gives the physician valuable information as to the state of the arteries.

Different types of heart disease have special features of the pulse associated with them. In atrial fibrillation the great character is irregularity. In cases in which the aortic valve is incompetent, the pulse has the peculiarity of rising very quickly and collapsing suddenly.

An instrument known as the sphygmograph has been devised, whereby the artery is made to register these waves. Another instrument known as the polygraph enables tracings to be taken from the pulse at the wrist and from the veins in the neck and simultaneous events in the two compared.

The pressure of the blood in various arteries is estimated by an instrument known as the sphygmomanometer. (See BLOOD-PRESSURE.)

PULSES are the seeds of the *Leguminosa* family. They include peas, beans and lentils and constitute a valuable source of food. Most contain around 20 grams of protein per 100 grams of dry weight but the biological value of this protein requires supplementation to ensure an adequate intake of first class, or essential, amino-acids (qv). They have been described as 'the poor man's protein', and a combination of pulse and cereal proteins may have a nutritive value comparable to that of animal protein. They are a good source of the B group of vitamins with the exception of riboflavine. (See also DIET.)

PUNCTATE BASOPHILIA (see BASOPHILIA.)

PUNCTUM (see EYE).

PUPIL (see EYE).

PURGATIVES are drugs or other measures which produce evacuation of the bowels.

Varieties and action: Purgatives are divided into several groups, according to the manner and degree of violence with which they act.

LAXATIVES are those which gently stimulate the bowels and render the motions slightly more frequent and softer without causing any griping. Most articles of food that leave a large indigestible residue upon which the intestine can contract, such as cabbage, brown bread, and oatmeal porridge, act in this way. Those fruits which contain rough seeds, sugar, and vegetable acids act similarly. Among the laxatives are honey, tamarinds, figs, raspberries, strawberries, prunes, stewed apples, senna and magnesia. Liquid paraffin also produces this effect.

SIMPLE PURGATIVES, or APERIENTS, produce one or more copious and slightly liquid movements, often accompanied or preceded by griping pains. Examples of this class are aloes, rhubarb, cascara sagrada, senna, castor oil.

DRASTIC PURGATIVES cause a violent action of the bowels, accompanied by considerable griping. In small doses many of them have a simple aperient action, while in excessive doses most are irritant poisons. Such are elaterium, colocynth, jalap, scammony, croton oil. Many of these produce very copious watery evacuations, and, since they remove a considerable quantity of water from the system, are known as *hydragogues*. These drastic purgatives are seldom used nowadays.

SALINE PURGATIVES are salts of the alkaline metals and alkaline earths. Such are sulphate of potassium, sulphate of sodium (Glauber's salt), sulphate of magnesium (Epsom salts), phosphate of sodium, bitartrate of potassium (cream of tartar), tartrate of potassium and sodium (Seidlitz powder), and citrate of magnesium. Taken in large doses, many of these salines also act as hydragogues.

Purgatives produce their effects either by stimulating the mucous membrane so that the amount of fluid in the intestine becomes larger, or by stimulating the muscular coat so that peristaltic contractions become more vigorous. Most purgatives have the double action, though one or other preponderates. Further, certain purgatives act all along the intestine, such as Epsom salts, whilst others, such as cascara, are almost devoid of action until they reach the large intestine. Castor oil, on the other hand, acts mainly on the small intestine.

Uses: The most common use of purgatives is to remove the contents of the bowels when their action is sluggish. (See CONSTIPATION.) In many cases of diarrhoea, due to the presence of irritating material in the intestine, a single dose of purgative medicine, such as castor oil, is given with the object of getting rid of the offending material, after which the diarrhoea ceases. In cases of inflammation affecting the bowels, saline purgatives are often given with the view of diminishing the congestion in the bowel-wall.

PURPURA is a disease characterized by the occurrence of purple spots upon the surface of the body, due to extravasations of blood in the skin, associated occasionally with haemorrhages from mucous membranes.

Causes: The condition is due either to an increased permeability of the smallest blood-vessels (ie. the capillaries) which allows blood to pass through their walls, or to a shortage of blood platelets which normally play an important part in sealing off any damage which may occur to the walls of the capillaries. The damage to the capillary wall may arise as a result of an infection, eg. septicaemia; a toxic factor, eg. certain drugs; or in scurvy.

A common cause of a lack of platelets in their auto-immune destruction in idiopathic thrombocytopenic purpura. Capillary damage is commonly due to anaphylactoid purpura which is an allergic condition, the increased permeability of the capillary wall being due to the individual coming in contact with, inhaling, or ingesting, some substance to which he is sensitized. Two special forms of anaphylactoid purpura are recognized. One is *Henoch's purpura*, in which the purpuric haemorrhages occur in the wall of the intestine, causing symptoms resembling an acute abdominal emergency. This form occurs in children and young adults. The other is *Schönlein's purpura*, in which the purpura occurs around the joints causing them to be painful and tender. This form principally affects young adults.

Symptoms: The complaint is usually ushered in by lassitude and feverishness. This is soon followed by the appearance on the surface of the body of the characteristic spots in the form of small red points scattered over the skin of the limbs and trunk. Their colour soon becomes deep purple or nearly black; but after a few days they undergo the changes which are observed in the case of an ordinary bruise, passing to a green and yellow hue and finally disappearing. When of minute size they are termed petechiae, when in patches of considerable size ecchymoses. They may come out in fresh crops over a lengthened period.

Treatment: The treatment of *secondary purpura* consists of that of the underlying cause: eg. scurvy. The treatment of *primary thrombocytopenic purpura* consists of the administration of one of the cortisone-like drugs: eg. prednisolone. In cases which do not respond to such therapy, removal of the spleen is often helpful, especially in children. In severe cases, with heavy loss of blood, blood transfusion may be necessary. The treatment of *anaphylactoid purpura* consists of the administration of antihistamine drugs. If these fail, then it is worth trying the effect of prednisolone. If, as is often the case, there is any anaemia, this must be treated by the administration of full doses of iron: eg. ferrous sulphate.

PUS, or MATTER, is a thick, white, yellow, or greenish fluid, which is found in abscesses, on ulcers, and on inflamed and discharging surfaces generally. Its colour and consistency are due to the presence, in great numbers, of pus corpuscles. These are derived mostly from the white corpuscles of the blood, and consist also of the superficial cells of granulation tissue or of a mucous membrane which die and are shed off in consequence of the inflammatory process. (See ABSCESS; PHAGOCYTOSIS.)

PUSTULE means a small collection of pus. (See ABSCESS.) Malignant pustule is one of the forms taken by woolsorters' disease. (See ANTHRAX.)

PUTREFACTION is the change that takes place in the bodies of plants and animals after death, whereby they are ultimately reduced to carbonic acid gas, ammonia, and other simple substances. The change is almost entirely due to the action of bacteria, and, in the course of the process, various offensive and poisonous intermediate substances are formed. In the case of the human body, putrescine, cadaverine, and other alkaloids are among these intermediate products.

The first sign of putrefaction is the appearance of a greenish tinge over the lower part of the abdomen, visible on the second or third day after death. This is not to be confused with the lividity seen on the back, due to the blood running down into the dependent parts, which is visible within eight or twelve hours. In from two to three weeks the body is greenish-brown throughout, the skin beginning to give way, and the features almost unrecognizable. By the end of one year, none of the organs is recognizable. After the lapse of four to seven years, bodies buried in gravel or sandy soil have lost all trace of the soft parts, the bones alone remaining.

When bodies decompose in water, particularly that drained from peaty soil, the skin becomes white and sodden and the changes take place more slowly. Sometimes, in these circumstances, instead of going through the usual changes, the body undergoes a process of saponification, and the tissues are converted into a mixture of soaps, fatty acids, and volatile substances known as *adipocere*. This does not readily undergo further changes, and so bodies lying in ponds or damp graves may become changed in the course of some months or years into this wax-like substance, after which they may be preserved with the smallest details of feature for many years.

Mummification may prevent putrefaction in the dry air of deserts, and even in the case of a body lying in a strong draught of air these changes may be indefinitely postponed by gradual drying. A similar result has been known to occur in the bodies of people who have taken antimony for a long period prior to death, the antimony deposited all through the body acting as an antiseptic.

PUTRID FEVER is an old name for typhus fever.

PUVA is a method of treating severe cases of psoriasis (qv) which do not respond to other forms of treatment. This consists of giving the patient a tablet of a psoralen preparation which sensitizes the skin cells to sunlight and then exposing him in a special cubicle to high-intensity long-wave ultraviolet radiation (UVA). Hence the name PUVA: a combination of P for psoralen and UVA. Initially this treatment is given twice a week. Although not curative, it has proved highly effective, but can only be carried out in specially equipped hospital departments.

PYAEMIA means a form of blood-poisoning in which abscesses appear in various parts of the body. (See BLOOD-POISONING.)

PYELITIS means inflammation of that part of the kidney known as the pelvis, which is connected with the ureter. It is now realized, however, that the infection is seldom restricted to the pelvis, but involves the kidney tissue as well. In other words the correct diagnosis is pyelonephritis.

The inflammation may spread upwards from the bladder or may follow on febrile diseases in which bacteria leave the body by the urine. One of the commonest organisms productive of this condition is the *Escherichia coli*, which produces a highly acid state of the urine accompanied by the presence of pus. Pyelitis sometimes occurs as a complication of pregnancy. There are generally symptoms of feverishness, general malaise, loss of weight, discomfort in the region of the loins, and frequency in passing water. Examination reveals the presence of the infecting organism and of pus in the urine.

Treatment: In some cases the administration of alkalis and the drinking of ample bland fluids are all that is required. As a rule, however, more active treatment is necessary and this consists of the administration of an antibiotic. As pyelitis may be due to some other condition of the kidney, such as a stone, a full investigation is necessary, as such cases will not clear up unless the underlying cause is removed.

PYELOGRAPHY is the term applied to the process whereby the kidneys are rendered radio-opaque, and therefore visible on an X-ray film. It constitutes a most important part of the examination of a patient with kidney disease. (See SODIUM DIATRIZOATE.)

PYELONEPHRITIS (see PYELITIS).

PYKNOLEPSY is the term applied to a type of epilepsy in which the only manifestation is a sudden and temporary loss of consciousness. There are no convulsions and the attacks tend to disappear in time.

PYLEPHLEBITIS means inflammation of the portal vein. It usually results from disease in the intestine and is part of a general blood-poisoning.

PYLOROSPASM means spasm of the pyloric portion of the stomach. This interferes with the passage of food in a normal, gentle fashion into the intestine and causes the pain that comes on from half an hour to three hours after meals and is associated with severe disorders of digestion. It is often produced by an ulcer of the stomach or duodenum.

PYLORUS is the lower opening of the stomach, through which the softened and partially digested food passes into the small intestine.

PYO- is a prefix attached to the name of various diseases to indicate cases in which pus is formed, such as pyonephrosis.

PYODERMA GANGRENOSUM: This is a disorder in which large ulcerating lesions appear suddenly and dramatically in the skin. It is the result of underlying vasculitis. It is usually the result of inflammatory bowel disease such as ulcerative colitis or Crohn's disease but can be associated with rheumatoid arthritis.

PYOGENIC is a term applied to those bacteria which cause the formation of pus and so lead to the formation of abscesses. Although many bacteria have this property, the most common cause of abscess is one of the rounded forms of bacterium (eg. streptococcus).

PYORRHOEA is the name given to any copious discharge of pus. For *Pyorrhoea alveolaris* see under TEETH, DISEASES OF.

PYREXIA means fever. (See FEVER.)

PYRIDOXINE, or vitamin B_6, plays an important part in the metabolism of a number of amino-acids. Deficiency leads to atrophy of the epidermis, the hair follicles, and the sebaceous glands, and peripheral neuritis may also occur. Young infants are more susceptible to pyridoxine deficiency than adults: they begin to lose weight and develop a hypochromic anaemia; irritability and convulsions may also occur. Liver, yeast, and cereals are relatively rich sources of it. Fish is a moderately rich source, but vegetables and milk contain little. The minimal daily requirement in the diet is probably about 2 mg.

PYRIMETHAMINE is an antimalarial drug which is particularly valuable as a prophylactic.

PYRO- is a prefix meaning anything connected with fire or produced by heating.

PYROGALLIC ACID is a substance derived from gallic acid and used in the treatment of psoriasis. It has the disadvantage of staining the skin a deep brown colour.

PYROSIS, or WATERBRASH, is a symptom of dyspepsia consisting of an irritable, burning pain in the throat, accompanied by the constant secretion of mouthfuls of saliva. (See DYSPEPSIA.)

PYURIA means the presence of pus in the urine, in consequence of inflammation situated in the kidney, bladder, or other part of the urinary tract. (See URINE.)

Q

Q FEVER is a disease of worldwide distribution due to the organism *Coxiella burneti*. It is characterized by fever, severe headache and often pneumonia. It was first described in 1937 amongst abattoir workers in Brisbane. The disease was given the name "Q" fever, the Q (?) referring to the unknown cause of the disease. The aetiology of the infection was later established by Burnet who cultured a micro-organism from the blood of an infected patient. This rickettsia-like organism was originally called *Rickettsia burneti* but was later renamed *Coxiella burneti* when Cox found that it had certain features which differentiated it from the true rickettsia.

The principal reservoir of human infection in Britain is probably cattle and sheep in which the infection is usually sub-clinical. The diagnosis is confirmed by the detection of serum antibodies to *Coxiella burneti*. The organism is sensitive to tetracycline.

QUADRICEPS is the large four-headed muscle occupying the front and sides of the thigh, which straightens the leg at the knee-joint and maintains the body in an upright position.

QUADRIPLEGIA means paralysis of the four limbs of the body.

QUADRUPLETS (see MULTIPLE BIRTHS).

QUARANTINE is the principle of preventing the spread of infectious disease by which people, baggage, merchandise, and so forth likely to be infected or coming from an infected locality are isolated at frontiers or ports till their harmlessness has been proved to the satisfaction of the authorities. (See INFECTION.)

Originally quarantine, as its name implies, involved detention for forty days; but, as this proved intolerable for people engaged in business, the time of detention is now calculated so as simply to cover the incubation period of the disease, the presence of which is suspected.

Numerous international conferences upon the subject have been held with the view of arriving at a uniform practice as regards quarantine in different countries. The diseases to which quarantine applies are cholera, yellow fever, plague, smallpox, typhus and relapsing fever.

The general practice with regard to quarantine is that when a serious disease breaks out in any country, the government of that country notifies surrounding governments as to the ports and other places that have become centres of infection. Any people travelling from these centres and attempting to enter another

Disease	*Patients*	*Contacts*
Chickenpox	6 days from the date of the appearance of the rash.	None.
Diphtheria	Until 3 consecutive throat and nose swabs are negative.	Until nose and throat swabs are bacteriologically clear.
German measles	5 days from the appearance of the rash.	None.
Measles	7 days after the appearance of the rash if the child appears well.	Infants who have not had the disease should be excluded for 14 days from the date of appearance of the rash in the last case in the house. Other contacts can attend school. Any contact suffering from a cold, chill or red eyes should be immediately excluded.
Mumps	9 days from the onset of the disease or 7 days from the subsidence of all swelling.	None.
Smallpox	Until the patient is pronounced free from infection.	21 days, unless recently vaccinated, when exclusion is unnecessary.
Whooping-cough	21 days from the beginning of the characteristic cough.	Infants who have not had the disease should be excluded for 21 days from the date of onset of the disease in the last case in the house.

Quarantine periods for the commoner infectious diseases.

country, are subject to measures prescribed in the appropriate Regulations. These measures vary with the disease involved; as often as not, today they merely involve keeping under the surveillance of the local medical officer through the incubation period of the disease in question.

QUASSIA is the wood of *Picrasma excelsa*, a large West Indian tree. Its virtues depend upon the presence of an active principle, quassin, which is excessively bitter and also irritating. The various preparations of the wood are mainly used as a bitter tonic. Quassia cups were for long to be found in many households. Made of quassia wood, they were filled with hot water. This resulted in a bitter water which was drunk as a 'bitter' to stimulate the appetite. These quassia cups could be used over and over again for several years, retaining their ability to produce a bitter extract. (See BITTERS.)

QUICKENING (see PREGNANCY).

QUILLAIA is the bark of *Quillaja saponaria*, or soapbark, a South American tree. Tincture of quillaia is used in cases of bronchitis, and for making emulsions, in doses of 4 millilitres.

QUINESTRADOL (PENTOVIS) (see OESTROGENS).

QUINESTROL (ESTROVIS) is a synthetic, long-acting oestrogen (qv). (See OESTROGENS.)

QUINIDINE is an alkaloid obtained from cinchona bark and closely related in chemical composition and in action to quinine. It is commonly used in the form of quinidine sulphate in doses of 200 to 600 mg. It is used in the treatment of the cardiac irregularity known as atrial fibrillation, being particularly useful in cases of recent onset.

QUININE is an alkaloid obtained from the bark of various species of cinchona trees. This bark is mainly derived from Peru and neighbouring parts of South America and the East Indies. For the story of its introduction see MALARIA. Other alkaloids and acid substances are also derived from cinchona bark, such as quinidine and cinchonine.

Quinine is generally used in the form of one of its salts, such as the sulphate of quinine, or dihydrochloride of quinine. All are sparingly soluble in water, much more so when taken along with an acid.

Action: Quinine lessens the activity of simple forms of life. It is therefore a powerful antiseptic. Its best-known action is in checking the recurrence of attacks of malaria, and this action it exerts by virtue of its destructive power against the malarial parasite in the blood. In fevers it acts as an antipyretic (qv).

In small doses it has a stimulating effect upon the stomach, although larger doses are capable of acting upon an irritable stomach to produce nausea and vomiting. Small doses have also a stimulating action upon the nervous system and a general tonic effect, whilst large doses cause decided depression of the respiration and the heart's action.

Among the other unpleasant effects, due to large doses, are ringing in the ears, temporary impairment of vision, and sometimes irritation of the kidneys: all these pass off when the drug is discontinued.

Uses: The most important use of quinine is its original one in malaria, attacks of which it quickly cuts short or prevents altogether, but it has largely been replaced by the more effective and less toxic anti-malarial drugs now available. (See MALARIA.) For intravenous injection, when this is necessary in cases of malaria, a soluble form of quinine, the dihydrochloride, is used in doses of 300 to 600 mg. Ammoniated solution of quinine given in teaspoonful doses in water is a favourite household remedy in feverish colds and other mild febrile attacks. Quinine and urea hydrochloride is employed as a local anaesthetic with a prolonged effect. Quinine hydrochloride has been used with urethane as a sclerosing agent in the treatment of varicose veins (qv).

QUINSY is a corruption of *cynanche*, and is an old name for a peritonsillar abscess (qv).

QUINTUPLETS (see MULTIPLE BIRTHS).

R

RABIES is an acute and fatal disease which affects animals, particularly carnivora, and may be communicated from them to man. Infection from man to man is very rare, but those in attendance on a case should take precautions to avoid being bitten or allowing themselves to be contaminated by the patient's saliva as this contains the causative virus.

Cause: The disease is in existence constantly among dogs and wolves in some countries, and from these it spreads widely now and then in epidemics. It also occurs in foxes, coyotes and skunks, as well as vampire bats. Thanks to quarantine measures, it has been practically stamped out in Great Britain since 1897. The last case of human infection contracted in Britain was in 1911. Since 1946, thirteen cases have been diagnosed in Britain, in all of which the infection was acquired overseas. There was one fatal case in England in 1981 in a woman who had been bitten in the hand by a rabid dog in India, a country in which dogs run wild and constitute a major public health rabies problem. Recent cases of rabies in dogs in this country demonstrate that continuing, indeed increasing, vigilance is necessary if the United

Kingdom is to be protected from the ravages of this dread disease. Particularly is such vigilance necessary in view of the way that the disease in animals is now spreading across Europe. Thus in France and West Germany 7,750 cases of rabies in animals were reported in 1975. In 1981 there were 19,549 cases of animal rabies in Europe, over 70 per cent of which were in the red fox. In Europe, in 1981 there were two cases of human rabies: one was a hunter bitten by his dog in East Germany; the other was the English woman referred to above. The global total of deaths is around 15,000 a year, mainly in India. In the whole of Western Europe, only Denmark and Britain are now free of rabies. The most worrying feature from the British point of view is that the current European epidemic of animal rabies, which started in Poland in 1939, is advancing at an annual rate of 30–60 kilometres and has now reached a point in France less than 40 kilometres from the English Channel coast line. Restrictions have accordingly been tightened up and under The Rabies Act 1974, which came into force in February 1975, all mammals, except farm livestock, brought into the country must come through designated ports (Dover [Eastern Docks], Harwich [Navy Yard Wharf], Hull, Liverpool, Southampton, and International Hoverport at Ramsgate) and airports (Birmingham, Edinburgh, Glasgow, Leeds, London [Gatwick and Heathrow], Manchester and Prestwick), have an import licence and undergo a compulsory six months' quarantine. Any animals brought in illegally may be destroyed on the spot, and the offender fined an unlimited amount, sentenced up to a year's imprisonment, or both. It also empowers the Government, in the event of the disease being confirmed in Britain again, to destroy foxes, control movement of domestic pets, ban hunts and dog and cat shows, and destroy stray animals.

It is highly infectious from the bite of an animal already affected, but the chance of infection from different animals varies. Thus only about one person in every four bitten by rabid dogs contracts rabies, whilst the bites of rabid wolves and cats almost invariably produce the disease. Bites on exposed parts, like the face, are more dangerous than those through the clothes. The disease is due to a virus which has a special affinity for attacking the nervous system. The test as to whether a dog, which has died, suffered from rabies, is to inject a preparation made from part of its brain into another animal, and to watch the latter for signs of the disease. In the brain of an affected animal, certain microscopic appearances known as *Negri bodies* can usually be found. The saliva of infected animals is highly infectious.

Symptoms: In animals there are two types of the disease: mad rabies and dumb rabies. In the former, the dog runs about, snapping at objects and other animals, unable to rest; in the latter, which is also the final stage of the mad type, the limbs become paralysed, and the dog crawls about or lies still.

In man the incubation period is usually six to eight weeks, but may be as short as ten days or as long as two years. The disease begins by mental symptoms, the person becoming irritable, restless, and melancholy. At the same time, feverishness and difficulty of swallowing gradually come on. After a couple of days or so, the irritability passes into a state of wildness or terror, and there is great difficulty in swallowing either food or drink. Even the mere sight of fluid may induce spasm of the muscles of the mouth and throat: hence the common name for the disease: hydrophobia (fear of water). Breathing, too, becomes difficult, because of spasm of the respiratory muscles. The flow of saliva is great, and therefore the patient is constantly spitting, and has a dry, short cough, which has given rise to the popular idea that he barks like a dog. A loud noise, a bright light, and particularly any attempt to drink are sufficient to throw the person into a convulsion. Convulsions and attacks of maniacal excitement become more frequent, and although between these the patient may be quite sensible and able to talk rationally, he becomes gradually weaker. Finally, about four days after the onset of the disease, the patient dies of exhaustion.

Treatment: The best treatment is, of course, preventive, and this may be attained by strict quarantine regulations and the slaughter of all animals bitten by, or coming into contact with, rabid dogs. The current regulations in the United Kingdom are a quarantine period of six months, and that the animal be given a dose of an inactivated rabies vaccine on entry into quarantine and another dose 28 days later. If a person has been bitten by a dog supposed to be rabid, the dog should not be killed at once, but should be carefully isolated for ten days; if, after this period it is still alive, it was non-infective at the time of biting.

Local treatment consists of immediate, thorough, and careful cleansing of the wound surfaces and surrounding skin with 20 per cent soap solution or any other detergent followed by flushing out with some antiseptic such as benzalkonium or cetrimide. Special attention should be paid to any deep fang punctures, which should be carefully probed with a swab-stick dipped in strong nitric acid. Immediate suture of lacerations should not be carried out.

This is followed by a course of rabies vaccine therapy. Only people bitten or in certain circumstances licked, either by a rabid animal or by one thought to be infected with rabies need treatment with rabies vaccine and antiserum and immunoglobulin (qv). This consists of injecting rabies antiserum or human antirabies immunoglobulin into the depth of the wound and also intramuscularly. The usual course of vaccine is six injections given intramuscularly on days 0, 3, 7, 14, 30, and 90. A person previously vaccinated against rabies who is subsequently bitten by a rabid animal should be given three to four doses of the vaccine. The vaccine is also used to give protection to those liable to infection, such as kennel workers and veterinary surgeons: two intramuscular injections four weeks apart, followed by a third a year later.

When the bitten person develops the disease, all that can be done is to quieten the convulsion by intravenous injections of a tranquilliser, and to keep him as comfortable as possible by good nursing.

RADIATION SICKNESS is the term applied to the nausea, vomiting, and loss of appetite which may follow the use of radiotherapy in the treatment of cancer and other diseases. The phenothiazine group of tranquillizers, such as chlorpromazine (qv), as well as the antihistamine drugs (qv), are of value in its prevention and treatment. Radiotherapy may also be accompanied by irritation and itching of the skin. To prevent this, or at least to reduce its incidence, the skin should be protected from all unnecessary irritation by avoiding, for example, tight collars, hot baths, brisk towelling, wet shaving and cosmetics. Should itching occur, this may be relieved by a weak solution of sodium bicarbonate (1 teaspoonful in a cup of warm water) applied to the skin and dabbed dry with cotton-wool. The application of a bland dusting powder, such as a baby powder, also helps.

RADIOACTIVE ISOTOPES (see ISOTOPES).

RADIOGRAPHY (see X-RAYS).

RADIO-IMMUNO ASSAY is a technique introduced in 1960 which enables the minute quantities of circulating hormones to be measured. A radio-immuno assay depends on the ability of an unlabelled hormone to inhibit, by simple competition, the binding of isotopically labelled hormone by specific antibodies. The requirements for a radio-immuno assay include adequate amounts of the hormone; a method for labelling the hormone with a radio active isotope; the production of satisfactory antibodies; and a technique for separating antibody-bound from free hormone. Radio-immuno assay is more sensitive than the best bio-assay for a given hormone and most sensitive radio-immuno assays permit the detection of picogram (pg = 10^{-12}g) and femtogram (fg = 10^{-15}g) amounts of material.

RADIONUCLIDE is another word for a radioactive isotope. (See ISOTOPES.)

RADIOTHERAPY is treatment by radium or other radioactive matter, including X-rays. For long, radium and X-rays were the only sources available. Developments in our knowledge of atomic energy, however, have changed the picture entirely, and we have now at our disposal radioactive isotopes (see ISOTOPES) and X-ray machines which have largely replaced radium, except in the case of certain tumours.

Supervoltage X-ray machines are now available capable of producing X-rays generated at up to 22 million electron volts (22 MeV). These include linear accelerators which produce X-rays at four or more million electron volts, and betatrons which produce X-rays at 22 million electron volts. The advantage of these supervoltage machines is that it is predominantly gamma-rays they produce, which are penetrating rays and can therefore be used to treat deep-seated tumours.

Almost equally high concentrations of gamma-rays can now be obtained from the use of certain radioactive isotopes, particularly cobalt and caesium. Thus a telecobalt machine is now in use which contains 2000 curies or more of radioactive cobalt (Co), an amount equivalent to 3000 grams of radium (an unheard-of amount in the pre-1939 days when the ordinary radium beam units contained only 10 grams of radium). Not only does this machine give a high concentration of gamma-rays (equivalent to that from a 3 million-volt X-ray machine), it is absolutely safe for both patient and operators, and allows the beam to be directed accurately on the tumour.

Other forms of radiant energy are now coming into use in radiotherapy. One of these is electron-beam therapy. The usual source of electrons, one of the particles in the atomic nucleus, is the betatron, which can produce either electrons or X-rays at energies ranging from 18 to 42 MeV. Whilst the effect of electrons in the tissues of the body is the same as that of X-rays, their great practical advantage is that their effect can be concentrated on the part being treated, without any adverse effect on the surrounding normal tissue. The other form of radiant energy now being used is neutron therapy. Neutrons of 6 MeV energy are obtained from a cyclotron. One of the advantages of neutron therapy is that even if a cell is only partially damaged by neutrons it never recovers, but inevitably dies.

RADIUM: The radiations of radium consist of: (1) alpha-rays, which are positively charged helium nuclei; (2) beta-rays, negatively charged electrons; (3) gamma-rays, similar to X-rays but of shorter wave-length.

At the present day the use of radium is largely restricted to the treatment of carcinoma of the neck of the womb, the tongue, and the lips.

Neither X-rays nor radium supersede active surgical measures when these are available for the complete removal of a tumour.

RADIUS is the outer of the two bones in the forearm. (See BONE.)

RAG-SORTERS' DISEASE is another name for anthrax. (See ANTHRAX.)

RANITIDINE is a drug that is proving of value in the treatment of duodenal ulcer (qv) by reducing the hyperacidity of the gastric juice. It is a histamine antagonist to the type-2 receptor.

RANULA is a swelling which occasionally appears beneath the tongue, caused by a collection of saliva in the distended duct of a salivary gland. (See MOUTH, DISEASES OF.)

RAPHE means a ridge or furrow between the halves of an organ.

RAREFACTION is the term applied to the diminution in the density of a bone as a result of withdrawal of calcium salts from it.

RASH (see ERUPTION).

RAT-BITE FEVER is an infectious disease following the bite of a rat. There are two causative organisms – *Spirillum minus* and *Actinobacillus muris* – and the incubation period depends upon which is involved. In the case of the former it is 5 to 30 days; in the case of the latter it is 2 to 10 days. The disease is characterized by fever, a characteristic skin rash and often muscular or joint pains. It responds well to penicillin.

RAUWOLFIA is a drug used in the treatment of high blood-pressure, and as a tranquillizer. It is derived from the root of *Rauwolfia serpentina*, a plant which grows widely in India, Ceylon, Burma, and Malaya. The active medicinal properties, which reside mainly in the root of the plant, have been recognized for centuries in India, where extracts of the root were used for the treatment of fevers, insomnia, and nervousness.

It is mainly used in the form of reserpine, which is an alkaloid obtained from the root of the plant. (See ESSENTIAL HYPERTENSION; TRANQUILLIZERS.)

RAY-FUNGUS is the organism that causes woody tongue. (See ACTINOMYCOSIS.)

RAYNAUD'S DISEASE, so called after Maurice Raynaud (1834–81), the Paris physician who published a thesis on the subject in 1862, is a condition in which the circulation becomes suddenly obstructed in outlying parts of the body. It is supposed to be due to spasm of the smaller arteries in the affected part, as the result of nervous influences, and its effects are increased both by cold and by various diseases involving the blood-vessels. It is predominantly a disease of women, the majority of cases occurring before the age of 40.

Symptoms: The condition is most commonly confined to the occurrence of dead fingers, the fingers or the toes, ears, or nose becoming white, numb, and waxy looking. This condition may last for some minutes, or may not pass off for several hours, or even for a day or two.

Treatment: People who are subject to these attacks should be careful in winter to protect the feet and hands from cold, and should always use warm water when washing the hands. In addition, the whole body should be kept warm, as spasm of the arterioles in the feet and hands may be induced by chilling of the body. Victims of this disease should be advised to give up smoking. Vasodilator drugs are helpful, especially the calcium antagonists (qv). In all cases which do not respond to such medical treatment, surgery should be considered in the form of sympathectomy: ie. cutting of the sympathetic nerves to the affected part. This results in dilatation of the arterioles and hence an improved blood supply. This operation is more successful in the case of the feet than in the case of the hands.

RAYON, OILED, consists of rayon fabric made waterproof with drying oils or oil-modified synthetic resins.

REACTIVE ARTHRITIS is an aseptic arthritis secondary to an episode of infection elsewhere in the body. It often occurs in association with enteritis caused by Salmonella and certain Shigella strains and in both yersinea and campylobacter enteritis. Non-gonococcal urethritis, usually due to clamydia, is another cause of reactive arthritis and Reiter's syndrome is a particularly florid form with mucocutaneous and ocular lesions. The synovitis usually starts acutely and is frequently asymmetrical with the knees and ankles most commonly affected. Often there are inflammatory lesions of tendon sheaths and entheses such as plantar faschitis. The severity and duration of the acute episode are extremely variable. Individuals with the histocompactibility antigen HLA-B27 are particularly prone to severe attacks.

RECTUM is the last part of the large intestine. It pursues a more or less straight course downwards through the cavity of the pelvis, lying against the sacrum at the back of this cavity. This section of the intestine is about 23 cm (9 inches) long. Its first part is freely movable and corresponds to the upper three pieces of the sacrum, the second part corresponds to the lower two pieces of the sacrum and the coccyx, whilst the third part, known also as the anal canal, is about 25 mm (1 inch) long, runs downwards and backwards, and is kept tightly closed by the internal and external sphincter muscles which surround it. The opening to the exterior is known as the anus. The structure of the rectum is similar to that of the rest of the intestine. (See INTESTINE.)

RECTUM, DISEASES OF: Owing to the fact that this part of the intestine is more exposed to external influences than the rest of the bowels, and that it forms the place of lodgment of the stools prior to the evacuation of the bowels, and is therefore often subject to considerable irritation, the rectum is specially liable to various diseases.

Peculiarities of the motions are treated under STOOLS, while PILES and FISTULA are described under these headings. DIARRHOEA and CONSTIPATION are also treated separately.

IMPERFORATE ANUS, or absence of the anus, may occur in newly born children, and, unless the condition is relieved by operation within a few days, the child dies.

ITCHING at the anal opening, or PRURITUS ANI, is often very troublesome. It may be due to slight abrasions, piles, the presence of threadworms, and anal sex. All stimulants, mustard and pepper must be avoided in the diet. After evacuation of the bowels, the part should be bathed with cotton-wool and warm or cold water; it is sometimes an advantage to add starch to the water. Toilet paper should not be used. In addition, the area should be bathed once or twice a day. Clothing should be loose and smooth – preferably cotton or linen next to the skin. Calamine lotion, containing 1 per cent phenol, or 0·1 to 0·5 per cent camphor, is soothing – applied as a compress on gauze at night and dabbed on during the day. The local application of Eurax or hydrocortisone ointment is often effective.

PAIN of an acute cutting character, at stool, is often due to the presence of a small ulcer or 'fissure', which, owing to movements of the sphincter, will not heal; it is treated by rubbing the ulcer with a caustic point or injecting into it a local anaesthetic of prolonged action. The pain soon disappears. Pain of an aching nature is not uncommonly caused by the presence of piles. (See also PROCTALGIA.)

ULCERATION may occur here in the course of tuberculous disease of the bowels, in dysentery, or even as the result of the constant irritation due to long-continued constipation. Ulcers in this locality cause a discharge of matter and often streaks of blood mixed with the motions. If the ulcer lasts a long time it may lead to narrowing and obstruction of the bowel.

ABSCESS in the cellular tissue at the side of the rectum, known from its position as an ischiorectal abscess, is fairly common. It may arise, like an abscess elsewhere, as the result of injury, exposure to cold, and other debilitating influences. In any case it is likely to produce a fistula. (See FISTULA.)

PROCTITIS, or inflammation of the rectum, due to sexually transmitted diseases has been on the increase in recent years. Thus, in 1977, homosexually acquired infection accounted for 28·7 per cent of the cases of gonorrhoea in the West End of London, where more than three-quarters of the cases of syphilis were acquired in this way.

PROLAPSE or protrusion of the rectum is sometimes found in children, usually between the ages of 6 months and 2 years. In slight cases, where a ring of bright red mucous membrane 12 or 25 mm (½ or 1 inch) in width protrudes as the result of straining at stool, the condition is generally easily curable. Any irritable condition of the bowels due to diarrhoea, constipation or worms, must be removed and the evacuations regulated by diet and laxatives, so as to avoid all straining. Each time the bowels move, the protruded portion must be returned by steady pressure with a cloth or sponge wrung out of cold water. If the bowel comes down when the child runs about, the wearing of a suitable pad is necessary, or the buttocks are strapped together and the child must lie down for some time each day. When the protruded part is very large and the condition does not yield to simple treatment it can be remedied by operation but this is not usually necessary, as the prolapse ceases to occur as the child grows older.

TUMOURS of small size situated on the skin near the opening of the bowel, and consisting of nodules, tags of skin, or cauliflower-like excrescences, are common, and may give rise to pain, itching, and watery discharges. These are easily removed if necessary. Polypi occasionally develop within the rectum, and may give rise to no pain, though they may cause frequent discharges of blood. Like polypi elsewhere, they may often be removed by a minor operation. (See POLYPOSIS.)

CANCER of the rectum is fairly common. In 1984, in England there were 5493 deaths from cancer of the rectum. It is a disease of later life, seldom affecting young people, and its appearance is generally insidious. The tumour begins commonly in the mucous membrane, its structure resembling that of the glands with which the membrane is furnished, and it quickly infiltrates the other coats of the intestine and then invades neighbouring organs. Secondary growths in most cases occur soon in the lymphatic glands within the abdomen and in the liver. The symptoms appear gradually and consist of diarrhoea, alternating with attacks of constipation, and, later on, discharges of blood or of thin blood-stained fluid from the bowels, together with increasing loss of weight and weakness, and pains about the lower part of the back and down the thighs. Upon examination, the tumour can be felt projecting from one side or in a ring-form into the interior of the bowel. These cases are usually far advanced before they give rise to much disturbance, but a lot can now be done to help them by surgical operation. In the majority of cases this consists of removal of the whole of the rectum and the distal two-thirds of the sigmoid colon, and the establishment of a colostomy (qv). Approximately 50 per cent of the patients who have this operation are alive and well after five years. In some cases in which the growth occurs in the upper part of the rectum it is now possible to remove the growth and preserve the anus so that the patient is saved the discomfort of having a colostomy.

RECURRENT LARYNGEAL NERVE is a branch of the vagus nerve which leaves the latter low down in its course, and, hooking round the right subclavian artery on the right side and round the arch of the aorta on the left, runs up again into the neck, where it enters the larynx and supplies branches to the muscles which control the vocal cords. The importance of this nerve is the fact that it is apt in its long course either to be injured by surgical procedures to the neck, by trauma to the neck, or to be pressed upon by enlarged lymph glands in the neck, by aneurysms of the aorta or right subclavian artery, resulting in defects of vocalization. These defects may therefore arise within the larynx itself or may arise from disease in the chest, which affects the left recurrent laryngeal nerve. If both recurrent laryngeal nerves are involved in the disease process or are injured, the vocal cords come to lie in the midline, causing embarrassment of the airway and this may necessitate some form of airway intervention, usually in the form of a tracheostomy.

RED LOTION is a lotion containing sulphate of zinc, compound tincture of lavender which gives it a red colour, and water. It is used as an astringent application to ulcers.

REDUX is a term applied to the reappearance of certain signs or symptoms which are absent at the height of a disease, and the reappearance of which indicates that the disease is passing off. Such are redux crepitations at the end of pneumonia.

REFLEX ACTION is one of the simplest forms of activity of the nervous system. (For the mechanism upon which it depends, see NERVES.) Reflex acts are divided usually into three classes. *Superficial reflexes* comprise the sudden movements which result when the skin is brushed or pricked, such as the movement of the toes that results from stroking the sole of the foot. *Deep reflexes* depend upon the state of mild contraction in which muscles are constantly maintained when at rest, and are obtained, as in the case of the knee-jerks, by sharply tapping the tendon of the muscle in question. *Visceral reflexes* are those connected with various organs, such as the narrowing of the pupil when a bright light is directed upon the eye, and the contraction of the bladder when distended by urine.

Faults in these reflexes, both in the direction of excess and of diminution, give valuable evidence as to the presence of nervous diseases and the part of the nervous system in which such disease is situated. Thus, absence of the knee-jerk, when the patellar tendon is tapped, means some interference with the sensory nerve, nerve-cells, or motor nerve upon which the act depends, as, for example, in poliomyelitis, or peripheral neuritis; whilst an excessive jerk implies that the controlling influence exerted by the brain upon this reflex mechanism has been cut off, as, for example, by a tumour high up in the spinal cord, or in the disease known as multiple sclerosis (qv).

The condition of the plantar reflex (obtained by stroking the skin of the sole of the foot) is an important point in diagnosing organic disease of the nervous system. The normal reflex consists in bending downwards of the toes towards the sole. In organic disease of the higher parts of the nervous system the great toe tends to bend upwards with spreading out of the other toes (extensor plantar response).

The reflex of the pupil to light is also of great diagnostic importance. The pupil quickly contracts when light falls upon the eye or when the eyes are directed suddenly to a near object. In certain serious diseases of the nervous system, especially in general paralysis and tabes dorsalis the contraction on looking at a near object remains, while the effect of light is lost (Argyll-Robertson pupil).

REFRACTION: The deviation of rays of light on passing from one transparent medium into another of different density. The refractive surfaces of the eye are the anterior surface of the cornea (which accounts for approximately two-thirds of the focusing or refractive power of the eye) and the lens (one-third of the focusing power of the eye). The refractive power of the lens can change, whereas that of the cornea is fixed. *Errors of refraction* (Ametropia) will occur when the focusing power of the lens and cornea do not match the length of the eye, so that rays of light parallel to the visual axis are not focused at the fovea centralis (see EYE). There are three types of refractive error: (i) *Hypermetropia* or long sightedness: the refractive power of the eye is too weak, or the eye is too short so that rays of light are brought to a focus at a point behind the retina. Long-sighted people can see well in the distance but generally require glasses with convex lenses for reading. Uncorrected long sight can lead to headaches and intermittent blurring of vision following prolonged close work, ie. *eye strain*. As a result of ageing the eye becomes gradually long sighted, resulting in many people's needing reading glasses in later life. This normal process is known as *presbyopia*. A particular form of long sightedness occurs after cataract extraction. (ii) *Myopia* (short sight or near sight): rays of light are brought to a focus in front of the retina because the refractive power of the eye is too great or the eye is too short. Short-sighted people can see close to but need spectacles with concave lenses in order to see in the distance. (iii) *Astigmatism*: the refractive power of the eye is not the same in each meridian. Some rays of light may be focused in front of the retina while others are focused on or behind the retina. Astigmatism can accompany hypermetropia or myopia. It may be corrected by cylindrical lenses (these consist of a slice from the side of a cylinder, ie. curved in one meridian and flat in the meridian at right angles to it).

REFRIGERANTS are substances which relieve thirst and give a feeling of coolness. The chief refrigerants are acidulous drinks such as lemon juice, weak mineral acids, and tartaric acid, in water. The parched condition of the mouth and throat that arises during hard work in a dry and dusty atmosphere is best relieved by water to which has been added some demulcent substance which forms a coating on the dried mucous membrane. Such liquids are obtained by mixing oatmeal or milk with water. (See also CITRIC ACID; IMPERIAL DRINK.)

REFRIGERATION ANAESTHESIA (see CRYMOTHERAPY).

REGIONAL HEALTH AUTHORITY (see NATIONAL HEALTH SERVICE).

REGIONAL ILEITIS (see under ILEITIS).

REGURGITATION is a term used in various connections in medicine. For instance, in diseases of the heart it is used to indicate a condition in which, as the result of valvular disease, the blood does not entirely pass on from the atria of the heart to the ventricles, or from the ventricles into the arteries. The defective valve is said to be incompetent, and a certain amount of blood leaks past it, or regurgitates back, into the cavity from which it has been driven. (See HEART DISEASES.)

The term is also applied to the return to the mouth of food already swallowed and present in the gullet or stomach.

REHABILITATION is the restoration to health and working capacity of a person incapacitated by disease, mental or physical, or by injury. It is a word that came into prominent use during the 1939–45 War, reflecting the growing awareness of the medical profession that the treatment of a sick or injured person does not end at the moment of recovery from the immediate effects of illness or injury. For example, a man with a fractured limb or spine has to recover full use not only of the injured part but of his whole body; and he has to recover confidence in his ability to work and enjoy life. (See DISABLED PERSONS; REMPLOY.)

REITER'S SYNDROME: For some 40 years the concurrence of polyarthritis, non-gonococcal urethritis and ocular inflammation has been called Reiter's Syndrome. The syndrome has over the years been associated with promiscuous sexual contact because urethritis is a common feature. The evidence for this is, however, circumstantial. It is now well recognized that urethritis can occur unrelated to sexual contact as a result of gastro-intestinal infection with yersinia enterocolitica. Possession of the HLA antigen B27 affects the severity of the disease and the prognosis, but the syndrome is not confined to patients with this antigen. (See REACTIVE ARTHRITIS.)

RELAPSE means the return of a disease during the period of convalescence.

RELAPSING FEVER, so-called because of the characteristic temperature chart showing recurring bouts of fever, is an infectious disease caused by spirochaetes. There are two main forms of the disease.

LOUSE-BORNE RELAPSING FEVER is an epidemic disease, usually associated with wars and famines, which has occurred in practically every country in the world. For long confused with typhus and typhoid, it was not until the 1870's that the causal organism was described by Obermeier. It is now known as the *Borrelia recurrentis*, a motile spiral organism 10 to 20 micrometres in length. The organism is transmitted from man to man by the louse, *Pediculus humanus*.

Symptoms: The incubation period is up to 12 days, usually 7 days. The onset is sudden, with high temperature, generalized aches and pains, and nose-bleeding. In about half the cases a rash appears at an early stage, beginning in the neck and spreading down over the trunk and arms. Jaundice may occur; and both the liver and the spleen are enlarged. The temperature subsides after five or six days, to rise again in about a week. There may be up to four such relapses (see the introductory paragraph above).

Treatment: Preventive measures are the same as those for typhus (qv). Rest in bed is essential, as are good nursing and a light, nourishing diet. There is usually a quick response to penicillin. The tetracyclines and chloramphenicol are also effective. Following such treatment the incidence of relapse is about 15 per cent. The mortality rate is low, except in a starved population.

TICK-BORNE RELAPSING FEVER is an endemic disease which occurs in most tropical and sub-tropical countries. The causative organism is *Borrelia duttoni*, which is transmitted by a tick, *Ornithodorus moubata*. David Livingstone suggested that it was a tick-borne disease, but it was not until 1905 that Dutton and Todd produced the definite evidence.

Symptoms: The main differences from the louse-borne disease are: (*a*) the incubation period is usually shorter, 3 to 6 days, but may be as short as 2 days or as long as 12; (*b*) the febrile period is usually shorter and the afebrile periods are more variable in duration, sometimes only lasting for a day or two; (*c*) relapses are much more numerous.

Treatment: Preventive measures are more difficult to carry out than in the case of the louse-borne infection. Protective clothing should always be worn in 'tick country'. Old, heavily infected houses should be destroyed. Curative treatment is the same as for the louse-borne infection.

RELATE NATIONAL MARRIAGE GUIDANCE: The idea of a marriage guidance council came from a group of doctors, clergy and social workers who were concerned for the welfare of marriage. It is based upon two major concepts: that marriage provides the best possible way for a man and woman to live and love together and rear their children, and that the counsellors share a basic respect for the unique personality of the individual and his (or her) right to make his (or her) own decisions. The organization consists of between 120 and 130 Marriage Guidance Councils throughout the country, comprising about 1250 counsellors. These Councils are affiliated to Relate National Marriage Guidance, which is responsible for the selection, training and continued supervision of all counsellors. Anyone seeking help can telephone or write for an appointment. No fees are charged, but those receiving help are encouraged to donate what they can. The address of Relate National Marriage Guidance is Herbert Gray College, Little Church Street, Rugby, Warwickshire CV21 3AP (0788 73241).

REMITTENT FEVER is the term applied to the form of fever in which, during remissions, the temperature falls, but not to normal.

REMPLOY is Britain's largest employer of severely disabled people, set up under the provisions of the 1944 Disabled Persons (Employment) Act.

1985 was Remploy's 40th anniversary year. The company currently has almost 9,000 severely disabled employees in 94 production units in Scotland, England and Wales, manufacturing over 100 different products and services. Sales during the year 1985 were in excess of £65 million. Full details may be obtained from Remploy Ltd, 415 Edgware Road, London NW2 6LR (01-452 8020).

RENAL DISEASES (see KIDNEYS, DISEASES OF).

RENIN is a protein-like substance extracted from the kidney which, when injected into animals, causes a rise of blood-pressure. This it does, apparently, by reacting with a substance normally present in the blood plasma to produce angiotensin. Angiotensin has been obtained in crystalline form, and it is angiotensin which causes the rise in blood-pressure. This work may have an important bearing on the problem of high blood-pressure in man.

RENNET is a substance prepared from the stomach of the calf, in order to curdle and partially digest milk. Its activity depends upon a ferment known as rennin. Rennet is used for the preparation of junket and in the making of cheese.

REPAIR of tissues after injury is described generally under WOUNDS, and the repair of special tissues which present various peculiarities is described under BONE; MUSCLES; NERVES, etc.

RESECTION is the name given to an operation in which a part of some organ is removed, as, for example, the resection of a fragment of dead bone.

RESERPINE is an alkaloid obtained from the root of Rauwolfia (qv), and is used as an antihypertensive and a tranquillizing agent.

RESINS are solid or semi-solid exudations from plants, which are insoluble in water, mostly soluble in alcohol or ether, soften or melt at moderate temperatures, and burn with a smoky flame. They are transparent when pure, but opaque when they contain water. They are non-conductors of electricity. Some of them are acids and combine with alkalis to form soaps. A *natural resin* is one that occurs as an exudation, such as mastic. A *prepared resin* is made from a drug, such as podophyllin, or from a natural oleoresin such as rosin which is obtained from various species of *Pinus*. *Oleoresins* may be either natural oleoresins, which are mixtures of volatile oils and resins generally obtained by incising trunks of trees, such as turpentine and copaiba; or prepared oleoresins which are concentrated liquid preparations made from drugs containing both volatile oil and resin, such as capsicum. *Gum resins* are natural mixtures of gums and resins, usually obtained as exudations from plants, such as myrrh and asafoetida. (See also ION EXCHANGE RESINS.)

RESOLUTION is a term applied to infective processes, to indicate a natural subsidence of the inflammation without the formation of pus. Thus a pneumonic lung is said to resolve when the material exuded into it is absorbed into the blood and lymph, so that recovery takes place naturally; an inflamed area is said to resolve when the inflammation fades away and no abscess forms; a glandular enlargement is said to resolve when it decreases in size without suppuration. Resolvents was an old term applied to procedures capable of assisting this process. (See BLISTERS; INFLAMMATION.)

RESONANCE means the lengthening and intensification of sound produced by striking the body over an air-containing structure. Decrease of resonance is called dullness and increase of resonance is called hyperresonance. The process of striking the chest or other part of the body to discover its degree of resonance is called percussion, and according to the note obtained, an opinion can be formed as to the state of consolidation of air-containing organs, the presence of abnormal cavities, and the dimensions and relations of solid and air-containing organs lying together. (See also AUSCULTATION.)

RESORCIN, or RESORCINOL, is a white, crystalline, antiseptic substance soluble in water, alcohol, and oils. It is mainly used in skin diseases which require a stimulating and antiseptic application.

RESPIRATION is the process in which air passes into and out of the lungs with the object of allowing the blood to absorb oxygen and to give off carbon dioxide and water. This occurs 18 times a minute in a healthy adult at rest, this being known as the respiratory rate. In other words we inspire more than 25,000 times a day and during this time inhale around 16 kg of air.

Mechanism of respiration: For the structure of the respiratory apparatus see AIR PASSAGES; CHEST; LUNGS. The air passes rhythmically into and out of the air passages, and mixes with the air already in the lungs, these two movements being known as inspiration and expiration.

INSPIRATION is due to a muscular effort which enlarges the chest in all three dimensions, so that the lungs have to expand in order to fill up the vacuum that would otherwise be left, and the air accordingly enters these organs by the air passages. There is no direct pull upon the lungs, each of which is simply suspended within the corresponding pleural cavity by its root, and made to fill this cavity in all conditions of the chest by the pressure of the outer air exerted through the nose, mouth, and air passages. The increase of the chest in size from above downwards is mainly due to the diaphragm, the muscular fibres of which, by their contraction, reduce its domed shape and cause it to descend, pushing down the abdominal organs beneath it. The increase from before back is mainly due to a tilting forwards of the lower end of the breast-bone, and of the lower rib cartilages. The increase from side to side can best be understood by examining a skeleton, noting the very oblique position of the lower ribs, and observing how greatly the capacity of the chest is increased when each is raised, in the manner of a bucket-handle, taking its fixed points at the spine and breast-bone. (See RIBS.)

The muscles which chiefly bring about these changes in ordinary quiet inspiration are the diaphragm, intercostal muscles, and levators of the ribs, whilst in forced or extraordinary inspiration, when a specially deep breath is taken, the sternocleidomastoid, serratus magnus, trapezius, and pectoral muscles are also brought powerfully into play. Many other muscles take part to a slight extent, steadying the spine and the upper and lower ribs, while even the muscles of the face and of the larynx are thrown rhythmically into activity, dilating the nostrils and the entrance to the larynx at each breath.

EXPIRATION is in ordinary circumstances simply an elastic recoil, the diaphragm rising and the ribs sinking into the position that they naturally occupy, when muscular contraction is finished. Expiration occupies a slightly longer period than inspiration. In forced expiration many powerful muscles of the abdomen and thorax are brought into play, and the act may be made a very forcible one, as, for example, in coughing.

Nervous control: Respiration is usually either an automatic or a reflex act, each expiration sending up afferent, sensory impulses to the central nervous system, from which efferent impulses are sent down various other nerves to the muscles that produce inspiration. It appears that there are several centres which govern the rate and force of the breathing, although all are presided over by a chief respiratory centre in the medulla oblongata, which is sometimes spoken of as the vital knot (*noeudvital*). Although this centre appears to be absolutely essential to life, it in turn is under the control of the higher centres in the cerebral hemispheres, through which the will acts, so that breathing can be voluntarily stopped, quickened, or otherwise changed at will. It would be impossible, however, to cause death by voluntarily holding the breath, because, as the blood becomes more venous, the vital centre in the medulla again assumes control and breathing starts again. Apart from changes due to will-power, the respirations follow one another rhythmically at the rate of about 18 per minute, being in general one for every four heart-beats.

Quantity of air: The lungs do not by any means completely empty themselves at each expiration and refill at each inspiration. An amount equivalent, in quiet respiration, to less than one-tenth of the total air in the lungs passes out and is replaced by the same quantity of fresh air, which mixes with the stale air in the lungs. This renewal, which in quiet breathing amounts to about 500 millilitres, is known as the *tidal air*. By a special inspiratory effort, one can, however, draw in about 3000 millilitres, this amount being known as *complemental air*. By a special expiratory effort, too, after an ordinary breath one can expel much more than the tidal air from the lungs, this extra amount being known as the *supplemental* or *reserve air*, and amounting to about 1300 millilitres. If one takes as deep an inspiration as possible and then makes a forced expiration, one breathes out the sum of these three, which is known as the *vitalcapacity*, and amounts to about 4000 millilitres in a healthy adult male of average size. These figures all apply to a man of average height. Figures for women are about 25 per cent lower. The vital capacity varies with size, sex, age and ethnic origin. The following formulae, incorporating age, height and sex, give an approximate guide to the vital capacity:

Men:
vital capacity (*in millilitres*)
= [27·63—(0·112 × age)] × height
(*in centimetres*)

Women:
vital capacity (*in millilitres*)
= [21·78—(0·101 × age)] × height
(*in centimetres*)

Over and above the vital capacity, the lungs contain air which cannot be expelled by the strongest possible expiration. This *residual air*, as it is known, which remains in the lungs even after death, amounts to another 1500 millilitres.

Tests of respiratory efficiency are being increasingly used to assess lung function in health and disease. The most widely used one is based on an analysis of a single forced expiration after a maximal inspiration. The volume expelled in the first second of expiration (known as FEV_1) correlates well with the respiratory efficiency. Normal values for FEV_1 vary with age, sex and, to a lesser extent, with the size of the body but, by and large, healthy persons can breathe out 15 per cent or more of vital capacity within the first second.

Abnormal forms of respiration: Apart from mere changes in rate and force, respiration is modified in several important ways, either involuntarily or voluntarily. *Sighing* is a long-drawn inspiration following a pause when breathing has been checked by mental preoccupation. This form of breathing also characterizes some conditions of extreme weakness of the nervous system, such as shock and diabetic coma. *Sobbing* is a series of convulsive inspirations, at each of which the larynx is partially closed; it follows grief or great exertion. *Snoring* (qv), or stertorous breathing, is due to a flaccid state of the soft palate causing it to vibrate as the air passes into the throat, or simply to sleeping with the mouth open, which has a similar effect. *Coughing* (qv) is a series of violent expirations, at each of which the larynx is suddenly opened after the pressure of air in the lungs has risen considerably; its object is to expel some irritating substance from the air passages. *Sneezing* (qv) is a single sudden expiration, which differs from coughing in that the sudden rush of air is directed by the soft palate up into the nose in order to expel some source of irritation from this narrow passage. *Cheyne-Stokes' breathing* (qv) is a type of breathing found in persons suffering from apoplexy, heart disease, and some other conditions, in which death is impending; it consists in an alternate dying away and gradual strengthening of the inspirations. Other disorders of breathing are found in LARYNGISMUS STRIDULUS and in ASTHMA (qv).

RESPIRATORY DISTRESS SYNDROME may occur in adults or new-born children. When it occurs in the latter it is known as hyaline membrane disease (qv). The adult respiratory distress syndrome consists of pulmonary oedema of non-cardiac origin. It is a complication of shock, systemic sepsis and viral respiratory infections. It was first described in 1967 and despite advances with assisted ventilation it remains a serious disease with a mortality of more than 50 per cent. The maintenance of adequate circulating blood volume, peripheral perfusion, acid base balance and arterial oxygenation is important and assisted ventilation should be instituted early. The aetiology is not understood though the process begins when tissue damage stimulates the autonomic nervous system, releases vaso-active substances, precipitates complement activation and produces abnormalities of the clotting cascade. The activation of complement causes white cells to lodge in the pulmonary capillaries where they release substances which damage the pulmonary endothelium.

RESPIRATORY SYNCYTIAL VIRUS, or RS VIRUS as it is usually known, is one of the myxoviruses (qv). It is the major cause of bronchiolitis and pneumonia in infants under the age of 6 months.

RESUSCITATION (see DROWNING, RECOVERY FROM).

RETCHING is an ineffectual form of vomiting. (See VOMITING.)

RETENTION OF URINE (see URINE, RETENTION OF).

RETICULOCYTES are newly formed red blood corpuscles, in which a fine network can be demonstrated by special staining methods.

RETICULO-ENDOTHELIAL SYSTEM consists of highly specialized cells scattered throughout the body, but found mainly in the spleen, bone marrow, liver, and lymph glands. Their main function is the ingestion of red blood cells and the conversion of haemoglobin to bilirubin. They are also able to ingest bacteria and foreign colloidal particles.

RETICULOSES is the term used to describe a group of conditions characterized by progressive widespread proliferation of the cells of the reticulo-endothelial system. The two most important members of this group are Hodgkin's disease (qv) and lymphosarcoma (qv).

RETINA (see EYE).

RETINA (DISORDERS OF): The retina can be damaged by disease that affects the retina alone, or by diseases affecting the whole body. *Retinopathy* is a term used to denote an abnormality of the retina without specifying a cause. Some retinal disorders are discussed below.

DIABETIC RETINOPATHY: Retinal disease occurring in patients with diabetes mellitus. It is the commonest cause of blind registration in Great Britain of people between 20 and 65 years of age. Diabetic retinopathy can be divided into several types. The two main causes of blindness are those that follow, first, development of new blood vessels from the retina, with resultant complications and, second, those following 'water logging' (oedema) of the macula. Treatment is by maintaining rigid control of blood-sugar levels combined with laser treatment for certain forms of the disease – in particular to get rid of new blood vessels.

HYPERTENSIVE RETINOPATHY: Retinal disease secondary to the development of high blood pressure. Treatment involves control of the blood pressure.

SICKLE CELL RETINOPATHY: People with sickle cell disease can develop a number of retinal problems including new blood vessels from the retina.
RETROLENTAL FIBROPLASIA: A disorder affecting low-birth-weight premature babies exposed to high oxygen pressures. Essentially new blood vessels develop which cause extensive traction on the retina with resultant retinal detachment and poor vision.
RETINAL ARTERY OCCLUSION, RETINAL VEIN OCCLUSION: These result in damage to those areas of retina supplied by the affected blood vessel. The blood vessels become blocked. If the peripheral retina is damaged the patient may be completely symptom free, although areas of blindness may be detected on examination of field of vision. If the macula is involved, visual loss may be sudden, profound and permanent. There is no effective treatment once visual loss has occurred.
SENILE MACULAR DEGENERATION ('senile' indicates age of onset and has no bearing on mental state) is the leading cause of blindness in the elderly in the western world. The average age of onset is 65 years. Patients initially notice a disturbance of their vision which gradually progresses over months or years. They lose the ability to recognize fine detail, eg. they cannot read fine print, cannot sew or recognize people's faces. They always retain the ability to recognize large objects such as doors and chairs. They are therefore able to get around and about reasonably well. There is no effective treatment in the majority of cases.
RETINITIS PIGMENTOSA: A group of rare, inherited diseases characterized by the development of night blindness and tunnel vision. Symptoms start in childhood and are progressive. Many patients retain good visual acuity, although their peripheral vision is limited. One of the characteristic findings on examination is collections of pigment in the retina which have a characteristic shape and are therefore known as 'bone spicules'. There is no effective treatment.
RETINAL DETACHMENT usually occurs because of development of a hole in the retina. Holes can occur because of degeneration of the retina, because of traction on the retina by the vitreous, or due to injury. Fluid from the vitreous passes through the hole causing a split within the retina. The inner part of the retina becomes detached from the outer part, the latter remains in contact with the choroid. Detached retina loses its ability to detect light with consequent impairment of vision. Retinal detachments are more common in the short sighted, in the elderly or following cataract extraction. Symptoms include spots before the eyes (*floaters*), flashing lights and a shadow over the eye with progressive loss of vision. Treatment by laser is very effective if caught early, at the stage when a hole has developed in the retina but the retina has not become detached. The edges of the hole can be 'spot welded' to the underlying choroid. Once a detachment has occurred, laser therapy cannot be used, the retina has to be repositioned. This is usually done by indenting the wall of the eye from the outside to meet the retina, then making the retina stick to the wall of the eye by inducing inflammation in the wall. This is done by freezing the wall. The outcome of surgery depends largely on the extent of the detachment and its duration. Complicated forms of detachment can occur due to diabetic eye disease, injury or tumour. Each requires a specialized form of treatment.

RETINOL is the official chemical name of vitamin A. (See VITAMIN.)

RETINOIC ACID is a synthetic vitamin A derivative. (See VITAMIN.)

RETINOPATHY (see RETINA, DISEASES OF).

RETRO- is a prefix signifying behind or turned backward.

RETROBULBAR NEURITIS: Inflammation of the optic nerve behind (rather than within) the eye. It usually occurs in young adults and presents with a rapid deterioration in vision over a few hours. Colour vision is also impaired. Usually vision recovers over a few weeks, but colour vision may be permanently lost. It can be associated with certain viral illnesses and with multiple sclerosis.

RETROFLEXION means bending of an organ so that its top is thrust backwards. Retroversion is a similar displacement in which the whole organ is turned backwards. These terms are particularly applied to the uterus.

RETROPHARYNGEAL ABSCESS is an abscess occurring in the cellular tissue behind the throat. It is the result in general of disease in the upper part of the spinal column.

REYE'S SYNDROME is a condition which occurs predominantly in young children following a virus infection of the upper respiratory tract or a viral infection such as chickenpox or influenza. The cause is not known, but there is some evidence that aspirin may play a part in its causation. It is of worldwide distribution, but relatively rare in Western Europe. The initial feature is severe, persistent vomiting and fever. This is followed by outbursts of wild behaviour, delirium and convulsions terminating in coma and death. The mortality rate is around 23 per cent, and 50 per cent of the survivors may have persistent mental or neurological disturbances. The younger the patient the higher the death rate and the more common the permanent residual effects.

RHABDOVIRUSES is a group of viruses which includes the rabies virus.

RHATANY, or KRAMERIA, is the root of *Krameria triandra*, a South American plant, which contains an astringent principle. It is mainly used in diarrhoea in the form of a tincture or extract, and to make lozenges for use in cases of relaxed throat.

RHESUS FACTOR (see BLOOD GROUPS).

RHEUMATIC FEVER is another term for acute rheumatism. (See RHEUMATISM.)

RHEUMATISM is a general term applied to a group of diseases, which have for their chief manifestations inflammatory or degenerative affections of the fibrous textures of joints, muscles, and other parts. The term is a very old one based upon the idea that the disease was of a moist nature leading to watery deposits in the joints. The parts affected may be the joints alone, either in acute or chronic form; or various other tissues, especially the fibrous tissues and nerves, may be affected, either with or without disorder in the joints. No satisfactory classification of this heterogeneous collection of diseases has yet been evolved, but the following, recommended by the Royal College of Physicians of London, is probably the best: (1) acute rheumatism (or rheumatic fever) and subacute rheumatism; (2) non-articular rheumatism; (3) gout; (4) chronic arthritis, which includes rheumatoid arthritis and osteoarthrosis. Gout is described elsewhere (see GOUT), and the remaining conditions will be noticed here.

ACUTE RHEUMATISM, or RHEUMATIC FEVER, is a general disorder accompanied by much pain in the joints, feverishness, and copious perspiration, with a tendency to spread in an erratic manner, and to involve the smooth membranes lining various cavities of the body, particularly the heart.

Causes: The nature of this disease is still unknown, but there appears to be a definite association with streptococcal infections. Certain predisposing causes are generally admitted. The disease is prevalent in the late autumn, October, and November in Britain, but in other countries reaches its chief frequency about March. It is rare before the age of 3 years, occurs most commonly in childhood and adolescence, and becomes increasingly less common after adult life is attained. If chorea is excluded, the disease is equally common in the two sexes. There is some evidence that the disease tends to occur in certain families and the suggestion has been put forward that there is a genetic constitution that favours the rheumatic response to infection with streptococci. The condition tends to occur more commonly in children with a high complexion and a reddish tint in their hair. The disease is more common among poor people. Any depressing cause acting upon the general health, such as overwork or anxiety, may precipitate an attack in people predisposed to them. Attacks of acute rheumatism may follow exposure to cold and damp and excessive fatigue. People who have once suffered from this disease are liable to a recurrence.

The relationship to diseases caused by the haemolytic streptococcus is particularly important. Thus, an attack of rheumatic fever is often preceded by a sore throat or tonsillitis due to this organism. This is especially apt to occur with recurrent attacks. Occasionally rheumatic fever follows an attack of scarlet fever, which is a disease due to the haemolytic streptococcus. Chorea (qv) is a manifestation of rheumatic fever; in 25 per cent of rheumatic children it is the first sign of the disease. In recent years there has been a marked decline in the incidence of the disease and in its severity in Britain and in other parts of the Western World, but it is still taking a heavy toll of health and heart disease in the Developing World, particularly Africa.

Symptoms: An attack of acute rheumatism usually begins with chilliness or rigors, followed by feverishness and a feeling of stiffness or pain in one or more joints, generally those of larger size, such as the knee, ankle, wrist or shoulder. The pain soon becomes intense and is accompanied by severe constitutional disturbance. The temperature is elevated: usually about 39·5°C (103°F); the pulse is rapid, full, and soft; the tongue is coated, and there are thirst, loss of appetite and constipation. At first the pain is confined to only one or two joints, but soon others become affected, very commonly similar joints on the two sides of the body. Flitting joint pains, as they are known, are very characteristic of the disease. The affected joints are red, swollen, hot and excessively tender. In mild cases one or two joints only are affected, but in severe cases scarcely a joint, large or small, may escape, and the pain, restlessness, and fever then render the patient's condition extremely miserable.

An attack of acute rheumatism is of variable duration, sometimes passing away in the course of a few days. The usual period during which the temperature remains elevated is a week or less, and, if the temperature subsides to normal and again rises, or if it continues elevated beyond ten days, some complication, such as involvement of the heart, may be suspected. Such cases may last for many weeks with relapses, in which all the former symptoms return and prolong the illness.

If no complication has arisen, there may be complete recovery in the course of about three weeks. Sometimes, when all the acute symptoms have disappeared, the joints remain swollen, stiff, and painful on movement, but this condition may also gradually pass away, or, on the other hand, the rheumatism may become chronic. In any case there always remains a liability to subsequent attacks.

In certain cases small subcutaneous nodules develop on the extensor aspect of certain joints, especially the back of the wrist, the back of the elbow, and the knee. They may also occur on the back of the neck. The significance of these rheumatic nodules, which are about the size of a split pea, is that they tend to occur in the more severe cases.

Complications: This disease derives much of its serious import from certain complications which are apt to arise during an attack. Among these the most frequent and the most serious is heart disease. This occurs in about 45 to 55 per cent of children with first attacks of acute rheumatism. If the heart is involved in a first attack of acute rheumatism, it is liable to become more seriously involved in subsequent attacks. Pericarditis (inflammation of the membrane covering the heart), endocarditis (inflammation of the lining membrane of the heart), and myocarditis (inflammation of the heart muscle) may all develop. (See HEART DISEASES.) The risk of cardiac complications seems to be greater the younger the patient, and, indeed, in children the joint pains are often so slight as to be overlooked, and the valvular disease may only be discovered accidentally at a later period of life. Pericarditis occurs less often, but is more serious as regards the patient's immediate prospect of recovery. Chorea (St. Vitus's dance) sometimes follows after the acute symptoms have subsided.

Treatment: Rest in bed is essential until all signs of activity of the disease have subsided. Movements of all kinds should be avoided so far as possible during the first few days. In view of the pain the child should be handled with particular care, and the weight of the bed-clothes should be kept off him by means of a cradle. The skin requires special care, with frequent sponging, in view of the excessive sweating that tends to occur. The diet should consist entirely of milk, glucose, and fruit juices in the acute stage of the disease.

Penicillin should be given for the first week, to kill off any haemolytic streptococci that may be present in the throat. Sodium salicylate forms the sheet anchor of drug treatment, the usual dose being equivalent to 120 mg per kg of body weight every day. Some authorities prefer aspirin (80 to 100 mg per kg of body weight). In severe cases one or other of the corticosteroid drugs may be given. In order to reduce the risk of permanent damage to the heart, it is essential that every patient with rheumatic fever should be kept at complete rest in bed for ten days following the return of the temperature to normal. It should be another two or three weeks before the patient is allowed out of bed. For some time following recovery special care should be taken in avoiding exposure to cold and damp, crowds, and over-exertion.

SUBACUTE RHEUMATISM is a name sometimes applied to mild attacks of acute rheumatism, in which the temperature does not exceed 38·3°C (101°F), and which respond quickly to treatment by sodium salicylate. These cases are often of long duration and they may be accompanied by endocarditis, especially in the case of children. The significance of these attacks is that, no matter how mild they may appear to be, they may involve the heart. Treatment should be instituted immediately by putting the patient to bed, and full doses of aspirin or sodium salicylate should be given. Experience in this country and in the United States has shown that the incidence of such recurrent attacks is reduced by giving children who are susceptible to, or who have had an attack of, rheumatic fever regular small daily doses of a sulphonamide drug or of penicillin over a long period.

NON-ARTICULAR RHEUMATISM includes all those forms of rheumatism which do not involve the joints. Classification is difficult as the cause is not known. Many different names have been given to the various manifestations of this group: eg. fibrositis, bursitis, myalgia, muscular rheumatism, neuritis, lumbago, sciatica, pleurodynia, panniculitis. Although the cause is obscure, there is no doubt about the practical importance of this group of diseases. In the United States of America it accounts for about 30 per cent of all rheumatic diseases, and in Great Britain the incidence is even higher.

Causes: Only certain predisposing factors are known. The actual cause is still to be found. The onset may be acute, as in certain cases of lumbago, or gradual. It may be generalized, eg. involving the muscles of the back and shoulders, or it may be localized. Exposure to cold or damp is a common predisposing factor. Undue exertion may precipitate an attack. In other cases it appears to be associated with a focus of infection somewhere in the body, eg. septic teeth, but the importance of this factor has been grossly over-rated in the past. The condition is much more apt to occur in middle-age than in young adults. Certain individuals are more likely to suffer from the condition than others, and it is in these susceptible individuals that the factors already mentioned are most likely to induce an attack.

Symptoms: These consist of pain and stiffness which range in intensity from the agonizing pain of acute lumbago, which literally immobilizes the victim for a time, to a vague sense of discomfort which the individual may have difficulty in localizing precisely. The pain and stiffness are usually worst after resting and tend to improve with exercise. Thus, they tend to be worst on awakening in the morning. Damp and cold weather make them worse, whilst they improve in dry warm weather. Tender spots can sometimes be felt in the affected muscles, and the detection of these is of importance from the point of view of treatment. There is seldom any wasting or atrophy of muscle and the joints are not involved. The general health is not affected.

Treatment: This depends upon the acuteness of the condition. If very acute, a period of rest in bed may be necessary, but as a rule this is not essential. Avoidance of strenuous physical exertion is advisable, but moderate exercise is advantageous as it prevents the affected muscles becoming stiff. For the relief of pain, heat in some form is used. This may consist of hot baths, hot packs, hot water bottles or diathermy. Warming the affected part gently in front of a gas-fire is as useful a way as any. In more severe cases some form of counter-irritation, eg. a mustard plaster, may be necessary. Electricity in the form of faradism, galvanism, or high-frequency currents is often useful. Massage is usually helpful. In severe cases analgesics are required, and the best of these is aspirin, with or without paracetamol. If localized tender spots are found, the injection into them of procaine often gives relief which is sometimes dramatic.

LUMBAGO: This is myalgia or fibrositis occurring in the strong and dense sinews of the erector spinae muscles of the back, and is considered separately because of its great frequency and importance in regard to occupation, and because it is readily distinguishable. (See LUMBAGO.)

SCIATICA AND BRACHIAL NEURITIS: The rheumatic processes may affect the fibrous tissues of various nerves, the nerves of the arm and the sciatic nerve running down the back of the thigh being especially liable to this affection. The causes described above under myalgia are also operative in producing neuritis, and, in the case of the nerves of the arm, overstrain at work, eg. in hammermen, plays an important part. The treatment of this condition is described under NEURALGIA. (See also SCIATICA.)

RHEUMATOID ARTHRITIS is one of the most crippling of all the rheumatic diseases.

Causes: The majority current concept at the moment is that it is a manifestation of autoimmunity (qv). The disease is one of temperate climates and is more common in women than in men. The majority of cases occur between the ages of 35 and 40. It is uncommon under the age of 25, and first attacks seldom occur after the age of 50. A form of rheumatoid arthritis known as Still's disease (qv) occurs in children. Another form occurs in association with psoriasis (qv).

Pathology: The first change in the affected joints consists of thickening of the synovial lining of the joint. This is followed by involvement of the articular cartilage, which becomes ulcerated, covered with granulation tissue, and ultimately destroyed in severe cases. There is an overproduction of connective tissue and in due course the joint becomes ankylosed and fixed. There is also rarefaction of the bone adjoining the joint, and marked wasting of the adjoining muscles. This last change is due, in part at least, to disuse: because of the painful state of the joint the individual uses it as little as possible.

Symptoms: The disease usually has a gradual onset. There is pain, swelling, and redness of the affected joints. The condition usually begins in the small joints of the hand, especially in the fingers. Later, almost any joint in the body may be involved, but the condition tends to spread from the smaller joints to the larger joints. Thus, the shoulder and the hip joint are usually affected last. Even mild attacks are usually accompanied by fever, and in acute attacks the rise in temperature may be quite high and accompanied by the rise in pulse-rate and all the other accompaniments of fever: eg. prostration, loss of appetite, sweating, and the like. With recurrent attacks the affected joints tend to become chronically swollen and fixed. The position in which fixation of the joint occurs depends upon the relative strength of the muscles around the joint. In the case of the hand this results in the characteristic deformity – with the hand deviated towards the little finger side. In comparison with the swelling of the joints, the wasting of the surrounding muscles shows up particularly markedly, and gives a

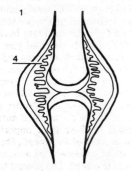

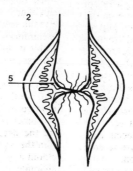

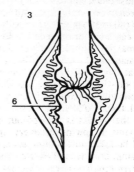

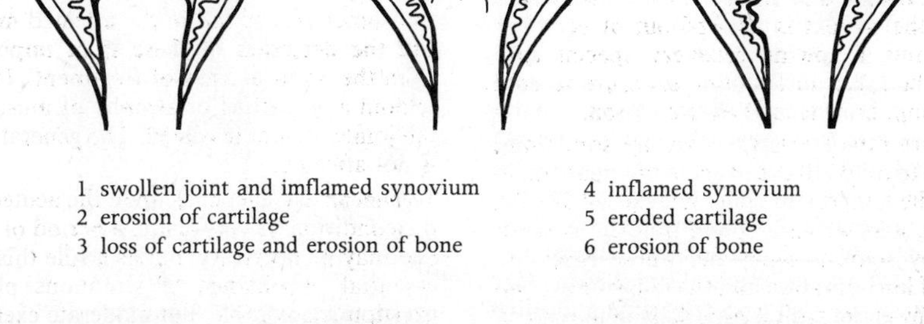

1 swollen joint and imflamed synovium
2 erosion of cartilage
3 loss of cartilage and erosion of bone

4 inflamed synovium
5 eroded cartilage
6 erosion of bone

Changes in a joint caused by rheumatoid arthritis.

characteristic appearance, which in the case of the fingers justifies the description of spindle-shaped. X-ray examination reveals the presence of well-marked changes in the joints, including widening of the joint space and decreased density of the bones adjoining the joints. The sedimentation rate (qv) is raised, and, though this is of little help in diagnosis, the course of the sedimentation rate over a period of time is a useful guide as to how the disease is responding to treatment. Other tests used in diagnosis and prognosis (qv) are the Rose-Waaler test, the latex test and the sheep cell agglutination test (SCAT). There is also some evidence that investigation of the HLA antigens (qv) may be of value. With recurring attacks the patient's general health tends to become affected; with anaemia, loss of weight, loss of appetite, and lassitude. The outlook, or prognosis, is satisfactory in so far as this is not a killing disease, but it is unsatisfactory in that, up to date, no effective treatment is available and the disease tends therefore to be chronic and recurrent. It has been estimated that a quarter of the patients show marked improvement approaching a cure, a half show slight or moderate improvement, and a quarter fail to improve, or become worse.

Treatment: It is now clear that cortisone is not a cure for the condition. Increasing experience has shown that its use is not without danger. Used with circumspection, under skilled supervision, it is undoubtedly a useful adjunct in the treatment of rheumatoid arthritis, but it by no means replaces the well-tried measures which are summarized in the remainder of this section.

These consist, in the first place, of rest, the degree of rest depending upon the severity of the condition. Rest, however, must never be absolute, even in the acute stages, as this may lead to unnecessary stiffness in the joints. It must be accompanied by exercises to keep the joints as mobile as possible. During the more acute phases, when it is necessary to keep the patient in bed, the affected joints should be splinted so as to prevent deformities developing. Heat, in the form of hot water bottles, wax baths, or diathermy, is useful in relieving pain and discomfort, and this may be supplemented by the administration of aspirin or other non-steroidal anti-inflammatory drugs. Spa treatment is also of value. Satisfactory results have been obtained from the use of certain salts of gold. Although gold does not produce a cure, it is the one agent which, apart from the cortisone group of drugs, has been shown to improve the condition. Its use, however, is not without risk, and it must therefore only be used under medical supervision. Penicillamine (qv) and chloroquine (qv) are two other potent drugs that are proving of value but, like gold, they must only be used under skilled medical supervison. Surgery is only required to correct any deformity which is crippling the patient, provided this crippling is confined to one or two joints. The general health of the patient must also be attended to by ensuring that he or she has an adequate nutritious diet, containing plenty of milk, fruit, and vegetables. Dental care is necessary, but it is now recognized that there is no justification for the wholesale extraction of teeth which was fashionable at one time. Removal to a dry, warm climate is beneficial, but economically this is seldom advice that can be followed by the affected individual. (See also STILL'S DISEASE.)

OSTEOARTHROSIS, or OSTEOARTHRITIS, is the most common disorder of joints and is estimated to be present in 80 to 90 per cent of people over the age of 60 years. It is characterized by gradual destruction of the central part of the cartilage lining the affected joint, whilst at the same time there is overgrowth of the outer part of the cartilage which ultimately results in the growth of bony spurs or osteophytes. The condition is probably a degenerative one, but it is accentuated or accelerated by trauma. Thus, it is liable to occur in a knee in which there has been cartilage trouble which has not been treated adequately. Obesity, accompanied as it so often is by faulty posture, results in abnormal stresses and strains being applied to the hip joints and knees, and this in due course results in osteoarthritic changes in these joints. There is some evidence that there may be a hereditary predisposition. The condition is more common in women than in men, and the joints mainly involved are the hip, the knee, and the shoulder joint. The terminal joints of the fingers are also quite a common site. Pain and stiffness in the affected joints are the usual manifestations of the disease. A creaking sensation (crepitus) is felt in moving the joint in the more advanced cases. In chronic cases the joint becomes enlarged. There is seldom any generalized disturbance such as fever or malaise. The diagnosis is confirmed by X-ray examination.

Treatment consists of rest and graduated exercises. When the joints are painful the local application of heat is beneficial: eg. hot towel packs or infra-red light. Aspirin or sodium salicylate also relieves the pain temporarily. If the individual is overweight, a reducing diet is necessary to bring the weight down. In the more advanced cases, surgery is often of value.

In advanced cases of the disease involving the hip, satisfactory results are now being obtained from replacement of the damaged hip by an artificial hip joint. Knee replacement operations are also being performed, but these have not yet attained the high standard of success achieved with the hip replacement operation performed by experienced orthopaedic surgeons in carefully selected cases.

People with rheumatism of any form, and their relatives, can obtain help and advice from Arthritis Care, 5 Grosvenor Crescent, London SW1X 7ER (01-235 0902).

RHEUMATOID ARTHRITIS (see RHEUMATISM).

RH FACTOR (see BLOOD GROUPS).

RHINITIS means inflammation of the mucous membrane of the nose. (See NOSE, DISEASES OF.)

RHINOPHYMA is the condition characterized by enlargement of the nose due to enormous enlargement of the sebaceous glands which may develop in the later stages of rosacea (qv).

RHINOPLASTY means the repair of the nose or modification of its shape by operation. This operation is performed by plastic and ENT surgeons alike. It may involve alteration of the bony skeleton of the nose and/or alteration of the septum (septorhinoplasty). It is mostly performed for cosmetic reasons. However, any disease process or injury which has caused defect in the nose may be repaired as well. The latter problem would usually involve the utilization of some form of skin flap, whereas this would not be required for cosmetic surgical purposes.

RHINOVIRUSES are a large group of viruses; to date around 80 distinct rhinoviruses have been identified. Their practical importance is that some of them are responsible for around one-quarter of the cases of the common cold.

RHIZOTOMY is the surgical operation of cutting a nerve root, as, for example, to relieve the pain of trigeminal neuralgia.

RHONCHI denotes the harsh cooing, hissing, or whistling sounds (wheezing) heard by auscultation over the bronchial tubes when they are the seat of infection. (See BRONCHITIS.)

RHUBARB is the root of *Rheum palmatum*, a plant originally derived from China and Tibet, and other species of Rheum. It has a gentle purgative action.

RHUS is a genus of trees and shrubs, some of which are used as astringents, while others, particularly *Rhus toxicodendron*, or poison oak, and *Rhus radicans*, or poison ivy, are poisonous. (See POISON IVY.)

RIBOFLAVINE is the *British Pharmacopoeia* name for what used to be known as vitamin B_2. Riboflavine belongs to a group of animal and plant pigments which give a greenish fluorescence on exposure to ultra-violet rays. It is present especially in milk, and is not destroyed during pasteurization. Other rich sources are eggs, liver, yeast and the green leaves of broccoli and spinach. It is also present in beer. Deficiency of riboflavine in the diet is thought to cause inflammation of the substance of the cornea, sores on the lips, especially at the angles of the mouth (cheilosis (qv)), and dermatitis.

The minimal daily requirement for an adult is 1·5 to 3 mg, but is greater during pregnancy and lactation.

RIBS are the bones, twelve on each side, which enclose the cavity of the chest. The upper seven are joined to the breast-bone by their costal cartilages and are therefore known as true ribs. The lower five do not reach the breast-bone, and are therefore known as false ribs. Of the latter, the 8th, 9th and 10th are joined by their costal cartilages, each one to the rib immediately above it, while the 11th and 12th are free from any such connection, and are therefore known as floating ribs. Each rib has a head, by which it is joined to the upper part of the body of the vertebra with which it corresponds, as well as to the vertebra immediately above. Next comes a narrow part known as the neck, and then a tubercle, by which the rib is joined to the transverse process of the corresponding vertebra. Finally, the greater part of the bone is made up of the shaft, which runs at first outwards and at the angle turns sharply forwards. On the lower margin of the shaft is a groove, which lodges the corresponding intercostal artery and nerve.

RICE-WATER is a useful diluent drink for invalids, similar to barley-water.

RICKETS is a disease of childhood characterized chiefly by a softened condition of the bones, and by other evidence of perverted nutrition.

Causes: This disease is the result of deficiency of vitamin D in the diet. Healthy bones cannot be built up without calcium (or lime) salts, and the body cannot utilize these salts in the absence of vitamin D. Want of sunlight and fresh air in the dwellings where the children are reared is also of importance. Once a common condition in industrial areas, it had almost disappeared in Great Britain, but there has been a recurrence of it in recent years that is giving rise to concern.

The changes that take place in the bones are due to an irregular process of bone formation. The periosteum, the membrane enveloping the bones, becomes inflamed, and in consequence the bone formed beneath it is defective in lime salts and very soft. At the growing ends of the bones there is an even more striking change. The epiphyseal plate of cartilage, from which growth takes place, is much thickened, the cellular elements in it much increased in number, and the bone which it produces markedly deficient in lime salts. The new bone shows a deficiency of lime amounting to 25 or 35 per cent, and this, too, notwithstanding the fact that there is abundance of lime in the body, as shown by its excessive excretion in the urine. The disease rarely occurs under the age of 6 months, from which it may be assumed that exposure to unsuitable conditions for several months is necessary before rickets ensues. It is most common between 1 and 2 years of age and is increasingly rare after the age of 3.

Symptoms: The symptoms of rickets most commonly attract attention about the end of the first year, and the disease rarely appears for the first time after the age of 5. The symptoms, which precede the outward manifestations of the disease, are marked disorders of the digestive and alimentary functions. The child's appetite is diminished; there is frequent vomiting and diarrhoea; or irregularity of the bowels appears, the evacuations being clay-coloured and unhealthy. In infants, convulsions are sometimes a symptom of rickets and disappear under the treatment appropriate to this disease. At the same time there is tenderness of the bones as shown by crying when the child is moved or handled. A little later it is noticed that there is delay in learning to sit up and walk, so that the child who has begun to walk loses this power.

Gradually changes in the shape of the bones becomes visible, first chiefly noticed at the ends of the long bones, as in those of the arm, causing enlargement at the wrists, or in the ribs, producing a row of knobs at the junction of their ends with the rib cartilages (rickety rosary). Because of their softened condition the bones also tend to become distorted and bent both by the action of the muscles and by the weight of the body resting upon them. Those of the legs are bent outwards and forwards and the child becomes bow-legged or knock-kneed, often to an extreme degree. The trunk of the body likewise shows various alterations and deformities owing to curvatures of the spine, flattening of the lateral curves of the ribs, and the projection forward of the breast-bone. (See CHEST DEFORMITIES.) The cavity of the chest may thus be contracted and interference produced with the development of the thoracic organs, whose functions thus become embarrassed. The liver is pushed outwards and the abdomen becomes protuberant (pot belly). The pelvis undergoes distortion which may reduce its capacity to such a degree that in females serious difficulties may arise later in life in the course of labour. The head of the rickety child is square with high 'intellectual' forehead; the individual bones of the cranium remain long ununited, while the soft fontanelle remains unclosed long after the end of the second year, the time by which it should have disappeared; the face is small and ill-developed; and the teeth appear late and fall out or decay early.

The disease usually terminates in recovery with more or less of deformity and dwarfing, the bones, although altered in shape, becoming ultimately firmly ossified. On the other hand, during the progress of the disease, various intercurrent ailments are apt to arise which may cause death, such as bronchitis and other chest complaints, meningitis, convulsions, laryngismus.

Treatment: The treatment of rickets is more hygienic and dietetic than medicinal. The specific remedy is vitamin D, given as a rule in the form of calciferol (vitamin D_2). A full diet is of course essential, with emphasis upon a sufficient supply of milk. Rickets practically does not occur in breast-fed children but it is a wise precaution to give breast-fed babies supplementary vitamin D. (See INFANT FEEDING.) After the child is weaned, the provision of suitable food is of the greatest importance, supplemented by the administration of some source of vitamin D. (See INFANT FEEDING.)

Deficiency of vitamin D in adults results in osteomalacia (qv).

RICKETTSIA is the general term given to a group of micro-organisms, which are intermediate between bacteria and viruses. They are the causal agents of typhus and a number of typhus-like diseases, such as Rocky Mountain spotted fever, Japanese River fever, and scrub typhus. These micro-organisms are usually conveyed to man by lice, fleas, ticks, and mites. VISCERAL RICKETTSIA is a disease transmitted by mites from an infected house mouse, which occurs in the USA, South Africa, Korea and USSR. The causal organism is *Rickettsia akari*. The incubation period is 7 to 14 days. The characteristic features are fever, headache, and a non-irritating rash on the face, trunk and extremities. The disease is non-fatal and responds rapidly to tetracyclines.

RIFAMPICIN is an antibiotic derived from *Streptomycesmediterranei*, which is proving of value in the treatment of tuberculosis and leprosy. It contains a dye which is excreted in the urine and gives it a red colour.

RIFT VALLEY FEVER is a virus disease, transmitted by mosquitoes, at one time confined to Sub-Saharan Africa and predominantly found in domestic animals, such as cattle, sheep and goats. The only human beings affected were veterinary surgeons, butchers and others exposed to heavy infection by direct contact with infected animals. These usually recovered. Thus in 1975, only four people died of it. In 1977, it suddenly flared up as a human infection in Egypt, involving 200,000 people and killing 600 of these. It recurred as a human disease in 1978 and 1979, and is now threatening to spread throughout the Middle East, and possibly farther afield. This human outbreak is attributed to a new virulent strain of virus. The illness in man is characterized by fever, haemorrhages, encephalitis (qv) and involvement of the eye. There is an efficient vaccine which protects both animals and human beings against the disease.

RIGOR means shivering. If prolonged, it is generally accompanied by raised temperature, and may be a sign of the onset of some acute febrile disease, such as influenza, pneumonia, or some internal inflammation. *Rigor mortis* is the name given to the stiffness that ensues soon after death. (See DEATH, SIGNS OF; MUSCLE.)

RIMA is a term, meaning a crack or fissure, applied to any narrow natural opening: eg. rima glottidis, the chink between the vocal cords.

RINGWORM, or TINEA, is the name given to inflammatory affections of the skin produced by a fungus. The main forms of ringworm in man are: (i) *Tinea capitis*, or ringworm of the scalp; (ii) *Tinea barbae*, or ringworm of the beard; (iii) *Tineacruris*, or ringworm of the groin, and also known as dhobie itch; (iv) *Tinea pedis*, or ringworm of the feet; (v) *Tinea corporis*, or ringworm of the body; (vi) *Tinea unguium*, or ringworm of the nails; (vii) *Tinea favosa*, favus, or honeycomb ringworm, affecting scalp; (viii) *Tinea versicolor*.

RINGWORM OF THE SCALP, a disease of childhood, is usually due to a human species of fungus, *Microsporum audouini*; some five per cent of cases are due to infection by microspora acquired from cats and dogs. Boys are more infected than girls, and in both it disappears spontaneously at adolescence, being excessively rare in adults. It is most contagious. The incidence of the disease fell rapidly in the 1920–30s, and by 1939 was a rare condition in many parts of the country. The typical appearance is that of circular patches of lustreless, greyish, broken hairs scattered over the scalp. The scalp itself is covered with fine greyish-white scabs. Under Wood's light (the rays of a mercury vapour lamp screened through a special glass) the infected hairs have a bright green colour, which is diagnostic.

Treatment: As in all other forms of ringworm, the outlook has been radically changed by the introduction of the antibiotic, griseofulvin (qv). When used under medical supervision, this is the most effective method of treatment yet discovered, curing the condition in a high proportion of cases. Treatment should be continued for four weeks or until there is complete cure. In order to prevent reinfection, the infected hairs should be removed either manually, or by clipping and shaving, after three weeks' treatment with griseofulvin. A daily application of an anti-fungal preparation is not essential but is of value in preventing the spread of infection to other parts of the scalp or to other children. The child should be excluded from school until cured.

RINGWORM OF THE BEARD is one of the forms of barber's rash. There is a form occurring in grooms and cattlemen, in which the infection is acquired from animals.

Treatment: This consists of the administration of griseofulvin (qv). If suppuration is also present, hot fomentations of 2 per cent sodium thiosulphate should be applied.

RINGWORM OF THE GROIN, or DHOBIE ITCH, is caused by a fungus of the same group as is responsible for ringworm of the foot: *Epidermophyton*. It occurs at any age, but is most common in young adult males. The eruption is a sharply defined, slightly raised reddish area, which begins in the inner aspect of the upper third of the thigh and tends to spread over the perineum. It is accompanied by considerable irritation at times.

Treatment: This consists of the administration of topical antifungal creams until the condition clears. Since a warm moist atmosphere encourages fungal growth, the groin should be kept dry and loose fitting underpants should be worn.

RINGWORM OF THE FOOT, or athlete's foot as it is often known, is one of the most common forms of ringworm at the present day. It is due to an *Epidermophyton*. Most common among adolescent and young adult males, the infection is usually acquired by walking with bare feet on infected floors: eg. hotel and school bathrooms, public swimming baths, and pithead baths. The eruption begins between the toes as a rule, but may also be found on the soles of the feet. There are two main forms of eruption: (*a*) the *vesicular*, in which the affected area is covered with small blisters – this form begins on the sole; (*b*) the *intertriginous*, in which the skin between the toes becomes white and sodden, and peels off, leaving a raw red area. Before beginning to treat this type of ringworm it is particularly important to demonstrate the fungus in material removed from the affected area, as a superficially similar appearance may be produced by other infecting organisms or even by excessive sweating alone.

Treatment: Careful hygiene of the feet, particularly for those who tend to perspire freely in the feet, is essential: (*a*) to prevent infection; (*b*) to aid in curing the condition once acquired; (*c*) to prevent relapses. Such hygiene consists of washing the feet every night in warm water, drying them thoroughly but carefully. A fresh pair of socks should be worn every day and rubber footwear is best avoided. Once the infection is acquired, the treatment depends upon the local condition. Treatment is with antifungal creams, such as clotrimazole, miconazole, or econazole. More severe inflammatory conditions may require creams which combine an antifungal agent and a corticosteroid. Dusting powders have no place in treatment except for cosmetic purposes, perhaps, and indeed some powders can cause skin irritation. More resistant cases may require oral griseofulvin.

RINGWORM OF THE BODY, which may occur with ringworm of the scalp, may be due to either a microsporum or a tricophyton. The eruption consists of circular discs, usually red in colour at first, but later tending to become pale in the centre, and blisters may appear in the surrounding ring. There is considerable itching.

Treatment is as for other forms of ringworm of the skin.

RINGWORM OF THE NAILS is not common but is most resistant to treatment. Several nails are usually affected, and they turn a greenish-grey colour, and become brittle, separated from the nail-bed, and thickened and, as a result, difficult to manicure.

Treatment consists of the administration of griseofulvin, but treatment may need to be continued for long periods: for up to six months or longer. Toe-nails are particularly resistant to griseofulvin.

FAVUS is due to a fungus of the genus, *Tricophyton*. It occurs on the scalp, skin, and nails, and consists of thick yellow cups of crust. It is rare in Great Britain. It responds to griseofulvin.
TINEA VERSICOLOR, due to *Malassazia furfur*, is characterized by thin, faint yellowish patches on the chest and abdomen. Treatment consists of the local daily application of lotion of selenium sulphide (qv). Ketoconazone orally is usually effective. It usually recurs despite treatment.
KERION, or TINEA KERION, is a complication of ringworm of the scalp. It takes the form of a boggy mass involving several hair follicles. Small beads of pus may be seen on the surface. Treatment consists of oral griseofulvin and, in very severe inflammation, oral corticosteroids.

RIPPLE BEDS are a modern development of the conventional air-bed (qv). Their essential feature is a mattress which is alternately pressurized by a compressor to create a gentle rippling effect along the entire length of the mattress. This provides a continuous massaging motion which stimulates the circulation and helps to maintain the nutrition of the skin, thereby reducing the risk of bed-sores (qv).

RISUS SARDONICUS is the term used for describing the facial appearance when the muscles of the forehead and the face go into spasm in tetanus, giving the effect of a sardonic grin.

RITODRINE is a drug that is used in the management of premature labour. It acts by suppressing the activity of the uterus. (See PREMATURE BIRTH.)

RNA is the abbreviation for ribonucleic acid, one of the two types of nucleic acid (qv) that exist in nature. It is present in both the cytoplasm and nucleus of the cells of the body, but principally in the former. With DNA (qv) it is an essential component of the genetic code. It exists in three categories known, respectively, as ribosomal (r), transfer (t), and messenger (m) RNA. Genetic information resides in the linear sequence of nucleotides (see NUCLEIC ACID) in DNA and is transcribed into messenger RNA before protein is synthesized. In the language of the computer, the genetic code consists of 64 three-letter code-words, or codons. The code in DNA is comparable to a tape which contains information written linearly in the form of these codons, each of which is the code for one of the 20 amino-acids (qv) from which proteins are made. The genetic information encoded in DNA is used to programme the manufacture of proteins in two stages.

In the first the information is transcribed from DNA on to a molecule of mRNA. In the second the messenger RNA-intermediary transports the information to the protein-manufacturing centres of the cell where the information is translated from the linear sequence of codons in the RNA into a linear sequence of amino-acids which are concurrently converted into protein.

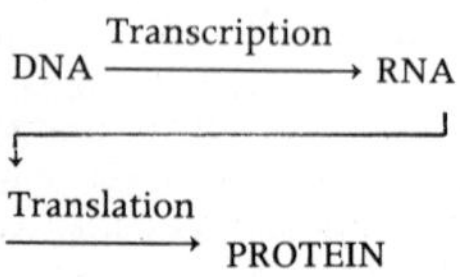

ROCHELLE SALT, SEIGNETTE SALT, and TARTRATED SODA are names for sodium potassium tartrate, a saline purgative which forms the chief constituent of Seidlitz powder. The dose of Rochelle salt as an aperient is 8 to 16 grams, or a heaped dessertspoonful.

ROCKY MOUNTAIN SPOTTED FEVER is a fever of the typhus group. It received its name from the fact that it was first reported in the Rocky Mountain States of USA. These are still the most heavily infected States, but it is now found in all parts of the United States. The causative organism is *Rickettsia rickettsi*, which is transmitted to man by tics. (See also TYPHUS FEVER.)

RODENT ULCER is a chronic form of ulcer, which is found chiefly about the nose and face of elderly people, and which gradually increases in size. It stands between a simple chronic ulcer and a cancer, being much slower in its growth than the latter. Treatment consists in cutting out the ulcer with the healthy skin for a little distance all round. It is also very amenable to treatment by X-rays, radium, and other forms of radiant energy.

ROMBERGISM is a term applied to marked unsteadiness in standing with the eyes shut. It is found as a symptom in some nervous diseases, such as peripheral neuropathy and tabes dorsalis.

ROOT FILLING or root-canal therapy is the treatment given when the nerve of a tooth has been exposed while the tooth is being prepared for a filling, or if it has died or become infected. The nerve debris is removed with thin files and, when the chamber is clear of infection, an inert radio-opaque material is inserted to seal off the root. This is generally effective.

RORSCHACH TEST is a method of investigating personality and disorders of personality. It was devised by a Swiss psychiatrist, Hermann Rorschach (1884–1922), who determined individuals' reactions to a series of symmetrical ink-blots, ten in number and standardized by him. The person investigated is shown the ink-blots in a defined order and is asked to describe what he sees. His descriptions and ideas about the blots are noted and an elaborate system of scoring is said to afford indications of the kind of personality and psychological make-up of the person investigated. Much work has been done on the test and it is thought highly of by experienced psychiatrists.

ROSACEA, or ACNE ROSACEA as it is sometimes known, is a condition in which there is chronic congestion of the flush areas of the face and forehead, leading to the formation of red papules. In the earlier stages the erythema, or redness of the skin, tends to wax and wane, being more marked after a meal or excessive drinking of alcohol or exposure to sunlight. Ultimately, however, the erythema becomes permanent, and may be accompanied by gross enlargement of the sebaceous glands (see SKIN), leading to the gross enlargement of the nose known as rhinophyma (qv) or grog blossoms.

Symptoms: In the milder forms there is simple redness, burning, and tingling of the nose, the redness lasting at first only for a few hours every day, but later tending to become permanent, and also to appear upon the cheeks, forehead and chin. In the severer form the nose becomes very red and the skin thick and lumpy, while the openings of the sebaceous glands are seen as quite wide pits. In exceptional cases, more commonly in men than in women, there may be enormous enlargement of the sebaceous glands of the nose, the condition known as rhinophyma.

Treatment: Tetracycline is the treatment of choice and most patients respond to 250 mg twice daily for a period of 3 to 6 months.

ROSEMARY is a plant giving a fragrant volatile oil which is used in the form of spirit of rosemary.

ROSEOLA is a term applied to any rose-coloured rash.

ROSE-WAALER TEST is a blood test which is proving of value in the diagnosis of rheumatoid arthritis. It is positive in over 70 per cent of patients with this disease, compared with only 4 per cent of people not suffering from rheumatoid arthritis.

ROSE-WATER is prepared by soaking rose-petals in water and distilling over part of the fluid. It is used as an ingredient of cold-cream, etc. Rose oil, or attar of rose, is prepared by distilling the fresh flowers of *Rosa damascena*. It is largely used in perfumery, and in lozenges, dentifrices and ointments.

ROTAVIRUSES are a group of viruses (so-called from their wheel-like structure: *rota* is Latin for wheel) which are a common cause of gastroenteritis in infants (see DIARRHOEA). They are rarely found in children over 6 years of age. They cause from 25 to 80 per cent of childhood diarrhoea in different parts of the world. In the United Kingdom they are responsible for 60 to 65 per cent of cases. They infect only the cells lining the small intestine. In the United Kingdom death from rotavirus is rare.

ROUGHAGE, or dietary fibre, has long been known to affect bowel function. How it does this is still not quite clear but the probability is that it achieves this through its capacity to hold water in a gel-like form. But fibre is not an inert substance as was long thought to be the case. It is digested and metabolized in the colon by the micro-organisms there. This digestive process alters the properties of dietary fibre, including an increase in the amount of bile acids in the stools. The full significance of these changes is not yet known. Many claims are being made for the value of dietary fibre in maintaining health and preventing disease. What does seem to be clear is that it plays a role in the prevention of constipation, diverticular disease (see DIVERTICULOSIS) and the irritable bowel syndrome (qv). There is also some evidence that it may reduce the incidence of cancer of the colon. Though bran is not the panacea it is made out to be by some, there seems little doubt that modern western diets do not contain as much roughage, such as wholemeal flour, as they should.

ROULEAUX is the term applied to the heaps into which red blood corpuscles collect as seen under the microscope.

ROUNDWORMS (see ASCARIASIS).

ROUS SARCOMA is a malignant tumour of fowls which is caused by a virus. This tumour has been the subject of much experimental work bearing upon the nature of cancer.

RUBBING (see MASSAGE; LINIMENTS).

RUBEFACIENTS (see BLISTERS AND COUNTER-IRRITANTS).

RUBELLA is another name for GERMAN MEASLES (qv).

RUE is a herb, *Ruta graveolens*, from which a volatile oil with irritating properties is produced.

RUGGER PLAYER'S EAR is a deformity of the ear which, when marked, may resemble a miniature cauliflower. It is usually the result of injury, most commonly in rugger players, in whom the requisite trauma to produce the condition occurs in the scrum. It also occurs in boxers. The repeated trauma of these two varieties of sports involves bleeding under the mucoperichondrium which lines the cartilege of the pinna. This results in some cartilagenous destruction and subsequent alteration of the shape of the pinna. If this injury is diagnosed accurately, the blood should be drained and the ear well strapped to prevent reaccumulation of this blood. With this technique, the cauliflower ear may be averted.

RUPTURE is a popular name for hernia. (See HERNIA.)

S

SACCHARIN is a soluble coal-tar product of white crystalline appearance. It has an extremely sweet taste, being prepared in various strengths so as to equal in sweetness from 300 to 500 times its own weight of cane-sugar. It escapes from the body unchanged, having practically no effect upon the tissues beyond its influence upon the sensation of taste. Accordingly it is used by diabetics, fat people and others to whom sugar is harmful. It tends to give a bitter flavour to drinks to which it is added.

SACCHAROMYCES is another name for yeast.

SACCHARUM is the Latin name for ordinary cane-sugar or beet-sugar. (See SUGAR.)

SACRUM is the portion of the spinal column near its lower end. The sacrum consists of five vertebrae fused together to form a broad triangular bone which lies between the two haunch-bones and forms the back wall of the pelvis.

SADISM (Marquis de Sade) is the term applied to a form of sexual perversion, in which satisfaction is derived from the infliction of cruelty upon another person.

SAFE PERIOD is that period during the menstrual cycle when fertilization of the ovum is unlikely to occur. Ovulation usually occurs about 15 days before the onset of the menstrual period. A woman is commonly believed to be fertile for about 11 days in each menstrual cycle: ie. on the day of ovulation and for 5 days before and 5 days after this. This would be the eighth to the eighteenth day of the usual 28-day menstrual cycle. Outside this fertile period is the SAFE PERIOD: the first week and the last ten days of the menstrual cycle. On the other hand, there is increasing evidence that the safest period is the last few days before menstruation. In the case of irregular menstruation it is not possible to calculate the safe period. In any event the safety is not absolute.

SAFETY OF DRUGS: The Medicines Act of 1968, which came into force in 1971, is a comprehensive measure replacing most of the previous legislation on the control of medicines for human and veterinary use. It is administered by the Health and Agriculture Ministers of the United Kingdom. It decreed the setting up of a Medicines Commission by the Ministers to give them advice generally relating to the execution of the provisions of the Act. On the advice of the Medicines Commission a series of expert advisory committees was set up. These are Standing Committees of independent experts, and consist of the Committee on Safety of Medicines, the Committee on the Review of Medicines, the Committee on Dental and Surgical Materials, the British Pharmacopoeia Commission which is responsible for the production of the *British Pharmacopoeia*, and the Veterinary Products Committee.

The Committee on Safety of Medicines (CSM) has the function of scrutinizing the efficacy, quality and safety of new drugs before clinical trial and before marketing, as well as the surveillance of each drug after marketing so that adverse reactions are monitored and documented, and warnings issued as required. Early clinical trial for a drug can only be carried out after a clinical trial certificate has been issued by the licensing authority: ie. all Ministers specified in the Act. In the case of human medicines the Minister acts through the Medicines Division of the Department of Health and Social Security.

The major defect in this carefully worked out system is the difficulty in obtaining reports of adverse reaction. The present evidence suggests that at most about 10 per cent of such reactions are reported. One method of trying to obtain this information is the yellow card system. It is so called because it is based on the distribution of yellow cards to all doctors and dentists, on which they are asked to report any adverse reaction they may encounter to a drug even though initially the evidence may not be 100 per cent certain. Even though the annual number of adverse reactions reported in this way has risen from 5052 in 1975 to 10,179 in 1980, there is ample evidence that this represents only a fraction of the adverse reactions that actually occur.

Two further committees in this safety screen are the Joint Committee on Vaccination and Immunization and the Adverse Reactions to Vaccines and Immunological Substances Committee. The function of the Committee on Review of Medicines is to review all medicinal products on the British market.

SAFFRON, or CROCUS, is a yellow powder derived from the dried stigmas and styles of the flower of *Crocus sativus*. It is used as a 'tonic' and colouring matter.

SAGITTAL is the term applied to a structure or section running from front to back in the body.

ST ANTHONY'S FIRE is an old name applied both to erysipelas and to ergot-poisoning.

ST VITUS'S DANCE is another name for CHOREA (qv).

SALABRASION is the removal of tattoos by superficial abrasion with table salt. (See TATTOOING.)

SAL AMMONIAC is another name for chloride of ammonium, which is widely used in cough mixtures and lozenges as an expectorant.

SALBUTAMOL is a drug that is proving of value, and safe, for the relief of spasm of the bronchi in asthma.

SALEP is a mucilaginous substance derived from the dried tubers of various species of orchid. It is used to allay irritation of the stomach and bowels, and in India constitutes an article of diet.

SALERATUS is another name for potassium bicarbonate.

SALICIN is an active principle derived from the bark of several species of poplar and willow trees. It is a crystalline powder of bitter taste and slight solubility. It has been used for the treatment of acute rheumatism, just as sodium salicylate is used.

SALICYLATE OF SODA is a white crystalline substance which is prepared from salicylic acid. It is very soluble in water, and has a sweet, mawkish taste, which to most people is very unpleasant.
Action: When taken internally in the course of acute fevers, and especially of acute rheumatism, it has the effect of reducing temperature, diminishing pain, and causing profuse sweating. Its action is similar to that of aspirin. When taken for some time, it causes fullness in the head, deafness, buzzing in the ears, curious disturbances of sight (so that the person may fancy he sees people in the room who are not there), and, if excessive doses be taken, great depression of the heart's action and of respiration.
Uses: The main use is in acute rheumatism, doses 600 mg, 1 g or more being given several times daily, according to circumstances. It not only diminishes pain and reduces temperature, but may help to cut short an attack of acute rheumatism. In other rheumatic conditions its use is also followed by great benefit.

SALICYLIC ACID is a white substance in fine crystals, of sweetish taste, and sparingly soluble in water.
Action: Salicylic acid is an antiseptic. Externally it is used in ointments to check various skin affections due to bacteria, and, since it has in addition a softening action on the surface of the skin, salicylic acid plasters are used to remove corns and various other superficial overgrowths.

SALINES are purgatives belonging to the class of salts which produce watery evacuations. (See PURGATIVES.) For normal or isotonic saline solution see ISOTONIC.

SALIVA is the fluid which is always present to some extent in the mouth, and is secreted in specially copious amount during a meal, or when the salivary glands are stimulated, as for example by an acid substance placed in the mouth. Saliva contains much mucus and a ferment known as ptyalin, which changes starch into dextrose and maltose (see DIGESTION); also many cells of different types. About 750 millilitres are produced daily.

The principal function of saliva is to aid in the initial processes of digestion. When food is taken into the mouth, an increased output of saliva is evoked. This saliva is essential for the process of mastication (qv), whereby food is reduced to a homogeneous mass before being swallowed. In addition, the ptyalin in the saliva initiates the digestion of starch in the food.

An excessive flow of saliva known as *salivation* occurs as the result of taking certain drugs over a considerable period. Salivation also occurs as the result of irritation in the mouth, as for instance, in the teething child, and from dyspepsia. Dribbling of saliva is a common symptom of bulbar paralysis. The converse state of lack, or deficiency, of saliva is known as xerostomia (qv).

SALIVARY GLANDS are the glands situated near, and opening into, the cavity of the mouth, by which the saliva is manufactured. They include the *parotid gland*, placed in the deep space that lies between the ear and the angle of the jaw; the *submandibular gland*, lying beneath the horizontal part of the jaw-bone; and the *sublingual gland*, which lies beneath the tongue.

Each gland is made up of branching tubes closely packed together, and supported by strong connective tissue. These tubes are lined by large cells that secrete the saliva, and from their interior lead ducts that unite with one another to form ultimately the large main ducts that open into the mouth. The appearance and character of the secreting cells vary in different glands. In the parotid gland they secrete a clear fluid containing the ferment, ptyalin; in the sublingual gland they mainly produce mucus, whilst the submandibular gland contains cells of both types.

SALMON PATCHES are small pink patches found in some new-born infants – on the eyelids, on the forehead between the eyes, and on the nape of the neck. Those on the first two of these three sites have usually faded by the baby's first birthday, but those on the nape of the neck may be more persistent. (See also BIRTH-MARKS.)

SALMONELLA INFECTIONS, or SALMONELLOSIS (see FOOD POISONING).

SALOL is a white, crystalline, tasteless substance with faint aromatic odour. It was used as an intestinal antiseptic at one time, but its main use now is in sun-screen lotions.

SALPINGITIS is inflammation situated in the Fallopian tubes.

SALPINGO- is a prefix indicating a connection with either the Fallopian (or uterine) tubes or the Eustachian (or auditory) tubes.

SALT is the substance produced by the replacement of the acidic hydrogen of an acid by a metal or basic radical. It is also a synonym for common salt or sodium chloride.

SALTPETRE (see NITRE).

SAL VOLATILE is another name for aromatic solution of ammonia, a liquid of burning taste and great stimulating powers. Its action depends upon various volatile oils, ammonia, and bicarbonate of ammonia which it contains. It is used as a stimulating expectorant in cough mixtures, and is valuable as a stimulant in faints. The dose is from half to one teaspoonful (1 to 5 millilitres) in a wineglassful of water. (See AMMONIA.)

SANDALWOOD OIL is a yellowish, fragrant-smelling oil with bitter taste obtained from the wood, *Santalum album*, by distillation. It has an antiseptic action and was at one time widely administered in doses of 0·3 to 1 ml for inflammation of mucous membranes, particularly those of the urinary organs. It is widely used in perfumery.

SANDFLY FEVER, also known as PHLEBOTOMUS FEVER, THREE-DAY FEVER, and PAPATACI FEVER, is a short, sharp fever occurring in many parts of the tropics and subtropics, including most of the Mediterranean littoral, due to a virus conveyed by the bite of a small hairy midge or sandfly (*Phlebotomus papatasi*). The incubation period is three to seven days.

Symptoms: There are headache, feverishness, general sensations like those of influenza, flushed face and bloodshot eyes, but no signs of catarrh. The fever passes off in three days, but the patient may take some time to convalesce.

Treatment: As there is no specific remedy, prophylaxis is important. This consists of the spraying of rooms with DDT or Gammexane; the application of insect repellents such as dimethyl phthalate to the exposed parts of the body (eg. ankles, wrists and face), particularly at sunset; and the use of sandfly nets at night. Once the infection is acquired, treatment consists of rest in bed, light diet and aspirin and codeine.

SANGUINEOUS means containing blood.

SANIES means an evil-smelling, thin discharge from a wound or ulcer.

SANITATION, or the science which aims at the prevention of disease, although only fully developed during the last hundred years, was recognized in ancient times. So well were its fundamental principles understood, that even in the Mosaic days isolation of infectious cases, disinfection of infected materials by burning, and regulations for the abatement of nuisances, were in force. The importance of adequate water supplies was appreciated even before the days of the Roman Empire, and the sewers of Nineveh point to the beginnings of the drainage systems of cities.

At first, preventive medicine took cognizance only of the preventable or infectious diseases, but in its vast ramifications at the present day it aims also at the improvement of the general health of the populace, by the mitigation of all external conditions which tend to disease in individuals. It is not a science independent or standing alone. It embraces a knowledge of medicine, bacteriology, engineering, meteorology, architecture and geology. It aims at the reduction of infectious diseases, but these have been its greatest advisers and teachers. The recurrent epidemics of cholera which formerly invaded Britain forced the hands of the populace to remedy their water supplies and remodel their systems of drainage. Smallpox and its long roll of victims forced on the compulsory adoption of Jenner's discovery of the value of vaccination. These sowed the seed, and other infectious diseases have brought it nearer maturity. Improved sanitation in matters of ventilation, sewerage, water supply, hospital accommodation, the abatement of nuisances and the inspection of meat has naturally followed from the first step in advance. Its value has been shown in the improved hygiene of the factory, where sanitation has been called in to save the workers from the dangers of their occupation, in meeting the demands of modern civilization, and in the improved conditions of life in dwellings and in general surroundings. It aims at correcting the evils arising from the aggregation of people in cities and towns. It benefits the country dweller and the resident in town by improved methods of sewage and refuse disposal.

Sanitary law: Numerous laws dealing with sanitary matters have been put in force in recent years. The general public health administration of the country is based, in England on the Public Health Act of 1875, and in Scotland on that of 1897, but into many Acts not primarily dealing with sanitation, sanitary provisions have been introduced, as in the various Factory and Workshop Acts. Special local Acts have also been obtained by various authorities, and almost every year some Act is passed by Parliament giving greater sanitary control.

In the various Public Health Acts, which constitute the basis of sanitary administration, machinery is provided for dealing with:

1. General nuisances and offensive trades. Offensive trades include the trades of blood boiler, blood drier, bone boiler, fat extractor, fat melter, fellmonger, glue maker, gut scraper,

rag and bone dealer, size maker, soap boiler, tallow melter or tripe boiler.
2. Scavenging and cleansing and the formation of scavenging districts.
3. The seizure of unsound food.
4. The general prevention and mitigation of infectious diseases, including the provision of isolation hospitals, ambulances, disinfecting stations and apparatus. (See INFECTION.)
5. The regulation of common lodging-houses and houses let in lodgings.
6. The provision of water and sewers and the formation of special districts for water supply and drainage.
7. The regulation of buildings.
8. The constitution of port sanitary authorities.
9. Prevention of pollution of rivers by sewage.
10. Regulations as to sale and adulteration of foods.
11. Dairies, cowsheds and milkshops Orders.
12. Various Acts for housing of working classes, including Town Planning Acts.
13. Tuberculosis Orders, Factory and Workshop Acts.
14. Cleansing of persons.
15. Notification of births. Children's and Midwives' Acts.
16. The control of air pollution, waste disposal, radioactivity, pesticides and noise.

Community Physician: Under the National Health Service Reorganization Act 1973, the post of Medical Officer of Health was abolished, and his duties were largely taken over by what are now known as Community Physicians. It is therefore now the Community Physician, designated as the Medical Officer for Environmental Health, who is required to acquaint himself with the general sanitary condition of his district, to suggest the steps he considers might be taken for its improvement, and to advise the local authority in all sanitary matters. He is expected to investigate all outbreaks of infectious disease, report upon them, and recommend and see carried into force such preventive measures as he deems necessary. He must, if it is advisable, or if he is directed by the sanitary authority, himself inspect any article exposed for food, and deal with it, if it is unsound. He advises also as to nuisances injurious to health. He is also expected to inform the Department of any outbreak of dangerous infectious disease.

Environmental Health Officer: The Environmental Health Officer, formerly known as the Public Health Inspector, and before that as the Sanitary Inspector, attends to the general sanitation of the district, investigates all conditions of nuisances, sees that the regulations and by-laws relating to offensive trades are observed, and that all unsound meat is dealt with. He takes, if authorized by the sanitary authority to do so, samples under the Sale of Food and Drugs Acts, and if these be found adulterated, he takes action under the Act. He reports to the Community Physician any infectious disease, coming under his notice, occurring in the district. He is required to preserve records of his inspections and actions.

Nuisances: A large number of objectionable processes are declared by the Public Health Acts to be 'Nuisances or injurious or dangerous to health'. Houses badly constructed or overcrowded, streets, ditches, water supplies, stables and byres, if foul and unclean, accumulations of filth, factories overcrowded, ill ventilated and filthy, furnaces not consuming their smoke as far as possible, overcrowded cemeteries, all constitute nuisances.

Every sanitary authority is required to have its district inspected for the detection of nuisances. Any person, however, who suspects the presence of a nuisance may complain to the sanitary authority, who will at once have the matter investigated. If the authority is convinced of the existence of a nuisance, a notice will be served on the person responsible, or, if the author cannot be found, on the owner or occupier of the premises, requiring the removal of the nuisance within a specified time. If the sanitary authorities fail to discharge their duty with reference to nuisances, individuals can appeal to the Department of Health and Social Security, who may issue an order to be enforced in a High Court of Justice, or may direct any police officer of the district to institute the ordinary legal proceedings in case of nuisances. The most expeditious method, however, for individuals to gain redress in case of default by the sanitary authority, is to complain direct to a justice, and the court may make orders and exact penalties, just as if the complaint had been made by the sanitary authority.

If the nuisance is then not removed, or is likely to recur, the sanitary authority may apply to a justice, who will require the presence of the person responsible before a court of summary jurisdiction. If satisfied that the nuisance exists, or is likely to recur, the court may at once decern (or decree), or may remit to a special inspector to report. When the court is satisfied of the existence of the nuisance, an order will be granted for its removal, and for the performance of such works as will prevent its recurrence. The court has the further power, if convinced that the nuisance arises from wilful fault or negligence, to fine the author of the nuisance. Where the author is not known, the local authority may be directed to remove the nuisance themselves. Special by-laws are also made by local authorities with reference to their own towns.

Houses and sites for building: The health of the community depends in a large measure on the condition of its housing. Several factors contribute to the healthiness of a dwelling. The site must be suitable, the ventilation and water supply adequate, the construction must ensure the absence of dampness, and the sewage and refuse must be efficiently removed.

Streets and open spaces: Streets not only act as thoroughfares for traffic, but also provide for ventilation and admission of sunlight to buildings, in addition to constituting the course for the main sewers and water-supply pipes. The width of the street is important with reference to the height of the houses along it. Too narrow a street with high buildings implies dingy, dark, ill-ventilated dwellings. Considerable powers have therefore been given to sanitary authorities under the various Public Health Acts to regulate the width of the street, the height of the buildings, and as to repair. More important still is the regulation dealing with the air-space required in the rear of the new house.

Air and ventilation: Pure atmospheric air contains a little over 20 per cent by volume of oxygen, about 78 per cent of nitrogen, and about 0·04 per cent of carbon dioxide, together with traces of water vapour and some inert gases. The carbon dioxide present is generally accepted as the standard of impurity, but this is only a guide. There is no evidence that the discomfort experienced in badly ventilated rooms is due to lack of oxygen or excess of carbon dioxide. It is more closely associated with heat stagnation due to excess of moisture and lack of air movement. The air is naturally purified by winds driving the impurities away and allowing fresher air to take its place; by rain removing dissolved gases and washing away suspended impurities; and by vegetable life absorbing carbon dioxide in the day-time and giving off oxygen. Fogs tend naturally to pollute it. It is vitiated by respiration, combustion, putrefactive processes of animal and vegetable matters, and by the products of trades and industries.

Water and water supplies: An adequate supply of water is necessary for every condition of life. Its importance has been recognized and appreciated from earliest times, and is closely bound up with the industrial activity and progress, as well as the health of communities. The increase in the purity of the supplies of this country has undoubtedly lessened the occurrence of water-borne epidemics of disease.

Refuse and sewage disposal: The subject of refuse and sewage disposal is concerned with removal from towns and from buildings of waste matters. These waste matters consist chiefly of two distinct kinds: the excreta and waste waters, commonly dealt with as one in the sewage (qv); and, secondly, the dry refuse. The dry refuse includes the dust, ashes and debris of vegetable and animal food from households, the sweepings of streets and the dust and mineral particles of trade processes. The liquid and solid excreta and the waste water of houses have to be dealt with in sewage disposal. All the dry refuse is usually removed by dust carts and street sweepers.

Food and disease: Foods are now rigidly inspected. Samples are taken for analysis, and if these are found to be adulterated the vendors or suppliers are prosecuted, and may be heavily punished. At every slaughterhouse, inspection of meat is carried through as a matter of routine, and no meat declared unsound is allowed to be sold. (See also ADULTERATION OF FOOD.)

Infectious diseases are due to the entrance into the body of certain bacteria or their toxins, or of viruses which multiply in the system, and can be given off from the person affected, and thus may be received into the body of other individuals, in whom they may reproduce the disease. Hence the diseases are known as infectious diseases.

The infectious diseases may be spread from a person in various ways.

1. By the breath, as, for example, in scarlet fever, measles and whooping-cough. In many cases the expired air gathers its infection from the throat.

2. By particles of skin and the dried purulent crusts of smallpox.

3. By excretions and secretions. The discharges from the throat and nose are highly infectious in scarlet fever, diphtheria and measles. The faecal excretions in enteric fever and cholera contain the infection. The purulent discharges of abscesses and pustules in certain diseases carry infection. The sputum of tuberculous patients contains the tubercle bacillus, or *Mycobacterium tuberculosis* as it is now known. The urine in enteric fever is infected, and can convey the disease. Milk, water and foods are often infected by excretions, defects in the drains allowing the excretions to soak through and infect the waters of wells, or the water used in washing and cleaning conveys the infection to the utensils in which the milk is received and the food cooked. These articles of diet may also be infected by direct contact with the excretions of a carelessly treated patient, resulting in localized epidemics of infectious disease. Contamination of food often occurs through the medium of flies. (See INSECTS IN RELATION TO DISEASE.)

If the person is susceptible to the disease, a period elapses after the organism is received, known as the incubation period, during which no symptoms develop, but during which the organism multiplies and produces its poison. This period varies with each disease. (See INCUBATION; INFECTION.)

METHODS OF PREVENTION may embrace removal of cases to hospital or isolation at home; disinfection of clothing, bedding and premises; isolation, if necessary, of persons who have been in contact with certain diseases; closure of schools if the disease is being spread by the school connection (see INFECTION); stoppage of milk supplies if these are infected, and injection of protective sera, as in those exposed to diphtheria, and the performance of vaccination upon persons who have come in contact with cases of smallpox.

Disinfection and disinfectants: Disinfection consists in the destruction of the organisms or other agencies of disease. It is accomplished by means of disinfectants, of which sunlight, fresh air and fire are the most efficient and natural. During epidemics, milk or water, if suspected of being infected, should be boiled. All cloths and the like, used to clean up discharges from infectious cases should, if possible, be destroyed, whilst, if the bedding and clothing are totally worthless or in a wretched condition, they may also be burned. Many of the ordinary disinfectants, though containing disinfectant materials, are used in such strength as only to act as deodorants, and so, while removing the noxious odours, particularly of excreta, do not destroy the infecting material and consequently give only a false sense of security. For the varieties and uses of disinfectants see DISINFECTION.

Radioactivity: There are stringent legislative controls on the transport, keeping and use of radioactive sources and materials and in the disposal of radioactive wastes. Premises in which such sources and materials are kept are required to be registered by the Secretary of State for the Environment under the Radioactive Substances Act, 1960, and the use of sources is controlled by the Ionising Radiation Regulations, 1968 and 1969.

Disposal of the dead: The chief object in the disposal of the dead is the speediest method by which the body can be dissolved into its simplest components. Two methods are in vogue in Britain: burial and cremation.

BURIAL, from a sanitary point of view, should take place in a loamy or sandy porous soil, well drained, and so situated as not to contaminate any water supply, and preferably removed from the neighbourhood of houses. The body should be confined in a thin, easily disintegrated coffin. Oak and lead coffins and brick vaults all violate the first principles of burial.

CREMATION is, perhaps, the best sanitary method of disposal, especially in cases of infectious disease, the germs of some of which can exist in the soil. The sanitary reason for it is powerful, but its adoption prevents the possibility of exhumation, and so might occasionally prevent the detection of crime. (For further details, see DEAD, DISPOSAL OF.)

SAPHENOUS is the name given to the two large superficial veins of the leg. The small saphenous vein which runs up the outside and back of the leg joins the deep veins at the bend of the knee; the great saphenous vein, the longest vein in the body, which has a long course from the inner ankle to the groin, is specially subject, with its branches, to become the site of varicose veins.

SAPO is the Latin name for soap.

SAPROPHYTE is the term applied to organisms which live usually upon decaying and dead matter and produce its decomposition.

SARCINA is a microscopic vegetable growth, which is found in the material vomited or drawn off by the stomach tube from a dilated stomach.

SARCO- is a prefix signifying flesh or fleshy.

SARCOIDOSIS is a chronic disease of unknown origin. It involves the skin, lymph nodes, eyes, salivary glands, lungs, heart and bones of the hands and feet. The Kveim Test is used to confirm the diagnosis. The disease is usually self limiting but occasionally treatment with corticosteroids is required.

SARCOMA (see CANCER.

SARCOPTES SCABIEI is the mite which causes scabies (qv).

SARSAPARILLA is the root of various species of *Smilax*. It is used in domestic medicine as a 'blood-purifier', and is an ingredient of many patent medicines. Its main use today is as a flavouring agent.

SASSAFRAS is a genus of laurel trees. The root bark of *Sassafras albidum* contains an oil, and its fluid extract was formerly much used in the treatment of various skin diseases. Mucilage derived from sassafras is also used in brochial and gastric affections.

SAUNA is a hot-air, steam or smoke bath, combined with ice-cold water bathing or douching. An old Finnish practice, practically every house or block of flats there has its sauna. Originally, these log cabins were heated by wood-burning stoves made of rough stones, but the modern sauna has an electric oven surrounded by stones. The sauna cabin has a tightly fitting door and narrow vents in the walls, but no windows. The bathers sit or lie naked, according to their preferences, on wooden benches. Before entering the sauna, with its temperature of 110°F, a cold shower is taken. Periodically the bathers come out and plunge into a nearby ice-cold lake or have another cold shower. At some stage of the sauna massage is given, or alternatively the bathers beat each other with birch twigs. After this a further session is spent in the heat, and the course ends with a cold bath. The bather should rest for twenty minutes or until he has ceased to sweat before beginning to dress. The precise therapeutic value of saunas may not be clear, though the Finns claim that they are a well-proven means of maintaining health. There is some evidence that they may be good for the skin, the upper air passages, weight reduction, and for the relief of rheumatic pains.

SCAB is the crust which forms on superficial injured areas. It is composed of fibrin, which is exuded from the raw surface, together with blood corpuscles and epithelial cells entangled in its meshes. Healing takes place naturally under this protection, and the scab dries up and falls off when healing is complete. Scabs appearing on the face without any previous abrasion are often of infectious nature. (See IMPETIGO.)

SCABIES is a skin disease caused by the *Sarcoptes scabiei* which resembles the cheese mite in appearance. It is a minute oval-shaped mite possessing four pairs of legs. It is just visible to the naked eye, the female measuring about 250 to 350 micrometres in length; the male is smaller. The female burrows in the skin, particularly that on the front of the wrist, the web and sides of the fingers, the buttocks, the genitals, and the feet, forming small tunnels in which she lays her eggs (25 to 30). The sides and legs may also be affected in the same way, though rarely the upper parts of the body. The eggs hatch in the burrows in four to five days, and it is the movement of the larvae which causes the intense itching which gives scabies its popular name of itch. The scratching caused by this itching is responsible for much of the eruption of scabies. The larvae ultimately leave the burrows and develop in the skin, a female becoming mature in about two weeks.

Scabies is rife among the population of Great Britain. Personal contact is the most important factor in keeping this infestation going. This is why it is so important that all members of a household in which a case occurs should be carefully examined, and treated if found to be infected. Less stress is now laid on dissemination of the mite by infested clothes and blankets.

Symptoms: The person complains of great itchiness and heat, felt particularly soon after he goes to bed, and preventing sleep in the early part of the night. The spaces between the fingers, the backs of the hands, and the front of the wrists are red and scabbed as the result of scratching, or the surface in these localities may even be much inflamed.

Treatment: The patient is scrubbed with soft soap in a hot bath, to open up the burrows. Immediately after drying, the official *British Pharmacopoeia* 25 per cent preparation of benzyl benzoate, known as Benzyl Benzoate Application BP, is applied to the whole surface of the body below the chin. A second and a third application is made at twelve-hourly intervals. The patient then has a bath, puts on clean underclothes, and has his bed clothes changed. In infants and young children, in whom benzyl benzoate may cause unpleasant stinging, monosulfiram or 1 per cent gamma benzene hexachloride may be used as an alternative.

SCALD HEAD is the old name for favus. (See RINGWORM.)

SCALDS (see BURNS AND SCALDS).

SCALP is the soft covering of the skull on the top of the head. It consists of five layers, which from the surface inwards are as follows: the skin, thickly furnished with hair; next a subcutaneous layer of fat, rendered tough and stringy by many bands of fibrous tissue passing through it to bind the skin and the third layer together; thirdly, a tough membrane composed of fibrous tissue, known as the epicranium; fourthly, a loose layer of connective tissue attaching the epicranium to the deepest layer, and permitting the free movements of which the scalp is capable; and, finally, another fibrous layer clinging closely to the skull, and known as the pericranium.

SCALPEL is a small, straight, surgical knife.

SCAPULA is the technical name for the shoulder-blade. (See SHOULDER-BLADE.)

SCAR is the name applied to a healed wound, ulcer or breach of tissue. A scar consists essentially of fibrous tissue, covered by an imperfect formation of epidermis in the case of scars on the surface of the skin. The fibrous tissue is produced by the connective tissue corpuscles that wander into the wound in the course of its repair (see WOUNDS), and is at first delicate in texture and richly provided with blood-vessels. Accordingly a scar at first is soft, and has a redder tint than the surrounding skin. Gradually this fibrous tissue contracts, becomes more dense, and loses its blood-vessels, so that an old scar is hard and white.

The more specialized textures are not repaired when a scar forms: thus on the skin-surface the scar does not reproduce hairs and sweat-glands, only the general epithelium growing over the wounded surface. Similarly in the case of internal organs, such as the stomach, no glands form in the scar. When muscles or nerves are wounded, however, new muscle- or nerve-fibres grow into the scar. Bone is repaired by a formation of fibrous tissue, which is produced just as in the soft parts, and later lime salts are deposited in the scars. (See BONE.)

The contraction that takes place in a scar has already been mentioned. The more quickly the surfaces of a wound are brought into contact with one another, the less fibrous tissue is produced for the union. Consequently a wound whose edges are accurately brought together and in which healing is rapid shows far less contraction afterwards, and leaves a fainter scar, than one in which the wound is allowed to gape, and in which healing is slow. Burns are therefore followed by very marked scars and great contraction, which often produces marked deformity of the part concerned. Similarly, when inflammation takes place, as when an operation wound becomes infected, or when such a disease as lupus is present, causing great irritation of the wound, a wide, unsightly scar results and causes much puckering of the surrounding skin as it contracts. Such scars are also of low vitality, stretch easily, so as to become still more evident, and if irritated, as, for example, by the pressure of a boot or badly fitting artificial limb, readily give way and produce an ulcer which is slow to heal. Unsightly scars, on the face for example, can often be removed by the plastic surgeon.

Scars are sometimes extremely painful, especially those which are left after the amputation of part of a limb. This is caused in general by the involvement of a sensory nerve in the hard contracting tissue of the scar. (See also KELOID.)

SCARIFICATION means the making of shallow cuts in the skin for the purpose of drawing blood.

SCARLET FEVER is caused by the erythrogenic toxin of the streptococcus. The symptoms of pyrexia, headache, vomiting and a punctate erythematous rash follow a streptococcal infection of the throat or even a wound. The rash is symmetrical and does not itch. The skin subsequently peels. In the latter half of the 19th century it was the commonest cause of death in children over the age of one year. The mortality was already decreasing by the year 1900 and had virtually ceased by 1965.

Symptoms: The period of incubation (ie. the time elapsing between the reception of infection and the development of symptoms) varies somewhat. In most cases it lasts only two to three days, but in occasional cases the patient may take a week to develop his first symptoms. The invasion of fever is usually short and sharp, with rapid rise of temperature to 40°C (104°F) or thereabouts in the first few hours. There also occur shivering, vomiting, headache, sore throat and marked increase in the rate of the pulse. In young children convulsions or delirium may also usher in the fever. The rash usually appears within 24 hours of the onset of fever. It is first seen on the neck, chest, arms and hands, but quickly spreads all over the body and legs. The rash consists of minute, thickly set, red points which coalesce to form a general redness. The rash tends to avoid the region of the nose and lips (circumoral pallor). Sometimes the redness is accompanied by small vesicles containing fluid. The rash is at its height in about two days and then begins to fade, being gone at the end of a week from its first appearance. The tongue at first is covered by thick, white, creamy fur through which, on the second day, red papillae project, giving the appearance of a white strawberry tongue. The fur is then gradually denuded, and by the fourth or fifth day the tongue is red, bare and glazed – red strawberry tongue. The interior of the throat is red and swollen, especially the uvula, soft palate and tonsils, and a considerable amount of secretion is found on the inflamed surfaces. The glands under the jaw are slightly swollen and tender. In favourable cases the fever falls distinctly about the third day, the symptoms at the same time rapidly improve and the rash fades. The throat becomes more comfortable, and peeling of the skin shows itself first about the cheeks and neck, and later spreads all over the surface of the body. The amount of peeling varies widely, and to a certain extent it tends to be worst in the more severe cases. In the mild cases being encountered in Britain today it is very slight.

Complications: The most common and serious of these is *inflammation of the kidneys*, or *glomerulonephritis*, which may arise during any period in the course of the fever, but is specially apt to appear in convalescence, while desquamation is in progress. Its onset is sometimes announced by a return of feverish symptoms, accompanied with vomiting and pain in the loins; but it often occurs insidiously. One of the most prominent symptoms is slight swelling of the face, particularly of the eyelids, which is rarely absent in this complication. The urine is diminished in quantity and of dark smoky or red appearance, due to the presence of blood and contains albumin. Microscopic examination reveals the presence of tube casts containing blood and epithelium. In favourable cases these symptoms may soon disappear, but they may, on the other hand, prove extremely serious – the risks being the suppression of urine, leading to uraemic poisoning and causing convulsions which may terminate fatally, or the rapid development of general dropsy, and death from this cause. If this complication ensues, it commonly does so about the third or fourth week after the beginning of the illness. Occasionally this condition does not wholly pass off, and consequently lays the foundation for chronic glomerulonephritis. (See GLOMERULONEPHRITIS.) Another complication is *suppuration of the ears*, due to the extension of the inflamatory process from the throat along the Eustachian tube into the middle ear. (See EAR, DISEASES OF.) Other maladies affecting the heart and lungs occasionally arise in connection with scarlet fever, the chief of these being *endocarditis*, which may lay the foundation of valvular disease of the heart later in life. Arthritis or *scarlatinal rheumatism* is another complication of the disease, producing swelling and pain in the smaller rather than in the larger joints. This complication usually occurs in the second week of illness.

Treatment: In view of the mild type of scarlet fever at present prevailing there is a tendency in Great Britain not to admit such cases to hospital unless they are particularly severe, the home conditions are unsatisfactory, or there is some risk to the public: eg. a member of the household works in a dairy and may therefore be responsible for infecting milk. Children who have been in contact with cases of scarlet fever are allowed to go to school provided they are sent home at the first suggestion of fever or malaise.

When the patient is treated at home, the sick-room should contain only such furniture as may be required, and the attendants should come as little as possible in contact with other members of the household. It is usual to keep the patient in bed for two weeks from the onset of the disease. All body or bed linen when removed should be placed at once in boiling water, or in some disinfecting fluid. All books, toys, etc., used by the patient during the illness should be destroyed if of no value, or alternatively, carefully disinfected. The chief sources of contagion are the discharges of ear, nose, and throat. The desquamating skin is not infectious.

As scarlet fever is predominantly a streptococcal infection, the sulphonamide drugs or penicillin should be given. Preference is now generally shown for penicillin, and this should be given in every case. As to general management during the progress of the fever, in favourable cases little is required beyond careful nursing and feeding. The diet should be light but nourishing, consisting mainly of milk foods. During the febrile stage plenty of fluid must be taken, which can be flavoured with fruit juices.

The treatment of the kidney complication is similar to that for acute glomerulonephritis. The management of the sore throat, enlarged glands and joint affections, is conducted on general principles.

SCHISTOSOMIASIS, also known as BILHARZIASIS, is one of the most important diseases in the tropics. The estimated global incidence is 200 million cases. The responsible parasites, *schistosomes* or blood flukes, which are responsible for the disease, occur in Egypt, the Middle East, many parts of tropical Africa, the Far East, and South America. The male is about 12 millimetres long. The female, which is about 24 millimetres in length, lies partly enclosed in a groove down the body of the male. The ova, or eggs, are provided with a sharp spike which is terminal in *S. haematobium* and lateral in *S. mansoni*. The schistosomes live in the portal vein and its branches. The ova ultimately reach either the bladder (*S. haematobium*) or the rectum (*S. mansoni* and *S. japonicum*), whence they are voided in the urine or faeces. The next stage of development takes place in certain snails. Human infection occurs by wading or bathing in infected water, the infection occurring through the skin, whence the immature schistosome ultimately reaches the portal vein.
SCHISTOSOMA HAEMATOBIUM is widely distributed throughout North Africa, including Egypt, East Africa, and South Africa. It is also found in the Middle East, Portugal and Cyprus. As the ova are excreted through the bladder, the main symptoms are cystitis and haematuria (ie. the passage of blood in the urine). In chronic cases there may be formation of stones in the bladder, and sometimes cancer develops in the bladder.
SCHISTOSOMA MANSONI is found predominantly in the Nile valley, East Africa, and West Africa. It is also found in Israel, Yemen, Central and South America and the Caribbean Islands. As the ova are mainly excreted through the rectum, the first manifestation of the disease is usually diarrhoea, with the passage of much blood in the stools. As with *S. haematobium* infections, there is often irritation of the skin or dermatitis, and there is always some anaemia, which may become severe. The spleen usually becomes enlarged, sometimes to a very considerable extent.
SCHISTOSOMA JAPONICUM is confined to the Far East, particularly the Yangtse valley, and South East Asia, particularly Indonesia. Here again the ova are found in the rectum, and the main manifestations of the infection are chronic dysentery, enlargement of the liver and the spleen, and anaemia.
Treatment: While prevention is the ideal way of coping with the disease, this is often difficult in practice. Drugs used in treating the disease include various preparations, such as metriphonate for *S. haematobium* infections, oxamniquine for *S. mansoni* infections, and praziquantel which is active against all three varieties.

SCHISTOSOME DERMATITIS (see BATHER'S ITCH).

SCHIZO- is a prefix signifying splitting.

SCHIZOPHRENIA (See MENTAL ILLNESS.)

SCHOTT TREATMENT is a system of treatment devised by a German physician for people suffering from disorders of the heart. The treatment is specially carried out at Nauheim in Germany, and consists in a combination of baths in spring-water containing brine or carbonic acid gas, with carefully graduated exercises, and suitable rules for the guidance of the daily life.

SCIATICA means pain in the distribution of the sciatic nerve. It is often accompanied by pain in the back, or lumbago. It may be due to a number of causes, such as a tumour in the spine or spinal column, tuberculosis of the spine, ankylosing spondylitis, (see SPINE, DISEASES AND INJURIES OF) or a tumour in one of the organs in the pelvis such as the uterus. In the majority of cases, however, it is due to a prolapsed intervertebral disc (qv) pressing on one or more of the nerve roots issuing from the lower part of the spinal cord that make up the sciatic nerve. The precise distribution of the pain will thus depend on which of the nerve roots are affected. As a rule, the pain is felt in the buttock, the back of the thigh and the outside and front of the leg, sometimes extending on to the top of the foot. In other cases the pain is felt in the buttock, the back of the thigh and the calf, and then along the outer border of the foot towards the little toe. What probably happens is that degenerative changes take place in the annulus fibrosus. (See SPINAL COLUMN.) Ultimately this ruptures, either as a result of some special strain such as is induced by heavy lifting, or spontaneously. The cushioning disc between the two neighbouring vertebral bodies slips through the rent in the annulus fibrosus, and presses on the neighbouring roots, thus causing the pain.

The condition usually occurs in adults under the age of 60. The pain may come on suddenly when the person concerned is undertaking some unusual effort, such as heavy lifting, and may be so severe that the victim faints and, when he comes to, he may be locked in one position. More commonly it comes on gradually and keeps on recurring over long periods of time. In these cases the amount of pain varies tremendously: from little more than a recurrent nuisance to a pain of almost unbearable intensity.

Treatment consists essentially of rest in bed in the early stages until the acute phase is over. Boards should be placed underneath the mattress to ensure adequate support for the back. Alternatively, the mattress may be put on the floor for the patient to sleep on. Anodynes, such as aspirin and codeine, are given to relieve the pain. A few days' rest in bed at the beginning of the trouble probably reduces the risk of further trouble. Expert opinion varies as to the desirability of wearing a plaster of Paris jacket or a specially made corset. Some contend that such support is advisable. Others contend that it is seldom necessary. Certainly a corset of this type is uncomfortable to wear, and there is a tendency for some victims of the disease to become too dependent on it. Equally, opinion differs as to the desirability of manipulation of the spine and operation. By and large the tendency in recent years has been for a reduction in the number of operations performed for prolapsed intervertebral disc.

SCIRRHUS is a hard form of cancer in which much fibrous tissue develops.

SCLERA (see EYE).

SCLERITIS (see EYE, DISEASE AND INJURIES).

SCLERODERMA is a condition in which the skin becomes hard –like leather – causing stiffening of the joints, and leading to gradual wasting of the muscles.

SCLEROSIS means literally hardening, and is a term applied to conditions in which portions of organs become hard and useless as the result of an excessive production of connective tissue. The term is especially applied to a change of this type taking place in the nervous system. (See MULTIPLE SCLEROSIS.) When a change of this nature takes place in other organs it is generally known as cirrhosis or fibrosis. (See CIRRHOSIS.) These conditions are generally attributed to some form of chronic inflammation.

SCOLIOSIS is the name applied to curvature of the spine consisting partly of a bend to one side, partly of a rotary twist. It may result from disease of the spine, but in weakly children it may arise from so slight a cause as a bad habit in standing or in leaning one arm on the table at lessons. It also arises from disease affecting one side of the chest, such as chronic pleurisy or tuberculosis. (See SPINE, DISEASES OF.)

SCOPARIUM is the tops of *Cytisus scoparius*, the common broom. It has a diuretic action.

SCOTOMA: An area of blindness in the field of vision.

SCRIVENER'S PALSY is another name for writer's cramp. (See CRAMP.)

SCROFULA, or STRUMA, is a state of constitutional weakness, generally exhibiting itself in early life, and characterized mainly by defective nutrition of the tissues, which renders them a ready prey to tuberculosis. The condition, as it manifests itself in disease of the glands in the neck, was formerly known in England as 'king's evil', from the belief that the touch of the sovereign could effect a cure. This superstition can be traced back to the time of Edward the Confessor in England, and to a much earlier period in France. Samuel Johnson was touched by Queen Anne in 1712, and the same supposed prerogative of royalty was exercised by Prince Charles Edward in 1745.

SCROMBOTOXIN POISONING occurs from eating poorly preserved scromboid fish such as tuna, mackerel and other members of the mackerel family. In such fish, a toxic histamine-like substance is produced by the action of bacteria or histidine, a normal component of fish flesh. This toxin produces nausea, vomiting, headache, upper abdominal pain, difficulty in swallowing, thirst, pruritus (qv) and sometimes urticaria (qv). The condition settles as a rule in 12 hours. Antihistamine drugs (qv) are sometimes of value in ameliorating the condition.

SCROTUM is the pouch of integument within which the testicles are suspended. It consists of a purse-like fold of skin, within which each testicle has a separate investment of muscle fibres, several layers of fibrous tissue, and a serous membrane known as the tunica vaginalis.

SCRUM-POX, or PROP-POX, is a popular name for a contagious affection of the face affecting Rugby football players. It is most likely to occur in forwards as a result of face-to-face contact with cases in the opposing side of the scrum. In one recent investigation, 47 of 48 cases were forwards. Other possible sources of infection are changing rooms and communal baths. The condition may take the form of impetigo (qv) or herpes simplex (qv).

SCURF, or DANDRUFF, is a popular name for the scaly condition that is often found on the scalp, and often precedes baldness. (See SEBORRHOEA.)

SCURVY, or SCORBUTUS, is a deficiency disease characterized by the occurrence of extravasations of blood in the tissues of the body, and due to an insufficiency of vitamin C, or ascorbic acid, in the diet.

Causes: In former times this disease was extremely common among sailors, and was responsible for a high mortality rate. It is now of rare occurrence at sea, its cause being well understood and its prevention readily secured by simple measures. Scurvy has also frequently broken out among soldiers on campaign, in beleaguered cities, as well as among communities in times of scarcity, and in prisons, workhouses and other public institutions. In all such instances it has been found to depend closely upon the character and amount of the food, the occurrence of serious illness, and a diet too limited, either in amount or variety. These conditions predispose to scurvy, but the essential cause lies in deprivation of fresh food and especially of fresh vegetables for a period of four to six months. The want of vitamin C, which is soluble in water and is found chiefly in citrus fruits, potatoes, green vegetables and black currants, is the essential deficient factor. Besides this essential defect, a diminution in the total amount of food, the large use of salted meat or fish, and all causes of a depressing kind, such as exposure, anxiety, bad hygiene, will contribute to the development of the disease.

Infants, too, may suffer from scurvy as the result of insufficiency of vitamin C in the diet.

Symptoms: The symptoms of scurvy come on gradually, and its onset is not marked by any special indications beyond a certain failure of strength, most manifest on making efforts. Breathlessness and exhaustion are thus easily induced, and there exists a corresponding mental depression. The countenance acquires a sallow or dusky hue; the gums are tender and the breath offensive almost from the first. These preliminary symptoms may continue for weeks, and in isolated cases may readily escape notice, but can scarcely fail to attract attention where they affect large numbers of men. Later the gums are livid, spongy, ulcerating and bleeding; the teeth are loosened and drop out; and the breath is excessively foetid. Extravasations of blood now take place in the skin and elsewhere. These may be small, like the petechial spots of purpura (qv), but are often large, and cause swellings of the muscles in which they occur, having the appearance of extensive bruises, and tending to become hard and brawny. These extravasations are most common in the muscles of the lower limbs; but they may be formed anywhere, and may easily be produced by very slight pressure upon the skin or by injuries to it. Bleeding into joints is a troublesome symptom because it produces stiffness later. In addition, there are bleedings from mucous membranes, such as those of the nose, eyes and alimentary or respiratory tracts, whilst effusions of fluid take place into the pleural, pericardial or peritoneal cavity. Painful, extensive, and destructive ulcers are apt to break out on the limbs. There is also a considerable amount of anaemia. The further progress of the malady is marked by profound exhaustion, with a tendency to fainting, and with various complications, such as diarrhoea and lung or kidney troubles, any of which may bring about a fatal result. On the other hand, even in desperate cases, recovery may be hopefully anticipated when the appropriate remedy can be obtained.

Treatment: No disease is more amenable to treatment, both as regards prevention and cure, than scurvy. This consists of the administration of vitamin C in adequate amounts, either in the form of tablets of ascorbic acid or foodstuffs rich in this vitamin. Potatoes, cabbages, tomatoes, swede turnips, many fresh fruits, especially black currants, oranges, grapefruit and lemons, are of great service for this purpose. Orange-juice or lemon-juice is often employed, either fresh or canned. The use, in a fresh state, of lime-juice in the British Navy, which has been practised since 1795, had the effect of virtually extinguishing scurvy in the Service, whilst similar regulations introduced by the British Board of Trade in 1865 had a like beneficial result in the mercantile marine. It is only when these regulations have not been fully carried out, or when the supply of lime-juice has become exhausted, that scurvy among sailors has been noticed in recent times. The anaemia and debility are best overcome by the continued administration of iron, aided by fresh air and other measures calculated to promote the general health.

SCYBALA is the name applied to the extremely hard condition which the stools assume in aggravated constipation.

SEA-SICKNESS is a characteristic set of symptoms experienced by many people when subjected to the pitching and rolling motion of a vessel at sea, of which depression, giddiness, nausea and vomiting are the most prominent.

Causes: Although the vast majority of people appear to be liable to this ailment at sea, they do not all suffer alike. Many endure distress of a most acute and even alarming kind, whilst others are simply conscious of transient feelings of nausea and discomfort. In long voyages, whilst many are affected with sea-sickness for the first few days only, others are tormented with it during the entire period, especially on the occurrence of rough weather. In short voyages, such as across the English Channel, not a few, of those susceptible, escape, whilst others suffer in an extreme degree, the sickness persisting long after arrival on shore.

A great number of theories have been advanced to account for the connection between the motion of a ship and sea-sickness. The conditions concerned in the production of the malady are apparently of complex character, embracing more than one set of causes. In the first place, the rolling or heaving of the vessel disturbs that feeling of the relation of the body to surrounding objects upon which our sense of security rests. The nervous system being thus subjected to a succession of shocks or surprises fails to effect the necessary adjustments for equilibrium. Giddiness, nausea and vomiting follow. Much importance has been laid by some upon the effects of the displacement of the abdominal viscera, especially the stomach, by the rolling of the vessel; but, while this may possibly operate to some extent, it can only be as an accessory cause. The same may be said of the influence of the changing impressions made upon the vision – which has been regarded by some as so powerful in the matter – since attacks of sea-sickness occur also in the dark, and in the case of blind persons. Other contributory causes may be mentioned, such as the feeling that sickness is certain to come, which may bring on the attack even before the vessel has begun to move. The sense of the body being in a liquid or yielding medium as it descends with the vessel into the trough of the sea, the varied odours to be met with on board ship, and circumstances of a like nature, tend also to precipitate or aggravate an attack. In the few rare instances where sea-sickness has proved fatal, *post-mortem* appearances have been almost entirely negative, and only such as are met with in death from syncope.

Symptoms: The symptoms generally show themselves soon after the vessel has begun to roll, by the onset of giddiness and discomfort in the head, together with a sense of nausea and sinking at the stomach, which soon develops into intense sickness and vomiting. At first the contents of the stomach only are ejected; but thereafter bilious matter, and occasionally even blood, are brought up by the violence of the retching. The vomiting is liable to exacerbations according to the amount of oscillation of the ship; but seasons of rest, sometimes admitting of sleep, occasionally intervene. Along with the sickness there is great physical prostration, as shown in the pallor of the skin, cold sweats and feeble pulse, accompanied with mental depression and wretchedness. In almost all instances the attack has a favourable termination, and it is extremely rare that serious results arise, except in the case of persons weakened by other diseases, although occasionally the symptoms are for a time sufficiently alarming.

Treatment: Innumerable preventives and remedies have been proposed, but most of them fall far short of the success claimed for them. No means has yet been discovered which can altogether prevent the occurrence of sea-sickness, nor is it likely any will be found, since it is largely due to the pitching movements of the vessel, which cannot be averted. Swinging couches or chambers have not proved of any practical utility. No doubt there is less risk of sickness in a large and well-ballasted vessel than in a small one; but, even though the rolling may be considerably modified, the ascending and descending movements which so readily produce nausea continue. None of the medicinal agents proposed possesses infallible properties; a remedy which suits one person will often wholly fail with another. Experience gained during the 1939–45 War has shown that the most satisfactory remedy is hyoscine hydrobromide, 0·6 to 0·3 mg. Other drugs which are proving of value in the prevention of sea-sickness include avomine, dramamine, ginger and marzine.

When the vessel is in motion, or even before starting, the recumbent position with the head low and the eyes closed (so that the motion of the ship and sea cannot be seen) should be assumed by those at all likely to suffer, and, should the weather admit, on deck rather than below – the body, especially the extremities, being well covered. Many people, however, find comfort and relief from lying down in their berths with a hot bottle to the feet, by which means sleep may be obtained, and with it a temporary abatement of the distressing giddiness and nausea. Individuals who tend to be constipated should ensure an adequate evacuation of the bowels before embarking. Should sickness supervene, small quantities of some light food ought to be swallowed if possible, in order to lessen the sense of exhaustion, which is often extreme, as well as to mitigate the pain or retching by giving the stomach something upon which it can contract. Alcohol usually tends to aggravate the sickness, but brandy has long had a reputation as a useful means of treatment in the early stages.

SEAT-WORM is another name for thread-worm. (See ENTEROBIASIS).

SEBACEOUS CYST is the term applied to a cyst in the skin formed as a result of blockage of the duct of a sebaceous gland.

SEBACEOUS GLANDS are the minute glands situated alongside of hairs and opening into the follicles of the latter a short distance below the point at which the hairs emerge on the surface. These glands secrete an oily material, and are especially large upon the nose, where their openings form pits that are easily visible. Some varieties of eczema, as well as acne, result from disorders of these glands. (See SKIN.)

SEBORRHOEA is a group of diseases of the skin in which the sebaceous or oil-forming glands are at fault. It manifests itself either by accumulation of dry scurf, or by the formation of an excessive oily deposit on an otherwise healthy skin.

Seborrhoeic dermatitis (or **eczema**), which is also known as SEBORRHOEA CAPITIS, is the form of seborrhoea which involves the scalp. In its mildest form it is little more than an exaggeration of the normal casting off of the superficial layers of the skin of the scalp (see SKIN), which manifests itself as the white scales popularly known as dandruff or scurf. In the more severe cases the amount of scaling is increased and is accompanied by redness of the scalp. This in turn may progress to such a stage that it is accompanied by a profuse discharge, sufficient to soak the victim's pillow at night. In these more severe cases the condition may spread to the forehead, eyebrows and back of the neck. There may indeed be involvement of these sites with minimal scalp disease.

Treatment in the milder cases consists of washing the hair twice weekly with spirit soap or a soapless shampoo. Shampoos containing tar extracts, for example Polytar, may be useful and they are also used to treat psoriasis of the scalp. Selenium sulphide shampoos are also of benefit, though no more so than others. In more severe cases, lotions containing combinations of corticosteroids and salicylic or salicylic acid and sulphur are effective.

SEBUM is the secretion of the sebaceous glands (qv). It acts as a natural lubricant of the hair and skin and protects the skin from the effects of moisture or excessive dryness. It may also have antibacterial action.

SECRETIN is a hormone secreted by the mucous membrane of the duodenum, the first part of the small intestine, when food comes in contact with it. On being carried by the blood to the pancreas, it stimulates the secretion of pancreatic juice.

SECRETION is the term applied to the material formed by a gland as the result of its activity. For example, saliva is the secretion of the salivary glands, gastric juice that of the glands in the stomach wall, bile that of the liver. (See GLANDS.) Some secretions consist apparently of waste material which is of no further use in the chemistry of the body. These secretions are often spoken of as excretions: for example, the urine and the sweat. (For further details, see SALIVA; URINE; ENDOCRINE GLANDS, and also under the headings of the various organs.)

SECUNDINES is another name for the afterbirth, consisting of the placenta and membranes expelled in the final stage of labour.

SECUNDUM ARTEM is a Latin expression meaning in a skilful professional manner.

SEDATIVES are drugs and other measures which soothe over-excitement of the nervous system, whether the effect of this excitement is pain, sleeplessness, delirium or muscular spasm. Those sedatives that soothe pain are generally spoken of as anodynes; sedatives in sleeplessness or delirium are known as hypnotics; sedatives of spasm are called antispasmodics. (See ANODYNES; COLIC; HEADACHE; HYPNOTICS; NEURALGIA; PAIN.)

SEDIMENTATION RATE, or ERYTHROCYTE SEDIMENTATION RATE to give it its full title, is a test for measuring the activity and progress of certain diseases. If blood is drawn and put into a test-tube the red blood corpuscles sink and leave a clear layer above. In disease the rate of sinking is increased and can be measured. The more active the disease, the higher the rate of sinking of red blood corpuscles.

SEIDLITZ POWDER, or COMPOUND EFFERVESCENT POWDER, is a mild purgative composed of Rochelle salt and bicarbonate of soda, which are wrapped together in a blue paper, and tartaric acid, which is wrapped in a white paper. The contents of each paper are dissolved separately in half a tumblerful or less of water; the two solutions are mixed and swallowed while effervescing.

SELENIUM SULPHIDE is used as a shampoo in the treatment of dandruff (qv) and seborrhoeic eczema (or dermatitis) of the scalp. In view of its potential toxicity it should only be used under medical supervision. It must never be applied to inflamed areas of the scalp, and it must not be allowed to get into the eyes, as it may cause conjunctivitis or keratitis. It is also used in the treatment of tinea versicolor. (See RINGWORM.)

SELF-POISONING has increased dramatically over the past 30 years and is now one of the commonest causes of acute admission to hospital. Drugs are usually taken in overdosage on impulse because of a crisis in coping with social or personal difficulties and most patients have previously been prescribed psychotrophic drugs. It is predominently a disease of young people, the mean age being in the 30s with a peak incidence in the 20s. There is a higher incidence of female patients. Despite the fact that 98 per cent of patients admitted with drug overdosage will recover, there were 1,875 deaths from suicide by overdose in 1984. There have been changes in the types of drugs used in deliberate self-poisoning. In 1962 barbiturates were used in 55 per cent of episodes whereas by 1977 they only accounted for 13 per cent. The benzodiazapines are now the most common drug used. The incidence of salicylate poisoning has declined but overdosage with paracetamol has become more common.

Admission to hospital for self-poisoning reached its peak in 1977 and the figures have been falling steadily almost every year since then. This is also true of the number of fatal suicidal poisonings. There may be more than one explanation for this decrease but the most likely cause is that since 1976 the annual number of prescriptions for hypnotics and tranquillisers have also fallen steadily. The tranquillisers which are so popular for overdoses are prescribed for the very patients who are most likely to wish to poison themselves. There was, in fact, a parallel decrease in the rate of carbon monoxide poisoning when carbon monoxide was removed from domestic gas.

Treatment: Emptying the stomach by gastric lavage is sometimes necessary but the risks of this procedure must be balanced against the toxicity of the ingested poison. The danger of gastric aspiration is the inhalation of stomach contents and it should not be attempted in drowsy patients unless there is good cough reflex or unless the airway can be protected by a cuffed tube. A tube should not be passed after corrosive poisoning. Emptying the stomach by gastric lavage is of doubtful value more than four hours after ingestion of a poison. There are, however, two exceptions, namely salicylates and tricyclic antidepressants. Salicylates may be recovered up to 24 hours and tricyclic antidepressants up to 8 hours after ingestion. Gastric lavage is seldom practical or desirable before the patient reaches hospital.

The more common poisons seen today include the amphetamine-related drugs, aspirin and other salicylates, tranquillisers, iron salts, lithium salts, morphine, paracetamol, phenothiazines, tricyclic antidepressants, carbon monoxide, paraquat and organophosphorus insecticides.

SELLA TURCICA is the deep hollow on the upper surface of the sphenoid bone in which the pituitary gland (qv) is enclosed.

SEMEIOLOGY is the part of medical science dealing with the symptoms and signs of disease.

SEMEN is the richly albuminous fluid in which spermatozoa are suspended.

SEMILUNAR CARTILAGES are two crescentic layers of fibro-cartilage on the outer and inner edges of the knee-joint, which form hollows on the upper surface of the tibia in which the condyles at the lower end of the femur rest. The inner cartilage is especially liable to be displaced by a sudden and violent movement at the knee. (See KNEE.)

SEMINAL VESICLE is one of the small paired sacs lying on either side of the male urethra (qv), which collect and store spermatozoa. (See TESTICLE.)

SENEGA is the root of *Polygala senega*, a small plant of the United States. It has an action as a stimulating expectorant, and its preparations are used in cough mixtures.

SENILITY (see AGE, NATURAL CHANGES IN).

SENNA is the leaves of various species of *Cassia senna*, being known as Tinnerelly senna and Alexandrian senna, according to its source. It is one of the most active of the simple laxative drugs, producing considerable griping if used alone. Senna is excreted in the urine, giving it a dark red or yellow colour. In the case of nursing mothers, some of the drug is excreted in the milk and may have a purgative effect upon the nursling. A standardized preparation of senna, Senokot, is now available which has none of the disadvantages of senna itself and is widely used for the management of constipation in old people.

SENSATION (see PAIN; TOUCH).

SENSITIZATION (see ALLERGY; ANAPHYLAXIS).

SEPSIS means poisoning by the products of the growth of micro-organisms in the body, and the general symptoms which accompany it are those of inflammation. (See INFLAMMATION.) It is prevented by the various procedures mentioned under ASEPSIS, and is neutralized, when it has occurred, by various substances. (See ANTISEPTICS.)

SEPTICAEMIA is a serious form of blood-poisoning due to the multiplication in the blood of bacteria – in fact, it is an infection of the blood. (See BLOOD-POISONING.)

SEQUELAE is the term applied to symptoms or effects which are liable to follow certain diseases. For example, bronchitis and other chest complaints may be sequelae of measles; heart disease is often a sequel of rheumatic fever; paralysis may follow diphtheria.

SEQUESTRUM is the name given to a fragment of dead bone cast off from the living bone in the process of necrosis. (See BONE DISEASES.) A sequestrum often remains in contact with, and partly enveloped by, newly formed bone, so that a sinus is produced, and a constant discharge goes on, till the dead bone is removed.

SEROUS MEMBRANES are smooth, transparent membranes that line certain large cavities of the body. The chief serous membranes are the peritoneum, lining the cavity of the abdomen; the pleurae, one of which lines each side of the chest, surrounding the corresponding lung; the pericardium, in which the heart lies; and the tunica vaginalis on each side, enclosing a testicle. The name of these membranes is derived from the fact that the surface is moistened by thin fluid derived from the serum of blood or lymph. Every serous membrane consists of a visceral portion, which closely envelops the organs concerned, and a parietal portion, which adheres to the wall of the cavity. These two portions are continuous with one another so as to form a closed sac, and the opposing surfaces are close together, separated only by a little fluid. This arrangement enables the organs in question to move freely within the cavities containing them. For further details see under PERITONEUM.

SERPENTARIA, or SNAKEROOT, is the root of various species of *Aristolochia* plants of the Southern United States. It has a stimulating action, and is used as a bitter in combination with other remedies in the treatment of indigestion.

SERPIGINOUS is a term used in connection with ulcers or eruptions that spread in a creeping manner.

SERUM is the fluid which separates from blood, lymph and other fluids of the body when clotting takes place in them. (See HAEMORRHAGE.) Blood plasma is the name given to the fluid of the blood circulating in the vessels, by which the corpuscles are carried along. As clotting takes place, fine threads of fibrin form from the fibrinogen contained in the plasma. These threads produce a network of increasing density in which the corpuscles are entangled, and, as a result, the fluid (serum) which is left outside this clot is clear, unmixed with corpuscles, and of a pale yellow colour.

The relation of these substances is shown below:

Blood = { Plasma { Serum = Fibrin } ; Corpuscles }

Fibrin + Corpuscles } = Clot

Serum is a clear, yellowish fluid and contains, in addition to water, about 7 per cent of albumin and globulin, with smaller quantities of salts, fat, sugar, urea, uric acid and other extractives, as well as minute amounts of other albuminous bodies, which are of great importance in the prevention of disease. (See IMMUNITY.) The chief salt in the serum is common salt.

Serum is derived from the lymph also, and the fluid which is found in effusions into the pleura and other cavities of the body is similar in composition.

The serum used for the administration of antitoxins in cases of diphtheria, tetanus, and other diseases, is generally derived from the blood drawn from horses which have been subjected to a long course of treatment. (See IMMUNITY; SERUM THERAPY.)

SERUM SICKNESS is a hypersensitivity reaction due to circulating antigen antibody complexes. It got its name because it was a not-uncommon reaction to the administration of foreign serum which used to be given as a form of passive immunity before the days of antibiotics. By definition it is a manifestation of sensitivity to serum but the same clinical and pathological picture can occur one to three weeks after the administration of drugs such as penicillin, streptomycin and sulphonamides. It is characterized by fever, arthralgia and lymphadenopathy and is usually self-limiting as it resolves when the supply of antigen is used up.

SERUM THERAPY is the treatment of disease by the administration of serum. It was originally conceived as a way of providing passive immunity. Before effective anti-bacterial drugs were available antitoxins were raised in animals, particularly horses, to a number of bacteria. The horse developed antibodies to the injected bacteria and the horse serum could then be used as a means of providing passive immunity. One of the problems with this form of therapy was the development of hypersensitivity. Horse serum was a foreign protein: antibodies were developed to this foreign protein and a disease called serum sickness developed. It was, in fact, a type-3 hypersensitivity reaction due to circulating antigen antibody complexes. More rarely anaphylaxis, which is a type-1 hypersensitivity reaction, developed as a result of administration of the foreign serum.

Human immunoglobulin is now used to provide passive immunity. Serum is collected from hyperimmunised human individuals, such as those convalescing from the specific infection, and the relevant immunoglobulin is isolated and used parenterally to provide passive immunity. Horse serum is still used to provide passive immunity for diphtheria but human tetanus antitoxin is now available and has largely replaced the horse serum antitoxin. Passive immunity for hepatitis, both hepatitis A and hepatitis B, can be provided by immunoglobulin obtained from convalescent serum. Snake venom antiserum (antivene) is still prepared from horse serum so that there is always a risk of producing serum sickness or anaphylactic shock. Snake venom antiserum must be specific for the species of snake involved if it is to be effective.

Passive immunisation against viruses is also available and passive immunisation against measles can be achieved by the administration of pooled human immunoglobulin. Similarly passive protection by normal human immunoglobulin can be given to women during the first four months of pregnancy who have been in contact with rubella and whose serum does not contain rubella antibody. After exposure to rabies the course of active immunisation is proceeded by a single injection of hyperimmune anti-rabies serum. Normal human immunoglobulin is used for protection against hepatitis A virus in travellers and occasionally for patients and staff in residential institutions to control outbreaks. Specific antibody preparations of known high titres against particular antigens, such as tetanus, rabies, vaccinia and hepatitis B, are now available. Zoster-immune globulin is also available for contacts with diseases in which varicella would present a special danger. These preparations are available through the Public Health Laboratory service.

SESAMOID BONES are rounded nodules of bone usually embedded in tendon. They are usually a few millimetres in diameter, but some are larger, such as the patella (qv), or knee-cap.

SETON is the name applied to a few strands of silk or thin strip of lint or gauze passed through the skin and underlying tissues by means of a large flattened needle, and left projecting at both ends.

SEX CHROMOSOMES: In the human being there are 23 pairs of chromosomes. Male and female differ in respect of one pair. In the nucleus of the female somatic cell the two members of the pair are identical and are called X-chromosomes. In the male nucleus there is one X-chromosome and another, unequal, dissimilar chromosome called the Y-chromosome. In the sex cells, after reduction division, all cells in the female will contain X-chromosomes. In the male, half will contain X-chromosomes and half Y-chromosomes. If, then, a sperm with an X-chromosome fertilizes an ovum (with, of course, an X-chromosome) the offspring will be female. If a sperm with a Y-chromosome fertilizes the ovum the offspring will be male. It is the sex chromosomes which determine the sex of an individual.

Sometimes during cell division chromosomes may be lost or duplicated, or abnormalities in the structure of individual chromosomes may occur. The surprising fact is the infrequency of such errors. About one in two hundred live-born babies has an abnormality of development caused by a chromosome and two-thirds of these involve the sex chromosomes. There is little doubt that the frequency of these abnormalities in the early embryo is much higher but because of the serious nature of the defect early spontaneous abortion occurs.

Chromosome studies on such early abortions show that half have chromosome abnormalities with errors of autosomes being three times as common as sex chromosome anomalies. Two of the most common abnormalities in such foetuses are triploidy with 69 chromosomes and trisomy of chromosome 16. These two anomalies almost always cause spontaneous abortion. Abnormalities of chromosome structure may arise because of:

(1) *Deletion:* where a segment of a chromosome is lost.

(2) *Inversion:* where a segment of a chromosome becomes detached and re-attached the other way around. Genes will then appear in the wrong order and thus will not correspond with their opposite numbers on homologous chromosomes.

(3) *Duplication:* where a segment of a chromosome is included twice over. One chromosome will have too little nuclear material and one too much. The individual inheriting too little may be non-viable and the one with too much may be abnormal.

(4) *Translocation:* where chromosomes of different pairs exchange segments.

(5) *Errors in division of centromere:* sometimes the centromere divides transversely instead of longitudinally. If the centromere is not central, one of the daughter chromosomes will arise from the two short arms of the parent chromosome and the other from the two long arms. These abnormal daughter chromosomes are called isochromosomes.

These changes have important bearings on heredity as the effect of a gene depends not only on its nature but on its position on the chromosome with reference to other genes. Genes do not act in isolation but against the background of other genes. Each gene normally has its own position on the chromosome and this corresponds precisely with the positon of its allene on the homologous chromosome of the pair. Each member of a pair of chromosomes will normally carry precisely the same number of genes in exactly the same order. Characteristic clinical syndromes, due to abnormalities of chromosome structure, are less constant than those due to loss or gain of a complete chromosome. This is because the degree of deletion, inversion and duplication is inconstant. However, translocation between chromosomes 15 and 21 of the parent is associated with a familial form of mongolism in the offspring and deletion of part of an X chromosome may result in Turner's syndrome.

Non-Disjunction: Whilst alterations in the structure of chromosomes arise as a result of deletion or translocation, alterations in the number of chromosomes usually arise as a result of non-disjunction occurring during maturation of the parental gametes. The two chromosomes of each pair (homologous chromosomes) may fail to come together at the beginning of meiosis and continue to lie free. If one chromosome then passes to each pole of the spindle, normal gametes may result but if both chromosomes pass to one pole and neither to the other, two kinds of abnormal gametes will be produced. One kind of gamete will contain both chromosomes of the pair and the other gamete will contain neither. Whilst this results in serious disease when the autosomes are involved, the loss or gain of sex chromosomes seems to be well tolerated. The loss of an autosome is incompatible with life and the malformation produced by a gain of an autosome is proportional to the size of the extra chromosome carried.

Only a few instances of a gain of an autosome are known. An additional chromosome 21 (one of the smallest autosomes) results in mongolism and trisomy of chromosome 13 and 18 are associated with severe mental, skeletal and congenital cardiac defects. Diseases resulting from a gain of a sex chromosome are not as severe. A normal ovum contains 22 autosomes and an X sex chromosome. A normal sperm contains 22 autosomes and either an X or a Y sex chromosome. Thus as a result of non-disjunction of the X chromosome at the first meiotic division during the formation of female gametes the ovum may contain two X chromosomes or none at all, whilst in the male the sperm may contain both X and Y chromosomes (XY) or none at all. (See aso CHROMOSOMES, HEREDITY.)

SEXUAL DYSFUNCTION: Inadequate sexual response may be due to a lack of sexual desire or to an inadequate performance, or it may be that there is a lack of satisfaction or orgasm. The lack of sexual desire may be due to any generalized illness or endocrine disorder or to the taking of drugs that antagonise endocrine function. Disorders of performance in men can occur during arousal, penetration and ejaculation. In the female dyspareunia and vaginismus are the main disorders of performance. Diabetes mellitus (qv) can cause a neuropathy which results in loss of erection. Impotence can follow nerve damage from operations on the prostate and lower bowel and can be the result of neurological diseases affecting the autonomic system. Disorders of satisfaction include, in men, emission without forceful ejaculation and pleasureless ejaculation. In women such disorders range from the absence of the congestive genital response to absence of orgasm.

Sexual dysfunction may be due to physical or psychiatric disease, or it may be the result of the administration of drugs. The main group of drugs likely to cause sexual problems are the anti-convulsants, psychotrophic drugs, the anti-hypertensive drugs and drugs such as metoclopramide that induce hyperprolactinaemia. The benzodiazepine tranquillisers can reduce libido and cause failure of erection. Tricyclic antidepressives may cause failure of erection and clomipramine may delay or abolish ejaculation by blockade of alpha-adrenergic receptors. The mono-amine oxidase inhibitors often inhibit ejaculation. The phenothiazides reduce sexual desire and arousal and may cause difficulty in maintaining an erection. Methyldopa causes impotence in over 20 per cent of patients on large doses. The beta-blockers and the diuretics can also cause impotence. The main psychiatric causes of sexual dysfunction include stress, depression and guilt.

SEXUALLY TRANSMITTED DISEASES (see VENEREAL DISEASES).

SHAKING PALSY is another name for Parkinsonism (qv).

SHELLFISH POISONING in the United Kingdom occurs in two main forms. Shellfish may be the cause of typhoid fever (see ENTERIC FEVERS) as a result of their contamination by sewage containing the causative organism. They may also be responsible for what is known as paralytic shellfish poisoning. This is caused by a toxin, or poison, known as saxotoxin, which is present in certain planktons which, under unusual conditions, multiply rapidly, giving rise to what are known as 'red tides'. In these circumstances this toxin accumulates in mussels, cockles and scallops which feed by filtering plankton. The manifestations of such poisoning are loss of feeling in the hands, tingling of the tongue, weakness of the arms and legs, and difficulty in breathing. There is also growing evidence that shellfish poisoning may be due to a virus infection. (See FOOD POISONING.)

SHELL-SHOCK was a form of war neurosis which presented one of the major medical problems in the 1914–18 War.

SHIGELLA is the name given to a group of rod-shaped, Gram-negative bacteria that are the cause of bacillary dysentery. (See DYSENTERY.)

SHINGLES is a popular name for herpes zos ter, which forms more or less of a belt round th body. (See HERPES.)

SHIN SPLINTS is the term applied by athlete to a condition characterized by pain over th inner border of the shin, which occurs in mos runners and sometimes in joggers. It is due t muscular swelling resulting in inadequat blood supply to the muscle: hence the pain. I usually disappears within a few weeks responding to rest and physiotherapy, with o without injections. In some cases, however, i becomes chronic and so severe that it occur even at rest. In such cases, relief is usuall obtained by a simple operation to relieve th stress and strain in the affected muscles. Tech nically it is known as the medial tibia syndrome.

SHOCK is a state of acute circulatory failure i which the cardiac output is inadequate to pro vide normal perfusion of the major organs. I represents a failure of blood flow rather than failure of blood pressure. While shock i accompanied by a fall in arterial blood pres sure, a fall in blood pressure is not necessaril indicative of shock. Shock can arise from variety of causes and produce variable clinica signs according to the state of deterioration o the underlying disease. Direct bedside mea surements of blood flow are not available s that physicians must usually rely on indirec evidence of inadequate perfusion. Shock i therefore a clinical syndrome and is character ized by systemic arterial hypotension (arteria blood pressure less than 80 mm of mercury sweating and signs of vasoconstriction. Thes signs include pallor, cyanosis, a cold clamm skin and a low-volume pulse. These may b associated with clinical evidence of poor tissu perfusion, such as mental apathy, confusion o restlessness and oliguria. In haemodynami terms shock is a state of circulatory failure asso ciated with a low cardiac output and hig peripheral resistance.

Shock results from many situations whic give rise to inadequate perfusion of tissues an organs. It may occur because of increased resis tance to blood flow, pooling or loss of blood o because of cardiac insufficiency, but the en result of impaired tissue perfusion is the same As perfusion depends on blood flow and no blood pressure the sphygmomanometer read ing is a poor indicator of circulatory failure.

The blood volume is approximately 5 litres The heart puts out this volume each minute, stroke volume of 70 ml being ejected 70 time per minute in the resting subject. Only 15 pe cent of the blood volume lies in the arterial be so that variations in arterial calibre have littl effect on the vascular capacity. The arteriole are extremely muscular vessels and the tone o the arteriolar muscle varies the blood flo enormously. Because the greatest decline i pressure occurs at this level the arterioles ar called resistance vessels. Over two-thirds of th circulating blood volume lies on the venous side of the circulation, particularly in the venules. Hence the venous system is called the capacitance system. The veins are less muscular than the arterioles but are also under autonomic nervous control. The pressure in veins is only about 7 mm of mercury. They have a relatively large diameter and correspondingly low resistance. The tension of venous musculature, although not great, has a critical influence on venous return and on venous pressure. Passive assumption of the erect posture will reduce the cardiac output by 25 per cent. Nervous adjustment through the sympathetic nervous system is intended to prevent pooling in the capacitance system. Failure of venous tone with pooling of blood in venules and capillaries is associated with a large fall in cardiac output and failure of the peripheral circulation. Failure of arteriolar tone, on the other hand, with consequent arteriolar dilatation is associated with hypotension but blood flow remains normal and there is only a transient decrease in the venous return to the heart. The normal regulatory mechanisms for the circulation, that is the Baro receptors and the autonomic innervation of the arterioles and venules, are geared to cope with the adjustments necessary in postural alterations, physical exercise and acute trauma. The adrenergic system regulates blood pressure, the distribution of blood, the capacity of the venous system and the force and rate of cardiac contraction. The autonomic nervous system can adequately compensate for 10 per cent alterations in blood volume, moderate systemic infections and a good deal of myocardial damage, by shunting away blood from visceral organs into cerebral, coronary and skeletal muscle beds. The haemodynamic response to shock inevitably produces inadequate perfusion of viscera in order to preserve circulation to the brain and coronary vessels. If this is prolonged the effects are disastrous. The ischaemic intestine permits the transfer of toxic bacterial products and proteins across its wall into the blood. Renal ischaemia prevents the maintenance of a normal electrolyte and acid base balance.

Shock may result from loss of blood or plasma volume. This may occur as a result of haemorrhage or severe diarrhoea and vomiting. It may also result because of peripheral pooling of blood due to such causes as toxaemia or anaphylaxis. The toxaemia is commonly the result of a septicaemia. Another form of shock is called cardogenic shock which is due to failure of the heart as a pump. It is most commonly seen as a result of myocardial infarction. The treatment of shock is dependent on its cause. If it is the result of haemorrhage or diarrhoea or vomiting, replacement of blood and lost electrolytes is of prime importance. If it is due to septicaemia the treatment of the infection is of paramount importance and in addition intravenous fluids and vasopressor drugs will be required.

SHORT-SIGHT is a condition in which objects near at hand are seen clearly, while objects at a distance are blurred. The condition is technically known as myopia. (See MYOPIA; SPECTACLES; VISION.)

SHOULDER is the joint formed by the upper end of the humerus and the shoulder-blade or scapula. The acromion process of the scapula and the outer end of the collar-bone form a protective bony arch above the joint, and from this arch the wide and thick deltoid muscle passes downwards, protecting the outer surface of the joint, and giving to the shoulder its rounded character. The joint itself is of the ball-and-socket variety, the rounded head of the humerus being received into the hollow glenoid cavity of the scapula, which is further deepened by a rim of cartilage. One tendon of the biceps muscle passes through the joint, grooving the humerus deeply, and being attached to the upper edge of the glenoid cavity. The joint is surrounded by a loose fibrous capsule, strengthened at certain places by ligamentous bands. The main strength of the joint comes from the powerful muscles that unite the upper arm with the scapula, clavicle and ribs.

SHOULDER-BLADE, or SCAPULA, is a flat bone, about as large as the flat hand and fingers, placed on the upper and back part of the thorax. Many of the large muscles that move the arm are attached to it. It is not in contact with the ribs, and its only attachment to the trunk of the body is through a joint between its acromion process and the clavicle on the tip of the shoulder and by the powerful muscles which suspend it from the backbone and ribs. With the arm hanging by the side the scapula extends from the second to the seventh rib, but, as the arm is raised and lowered, it slides freely over the back of the chest. From the hinder surface of the bone springs a strong process, the spine of the scapula, which arches upwards and forwards into the acromion process. The latter forms the bony prominence on the top of the shoulder, where it unites in a joint with the outer end of the clavicle.

SIALAGOGUES are substances which produce a copious flow of saliva.

SIAMESE TWINS, or CONJOINED TWINS, is the term applied to twins who are united bodily but are possessed of separate personalities. Their frequency is not known, but it has been estimated that throughout the world six or more conjoined twins are born every year who are capable of separation. The earliest case on record is that of the 'Biddendon Maids' who were born in England in 1100. The 'Scottish Brothers' lived for 28 years at the court of James III of Scotland. Perhaps the most famous, however, were Chang and Eng, who were born of Chinese parents in Siam in 1811. It was they who were responsible for the introduction of the term, 'Siamese twins', which still remains the popular name for 'conjoined twins'. They were joined together at the lower end of the chest bone, and achieved fame by being shown in Barnum's circus in the United States. They subsequently married English sisters and settled as farmers in North Carolina. They died in 1874.

The earliest attempt at surgical separation is said to have been made by Dr Farius of Basle in 1689. The first successful separation in Great Britain was in 1912. Both twins survived the operation and one survived well into adult life. This is said to be the first occasion in which both twins survived the operation. The success of the operation is largely dependent upon the degree of union between the twins. Thus, if this is only skin, subcutaneous tissue and cartilage, the prospects of survival for both twins are good, but if some vital organ such as the liver is shared the operation is much more hazardous.

SIBLING is a brother or sister.

SICK-HEADACHE (see HEADACHE).

SICKLE-CELL ANAEMIA is a form of anaemia in black people, so-called because of the sickle shape of the red blood cells. The fundamental abnormality is the presence of an abnormal form of haemoglobin. This leads to the sickle shape of the red blood cell. Such a cell is more fragile than the normal red blood cell, and it is this fragility of the cell which is responsible for the anaemia. Advice can be obtained from the Sickle Cell Society, Green Lodge, Barretts Green Road, London NW10 (01-961 7795).

SICKNESS (see VOMITING; SEA-SICKNESS).

SICK-ROOM (see NURSING).

SIDEROSIS is the name given to chronic fibrosis (qv) of the lungs occurring in iron-workers and due to the inhalation of fine iron particles. The term is also applied to the condition in which there is an excessive deposit of iron in the tissues of the body.

SIGHT (see VISION).

SILICA is a major constituent of the earth's crust. Its main danger to health arises from free silica, present mainly as quartz and flint and as an important constituent of granite, sandstone and slate. (See SILICOSIS.)

SILICONES are organic compounds of silicon, with a structure of alternate atoms of silicon and oxygen with organic groups, such as methyl and phenyl attached to the silicone atoms. As they produce a flexible and stable water-repellent film on the skin, they are used as barrier creams (qv).

SILICOSIS constitutes the most important industrial hazard in those industries in which silica is encountered: ie. the pottery industry, the sandstone industry, sand-blasting, metal grinding, the tin-mining industry, anthracite coal mines. It is a specific form of pneumoconiosis (qv) caused by the inhalation of free silica. Among pottery workers the condition has for long been known as potter's asthma, whilst in the cutlery industry it was known as grinder's rot. For the production of silicosis the particles of silica must measure 0·5 to 5 micrometres in diameter and they must be inhaled into the alveoli of the lungs, where they produce fibrosis. This diminishes the efficiency of the lungs, which manifests itself by slowly progressive shortness of breath. The main danger of silicosis, however, is that it is liable to be complicated by tuberculosis. The incidence of silicosis is steadily being reduced by various measures which diminish the risk of inhaling silica dust. These include adequate ventilation to draw off the dust; the suppression of dust by the use of water; the wearing of respirators where the risk is particularly great and it is not possible to reduce the amount of dust: eg. in sand-blasting; periodic medical examination of workpeople exposed to risk. In 1976, there were 171 notified cases.

SILK, OILED, consists of silk fabric made waterproof with drying oils or oil-modified synthetic resins.

SILVER is used in medicine externally in the form of three of its salts. *Silver nitrate*, also known as lunar caustic, is a caustic that is used to destroy warts. It is also bactericidal, and in this rôle it is used as a 0·2 to 0·6 per cent solution as eye-drops, particularly as a preventive of ophthalmia neonatorum, (see EYE DISEASES AND INJURIES), but for this purpose it is largely being replaced by antibiotics and the sulphonamides. *Silver protein*, also known as Protargol, is prepared by the interaction of a silver compound and gelatine in the presence of an alkali. It has antibacterial properties and is used as eye-drops in the treatment of conjunctivitis. *Mild silver protein*, also known as Argyrol, contains a higher percentage of silver than silver protein, but is less irritating to the tissues. It is used as a 20 per cent solution in the treatment of conjunctivitis and for the prevention of ophthalmia neonatorum (though here it is largely being replaced by antibiotics and the sulphonamides). As a 50 per cent solution it is used in the treatment of corneal ulcers. (See EYE DISEASES.) All silver salts, if used for any length of time, are liable to produce discoloration of the skin; the condition known as argyria (qv).

SIMMONDS' DISEASE, or PITUITARY CACHEXIA, is a rare condition in which wasting of the skin and the bones, impotence, and loss of hair occur as a result of destruction of the pituitary gland.

SINGER'S NODULE is a small excrescence on the vocal cords which causes hoarseness. This tends to develop in people who abuse their voices, eg. singers, people who shout excessively.

SINGULTUS is the Latin term for hiccup.

SINUS is a term applied to narrow cavities of various kinds, occurring naturally in the body, or resulting from disease. Thus it is applied to the air-containing cavities which are found in the frontal, ethmoidal, sphenoidal and maxillary bones, and which communicate with the nose. The function of these paranasal sinuses, as they are known, is doubtful, but they do lighten the skull and add resonance to the voice. They enlarge considerably around puberty and in this way are a factor in the alteration of the size and shape of the face. The term is also used in connection with the wide spaces through which the blood circulates in the membranes of the brain. Cavities which are produced when an abscess has burst but remain unhealed, are also known as sinuses. (See ABSCESS; FISTULA.)

SINUSITIS is inflammation of a sinus. It is usually applied to inflammation of the sinuses in the face. (See NOSE, DISEASES OF.)

SINUSOIDAL CURRENT (see ELECTRICITY IN MEDICINE).

SJOGREN'S SYNDROME: Sjogren described the association of dryness of the mouth (xerostomia) and dryness of the eye (kerato conjunctivitis sieca) with rheumatoid arthritis. It occurs in approximately 10 per cent of patients with rheumatoid arthritis but it can occur, and frequently does so, independently of rheumatoid disease. The lack of tears gives rise to symptoms of dryness and grittiness of the eyes. The dry mouth can occasionally be so severe as to cause a dysphagia. The disease is due to the auto-immune destruction of the salivary glands and the lacrimal glands. The disorder is usually associated with specific HLA antigen. The treatment is unsatisfactory and is limited to oral and ocular hygiene as well as the provision of artificial tears in the form of cellulose eye drops.

SKATOL is a strongly smelling, crystalline substance contained in the stools, produced by decomposition of protein material.

SKELETON is the comprehensive term applied to the hard structures that support or protect the softer tissues of the body. Many animals are possessed of an exoskeleton, consisting of superficial plates of bone, horn, or the like; but in man the skeleton is entirely an endoskeleton, covered everywhere by soft parts, and consisting mainly of bones, but in places also of cartilage. The chief positions in which cartilage is found in place of bone are the larynx and the front of the chest. (For the details of the skeleton, see BONE.)

SKIAGRAM is the name applied to a photograph – strictly speaking a 'shadowgraph', for this is what it is – made by X-rays.

SKIN is the membrane which envelops the outer surface of the body, meeting, at the various orifices of the body, with the mucous membrane which lines the internal cavities. The skin consists of two distinct layers which differ entirely in structure and in origin. These are (*a*) *the epidermis*, also known as *scarf-skin, cuticle*, or *epithelium*, which is a cellular covering formed from the outer layer of the embryo; and (*b*) *thecorium*, also known as the *cutis vera, true skin*, or *dermis*, which is a fibrous covering developed from the middle embryonic layer.

(*a*) **The epidermis** is the cellular layer which covers the outer surface of the body, varying in thickness from 1 mm on the palms and soles to 0·1 mm on the face. It is composed of four layers, which, from the surface inwards, are as follows:

(1) THE HORNY LAYER, or STRATUM CORNEUM, made up of several thicknesses of flat cells, forming an impervious covering pierced only by the openings of the sweat-glands and by the hairs. The flat cells are rubbed off the surface constantly as minute white scales, being replaced by growth from below.

(2) THE CLEAR LAYER, or STRATUM LUCIDUM, in which the cells are firmly fixed together into a kind of membrane.

(3) THE GRANULAR LAYER, or STRATUM GRANULOSUM, in which the cells are undergoing a change in form and substance from those of the fourth layer to those of the two on the surface.

(4) THE MALPIGHIAN LAYER, or GERMINATIVE ZONE, as it is sometimes known, which is made up of the STRATUM SPINOSUM (or PRICKLY CELL LAYER) and the STRATUM BASALE, in which the cells are soft, tender and living. These cells live in several rows, the deepest (the stratum basale) being set directly upon the uneven surface of the true skin, which is richly supplied with blood-vessels that nourish the cells. These cells divide continually and as they multiply they are pushed upwards to supply the constant wear and tear on the surface of the horny layer. There are no blood-vessels in the epidermis, but fine sensory nerves terminate between the cells of the Malpighian layer. These cells are joined together by cement substance and by minute processes that are continued from each cell into its neighbours. The cells in the stratum basale include the melanocytes which are responsible for the production of melanin, the pigment responsible for suntan. (See MELANIN; SUNBURN.)

NAILS are analogous to the horny layer, but the cells of which they are composed are harder and more adherent. Beneath the nail is the nail bed, which is made up of the germinative zone together with the corium. Underneath the greater part of the nail the corium has a very liberal blood supply, which gives the nail its

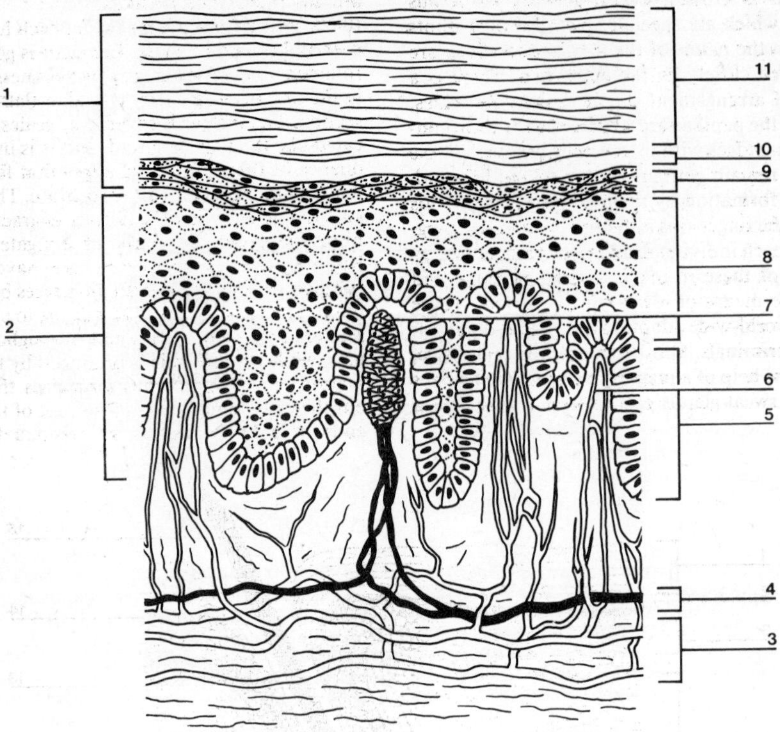

1 horny zone
2 germinative zone
3 blood vessels
4 nerves
5 stratum basale
6 vascular papilla of corium
7 oval corpuscle in corium (tactile)
8 stratum spinosum
9 stratum granulosum
10 stratum lucidum
11 stratum corneum

Vertical section of epidermis and corium.

pink colour. Towards the root of the nail, however, the nail becomes denser and the corium has a less liberal blood supply. As a result the nail is whiter. This is the part known as the lunule, which is most evident in the thumb, and gradually becomes covered by the nail fold towards the little finger where the lunule is usually hidden completely. The stratum corneum of the nail fold is prolonged over the nail as a thin fold known as the eponychium. All growth of the nail occurs at its root. Finger nails grow at an average rate of 0·5 mm a week. There is a gradual slowing of the rate with age, and a slight variation from finger to finger, the longer the finger the faster the rate of growth. Growth is quicker in summer than in winter. Toe nails grow more slowly than finger nails – at about a fourth of the rate of the latter.

A *blister* is a collection of fluid separating the Malpighian layer from the superficial ones.

(b) **The corium** is the fibrous layer which forms the chief part of the bodily covering. It varies greatly in thickness from about 0·5 to 3 mm, being coarser on the back than on the front of the body, and thicker in men than in women. It contains many nerves, which play an important part in affording sensations of touch, pain and temperature, and blood-vessels which, in addition to nourishing the skin, are largely concerned in regulating the temperature of the body. The corium bears also the hairs which pierce the epidermis, and the sweat-glands, whose ducts also penetrate the epidermis to reach the surface. Beneath the corium lies a loose fibrous layer of subcutaneous tissue which joins the skin to deeper parts and contains more or less fat, according to the stoutness of the person.

The fibrous tissue of the corium is composed of interlacing bundles of white fibrous tissue that form a dense feltwork. Here and there, elastic fibres are mixed with the others, and these serve to give the skin pliability, and at the same time to keep it always stretched. On the surface the network is very fine and close, and the skin is raised up into projections, known as papillae, which fit into corresponding depressions on the under-surface of the epidermis, and thus render the two inseparable. The corium is crossed everywhere by numerous folds, which are specially plentiful over joints and on the palms of the hands, and which are followed closely by the epidermis. There is a special arrangement on the palms and soles, where the papillae are so placed as to form continuous ridges with intervening grooves. These ridges remain permanent throughout life, and, as the formation by them of whorls and loops upon the finger-tips is distinctive and unchanging in each individual, an impression, or fingerprint, of these in ink is a most effective and reliable means of identifying a person. Hence their world-wide adoption as a means of identifying criminals. On the summit of each ridge, with the help of a magnifying glass, the orifices of the sweat-glands can be seen arranged in a row.

The endings of the sensory nerves in the skin are described under NERVES.

HAIRS spring from the true skin, each having a root and a stem or shaft. The stem is generally rounded, and varies greatly in thickness, while in the case of curly hair it is oval or flattened in section. The surface is covered by scales, imbricated like the tiles on a roof, and it is in consequence of their projecting edges that felted or matted hair is so difficult to separate. The chief part of the stem is of a fibrous character, the fibres being composed also of elongated cells. Running up the centre, some hairs have a pith composed of soft cells with air-spaces between them. The varying tint of hair is due to pigment scattered in varying amount throughout the hair, while a white hair is produced by the formation of very numerous air-spaces throughout the cells composing it. The root of the hair ends in a knob, and is set upon a fibrous

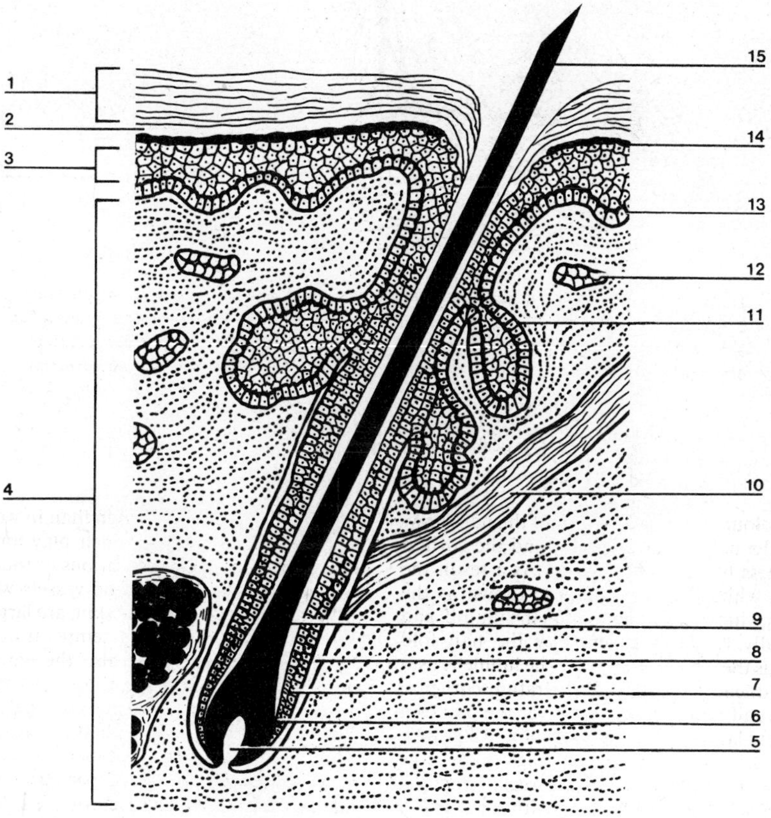

1 stratum corneum
2 stratum lucidum
3 stratum spinosum
4 corium
5 papilla of hair
6 bulb of hair
7 dermic coat, outer root-sheath
8 dermic coat, inner root-sheath
9 medulla of hair
10 arrector pili muscle
11 sebaceous gland
12 vessel
13 stratum basale
14 stratum granulosum
15 cortex of hair

Section through the skin showing the epidermis and corium, a hair in its follicle, the arrector pili muscle which raises the hair, and sebaceous glands opening into the hair follicle.

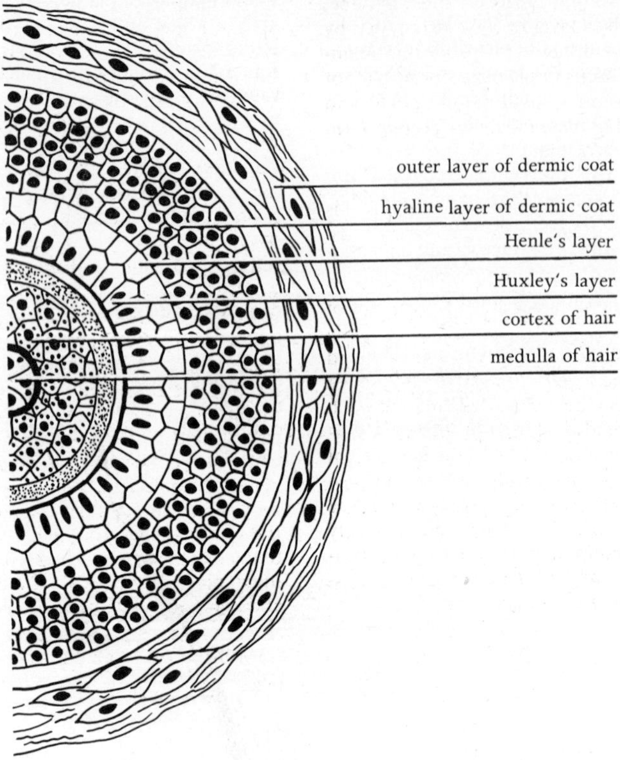

Transverse section through half of a hair follicle.

papilla, from which the hair appears to derive its principal nutriment. This root is set deep in the corium, and is the growing part of the hair which pushes the older part of the hair out through the epidermis. In the scalp each hair grows steadily and continuously for three to five years at a rate of a little over 0·3 mm daily. Growth then ceases and after three to four months the hair is shed. In the latter half of this resting period the follicle forms a new hair which replaces the old one. The average daily moult varies from 50 to 100 hairs. The tube which contains the part of the hair embedded in the skin is known as the hair follicle and is lined by a fibrous coat derived from the true skin and a cellular coat developed from the cuticle, each of which consists of three layers. When a hair is roughly pulled out, the clear membrane that is often found surrounding it is part of the cellular root sheath. The follicle does not run straight down into the skin, but has a considerable obliquity, so that the part of the hair above the surface has a natural slope to one side. Attached to the underside of each sloping hair-follicle, near its deep end, is a small muscle, whose other end is attached to the surface of the true skin a little distance off. These muscles have the action of raising the hair, and also of producing goose-flesh, when stimulated to contract by the influence of cold or of fear.

GLANDS are found in immense numbers in the skin, and are of two kinds: *sebaceous glands*, which secrete a fatty substance, and *sweat glands*, which secrete a clear, watery fluid.

The *sebaceous glands* lie in the true skin, and open into the follicles of the hairs a little way from the surface. Each consists of a bunch of small sacs, within which fatty material is produced. The secretion reaches the surface by the hair-follicle, and serves to lubricate the hair and give pliability to the surface of the skin.

Sweat glands, or sudoriparous glands, are very numerous (there are around 3 million of them), are found all over the surface of the body at a slightly deeper level than the sebaceous glands, and have no connection with the hairs. Each consists of a long tube, coiled up into a ball, from which a duct leads in a zigzag manner up towards the surface. The outlets of these ducts can just be seen with the naked eye as minute openings (pores), though with a magnifying glass they are readily visible. The number is said to vary from 400 in a square inch, on the lower limbs and back, to 2800 in the same area on the palm of the hand. The structure of these glands is simple. Each is a coiled-up tube, which is lined by a layer of cells surrounded by muscle fibres, and these again by a thin membrane. In the fibrous tissue between the coils of the glands run many small blood-vessels, and from the blood in these the materials that form the sweat are extracted.

Functions of the skin: The main use of the skin is a *protective* one. It covers the underlying muscles, both protecting them from injury and, especially by virtue of the layer of fat immediately beneath the skin, warding off extremes of temperature. The epidermis forms a highly impenetrable surface, its horny character and elasticity being well calculated to resist wounds; whilst the sebaceous matter with which it is provided renders it almost waterproof. Thus poisons, drugs, and the like are not absorbed in any appreciable amount through the unbroken skin, unless combined with some fatty material, as in ointments, and diligently rubbed in, or alternatively by molecular diffusion. This latter method is known as the Transdermal Therapeutic System.

Secretion is an important function of the skin, the two secretions being sebaceous material and perspiration. Of these, the former is a lubricant for the hair and skin, the latter is treated of under PERSPIRATION.

Heat regulation is one of the most important functions of the skin. Man is a warm-blooded animal, that is to say, his temperature remains constant in health between 36·7° and 37·2°C (98° and 99°F), no matter what the temperature of the surrounding medium may be. In order to maintain this constancy, it is evident that he must be provided with some means of quickly developing heat which will come into action when the body is cooled down by exposure to cold, and also some mechanism which can quickly get rid of heat when necessary. The main source of heat in the body lies in the muscular tissue, which develops heat every time a contraction takes place. The skin also plays a prominent part in this connection. When cold air or water come into contact with the surface, the skin blanches, the numerous blood-vessels of the true skin contracting and thus preventing much blood from circulating through the skin, and being thereby unduly cooled. On the other

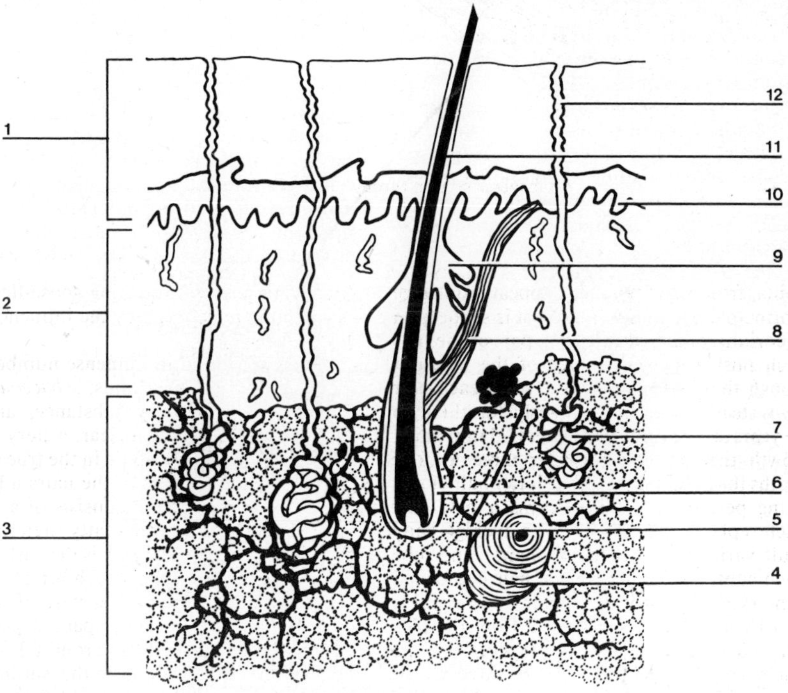

1 epidermis
2 corium
3 subcutaneous fatty tissue
4 oblique section through a lamellated corpuscle
5 papilla of hair
6 hair follicle
7 body of sweat gland
8 arrector pili muscle
9 sebaceous gland
10 papilla of corium
11 hair
12 duct of sweat gland

Schematic vertical section of skin.

hand, when the surface is exposed to a temperature approaching that of the body, say one of 26·7° or 32·2°C (80° or 90°F), or when an excessive amount of heat is produced by great muscular efforts, the blood-vessels of the surface dilate, the skin reddens as much blood comes to the surface, and there is a copious secretion of perspiration, which produces great cooling as it evaporates from the surface. These actions of narrowing and dilatation of vessels, and of sweat secretion, are brought about through reflex nerve influence. When the temperature rises so high that these processes are unable to take place, very serious results ensue. (See HEAT-STROKE.) It can be readily understood why the body tolerates high temperatures at a dry heat much better than continued moist heat, since evaporation of the perspiration takes place more readily the drier the surrounding air, and thus produces more rapid cooling.

Respiration is a function of the skin which in man is not of so great importance as in the lower animals. In the frog, the lungs and skin are of equal importance as breathing organs, although in man the amount of carbon dioxide given off by the skin is only about $\frac{1}{150}$ or $\frac{1}{200}$ of the amount given off by the lungs. It is probable however, that much of the organic matter which gives to impure air its disagreeable smell and contributes to its poisonous properties is given off by the skin.

Social function: The skin, it has been said, also provides a major pathway for social communication, by virtue of its vascular responses associated with signalling of emotional states, muscular responses of expression, creating a complex sign language, and by the equally subtle possibilities of tactile communication. In primates, it has been noted, the skin forms a signalling system related to complicated instinctive behaviour patterns, but 'how far the signals mediated in man by facial expression and other factors causing alterations in skin appearance are linked to instinctive behaviour patterns rather than to conditioned behaviour is debatable in adults, although studies in children indicate the fusion of these two elements in a complex fashion'.

SKIN DISEASES: These form a large and important class. They are very extensive, owing to the varied forms of change which the skin texture may undergo, and to the different structures in the skin which may be specially affected. Skin diseases are of great importance, not only from the fact that they have an influence on the general health, but also because these diseases are often the expression of constitutional conditions, inherited or acquired, the recognition of which is essential to their effectual treatment.

CANCER of the skin occurs in various forms. *Rodent ulcer* (qv), or basal cell epithelioma responds well to treatment. Cure is obtained in 98 per cent of cases if treated early. Anyone over the age of 50 with a persistent superficial crusted ulcer on the cheek or the side of the nose which has not healed over a period of months should seek medical advice in case it is a rodent ulcer. *Squamous cell carcinoma* which usually starts as a hard nodule, is usually the result of long excessive exposure to sunlight. *Malignant melanoma* (see MELANOMA) develops in a pigmented spot. Cancer of the skin may also be induced by exposure to tar, pitch, bitumen, the mineral oils, and X-rays.

(See also ACNE; BOILS; BROMIDROSIS; DERMATITIS; ECTHYMA; ECZEMA; ERYSIPELAS; ERYTHEMA; ERYTHRASMA; HERPES SIMPLEX; HERPES ZOSTER; HYPERIDROSIS; ICHTHYOSIS; IMPETIGO; ITCHING; KERATOSIS; LEUCODERMA; LICHEN; LUPUS; MOLLUSCUM CONTAGIOSUM; NAPKIN RASH; NEURODERMATOSES; PEMPHIGUS; PITYRIASIS ROSEA; POMPHYLYX; PRURIGO; PRURITUS; PSORIASIS; RINGWORM; ROSACEA; SEBORRHOEA; URTICARIA; WENS.)

SKIN-GRAFTING is an operation in which large breaches of surface due to wounding or ulceration are closed by transplantation of skin from other parts. There are three methods by which this is done. Most frequently the epidermis only is transplanted, according to a method introduced by Reverdin and by Thiersch, and known by their names. For this purpose, a broad strip of epidermis is shaved off the thigh or upper arm, after the part has been carefully purified, and is transferred bodily to the raw or ulcerated surface, or is cut into smaller strips and laid upon it. By a second method, small pieces of the skin in its whole thickness are removed from the arm and thigh, or even from other people, and are implanted and bound upon the raw surface. This method has the disadvantage that the true skin must contract at the spot from which the graft is taken, leaving an unsightly scar. When very large areas require to be covered, a third method is sometimes adopted, as follows. A large flap of skin, amply sufficient to cover the gap, is raised from a neighbouring or distant part of the body, in such a way that it remains attached along one margin, so that blood-vessels can still enter and nourish it. It is then turned so as to cover the gap; or, if it be situated on a distant part, the two parts are brought together and fixed in this position till the flap grows firmly to its new bed. The old connection of the flap is then severed, leaving it growing in its new place.

SKULL is the collection of 22 flat and irregularly shaped bones which protect the brain and form the face. The names of the individual bones composing the skull are given under BONE.

Arrangement of the bones: In early life the brain and organs of special sense are enclosed in a case which is formed partly of cartilage, partly of fibrous membrane. At various parts of this investment, ossification begins early in life, and the bone gradually spreads outwards from each of these centres. Certain of the bones so formed fuse together in early childhood, thus constituting the twenty-two bones of the adult skull, which maintain their independence throughout the greater part of life. In old age, however, the bones fuse so completely that the cranium comes to be a solid bony case. Even before this happens, the bones are fastened to one another by sutures so tightly that their separation without breaking is very difficult. The sutures are joints in which each edge is locked with the edges of neighbouring bones by exactly fitting projections and depressions, resembling a complicated mortise-work. Occasionally small bones develop in the sutures between the ordinary, named ones, these extra bones being known as sutural bones.

The growth of the bones spreads outwards, as already stated, from certain centres, and at the time of birth the growth of several bones has not been quite completed, so that an infant's head presents six soft spots or fontanelles where the brain is covered only by skin and membranes, and at some of which the pulsations of its blood-vessels can be seen. One of these spots, the anterior fontanelle, situated on the top of the head, does not completely close till the child is 2½ years old. Another change takes place as age advances, consisting in the development of an outer and inner hard table in each of the cranial bones, the tables being separated by a layer of cancellous bone (*diplöe*), and in some positions by spaces containing air, which communicate with the respiratory passages. (See SINUS.) This change begins at the age of 10 years, and leads to great thickening and increased strength in the skull.

Parts of the skull: The skull consists of two distinct parts: the cranium, which encloses the brain and consists of eight bones; and the face, which forms a bony framework for the eyes, nose, and mouth, and is composed of fourteen bones. These two parts can be detached from one another. The lower jaw is connected with the base of the cranium by a movable joint on each side, and when the bones are bare of soft parts there is no union between them. The ear, which lies just behind and above this joint, is enclosed in the substance of the temporal bone, lying beneath the brain and separated from it in places only by a very thin shell of bone. The interior of the cranium is moulded so as to form a support for the brain. Its base is divided by bony ridges into three fossae, which from before back support the frontal lobes, the temporosphenoidal lobes, and the cerebellum. Further, the inner surface of the bone shows grooves and hollows corresponding to the convolutions and blood-vessels of the brain. The bones, especially on the base of the skull, are pierced by many small canals (*foramina*) which transmit nerves, blood-vessels and the like. Of these, the largest is the foramen magnum, through which the medulla oblongata and the spinal cord are continuous with one another.

Shape of the skull: In the lower animals, the cranium is placed in the back part of the head, and the face looks upwards to a great extent as well as forwards. In man, as a consequence of the great development of the cerebral hemispheres of the brain, in connection with his mental activity, the cranium extends above, as well as behind, the face, which therefore looks straight forwards. One method of classification is obtained by taking what is known as the cephalic index: ie. the percentage that the skull's breadth forms of its length. Long-headed peoples, like the Australian aborigines, are known as *dolichocephalic*; peoples with rounded heads, like most European races, are called *mesocephalic*; while races with broad heads, like some American Indians, are said to be *brachycephalic*.

Age makes considerable changes in the skull. The persistence of soft spots in the skull during the first two years of life, as well as the gradual obliteration of the sutures in later life, have been already mentioned. In children the size of the cranium is large compared with that of the face, which measures only one-eighth of the whole head, but increases till in adult life cranium and face are of almost equal proportions. In old age the face once more decreases, owing largely to loss of the teeth and consequent absorption of their bony sockets, which allows the cheeks to sink inwards and gives the appearance known as nut-cracker jaws. A similar result is produced earlier in life by premature extraction of the teeth. The child's head is gently rounded, and does not show the prominences above the eyebrows and behind the ears, due to the presence of air-cells at these localities in the full-grown skull. Further, the skull is thinner in childhood, does not show the heavy ridges for attachment of muscles displayed in later life, and is more vertical on the front and sides.

Sex also makes some differences, so that, as a rule, though not invariably, the skull of a woman can be told from that of a man. In the woman the characters resemble those of the child, the skull being lighter, smoother, and having less marked prominences. The woman's skull has on an average nine-tenths the capacity of the male skull.

Deformities result from various causes. The head is rarely symmetrical, one side almost always bulging more than the other. Premature closure of one of the sutures leads to increased growth at other sutures. Thus if the suture running from before backwards on the vertex of the head (sagittal suture) close too early, the result is a very long boat-shaped head. Some races, as, for example, the flat-head Indians of North America, show striking deformities of the head produced by applying boards and bandages in infant life.

SLAPPED CHEEK DISEASE (see ERYTHEMA).

SLEEP is a periodic resting condition of the body, and especially of the nervous system. It is more than rest. It is a phase that ensures that the whole body, including the nervous system, can recuperate. It has been shown in animals that the formation of protein is more active during sleep, and the same presumably holds in man. It is the brain that controls sleep, and the benefit of sleep is most obvious for the brain. The highest rate of synthesis, or formation, of brain protein takes place during sleep.

Causes of sleep: There is a natural rotation of sleeping and waking every twenty-four hours, and sleep comes on commonly during the night when little work can be done. Sleep is not, however, a necessary consequence of darkness, as is proved by those people who have to work in the night and sleep by day, and who speedily adapt themselves to this condition. Many people, too, such as sailors, gain the power of sleeping as soon as they turn in, and for them short four-hourly periods of sleep and work become natural.

Many theories have been advanced as to the cause of sleep. One theory is that sleep is due to cerebral anaemia, or a poor blood supply to the brain. Against this is the fact that it has been shown that the total blood flow through the brain is not altered during sleep. On the other hand, this does not exclude the possibility that there may be local alterations in certain parts of the brain, such as the midbrain which is known to be concerned with the process of sleeping.

Another theory is the chemical one that sleep is due to want of oxygen in the nerve centres. It has been shown that, of the oxygen taken in during the twenty-four hours, 67 per cent is taken in during the twelve hours of day and 33 per cent during the twelve hours of night, while of the carbon dioxide given off, 58 per cent is the amount by day and 42 per cent by night. It is also well known that vitiated air containing an excess of carbon dioxide is capable, like many other substances, of causing drowsiness followed by unconsciousness. But these facts – while making it plain that want of oxygen or the presence of carbon dioxide and other products of activity in the tissues may cause sleep – do not explain why sleep comes on regularly in people who are not exhausted by their day's work, nor why many people are able to compose themselves and fall asleep at any time they find convenient.

A third theory raises the question as to whether the mind remains active during the period of sleep. This theory brings forward the fact that all sensations, volitions, and other acts of consciousness are accompanied by chemical disturbances in the brain-cells that stimulate the mind to activity. When external impressions are cut off by closing the eyes and otherwise composing oneself for sleep, the mind ceases to be stimulated, and tranquil sleep ensues. What might be described as a slightly less fanciful variation of this theory is that during waking hours there is an accumulation in the brain of a sleep-inducing substance, and that after a period of time this ultimately induces sleep. None of these theories explains the direct cause of sleep, although each probably accounts for the main cause in different circumstances.

Sleep is not one steady process of gradually deepening sleep, as was at one time thought. It consists of several cycles of alternation between two stages: NREM (*Non-Rapid-Eye Movement*) or orthodox sleep, and REM or paradoxical sleep. On falling asleep we pass straight into the orthodox phase which lasts for about an hour or so. This is followed by the REM, so called because it is accompanied by *Rapid Eye Movement* (hence the abbreviation, REM) which lasts for two or fifteen minutes. This is the stage during which dreaming occurs. When it is over we pass back into the orthodox stage and so we alternate during the night, the orthodox stages tending to last longer in the earlier stages of sleep. By and large, however, orthodox sleep occupies about three-quarters of the sleep period in adults. In infants, however, it occupies only about half of the sleep period.

When sleep comes on, the eyes are closed as a rule, though in man, even when they are left open, the sense of sight is quickly lost as the sleep deepens. The pupils contract, also, during sleep, and dilate widely as the person awakes. Hearing is lost more slowly, and a person can be wakened even from deep sleep by a loud noise. In natural sleep, touch remains the least affected of the senses, and even the lightest touch will awaken many people from deep sleep. This does not hold good for sleep caused by drugs, many of which have a special effect in dulling general sensation, though much less effect upon the sense of hearing. With regard to the onset of sleep as it affects the mind, will-power is the first faculty to go and the last to appear in wakening. The association of ideas and power of reasoning next disappear, and people are often worried in light sleep by some simple idea which they cannot explain or understand. Memory and imagination remain longest, and, in dreams, the mind is presented with a series of bright, unconnected pictures, all jumbled together, which it does not attempt to explain. The part of the brain which regulates the power of movement is late in falling asleep, sleeps only lightly – since people may turn and make various other movements without waking – and usually wakens before the intellectual faculties and the special senses.

Other parts of the body, as well as the brain, rest during sleep. Thus the kidneys secrete less urine, the stomach secretes less gastric juice, the liver secretes less bile, the heart beats less strongly, the blood-pressure falls, and the respirations are slower and shallower than in the waking state. The skin becomes flushed with blood, so that it is specially necessary to keep the surface well covered during sleep in order to avoid chills. Some parts of the body never have a continued rest throughout life. Thus the heart, during the course of the two to three thousand million beats which it makes throughout an average life, never ceases longer than the fraction of a second that intervenes between each pair of beats, and, in each of these brief intervals, it recuperates itself for its next effort. Similarly the vital centres in the brain may be said never to sleep.

The amount of sleep suitable at different ages varies considerably as it also does from individual to individual. Some people keep going quite happily with five hours a night; others need eight hours or even more. Young people sleep easily but with increasing age sleep becomes more difficult. It becomes more broken and also less deep. At the same time there is a tendency for the elderly to require less sleep. (See also CHILDREN, PECULIARITIES OF.)

Dreams: The mind, like the vital centres, is probably never completely inactive during sleep, but is constantly receiving slight impressions which produce only a faint and quickly forgotten sensation. This is borne out by the fact that a sleeper may be awakened, not only by a loud sound or light touch, but by the ceasing of a continuous sound, as when machinery stops. A sleeper is also especially easily awakened by some sound or other sensation that he expects, and, in further proof of this constant wakefulness of the mind, may be mentioned the fact that many people have the power of wakening after having slept for a period which they have previously determined. It has been already stated that the different parts of the brain and the different faculties of the mind go to sleep usually in a certain order. When the higher intellectual faculties of will and reason have become dulled, but deeper sleep does not at once come on, memory and imagination become increasingly vivid, so that brilliant pictures are presented to the mind. Often these are mingled with misinterpreted sensations from the surface of the body or from disordered internal organs, which serve to give them an unpleasant tinge. For example, dyspepsia may give rise to sensations of falling over precipices, of vague depression, or of other unpleasant experiences which are in part memories of past events. Again, a wakeful memory and imagination may be associated with wakefulness of the motor portion of the brain, as when the person dreams that he is making desperate efforts to achieve some object or to escape pursuit, and his limbs go through movements associated with the ideas presented in his dream. Any sensation received from the surface of the body or from a disordered organ may suffice to produce the condition of partial sleep in which dreams occur, or it may become sufficiently strong to awaken the sleeper altogether. Again, the impression of the dream may produce so great an effect upon consciousness that the dream is remembered on waking, or it may fade so completely that only a sense of something forgotten is present, and a feeling that the slumber has been unrefreshing to the weary mind. Much attention has been paid to dreams with the object of finding out repressed memories responsible for mental unrest in the person concerned. These often become more evident during sleep than in the waking hours, and, if the dreams are remembered, they give a guide to the identity of the disturbing memories. Appearances seen and things felt or heard in dreams often have a symbolic meaning; and the interpretation of this by those who practise psychotherapy often plays an important part in treatment. Dreams are usually in black and white, but occasionally in colour.

Night terrors occur in nervous children and are allied to dreaming. The child goes to sleep after a day of unusual excitement or fatigue, or perhaps after partaking of some indigestible meal, and in a short time, when sleep should be sound and dreamless, he awakens with a start and in a state of terror. Frequently the child screams with fear, cannot be pacified, and for several minutes does not seem to recognize those near him. When quieted, he can often give no reason for his fear, or he may attribute his behaviour to a dream. Children who suffer in this way should be guarded from excitement and fatigue, and, should the night terrors, or nightmares, persist, may well be taken to a child-guidance clinic or to a child psychologist.

Somnambulism, or habitual sleep-walking, is an imperfect form of sleep, in which the muscular apparatus, and the portion of brain controlling it, remain awake though the intellectual faculties are buried in slumber. In children it is not uncommon as an isolated phenomenon and is seldom of any significance, especially if it is ignored. Occasionally it may be associated with something that is worrying the child, either at home or at school. This is usually revealed by discreet enquiry, and relatively easily settled. In adults it may be a manifestation of a hysterical personality (see HYSTERIA) precipitated by some mental stress or strain though this may be difficult to ascertain in the hysteric. While the somnambulistic state persists the individual is unaware of his actions though he may see and avoid objects in his path, or may hear and answer questions, though seldom with coherence. It is almost unknown for somnambulists to injure themselves. On awakening they remember nothing of the episode.

Paralysed wakefulness is a condition of which people sometimes complain. This is the converse of somnambulism, the person waking from sleep to full consciousness and finding himself unable to make any movement for several seconds or minutes. In this condition the motor part of the brain seems to lag behind the intellectual and sensory part in waking up, but the condition is a transitory and unimportant one, though it can be quite terrifying for the victim.

Insomnia, or sleeplessness, is a condition that often causes annoyance, and by depriving the person of natural rest produces interference with the full activity during the day-time. When it becomes a habit, it may form a serious menace to health.

It may be due to a variety of causes, and these may act so effectively as to keep the person awake altogether, or they may serve, when present in a lesser degree, to produce one of the forms of dreaming and unrefreshing slumber already mentioned. In the first place, there are some people of a nervous temperament whose sleep is much more liable to be interrupted by trivial causes than that of their more phlegmatic neighbours. In temporary cases of sleeplessness or dreaming, in which the affected person suffers from a disturbed night now and then, the cause is usually to be sought in some external source of irritation. A slight degree of pain, too light a bed-covering leading to general coldness, or even the presence of cold feet may be quite enough to prevent the brain from attaining the necessary degree of repose. Indigestion, due to eating a heavy meal shortly before retiring to rest, or some other internal disorder may act in a similar manner, even although there be no severe pain. In cases of habitual sleeplessness, a voluntary limitation of the hours of sleep, combined with overstudy, worry, or grief, is often instrumental in forming a bad habit which it is exceedingly hard to break. The brain in these cases remains fully active, despite the best endeavours of the sleepless person to compose himself for rest. A similar state of matters is often set up by poisonous materials circulating in the blood, as in fevers, malaria, gout, intemperance, and over-indulgence in tobacco. Another cause of sleeplessness or dreaming is found in persons suffering from depression who are often affected in such a way that they fall asleep on retiring to rest, enjoy only a light and partial slumber for an hour or two, and then lie wide awake till morning.

Treatment of disordered sleep: This varies greatly, depending indeed entirely upon the cause. A greater amount of exercise during the day, and care with regard to the diet may be sufficient in some of the slighter cases to remedy insomnia. In other cases a hot drink, eg. milk, just before retiring is an excellent sedative. In old people a hot whisky is often a most effective nightcap. As cold feet is a not uncommon cause of insomnia in old people, the wearing of bed-socks may ensure a good night's sleep. A comfortable warm bed can be better than any hypnotic. Where any known cause of pain or irritation exists, this must of course be remedied. Headache is not uncommonly a cause of sleeplessness, and the relief of this condition is then requisite and often sufficient to restore natural sleep. (See HEADACHE.) When a mental cause is at the root of the condition, the habit of overstudy, business worry, and the like which was originally responsible for the want of sleep, must be abandoned. Some change of occupation in the later part of the evening, such as reading some simple book or engaging in conversation, often helps to quiet the overworked brain. Cases which resist these simple means often yield to hypnotics. (See HYPNOTICS.) In cases in which the nervous system is thoroughly run down, treatment of a bracing nature is required. (See NEURASTHENIA.) Finally, any bad habits, like intemperance and excessive smoking, require appropriate treatment.

Coma is the name applied to a state of deep sleep from which the person cannot be roused. (See COMA.) The condition may be due to apoplexy, compression or concussion of the brain, poisoning by excess of alcohol or by narcotic poisons such as opium. (See OPIUM.)

Apparent death is a condition deeper than coma, in which persons are to all appearance dead. Cases have occurred of supposed death in which the person has been in a deep sleep or trance, from which some sudden shock has awakened him after several hours or even days. In all such cases, however, careful examination would reveal signs of life. (See CATALEPSY; DEATH, SIGNS OF.)

SLEEPING SICKNESS, or **AFRICAN TRYPANOSOMIASIS** is a disease occurring in West, East, Central and South Africa, between 14°N and 25°S latitude, and characterized by increasing weakness, lethargy, and a constant tendency to sleep, with gradual emaciation and finally death. It is one of the group of diseases caused by the presence in the blood of minute parasites known as *trypanosomes.* The discovery of these parasites in the blood in cases of sleeping sickness was first made in 1902. Later it was shown that this parasite is transmitted by various forms of the tsetse fly. The disease also occurs in cattle, when it is known as nagana. The most important species of trypanosomes are *Trypanosoma gambiense*, which only affects man, and *Trypanosoma rhodesiense*, which affects mainly man. *Trypanosoma brucei, Trypanosoma vivax*, and *Trypanosomacongolense* are all found in wild animals and are fatal to cattle and other domestic animals, but harmless to man. The tsetse flies responsible for the transmission of the disease are *Glossina morsitans* in the case of *Trypanosoma rhodesiense*, and *Glossina morsitans, Glossina swynnertoni*, and *Glossina palpalis* in the case of *Trypanosoma gambiense.*

Other forms of the disease transmitted by other insects are also known, such as a disease occurring in Central and South America called *American trypanosomiasis*, or Chagas' disease (qv).

The parasite, when introduced into the blood, produces its effects by developing in the small blood-vessels and in the lymphatic glands, around which its presence causes inflammation.

Symptoms: A few days after the person has been bitten by the fly, fever accompanied by a slight rash develops. This fever subsides but recurs at irregular intervals of a few days or weeks. Gradually the fever becomes more pronounced, and in time the patient becomes weakened and anaemic. The glands of the neck and other parts of the body become enlarged and tender, and this state may last for months or even for years. Some cases appear to recover at this stage even after an illness of many months, and the parasite may disappear altogether from the blood. In most cases, however, the stage known as sleeping sickness gradually appears, although the lethargy may not set in for as long as seven years after the original infection. The patient now becomes disinclined for exertion, is slow mentally and weak physically, often complains of headache, and has an increasing tendency to sleep, although at first he is able to engage in conversation and to take his food. As time goes on, the weakness increases and the patient becomes more and more emaciated, bed sores form, and death finally takes place from weakness or from some intercurrent disease. The later symptoms appear to be due to the development of the parasites in the minute blood-vessels of the brain, around which, in consequence, inflammatory changes occur, with disorganization of the nervous tissues.

Treatment: For the prevention of sleeping sickness the chief essential is the avoidance of the flies which carry the disease. Fortunately, the occurrence of the flies is very definitely localized to certain regions, and, when such regions have to be traversed, the journey is made during the night-time when the flies do not feed. Those who live in fly-infested regions should have their houses and persons carefully protected against the fly. The wearing of long trousers and long-sleeved shirts gives some protection, as does the use of insect repellents such as dimethyl phthalate (qv). As the flies are mostly found close to streams, much has been done in certain localities by clearing the neighbourhood of streams in infested districts of all vegetation which would shelter the flies. The use of insecticides is proving more difficult than in the case of certain other insect-borne diseases, but promising results are being obtained from the hand-spraying of belts of vegetation bordering roads and tracks, and from aerial spraying of larger areas.

Suramin is the drug of choice in the treatment of *Trypanosoma rhodesiense* infections, and pentamidine in the treatment of *Trypanosoma gambiense* infections. Melarsoprol, a trivalent melaminyl arsenical, has replaced tryparsamide in the treatment of advanced cases of the disease, but it is a drug which must be administered with great care on account of its toxicity.

SLEEPY SICKNESS is a popular name for encephalitis lethargica. (See ENCEPHALITIS.)

SLING means a hanging bandage for the support of injured or diseased parts. Slings are generally applied for support of the upper limb, in which case the limb is suspended from the neck. The lower limb is also frequently supported in a sling from an iron cage placed upon the bed on which the patient lies. In the latter case the object of slinging the limb is usually to aid the circulation, and so quicken the healing of ulcers on the leg.

In the case of the upper limb, the sling is made from Esmarch's triangular handkerchief bandage, formed by cutting a yard of calico diagonally from corner to corner into two triangular pieces. There are four varieties of sling.

Sling for the wrist is made by folding the bandage up into a narrow cravat, laying the wrist upon the centre, and carrying one end up each side of the neck, behind which the two are tied.

Sling for the forearm is applied as follows: the unfolded triangle is laid with one end over the shoulder of the sound side, the centre of the base at the wrist of the injured limb, and the point of the bandage at the elbow of the injured limb. The other end is carried up in front of the injured limb, over the shoulder, and the two ends are tied behind the neck. The point is finally pinned neatly round the elbow.

Sling for the elbow is applied in much the same way, with this exception: that the point of the triangle is placed under the wrist, while the centre of the base supports the elbow. The bandage is completed by turning the point up over the wrist and pinning it to the part of the bandage above.

Sling for the shoulder is applied, as in the case of the sling for the elbow, with the centre of the base at the elbow, and the front end is carried over the opposite shoulder. The other end passes up behind the upper arm and across the back, the two ends being tied upon the sound shoulder. The object of this sling is to support, while avoiding pressure on the injured shoulder, as in fracture of the collar-bone. (See FRACTURES.)

SLIPPED DISC is the popular name for a prolapsed intervertebral disc (qv).

SLOUGH means a dead part separated by natural processes from the living body. The term is applied to hard external parts which the lower animals cast off naturally in the course of growth, like the skin of snakes or the shell of crabs. In man, however, the process is generally associated with disease, and is then known as gangrene. (See GANGRENE.) Sloughs may be of very small size, as in the case of the core of a boil, or they may include a whole limb, but in general a slough involves a limited area of skin or of the underlying tissues. The process of separation of a slough is described under gangrene.

SMALLPOX, so called to distinguish it from syphilis, the great pox (pox being the plural of pock, the Old English term for a pustule (qv)), is also known as VARIOLA (from *varus*, the Latin for pimple). It is an acute, highly infectious disease due to a virus.

Until recent times it was one of the major killing diseases. In the 1960s the World Health Organization undertook an eradication scheme by means of mass vaccination. As a result, the last naturally occurring case was recorded in October 1977, and on May 8, 1980, the World Health Assembly solemnly agreed a Resolution confirming that smallpox has finally been eradicated from the world. This was indeed a historic occasion; the first occasion on which man has attempted to eradicate a disease and has succeeded in so doing. The public lack of interest in it is explained by the fact that so few of those living today have had any experience of it – even doctors.

Since 1960, there have been only 141 reported cases, with 28 deaths, in England and Wales, and not a single naturally occurring case since 1973. (See VACCINATION.)

SMEGMA is a thick, cheesy secretion formed by the sebaceous glands of the glans penis. A bacillus, closely resembling the tubercle bacillus morphologically, develops readily in this secretion.

SMELL: The sense of smell is picked up in what is known as the olfactory areas of the nose. Each of these is about 3 square centimetres in area and contains 50 million olfactory, or smelling, cells. They lie, one on either side, at the highest part of each nasal cavity. This is why we have to sniff if we want to smell anything carefully, as in ordinary quiet breathing only a few eddies of the air we breathe in reaches an olfactory area. From these olfactory cells the olfactory nerves (one on each side) run up to the olfactory bulbs underneath the frontal lobe of the brain (qv), and here the impulse is translated into what we describe as smell.

SMELLING SALTS (see AMMONIA).

SMOKING (see TOBACCO).

SNAKE-BITE (see BITES AND STINGS).

SNARE is a wire loop used by the ear, nose, and throat surgeon for removing polypi from the nose.

SNEEZING means a sudden expulsion of air through the nose, designed to expel irritating materials from the upper air passages. In sneezing, a powerful expiratory effort is made, the vocal cords are kept shut till the pressure in the chest has risen high, and air is then suddenly allowed to escape upward, being directed into the back of the nose by the soft palate. One sneeze projects 10,000 to 100,000 droplets a distance of up to 10 metres at a rate of over 60 kilometres an hour. As such droplets may contain micro-organisms, it is clear what an important part sneezing plays in transmitting infections such as the common cold. Though usually transitory, sneezing may persist for days on end – up to 204 days have been recorded.

Sneezing may be caused by the presence of irritating particles in the nose, such as snuff, the pollen of grasses and flowers. It is also an early symptom of colds, influenza, measles, and hay-fever, being then accompanied or followed by running at the nose.

SNORING is usually attributed to vibrations of the soft palate, but there is evidence that the main fault lies in the edge of the posterior pillars of the fauces (qv) which vibrate noisily. Mouth breathing is necessary for snoring, but not all mouth-breathers snore. The principal cause is blockage of the nose, such as occurs during the course of the common cold or chronic nasal catarrh. Such blockage also occurs in some cases of deviation of the nasal septum or nasal polypi. (See NOSE, DISEASES OF.) In children, mouth-breathing, with resulting snoring, is often due to enlarged tonsils and adenoids. A further cause of snoring is loss of tone in the soft palate and surrounding tissues due to smoking, overwork, fatigue, obesity, and general poor health. One in eight people are said to snore regularly. The intensity, or loudness, of snoring is in the range, 40 to 69 decibels. (Pneumatic drills register between 70 and 90 decibels.)

Treatment therefore consists of the removal of any of these causes of mouth-breathing that may be present. Should these not succeed in preventing snoring, then measures should be taken to prevent the victim from sleeping lying on his back, as this is a habit which strongly conduces to snoring. Simple measures include sleeping with several pillows so that the head is raised quite considerably when asleep. Alternatively, a small pillow may be put under the nape of the neck. If all these measures fail, there is much to be said for the old traditional method of sewing a hair-brush, or some other hard object such as a stone, into the back of the snorer's pyjamas. This means that if he does turn on to his back while asleep, he is quickly awakened and therefore able to turn on his side again. (See also STERTOR.)

SNOW BLINDNESS results from exposure to ultraviolet light reflected from snowfields. It causes pain, photophobia and watering of the eyes. Examining the eye shows that there are hundreds of punctate areas of corneal epithelial damage. The symptoms and appearance are exactly the same as in *Arc Eye*, acquired by using an arc welder without adequate eye protection. (See EYE, DISEASE AND INJURIES, *radiant energy injuries*). Treatment is to keep the eye covered with a pad for twenty-four hours.

SNUFFLES is the name applied to noisy breathing in children due to the constant presence of nasal discharge. (For treatment, see NOSE, DISEASES OF.)

SOAP is a substance made by boiling a fat or oil with an alkali. The most commonly used oil is olive oil, and the most frequent alkali is caustic soda. In the process of manufacture the fatty acids of the oil unite with the alkali, glycerin separating out. In soft soap or green soap, caustic potash is used in place of soda; marine soap

is made with coconut oil; curd soap has tallow for its fat: while many toilet soaps have palm oil or almond oil. Barilla soap is made from soda got by burning plants; in superfatted soaps care is taken that the fatty part is in excess, so that no crude alkali is left to irritate the skin; whilst glycerin soaps have a specially emollient action. Medicated soaps of various kinds are prepared, the chief drugs added to soap being of an antiseptic nature, such as carbolic acid, coal-tar, formalin, hexachlorophane, terebene.
Uses: The chief use of soap is, mixed with water, as a cleansing agent. Internally, hard soap is often used to make up the bulk of pills containing very active ingredients. As a purgative enema, soap is used made up into a strong solution in warm water. Soap liniment, better known as 'opodeldoc', is used as a popular remedy for stiffness or sprains.

SOCIAL CLASSES: As factors such as the cause of death and the incidence of diseases vary in different social strata, the Registrar-General evolved the following social classification, which has now been in official use for many years:
Class I Professional occupations, such as lawyers, clergymen, and commissioned officers in the Armed Forces.
Class II Intermediate occupations, such as teachers.
Class III Skilled occupations, such as mineworkers, transport workers, and clerical workers.
Class IV Partly skilled occupations, such as agricultural workers.
Class V Unskilled occupations, such as building and dock labourers.

SODA (see ALKALI; SODIUM).

SODIUM is a metal, the salts of which are white, crystalline, and very soluble. The fluids of the body contain naturally a considerable quantity of sodium chloride.
SODIUM CARBONATE, commonly known as SODA or WASHING SODA, has a powerful softening action upon the tissues.
SODIUM BICARBONATE, or BAKING SODA, is used as an antacid in relieving indigestion associated with increased acidity of the gastric secretion. It is taken in doses of 600 or 1,200 mg, as a rule. The citrate and the acetate of sodium are used as diuretics and in the treatment of inflammatory conditions of the kidneys and bladder, though the corresponding potassium salts are more often used.

SODIUM CALCIUMEDETATE is the calcium complex of diamine tetra-acetic acid, which is proving of value in the treatment of lead poisoning and of chrome ulceration.

SODIUM CHLORIDE is the chemical name for common salt.

SODIUM CROMOGLYCATE (INTAL) is the main drug used in the prophylaxis of asthma. It is administered by inhalation and can reduce the incidence of asthmatic attacks but is of no value in the treatment of an acute attack. It acts by preventing the release of pharmacological mediators of bronchospasm, particularly histamine, by stabilising mastcell membranes. It is thus of particular use in patients whose asthma has an allergic basis. The dose frequency is adjusted to the patient's response but is usually administered by inhalation four times daily.

SODIUM DIATRIZOATE is an organic iodine salt that is radio-opaque and is therefore used as a contrast medium to outline various organs in the body in X-ray films. It is given intravenously. Its main use is in pyelography (qv), that is in rendering the kidneys radio-opaque, but it is also used to outline the blood-vessels (angiography) and the gall-bladder and bile ducts (cholangiography).

SODIUM HYPOCHLORITE is a disinfectant by virtue of the fact that it gives off chlorine. For domestic use, as, for example, for sterilizing baby feeding bottles, it is available in a variety of proprietary preparations. (See also CHLORINATED LIME.)

SODIUM SULPHATE (see GLAUBER'S SALT).

SODIUM VALPROATE is a drug that is proving of value in the treatment of some cases of epilepsy which will not respond to any of the other drugs used for the treatment of this condition. It must be used with care as it may cause liver damage.

SOFTENING OF THE BRAIN (see APOPLEXY; BRAIN, DISEASES OF).

SOFT SORE, or CHANCROID, is an infective venereal ulceration due to the *Haemophilus ducreyi*, which is common in the tropics and subtropics. It is a local condition, not spreading beyond the glands in the neighbourhood of the original ulcer, although there is always a possibility that syphilis may be contracted along with this disease and may show itself later. The condition begins within a few hours after infection as a pimple which enlarges rapidly and ulcerates. The glands in the groin speedily become affected, and as these may soften and ulcerate, the condition sometimes results in a tedious illness. In England 49 cases were reported in the year ending June 30, 1980.
Treatment consists in the administration of full doses of one of the sulphonamides by mouth. The affected glands are not drained, but if they become fluctuant the pus may be aspirated with a needle and syringe. In resistant cases, streptomycin or tetracycline may be tried.

SOLAPSONE is a sulphone derivative which is used in the treatment of leprosy. It can be given by mouth or by injection.

SOLARIUM is a room enclosed by glass in which sun baths are taken while protection is afforded from the weather.

SOLDIER'S HEART, or DISORDERED ACTION OF THE HEART (DAH), or EFFORT SYNDROME, is a term applied to a set of symptoms arising under conditions of great anxiety and unusual physical strain, and consisting of palpitation, shortness of breath, speedy exhaustion, depression, and irritability. The condition received its name from the frequency with which it was noticed during the 1914–18 War. (See HEART DISEASES.)

SOLOMON'S SEAL is a popular name for *Polygonatum officinale*. The fluid extract has astringent properties and is used as an application to bruises.

SOLUTION or LIQUOR as it used to be known, is a liquid preparation containing one or more soluble drugs, usually dissolved in water.

SOMATIC means relating to the body, as opposed to the mind.

SOMNAMBULISM means sleep-walking. (See SLEEP.)

SOPORIFICS are measures which induce sleep. (See HYPNOTICS.)

SORDES is the thick offensive material which gathers on the lips, teeth, and tongue of people who are very weak from fever or other cause. In healthy people the constant movements of the tongue and lips serve to keep them free of growing bacteria, remnants of food, and cells cast off from the mucous membrane of the mouth, which in the enfeebled state collect and form a brown or black putrefying deposit.
Treatment: The lips, tongue, and teeth should be wiped occasionally with a rag dipped in borax and honey, or glycerin of borax, and the rag then burned. Syringing out the mouth with bicarbonate of soda solution, one teaspoonful to a tumblerful of warm water, is also helpful in very weak people. If the person is strong enough, he may rinse his mouth with a weak solution of permanganate of potassium in water, diluted to a pale pink colour.

SORE is a popular term for ulcer (qv).

SORE THROAT (see THROAT, DISEASES OF; TONSILLITIS).

SOTALOL (BETA-CARDONE, SOTACOR) (see ADRENERGIC RECEPTORS).

SOUND is a rod with a curve at one end used mainly for passing into the bladder to determine whether a stone is present or not. (See BLADDER, DISEASES OF.)

SOUR MILK (see LACTIC ACID BACILLI).

SOUTHEY'S TUBES are long, fine tubes for drawing off fluid slowly from cases of oedema. (See ASPIRATION.)

SOYA BEAN is the bean of *Glycine soja*, a leguminous plant related to peas and beans. The outstanding characteristic of the soya bean is its high protein and fat content. There is an almost complete absence of starch, but a large amount of mineral matter. Soya flour contains 40 per cent of protein and 20 per cent of fat. It yields 470 Calories per 100 grams as compared with 370 Calories for white wheat flour. Soya flour contains 0·2 per cent of calcium (about ten times as much as in white flour). It also contains a variable but large amount of iron: 6·7 to 30 mg per 100 grams of soya flour compared with 1 mg in white flour and 3 mg in 100 grams of wholemeal flour. It is a good source of thiamine and riboflavine, and of vitamin A in the form of carotene. (See BEANS.)

SPANISH FLY is a popular term for cantharides, which is used as a blistering agent. (See CANTHARIDES.)

SPASM means an involuntary, and, in severe cases, painful contraction of a muscle or of a hollow organ with a muscular wall. Spasm may be due to affections in the muscle where the spasm takes place, or it may originate in some disturbance of that part of the nervous system which controls the spasmodically acting muscles. Spasms of a general nature are usually spoken of as convulsions; spasms of a painful nature are known as cramp when they affect the muscles of the limbs, and as colic when they are situated in the stomach, bowels, or other organs of the abdomen. Spasm of the heart receives the name of breast-pang or angina pectoris, and is both a serious and an agonizing condition. When the spasm is a prolonged firm contraction, it is spoken of as tonic spasm; when it consists of a series of twitches or quick alternate contractions and relaxations, it is known as clonic spasm. Spasm is a symptom of many diseases.

SPASMODIC TORTICOLLIS is the term applied to a chronic condition in which the neck is rotated or deviated laterally, forwards, or backwards, often with additional jerking or tremor. It is a form of focal dystonia, and should not be confused with the far commoner transient condition of acute painful wry-neck. (See DYSTONIA.)

SPASMOLYTICS are remedies which diminish spasm. They may achieve this in one of three ways: (*a*) by interfering with the transmission of the nerve impulses that are causing the spasm; (*b*) by a direct action on the affected muscle; (*c*) by depressing the central nervous system.
Varieties: In the past many of the favourites in this field, such as oil of cinnamon, oil of cloves, oil of peppermint, and valerian, achieved their

reputation by virtue of their depressing effect on the sensitivity of the nerve endings. Others, such as lobelia and stramonium, often in the form of cigarettes to be inhaled, achieved a wide reputation as asthma cures.

Today, a more scientific approach is maintained, though there is still much to be said for the use of preparations, such as oil of cinnamon or of peppermint for the relief of mild spasm of the gut, and not a few asthmatics have implicit faith in the relieving power of lobelia or stramonium. The most widely used spasmolytics today are atropine and its derivatives, or its many synthetic substitutes. These act by paralysing the action of the parasympathetic nerve fibres that induce contraction of smooth muscle. They are most widely used in relieving spasm in the alimentary and renal tracts. For the relief of the spasm of asthma adrenaline and ephedrine are still great standbys, though isoprenaline and other similarly acting drugs are being used to an increasing extent. All these act through the sympathetic nervous system.

Of the spasmolytics acting directly on muscle, the best known group is the nitrites – amyl nitrite and glyceryl trinitrate – which are the great standby for the relief of the spasm that induces angina pectoris. Other drugs that act in this way are theophylline and aminophylline. If the spasm is really severe, and therefore painful enough, general depression of the brain may be necessary by means of general anaesthetics. In less severe cases, the lesser degrees of depression of the brain induced by hypnotics may have a spasmolytic action, and, though it should seldom be used for this purpose because of its habit-forming propensities, even alcohol could rank as a spasmolytic.

SPASMOPHILIA is a term applied to a condition affecting certain people, especially in childhood, in which the motor nerves are unusually sensitive to irritation. Such patients show an abnormal tendency to convulsions and spasms on very slight cause.

SPASMUS NUTANS is the term for describing the rhythmic nodding of the head sometimes seen in infants during the first year of life.

SPASTIC is a term applied to any condition showing increased muscle tone: eg. spastic gait. This is specially associated with some disease affecting the upper part of the nervous system connected with movement (upper neuron), so that its controlling influence is lost and the muscles are in a state of over-excitability.

SPATULA is a flat, knife-like instrument used for spreading plasters and ointments, and also for depressing the tongue when the throat is being examined.

SPECIAL HEALTH AUTHORITY (see NATIONAL HEALTH SERVICE).

SPECIFIC is a term used in various ways. It is applied to remedies which appear to have a definitely curative effect in certain disease, as, for example, to sodium salicylate, which is said to be specific in rheumatism, or to quinine, which is a specific for malaria. Again, it is applied to bacteria and other agents which form the chief cause of certain diseases, though there may be other minor contributing causes: for example, the comma bacillus is the specific cause of cholera, the sarcoptes parasite is the specific cause of scabies. The term is also used to designate diseases that have an identity of their own, have a definite cause, and do not consist merely of a group of symptoms: for example, scarlet fever, measles, typhoid fever are specific as compared with vague ailments such as enlargement of the glands in the neck, diarrhoea, or dyspepsia. The word specific is also sometimes used as a euphemism for venereal disease.

SPECTACLES can be worn for a variety of reasons including correction of a refractive error, correction of a squint, for protection (from foreign bodies or, with tinted lenses, from bright light), or occasionally to hold a prosthesis.

SPECULUM is an instrument designed to aid the examination of the various openings on the surface of the body. Many specula are provided with small electric lamps so placed as to light up the cavity brilliantly.

SPEECH, DISORDERS OF: Speech is the ability to express oneself orally, using exclamations, words and sentences. A child needs to know how to do this and difficulties may occur either through problems during pregnancy, at birth, childhood illnesses or delayed development. For example, a child with severe cleft lip and palate may need to undergo surgery before being able to produce speech which is intelligible to his family. This may discourage talking, and language development may fall behind. In another instance, a child with recurrent ear infections may find it less easy to listen to others and therefore his experience of spoken language is limited. In rare cases a child may develop normally except for the sole area of language development. The result is *childhood dysphasia* and he may need specialist education if he is to develop his full potential.

Adults may lose the ability to talk having acquired it in early childhood in the usual way. This is usually due to a stroke (see DYSPHASIA, STROKE), or to a head injury. They may also have difficulty in articulating words as the result of illness (see DYSARTHRIA). Stammering may persist into adulthood (see STAMMERING). Children and more often adults, particularly those who use their voices during working hours to a great extent (eg. teachers) may be prone to hoarse voice (see DYSPHONIA).

A very small minority of adults will undergo an operation for removal of the larynx and may need help in using other methods to communicate (see LARYNGECTOMY).

Increasing recognition is being given to those children and adults who are intellectually handicapped and of the impairment of articulation and language which often occurs. Social skills and communication in general are often impaired with those who are severely psychiatrically disturbed. (See also VOICE AND SPEECH.)

SPEECH THERAPY is a small independent graduate profession. Speech therapists assist, diagnose and treat the whole spectrum of acquired or developmental communication disorders. They work in medical and education establishments often in an advisory or consultative capacity. The medical conditions in which speech therapy is employed include: dysgraphia, dyslexia, dysathria, dysphasia, dysphonia, dyspraxia, autism, Bell's palsy, cerebral palsy, deafness, disordered language, delayed speech, disordered speech, Down's syndrome, laryngectomy, macroglossia, mental subnormality, motor neurone disease, malformations of the palate, Parkinsonism, psychiatric disorders, stammering, stroke and disorders of voice production.

It is a caring profession; most speech therapists work for the National Health Service in community clinics and hospitals. They may also work in schools or in units for the handicapped, paediatric assessment centres, language units attached to primary schools, adult training centres and day centres for the elderly.

A speech therapist undergoes a four-year degree course which covers the study of disorders of communication in children and adults, phonetics and linguistics, anatomy and physiology, psychology and many other related subjects. Further information on training can be obtained from the College of Speech Therapists, 6 Lechmere Road, London NW2 5BU.

If the parents of a child are concerned about their child's speech, they may approach a speech therapist for assessment and guidance. Their General Practitioner will be able to give them local addresses or they should contact the District Speech Therapist. Adults are usually referred by hospital consultants.

The College of Speech Therapists keeps a register of all those who have passed a recognised degree or equivalent qualification in speech therapy. It will be able to direct you to your nearest NHS or private speech therapist.

SPERMATIC is the name applied to the blood-vessels and other structures associated with the testicle.

SPERMATORRHOEA is the passage of semen without erection of the penis or orgasm.

SPERMATOZOON (plural: SPERMATOZOA) is the male sex or germ cell which unites with the ovum to form the embryo or foetus. It is a highly mobile cell approximately 4 micrometres in length, much smaller than an ovum, which is about 35 micrometres in diameter. Each millilitre of semen (qv) contains on average about 100 million spermatozoa, and the average volume of semen discharged during ejaculation in sexual intercourse is between 2 and 4 ml. Once ejaculated during intercourse it travels at a rate of 1·5 to 3 millimetres a minute and remains mobile for several days after insemination, but quickly loses its potency for fertilization. As it takes only about 70 minutes to reach the ovarian end of the uterine tube, it is assumed that there must be factors other than its own mobility, such as contraction of the muscle of the womb and uterine tube, that speed it on its way. (See also FOETUS.)

SPHAGNUM MOSS, or peat or bog moss, has been used as a wound dressing from time immemorial. A skeleton from the Bronze Age in Scotland showed a large pad of sphagnum moss applied to what had been a chest wound. It was used on a large scale as a wound dressing in the 1914–18 War. It is widely distributed in Scotland, Ireland and Western England. Its main value lies in its great absorptive powers: it can absorb up to seven times its weight of water. It is deodorizing and does not allow discharges from wounds to pass through it as does cotton wool.

SPHENOID is a bone lying in the centre of the base of the skull, and supporting the others like a wedge or keystone. (See SKULL.)

SPHINCTER means a circular muscle which surrounds the opening from an organ, and, by maintaining a constant state of moderate contraction, prevents the escape of the contents of the organ. Sphincters close the outlet from the bladder and rectum, and in certain nervous diseases their action is interfered with, so that the power to relax or to keep moderately contracted is lost, and retention or incontinence of the evacuation results.

SPHYGMOGRAPH is an instrument for recording the pulse. (See PULSE.)

SPHYGMOMANOMETER is the name of an instrument for measuring blood-pressure in the arteries. It usually consists of a pneumatic armlet, the interior of which communicates by a rubber tube with an air-pressure pump and a gauge. The armlet is bound about the upper arm and pumped up sufficiently to obliterate the pulse as felt at the wrist or as heard in the artery at the bend of the elbow. The pressure registered on the gauge at this point is regarded as the pressure of the blood at each heart-beat (systolic pressure). The pressure at which the sound heard in the artery suddenly changes its character marks the diastolic pressure.

SPINA BIFIDA is one of the commonest of the congenital malformations. There are marked regional variations. It takes two main forms. SPINA BIFIDA OCCULTA is much the commoner of the two and consists of a defect in the posterior wall of the spinal wall, usually in the lumbar region. As a rule it has no deleterious effects unless the underlying spinal cord is affected. It has been said that one in every ten individuals has such a defect.

SPINA BIFIDA CYSTICA, the other form, is a much more serious condition. Here the defect in the spinal canal is accompanied by protrusion of the spinal cord which, in turn, may take one of two forms. One is a *meningocele*, in which the meninges (qv), containing cerebrospinal fluid, protrude through the defect. The other is a *meningomyelocele*, in which the protruding sac contains spinal cord and nerves. This is much the more serious condition of the two and, unfortunately, much the commoner, accounting for 90 per cent of all cases. The over-all incidence of spina bifida cystica varies from one part of the country to another, but in England and Wales, in 1966, 1206 babies were born alive with this condition, representing a rate of 1·4 per 1000 births. This compares with a rate of 4·1 per 1000 births in rural areas of South Wales. The cause is not known but there is a strong genetic factor. Thus, a couple who have had one baby affected with spina bifida have a 5 to 8 per cent chance that any subsequent babies they have will have a major malformation of the central nervous system. If they have already had two or more affected infants, the risk of any further having a similar condition is about 1 in 4 to 1 in 8. Tests are now available, whereby severe cases of spina bifida (and anencephaly) can be recognized in the unborn child during pregnancy. In 1984 there were 378 children born with spina bifida in England and Wales.

The usual site of the defect is in the lumbosacral, or lower, part of the spine. When the baby is born the protruding sac is quite soft, but if it is a meningomyelocele, as it usually is, the baby's condition rapidly deteriorates, with the development of paralysis and incontinence, and a high risk of meningitis. This is why it is now recommended that the baby should be operated on as soon as possible – preferably in a special centre. Many of these babies also have hydrocephalus (qv). So successful are the results of operation on carefully selected cases in special centres that it is now claimed that 'the majority of adequately treated children with spina bifida associated with hydrocephalus will grow up with a normal intelligence, although the average intelligence of the whole group falls below the 100 IQ figure which applies to the general population'. The emphasis here, however, is on 'carefully selected cases', and 'adequately treated' and 'special centre'. Indeed, the decision as to how to deal with a severe case of spina bifida can be one of the most heart-rending and difficult in the whole of medicine.

There is a growing volume of evidence of the value of vitamin supplements preceding and during pregnancy in reducing the incidence of this pathetic congenital abnormality.

Parents of children with spina bifida or hydrocephalus are recommended to join the Association for Spina Bifida and Hydrocephalus, 22 Upper Woburn Place, London WC1H 0EP (01–388 1382), which has branches in all parts of the country, or The Scottish Spina Bifida Association, 190 Queensferry Road, Edinburgh EH4 2BW (031–332 0743). In this way they will receive continuing help, advice and encouragement.

SPINAL COLUMN, also known as the SPINE, CHINE, BACKBONE, and VERTEBRAL COLUMN, forms an important part of the skeleton, acting both as the rigid pillar which supports the upper parts of the body and as a protection to the spinal cord and nerves arising from it. The spinal column is built up of a number of bones placed one upon another, which, in consequence of having a slight degree of turning-movement, are known as the vertebrae. The possession of a spinal cord supported by a vertebral column distinguishes the higher animals from the lower types, and gains for them the general name of vertebrates. Of the vertebrates, man alone stands absolutely erect, and this erect carriage of the body gives to the skull and vertebral column certain distinctive characters.

The human backbone is about 70 cm (28 inches) in length, and varies little in full-grown people; differences in height depend mainly upon the length of the lower limbs. The number of vertebrae is 33 in children, although in adult life 5 of these fuse together to form the sacrum, and the lowest 4 unite in the coccyx, so that the number of separate bones is reduced to 26. Of these there are 7 in the neck, known therefore as *cervical vertebrae*; 12 with ribs attached, in the region of the thorax, and known as *thoracic* or *dorsal vertebrae*; 5 in the loins, called *lumbar vertebrae*; 5 fused to form the *sacrum*; and 4 joined in the *coccyx*. These numbers are expressed in a formula thus: C7, D12, L5, S5, Coc4=33. The formula in different animals varies considerably, but throughout the class of mammalia the number of cervical vertebrae is almost constantly seven, even in long-necked animals like the giraffe and short-necked animals like the whale. Although the vertebrae in each of these regions have distinguishing features, all the vertebrae are constructed on the same general plan. Each has a thick, rounded, bony part in front, known as the body, and these bodies form the main thickness of the column. Behind the body of each is a ring of bone, the neural ring, these rings placed one above another forming the bony canal which lodges the spinal cord. From each side of the ring a short process of bone known as the transverse process stands out, and from the back of the ring a larger process, the spinous process, projects. These processes give attachment to the strong ligaments and muscles which unite, support, and bend the column. The spines can be seen or felt beneath the skin of the back lying in the centre of a groove between the muscular masses of the two sides, and they give to the column its name of the spinal column. One of these spines, that of the 7th cervical vertebra, is especially large and forms a distinct bony prominence, where the neck joins the back. Between the bodies of the vertebrae lies a series of thick discs of fibro-cartilage known as intervertebral discs. Each disc consists of an outer portion, known as the annulus fibrosus, and an inner core, known as the nucleus pulposus. To these 23 discs the upper part of the spine owes much of its pliability, as well as a great deal of its resiliency and power of diminishing the effect of jars and blows communicated through the feet or head. There is also a small joint at each side upon the ring of the vertebra so that each vertebra comes in contact with the one above and the one beneath in three places.

The first and second cervical vertebrae are modified in a very special manner. The first vertebra, known as the atlas, is devoid of a body, but has a specially large and strong ring with two hollows upon which the skull rests, thus permitting of nodding movements. The second vertebra, known as the axis, has a pivot upon its body which fits into the first vertebra and thus permits of free rotation of the head from side to side.

An important feature of the spinal column, and one especially marked in human beings, is the presence of four curves from behind forwards. Thus the cervical vertebrae are arranged with a curve whose hollow looks backwards, the dorsal vertebrae have a marked curve with the hollow forwards; in the lumbar region the hollow is directed backwards, while the sacrum and coccyx form a marked hollow to the front. The effect of the dorsal and sacral curves is greatly to increase the size of the cavities of chest and pelvis, while the compensating curves of the neck and loins serve to keep the general axis of the spinal column in a vertical line. The curves have also an action very similar to that of the springs of a vehicle, in minimizing jolting and jarring of the internal organs. There is usually a very slight curve to one side in the upper dorsal region, resulting from the greater development and use of one arm.

The neural rings placed one above another form a canal, which is wide in the neck, smaller and almost round in the dorsal region, and wide again in the lumbar vertebrae. This canal lodges the spinal cord, and the nerves that issue from the cord pass out from the canal by openings between the vertebrae which are produced by notches on the upper and lower margins of each ring. The intervertebral foramina formed by these notches are so large in comparison with the nerves passing through them that there is no chance of pressure upon the latter, except in very serious injuries which dislocate and fracture the spine.

SPINAL CORD is the lower portion of the central nervous system which is situated within the spinal column. Above, it forms the direct continuation of the medulla oblongata, this part of the brain changing its name to spinal cord at the *foramen magnum*, the large opening in the base of the skull through which it passes into the spinal canal. Below, the spinal cord extends to about the upper border of the second lumbar vertebra, where it tapers off into a fine thread, known as the filum terminale, that is attached to the coccyx at the lower end of the spine. The spinal cord is thus considerably shorter than the spinal column, being only 37 to 45 cm (15 to 18 inches) in length, and weighing around 30 grams. In its course from the base of the skull to the lumbar region the cord gives off thirty-one nerves on each side, each of which arises by an anterior and a posterior root that join before the nerve emerges from the spinal canal. The openings for the nerves formed by notches on the ring of each vertebra have been mentioned under SPINAL COLUMN. To reach these openings the upper nerves pass almost directly outwards, whilst lower in the series their obliquity increases, until below the point where the cord terminates there is a sheaf of nerves, known as the cauda equina, running downwards to leave the spinal canal at their appropriate openings.

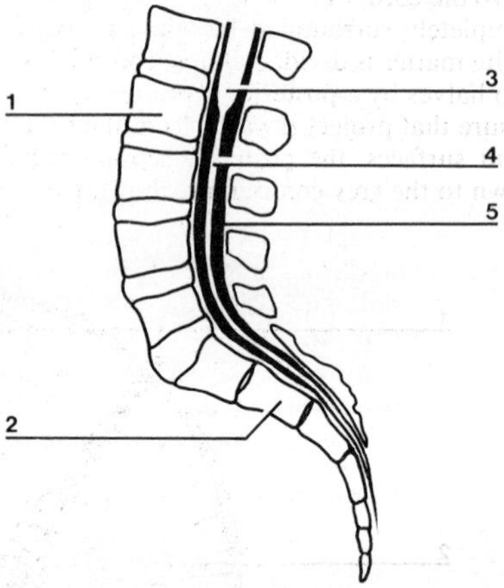

1 second lumbar vertebrae
2 second sacral vertebrae
3 spinal medulla or cord
4 filum terminale
5 subarachnoid space, containing cerebo-spinal fluid

Diagram of the lower end of the spinal cord.

In shape the cord is a cylinder, about the thickness of the little finger, and slightly flattened from before backwards. It has two slightly enlarged portions, one in the lower part of the neck, the other at the last dorsal vertebra, and from these thickenings arise the nerves that pass to the upper and lower limbs. (See

NERVES.) The spinal cord, like the brain, is surrounded by three membranes, the dura mater, arachnoid mater, and pia mater, from without inwards. The arrangement of the dura and arachnoid is much looser in the case of the cord than their application to the brain. The dura especially forms a wide tube which is separated from the cord by fluid and from the vertebral canal by blood-vessels and fat, this arrangement protecting the cord from pressure in any ordinary movements of the spine.

IN SECTION, the spinal cord consists partly of grey, but mainly of white, matter. It differs from the upper parts of the brain in that the white matter in the cord is arranged on the surface, surrounding a mass of grey matter, while in the brain the grey matter is superficial. The arrangement of grey matter, as seen in a section across the cord, resembles the letter H, each half of the cord possessing an anterior and a posterior horn, and the masses of the two sides being joined by a wide posterior grey commissure. In the middle of this commissure lies the central canal of the cord, a small tube which is the continuation of the ventricles in the brain. The horns of grey matter reach almost to the surface of the cord, and from their ends arise the roots of the nerves that leave the cord, but elsewhere the grey matter is completely surrounded by white matter. The white matter is divided almost completely into two halves by a posterior septum and anterior fissure that project inwards from the back and front surfaces, the posterior septum reaching down to the grey commissure, but the anterior fissure being separated from it by a small anterior white commissure that joins the white matter of the two sides together. The white matter is further divided into three columns, on each side, by the horns of grey matter and the nerve roots passing from them to the surface; these are known as the anterior, lateral, and posterior columns.

Minute structure: The *grey matter* is found upon microscopic examination to consist largely of neuroglia, the connective tissue of the central nervous system, which is made up of small cells with long branching processes. This neuroglia forms a sort of felt-work, in the meshes of which lie numbers of multipolar nerve-cells and the nerve-fibres that spring from them and unite one cell to another or pass out into the nerves. The *whitematter* consists almost entirely of bundles of nerve-fibres provided in general with a medullary sheath, the white colour being due to the collective appearance of these sheaths. (See NERVES.) There is also in the white matter a small quantity of supporting connective tissue. Most of the nerve-fibres run vertically, so that a cross-section of the cord shows them as a collection of dots, each surrounded by a clear space. Blood-vessels are found in the cord both in grey and in white matter.

Functions: The cord is, in part, a receiver and originator of nerve impulses, and in part merely a conductor of such impulses along fibres which pass through it to and from the brain. The presence of centres in the cord, capable of receiving sensory impressions and originating

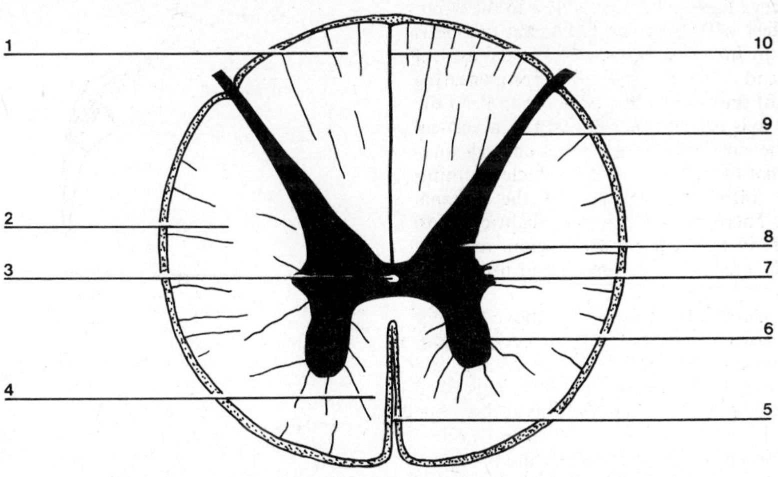

1 posterior white column
2 lateral white column
3 central canal
4 anterior white column
5 anterior median tissue
6 anterior horn
7 lateral horn
8 thoracic nucleus
9 posterior horn
10 posterior median septum

Transverse section through the spinal cord in the thoracic region. Magnified eight times.

motor impulses, is proved by several facts. Thus, it has been calculated that the number of nerve-fibres entering or leaving the cord by the spinal nerves is twice as great as the number of fibres contained in the upper end of the cord, where it is continued into the brain. Again, if the cord is severed in the dorsal region, as by a fracture of the spine, the centres which govern the evacuation of the bladder and bowel do not lose their power of controlling these organs immediately upon being severed from the brain. Many of these centres are known to exist in the cord, such as centres for regulating the size of the blood-vessels, for altering the size of the pupil of the eye, for sweating, for breathing. Over most, if not all, of these centres, however, the brain exerts a controlling influence, and before any incoming sensation can produce an effect upon consciousness, it is in all probability necessary that it should obtain a clear passage up to the brain.

Many of these centres act in a rhythmical or *automatic* way. Other cells of the cord are capable of originating movements in response to impulses brought direct to them through sensory nerves, such activity being known as *reflex* action. (For a fuller description of the activities of the spinal cord, see NERVES.)

By observing the process of degeneration that takes place when nerve-fibres are cut off by disease or injury from the cells to which they belong, and by observing also the manner in which the fibres in different portions of the cord develop, it has been found possible to divide the three white columns of the cord into tracts, in each of which the fibres have a special function. Thus the posterior column consists of the *fasciculus gracilis* and the *fasciculus cuneatus* both conveying sensory impressions upwards. The lateral column contains the ventral and the dorsal spino-cerebellar tracts passing to the cerebellum, the crossed pyramidal tract of motor fibres carrying outgoing impulses downwards together with the rubrospinal, the spino-thalamic, the spino-tectal, and the postero-lateral tracts. And, finally, the anterior column contains the direct pyramidal tract of motor fibres and an anterior mixed zone. The pyramidal tracts have the best-known course. Starting from cells near the central sulcus on the brain (see BRAIN), the motor nerve-fibres run down through the internal capsule, pons, and medulla, in the lower part of which many of those coming from the right side of the brain cross to the left side of the spinal cord, and vice versa. Thence the fibres run down in the crossed pyramidal tract to end beside nerve-cells in the anterior horn of the cord. From these nerve-cells other fibres pass outwards to form the nerves that go direct to the muscles. Thus the motor nerve path from brain to muscle is divided into two sections of neurons, of which the upper exerts a controlling influence upon the lower, while the lower is concerned in maintaining the muscle in a state of health and good nutrition, and in directly calling it into action.

SPINE AND SPINAL CORD, DISEASES AND INJURIES OF: These are considered together, because the chief danger of interference with the spinal column lies in the risk of injury to the spinal cord and nerves. Only some of the chief diseases will be dealt with.

LATERAL CURVATURE OF THE SPINE, or SCOLIOSIS, consists chiefly in bending of the spine over to one side, although, in consequence of the vertebrae being broader in front than behind, this is accompanied by a certain amount of twisting of the vertebrae round their vertical axis. The shape of the chest becomes, in consequence, markedly altered, the ribs on one side projecting behind at their angles, and causing the shoulder-blade to be very prominent, while on the other side the chest is flattened. (See CHEST DEFORMITIES.) The shoulder of the bulging side is usually considerably elevated. This condition may be started by slight injuries of the spine, by rickets in early life, by diseases in the chest, such as pleurisy, which cause partial collapse of one side, or by weakness of the muscles, such as occurs in certain diseases of the nervous system: for example, cerebral paralysis (qv). *Idiopathic scoliosis*, so called because the cause is not known, is a familial condition which occurs at two different ages. The infantile type occurs more commonly in boys and the curve is usually to the left. The curve usually develops during the first year of life. The vast majority (90 per cent) of these recover spontaneously. Those which prove to be progressive require active treatment with what is known as the Milwaukee brace and plaster of Paris. The adolescent type occurs predominantly in girls and the curve is usually to the right. Occasionally a similar type may occur at the age of 5 or 6. As often as not it arises in an otherwise apparently healthy girl. This type does not disappear spontaneously, and treatment, which should be instituted as early as possible, may be prolonged and quite often involves spinal fusion.

BACKWARD CURVATURE OF THE SPINE, KYPHOSIS, or HUMP-BACK, may be due to various causes. One cause is tuberculosis of the spine, first described by the famous surgeon, Percivall Pott (1714–88), after whom it is also called *Pott's disease*. This results in destruction and collapse of one or more vertebrae with posterior angulation of the spine. Other causes are what is known as a compression fracture of the spine following an accident, spondylitis (qv), rickets (qv) and conditions which cause decalcification, or softening of the bones such as osteomalacia (qv). The round shoulders of the adolescent due to faulty posture and lack of exercise, is a form of more generalized kyphosis.

The symptoms of Pott's disease are not well marked in the early stages. There is a general loss of health and strength, and the person becomes easily tired. The affected part of the spine is tender when pressure is made on the back, and the child holds himself stiffly. If the neck be diseased the head is not turned from side to side, and the child often supports the chin on his hand. If the back be the part concerned, the child holds himself very erect, and when he wishes to pick something off the floor, goes down upon his knees rather than bend the back. When the lumbar region of the spine is diseased a not uncommon result is a psoas abscess which burrows towards the back or into the groin.

Treatment of Pott's disease is essentially that applicable to tuberculous disease affecting any other organ, consisting of chemotherapy combined with good food and fresh air. (See TUBERCULOSIS.) So effective is chemotherapy that, in the case of children anyhow, admission to hospital may not be necessary, and the child may often be treated as an outpatient. Even plaster-of-Paris jackets are seldom considered necessary nowadays, and surgical treatment is only required in a small majority of cases. In the case of the other forms of the condition the treatment is that of the causative condition. In the case of the round-shouldered adolescent, this involves gymnastics, adequate exercise and fresh air and instructions to maintain an erect posture.

COMPRESSION OF THE CORD may arise from various causes. The seriousness of most diseases affecting the spine is, in fact, measured by their tendency to interfere with the spinal cord. This condition may be caused suddenly by a severe crush or blow upon the back, which produces a fracture of the spine with displacement of the fragments. Or it may come on slowly, and is then in the great majority of cases due to Pott's disease (see above). Compression of the cord in the neck is speedily fatal as a rule, owing to the involvement of important vital centres; but when it occurs in the region of the chest, the person may live a long time a more or less invalid life.

Symptoms comprise interference with sensation below the level of compression, and, in chronic cases, pain round the body at this level; more or less complete rigidity and paralysis of the lower limbs; interference with the functions of the bladder and rectum, and a special tendency to bed sores in the paralysed parts.

Treatment, in cases due to accident, is not as a rule hopeful, since the spinal cord is generally lacerated, as well as compressed, by the damage to the spine. But cases which come on slowly, for example as the result of Pott's disease, often yield to treatment. This consists in prolonged rest and support to the spine; whilst brilliant results are often obtained, even after several months of complete paralysis, by an operation designed to remove the bone or inflammatory product which is pressing upon the cord. Apart from the question of recovery, these cases require special care and watchfulness in nursing because of the great tendency that is present to the formation of bed sores, and because the patient loses to a great extent the power of voluntary control over the bladder and bowels, so that septic inflammation of the bladder and kidneys is very apt to ensue and to terminate the patient's life. Modern methods of rehabilitation, however, have done much to ensure that, paralysed though they may be, many of the victims of severe damage to the spinal cord can return to a useful life in the community.

SPONDYLITIS, or inflammation of the vertebrae of the spine, may occur at any age, but the most important form is *ankylosing spondylitis*, also known as bamboo spine and poker spine. This is a disease predominantly of young men between the ages of 20 and 40. It is characterized in the early stages by low back pain and stiffness that are aggravated by rest and relieved by exercise. Unless treated in the early stages, it tends to run an inexorable course, leading in the end to complete fixation of the spine as a result of bony ankylosis between the vertebrae.

Treatment consists of deep X-ray therapy and, if given early in the disease, the results are excellent. Even in the later stages it may give considerable relief and slow the progress of the disease. Promising results are also being obtained from the use of the non-steroidal anti-inflammatory drugs. Physiotherapy, consisting of mobilizing and postures, constitutes an essential part of treatment and must be maintained throughout life.

A National Association for Ankylosing Spondylitis has been formed which is open to those with the disease, their families, friends and doctors. Those interested should apply to the secretary, 5 Grosvenor Crescent, London SW1X 7ER (01–235 9585).

SPONDYLOLISTHESIS is a congenital defect of the spine, usually the fifth lumbar vertebra. This results in slipping forward of the affected vertebra which induces backache. This usually responds to treatment with a spinal support, but in more severe cases an operation may be necessary.

SPONDYLOSIS is a degenerative lesion of the spine, often leading on to ankylosis (qv). It may also be the cause of stress fractures (qv) in sport. A long period of rest is necessary to allow the fracture to reunite, and in some cases surgical intervention may be necessary to achieve union.

CERVICAL SPONDYLOSIS is the form of spondylosis confined to the vertebrae of the cervical spine (the spine in the neck) and is characterized by degenerative changes in the intervertebral discs. These changes produce pain and stiffness in the neck, pain in the arms and, in the more advanced cases, weakness in the legs. Most men over 50 and women over 55 have X-ray evidence of cervical spondylosis, but it is only in a few that these changes cause trouble. Treatment consists of resting the muscles of neck, which may involve the wearing of a plastic collar, and physiotherapy. In the most severe cases a surgical operation may be necessary to reduce pressure on the spinal cord.

MENINGITIS, or inflammation of the membranes surrounding the cord, is dealt with under MENINGITIS.

MYELITIS, or inflammation situated in the spinal cord itself, may be of an acute or chronic nature, and gives rise to symptoms much resembling those of compression though unaccompanied by pain. A special form of myelitis is poliomyelitis, affecting only the grey matter of the cord. (See POLIOMYELITIS.)

SCLEROSIS is a very chronic condition of the cord in which certain parts become increasingly hard in consequence of disappearance of the white nerve-fibres and their replacement by an overgrowth of the connective tissue of the cord. This change is due to various causes, and the symptoms which it produces depend mainly upon the particular tracts of fibres that are affected. Sclerosis in the posterior part of the cord, for example, produces the disease known as tabes dorsalis (see TABES DORSALIS); whilst another disease, known as multiple sclerosis, in which the degenerated patches are scattered through the nervous system, affects mainly the lateral portions of the cord. (See MULTIPLE SCLEROSIS.)

PROGRESSIVE MUSCULAR ATROPHY is the chief member of a group of diseases in which the main characteristic is loss of power and muscular wasting, due to a gradual degeneration in the grey matter of the spinal cord and brain. (See PARALYSIS.)

SYRINGOMYELIA is a disease in which fissures and cavities exist in the cord together with an overgrowth of the supporting neuroglia. (See SYRINGOMYELIA.)

INJURIES TO THE SPINE AND CORD are of various grades of severity. *Sprains* of the back due to a twist and leding to tearing of muscles and ligaments, and to deep-seated effusion of blood, may be productive of long-continued pain and even of a considerable amount of paralysis. In most cases this is probably due to some injury of the spinal nerves, but the symptoms pass off in general with rest and time. *Fracture of the spine* has been mentioned under the heading of COMPRESSION. *Concussion of the cord* is a term which includes a number of possible injuries that may have been inflicted upon the cord by severe jarring or shaking of the body.

SPINNER'S FINGER is a cricket injury. Bowlers are liable to develop callosities (qv) of the fingers of the bowling hand. These tend to crack, and this is the condition known as spinner's finger.

SPIRAMYCIN is an antibiotic isolated from *Streptomycesambofaciens*, which is useful in the treatment of certain cases of staphylococcal infection.

SPIRILLUM is a form of micro-organism of wavy or spiral shape. (See BACTERIOLOGY.)

SPIRIT is a strong solution of alcohol in water. (See ALCOHOL.) Proof spirit is one containing 57 per cent of alcohol by volume or 49 per cent by weight, and is so named because it can stand the proof of just catching fire. Rectified spirit contains 90 per cent of alcohol by volume or over 85 per cent by weight. Proof spirit is generally used in the preparation of tinctures. Spirits of various drugs contain a solution of any given drug in rectified spirit. Among the most commonly used spirits are spirit of chloroform (also known as chloric ether), sweet spirit of nitre (spirit of nitrous ether), aromatic spirit of ammonia (sal volatile), spirit of ether, spirit of Cologne (eau-de-Cologne), spirit of camphor, and spirit of various volatile oils. Methylated spirit (also known as wood naphtha or wood spirit) is distilled from wood. When taken internally, it is a dangerous poison producing neuritis with great readiness, and especially neuritis of the optic nerves which may result in blindness. Mineralized or denatured methylated spirit is one to which crude pyridine and mineral naphtha have been added in small proportions, together with a minute quantity of methyl violet for colouring, to prevent its being drunk.

The term spirit is also used popularly in a loose application to various active substances: eg. spirit of turpentine (oil of turpentine), spirit of hartshorn (ammonia in water), spirit of nitre (nitric acid), Mindererus spirit (liquor ammonii acetatis), and spirit of salt (hydrochloric acid).

Uses (for internal uses, see ALCOHOL): Externally, methylated spirit or eau-de-Cologne is used to sprinkle on the skin or to apply on lint, as an evaporating lotion for its cooling and soothing effect. (See LOTIONS.) Methylated spirit is also used to harden the skin for the prevention of bed sores and foot soreness. The spirits of the various oils form a convenient method of administering these oils as expectorants, or for colic, flatulence, etc. (See OILS.)

SPIRITS consist of medicinal substances or flavouring agents dissolved in alcohol.

SPIROCHAETE is an order of bacteria which has a spiral form.

SPIROCHAETOSIS ICTEROHAEMORRHAGICA (see LEPTOSPIROSIS).

SPIRONOLACTONE (ALDACTONE, DIATENSAC, SPIROCTAN) belongs to the group of substances known as spirolactones. These are steroids similar to aldosterone (qv) in structure which competitively act as inhibitors of it. They can thus antagonise the action of aldosterone in the renal tubules. As there is evidence that there is an increased output of aldosterone in oedematous conditions, such as congestive heart failure, which accentuates the oedema, spironolactone is used, along with other diuretics, in resistant cases of oedema – to antagonise the fluid-retaining action of aldosterone. (See DIURETICS.)

SPLANCHNIC means anything belonging to the internal organs of the body as distinguished from its framework.

SPLEEN is an organ deeply placed in the abdomen.

Position and size: The spleen lies behind the stomach, high up on the left side of the abdomen, and corresponds to the position of the 9th, 10th, and 11th ribs, from which it is separated by the diaphragm. It is a soft, highly vascular, plum-coloured organ, and has a smooth surface, being almost completely covered by peritoneum. There are two wide peritoneal ligaments that support the spleen, the one attaching it to the stomach, the other to the kidney. Through the latter ligament the large vessels that supply the spleen with blood make their way. The size of the spleen varies widely. It is usually about 12·5 to 15 cm (5 to 6 inches) in length, and weighs about 170 grams or more, but these dimensions depend upon the amount of blood contained in it, for it contracts from time to time, and after meals is much smaller than at other times. In diseased conditions the organ may reach a weight of 8 to 9 kg.

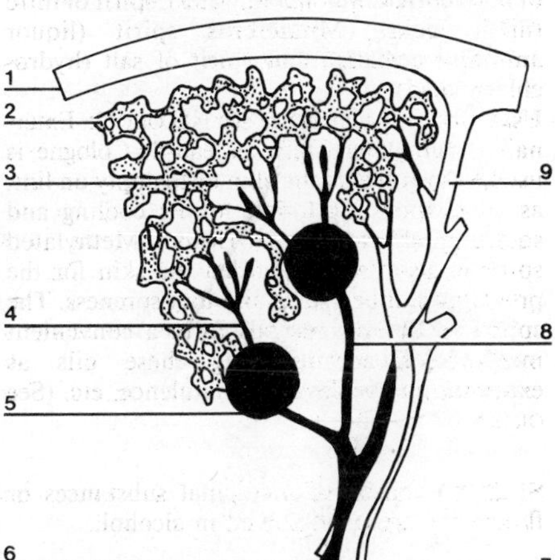

1 capsule
2 venous sinuses
3 arterial capillaries ending in sinuses
4 small arteries
5 Malphigi capsules
6 artery
7 vein
8 central artery of Malphigi corpuscle
9 trabecula of capsule

Diagram of spleen.

Structure: The spleen is enveloped by peritoneal membrane like the stomach and intestines, and this smooth coat greatly facilitates its movements. Beneath the peritoneum is a strong elastic tunic, composed partly of fibrous tissue containing many elastic fibres, and partly of unstriped muscle. This elastic coat allows of the free expansion and contraction of the organ according to the varying amount of blood present in it. From the inner surface of the membrane fibrous partitions known as trabeculae run down into the substance and form a network in which the dark spleen pulp is contained. If the spleen is cut open and the pulp washed away, these trabeculae stand out as shaggy projections on the cut surface. The pulp consists of delicate connective tissue fibres passing between the various trabeculae and of white and red blood corpuscles lying in this meshwork. Round the smaller arteries there are condensed areas of this pulp formed of developing white blood corpuscles, and known as Malpighian bodies or corpuscles.

BLOOD-VESSELS pass to the spleen, and are so large compared with the size which would be necessary in order simply to carry nutritive material to the spleen as to render it clear that the organ has some important action connected with the maintenance of the blood. The arteries which enter the spleen at the hilum become smaller and smaller till they end in capillaries, which open freely into the pulp. The blood thus escapes readily into the substance of the spleen, and, after passing through its meshwork, is collected by veins that unite into larger trunks till they form the splenic vein, which leaves the organ and joins the portal vein. There are also numerous lymphatics in the organ, which run in the trabeculae or surround the veins.

Functions: The organ produces lymphocytes and acts as a reservoir of red blood cells for use in emergencies. It is also one of the sites for the manufacture of red blood cells in the foetus, but not after birth. Useless or worn-out red and white blood corpuscles and blood platelets are broken up by this organ. This results in the production of bilirubin (qv), which is conveyed to the liver, and of iron, which is used in the bone marrow for the production of new red blood cells. Nevertheless the spleen does not appear to be absolutely essential to life, since its removal is followed by increase in size of the lymphatic glands all over the body, and does not necessarily interfere with health.

SPLEEN, DISEASES OF: In certain diseases associated with marked changes in the blood, such as leukaemia, and malaria, the spleen becomes chronically enlarged. In some of the acute infectious diseases, it becomes congested and acutely enlarged: for example, in typhoid fever, anthrax, and infectious mononucleosis. Rupture of the spleen may occur, like rupture of other internal organs, in consequence of extreme violence, but in malarious countries, where many people have the spleen greatly enlarged and softened as the result of malaria, rupture of this organ occurs now and then as the result of some quite trivial blow upon the left side. The spleen, in consequence of its structure, bleeds excessively when torn, so that this accident is generally followed by collapse, signs of internal haemorrhage – and death if not dealt with promptly by operation.

SPLENECTOMY means removal of the spleen. This operation may be necessary if the spleen has been severely injured or in the treatment of the severe form of acholuric jaundice or autoimmune thrombocytopenic purpura. (See PURPURA.)

SPLENIC ANAEMIA (also known as BANTI'S DISEASE) is a chronic disease, of unknown cause, characterized by enlargement of the spleen and anaemia. The condition usually begins before the age of 30 years. There is no specific treatment, but some cases respond to removal of the spleen. In the majority of cases, however, all that can be done is to maintain, so far as possible, the general health of the patient and to treat the anaemia with full doses of iron. Blood transfusion is necessary if haemorrhage occurs.

SPLENOMEGALY means enlargement of the spleen beyond its normal size.

SPLINTER HAEMORRHAGES are linear bleeds under the finger nails. Although they may result from injury they are a useful physical sign of infective endocarditis.

SPLINTS are supports for an injured or wounded part. They are most commonly employed in cases in which a bone is fractured, and consist then of some rigid substance designed to take the place of the broken bone in maintaining the shape of the limb, as well as to keep the broken ends at rest and in contact, and thus to ensure their union. Splints are most commonly made of wood either shaped to the limb or consisting merely of strips of wood about the width of the injured limb, and carefully padded with wool or similar soft material. Splints are also made of metal, poroplastic felt, leather, and cotton stiffened with plaster of Paris, as well as other materials. Splints may be improvised for first-aid out of walking-sticks, rifles, broom-handles, branches, folded-up newspapers, and in fact anything of suitable length and rigidity. (See FRACTURES.)

SPONDYLITIS is another name for arthritis of the spine. (See SPINE AND SPINAL CORD, DISEASES OF.)

SPONDYLOLISTHESIS (see SPINE AND SPINAL CORD, DISEASES OF).

SPONDYLOSIS (see SPINE AND SPINAL CORD, DISEASES AND INJURIES OF.)

SPORADIC is the term applied to cases of disease occurring here and there, as opposed to epidemic outbreaks.

SPORTS INJURIES, PREVENTION OF: There are four basic rules for the prevention of sports injuries. (1) Be fit for the sport or game. (2) Obey the rules, written and unwritten. (3) Wear the right clothes and shoes. (4) Use common sense. The first of these is obvious. In amplification of the others, Dr John Williams, Medical Director of the Regional Sports Injuries Centre, Farnham Park Rehabilitation Centre, Slough, makes some cogent comments in his book, *Injury in Sport*. 'Obedience to the rules of the game (the spirit as well as the letter) is an essential component of injury prevention.' 'Reckless play is a not uncommon cause of injury.' 'It is the self-discipline of each individual player that finally determines whether sport will be safe or not. Since self-discipline is an essential component of sport, he who cannot discipline himself must be regarded as a menace on the sports field and if necessary permanently banned.'

Emphasis is laid on the importance of correct clothing and footwear. Clothing is often made of unsuitable material. Worn-out shoes and laces, jagged trouser buckles and sweat-rotted collars can all cause serious injury. The design of shoes may be faulty (eg. the wrong siting of studs on football boots), or inappropriate (eg. the same pair of shoes would not be suitable for running both on tartan track and asphalt road). A warning is given against advertisements that claim sports gear is in some way medically tested. Natural materials are better than man-made for clothes and footwear because of their absorbent and sweat evaporation qualities. When man-made fibres are worn, open weave is recommended.

All sportsmen should be immunized against tetanus (qv), and maintain this immunity by receiving regular booster injections every three years.

SPOTS BEFORE THE EYES can arise from a variety of causes including inflammation and bleeding in the eye, or preceding a retina detachment. They may also occur for a variety of totally harmless reasons.

SPOTTED FEVER (see MENINGITIS, EPIDEMIC CEREBROSPINAL; TYPHUS FEVER).

SPRAINS are injuries in the neighbourhood of joints, consisting usually in tearing of a ligament with effusion of blood. (See JOINTS, DISEASES OF.)

SPRAYS (see INHALATIONS).

SPRUE, or PSILOSIS, is a disease of uncertain origin, characterized by diarrhoea with the passage of large, fatty stools, anaemia, sore tongue, and loss of weight. The name was first given to the condition in 1879 by Sir Patrick Manson, and it was then considered to be a disease of tropical climates. Subsequent investigations have shown that a similar condition occurs in individuals who have never been in the tropics. To this latter condition the name of non-tropical sprue is usually given. The following description applies predominantly to the condition as it occurs in the tropics.

Causes: Many theories have been advanced concerning the cause of sprue, but the general consensus of opinion today is that it is due to an inborn error of metabolism characterized primarily by inability to absorb fats from the intestine. This explains the bulky, frothy stools due to excess of fat. Subsequently there is interference with the absorption of carbohydrate, vitamins and minerals. The poor absorption of vitamins is responsible for the anaemia and sore tongue, whilst the decreased absorption of calcium is responsible for the low level of calcium in the blood. One advantage of this theory is that it correlates three somewhat similar conditions: (1) tropical sprue; (2) non-tropical sprue; (3) coeliac disease (qv) which is a condition found in children. In all these the fundamental cause is the same. In children with coeliac disease the error of metabolism is so marked that the condition appears early in life. In adults the error is less marked and requires either some precipitating factor to provoke it, or else the normal ageing process. In the case of tropical sprue these precipitating factors are one or more of the following: an attack of dysentery; the strain of living in a hot, damp climate; dietetic indiscretions; the highly spiced diet so commonly eaten by Europeans in the tropics.

Tropical sprue is found chiefly in India, Burma, Malaysia, Indonesia and China. It also occurs in the Southern States of USA, the West Indies, and South America. It is more common in Europeans than in natives, and is more common in women than in men. As a rule it occurs after long residence in the tropics, and the onset is usually after the rains. There is quite often a preceding history of dysentery.

Symptoms: The onset may be gradual or rapid. Initially there are weakness, soreness of the tongue, difficulty in swallowing, indigestion, and diarrhoea. The diarrhoea is usually worst in the morning, and the stools are pale, bulky, and frothy. The appetite is usually poor. There is a marked degree of anaemia, usually of the macrocytic type: ie. there is a high colour index. The tongue is smooth and red. Gastric acidity is low. Other characteristic findings are that the rise in the blood sugar level following the taking of sugar is less than normal, and there is an increase in the amount of fat in the stools. In untreated cases the patient steadily loses weight and becomes emaciated. Death is usually due to exhaustion and some inter-current infection. The prognosis depends largely upon the stage at which treatment is begun.

Treatment: The essentials of treatment are rest in bed, a high-protein diet, and treatment of the anaemia and any other deficiency that may be present. It is usual to start the diet with skimmed milk and gradually add other items such as meat. Some authorities, on the other hand, recommend beginning with a diet consisting largely of beef. Whichever diet is used, the essential fact to be borne in mind is that the patient cannot tolerate fats, but that a high caloric intake is necessary to ensure that the patient is adequately nourished. This can best be done by a diet consisting predominantly of protein. For the anaemia folic acid and cyanocobalamin are required. Large doses of the vitamin B complex are also helpful: eg. Marmite. As the blood calcium level is also diminished, vitamins A and D should be given, and it is sometimes useful to supplement this by calcium lactate. As has already been pointed out, convalescence is often prolonged, resulting sometimes in marked depression on the part of the patient. Satisfactory results are seldom obtained unless the patient is sent home to a temperate climate. An individual who has had sprue should never return to residence in the tropics unless it is absolutely essential.

Non-tropical sprue or gluten enteropathy is due to a hypersensitivity to gluten and the treatment is a gluten-free diet.

SPUTUM means material spat out of the mouth. It may consist of saliva from the mouth, of mucous secretions from the throat or back of the nose, but is generally expectorated by coughing from the lower air passages. (See EXPECTORATION.)

SQUILL is the sliced bulb of *Urginea maritima*, a plant from the shores of the Mediterranean. It contains several substances which exert an irritating, or, in small doses, a stimulating effect upon the kidneys and the mucous membrane of the stomach and bronchial tubes.

Uses: The tincture, syrup, and vinegar of squills are now used mainly as constituents of expectorant (or cough) mixtures. Squill is also a constituent of Guy's pill which is used in the treatment of oedema due to heart failure.

SQUINT (OR STRABISMUS): A condition in which the visual axes of each eye are not directed simultaneously at the same fixation point (ie. each eye is not pointing at the same object at the same time). Squints may be: (a) Paralytic, where one or more of the muscles, or their nerve supply is damaged; this type usually results in double vision. (b) Non-paralytic, where the muscles and nerves are normal. It is usually found in children. This type of squint can either result in poor vision, or occasionally may result from poor vision. Squints may be convergent (where one eye 'turns in') or divergent (one eye 'turns out'). Vertical squints can also occur but are less common. All squints should be seen by an eye specialist as soon as possible. Some squints can be corrected by exercises or spectacles; others require surgery.

STABS (see WOUNDS).

STAMMERING is a disruption of the forward flow of speech. The individual knows what he wants to say but he temporarily loses his ability to execute linguistically formulated speech. Stammering is characterised by a silent or audible involuntary repetition/prolongation of an utterance, be it a sound, syllable or word.

Sometimes it is accompanied by accessory behaviours, or speech-related struggle. Usually there are indications or the report of an accompanying emotional state, involving excitement, tension, fear or embarrassment.

Idiopathic stammering begins sometime between the onset of speech and puberty, mostly between 2 and 5 years of age. Acquired stammering at a later age due to brain damage is rare. The prevalence of stammering (the percentage of the population actually stammering at any point in time) is approximately 0·9 per cent. Three times as many boys as girls stammer. About 70 per cent of stammering children recover with little or no therapy. Stammerers have not been shown to demonstrate differences in personality from non-stammerers. There are however, indications that at least some stammerers show minimal differences from fluent speakers in cerebral processing of verbal material.

There is a genetic predisposition towards stammering. The risk of stammering among first-degree relatives of stammerers is more than three times the population risk. In 77 per cent of identical twins either both stammer or both are fluent. Only 33 per cent of non-identical twins agree in this way. As there are identical twins who differ for stammering, environmental factors must be important for some stammerers. There are relatively large numbers of stammerers in highly competitive societies, where status and prestige are important and high standards of speech competence are valued.

Different treatments have been demonstrated to produce considerable benefit, their basic outline being similar. A long period of time is spent in training stammerers to speak in a different way (fluency shaping techniques). This may include slowing down the rate of speech, gentle onset of utterance, continuous flow with correct juncturing, etc. When the targets have been achieved within the clinic a series of planned speech assignments outside the clinic is undertaken. In these assignments, and initially in everyday situations, the fluency enchancing techniques have to be used conscientiously. Gradually speech is shaped towards normality requiring less and less effort. Therapy may also include some work on attitude change (ie. helping the client to see himself as a fluent speaker) and possibly general communicative skills training.

STANNOSIS is the form of pneumoconiosis (qv) caused by the inhalation of stannous (tin) oxide, which occurs in tin ore mining.

STANOZOLOL (STROMBA) (see ANABOLIC STEROIDS).

STAPHYLOCOCCUS is a bacterium which under the microscope appears in small masses like bunches of grapes. It is one of the commonest infectious micro-organisms and is found, for example, in the pus discharged from boils.

STARCH is a substance belonging to that group of carbohydrates known as the amyloses. It is the form in which utilizable carbohydrate is stored in granules within the seeds and roots of many plants. It is converted into sugar when treated with heat in presence of a dilute acid. It is changed largely into dextrin when exposed to a considerable degree of dry heat, as in toasting bread; and a similar change into dextrin and malt-sugar takes place under the action of various ferments such as the ptyalin of the saliva. Starch forms a chief constituent of the carbohydrate foods (see DIET), and in the process of digestion the above-mentioned change takes place to prepare it for absorption. It is also slowly broken down in the process of cooking.

Starch is used externally to form a poultice for softening the skin in skin diseases. (See POULTICES.) It is also used as a constituent of dusting powders for application to chafed or irritable areas of the skin. (See CHAFING.) Starch enema is administered in inflammatory conditions of the bowel. (See ENEMA.)

STARVATION: Partial starvation, as a method of treatment, is used in certain diseases associated with previous excess of food, particularly obesity. (See OBESITY.) When a person is completely deprived of food for a time, not only is there great loss of weight but the chemical processes of the body are altered, and a poisoning effect is produced by the formation of acetone and other ketone bodies. In cases of slow starvation, the vitality of the tissues is reduced and they become more liable to tuberculosis and other diseases. (See also FASTING.)

STASIS is a term applied to stoppage of the flow of blood in the vessels or of the food materials down the intestinal canal. (For Blood Stasis, see CIRCULATION, DISORDERS OF.)

STAVESACRE is the seeds of *Delphinum staphisagria*, which are crushed and made into an ointment for use as a parasiticide.

STEATORRHOEA is any condition characterized by the passing of stools containing an excess of fat. (See MALABSORPTION SYNDROME.)

STENOSIS is a term applied to a condition of unnatural narrowing in any passage or orifice of the body. The word is specially used in connection with the four openings of the heart at which the valves are situated. (See HEART DISEASES.)

STEPPAGE GAIT is the name given to the peculiar walk characteristic of neuritis affecting the muscles of the leg and causing dropfoot. The feet are lifted high so that the toes may clear the ground.

STEREOGNOSIS means the faculty of recognizing the solidity of objects, and thus their nature, by handling them.

STEREOTAXIS is the procedure whereby precise localization in space is achieved. It is applied to that branch of surgery known as *stereotactic neurosurgery*, in which the surgeon is able to localize precisely those areas of the brain on which he wishes to operate.

STERILIZATION means either (1) the process of rendering various objects, such as those which come in contact with wounds, and various foods, free from microbes, or (2) the process of rendering a person incapable of producing children.

The manner of sterilizing bedding, furniture, and the like, after contact with a case of infectious disease, is given under DISINFECTION, whilst the sterilization of instruments, dressings, and skin surfaces, necessary before surgical procedures, is mentioned in the same article and also under ANTISEPTICS, ASEPSIS, and WOUNDS. For general purposes, one of the cheapest and most effective agents is boiling water or steam.

Use of sterilization: Milk is the chief article of food that calls for special sterilization. With regard to other foods, ordinary cooking has this for one of its chief objects.

Method of sterilization: One of the most effective modes is simply to boil the milk for a prolonged period in a covered pan; but this changes its taste considerably, and is therefore unsuitable for children and invalids, who tend to drink large amounts of milk.

Another method is to place the milk in a flask or bottle of which the neck is closed by a plug of cotton-wool, and set it in a pot of water, from the bottom of which it is separated by a triangle of wire or other means. The pot is placed on the stove and the water boiled for three-quarters of an hour, by which time the milk is sufficiently sterilized without appreciably affecting its taste. Many forms of sterilizer are on the market, but all depend upon this principle of having an inner vessel or set of bottles suspended within an outer pot containing water, which is boiled for three-quarters of an hour to one hour. Care must be taken that the milk is not uncovered, after being sterilized, until just before it is to be used.

Pasteurization is a slightly different method of treatment, which is sufficient to destroy the microbes that cause gastroenteritis, as well as those of many other diseases such as tuberculosis and typhoid fever, while preserving the natural state of the milk. (See PASTEURIZATION.)

Koch's method of sterilization is used in bacteriological investigation, where even the spores of bacteria must be destroyed. It is carried out by steaming the objects to be sterilized on three successive days. (See BACTERIOLOGY.)

BACTERIOLOGICAL STERILIZATION may be effected in many ways, and different methods are used in different cases, for it is evident that processes applicable to clothing or to a room may be quite unsuited for the sterilization of food.

SEXUAL STERILIZATION is being used to an increasing extent. In women it is performed by ligating, or cutting, and then tying the Fallopian tubes (qv), the tubes that carry the ovum from the ovary to the uterus. Alternatively the tubes may be sealed off by means of plastic and silicone clips or rings. It is usually performed through a small incision, or cut, in the lower abdominal wall. It has no effect on sexual or menstrual function, and, unlike the comparable operation in men, it is immediately effective. The sterilization is almost always permanent, but occasionally, for some unknown reason, the two cut ends of the Fallopian tubes reunite, and pregnancy is then again possible. Removal of the uterus and/or the ovaries also causes sterilization, but such procedures are only used when there is some special reason, such as the presence of a tumour.

The operation for sterilizing men is known as vasectomy (qv).

STERNUM is another name for the breastbone.

STERNUTATORIES are substances that provoke sneezing.

STEROID is the group name for compounds that resemble cholesterol chemically. The group includes the sex hormones, the hormones of the adrenal cortex, and bile acids.

STERTOR is a term applied to noisy breathing resembling snoring. It is due usually to flapping of the soft palate between a stream of air entering by the nose and one entering by the mouth. In ordinary snoring (qv) this results from the habit of sleeping with the mouth open, and in certain serious disorders it arises from paralysis of the soft palate. Some of these conditions affecting the nervous system and thus leading to paralysis of the soft palate are: apoplexy, suffocation, concussion of the brain, drunkenness, poisoning by opium or by chloroform. (For the means of distinguishing between these conditions see OPIUM POISONING.) In some of these paralytic conditions the snoring is very loud, and the noise is due then, not to flapping of the soft palate, but to lolling back of the tongue against the back of the throat as the patient lies on his back. In this case the breathing is at once relieved by pulling forward the lower jaw, by pulling the tongue out of the mouth, or by turning the patient upon one side, as is done, for example, in suffocation due to drowning.

Stertorous breathing is not to be confused with *sniffing* breathing produced by paralysis of the muscles that should hold the nostrils still and open; nor with *puffing* breathing due to paralysis of the muscles in the cheeks and lips; though all three conditions may be produced by the same causes. Nor must it be mistaken for *stridor*, or crowing breathing, due to spasmodic narrowing in the larynx (see LARYNGISMUS); nor for the prolonged, noisy, *wheezing* breathing of asthma produced by narrowing of the bronchial tubes.

STERULE is a glass capsule containing a sterile solution for hypodermic administration.

STETHOSCOPE is an instrument used for listening to the sounds produced by the action of the lungs, heart, and other internal organs. (See AUSCULTATION.)

STEVENS-JOHNSON SYNDROME: This is a form of erythema multiforme which is characterized by annular lesions which can develop into blisters. In addition to the skin lesions in this syndrome there is severe involvement of the eyes and the mucosa, giving rise to ulceration. It is commonly a hypersensitivity reaction to drugs particularly the sulphonamide group of antibiotics.

STHENIC is a term applied to certain diseases, especially fevers, to indicate that they are not associated with prostration.

STIBOCAPTATE is an organic antimony compound which is used in the treatment of schistosomiasis (qv).

STIFFNESS is a condition which may be due to a change in the joints, ligaments, tendons, or muscles, or to the influence of the nervous system over the muscles of the part affected. Stiffness is associated with various forms of rheumatism. Stiffness of the neck muscles resulting in bending backward the head, and of the hamstring muscles, causing difficulty in straightening the lower limbs, is a sign of meningitis. Stiffness or spasticity also occurs in certain diseases of the central nervous system.

STIGMA means any spot or impression upon the skin. The term, stigmas of degeneration, is applied to physical defects that are found in mentally defective persons. (See MENTAL ILLNESS.)

STILBOESTROL (PABESTROL) is a synthetic oestrogen. Its physiological actions are closely similar to those of the natural ovarian hormone, and it has the great merit of being active when taken by mouth. An interesting property of stilboestrol is seen in the relief it affords when given to patients suffering from cancer of the prostate, inducing in some cases, it appears, regression of the primary tumour and of secondary deposits in bone. (See OESTROGEN.)

STILBOESTROL DIPHOSPHATE (HONVAN) (see OESTROGEN).

STILET, or STILETTE, means the delicate probe or the wire used to clear a catheter or hollow needle.

STILLBIRTH: A stillborn child is 'any child which has issued forth from its mother after the twenty-eighth week of pregnancy and which did not at any time after being completely expelled from its mother, breathe or show any other sign of life'. In England, in 1986, the number of stillbirths was 3,549. (See PERINATAL MORTALITY.)

STILL'S DISEASE, or JUVENILE RHEUMATOID ARTHRITIS, is a disease of childhood first described by Sir Frederic Still (1868–1941). The characteristic of the disease is that the arthritis is usually symmetrical. It tends to start in the fingers, which become spindle-shaped due to the swelling of the affected joints. It then spreads to involve other joints, practically always in a symmetrical manner, including the wrists, elbows, knees and ankles. Occasionally, only one joint, such as the knee, may be involved initially. The onset may be abrupt, with high temperature, or gradual. The cervical spine is often involved, leading to stiffness of the neck, and some of these cases go on to ankylosing spondylitis (qv). As a result of the child not moving the affected joints because of the pain this causes, there is marked wasting of the muscles. The heart is seldom involved, but there is often a characteristic rash. The age of onset is usulally between 2 and 5 years, and the disease is marked by repeated recurrences. The disease is usally self-limiting, but tends to relapse and may persist for several years. Treatment is as for rheumatoid arthritis in the adult (qv).

STIMULANTS are drugs and other agents employed to call forth special powers of the body or of individual organs in order to effect some special purpose or to offer resistance to some acute attack of disease. The use of stimulants presupposes a certain amount of reserve power on the part of the body or of the organ stimulated, which is lying dormant and requires an appropriate stimulus before it can be brought into action. In its broadest sense, the term stimulant includes all remedies which are not simply foods destined to supply the wear and tear of the body and to provide it with a store of energy-producing material. It also excludes remedies which have a sedative action upon the nervous system or other organs, and remedies which act directly upon the causes of disease without any reference to the body, such as antiseptics.

(For drugs which stimulate the intestines, see PURGATIVES; for those that stimulate the liver, see CHOLAGOGUES; for those that stimulate the kidneys, see DIURETICS.) Many substances, such as aromatics, spices, and bitters, stimulate the function of the stomach.

STINGS (see BITES AND STINGS).

STITCH is a popular name for a sharp pain in the side. It is generally due to cramp following unusually hard exertion (see CRAMP), but care must be taken that this trivial condition is not taken for pleurisy or for a fractured rib.

(For the stitches used to unite the edges of wounds, see WOUNDS.)

STOKES-ADAMS SYNDROME is a term applied to a condition in which slowness of the pulse is associated with attacks of unconsciousness, and which is due to a state of heart-block.

STOMA: A stoma refers to an opening constructed when the bowel has to be brought to the skin surface to convey gastrointestinal contents to the exterior. It is derived from the Greek word meaning mouth. In the United Kingdom there are about 100,000 patients with a colostomy, 10,000 with an ileostomy and some 2,000 with a urostomy in which the ureters are brought to the skin surface. They may be undertaken because of malignancy of the colon or rectum or as a result of inflammatory bowel diseases such as Crohn's disease. Urostomies usually take the form of an isolated loop of ilium into which the ureters have been implanted and which in its turn is brought to the skin's surface. This is undertaken because of bladder cancer or because of neurological diseases of the bladder. The stomas drain into appliances such as disposable plastic bags. Most of the modern appliances collect the effluent of the stoma without any leak or odour.

Patients with stomas often find explanatory booklets helpful. *Living with your Colostomy* and *Understanding Colostomy* are examples.

STOMACH: The stomach is a dilated portion of the alimentary canal, which in man has a shape somewhat resembling a pear. The larger end, known as the fundus, lies in the hollow of the left side of the diaphragm, and at one side of this is the opening from the gullet. The greater part of the stomach, into which the gullet opens, is known as the cardiac part, whilst the lower and narrower portion is known as the cardia, or cardiac orifice, and the pylorus. The stomach is slightly flattened from before backwards, and the two edges are known as the lesser curvature, which runs from one opening to the other direct, and the greater curvature, which sweeps round the fundus from the cardia to the pylorus.

Size and position: The stomach hangs freely suspended in the upper and left part of the abdomen, so that changes in position and shape take place readily according to the amount of food it contains. On the surface, the stomach corresponds to the ribs on the left side from about the fifth to the ninth, and extends below their protecting margin about halfway down to the navel, while the person is recumbent, and slightly below the navel when he stands up. The fundus lies immediately below the heart and base of the left lung, separated from them only by the diaphragm and their enveloping membranes. This explains the embarrassment of the heart's action and of breathing sometimes experienced by dyspeptics. The stomach is attached at the cardiac opening to the gullet, and at this point it is further secured to the diaphragm by a ligament. A broad band of peritoneum (small omentum) attaches the lesser curvature to the under surface of the liver, and a similar peritoneal fold unites its hinder surface to the spleen. The pyloric end, like the cardiac opening, is to a great extent fixed in position, but the greater curvature is quite freely movable.

The greatest length of the stomach from the fundus to the greater curvature near the pylorus is about 30 cm (12 inches), and the greatest breadth does not exceed 10 to 12·5 cm (4 to 5 inches). The capacity varies greatly in different people, but is usually about 1 to 1½ litres in adults. At birth its capacity is around 30 millilitres.

Structure: The stomach possesses four coats similar to those of the intestine. From within outwards, these are a lining of mucous membrane, a submucous layer, a muscular coat, and a peritoneal coat.

MUCOUS MEMBRANE lines the interior of the stomach and is of smooth, soft texture, though raised up into ridges when the stomach is empty. The surface can be seen with the naked eye to be thickly covered by minute pits into each of which several tube-shaped glands are found, on microscopic section, to open. The mucous membrane in fact consists almost entirely of these glands placed side by side, and supported by a small quantity of connective tissue and by fibres of unstriped muscle. The surface of the mucous membrane is composed of a single layer of columnar cells, and these also line the pits referred to. Each gland is composed of large cubical cells so arranged as to form a tube, open at the upper end where it meets the pit, and closed beneath. These cells secrete the gastric juice which exudes from all the minute tubes as digestion is proceeding. In the cardiac end of the stomach there are other larger cells in addition, mingled with those just described, and the large cells are supposed to secrete the acid of the gastric juice. Between the tubular glands lies some supporting connective tissue in which run numerous blood-capillaries and lymph-vessels.

SUBMUCOUS COAT is a loose connective tissue layer which joins the mucous coat to the muscular coat, and in which the large blood-vessels of the stomach run. The loose arrangement of its fibres allows the mucous membrane to glide freely over the muscular coat in the movements and variations in size of the stomach.

MUSCULAR COAT is of considerable thickness in the stomach, and is of great importance in varying the size of the organ according to the amount of food it contains, in making the peristaltic movements which mix the food with the digestive juice, and finally in expelling the softened food from the stomach into the small intestine. This coat consists of three layers: an outer one in which the fibres run lengthwise, a middle one where they are circular, and an inner layer in which they run obliquely across the stomach.

PERITONEAL COAT is similar to the peritoneum covering the other organs of the abdomen. (See PERITONEUM.)

BLOOD-VESSELS: The stomach is abundantly supplied with blood from the coeliac trunk, a short, wide artery which comes directly from the aorta and also gives branches to the liver, pancreas, and spleen. There is a large arterial arch round either curvature, and from these two arches smaller branches run into the wall of the stomach and reach the submucous coat, from which minute branches are distributed to the other coats. The blood is collected by veins which ultimately return it to the portal vein.

NERVES: The stomach is richly supplied with nerves both from the brain and from the autonomic system. The tenth cranial nerve (vagus) of each side has a long course down the side of the gullet (hence its name: vagus or wanderer), and after giving branches to the larynx, heart, lungs, and other organs, terminates in the stomach, which has therefore important nervous connections with these vital organs. Other branches come from the solar (or coeliac) plexus of the sympathetic system. These nerves form a plexus in the submucous coat and another in the muscular coat, which exert a powerful influence over the secretions and movements of the organ, although these functions are, in the main, carried out automatically.

Functions of the stomach: The part played by the stomach in digestion consists in storing, warming, and softening the food, as well as partially digesting it, and then in passing it on in small quantities to the intestine, where the more important digestive processes that prepare it for absorption take place. The action of the gastric juice upon the food has been described under DIGESTION. The action of the muscular coat of the stomach is also very important. The movements, as seen by the aid of X-rays, consist of a series of waves, each of which takes about half a minute to pass along the stomach. These movements have also the effect of separating the more fluid parts from lumps still left in the later stages of digestion which are retained in the cardiac part of the stomach while the pylorus relaxes as each wave reaches it to allow some of the softened mass to pass through into the small intestine. This muscular movement takes place in health without causing any sensation, but in irritable conditions of the stomach, when digestion is not proceeding naturally, it may increase in force and give rise to irregular spasms which come and go, and which are attended by much pain. (See DYSPEPSIA.)

STOMACH, DISEASES OF: Only the more common and serious varieties of gastric disease can be considered here. The majority of them exhibit as their most marked and sometimes their only feature, the symptoms of dyspepsia. (See DYSPEPSIA.)

ACUTE GASTRITIS: **Causes**: Of these, the most important are: (1) Dietetic indiscretions: eg. a large indigestible meal, or the excessive

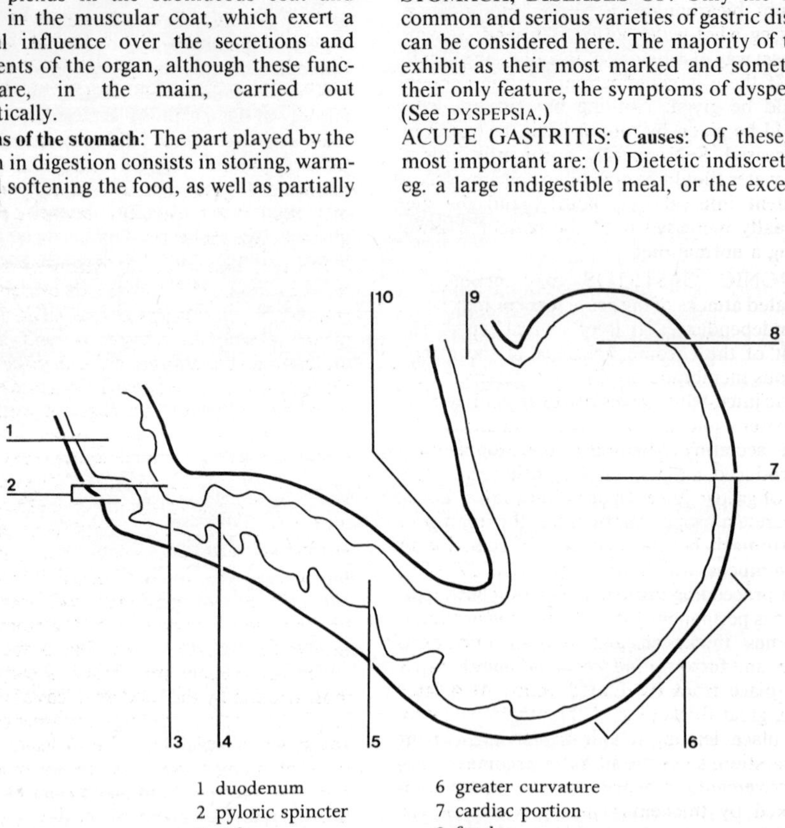

1 duodenum
2 pyloric spincter
3 pylorus
4 pyloric canal
5 pyloric portion
6 greater curvature
7 cardiac portion
8 fundus
9 cardiac orifice
10 lesser curvature

The interior of the stomach.

consumption of alcohol; (2) food poisoning; (3) infections: eg. influenza, septicaemia; (4) toxins: eg. uraemia; (5) the swallowing of poisons: eg. acids, alkalis.

Symptoms: The chief change the stomach undergoes affects its mucous membrane, which is in a state of congestion, either throughout or in parts. The symptoms are those well known as characterizing an acute 'bilious attack', consisting in loss of appetite, sickness or nausea, and headache, frontal or occipital, often accompanied with giddiness. The tongue is furred, the breath foetid, and there is pain or discomfort in the region of the stomach, with sour eructations, and often vomiting, first of food and then of bilious matter. An attack of this kind tends to subside in a few days, especially if the exciting cause is removed. Sometimes, however, the symptoms recur with such frequency as to lead to the more serious chronic form of the disease.

Treatment: The patient must be kept in bed. If the irritant causing the gastritis has not been got rid of by vomiting, vomiting should be induced by giving the patient 280 ml (half a pint) of water, containing a teaspoonful of sodium bicarbonate, to drink. Hot applications, eg. a hot-water bottle, to the abdomen are the best way of relieving pain and easing vomiting. If there is constipation a saline aperient should be given. Nothing but sips of water should be given by mouth until the vomiting has ceased. Subsequently warm milk diluted with water should be given in small amounts at frequent intervals, eg. hourly, and the diet gradually increased until the patient is again taking a normal diet.

CHRONIC GASTRITIS may arise after repeated attacks of the acute form or may come on independently. It is of several types. The result of the chronic irritation of the gastric mucous membrane may be an excessively acid gastric juice, which gives rise to an acid dyspepsia. After a long period of irritation an atrophy of the secreting structures of the stomach may be produced, and there is then little or no secretion of gastric juice. In addition to this failure to secrete a proper gastric juice, the interior of the stomach becomes constantly coated with tough mucus, which further prevents digestion from proceeding normally. The mucous membrane is permanently in a state of congestion, it becomes thickened and thrown into deep ridges and furrows, and frequent haemorrhages take place from its dilated veins. At a later stage, great thickening of the other coats may take place, leading to still further impairment of digestion, since the stomach becomes small, its movements impeded, and the outlet often blocked by thickening in the region of the pylorus.

Causes: Chronic gastritis is more common in women than men, and its incidence increases with age. A high proportion of its victims have a long-standing iron-deficiency anaemia. (See ANAEMIA.) Overeating and alcoholic excess are two common causes. It may be the result of some other disease such as cirrhosis of the liver or heart failure.

Symptoms: The symptoms are those of dyspepsia in an aggravated form (see DYSPEPSIA), of which loss of appetite, discomfort and pain after food, with distension and frequent vomiting, are the chief.

Treatment: This consists essentially of ensuring that the affected individual is having a bland diet which is well cooked and that meals are taken regularly. Careful chewing of food must be insisted upon, and this is often facilitated by not drinking with meals. Alcohol and smoking should be avoided. Particular care must be taken not to eat coarse foods, fruit skins or pips, or pickles or sauces. Neither bitters nor alkaline mixtures should be taken until careful dieting has been given a full trial. Any underlying cause for the gastritis should be treated. Careful dental treatment is necessary if there is any evidence of dental sepsis or if there are not sufficient teeth to ensure adequate chewing of food.

ULCER OF THE STOMACH, GASTRIC ULCER, is of frequent occurrence, and may be a disease of much gravity. It occurs more often than is generally supposed, the result of necropsies showing that one person in every twenty or thereabout suffers from gastric ulcer at some period of life.

Causes: These are not fully understood, but the following points may be regarded as generally admitted: (1) gastric ulcer is more common in men than in women; (2) it becomes more frequent as age increases.

It is held that when any degenerative change takes place in the mucous membrane of the stomach the part is less able to resist the action of the gastric juice upon it, and is apt to undergo disintegration all the more readily. Hence an ulcer is formed. Prostaglandins are necessary to promote the mucous protection of the stomach. As the non-steroidal anti-inflammatory drugs are prostaglandin inhibitors, they predispose to the development of gastric ulcers. This ulcer is usually of small size (15 to 25 mm in diameter), of round or oval form, and tends to advance, not superficially, but to penetrate through the coats of the stomach. Its most usual site is upon the posterior wall towards the upper or lesser curvature of the stomach and near to the pyloric orifice. This is the point at which the mucous membrane is subjected to most friction by the food as it leaves the stomach. The ulcer may undergo a healing process at any stage, in which case it may leave but little trace of its existence. On the other hand, its scar may produce such an amount of contraction as to lead to narrowing of the pylorus, and later dilatation of the stomach. Also, perforation may take place, which, if not quickly operated upon, may be rapidly fatal, unless previously the stomach has become, as it may, adherent to another organ, by which the dangerous effects of this occurrence may be averted. It may also lead to severe bleeding, the condition known as haematemesis (qv). Usually there is only one ulcer, but sometimes there are more.

Symptoms: The symptoms to which this disease gives rise are sometimes indefinite and obscure, and in some cases the diagnosis has been first made by the sudden occurrence of a perforation. First among the symptoms is *pain*, which is usually worse before food. This pain is situated either in front, at the lower end of the breast-bone, or behind, about the middle of the back. It is often severe, and is usually accompanied with much tenderness to touch, and also with a sense of oppression and inability to wear tight clothing. Accompanying the pain there may be vomiting, particularly in more advanced cases. This tends in some measure to relieve the pain and discomfort, and in many instances the patient rather encourages this act. *Vomiting of blood* (haematemesis) occurs in about 25 per cent of cases and is most important diagnostically. It may show itself either to a slight extent, and in the form of a brown or coffee-like mixture, or as a copious discharge of pure blood of dark colour and containing clots. The source of the blood is some vessel or vessels which the ulcerative process has ruptured. Vomiting of blood, however, does not always indicate the presence of a gastric ulcer. Blood is also found mixed with the stools, rendering them dark and tarry-looking (melaena). There is usually constipation. X-ray examination gives little evidence of the presence of an acute ulcer, beyond showing that there is much irritation near the pyloric opening, with spasm in the rest of the stomach; but in chronic cases the deep ulcer often fills up with the barium that has been administered for the examination, and its outline can then be readily seen.

The course of a case of gastric ulcer is very variable. In some instances it is acute, making rapid progress to a favourable or unfavourable termination. In others, however, the disease is chronic, lasting for months or years, and in those cases where the ulcers are multiple or of extensive size, incomplete healing may take place and relapses of the symptoms occur from time to time. Ulcers are sometimes present and yet give rise to no marked symptoms, and one occasionally meets with cases where fatal perforation has suddenly taken place and where *post-mortem* examination reveals the existence of a long-standing ulcer which has furnished little or no evidence of its presence during life. Again, an unsuspected ulcer may run a favourable course, and the contraction of its scar may, at a later period of life, cause interference with the exit of food by the pylorus and consequent dilatation of the organ, and thus give the only evidence that an ulcer has at one time been present.

Although the majority of cases of gastric ulcer respond satisfactorily to a course of medical treatment, the relapse rate is high. This, however, has been reduced since the introduction of carbenoxolone and the histamine antagonists such as cimetidine and ranitidine in treatment. Further, as already noted, there is also the possiblity of three serious complications developing: (i) haemorrhage; (ii) perforation; (iii) obstruction of the pylorus as a result of contraction of the wall of the stomach produced by the ulcer.

Duodenal ulcer, in which a condition similar to gastric ulcer is found just beyond the pyloric opening, has symptoms like those of gastric ulcer, but is six to twelve times more common in males than females, and tends to occur at an earlier age. (See DUODENAL ULCER.)

Treatment: The mainstay of treatment is a derivative of liquorice known as carbenoxolone and the histamine receptor antagonists. This has largely replaced all other drugs. So effective is it that in many cases admission to hospital is no longer necessary. Attention to the diet, however, is still advisable.

The essentials of an effective diet are small feeds every two hours, starting off with milk, or equal parts of milk and cream, and gradually working up to a diet which the individual can take while going about his daily work. In practice, this means breakfast, lunch and dinner (or supper) with a glass of milk in mid-morning, mid-afternoon, and at bedtime. Highly spiced foods should be avoided. Alcohol should be taken in strict moderation and only with food – preferably in the form of light wines. Smoking should be given up.

When haemorrhage occurs, it is treated by complete rest in bed, morphine, and small two-hourly feeds of diluted milk for the first twenty-four hours. When much blood has been lost a transfusion may be necessary. In the event of perforation, treatment is by an immediate operation in which the peritoneal cavity is cleansed and the opening in the stomach wall stitched together. Most surgeons consider that such an operation must be performed at the earliest possible moment in order to afford good hope of recovery.

Surgical treatment, usually in the form of removal of that part of the stomach containing the ulcer, is indicated: (i) in the presence of perforation of the ulcer; (ii) in the presence of severe pyloric obstruction; (iii) in the absence of satisfactory response to medical treatment.

CANCER OF THE STOMACH is the second most common form of cancer in men. In 1984 there were 10,340 deaths (6,157 men; 4,183 women) from cancer of the stomach in England. In all except the oldest age-groups its incidence has been falling in England and Wales over the last forty years. It occurs for the most part in persons at or after middle life, and is more common in men and in individuals belonging to blood group A. (See BLOOD GROUPS.)

The most common parts affected are at the outlet (or pylorus) and along the lesser curvature, but the disease may spread widely in the stomach wall. When it is situated in the neighbourhood of the pylorus, a stricture may be produced as the disease advances. The growth spreads in the submucous tissue, but as it progresses it tends to ulcerate through the mucous membrane, and in this process bleeding and vomiting of blood may occur. The early symptoms of this disease are in many instances so indefinite as to render the diagnosis for a long time conjectural. They are mostly those of dyspepsia, with more or less pain, discomfort, and vomiting, particularly after meals. The vomited material is often of coffee-ground appearance, due to admixture with blood, but copious haematemesis is less frequent than in cases of gastric ulcer. The patient loses flesh and strength, and soon comes to acquire the cachectic aspect commonly associated with cancer. (See CANCER.) The diagnosis is rendered all the more certain when, as is often the case, a tumour can be detected on examination over the region of the stomach; but where no such evidence is obtained, the nature of the disease is left to be made out by fibroscopy (qv) and by X-ray examination. Cases of cancer of the stomach advance with more or less rapidity to a fatal termination. Treatment can usually be only palliative, but much relief may be afforded by a careful attention to diet, by the treatment applicable to dilatation of the stomach, and by the use of morphine and other drugs which relieve pain. In early cases an operation can sometimes be performed by which the disease is completely removed, or, when this cannot be carried out, vomiting, pain, and other symptoms of obstruction are relieved by making a communication between the stomach and a loop in the small intestine (gastro-enterostomy).

CONGENITAL PYLORIC STENOSIS is a congenital defect that occurs once in every 300 births. It is much more common in baby boys than baby girls, about 85 per cent of cases occurring in boys. It consists of marked hypertrophy, or enlargement of the muscles round the pylorus (qv): the opening from the stomach into the duodenum. The baby appears healthy at birth but within a fortnight he starts vomiting towards the end of his feed. The vomiting is described as projectile because the baby shoots the food out in one forceful volley. As the baby feeds, movements of the distended stomach can be seen moving across from left to right (*visible gastric peristalsis*), and the hypertrophied pylorus can be felt as a tumour or swelling. If surgical facilities are available operation is the recommended treatment. In mild cases, or if proper surgical facilities are not available, medical treatment with atropine methonitrate may be tried. If diagnosed and treated early, the results are excellent.

STOMACH TUBE is a soft rubber or plastic tube with rounded end, and usually about 75 cm (30 inches) in length, which is used for washing out the stomach when it contains some poisonous material, or when it is dilated and filled with fermenting food. (See WASHING OUT STOMACH.) A narrower tube, 90 cm (36 inches) in length, is used for the purpose of obtaining a sample of gastric juice for examination. (See also TEST MEAL.) Such a tube can also be allowed to pass out of the stomach into the duodenum so that the contents of the upper part of the small intestine are similarly obtained for analysis.

STOMATITIS means inflammation of the mouth. (See MOUTH, DISEASES OF.)

-STOMY is a suffix signifying formation of an opening in an organ by operation: eg. colostomy (qv).

STONE (see CONCRETIONS; BLADDER, DISEASES OF; GALL-STONES).

STOOLS, or FAECES, consist of the remainder of the food after it has passed through the alimentary canal and been subjected to the action of the digestive juices, and after the nutritious parts have been absorbed by the intestinal mucous membrane. The stools also contain various other matters, such as pigment, derived from the bile, and large quantities of bacteria which are the main component of human stools. The stools are passed once daily by most people, but infants have several evacuations of the bowels in twenty-four hours. To some people the habit of opening the bowels only once or twice a week seems to be quite natural, though such cases are not common.

The *colour* of the stools is naturally of a dark brown, due to a pigment known as stercobilin, derived from the bile. This colour may be changed to green by the action of certain bacteria when decomposition is proceeding to a greater extent than usual in the bowels, and a deep green colour is also produced by some vegetables, such as spinach. White stools, having an appearance like that of clay or putty, are found in cases where the outlet of bile into the small intestine is stopped, and where jaundice is consequently present. When an excess of fat is taken in the food, as in the case of children fed on great quantities of cream, the digestive organs are unable to deal with it, and much of it is passed in the stools, giving the stools in these circumstances also a whitish colour. Black or slate-grey stools are produced when certain drugs are taken, as, for example, iron and bismuth; and a tarry blackness known as malaena is sometimes imparted to them when bleeding takes place from the stomach, the iron in the blood being acted upon by the sulphuretted hydrogen always present in the stools to produce the black sulphide of iron. Bright yellow stools are produced in diarrhoea, when the bile is passed almost unchanged, and a similar colour is caused by rhubarb, senna, and some other drugs. Mucus in the stools, whether in strings, or mixed with the food remnants, or in the form of membranes coating the hardened stools, is almost always a sign of irritation or inflammation in the mucous membrane low down in the bowel (colitis). Red blood in the stools signifies some diseased condition situated near the lower end of the bowel, such as an ulcer or piles. When the blood proceeds from a point higher up, such as an ulcer of the stomach, it is changed by the action of the digestive juices as already described.

Incontinence of the bowels, or inability to retain the stools, is found in several diseases of a prostrating nature in which the sphincter muscles, that naturally keep the bowel closed, relax. It is also a symptom of disease in, or injury to, the spinal cord.

Pain at stool is a characteristic symptom of a fissure at the anus or of inflamed piles, and in such cases is of a very sharp nature. Pain of a duller character associated with the movements of the bowels is often caused by inflammation in the other pelvic organs.

CONSTIPATION and DIARRHOEA are considered under separate headings.

STOUTNESS (see OBESITY).

STRABISMUS (see SQUINT).

STRAMONIUM is the leaf of *Datura stramonium* (thorn-apple, devil's apple, Jimson weed). It contains an alkaloid named daturine, which is almost identical with atropine, and upon which its action depends. Certain preparations of stramonium are used similarly to those of atropine or of belladonna for various conditions. (See ATROPINE.)

STRANGURY is a condition in which there is constant desire to pass water, accompanied by a straining sensation, though only a few drops can be voided. It is a symptom of inflammation situated in the kidneys, bladder or urinary passages.

STRAPPING means the application of strips of adhesive plaster, one overlapping the other, so as to cover a part and make pressure upon it. This method of treatment is used in cases of injury or disease when it is desired to keep a part at rest: for example, strapping may be applied to the chest in cases of pleurisy and fracture of the ribs. Also, it is often used to prevent the movement of joints which are sprained or otherwise injured.

STREPTOCOCCUS is a variety of bacterium which under the microscope has much the appearance of a string of beads. It is responsible for erysipelas and other virulent forms of inflammation. (See BACTERIOLOGY.)

STREPTOKINASE is an enzyme produced by certain streptococci, which has the property of removing blood clot and inflammatory material. It is now available on a commercial scale and is being used in the treatment of bruises and inflammatory conditions in order to facilitate the absorption of extravasated blood and inflammatory exudates. It is also being used to try and overcome the ill effects produced by the formation of clots (emboli or thrombi) in large blood-vessels.

STREPTOMYCIN is an anti-bacterial substance obtained from the soil mould, *Streptomyces griseus*. It was first isolated in 1944 by Dr Waksman in the United States of America. It was the first antibiotic to be effective against the tubercle bacillus.

Streptomycin has two disadvantages. The most important of these is the tendency of organisms to become resistant to it. This means that the administration of this antibiotic must be carefully supervised to ensure that correct dosage is being used. The other disadvantage is that streptomycin produces toxic effects, especially disturbance of the vestibular and hearing apparatus. This may result in deafness, giddiness, and tinnitus (qv). Whilst in many cases these toxic manifestations disappear when the antibiotic is withdrawn, they may be permanent. For this reason therefore streptomycin must always be used with special care.

STRESS FRACTURES are comparatively common in sportsmen. They tend to occur when an undue amount of exercise is taken: an amount of exercise which an individual is not capable of coping with in his (or her) state of training. The main initial feature is pain over the affected bone. This is usually insidious in onset, and worse at night and during and after exercise. It is accompanied by tenderness, and a lump may be felt over the affected site. X-ray evidence of them only appears after several weeks. Treatment consists of rest, some form of external support, and in the initial stage analgesics (qv) to deaden or kill the pain.

STRETCHERS (see INJURED, REMOVAL OF).

STRIAE ATROPHICAE is the term applied to atrophied strips of skin where this has been excessively stretched, as, for example, in pregnancy, when the greyish atrophied strips are known as STRIAE GRAVIDARUM.

STRICTURE means a narrowing in any of the natural passages of the body, such as the gullet, the bowel, or the urethra. It may be due to the development of some growth in the wall of the passage affected, or to pressure upon it by such a growth in some neighbouring organ, but in the majority of cases a stricture is the result of previous ulceration on the inner surface of the passage, followed by contraction of the scar. (See INTESTINE, DISEASES OF; THROAT, DISEASES OF; URETHRA, DISEASES OF.)

STRIDOR is a noise associated with inspiration due to narrowing of the upper airway, in particular the larynx.

STROKE is sudden insensibility or bodily disablement connected with some diseased condition of the brain.

Causes: In subjects of heart disease, a clot may form in the cavities or on a valve of the heart, and being carried away by the blood-stream may lodge in a vessel of the brain so as to form a plug which prevents blood from reaching the part supplied by the vessel in question. The occurrence of this *embolism* is sudden and produces all the symptoms of stroke. When it occurs, the prospect of improvement is better than when the apoplectic symptoms are due to haemorrhage. In elderly people whose blood-vessels are extensively diseased and whose circulation is feeble, a type of stroke, of more gradual onset, may appear in consequence of the blood clotting in the interior of the vessels, this process being known as *thrombosis*.

The most important occasion of stroke is *haemorrhage* into the brain by the rupture of blood-vessels. The blood-vessels of the brain, like those in other parts of the body, are liable to undergo degenerative changes after middle life. These changes affect the minute arteries as well as the larger vessels, rendering their texture fragile, and at the same time impairing their function in maintaining the healthy nutrition of the brain. Hence, in the immediate vicinity of the diseased blood-vessels the substance of the brain itself undergoes degeneration and becomes softened. The small vessels having thus lost the natural support of the surrounding tissues, and being here and there distended into aneurysms by disease, are liable to give way, and blood escapes into the brain. The haemorrhage may be slight in amount and in parts of the brain where its presence gives rise to little disturbance; but where a large blood-vessel has ruptured, and more especially where the blood has been extravasated in or around the important structures at the base of the brain, the result is a stroke or apoplexy, as described below, and death not infrequently follows within a short period. In favourable cases, in which a certain measure of recovery takes place, the effused blood undergoes gradual absorption, or becomes enveloped in a sort of capsule formed by the surrounding brain substance, and ceases to cause further disturbance. But even in such cases some degree of paralysis remains. Stroke in a young person is usually due to a subarachnoid haemorrhage resulting from the rupture of a congenital aneurysm.

Stroke is usually a disease of advanced life. Nevertheless it may occur at any period of life, and cases of true stroke in very young children have, for example, sometimes followed whooping-cough. It is more common in men than in women. What has from early times been described as the apoplectic habit of body, consisting of a stout build, a short neck, and florid complexion, is now generally discredited, it being admitted that stroke occurs about as often in thin and spare persons who present no such peculiarity of conformation. A hereditary tendency is acknowledged as one of the predisposing causes of stroke. Important contributory factors are degenerative changes in the heart and blood-vessels and raised blood-pressure. With respect to the exciting causes of a stroke or apoplexy, it may be stated generally that whatever tends directly or indirectly to increase the tension within the cerebral blood-vessels may bring on an attack. Hence, such causes as severe exertion of body or mind, violent emotions, much stooping, and sudden shocks to the body, may precipitate the attack in a susceptible individual. Many cases in elderly people occur while some violent exertion is being made, such as hurrying to catch a train or during straining at stool.

Symptoms: Strokes vary both as regards their intensity, the particular symptoms shown, and the after-effects, but well-marked cases present the following symptoms. The person attacked becomes, more or less suddenly, deprived of consciousness and all power of voluntary motion. He lies as if in a deep sleep, with a flushed face, a slow pulse, stertorous breathing, accompanied with puffing of the cheeks during expiration, and with the pupils of the eyes insensible to light and contracted or unequal. This state in many respects resembles the coma of narcotic poisoning, and is unfortunately too often mistaken by unskilled people for alcoholic intoxication. The symptoms and history of the case, however, are usually sufficient to enable a correct diagnosis to be made.

The presence of complete paralysis down one or other side is a point which in general differentiates stroke from narcotic poisoning and alcoholic intoxication, the paralysis being demonstrable even during unconsciousness by lifting the limbs and noting the characteristic suddenness and helplessness with which those on the affected side fall when not supported. The fact that in either of the last-named conditions the person can generally be partially roused, while in stroke unconsciousness is complete, is also valuable. Assistance is also gained by observing the state of the pupils, which are usually unequal, whereas in narcotic poisoning they are usually much contracted, while in alcoholic intoxication they are widely dilated.

In this condition of insensibility death may occur within a few hours, or there may be a gradual return to consciousness, in which case it is usually found that the result of the attack remains in the form of paralysis of one side of the body (hemiplegia), while occasionally there may also be noticed some impairment of the mental powers, pointing to damage done to the brain. (See PARALYSIS; APHASIA.)

Stroke may occur without unconsciousness, a sudden paralysis of one side of the body being the only manifestation. Occasionally, when the haemorrhage takes place gently, the symptoms are gradually developed over a period of several hours (*ingravescent stroke*). Sometimes premonitory symptoms occur. Persistent headache of a dull throbbing character, a sense of fullness in the head, vomiting, giddiness, noises in the ears, slight confusion of mind, and numbness of a limb or of one side of the body are among the more important premonitory symptoms; and these may exist for a variable length of time before the attack comes on.

The effects of a stroke or apoplexy, as regards the paralysis which remains after the immediate attack is over, are described under *Hemiplegia* in the article on PARALYSIS.

Treatment: A knowledge of these facts is of the utmost importance in the treatment of stroke, as obviously much can be done in the way of warding off a stroke when it appears to threaten, and of preventing a recurrence in cases where there have been previous attacks. With respect to the treatment of stroke, little can be done during the state of unconsciousness, apart from skilled nursing. The great importance of absolute quiet, with the body in the recumbent position and the head supported on a low pillow, cannot be too strongly emphasized. Care must be taken that the patient receives nothing of a stimulant nature, which would tend to raise the general blood-pressure and increase the haemorrhage in the brain. If the blood-pressure is very high, the administration of hypotensive drugs may be of value. (See ESSENTIAL HYPERTENSION.)

The patient must be carefully watched, and symptoms treated as they arise. In the after-treatment of the resulting paralysis much may be done to prevent stiffness and to preserve the power of the muscles in the weakened limbs by physiotherapy, including exercises, massage and electrical treatment, and continuing reassurance.

STROMA is the name applied to the tissue which forms the framework and covering of an organ.

STRONGYLOIDIASIS is the disease produced by *Strongyloidesstercoralis*, a small nematode, which is found throughout the tropics, particularly in the Far East. It produces a characteristic itching skin rash, known as 'creeping eruption', as well as severe diarrhoea which, like hookworm, may lead to severe anaemia and prostration. The drug used in its treatment is thiabendazole.

STROPHANTHUS is the seed of an East African climbing plant, *Strophanthus kombé*, from which the natives made Kombé arrow-poison. From these seeds an active principle, strophanthin, can be separated, and upon this substance the activity of the drug depends. Its action upon the heart is almost identical with that of digitalis. (See DIGITALIS.) Strophanthin-K must be distinguished from ouabain, which is strophanthin-G.

Uses: It is specially in cases of heart disease in which the heart is beating feebly and the pulse weak and irregular – ie. cases of atrial fibrillation – that strophanthus is used. The effects of this drug, like those of digitalis, are often remarkable. (See also OUABAIN.)

STROPHULUS, or RED GUM, is a rash consisting of numerous small red pimples, which appears in young children usually about teething-time, and is associated with excessive sweating. It is relieved by light clothing, the exclusion of nylon and by frequent use of some astringent dusting powder.

STRUMA is an old term which was applied to swellings in the neck: either tuberculous glands or enlargement of the thyroid gland. In the former sense it is equivalent to scrofula. (See SCROFULA.) (For the second meaning, see GOITRE.) The term strumous is equivalent to tuberculous.

STRYCHNINE is an alkaloid derived from *Strychnos nux-vomca*, the seeds of an East Indian tree, as well as from the seeds of several other closely allied trees and shrubs. It is a white crystalline body possessed of an intensely bitter taste, more bitter perhaps than that of any other substance, and it is not very soluble in water. It stimulates all parts of the nervous system, and was at one time widely used for this purpose. Today, however, its use has largely been given up, though it is still found as a constituent of some so-called 'tonics'.

STRYCHNINE POISONING is fortunately of rare occurrence. It shows itself in convulsions, which come on very speedily after the person has taken the poison. These convulsions are brought on by slight causes, and the sufferer becomes quite flaccid between them. The mental faculties remain unaffected, and the symptoms end in death or recovery within a few hours. These symptoms serve to distinguish strychnine poisoning from tetanus or lock-jaw, the only malady which it resembles. (See TETANUS.)

Treatment: The patient should be kept quiet by himself in a darkened room, all noise and disturbance being reduced to a minimum. At the earliest moment a benzodiazepine is injected intravenously in a large enough dose to stop the convulsions and put the patient to sleep. If the patient is seen early enough after taking the poisonous dose, potassium permanganate, tannic accid, or charcoal may be given by mouth. To wash out the stomach or to induce vomiting in a patient with convulsions is not free from risk. If the muscles of respiration are fixed in spasm, artificial respiration is needed.

STUPE is a hot fomentation with turpentine sprinkled on it. (See FOMENTATIONS.)

STUPOR (see UNCONSCIOUSNESS).

STUTTERING (see STAMMERING).

STYE (see EYE, DISEASE AND INJURIES OF).

STYPTICS are applications which check bleeding, either by making the blood-vessels contract more firmly or by causing rapid clotting in the blood. Some possess both modes of action.

Varieties: Many substances have this action on account of their chemical or physical properties. Among them may be mentioned ice; hot

water at 49°C if brought directly in contact with the bleeding surface; perchloride of iron; acetate of lead and Goulard's water; nitrate of silver; sulphate of copper; sulphate of zinc; alum; tannin; hazeline; ergot; adrenaline; and Russell-viper venom.
Uses: The use of styptics is described under HAEMORRHAGE.

SUB- is a prefix signifying under, near, or moderately.

SUBACUTE COMBINED DEGENERATION OF THE CORD is a degenerative condition of the spinal cord which most commonly occurs as a complication of pernicious anaemia. (See ANAEMIA.)

SUBACUTE SCLEROSING PANENCEPHALITIS is a rare complication of measles due to infection of the brain with the measles virus. It develops two to eighteen years after the onset of the measles, and is characterized by mental deterioration leading on to convulsions, coma and death. The annual incidence in Britain is about 1 per million of the childhood population. The risk of its developing is five to twenty times greater after measles than after measles vaccination.

SUBARACHNOID HAEMORRHAGE is a haemorrhage into the subarachnoid space. It is usually the result of rupture of an aneurysm on the circle of Willis (qv).

SUBARACHNOID SPACE is the space between the arachnoid and the pia mater, two of the membranes covering the brain (qv).

SUBCLAVIAN is the name applied to a large artery and vein which pass to the upper arm between the collar bone and the first rib.

SUBCONSCIOUS is a state of being partially conscious, or the condition in which mental processes occur and outside objects and events are perceived with the mind nearly or quite unconscious of them. Such subconscious impressions or events may be forgotten at the time but may nevertheless exert a continued influence over the conscious mind, or may at a subsequent time come fully into consciousness. Much importance is attached to the influence of painful or unpleasant experiences which, though forgotten, continue to influence the mind, and these are held to be largely responsible for neurasthenic and similar states. This injurious influence is removed when the subconscious impressions come fully into consciousness and are then remembered and clearly seen in their relative importance.

SUBCUTANEOUS means anything pertaining to the loose cellular tissue beneath the skin: eg. a subcutaneous injection. (See HYPODERMIC INJECTION.)

SUBINVOLUTION is a term used to indicate that the womb has failed to undergo the usual involution, or decrease in size, which naturally takes place within one month after a child is born.

SUBJECTIVE is a term applied to symptoms, and sensations, perceived only by the affected individual. For example, numbness is a purely subjective sensation, whilst the jerk given by the leg on tapping the tendon of the knee is an objective sign.

SUBLIMATION is the conversion of a solid substance into a vapour and its recondensation. The term is also used in a mental sense for the process of converting instinctive sexual desires to new aims and objects devoid of sexual significance.

SUBLUXATION means a partial dislocation, and is a term sometimes applied to a sprain.

SUCCINYLSULPHATHIAZOLE is a sulphonamide drug which is absorbed only slowly from the intestine, and on that account used in the treatment of intestinal infections.

SUCCUSSION is a method of examination by shaking the body of a patient in order to elicit splashing sounds, with a view to determining the presence of gas and fluid in a cavity such as the interior of the stomach or the pleural cavity.

SUCKLING (see INFANT FEEDING; BREASTS, DISEASES OF).

SUCRALFATE is a drug that is proving of value in the treatment of peptic ulcer (qv).

SUCROSE, or CANE SUGAR (see SUGAR).

SUDAMINA are small vesicles which appear underneath the surface layer of the skin during diseases associated with constant perspiration: eg. rheumatic fever.

SUDDEN INFANT DEATH SYNDROME (see COT DEATH).

SUDORIFICS are drugs and other agents which produce copious perspiration. (See DIAPHORETICS.)

SUFFOCATION (see ASPHYXIA; CHOKING).

SUGAR is a substance containing carbon, hydrogen, and oxygen, and belonging therefore to the chemical group of carbohydrates. This group includes three subdivisions:

(1) Monosaccharides ($C_6H_{12}O_6$)
eg. Glucose, or dextrose, or grape sugar.
Fructose, or laevulose, or fruit sugar.
Galactose.
(2) Disaccharides ($C_{12}H_{22}O_{11}$)
eg. Sucrose, or cane sugar, or beet sugar.
Lactose or milk sugar.
Maltose or malt sugar.
(3) Polysaccharides ($C_6H_{10}O_5$)
eg. Starch.
Glycogen or animal starch.

Glucose, also known as grape sugar because it is found in various kinds of fruit, including grapes, is the form of sugar produced by the tissues and excreted in large amount by the kidneys in diabetes mellitus.

Sucrose is widely distributed through the vegetable kingdom, though it is specially plentiful in the juice of the sugar-cane, beetroot, and maple. When taken as a food, it is converted by the digestive juices into glucose before it is absorbed, this process being known as inversion. It is a valuable food, being utilized in the production of heat and energy, although it is also to a certain extent a tissue-builder so far as fat is concerned. It is to be avoided by people who tend to get fat as well as by diabetics.

Lactose is found in milk, and it is to the fermentation of this sugar and consequent production of lactic acid by certain bacteria that the souring of milk is due. The extent to which it is present in the milk of different animals is mentioned under INFANT FEEDING. It has little sweetening power compared with cane sugar, but it is used sometimes as a laxative.

Maltose is produced by the action of the ferment, diastase, upon the starch contained in barley, and also by the ferments of the saliva and pancreatic juice, and is still further changed by the intestinal ferments into glucose before it is absorbed.

Invert sugar is a natural mixture of dextrose and laevulose resulting from a chemical decomposition of cane sugar or of starch.

Starch is mentioned under a separate heading, and its use as a food under DIET and CEREALS.

The energy-producing value of sugars generally is taken as being, on the average, 4 Calories for each gram of sugar.

SUGAR OF LEAD (see LEAD).

SUGGESTION TREATMENT (see PSYCHOTHERAPY).

SUICIDE (see under MENTAL ILLNESS).

SULCUS is the term applied to any groove or furrow, but especially to a fissure of the brain.

SULFADOXINE is a long-acting sulphonamide (qv) with a range of action comparable to that of sulphamethoxypyridazine (qv). Along with pyrimethamine it is used in the prophylactic, or preventive, treatment of malaria. (See FANSIDAR.)

SULFAMETOPYRAZINE is a long-acting sulphonamide. Given in one weekly dose of 2 grams it is proving of value in preventing relapses during the winter in patients with chronic bronchitis.

SULINDAC (CLINORIL) is a recently introduced drug that is proving of value in the treatment of rheumatic conditions. (See NON-STEROIDAL ANTI INFLAMMATORY DRUGS.)

SULPHACETAMIDE is one of the sulphonamides. Its main use today is in the form of eye drops of the sodium salt used locally in the treatment of infections of the eye.

SULPHADIAZINE is one of the sulphonamides. It is a highly active drug and in moderate dosage produces a high and persistent blood concentration. It is relatively non-toxic and is particularly useful in the treatment of meningitis.

SULPHADIMETHOXINE is one of the long-acting sulphonamides, only one dose of which is required daily.

SULPHADIMIDINE is comparable in activity to sulphadiazine, and has the advantage of being even more non-toxic and of producing higher blood concentrations.

SULPHAEMOGLOBIN is an abnormal pigment sometimes found in the blood as a result of the interaction of certain drugs derived from aniline, such as phenacetin and acetanilide.

SULPHAFURAZOLE is a sulphonamide which has a wide range of anti-bacterial action. In view of its high solubility, it is particularly useful in infections of the urinary tract.

SULPHAGUANIDINE is a sulphonamide which is not readily absorbed from the intestine, and is therefore of value in the treatment of bacillary dysentery.

SULPHAMERAZINE is a sulphonamide which is absorbed rapidly from the gut and is excreted slowly by the kidneys. The concentration of the drug in the blood therefore remains high for a long time, and so its action against bacterial infection is correspondingly maintained. Its therapeutic use is similar to that of sulphadiazine.

SULPHAMETHOXAZOLE is one of the long-acting sulphonamides. It is related to sulphafurazole, has a duration of action of 12 hours, and is said to be particularly effective against streptococci.

SULPHAMETHOXYPYRIDAZINE is one of the new long-acting sulphonamides, only one dose of which is required daily.

SULPHAMEZATHINE is another term for SULPHADIMIDINE (qv).

SULPHANILAMIDE, or *p*-amino-benzene-sulphonamide, is a drug the discovery of which is one of the most important in medicine in the twentieth century. It was the first of the sulphonamide drugs. In 1935 the German chemist, Gerhard Domagk, announced the discovery of the effect of prontosil on streptococci. It was later found that this action was due to conversion in the body of prontosil into sulphanilamide, which acts by inhibiting the growth of various bacteria, especially the ubiquitous and dangerous *Streptococcus haemolyticus*. Although many other sulphonamides with various advantages have been subsequently introduced, sulphanilamide is still used to a certain extent. (See also SULPHONAMIDE.)

SULPHAPHENAZOLE is one of the long-acting sulphonamides.

SULPHASALAZINE is a sulphonamide which is proving of value in the treatment of ulcerative colitis.

SULPHASOMIZOLE is one of the long-acting sulphonamides.

SULPHINPYRAZONE is a derivative of phenylbutazone (qv) which is proving of value in the treatment of gout.

SULPHONAMIDE: A drug having the sulphonamide grouping $-SO_2NH_2$. In 1935, Gerhard Domagk, a German chemist, announced the discovery of the effect of prontosil on streptococci. Subsequent work showed that this action was due to the conversion in the body of prontosil to sulphanilamide. The action of the sulphonamides is bacteriostatic and not bactericidal: ie. they do not directly kill the bacteria but so interfere with their growth that they are unable to multiply. This action of the sulphonamides is now believed to be due to the similarity of their chemical structure to that of *p*-aminobenzoic acid. This latter substance is essential for the growth of many bacteria. If the bacteria are surrounded by a sulphonamide in greater concentration than *p*-aminobenzoic acid, then the bacteria take up the sulphonamide. This interferes with their development and they therefore never mature; nor are they able to reproduce themselves. Although the sulphonamides are being replaced to an increasing extent by penicillin, which is active against many of the same organisms, they are still a useful addition to our ability to control diseases due to bacterial infection.

SULPHONES are a group of drugs allied to the sulphonamides. They are used in the treatment of leprosy. The members of this group include dapsone.

SULPHONYLUREAS are sulphonamide derivitives which lower the blood sugar when they are given by mouth by enhancing the production of insulin. They are effective only when some residual pancreatic beta cell function is present. All may lead to a hypoglycaemia if given in overdose and this is particularly common when long-acting sulphonylureas are given to elderly patients. Tolbutamide (Pramidex, Rastinon) was the first of the sulphonlyurea drugs. It has a short duration of action and is usually given twice daily. Chlorpropamide (Diabenese, Melitase) has a more prolonged action and only needs to be given once daily. Other oral hypoglycaemic agents of this family include glibenclamide (Daonil, Euglucon), which has a duration of action intermediate between tolbutamide and chlorpropamide. Other sulphonlyureas include acetohexamide (Dimelor), glibornuride (Glutril), Gliclazide (Diamicron), glipizide (Glibenese, Minodiab), gliquidone (Glurenorm) and tolazamide (Tolanase). Glymidine (Gondafon) is a related compound with a similar action to the sulphonylureas. It is particularly useful in patients who are hypersensitive to sulphonylureas.

Sulphonylureas are best avoided in patients who are overweight as they tend to stimulate the appetite and aggravate obesity. They should be used with caution in patients with hepatic or renal disease. Side-effects are infrequent and usually not severe, the most common being epigastric discomfort with occasional nausea, vomiting and anorexia. In about 10 per cent of patients chlorpropamide and tolbutamide may cause facial flushing after drinking alcohol (see DIABETES MELLITUS). Some patients are hypersensitive to oral hypoglycaemic agents and develop rashes which may progress to erythema multiforme and exfoliative dermatitis. These reactions usually appear in the first 6 to 8 weeks of treatment.

SULPHUR is a non-metallic element. Crude sulphur is obtained in volcanic districts, and from it sublimed sulphur is prepared by heating. This sublimed sulphur is either run into moulds as rolled sulphur, or allowed to deposit as flowers of sulphur, which consists of a fine gritty powder and is the most commonly used form. The sublimed sulphur may be boiled with slaked lime and treated with hydrochloric acid, when the sulphur settles down in the form of a fine greyish-yellow powder –precipitated sulphur.

Action: The action of sulphur depends partly upon the grittiness of the flowers of sulphur, and mainly upon the readiness with which sulphur enters into chemical combinations to form sulphides and sulphates. In consequence of this property, it has disinfectant and antiparasitic powers. When taken internally, the sulphides that are formed stimulate the action of the bowels, and, being excreted partly from the surface of the skin and mucous membranes of the air passages, they also stimulate these.

Uses: Sulphur is burned in order to produce sulphurous acid gas, which is used as a disinfectant. (See DISINFECTION.) Externally, sulphur ointment is an old remedy against the minute parasite that is responsible for the itch; and milk of sulphur is used in lotions for acne on the face. Sulphur is also used in baths for its stimulating action on the skin in cases of skin disease and rheumatism. For this purpose either plain sulphur or, more commonly, sulphurated potash is added to hot water. Internally, sulphur is a time-honoured remedy for constipation, in doses of a teaspoonful or thereabout made into a paste with treacle. It may be used for the same purpose in the more palatable form of lozenges, several of these being taken at one time, and has a gentle laxative action. In old people who suffer from rheumatism and who are liable to constipation and to bronchitis, sulphur has been long used in combination with various anti-rheumatic drugs in the confection known as Chelsea Pensioner. (See CONFECTIONS.)

SULPHURIC ACID, or OIL OF VITRIOL, is, in its undiluted state, one of the most powerful of the mineral acids. It is a heavy, colourless liquid of oily consistence and is largely used in various manufacturing operations, so that poisoning by sulphuric acid is not uncommon. It chars any organic substance with which it is brought in contact, and acts as a violent corrosive poison. The treatment of sulphuric acid poisoning is that for corrosive poisons generally: eg. to administer weak alkalis such as baking soda, whitening, magnesia, or soap in water, and to apply oil to the injured surfaces.

Uses: Dilute sulphuric acid, or aromatic sulphuric acid containing cinnamon and ginger, and commonly known as elixir of vitriol, is used in cases of diarrhoea for its astringent properties, in doses of 5 or 20 drops well diluted in water. A lemonade is also made, containing small quantities of sulphuric acid, for use by lead-workers; since it forms an insoluble sulphate with lead, and thus prevents absorption of any lead which may be accidentally swallowed at work.

SULPHURIC ETHER is a name sometimes applied to the ether used for cleansing purposes, because sulphuric acid is employed in its preparation. (See ETHER.)

SULPHUROUS ACID is a saturated solution of sulphur dioxide. It has an extremely pungent odour and strong disinfectant power.

SULPIRIDE (DOLMATIL) (see ANTI-PSYCHOTIC DRUGS).

SUMMER DIARRHOEA (see DIARRHOEA; INFANT FEEDING).

SUNBURN includes the various effects produced on the skin by the sun's rays. The effects produced on the skin by sunlight are predominantly due to the ultra-violet rays. They are more marked in fair-skinned than in dark-skinned people, and consist predominantly of darkening, or tanning, of the skin as a result of the production in the skin of a dark pigment known as melanin (qv), which protects the skin against the deleterious effects of continued exposure to ultra-violet rays. In addition there is thickening of the superficial layer of the skin (qv). This production of melanin is preceded by reddening of the skin due to dilatation of the blood-vessels of the skin, and it is this action on the unprotected white skin that is responsible for the painful manifestations of sunburn, using this word in the strict sense of the term. With substantial long-continued exposure to sunlight there is an increase in the risk of skin cancer. In northern Europe the sensitivity of the skin to sunshine decreases during the late spring and early summer, to increase again in the autumn. This is probably a result of increasing exposure to the sun inducing thickening of the superficial layers of the skin and increasing their content of melanin.

The first manifestation of sunburn, the reddening of the skin, begins to develop in a few hours. This persists for about two days, when it is gradually replaced by tanning or darkening of the skin which gradually develops in extent and depth, depending on how long the body is exposed to the sun's rays and the intensity of the sunlight. The effect of the sun in this respect is much diminished by cloud, and increased by snow. This latter effect is the result of reflection of the ultra-violet rays by the snow, and explains why particular care must be exercised when exposing oneself to the sun in snowy conditions, as on a skiing holiday. There is probably little extra risk of sunburn from exposure to the sun at sea as the surface of the sea does not reflect ultra-violet rays to any appreciable extent.

Symptoms: If the body is over-exposed to the sun, the initial reddening of the skin increases. The skin begins to itch and tingle, becomes swollen, and then blisters begin to form, with peeling of the skin. The speed with which these changes occur, and their extent, depend upon the individual susceptibility of the skin and also the degree and extent of exposure to the sun, but in severe caes the effects may be extensive enough to cause a general upset accompanied by fever.

Prevention: All these unpleasant effects of sunburn can be avoided by gradual exposure of the body to the sun. How gradual this should be depends on the susceptibility of the individual's skin to sunlight, and the intensity of the sun's rays. For the first few days such exposure should not exceed an hour or so, and initially only part of the body should be exposed. Those who are proposing to sunbathe in warm climates, as around the Mediterranean, would be well advised to 'get into training' by preliminary sunbathing in the garden at home. It is the parts of the body that are normally not exposed to the sun that are most susceptible to sunburn.

Other preventive measures include the sensible use of 'beach umbrellas', and other shades. Oiling of the skin is an ancient practice that has stood up well to the test of time. There is now a wide range of sunscreen preparations on the market, the active constituents of which include titanium dioxide and zinc oxide. Care, however, must be exercised in the choice of these, as there is by no means invariably a direct correlation between price and efficacy. A

basic formula which seems to be standing up to the test of time is 5 per cent para-aminobenzoic acid in 70 per cent ethanol. A more complicated prescription for those who are particularly sensitive to sunlight is 5 per cent para-aminobenzoic acid, 2·5 per cent amyl dimethylaminobenzoate, and 70 per cent ethanol. Another useful preparation is mexenone cream BPC (qv). The French swear by a preparation of horse-chestnut known as Esculoside.
Treatment: Once sunburn, as opposed to suntan, has developed, the affected individual must keep in the shade. The itching and tingling of the skin may be relieved by applying calamine lotion, calamine lotion containing 1 per cent phenol, or 2·5 per cent solution of coal tar. In milder cases the dabbing on of an evaporating fluid such as eau-de-Cologne, elderflower water, or rose water may be helpful, as may be sponging the affected skin with an astringent such as Goulard's water (qv) or hazeline (qv). (See also MELANOMA.)

SUNLIGHT (see LIGHT TREATMENT).

SUPER- is a prefix signifying above or implying excess.

SUPERFOETATION is the condition in which there is fertilization of a second ovum in a woman already pregnant.

SUPERINVOLUTION is the process by which the womb decreases in size after childbirth, when, instead of stopping at the point when the womb reaches its usual size, more or less complete wasting away of this organ takes place.

SUPINATION means the turning of the forearm and hand so that the palm faces upwards.

SUPPOSITORY is a small conical mass made of oil of theobroma, to which white beeswax is sometimes added, or glycerin-jelly, and containing drugs intended for introduction into the rectum. This method of using drugs, which is more popular on the Continent than in the United Kingdom, may be chosen for various reasons. For example, the suppository, as in the case of soap or glycerin suppositories, may be used to produce an aperient action. Other suppositories, such as those of morphine, are used to quiet pain and check the action of the bowels. Others are used for the sake of their influence on neighbouring organs.
Method of use: The suppository is placed with its pointed end against the anus and with a firm but gentle screwing movement is pushed upwards. With the point of the forefinger, it must be pushed onwards for about 25 mm (1 inch), past the sphincter muscle, otherwise it will not be retained. It must be quickly introduced, as the material of which it is composed rapidly softens when brought into contact with the body. It may be retained in position by crossing the legs or lying on the side. To facilitate insertion it may be lubricated with a small amount of olive oil before insertion.

SUPPURATION means the process of pus formation. When pus forms on a raw surface the process is called ulceration, whilst a deep-seated collection of pus is known as an abscess. (For more detailed information, see ABSCESS; INFLAMMATION; PHAGOCYTOSIS; ULCER; WOUNDS.)

SUPRA- is a prefix signifying above or upon.

SUPRAPUBIC operation is one in which the abdomen is opened in its lower part, immediately above the pubic bones. (See LITHOTOMY.)

SUPRARENAL GLANDS, also known as ADRENAL GLANDS, are two organs situated one upon the upper end of each kidney. Each measures about 5 cm (2 inches) in length from above downwards, rather less than that from side to side; and each is about 6 mm (¼ inch) thick. The two together weigh about 7 grams.
Structure: Each suprarenal gland has an enveloping layer of fibrous tissue. Within this the gland shows two distinct parts: an outer, firm, deep-yellow, *cortical* layer, and a central, soft, dark-brown, *medullary* portion. The cortical part consists of columns of cells running from the surface inwards, whilst in the medullary portion the cells are arranged irregularly and separated from one another by large capillary blood-vessels. Both the blood vessels and the nerves of the suprarenal glands are large and numerous, considering the small size of the organ.
Functions: It has long been known that removal of the suprarenal glands in animals is speedily followed by great muscular prostration and death in a few days. In human beings, disease of the suprarenal glands is apt to bring on Addison's disease, in which the chief symptoms are increasing weakness and bronzing of the skin. The medulla of the glands produces a substance –adrenaline – the effects of which closely resemble those brought about by activity of the sympathetic nervous system: dilated pupils, hair standing on end, quickening and strengthening of the heart-beat, immobilization of the gut, increased output of sugar from the liver into the blood-stream. From the cortex of the gland are produced a series of hormones which play a vital, though as yet incompletely elucidated, rôle in the metabolism of the body. Some (such as aldosterone) control the electrolyte balance of the body, others are concerned in carbohydrate metabolism, whilst others again are concerned with sex physiology. Cortisone is the most important hormone of the adrenal cortex and is essential for life. (See ADRENALINE; ADDISON'S DISEASE; CORTISONE.)

SURAMIN is the *British Pharmacopoeia* name for a drug which has been much used, and with success, in the treatment of trypanosomiasis (qv).

SURFACTANT is a surface-active agent lining the alveoli of the lungs, which plays an essential part in respiration (qv) by preventing the alveoli collapsing at the end of expiration. Absence, or lack, of surfactant is one of the factors responsible for hyaline membrane disease (qv), and it is now being used in the treatment of this condition by means of instillation into the trachea.

SURMA is a fine powder which is applied to the inner surface of the eyelids in the same way as mascara is applied to the outer surface. Its name is derived from the Urdu for antimony, but in practice it may contain salts of antimony, zinc, and lead. Lead sulphide (galena) is the most common constituent, often combined with camphor or menthol to induce watering of the eyes. It is used by Asians, mainly as a cosmetic, but also to relieve eyestrain. It has been shown to induce lead poisoning in Asian children. Since January 1979 the use and sale of surma and other lead-containing cosmetics have been prohibited in Great Britain.

SURROGATE is a term applied in medicine to a substance used as a substitute for another.

SUSPENDED ANIMATION (see DEATH, SIGNS OF; SLEEP).

SUTURE is the name given either to the close union between two neighbouring bones of the skull, or to the series of stitches by which a wound is closed. (See WOUNDS.)

SWAB is a term applied to a small piece of gauze, lint, or similar material used for wiping out the mouth of a helpless patient or for drying out a wound. The term is also applied to a tuft of sterilized cotton-wool wrapped round a wire and enclosed in a sterile glass tube used for obtaining matter or membrane from the throat, from wounds, or the like, in order that this may be subjected to bacteriological examination.

SWAN-GANZ CATHETER is a flexible tube with a double lumen and a small balloon at its distal end. It is introduced into a vein in the arm and advanced until the end of the catheter is in the right atrium. The balloon is then inflated with air through one lumen and this enables the blood stream to propel the catheter through the right ventricle to the pulmonary artery. The balloon is deflated and the catheter can then record the pulmonary artery pressure. When the balloon is inflated the tip is isolated from the pulmonary artery and measures the left atrial pressure. These measurements are important in the management of patients with circulatory failure as under these circumstances the central venous pressure or the right atrial pressure is an unreliable guide to fluid replacement.

SWEAT (see PERSPIRATION).

SWEAT GLANDS (see SKIN).

SWEETBREAD is a popular term applied to several glands used for food, including the thymus gland of young animals (neck sweetbread), the pancreas (stomach sweetbread), and the testis.

SWEET SPIRIT OF NITRE, also known as NITROUS ETHER SPIRIT, consists of a mixture of water, alcohol, acetaldehyde, and various nitrous bodies. Like other drugs containing nitrites, sweet spirit of nitre has an action in checking spasm of all sorts and in dilating the blood-vessels. (See GLYCERYL TRINITRATE.) In certain circumstances it is a diaphoretic, causing copious perspiration and thus reducing feverishness. In other circumstances it acts as a diuretic, increasing the action of the kidneys. When kept in unstoppered bottles, it rapidly loses strength. To be of any value, it must be used fresh.

SYCOSIS is a skin disease in which the hair follicles, especially of the chin, are inflamed, forming pustules round the hairs, surrounded by a swollen and reddened area of skin. The disease is directly due to infection of the hair follicles with staphylococcus or ringworm. The infection is generally attributed to a barber's utensils, and the condition is sometimes known as barber's itch, foul shave, or ringworm of the beard. (For treatment, see IMPETIGO; RINGWORM.)

SYMPATHETIC is a term applied to certain diseases or symptoms which arise in one part of the body in consequence of disease in some distant part. Inflammation may arise in one eye, in consequence of injury to the other, by the spread of organisms along the lymphatic channels connecting the two, and is then known as sympathetic inflammation. Pain also may be of a sympathetic nature. (See PAIN.)

SYMPATHETIC SYSTEM is part of the autonomic nervous system (qv). It consists of scattered collections of grey matter known as ganglia, united by an irregular network of nerve-fibres, those portions where the ganglia are placed most closely and the network of fibres is specially dense being known as plexuses. The chief part of the sympathetic system consists of two ganglionated cords that run through the neck, chest, and abdomen, lying close in front of the spine. (For further details, see NERVES.)

SYMPATHOMIMETIC DRUGS are those producing an effect comparable to those produced by stimulation of the sympathetic nervous system: eg. adrenaline (qv).

SYMPTOM is a term applied to any evidence of disease. The term, physical sign, is generally applied to evidence of disease of which the patient does not complain but which is elicited upon examination. For the symptoms indicative of the various diseases see under the headings of each disease.

SYN- is a prefix signifying union.

SYNAPSE is the term applied to the anatomical relation of one nerve-cell with another which is effected at various points by contact of their branching processes. The state of shrinkage or relaxation at these points (synapses) is supposed in some cases to determine the readiness with which a nervous impulse is transmitted from one part of the nervous system to another. Many drugs act upon the nervous system through their effect in closing or widening these junctions.

SYNCOPE, or fainting, is a loss of consciousness due to a fall in blood pressure. This may result because the cardiac output has become reduced or because the peripheral resistance provided by the arterioles has decreased. The simple faint or vaso-vagal attack is a result of a failure to maintain an adequate venous return of blood to the heart. This is likely to occur after prolonged periods of standing, particularly if one is standing still or if the climatic conditions are hot. It can also result from an unpleasant or painful experience. Pallor, sweating and a slow pulse are characteristic. Recovery is immediate when the venous return is restored by lying flat. Syncope can also result when the venous return to the heart is impaired as a result of a rise in intra-thoracic pressure. This may happen after prolonged vigorous coughing, the so-called cough syncope, or when elderly men with prostatic hypertrophy strain to empty their bladder. This is known as micturition syncope. Syncope is particularly likely to occur when the arterial blood pressure is unusually low. This may result from overtreatment of hypertension with drugs or it may be the result of diseases, such as Addison's disease, which are associated with low blood pressures. It is important that syncope is distinguished from epilepsy.

SYNDACTYLY is the condition which a child is born with, in which two or more fingers or toes are fused together to a varying extent. The condition is popularly known as webbed fingers or toes (qv).

SYNDROME is a term applied to a group of symptoms occurring together regularly and thus constituting a disease to which some particular name is given: eg. *Cushing's Syndrome* comprising obesity, hypertension, purple striae and osteoporosis; *Korsakoff's Syndrome*, of loss of appreciation of time and place combined with talkativeness, forming signs of alcoholic delirium.

SYNECHIAE: Adhesions between the iris and adjacent structures, eg. cornea, lens. They usually arise as a result of inflammation of the iris.

SYNGANOSIS is a disease of the lungs caused by roundworm known as *Syngamus laryngeus* (or *Mammomonogamus laryngeus*). It occurs in the Caribbean and may affect tourists as well as natives. It is characterized by a chronic persistent cough, sometimes accompanied by fever, blood in the sputum and loss of weight. It may end by the spontaneous coughing up of the red wriggling worm. If this does not occur, the worm may be removed through a bronchoscope (qv). Should this fail, the administration of thiabendazole effects a cure. The mode of transmission to man is not known.

SYNOSTOSIS is the term applied to a union by bony material of adjacent bones normally separate.

SYNOVIAL MEMBRANE forms the lining of the soft parts that enclose the cavity of a joint. (See JOINTS.)

SYNOVITIS means inflammation of the membrane lining a joint. It is usually painful and accompanied by effusion of fluid within the synovial sac of the joint. It is found in acute rheumatism, various injuries and inflammations of joints, and in the chronic form in tuberculosis. (See JOINTS, DISEASES OF.)

SYNTHETIC is a term applied to substances produced by chemical processes in the laboratory or by artificial building up.

SYPHILIS is a contagious disease of slow development, which, at its start, shows a characteristic sore at the site of infection, later brings on constitutional effects resembling those of other infectious diseases, and at a still later period produces certain changes in the central nervous system, the arteries and elsewhere. Because, in the majority of cases the disease is acquired as a result of sexual intercourse with an infected individual, it is classed as one of the *venereal* diseases, or sexually transmitted diseases as they are now known. Syphilis affects only human beings, though it has been experimentally produced in anthropoid apes.

The disease seems to have first attracted public attention about or soon after the year 1494 in consequence of a severe and widespread outbreak among the French soldiers then occupied in the siege of Naples. An association with martial activity has persisted ever since. Thus it has been estimated that during the 1914–18 War a quarter of the armies in Europe were incapacitated by syphilis and gonorrhoea. For long it was known as the Neapolitan disease, French Pox, or Great Pox; and, in consequence probably of the licentiousness and the want of cleanliness that then prevailed, it spread in epidemic form. Later, it came to be called syphilis, the name being derived from that of the chief character in a Latin poem published by Fracastoro in 1530. It has been suggested that the disease existed in ancient times among the natives of America, and that the infection was brought to Europe by the followers of Columbus, but there are also grounds for supposing that the disease occurred among the Eastern races in ancient times, although it was most likely often confounded with leprosy and tuberculosis. Today, according to the World Health Organization, around 40 million new cases are notified annually in the world, and, according to many, this is an underestimate.

Causes: The causative organism is the *Treponema pallidum*, a long, thread-like wavy organism with pointed tapering ends. It is found in large numbers in the sores in the primary stage of the disease and in the skin lesions in the secondary stage.

The number of cases of syphilis reported in England in the year ending June 30, 1986, was 3,000. The number of deaths from the disease in England in 1984 was 73, of which five deaths were due to congenital syphilis.

Syphilis may be ACQUIRED from people already suffering from the disease, or it may be CONGENITAL. The acquired form is usually got by sexual intercourse, but it may also result from kissing or from contact with a sore upon another person through some wound or abrasion. The epithelium covering the general surface of the skin seems to be an efficient protection, but the infective material apparently has the power of penetrating mucous membranes. Not only may the disease be spread as a venereal affection, but cups, spoons, towels, sponges, sheets, which have been used by the diseased, have been known to convey the contagion to others, although fortunately such inanimate articles appear to retain their infectiveness only for a short time. The acquired form of the disease is infectious from contact with sores, both in its primary and secondary stages; whilst infants suffering from the congenital form are also highly infectious. Accordingly any one frequently handling such an infant runs great risk of infection, although the mother may handle the babe with impunity (Colles' Law).

Symptoms: The *acquired form* of the disease is commonly divided into three stages –PRIMARY, SECONDARY, and TERTIARY, although in many cases the tertiary stage is wanting, whilst in others there is no dividing line between the secondary and tertiary symptoms. To certain late affections, which may appear after the lapse of several years, such as general paralysis, the terms parasyphilis and QUATERNARY syphilis are sometimes applied. The disease presents great variations of intensity, being occasionally of a 'malignant' type, in which widespread ulceration speedily comes on and even causes death; and in other cases showing little more than a slight skin eruption, although probably it exerts, even in such mild cases, a highly prejudicial effect upon the constitution. There are several laboratory tests for confirming the diagnosis.

The incubation period ranges from 10 to 90 days, though most frequently it occupies about four weeks. Then a small ulcer appears at the site of infection, which is accompanied by a typical cartilaginous hardness of the tissues immediately round and beneath it, and characterized by its resistance to all healing treatment. This, which is known as the PRIMARY SORE (or *chancre*), may be very much inflamed, or it may be so small and occasion so little trouble as to pass almost or quite unnoticed. A few days after this sore has appeared, the lymphatic glands in its neighbourhood, and later those all over the body, become swollen and hard. This condition lasts for several weeks as a rule, and then the sore slowly heals and the glands subside. After a variable period, which, however, may in most cases be placed at about two months from the date of infection, the SECONDARY SYMPTOMS appear and resemble the symptoms of an ordinary fever in so far as they include rise of temperature and feverishness, loss of appetite, vague pains through the body, and a faint red rash seen best upon the front of the chest. The rash may also show other characters. Other symptoms often present at this stage, including falling out of the hair, bloodlessness, the appearance of sores in the mouth and throat (mucous patches), fleshy-looking masses round the genitalia (*condylomatua lata*), headache with, occasionally, mental deterioration, and painful swellings on the bones due to periostitis. There is also general enlargement of the lymphatic glands. The duration of this stage is largely dependent upon the efficiency with which it is treated.

In untreated or inadequately treated cases manifestations of the TERTIARY STAGE develop after the lapse of some months or years. These consist in the growth, here and there throughout the body, of masses of granulation tissue known as *gummas*. These gummas may appear as hard nodules in the skin, or form tumour-like masses in the muscles, or cause great thickening of bones, or they may develop in the brain and spinal cord, where their presence causes very serious symptoms. Those which lie beneath the skin or a mucous membrane may break down and form deep ulcers with characteristic thickened, sharply cut edges. These often leave rounded brownish scars when they heal. Gummas yield readily, as a rule, to appropriate treatment, and generally disappear speedily when this is secured.

Still later effects are apt to follow, such as disease of the arteries, leading to aneurysm (see ARTERIES, DISEASES OF; ANEURYSM), to apoplexy, and to early mental failure (see MENTAL ILLNESS); also certain nervous diseases, of which tabes dorsalis and general paralysis are the chief.

The *congenital form* of syphilis, of which there were 80 cases in England in 1983, may affect the child before birth, leading then as a rule to miscarriage, or to a stillbirth if born at full time. Or he (or she) may show the first symptoms a few weeks after birth, the appearances then corresponding to the secondary manifestations of the acquired form. The child, apparently at first quite healthy, begins to waste, so that the skin appears loose and wrinkled. Eruptions develop and the breathing is of a snuffling character, in consequence of inflammation in the mucous membrane of the mouth and nose. Deafness is also a common result of inflammation of the inner ear. On the other hand, no symptoms may appear till later in life, when the nose becomes sunken and broad at the bridge, and the eyes are dull as the result of the inflammation affecting the cornea (keratitis) or iris (iritis). These changes often appear about the age of 12 or 14, causing dimness of vision. When the permanent teeth appear, the central incisors are often notched at the edge (Hutchinson's teeth).

Treatment: Any person who suffers from this disease forms a source of infection to those around, and it is his duty to take precautions that he may not spread it. He should bear in mind the fact that, whilst the natural secretions of the body are harmless, the discharge from any sore or abraded surface is highly contagious.

For generations, salts of mercury were the traditional drugs for the treatment of syphilis, given by mouth or by inunction, and later by intramuscular injection. Following the discovery by Ehrlich, in 1910, of the anti-syphilitic action of organic arsenical preparations, these became the essential part of the treatment of the condition, supplemented by bismuth salts.

For nearly forty years the organic arsenical preparations, in one form or another, constituted the first line of attack on syphilis. During the last thirty years, however, they have been replaced by penicillin which, used in the correct dosage, is now accepted as the drug of choice in the treatment of syphilis in all its stages. Typical of its efficacy is the fact that, whilst in one investigation, of 534 offspring of 200 mothers with untreated syphilis, 254 (47·6 per cent) had congenital syphilis, no case of congenital syphilis was found whenever a hitherto untreated syphilitic woman received a full course of penicillin and had completed this at least a fortnight before delivery.

The successful introduction of penicillin, however, has not altered the three essential bases of successful treatment: (1) treatment must be instituted as soon as possible after infection is acquired; (2) a full course of treatment is essential in every case, no matter how mild the disease may appear to be; (3) periodic blood examinations must be carried out on every patient for at least two years after he or she has been apparently cured.

SYRINGE is an instrument for injecting liquids into the body. Syringes vary considerably in shape and size according to the purpose for which they are used. (For the method of using a hypodermic syringe, see HYPODERMIC.)

SYRINGOMYELIA is a rare disease affecting the spinal cord, in which are found irregular cavities surrounded by an excessive amount of the connective tissue of the central nervous system. These cavities encroach upon the nerve tracts in the cord, producing especially loss of the sense of pain or of that for heat and cold in parts of the limbs, although the sensation of touch is retained. Another symptom sometimes present is wasting of certain muscles in the limbs. Changes affecting outlying parts like the fingers are also found. On account of their insensitiveness to pain, the fingers, for example, are often burnt or wounded, and troublesome ulcers, or loss of parts of the fingers, result. The condition of the spinal cord is probably present at birth, though the symptoms do not usually appear till young adulthood is reached. The disease is slowly progressive, though sudden exacerbations may occur after a cough, a sneeze, or sudden straining. Treatment consists simply in the maintenance of general good health.

SYRUP, formed of a mixture of sugar and water, is a fluid often used for the administration of drugs. It is employed partly on account of its pleasant taste, and largely also because it retards changes in drugs which deteriorate on exposure to the air.

SYSTOLE means the contraction of the heart, and alternates with the resting phase, known as diastole. The two occupy, respectively, about one-third and two-thirds of the cycle of heart action.

T

TABES means, literally, a wasting disease, and is an old name applied to various diseases, such as tabes dorsalis and tuberculosis accompanied by enlargement of glands. At present the name *tabes dorsalis* is used for locomotor ataxia and *tabes mesenterica* is used for tuberculosis affecting the glands in the abdomen: two diseases totally different in their nature and cause.

TABLET is the name given to a solid disc-like preparation made by compression and containing drugs mixed usually with sugar and other indifferent material. Tablets are widely used because of their convenience and accurate dosage. The word, 'tabloid', indicates a proprietary preparation.

TACHE CEREBRALE is a sign often observed in meningitis. It consists in the production of a bright-red line of congestion when the fingernail is drawn across the patient's skin – for example, across his abdomen.

TACHYCARDIA means a rapid pulse rate. (See HEART DISEASES.)

TACHYPNOEA means unusual quickness of breathing.

TAENIASIS is the disease caused by taeniae, or tapeworms. Their shape is modified to present as large an absorbing surface as possible to the digested food passing down the intestine, so that they are flat, white and long (up to 12 metres [40 feet] in length), like a piece of tape, as their name implies. Each consists of a head, the size of a small pin's head, provided with suckers, and sometimes with hooklets, for adhesion to the bowel wall, and from this head segments are produced that gradually increase in size and develop ova the farther they recede from the head. The mature segments at the extremity of the worm are crammed full of ova, and are constantly splitting off to be discharged in the stools. When these mature segments, or proglottides, are discharged, they fall upon the ground, and the ova they contain are afterwards conveyed either by food or drink into the stomach of an intermediate host, which may be a pig, ox or cattle, in the case of different parasites. The geographical distribution of different tapeworm infestation depends largely upon the eating habits of the inhabitants. Thus *Taenia saginata*, or the beef tapeworm, is found in beef-eating areas, especially in Europe and Mohammedan countries. *Taeniasolium*, the pork tapeworm, is found most commonly in Germany and the Slav countries. *Echinococcus granulosus* is found where dogs are widely used, as in Iceland or sheep-rearing countries such as Australia, New Zealand and Argentina. When the ova reach the stomach of the intermediate host their capsule is dissolved, the embryos escape and find their way through the wall of stomach or intestine into the blood-vessels, by which they are carried to distant parts of the body. In the case of TAENIA SOLIUM the intermediate host is the pig, in the case of TAENIA SAGINATA it is cattle. In the muscles of these animals the embryos of the worm become encysted and remain so till they die, or till the animal's flesh happens to be eaten by the proper host, when they develop again into a new tapeworm in his intestine. The flesh of a pig thus infected shows plainly the encysted embryo (known as *Cysticercus cellulosae*), and is called measly pork. DIPHYLLOBOTHRIUM LATUM is seldom met with, except in the north of Europe and Asia, and the intermediate hosts are several varieties of fish. In the case of the tapeworm known as *Echinococcus granulosus*, relations are reversed, and man plays the rôle of intermediate host, the host of the mature tapeworm being the dog, from which the human being derives the embryo worm by allowing the dog to lick his hands and face, or to contaminate his food. Although the worm in the dog is very small (having only three segments, as a rule), the encysted form in man, known as a hydatid cyst, may reach a large size, situated in the liver, lungs, kidney or brain.

In the case of infestation with *Taenia saginata* there may be no symptoms or signs at all, and the 'host' only becomes aware that he is infested, when he sees the tapeworm, or rather part of it, in the stools. In the case of *Taenia solium*, the outlook is more serious because the eggs, when swallowed, are liable to migrate into the tissues of the body, as they do in the pig, and cause cysts. If these occur in the muscles they may cause little trouble but, if they occur in the brain, they can prove very serious.

Hydatid cysts often grow to a great size, budding off in their interior smaller cysts, which may have still smaller ones within them, the final contents of the smallest cysts being a salt, watery fluid and numerous heads of echinococci, each provided with a circle of hooks, and each capable, under proper conditions, of forming a new worm. The symptoms produced by a hydatid cyst depend mainly upon the effects of its size and consequent pressure. Very small cysts in the brain may produce serious results, like those of a tumour, whilst in the liver a cyst may grow to the size of a man's head before causing much trouble.

Treatment of tapeworm infestation consists of the administration of mepacrine, niclosamide or dichlorophen, followed by a purgative. Castor oil must not be used for this purpose. During treatment the stools must be carefully examined for the head of the tapeworm. Unless the head is passed in the stools, the worm will grow again. The treatment of hydatid cyst is surgical: ie. the cyst must be removed by operation.

TALAMPICILLIN (see PENICILLIN, ANTIBIOTIC).

TALC is a soft mineral consisting of magnesium silicate. It is much used as an ingredient of dusting powders.

TALIPES is the technical name for club-foot (qv).

TALUS is the somewhat square-shaped bone which forms the lower part of the ankle-joint and unites the leg bones to the foot.

TAMARIND is the preserved pulp of the fruit of *Tamarindusindica*, a West Indian tree. It contains a large amount of vegetable acid, and has a laxative action.

TAMOXIFEN is a drug that is proving of value in the treatment of some cases of cancer of the breast.

TANNIN, or TANNIC ACID, is an uncrystallizable white or yellowish-white powder, which is soluble in water or glycerin. It is extracted from oak galls in large amount, but it is also present in almost all vegetable infusions. Tannic acid, when brought in contact with any mucous membrane, acts as an astringent and diminishes its secretion. It coagulates albuminous substances and thus hardens animal food with which it is mixed, and also leads to rapid clotting of blood with which it is brought in contact.

Uses: Tannin is used as a styptic to apply directly to bleeding wounds or surfaces with which it can be brought in contact, as the mouth, interior of the stomach, or of the rectum, and since its action in coagulating albumin is powerful, it speedily causes a clot to form. It is applied to relaxed mucous membranes, employed, for instance, in lozenges when the throat is relaxed, or applied in ointment for piles. Glycerin of tannin is a convenient method of applying this substance as an astringent, by painting, to the throat. Tannin is used to check diarrhoea, administered either in the form of some vegetable astringent infusion, or in a chemical combination which is not destroyed in the stomach, such as acetannin or albumin tannate.

As tannin neutralizes many poisonous alkaloids, it is often administered as an antidote to vegetable poisons.

Many vegetable astringents owe their usefulness to the tannin they contain, as, for example, catechu, kino, and rhatany.

TAPEWORM (see TAENIASIS).

TAPPING is the popular name for the withdrawal of oedema fluid from the cavities or the subcutaneous tissues of the body. (See ASPIRATION.)

TAR, or PIX LIQUIDA, is a thick, dark, oily substance obtained by the destructive distillation of several species of pine-tree. It is slightly soluble in water, more readily so in alcohol, oils, and strong alkaline solutions. Other tars of similar physical and medicinal properties are obtained from other woods, as well as from coal, shale, and peat. Tar is a substance of complex chemical composition, varying not only according to the source from which it is derived, but still more with the temperature at which it has been distilled. Generally speaking, wood-tar contains resin, creosote, and turpentine in considerable quantities, also benzol, carbolic acid, acetic acid, wood-spirit or methyl alcohol, methyl acetate, acetone, and wood-naphtha. The aniline dyes, many antipyretic bodies, saccharin, and various other medicinal substances and disinfectants are obtained indirectly from coal-tar.

Action: In consequence of the numerous medicinally active bodies it contains, tar exerts many marked effects upon the body. By reason of the creosote, carbolic acid, and methyl alcohol that it contains, it possesses an antiseptic and preservative power. Certain of its ingredients are of an irritating nature, and tar therefore stimulates the action of any skin surface with which it is brought in contact, as well as the respiratory and other mucous membranes by which it is excreted after being taken internally.

Uses: Externally, tar is one of the most efficient preservatives of animal and vegetable tissues that we possess. For its germicidal action and stimulating properties it is used in chronic skin diseases, particularly psoriasis and dry eczema. To this end it is employed most commonly in the form of tar ointment. An alcoholic extract known as coal tar solution is also used to cleanse areas of skin affected by the disease.

TARAXACUM, or DANDELION, is a very old remedy for dyspepsia. The fresh milky juice of the flower-stalks is also sometimes used as a remedy for warts.

TARSUS is the region of the instep with its seven bones, the chief of which are the talus supporting the leg-bones and the calcaneus or heel-bone, the others being the navicular, cuboid, and three cuneiform bones.

TARTAR is a concretion that forms on the teeth near the margin of the gum, consisting chiefly of phosphate of lime deposited from the saliva. Mixed with this are food particles, and in it flourish numberless bacteria. It is important that it should be prevented from forming by regular brushing of the teeth, or removal after it has formed by regular visits to the dentist, because it gives rise to wasting of the gums and loosening of the teeth.

TARTAR EMETIC is another name for antimony potassium tartrate, a drug used in the treatment of schistosomiasis. (See SCHISTOSOMIASIS.)

TARTARIC ACID is almost identical with citric acid in appearance, chemical properties, and medicinal uses. Tartaric acid is obtained from grapes, whilst citric acid is contained in many fruits like the lemon, lime, and orange. (See CITRIC ACID.)

TASTE (see TONGUE).

TATTOOING has been a cult, or fashion, since the earliest days of history. Apart from the mixed motifs for its use, it has a definite therapeutic indication in matching the colour of skin grafts. It is performed by implanting particles of colour pigment into the deeper layer of the skin known as the corium (see SKIN). This is done by means of a needle or needles. The pigments commonly used are carbon for black, cinnabar (red mercuric sulphide) or cadmium salts for red, chrome salts for greens and yellows, cobalt for blue, ferric (iron) salts for browns, pinks and yellows, and titanium for white. The main medical hazard of tattooing is infection, particularly of the liver, which may be fatal. The tattooed person may also become allergic to one of the pigments used, particularly cinnabar. Removal, which should be done

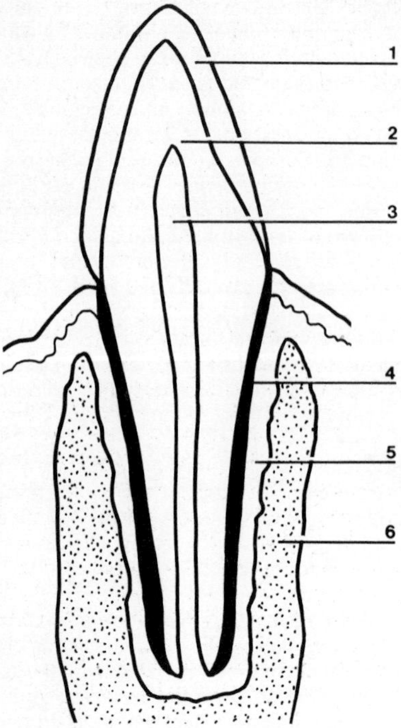

1 enamel
2 dentine
3 pulp cavity
4 cement
5 dental periosteum
6 bone of jaw

Vertical section through incisor tooth.

by a plastic surgeon, always leaves a residual scar, and often needs to be followed by a skin graft. Removal is not allowed under the National Health Service unless there is some medical reason: for example, allergic reactions to it. Other methods of removal are by cryosurgery (qv), dermabrasion (qv) and salabrasion (qv). These, too, must only be carried out under skilled medical supervision. Promising results are also being obtained from the use of laser (qv), a method that appears to produce less scarring than other methods, if it is carried out under expert medical supervision.

In order to reduce the health hazards, tattooists, along with acupuncturists, cosmetic skin-piercers and hair electrolysers, are required, under the Local Government (Miscellaneous Provisions) Act 1982, to register their premises with health and local authorities before starting business. The practitioners have to satisfy the authorities that adequate precautions have been taken to prevent the transmission of infections, such as hepatitis.

TAXIS is the method of pushing back, into the abdominal cavity, a loop of bowel which has passed through the wall in consequence of a rupture.

TEARS (see EYE).

TEETH are hard organs developed from the mucous membranes of the mouth and embedded in the jawbones. They are used to bite and grind food and to aid clarity of speech. In some animals the teeth may be modified in shape to enable them to be used as weapons.

Structure: Each tooth is composed of enamel, dentine, cement, pulp and periodontal membrane.

Enamel is the almost translucent material which covers the crown of a tooth. It is the most highly calcified material in the body, 96–97 per cent being composed of calcified salts. It is

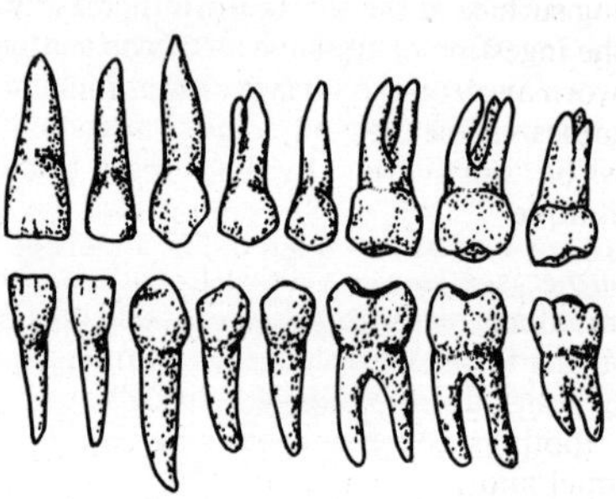

The permanent teeth of the right side.

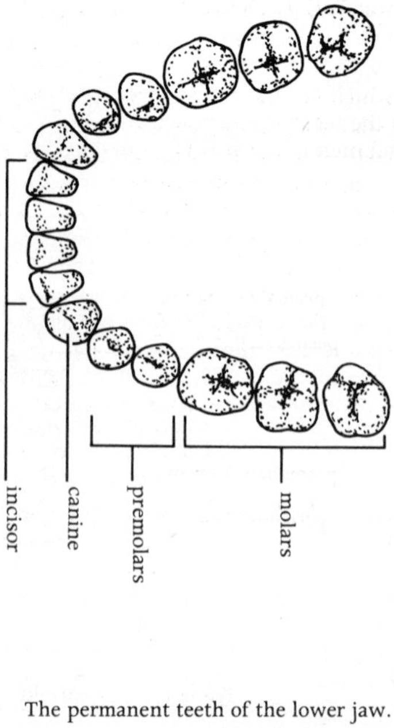

The permanent teeth of the lower jaw.

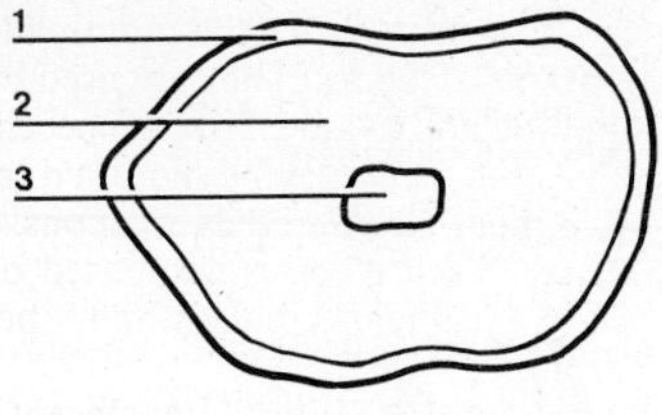

Transverse section across the crown of a tooth.

arranged from millions of long six-sided prisms set on end on the dentine. It is thickest over the biting surface of the tooth. With increasing age or the ingestion of abrasive foods the teeth may be worn away on the surface so that the dentine becomes visible. The outer sides of some teeth may be worn away by bad tooth-brushing technique.

Dentine is a dense yellowish-white material from which the bulk and the basic shape of a tooth are formed. It is like ivory and it is harder than bone but softer than enamel. The crown of the tooth is covered by the hard protective enamel and the root is covered by a bonelike substance called cement. Dentine is formed from cells which produce cylinders of calcified material in the centre of which are tubules which contain protoplasmic processes which are extensions of the cells. These processes can transfer pain from the enamel to the sensitive pulp in the centre of the tooth. Dentine is formed from inorganic and organic matter. The composition is approximately 75 per cent inorganic salts and 25 per cent organic matter and water. Decay can erode dentine faster than enamel.

Cement or CEMENTUM is a thin bonelike material which covers the roots of teeth and helps hold the teeth in the bone. Fibres of the periodontal membrane are embedded in the cement and the bone. When the gums recede, part of the cement may be exposed and the cells die. Once this has happened, the periodontal membrane can no longer be attached to the tooth and, if sufficient cement is destroyed, the tooth support will be so weakened that the tooth will become loose.

Pulp: This is the inner core of the tooth and is composed of a highly vascular, delicate fibrous tissue with many fine nerve fibres. The outer layer is formed by the odontoblasts which formed the dentine and are now dormant unless required to lay down a further thickness of dentine in response to a destructive stimulus at the outer edge of the dentine. The pulp is the tissue remaining after the tooth has been formed and may have helped in its eruption. The pulp is very sensitive to temperature variation and touch. If the pulp becomes exposed it will become infected and usually cannot overcome this. Root-canal treatment or extraction of the tooth may be necessary.

Periodontal membrane: This is a layer of fibrous tissue arranged in groups of fibres which surround and support the root of a tooth in a bone socket. The fibres are interspersed with blood-vessels and nerves. Loss of the membrane leads to loss of the tooth. The membrane can release and re-attach the fibres to allow the tooth to move when it erupts or is being moved by orthodontic springs.

Arrangement and form: Teeth are present in most mammals and nearly all have two sets: a temporary or milk set followed by a permanent or adult set. In some animals, like the toothed whale, all the teeth are similar, but in man there are four different shapes: incisors, canines (eyeteeth), premolars (bicuspids), and molars. The incisors are chisel shaped and the canine is pointed. Premolars have two cusps on the crown (one medial to the other) and molars have at least four cusps. They are arranged together in an arch in each jaw and the cusps of opposing teeth interdigitate. Some herbivores have no upper anterior teeth but use a pad of gum instead. As each arch is symmetrical, the teeth in an upper and lower quadrant can be

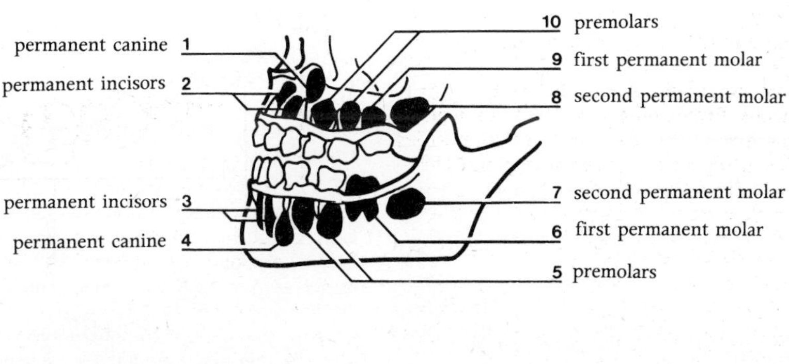

Teeth of a six-year-old child. The permanent teeth are coloured black.

used to identify the animal. In man the quadrants are the same, ie. in the child there are two incisors, one canine and two molars (total teeth 20). In the adult there are two incisors, one canine, two premolars and three molars (total 32). This mixture of tooth form suggests that man is omniverous. Anatomically the crown of the tooth has mesial and distal surfaces which touch the tooth next to it. The mesial surface is the one nearer to the centre line and the distal is the further away. The biting surface is called the incisal edge for the anterior teeth and the occlusal surface for the posteriors.

Development: The first stage in the formation of the teeth is the appearance of a downgrowth of epithelium into the underlying mesoderm. This is the dental lamina, and from it ten smaller swellings in each jaw appear. These become bell shaped and enclose a part of the mesoderm, the cells of which become specialized and are called the dental papillae. The epithelial cells produce enamel and the dental papilla forms the dentine, cement and pulp. At a fixed time the teeth start to erupt and a root is formed. Before the deciduous teeth erupt, the permanent teeth form, medial to them. In due course the deciduous roots resorb and the permanent teeth are then able to push the crowns out and erupt themselves. If this process is disturbed, the permanent teeth may be displaced and appear in an abnormal position or be impacted.

Eruption of teeth is in a definite order and at a fixed time, although there may be a few months leeway in either direction which is of no significance. Excessive delay is found in some congenital disorders such as cretinism. It may also be associated with local abnormalities of the jaws such as cysts, malformed teeth and supernumerary teeth.

The usual order of eruption of deciduous teeth is:

Middle incisors	6–8 months
Lateral incisors	8–10 "
First molars	12–16 "
Canines (eye-teeth)	16–20 "
Second molars	20–30 "

The usual order of eruption of permanent teeth is:

First molars	6–7 years
Middle incisors	6–8 "
Lateral incisors	7–9 "
Canines	9–12 "
First and second premolars	10–12 "
Second molars	11–13 "
Third molars (wisdom teeth)	17–21 "

TEETH, DISEASES OF: Teeth are important for appearance and speech and in the proper preparation of the food for its onward journey into the stomach. With modern foods biting and chewing are less important. Damage to the teeth can be painful.

TEETHING, or the process of eruption of the teeth, may be accompanied by symptoms which are particularly distressing in the child. There may be irritability, salivation, loss of sleep and a failure to feed. The child will tend to rub or touch the painful area. To a lesser extent this may also occur in the adult as the third molars try to erupt. Relief may be obtained in the child by allowing them to chew on a hard object such as a toy or rusk. If this is not sufficient, then various tinctures and pastes can be applied to the reddened area of gum. These remedies may contain salicilates or local anaesthetics.

TOOTHACHE is the pain felt when there is inflammation of the pulp or periodontal membrane of a tooth. It can vary in intensity and may be recurring. The commonest cause is caries when the cavity is close to the pulp. Once the pulp has become infected, this is likely to spread from the apex of the tooth into the bone to form an abscess (gumboil). A lesser but more long-lasting pain is felt when the dentine is unprotected. This can occur when the enamel is lost due to decay or trauma or because the gums have receded. This pain is often associated with temperature change or sweet foods. General debility makes a person more aware of minor discomforts. Expert dental advice should be sought early before the decay is extensive, even though the pain has disappeared temporarily. If a large cavity is accessible, temporary relief may be obtained by inserting a small piece of cotton wool soaked in one of the essential oils such as oil of cloves. A paste made from oil of cloves and zinc oxide powder is longer lasting but may make the pain more severe if the pulp is exposed and infected. Such a tooth requires root-canal therapy or extraction.

CARIES OF THE TEETH or dental decay is very common in the more affluent countries and is commonest in children and young adults. Increasing awareness of the causes has resulted in a considerable improvement in dental health, particularly in the last ten years. This has coincided with a rise in general health. Now 50 per cent of five-year-old children are caries free and of the others 10 per cent have half of the remaining carious cavities. Since the start of the National Health Service the emphasis has been on saving teeth. In south-east England, which has a high ratio of dentists for the population, less than 5 per cent of the people under 45 years have dentures. Now edentulous patients are mainly found among the elderly who had their teeth removed before 1948.

The precise cause of caries is still uncertain but the acidic theory is most widely held. Acid is produced by oral bacteria from dietary carbohydrates, particularly refined sugar, and this dissolves part of the enamel. The dentine is eroded more quickly as it is softer and the first time the person is aware of trouble is when the now hollow tooth collapses. Decay usually starts in a part of the tooth where cleaning is difficult, ie. in the pits and fissures of the crown

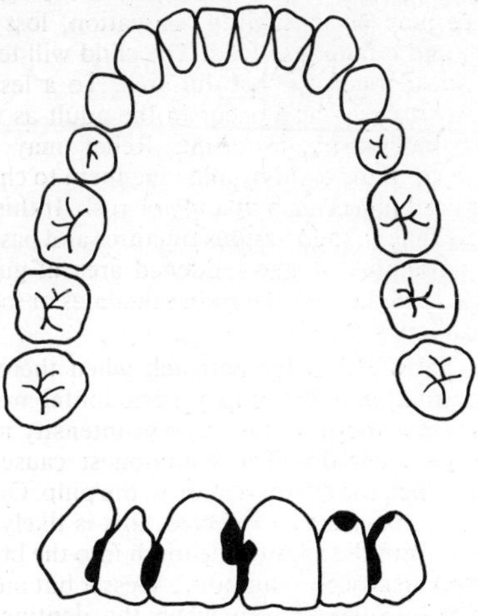

(Above) Natural crevices on healthy back teeth in which food collects. (Below) Front teeth of upper jaw showing places between teeth where food has collected and led to decay.

and between two teeth. The exposed smooth surfaces are usually protected as they are easily cleaned during normal eating and by brushing. Irregular and overcrowded teeth are more at risk from decay as they are difficult to clean. Primitive people who chew coarse foods rarely get caries. Fluoride in the drinking water at the rate of about 1 part per million is associated with a reduction in the caries rate. Prolonged severe disease in infancy is associated with poor calcification of the teeth, making them more vulnerable to decay. As the teeth are formed and partly calcified by the time of birth, the diet and health of the mother are also important to the teeth of the child. Pregnant mothers and children should have a good balanced diet with sufficient calcium and vitamin D. A fibrous diet will also aid cleansing of the teeth and stimulate the circulation in the teeth and jaws. The caries rate can be reduced by regular brushing with a fluoride toothpaste two or three times per day and certainly before going to sleep. This can be carried out with a brush and a tooth powder or paste. Powders tend to be more abrasive and, if used too often and with too much force, can wear the teeth away. Confectionary should be avoided between meals. The provision of sweet or sugary juices in a pacifier or bottle to help an infant sleep will rapidly lead to the loss of the upper front teeth.

The dental health of children has improved greatly in the past fifteen years in most industrial countries. This appears to be due to a number of factors. Public awareness of the need to brush and clean the teeth has greatly increased. Toothpastes now contain additives which reduce the formation of plaque and fluoride will strengthen the enamel up to 50 per cent. Fluoride in the water, whether it occurs naturally or is added, is associated with a lower caries rate. Fluoride is also available in tablet form for children but probably the most common source of the ion is in toothpaste.

IRREGULARITY OF THE PERMANENT TEETH may be due to an abnormality in the growth of the jaws or to the early or late loss of the deciduous set. Most frequently it is due to an imbalance in the size of the teeth and the length of the jaws. Some improvement may take place with age but many will require the help of an orthodontist (specialist dentist) who can correct many mal-occlusions by removing a few teeth to allow him to move the others into a good position by means of springs and elastics on various appliances which are worn in the mouth.

LOOSENING OF THE TEETH may be due to an accident or inflammation of the gum. Teeth loosened by trauma may be replaced in the socket, even if knocked right out. If they are then splinted to the neighbouring teeth for a few weeks they may re-attach themselves to the bone. If the loosening is due to periodontal disease the prognosis is less favourable. The removal of any calculus and the use of some antiseptic mouthwashes will help.

DISCOLORATION of the teeth may be intrinsic or extrinsic, ie. the stain may be in the calcified structure or stuck on to it. Intrinsic staining may be due to jaundice or the antibiotic tetracycline. Dark teeth are due to blood-breakdown products entering the dentinal tubules as a result of some trauma that has damaged the pulp. It may be possible to bleach such teeth but it usually needs to be repeated frequently. Extrinsic stain may be due to tea, coffee, tobacco, pan (a mixture of chuna and betel nuts wrapped in a leaf), iron-containing medicines or excess fluoride. Some of these can be removed by brushing with an abrasive paste but where the stain is within the tooth or the surface of the tooth is damaged, an artificial crown or veneer may be required.

GINGIVITIS or inflammation of the gums may occur as an acute or chronic condition. In the acute form it is often part of a general infection of the mouth and principally occurs in children or young adults and resolves after ten to fourteen days. The chronic form occurs later in life and tends to be progressive. There is moderate pain but the gums appear congested, bleed easily and may be ulcerated. Later calculus appears on the teeth. Eating may be difficult if the ulceration is extensive. Various micro-organisms may be found on the lesions including anaerobes. Treatment is initially supportive but the mouth should be kept as clean and moist as possible. Antiseptic mouthwashes may help and once the painful stage is past, the gums should be thoroughly cleaned and any calculus removed. In severe conditions an antibiotic may be required.

PERIODONTAL DISEASE is the spread of gingivitis to involve the periodontal membrane of the tooth and in its florid form used to be called pyorrhoea. In this, the membrane becomes damaged by the inflammatory process and a space or pocket is formed into which a probe can be easily passed. As the pocket becomes more extensive the tooth loosens. Although neglect hastens the process, the cause is still largely unknown. The production of calculus from plaque increases the trauma on the gingival margins and the injection of micro-organisms. The loss of the periodontal membrane also leads to the loss of supporting bone. Chronic inflammation soon occurs and is difficult to eradicate. The effect of chewing on mobile teeth is debatable but some shedding of bacteria into the bloodstream occurs and this may affect damaged organs such as heart valves after rheumatic fever. Acute flare-ups of the disease may occur when the patient is unwell and also during pregnancy. Pain is not a feature of the disease but there is often an unpleasant odour (halitosis). The gums bleed easily and there may be dyspepsia. Treatment is largely aimed at stabilizing the condition rather than curing it. This is done by meticulous care of the mouth and teeth and the removal of calculus. Where there is excess tissue, the edge of the gums can be reshaped by surgical means, but attempts at replacing bone have only been partially successful.

DENTAL ABSCESS or ALVEOLAR ABSCESS is an infection that arises in or round a tooth and spreads to involve the bone. It may occur many years after a blow has killed the pulp of the tooth or more quickly after caries has reached the pulp. At first the pain may be mild and intermittent but eventually it will become severe and a swelling will develop in the gum over the apex of the tooth. The tooth may be sensitive to hot and cold at first, then will not respond but will feel extruded from the socket and be tender when touched. The swelling will enlarge until it feels like a bag of fluid, then may burst to discharge pus and will be more comfortable for a time. The discharge may become chronic. A radiograph of the tooth will show a round clear area at the apex of the tooth. Treatment may be by painting the gum with a mild counter-irritant such as a tincture of aconite and iodine in the early stages but later root-canal therapy or apicectomy may be required. If a swelling is present, it may need to be drained and antibiotics given. Where the tooth is beyond repair or of little use, then extraction may be preferable.

INJURIES TO TEETH are common. The more minor injuries include crazing and the loss of small chips of enamel, and the major ones include a broken root and avulsion of the entire tooth. A specialist dental opinion should be sought as soon as possible. The exposure of dentine will be painful for some weeks but can be easily treated by covering the tooth with a substance that does not easily conduct heat. Nail varnish or chewing gum will help for a few hours at least. When the pulp is exposed, it will almost certainly have to be removed before it becomes infected. A tooth that has been knocked out can be re-implanted if it is clean and replaced within a few hours. It will then require splinting in place for 4–6 weeks. Tinfoil can be used as a temporary splint. If the tooth was on the ground, then prevention of infection, including tetanus, will be necessary.

PREVENTION OF DENTAL DISEASE: As with other matters, prevention is better than cure. Children should be taught at an early age to keep their teeth and gums clean and to avoid refined sugars between meals. It is better to finish a meal with a drink of water rather than a sweetened drink. Sweetened drinks are particularly harmful just before going to sleep. Fluoride in some of its forms is useful in the reduction of dental caries and a vaccine now being developed may be useful. Overcrowding of the teeth, obvious maldevelopment of the jaw and persistent thumbsucking into the teens are all indications for seeking the advice of an orthodontist. Generally adults have less trouble with decay but more with periodontal disease and, as its onset is insidious, regular dental inspections are desirable. Dentures are also not without problem and should be checked at least every five years. If worn day and night, there is a risk of developing thrush under the denture and damaging the gum and mucous membrane.

TEETH GRINDING, or BRUXISM as it is technically known, is quite common in children during sleep, when it is of no significance unless really persistent. During the day it may be an attention-seeking device, often perpetuated by the anxiety which it elicits in the parents. There is no treatment for it and if ignored it will stop, though any genuine anxiety or worry on the part of the child should be dealt with. It is more common and persistent in mentally retarded children.

In adults it is usually associated with stress or anxiety, but may be due to some local condition in the mouth such as an unsatisfactory filling. It may also be caused by certain drugs, including fenfluramine and levodopa. More rarely it may be due to brain disease. Some families seem to be more prone to teeth grinding than others. If not controlled, it produces excessive wear of the enamel covering of the teeth. Treatment consists of alleviation of any condition in the mouth, and it may be useful to wear a splint covering the teeth of one jaw at night. Treatment should also be aimed at the alleviation of anxiety and stress.

TEETHING (see TEETH, DISEASES OF).

TEICHOPSIA: This refers to zigzag lines that patients with migraine often experience as an aura preceding an attack.

TELANGIECTASIS means an abnormal dilatation of arterioles and capillaries, forming sometimes a tumour or TELANGIOMA.

TEMAZEPAM (EUHYPNOS, NORMISON) is a relatively quick-acting hypnotic of short duration so that there is little or no 'hangover' the next morning. It is a derivative of diazepam (qv). (See BENZODIAZEPINES.)

TEMPERAMENT is a term that includes those vague general peculiarities of mind and body that render some people more liable than others to be affected by particular diseases.

TEMPERATURE of the body is a subject of great importance. Animals are generally divided as regards their temperature into two classes: *cold-blooded animals*, including reptiles, amphibians, fish, and invertebrates generally, whose temperature varies to a great extent according to that of the surrounding medium; and *warm-blooded animals*, including mammals and birds, whose temperature remains almost constant, no matter how the surrounding temperature falls or rises. In warm-blooded animals, this constancy of body temperature is effected by a perpetual balancing of the various forces which produce heat and give off heat. The chief heat producer in the body is the oxidizing action that takes place on muscular contraction, and the chief cooling agents are the skin and lungs, which act by the exposure of the blood circulating in them to the air, and by the evaporation of moisture from their surfaces. The temperature of different warm-blooded animals varies considerably; in man it is somewhere between 36·7° and 37·2°C (98° and 99°F). It varies in different people but is generally stated to be about 37°C (98·4°F). Even in a given healthy individual the temperature is constantly changing, being lowest in the early morning and highest in the evening. The chief reason for this change is to be found probably in the variations as regards activity at different periods of the day. The temperature also varies in different parts of the body, that of the skin being about half a degree lower than that taken within the hollow organs of the body; and in stout people this difference between the surface and the interior is still more marked. In parts exposed to cold or provided with a feeble blood supply, such as paralysed limbs, the temperature may sink very low.

Temperature in disease: The maintenance of a nearly steady temperature is the result of a constant process of balancing between heat-production and heat-loss, controlled probably by a special centre in the nervous system. In disease, one or other of these processes may be impaired or the controlling mechanism may be thrown completely out of gear. The general temperature may rise as high as 43·3°C (110°F), or sink to 32·2°C (90°F) for a time; but the risk to life is great when it passes above 41°C (106°F) or below 35°C (95°F).

Fall of temperature may be due to many causes. Thus it generally accompanies great loss of blood, starvation, and the collapsed condition which sometimes results from severe attacks of fever, peritonitis, and other devitalizing acute diseases. Certain chronic diseases are generally accompanied by a subnormal temperature; of these, myxoedema is the most outstanding.

Rise of temperature is a characteristic of acute diseases, and of diseases due to micro-organisms, the poisonous products of which lead to increased waste of the tissues. Injuries to the nervous system, even unpleasant sensations in children and nervous people, may have a similar effect. In people dying in a feverish condition, the temperature often rises very high immediately before death, owing probably to failure of the circulation and other conditions which diminish the body heat. Rapid rise of temperature in such a case is therefore an ominous sign.

Many diseases have a characteristic course of temperature, so that in hospital a glance at the temperature chart is often sufficient to acquaint a physician with the disease from which the patient is suffering. Thus pneumonia, enteric fever, measles, and malaria show, as a rule, quite recognizable temperature records.

High temperature in some diseases is a much less serious feature than in others. Thus in enteric fever or pneumonia 40·5°C (105°F) is an ordinary temperature, whilst in rheumatic fever and diphtheria the temperature generally ranges between 38·3° and 39·5°C (101° and 103°F), so that in these diseases a temperature of 40°C (104°F) gives cause for anxiety.

In most diseases the temperature gradually abates as the patient recovers, but others, for example pneumonia and typhus fever, end rapidly by a *crisis* in which the temperature falls, perspiration breaks out, the pulse becomes slower, and the breathing quieter. The reason for the sudden change lies probably in the fact that in favourable cases, after the disease has lasted a certain time, the resisting power of the body becomes able fully to neutralize the poisons produced by the organisms of the disease. This crisis is often preceded by an increase of all the symptoms, including an epicritical rise of temperature.

Record of temperature: Temperature is generally measured by a thermometer. Those intended for clinical use possess a long, narrow bulb, an index registering from 35° to 43·3°C (95° to 110°F), and are made so that the column of mercury does not fall back into the bulb till it is shaken down.

There are two scales in common use: the Fahrenheit scale and the Centigrade or Celsius scale. Hitherto, in Britain the term Centigrade has been preferred, but under the new International System of Units (see WEIGHTS AND MEASURES) the term Celsius is recommended. The difference consists in this, that in the Centigrade scale the freezing-point of water is marked 0° and the boiling-point 100°, while in the Fahrenheit scale these are 32° and 212°, respectively. Accordingly 100 divisions on the Centigrade scale are equivalent to 180 divisions on the Fahrenheit scale, and 1 degree C equals 1·8 degrees F. To convert from degrees F to degrees C the following formula may be used:

$$n°\text{Fahr} = [(n-32) + \frac{5}{9}]\ \text{C},$$

and to convert from degrees C to degrees F the following:

$$n°\text{C} = [(n \times \frac{9}{5} + 32]\ \text{Fahr}.$$

The Réaumur scale, in which the freezing-point is 0° and the boiling-point 80°, is also used in some countries, eg. France, though not for scientific purposes.

As to the part of the body where the temperature is taken, the mouth is preferable, the bulb of the thermometer being placed beneath the tongue. The thermometer must be carefully washed with cold water before use, so that it does not convey infection, and care taken to ensure that the mercury is shaken down to below 35·5°C (96°F). The patient must be directed to keep the mouth shut but not to bite the thermometer with the teeth, and breathe through the nose. It is essential to ensure that the patient has not just had a hot drink. The thermometer must be kept in the mouth for at least three minutes. After use the thermometer must be thoroughly rinsed under running cold water and the mercury shaken down. When taken in the armpit the skin should be wiped dry, the bulb of the thermometer placed as high as possible, and the arm tightly folded across the chest. To obtain a correct reading, it is necessary to leave the thermometer in place for at least five minutes, because the skin surfaces do not at once represent the internal temperature of the body. Occasionally the temperature is taken by inserting the thermometer bulb about 5 cm (2 inches) into the rectum, a method which gives the most correct result of all, and is the most satisfactory in infants.

To keep a record, a piece of paper ruled with vertical lines to represent the periods at which the temperature is taken, and with horizontal lines corresponding to degrees, is used. A large dot is marked in the proper place each time the temperature is taken and the successive dots are afterwards joined by straight lines.

Treatment of high temperature is mentioned under ANTIPYRETICS; COLD, USES OF; FEVER.

TEMPLE is the side of the head above the line between the eye and ear. The term, temporal, is applied to the muscles, nerves, and artery of this region. The hair usually begins to turn grey first at the temples.

TENDERNESS is the term usually applied in medical nomenclature to pain experienced when a diseased part is handled, the term, pain, being reserved for unpleasant sensations felt apart from any manipulation.

TENDON, SINEW, or LEADER, is the cord that attaches the end of a muscle to the bone or other structure upon which the muscle acts when it contracts. Tendons are composed of bundles of white fibrous tissue arranged in a very dense manner, and are of great strength. Some are rounded, some flattened bands, whilst others are very short, the muscle-fibres being attached almost directly to the bone. Most tendons are surrounded by sheaths lined with membrane similar to the synovial membrane lining joint-cavities. In this sheath the tendon glides smoothly over surrounding parts. The fibres of a tendon pass into the substance of the bone and blend with the fibres composing it. One of the largest tendons in the body is the tendo Achilles, or tendo calcaneus as it is now known, which attaches the muscle of the calf to the calcaneus or heel-bone.

Tendon injuries are one of the hazards of sports. They usually result from indirect violence, or overuse, rather than direct violence. *Rupture* usually results from the sudden application of an unbalanced load. Thus complete rupture of the Achilles tendon is common in taking an awkward step backwards playing squash. There is sudden pain, the victim is often under the impression that he received a blow. This is accompanied by loss of function, and a gap may be felt in the tendon. *Partial rupture* is also accompanied by pain, but there is no breach of continuity or complete loss of function. Treatment of a complete rupture usually means surgical repair followed by immobilization of the tendon in plaster of Paris for six weeks. Partial rupture usually responds to physiotherapy and immobilization, but healing is slow.

Tendinitis, or inflammation of a tendon, is usually due to misuse or overuse. The tendon is swollen, tense and tender. Much of the pain is due to raised pressure within the tendon. This may be relieved in severe cases by decompression by surgical means. In most cases, however, conservative treatment such as aspirin, rest, and physiotherapy, especially ultrasonics, is adequate, though the response is usually slow. In the case of the Achilles tendon, much relief may be obtained by providing a heel pad so that the range of movement is restricted.

In *peritendinitis* it is the tissues around the tendon that are involved. This occurs as a result of overuse, and causes pain and swelling around the tendon, often accompanied by creaking in movement. The condition can be quite crippling and develop quite quickly following a bout of excessive or unaccustomed exercise. It usually responds satisfactorily to rest (including splinting), injection into the tissues around the tendon (not in the tendon) of hyaluronidase (qv) in a local anaesthetic, heparin, a heparinoid preparation (qv), or a corticosteroid (qv). In some cases it becomes chronic, and surgical treatment may be called for.

TENDOVAGINITIS means inflammation of a tendon and of the sheath enveloping it.

TENESMUS is a term applied to a symptom of disease affecting the lower part of the large intestine, such as dysentery, piles, or tumour. It consists of a constant sense of weight about the lower bowel and desire to go to stool, coupled with straining at stool and the passage of little but mucus and perhaps some blood.

TENNIS ELBOW (see ELBOW).

TENO- is a prefix denoting some relation to a tendon.

TENOSYNOVITIS, or TENOSITIS, means inflammation of a tendon.

TENOTOMY means an operation in which one or more tendons are divided, usually with the object of remedying some deformity.

TENTORIUM is a wide process of dura mater forming a partition between the cerebrum and cerebellum and supporting the former.

TENTS are instruments used for dilating narrow openings. The tent consists of some substance, like sea-tangle or sponge, which shrivels up when dried, and expands powerfully as it absorbs moisture. It is introduced dry into the opening it is to dilate, and expands in the course of some hours without producing pain.

TERATOGENESIS is the production of physical defects in the foetus. It is understandable that a drug may interfere with a mechanism that is essential for growth and result in arrested or distorted development of the foetus and yet cause no disturbance in adults, in whom these growth processes have ceased to be relevant. Thus the effect of a drug upon a foetus may differ qualitively as well as quantitively from its effect on the mother. The susceptibility of the embryo will depend on the stage of development it has reached when the drug is given. The age of early differentiation, that is from the beginning of the third week to the end of the tenth week of pregnancy is the time of greatest susceptibility. After this time the likelihood of congenital malformation resulting from drug treatment is less, although the death of the foetus can occur at any time as a result of drugs crossing the placenta or as a result of their effect on the placental circulation. The term teratogenesis has come into common usage since the thalidomide disaster.

Thalidomide was an effective non-barbiturate hypnotic which had passed stringent tests before being released for general use. In spite of this it produced a number of congenital defects, esecially of the limbs, in children born to mothers who had taken the drug while pregnant. As soon as this was discovered the drug was withdrawn from use. Subsequently the government set up a Committee of Drug Safety to try and ensure that there was no recurrence of such a distressing episode with subsequent drugs. Even the most stringent precautions, however, cannot ensure the complete elimination of this risk. Fortunately the risk is a remote one, but it is now realised that no drug should be given to a pregnant woman, particularly during the first few months of pregnancy, unless it is absolutely essential for her health or that of her unborn child. There is no satisfactory test on animals that will clear a drug of the possibility of producing congenital malformation in man. Indeed drugs such as aspirin, caffein, insulin and thyroxine cause foetal abnormalities in some animal species but there is no evidence that they do so in man. Furthermore, the problem must be kept in perspective and it should be appreciated that only 1 per cent of congenital malformations are the results of environmental factors, which include not only drugs but infections such as German measles and irradiation. The risk that any random pregnancy will end in some serious malformation is about 1 in 40. Of drugs in current use there is circumstantial evidence that the alkylating agents and antimetabolites used in the treatment of reticulosis and leukaemia are teratogenic. There is some evidence that oral hypoglycaemic agents and antihistamine agents may also be responsible for a few congenital malformations.

TERATOMA is a tumour that consists of partially developed embryonic tissues. The most common sites of this tumour are the ovary and the testicle.

TERBUTALINE is a drug that is proving of value in the treatment of asthma. It is given by injection under the skin or by inhalation. It is a beta adrenoreceptor agonist.

TEREBENE is a clear, colourless fluid, with an odour like fresh pine sawdust, prepared by the action of sulphuric acid upon turpentine. It is used as an expectorant in bronchitis.

TERTIAN FEVER is the name applied to that type of malaria in which the fever reappears every other day. (See MALARIA.)

TESTICLE: The testes, or testicles, are the two male sexual glands. Each is developed in the corresponding loin, but before birth they descend through openings in the lower part of the front of the abdomen into a fold or pouch of skin known as the scrotum. This fold is strengthened by a layer of muscle fibres and fibrous tissues, and within it each testicle possesses a separate covering known as the tunica vaginalis. This tunic is a double layer of serous membrane similar in structure to the peritoneum or pleura, and it is derived from the peritoneum while the testicle is still within the abdomen. Occasionally, as the result of defective development, a more or less open channel of communication is left between the peritoneum and tunica vaginalis, and down this channel a hernia is liable to form in childhood or later. Throughout life, the openings in the abdominal wall remain, but each inguinal canal should be just large enough to allow the passage of one of the two spermatic cords, each of which is composed of the vas (or ductus) deferens, together with the blood-vessels, nerves, and lymphatics proceeding to the gland. Within the tunica vaginalis lies a dense fibrous coat known as the tunica albuginea, which affords protection to the gland. On microscopic examination, each testicle is found to consist of a series of minute tubes, from eight hundred to one thousand in number, supported by fibrous tissue in which the nerves and blood-vessels run, and lined by cells from which the spermatozoa are formed. Around 4·5 million spermatozoa are produced per gram of testicle per day. These tubes communicate with one another near the centre of the testicle, and are connected by a much convoluted tube, the epididymis, with the ductus, or vas deferens, which enters the abdomen, and passes on to the base of the bladder. This duct, after joining a reservoir known as the seminal vesicle, opens, close to the duct from the other side of the body, into that part of the urethra which is surrounded by the prostate gland. Owing to the convulutions of these ducts leading from the testicles to the urethra, and their indirect route, the passage from testicle to urethra is over 6 metres (20 feet) in length. In addition to producing spermotozoa, the testicle also forms an internal secretion which is responsible for the development of male characteristics. This hormone has been isolated and is known as testosterone.

TESTICLE, DISEASES OF: The pouch of skin, or scrotum, in which the testicles lie is liable to various general skin diseases, but particularly

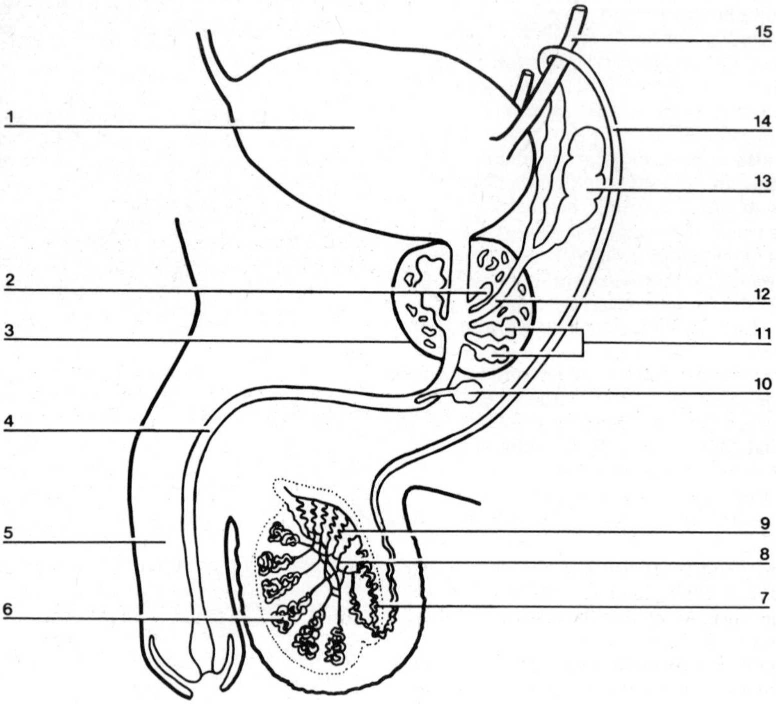

1 urinary bladder	6 convoluted seminiferous tubule	11 prostatic follicles
2 prostrate utricle	7 canal of the epydidymus	12 ejaculatory duct
3 capsule of prostate	8 rete testis	13 seminal vesicle
4 urethra	9 efferent ductules	14 vas (ductus) deferens
5 penis	10 bulbo-urethral gland	15 ureter

Diagram of the male sex organs.

to eczema, which in many cases is often difficult to cure. Cancer of the skin in this region is specially common among chimney-sweeps, shale workers and cotton spinners, the result of chronic irritation by a carcinogenic agent in soot and paraffin products. Hernia, which in some cases passes into the scrotum, is treated under a special heading. (See HERNIA.) Sometimes, owing to defective development, the testicles are retained within the abdomen.

HYDROCELE is a local dropsy affecting one tunica vaginalis, and distending that side of the scrotum with fluid. (See HYDROCELE.)

VARICOCELE is a condition in which the veins of the spermatic cord, especially on the left side, become unusually numerous and distended, the causes being much the same as those of varicose veins in other parts. The chief symptom is a dragging sensation in the testicle, which in some cases becomes at times very painful. This symptom is specially marked in warm weather and after exertion, the mass of veins at such a time becoming very distinct and resembling a 'bag of worms', though they empty quickly when the person lies down. Cold sponging of the part, careful regulation of the bowels, and the support of a suspensory net bandage afford all the treatment that is necessary in many cases; but an operation may sometimes be advisable.

INFLAMMATION of an acute type (orchitis) may arise in people suffering from cystitis, stone in the bladder, and various forms of inflammation in the urinary organs, the most common cause of all being gonorrhoea. It may follow also upon some cases of mumps. The symptoms are intense pain and swelling with redness of the skin over the affected testicle; and the usual treatment consists of rest in bed, support of the scrotum with a suspensory bandage or wads of cotton-wool, the administration of analgesics (in some cases the pain may be so severe that morphine is necessary), and the administration of antibiotics if there is some definite causative micro-organism. In some cases the condition goes on to the formation of an abscess which bursts through the skin with immediate relief of pain. The condition is then treated as an abscess elsewhere.

TORSION, or twisting or rotation, of the testes, or, strictly speaking, of the spermatic cord, is a relatively common occurrence in adolescent and young adult males. It can occur during sleep, at rest, while playing games or doing hard physical work. About half the cases occur in the early hours of the morning during sleep. It is more liable to happen more often in the colder, than the warmer, months of the year. It makes itself felt by pain of varying severity – from slight to excruciating – either in the lower part of the abdomen or in the scrotum. In time the pain diminishes or disappears. The testes become hard and swollen. Treatment consists of immediate undoing of the torsion. If this is done within a few hours no harm ensues as a rule, but it should be followed within six hours by surgical operation to ensure that the torsion has been successfully undone and to fix the testes so that there should be no recurrence.

TUBERCULOSIS occurs in the testicle occasionally, especially when some other organ, such as the bladder, is already the seat of the disease. It causes practically no pain, and is therefore often far advanced before it attracts attention. It responds well to chemotherapy with streptomycin, paraaminosaliylic acid and/or isoniazid.

TUMOURS of the testes occur in around 600 males annually in Britain. They represent the second commonest form of malignant growth in young males. There are two types: seminomas and teratomas (qv). When adequately treated the survival rate for seminomas is 95 per cent, whilst that for teratomas is 50 per cent.

INJURIES of the testicles are relatively rare. A severe blow may lead to shock and symptoms of severe collapse for a time, and may cause an effusion of blood into the tunica vaginalis. These symptoms are usually relieved by rest in bed.

TEST MEAL is a term originally applied to a meal given for the purpose of testing the digestive powers. At the present day the original gruel meal has been replaced by the injection of histamine (qv), which is a powerful stimulator of gastric juice. In this *histamine test*, as it is known, samples of the fasting gastric juice are withdrawn through a Ryle's tube (see STOMACH TUBE) before and after a subcutaneous injection of histamine. A modification of this test is the *augmented histamine test*, in which a larger dose of histamine is injected preceded by a dose of an antihistamine drug. This allows a larger dose of histamine to be given because the antihistamine counteracts its unpleasant effects, and the response to the larger dose provides a more accurate picture of the degree of acidity of the gastric juice. Other tests that have been introduced, and named, respectively, after the stimulating substance used, are the *ametazole test*, the *pentagastrin test*, and the *insulin test*.

Tubeless test meals, so-called because they do not involve the passage of a stomach tube, have been evolved. These depend upon the dissociation of a cation-exchange resin (see ION EXCHANGE RESINS) by the hydrochloric acid in the gastric juice. The cation is then absorbed and the amount excreted in the urine is measured. The restanus, with 22 deaths. In 1980, there were 18 cases, with 4 deaths.

TESTOSTERONE (TESTORAL) is the name given to the male sex hormone secreted by the testes. It has also been prepared synthetically and has the formula CHO_2. In true eunuchoid conditions it has the power of restoring male sexual characteristics. (See ANDROGENS.)

TESTOSTERONE ENANTHATE (PRIMOTESTON DEPOT) (see ANDROGENS).

TESTOSTERONE ESTERS (SUSTANON) (see ANDROGENS).

TESTOSTERONE PHENYLPROPIONATE (see ANDROGENS).

TESTOSTERONE PROPIONATE (VIRORMONE) (see ANDROGENS).

TESTOSTERONE UNDECANOATE (RESTANDOL) (see ANDROGENS).

TEST-TUBE is a tube of thin glass closed at one end, which is used for observing chemical reactions or for bacterial culture.

'TEST-TUBE BABY' (see EMBRYO TRANSFER).

TETANUS, or LOCKJAW, is a disorder of the nervous system, consisting in a greatly increased excitability of the spinal cord and manifesting itself by painful and lengthened spasm of the voluntary muscles throughout the body. The disease was well known in former wars, and Hippocrates (400 BC) refers to its rapidly fatal character.

Causes: The onset of the disease generally follows a wound, especially a deeply punctured, lacerated, or gunshot wound, usually appearing some 4 or 5 days after the wound has been inflicted, although it may be delayed for 3 or 4 weeks, by which time the wound is likely to be completely healed up. The presence in a wound of some foreign body, such as a splinter of wood or a portion of a bullet, seems to favour the onset of tetanus.

The direct cause of tetanus was discovered in 1889 by Kitasato, a Japanese observer, to be a bacillus: *Clostridium tetani*. This organism has a characteristic appearance, being long and bearing often at one end a large spore which gives to it a drumstick outline. It inhabits earth and dust, living especially a little distance below the surface in places where the manure of horses and cattle is collected. Hence it is found especially in the neighbourhood of stables, and is liable to infect wounds soiled with heavily manured earth. The bacillus develops a poison or toxin in the wound, and this, being absorbed, finds its way up the motor nerves to the spinal cord, which it renders excessively sensitive, so that its cells are excited by mild stimuli that under ordinary conditions would produce no reaction. After death, patients who have died of tetanus show very few lesions except congestion of the brain and spinal cord and degenerative changes in the cells of the latter.

In England and Wales, in 1974–78, there were 86 cases of tetanus, with 22 deaths. In 1984, there were 6 cases.

Symptoms: The onset of tetanus usually occurs within two days to three weeks of the wound responsible for the introduction of the infection. This is not necessarily an incubation period in the strict sense of the term because the causative organism may be dormant in the tissues of the body before producing toxin. The importance of this is that, whilst generally speaking, it is a fact that the longer the period between the wound and the onset of tetanus, the better the outlook, there are occasions when a delayed onset of the disease is acute and dangerous because a hitherto dormant strain of the organism has suddenly started to produce large amounts of toxin. The first signs of the disease usually show themselves as stiffness in the muscles near the wound, followed later, no matter where the wound is situated, by stiffness about the muscles of the jaw, causing difficulty in opening the mouth, which soon increases to *lockjaw* or trismus. This is accompanied by spasm in neighbouring muscles, and the drawn features and exposed teeth give to the countenance the peculiar expression known as *risus sardonicus*. The rigidity extends to the muscles of the neck, back, chest, abdomen, and extremities, and the body may assume a bent attitude, either backward (*opisthotonos*), forward (*emprosthotonos*), or laterally (*pleurosthotonos*). This general muscular rigidity, which at first is not constant but occasionally undergoes relaxation, is accompanied by frequently recurring convulsive seizures, which are readily excited by the slightest irritation, such as from a draught of cool air, a bright light, the closing of a door. In such attacks there is great suffering and the expression of the face is indicative of agony. The function of respiration may be seriously involved and asphyxia threaten or actually take place. The temperature sometimes rises to a high degree, and copious perspiration is also a constant symptom. These acute symptoms may subside after a few days and the patient gradually recover. On the other hand, the symptoms may increase in severity and death ensue either by asphyxia from prolonged spasm of the respiratory muscles, or exhaustion consequent on the violence of the symptoms, together with the absence of sleep. Throughout the whole course of the illness the mind is clear, and the patient waits with anxiety for the next convulsive attack. In milder cases the symptoms are less severe, the course more chronic, and recovery more common.

Tetanus sometimes occurs in new-born children, showing itself within a week of birth by obvious difficulty in the acts of sucking and swallowing, and, by the supervention of lockjaw, together with prolonged contraction of the muscles of the limbs and body, accompanied by convulsive seizures. *Local cases* of tetanus occur in which the muscles of a limb in the neighbourhood of the wound show spasms, but these do not become general, or they pass off after appearing to a slight extent. Such cases often show stiffness for several months.

The symptoms of strychnine poisoning bear a strong resemblance to those of tetanus, but in the former case they are more acute, less prolonged than the spasms of tetanus, come on after something has been swallowed, and end either in death or in recovery within a few hours. Hydrophobia (rabies), too, resembles tetanus in some respects.

The outcome depends upon various factors, including the virulence of the toxin, the age of the patient, his state of immunity and the availability of expert medical and nursing attention. The very young and the old do badly. The mortality is often said to be 40 per cent, but among the 59 cases treated in the Leeds Tetanus Unit in the decade, 1966–76, the mortality rate was only 13 per cent, all but one of the eight deaths occurring in patients over the age of 50. As an expert in this field has said, in the absence of the highest medical and nursing skill, tetanus is a highly fatal disease.

Prevention: The outlook in tetanus has been entirely altered by the introduction of tetanus antitoxin and of tetanus toxoid. The latter provides effective protection against the disease. Tetanus immunization is now an accepted part of the immunization programme for children in the United Kingdom. (See VACCINE.) Sportsmen using muddy playing fields are especially vulnerable and should have effective immunization, as should regular gardeners. Some authorities recommend booster injections of vaccine at intervals of ten years to maintain protection against the disease.

Whilst antitoxin is of primary value from the point of view of treatment, it is of prophylactic value if given immediately after an individual has received a wound which may be contaminated with the tetanus organism.

Treatment: Tetanus tends especially to follow wounds infected by stable refuse, by street dust, or by the deeper soil thrown up by shells on the battlefield. In all such cases, 1500 international units of antitoxin must be injected subcutaneously as soon as possible, unless it is definitely known that the individual has been completely immunized by a previous course of toxoid.

If the wound is only slight, all that may be required may be a dose of tetanus toxoid (0·5 ml) with or without an intramuscular injection of 1·2 mega units of benzathine penicillin. Other antibiotics active against *Cl. tetani* are benzylpenicillin, erythromycin and tetracycline, as is also metronidazole. In addition careful cleaning of the wound is required. All these are preventive measures. In actual treatment expert opinion differs as to whether or not antibiotics and tetanus antitoxin should be given routinely. If the latter is given, particular care must be taken as to whether or not the patient suffers from asthma or any other allergic condition, as he may be allergic to the horse serum in which the antitoxin is contained, and react in a violent manner, which might even prove fatal. Tetanus immunoglobulin (see IMMUNOGLOBULIN) is now available and an injection of 250 units provides immunity for four weeks.

Various drugs, which diminish the reflex excitability of the spinal cord and relax spasm, help in relieving the patient's sufferings and in carrying him over the period during which the toxin of the disease is being excreted. These include thiopentone, barbiturates, paraldehyde, and tubocurarine. Quietness around the patient, a darkened room, and the absence of all noise and excitement are of great importance in preventing convulsions, and the patient must receive stimulating fluid nourishment.

TETANY is a condition characterized by spasm of muscle usually caused by a fall in the ionic calcium of the blood. This fall in ionic calcium results in hyperexcitability of the muscles, which are thus liable to go into spasm on the slightest stimulus. This is well demonstrated in two of the classical signs of the disease: *Chvostek's sign*, in which the muscles of the face contract when the cheek is tapped over the facial nerve as it emerges on the cheek; *Erb's sign*, in which muscles go into spasm in response to an electrical stimulus which normally causes only a contraction of the muscle. Tetany is most common in infants, in whom it may arise as a result of rickets, excessive vomiting, or certain forms of nephritis. It may also be due to lack of the active principle of the parathyroid glands. Overbreathing may also cause it. Treatment consists of the administration of calcium salts, and in severe cases this is done by giving calcium gluconate intravenously or intramuscularly. High doses of vitamin D are also required: calcitriol is the most active preparation.

TETRACYCLINES are a group of antibiotics which include chlorteracycline, oxytetracycline, tetracycline, demethylchlote tracycline, methacycline, lymecycline, minocycline, and clomocycline. Chlortetracycline, which is derived from *Streptomyces aureofaciens*, was the first to be discovered, followed by oxytetracycline which is derived from *Streptomyces rimosus*. Subsequently it was discovered that the active constituent of both these antibiotics was tetracycline, which can be prepared on a large scale by the catalytic hydrogenation of chlortetracycline. Methacycline, lymecycline, and clomocycline are subsequently discovered derivatives.

From the point of view of antibacterial activity, all the preparations are virtually identical, being active against both Gram-negative and Gram-positive bacteria, as well as certain rickettsiae (qv) and chlamydia including those causing Q fever, trachoma, psittacosis, and lymphogranuloma inguinale.

It is this wide range of activity, which has given them the name of broad-spectrum antibiotics, combined with the fact that they are given by mouth, that has made them such a useful contribution to the treatment of infective diseases. They must be used with discrimination in young children as they are liable to produce permanent discoloration of the teeth.

TETRALOGY OF FALLOT is the most common form of cyanotic congenital heart disease. The tetralogy consists of: (*a*) stenosis of the pulmonary valve; (*b*) a defect in the septum separating the two ventricles; (*c*) the aorta overrides both ventricles; (*d*) marked hypertrophy of the right ventricle.

TETRAMINE is a preparation which is of value in the treatment of certain forms of malignant disease, including Hodgkin's disease and chronic leukaemia.

THALAMUS is one of two masses of grey matter lying on either side of the third ventricle of the brain. It is an important relay and coordinating station for sensory impulses such as those for sight. (Plural: Thalami.)

THALASSAEMIA, also known as Cooley's anaemia, is a condition characterized by severe anaemia, due to the individual having an abnormal form of haemoglobin in his blood. It is a genetically inherited disease which is widely spread across the Mediterranean through the Middle East and into the Far East. It has a particularly high incidence in Greece and in Italy.

THENAR EMINENCE is the projecting mass at the base of the thumb: what is popularly known as the ball of the thumb.

THEOBROMINE is the alkaloidal principle upon which the stimulating action of cocoa and chocolate depends. (See CHOCOLATE.)

THEOPHYLLINE is an alkaloid similar to theobromine and occurs in small amounts in tea. It is a diuretic, usually administered in the form of theophylline and sodium acetate or of theophylline with ethylenediamine (aminophylline).

THERAPEUTICS is the general name applied to the science and art of healing.

THERAPY means the treatment of disease.

THERIAC means an antidote or substance given to neutralize poison. The name was specially given to Venice treacle, a celebrated mixture of 64 drugs prescribed in olden times as an antidote for poisons and a preventive of disease.

THERMO- is a prefix implying some relation to heat.

THERMOGRAPHY is a method of detecting cancer of the breast. It is based on the fact that abnormally hot areas of skin occur in an area of cancer. The process records such changes in temperature in a record known as a thermogram. Unfortunately, such hot areas of skin are caused by a number of other conditions. It is therefore a diagnostic method that can be used only as a rough screening procedure, but to this extent it is proving of some value in the early detection of cancer of the breast.

THERMOMETER SCALES (see TEMPERATURE).

THERMOPHORE is the name applied to a box or rubber bag filled with a mixture of glue, acetate of soda, chloride of soda, and sulphate of calcium. When it is placed in hot water for some time it has the property of retaining its heat for several hours and is used as a warm application.

THIABENDAZOLE is a drug that is proving of value in the treatment of various parasitic infections, including those due to guinea-worm and certain nematodes, as well as strongyloidiasis (qv).

THIACETAZONE was introduced into medicine by Domagk, the discoverer of the original sulphonamide, for the treatment of tuberculosis. It is also proving of value in the treatment of leprosy. It is administered by mouth.

THIAMBUTOSINE is a diphenylthiourea that is proving of value in the treatment of patients with leprosy who are intolerant of, or hypersensitive to, dapsone.

THIAMINE is the *British Pharmacopoeia* name for vitamin B_1. Also known as ANEURINE, it is found in the husks of cereal grains. Its deficiency may be produced by too careful milling of rice in the East, or by a diet of white bread to the exclusion of brown bread and other cereal sources of this vitamin. The resulting disease is a form of neuritis with muscular weakness and heart failure, common in Japan and other parts of the East and known as beriberi (qv). Vitamin B_1 has been isolated in crystalline form, and a minute dose of this rapidly cures the symptoms of beriberi. The best sources of this vitamin are wholemeal flour, bacon, liver, egg-yolk, yeast and the pulses. The daily requirement is dependent, among other things, upon the total food intake, and has been estimated to be in the region of 0·5 mg of thiamine per 1000 Calories, increased during pregnancy to 2 mg daily as a minimum.

THIAZIDES (see BENZOTHIADIAZINES).

THIERSCH'S GRAFT is the term given to a method of skin-grafting in which strips of skin are shaved from a normal area and placed on the abnormal area to be grafted. (See SKIN-GRAFTING.)

THIGH is the portion of the lower limb above the knee. The thigh is supported by the femur or thigh-bone, the longest and strongest bone in the body. This fits by a rounded head at its upper end into the acetabulum, a hollow at the side of the pelvis, and at the lower end two large rounded condyles or knuckles rest upon the head of the tibia, and, along with the patella, or knee-cap, form the knee-joint. A large four-headed muscle, the quadriceps, forms most of the fleshy mass on the front and sides of the thigh and serves to straighten the leg in walking and to maintain the erect posture of the body in standing. At the back of the thigh, lie the hamstring muscles; and on the inner side the adductor muscles, attached above to the pelvis and below to the femur, pull the lower limb inwards. The large femoral vessels emerge from the abdomen in the middle of the groin, the vein lying to the inner side of the artery. These pass downwards with an inclination inwards deeply placed between the muscles, and at the knee they lie behind the joint. The great saphenous vein lies near the surface and can be seen towards the inner side of the thigh passing up to the groin, where it joins the femoral vein. The femoral nerve accompanies the large vessels and controls the muscles on the front and inner side of the thigh; while the sciatic nerve, about the thickness of a lead pencil, lies close to the back of the femur and supplies the muscles at the back of the thigh and muscles below the knee.

Deep wounds on the inner side of the thigh are dangerous by reason of the risk of damage to the large vessels. Pain in the back of the thigh is often due to inflammation of the sciatic nerve. (See SCIATICA.) The veins on the inner side of the thigh are specially liable to become dilated. (See VARICOSE VEINS.)

THIOPENTONE SODIUM is the *British Pharmacopoeia* name for a commonly used intravenous anaesthetic. Its main use is for inducing anaesthesia, which it does rapidly and painlessly.

THIORIDAZINE (MELLERIL) is a tranquillizer that is proving of value as an antipsychotic drug. (See ANTI-PSYCHOTIC DRUGS.)

THIOSULPHATE OF SODIUM, or sodium hyposulphite, is much used in photography as a solvent of silver, and in medicine is used, in conjunction with sodium nitrite, in the treatment of cyanide, or prussic acid, poisoning. (See PRUSSIC ACID POISONING.)

THIOTEPA is one of the alkylating agents that is proving of value in the treatment of certain forms of malignant disease, including cancer of the breast and ovary. (See CYTOTOXIC DRUGS.)

THIOURACIL has the property of interfering with the synthesis of thyroxine in the thyroid gland. It was therefore intoduced, with success, for the treatment of thyrotoxicosis, and is now widely used for this purpose, as the propyl salt. The use of thiouracil is not without its risks, but these are negligible provided the drug is only used under medical supervision. Thiouracil is used in one of two ways: (*a*) to control thyrotoxicosis, and for this purose it usually needs to be taken for long periods; (*b*) as a preoperative measure in cases in which it has been decided that operation is necessary.

THIRST, like appetite, is an instinctive craving for something necessary to the continuance of bodily activity. The sensation of thirst is generally referred to the back of the throat, because, when there is a deficiency of water in the system, the throat and mouth especially become parched by evaporation of moisture from their surface. The mere swallowing of water, however, is not sufficient to abolish thirst, as appears in cases where a fistulous opening into the gullet exists, through which the water escapes. Thirst is increased by heat, and is a constant symptom of fever; it is also present in diseases which remove a considerable amount of fluid from the system, such as diarrhoea, diabetes mellitus, and after great loss of blood by haemorrhage. A desire for water is also a feature of many conditions associated with great exhaustion.

THORACIC DUCT is the large lymph-vessel which collects the contents of the lymphatics proceeding from the lower limbs, the abdomen, the left arm, and left side of the chest, neck, and head. It is about the size of a goose quill, is provided with numerous valves, and opens into the veins at the left side of the neck. (See GLANDS; LYMPHATICS.)

THORACOCENTESIS means the withdrawal of fluid from the pleural cavity. (See ASPIRATION.)

THORACOPLASTY is the operation of removing a varying number of ribs so that the underlying lung collapses.

THORAX is another name for the chest.

THORN-APPLE is a popular name for stramonium. (See STRAMONIUM.)

THREADWORM (see ENTEROBIASIS).

THREE-DAY FEVER (see SANDFLY FEVER).

THRILL is a tremor or vibration felt on applying the hand to the surface of the body. It is felt particularly over the region of the heart in conditions in which the valve openings are narrowed or an aneurysm is present.

THROAT is, in popular language, a vague term applied indifferently to the region in front of the neck, to the larynx or organ of voice, and to the cavity at the back of the mouth. The last-mentioned use of the word, to denote the pharynx or cavity into which the nose, mouth, gullet, and larynx all open, is the correct one. (See PHARYNX. Information will also be found under LARYNX; NECK; TONSILS; NOSE.)

THROAT, DISEASES OF (see CHOKING; CLERGYMAN'S SORE THROAT; CROUP; CUT-THROAT; DIPHTHERIA; LARYNGISMUS; LARYNGITIS; MOUTH, DISEASES OF; NOSE, DISEASES OF; PHARYNGITIS; TONSILLITIS).

FOREIGN BODIES sometimes lodge in the throat, being either of the nature of food which has been swallowed in too large or too hard pieces, or of the nature of indigestible substances like coins which children are apt to place in the mouth. Bodies which lodge in the respiratory part of the throat, ie. at the entrance to, or in the cavity of, the larynx, set up immediate symptoms of choking (qv).
INJURIES OF THE THROAT from without have been briefly referred to under CUT-THROAT.

THROMBIN (see COAGULATION).

THROMBOANGIITIS OBLITERANS, also known as BUERGER'S DISEASE after the American surgeon who gave the first coordinated description of it in 1908, is an inflammatory disease involving the blood-vessels of the limbs, particularly the lower limbs. The cause is not known, but the use of tobacco is an important factor in its causation. It is almost entirely confined to men, and is more common in Jews than in Gentiles. Pain is the outstanding symptom, accompanied by pallor of the affected part. Sooner or later ulceration and gangrene tend to develop in the feet or hands. There is no specific treatment, but, if seen in the early stages, considerable relief may be given to the patient.

THROMBOCYTE (see PLATELETS).

THROMBOCYTOPENIA is the disease characterized by absence, or marked diminution, of platelets (or thrombocytes) in the blood. (See PLATELETS.)

THROMBOPHLEBITIS is the condition characterized by inflammation of the veins combined with clot formation. (See VEINS, DISEASES OF.)

THROMBOSIS means the formation of a blood-clot within the vessels or heart during life. The process of clotting within the body depends upon the same factors as in clotting of blood outside the body, involving the fibrinogen and lime salts circulating in the blood, as well as blood platelets. The indirect cause of thrombosis is usually some damage to the smooth lining of the blood-vessels brought about by inflammation, or the result of atheroma, a chronic disease of the vessel walls. The blood is also specially prone to clot in certain general conditions such as anaemia, the ill health of wasting diseases like cancer, and in consequence of the feeble circulation of old age.

Thrombosis may occur in the heart and terminate some chronic wasting disease; it often takes place in the vessels of the brain and thus causes apoplexy in people whose arteries are much diseased. It is sometimes a salutary thing, as in aneurysm, where the deposition of a clot within the sac forms the natural cure of this condition.

Thrombosis of a coronary artery of the heart is a very serious condition which affects, as a rule, middle-aged or elderly people, appearing suddenly during rest and causing great pain in front of the chest or upper part of the abdomen, with pallor, feeble pulse, breathlessness, and sometimes vomiting. These symptoms may last for several hours or days, the pain being lessened by injections of morphine; but recovery takes place from about one-half of such attacks after a period of carefully supervised rehabilitation. (See also ARTERIES, DISEASES OF; CLOT; COAGULATION; CORONARY THROMBOSIS; APOPLEXY.)

THROMBOXANE is a substance produced in the blood platelets (see PLATELETS) which induces aggregation of platelets and thereby thrombosis (qv). It is also a vasoconstrictor (qv).

THROWER'S FRACTURE is a fracture of the humerus caused by the muscular force generated in a hard throw.

THRUSH is a type of inflammation affecting particularly the mouth of weakly children and causing a patchy white appearance on the lips, tongue, or palate. It is caused by the growth of a fungus on the surface of the mucous membrane. (See MOUTH, DISEASES OF.)

THUMB-SUCKING, or FINGER-SUCKING, is a universal habit in infancy. It is a harmless habit and nothing should be done to prevent it. On no account should any attempt be made to 'cure' it by giving the child a so-called 'dummy' to suck: a reprehensible habit that cannot be too strongly condemned. After the age of 1 year it is usually indulged in on going to sleep. It is usually gradually given up during the pre-school period, but quite often persists after school age especially if the child is tired, lonely or unhappy. In these cases the remedy is to deal with the cause. On no account should threats be used to try and stop the habit. These only tend to make matters worse by inducing the child to persist in the habit in order to attract attention. On the other hand, if the habit is persistent and excessive after the age of 3 the child may be helped to stop it by being appealed to on the grounds that he is getting too old for such a baby habit. There is no evidence that in the vast majority of children it has any effect on the shape of the mouth. Indeed, there is evidence that children who suck their thumbs are more likely to be free of caries of the teeth than those who are not thumb-suckers.

THYMOL is a white, crystalline substance derived from oil of thyme and other volatile oils. It has an antiseptic action. It is also used either alone or in combination with menthol as a local application for the relief of pruritus (ie. itching of the skin).

THYMUS GLAND: The thymus gland was given its name by Galen in the second century AD because of its resemblance to a bunch of thyme flowers. It has two lobes and lies in the upper part of the chest. Each lobe is made up of a number of lobules divided into an outer portion, or cortex, and a central portion, or medulla. The cortex resembles lymphoid tissue and is made up of masses of small round cells called thymocytes. It is an area of intense lymphopoiesis and the rate of production of new cells is five times greater than that in lymph nodes and other lymphoid tissues. The medulla is more loosely cellular and consists of a stroma which contains far fewer lymphocytes than in the cortex but also contains epithelial cells and Hassall's corpuscles.

The thymus gland is now established as a vital part of the immunological system. Until 1960 the function of the thymus was completely unknown. Stem cells from the bone marrow come to the thymus where they develop into immunologically competent cells. They are then seeded out to the rest of the lymphoid tissue. There are two distinct populations of lymphocytes. One is dependent of the presence of the thymus (T lymphocytes) and the other is independent of the thymus (B lymphocytes). Both are concerned with immune responses. They differ in their distribution and in their life span. The thymus-dependent lymphocyte is a cell which in the absence of antigenic stimulation circulates through the blood, lymph nodes and back into the circulation again over a period of more than 10 years. It performs a policing role, awaiting recognition of foreign material which it is able to identify as such. It reacts by multiplication and transformation and these are the ingredients of the immune response. B lymphocytes are produced in the bone marrow and are concerned with the production of the circulating humoral antibodies.

The most common clinical disorder associated with abnormality of the thymus is myasthenia gravis (qv). Ten per cent of patients with myasthenia gravis will have a tumour of the thymus whilst the remainder will have inflammatory changes in the thymus called thymitis.

THYROCALCITON is a hormone produced by the thyroid gland which helps to control the metabolism of calcium.

THYROID CARTILAGE is the largest cartilage in the larynx and forms the prominence of the Adam's apple in front of the neck. (See LARYNX.)

THYROID GLAND is a highly vascular organ situated in front of the neck. It consists of a narrow isthmus crossing the windpipe close to its upper end, and joining together two lateral lobes which run upwards, one on each side of the larynx. The gland is therefore shaped somewhat like a horseshoe, each lateral lobe being about 5 cm (2 inches) long and the isthmus about 12 mm (½ inch) wide, and it is firmly bound to the larynx. The weight of the thyroid gland is about 28·5 grams (1 ounce), but it is larger in females than in males, undergoes in many women a periodic increase at each time of menstruation, and often reaches an enormous size in the condition known as goitre (qv).

Minute structure: The gland is enveloped in a layer of fibrous tissue and possesses a rich blood supply. It is composed of multitudes of closed vesicles, each formed by a layer of cubical cells and containing a thick yellow fluid (colloid). Round the vesicles there is a dense network of capillary blood-vessels, whilst the finest lymphatic vessels communicate with the interior of these vesicles.

Function: The chief function of the thyroid gland is to produce a hormone rich in iodine. The main active ingredient of this hormone is thyroxine, and its probable mode of manufacture is:

This hormone, or secretion, which passes directly from the thyroid into the bloodstream, is de-iodinated in the body cells to triiodothyronine which exerts the physiological action of the thyroid hormone. The hormone is one of the most important in the body and controls the rate of metabolism. Thus, if it is deficient in children they fail to grow, a condition known as CRETINISM (qv). If the deficiency develops in adult life, the individual becomes obese, lethargic, and develops a coarse skin, a condition known as MYXOEDEMA (qv). Overaction of the thyroid, or HYPER-THYROIDISM, results in loss of weight, rapid heart action, and a highly strung nervous temperament.

The production of the thyroid hormone is controlled by a hormone of the pituitary gland – the thyrotrophic hormone.

THYROID GLAND, DISEASES OF (see CRETINISM; GOITRE; GRAVES' DISEASE; MYXOEDEMA).

THYROTOXIC ADENOMA is a variety of thyrotoxicosis in which one of the nodules of a multinodular goitre becomes autonomous and secretes excess thyroid hormone. The symptoms that result are similar to those of Graves' disease (qv), but there are minor differences. The first difference is that these autonomous adenomas tend to occur in long-standing nodular goitres so that the patients are older than those with Graves' disease. The symptoms of hyperthyroidism therefore tend to be more cardio-vascular, such as atrial fibrillation and heart failure. Exophthalmos and pre-tibial myxoedema do not occur as these are auto-immune manifestations of Graves' disease and toxic adenomas do not have an auto-immune basis.

Treatment: The first line of treatment is to render the patient euthyroid by treatment with antithyroid drugs. Then the nodule should be removed surgically or annihilated by radioactive iodine treatment.

THYROTOXICOSIS (see GRAVES' DISEASE).

THYROXINE is a crystalline substance, containing iodine, isolated from the thyroid gland and possessing the properties of thyroid extract. It has also been synthesized. It is used in cases of defective function of the thyroid, such as cretinism, and myxoedema.

TIAPROFENIC ACID (SURGAM) (see NON-STEROIDAL ANTI-INFLAMMATORY DRUGS).

TIBIA is the larger of the two bones in the leg. One surface of the tibia lies immediately beneath the skin in front and towards the inner side of the leg, forming the shin. Fractures of this bone are accordingly very liable to wound the skin and become compound. The thigh-bone rests upon the larger upper end of the tibia at the knee-joint, whilst below, the tibia and fibula together enter into the ankle-joint, the two bosses or malleoli at the ankle belonging, the inner to the tibia, the outer to the fibula.

TIC is the term applied to the habit spasm which forms a personal peculiarity in neurotic subjects. (See CRAMP.)

TICARCILLIN (see ANTIBIOTIC).

TIC DOULOUREUX is another name for facial, or trigeminal, neuralgia due to some affection of the fifth cranial nerve, and characterized by pain, situated somewhere about the temple, forehead, face, or jaw, and sometimes by spasm in the muscles of the affected region. (See TRIGEMINAL NEURALGIA.)

TICK is the general name given to a group of arachnid insects, some of which act as transmitters of diseases.

Ticks are blood-sucking arthropods which are responsible for transmitting a wide range of diseases to man, including Rocky Mountain spotted fever. African tick typhus and fièvre boutonneuse (see TYPHUS FEVER). Apart from being transmitters of disease, they cause intense itching and may cause quite severe lesions of the skin. The best repellents are dimethyl phthalate and diethyltoluamide. Once bitten, relief from the itching is obtained from the application of calamine lotion. Tick-bites are an occupational hazard of shepherds and gamekeepers. (See BITES AND STINGS.)

TIMOLOL MALEATE (BETIM, BLOCADREN) is a beta-adrenoceptor-blocking drug which is proving of value in the treatment of angina pectoris, myocardial infarction, and hypertension. It is also used in the treatment of glaucoma. (See ADRENERGIC RECEPTORS.)

TINCTURE is an alcoholic solution, generally of some vegetable substance.

TINEA is the technical name for ringworm. (See RINGWORM.)

TINNITUS means a noise heard in the ear without any external cause. It is a frequent accompaniment of deafness.

Tinnitus is common, affecting about one in six adults at some time in their life. Only one third of these consult a doctor and in less than one per cent does the tinnitus interfere with leading a normal life. The cause is damage to the auditory pathway and the most common part of the pathway to be damaged is the cochlea. It may be the result of drugs, particularly aspirin, chloroquine and quinine. Investigation is necessary to exclude any underlying cause but in most cases no cause can be found, and the management depends on relieving the effects of tinnitus on the patient because it is not usually possible to abolish the tinnitus altogether. Drugs such as carbamazepine (Tegretol), tocainide amide (Tonocard) and mexiletine (Mexitil) may have some beneficial effect, although none of these drugs has been licensed for use in tinnitus. The use of tinnitus maskers and hearing aids can suppress tinnitus by masking it with other sounds which the patient learns to listen to. Hearing aids suppress tinnitus by amplifying background noise. If the underlying cause is otosclerosis or Menière's disease surgery may be helpful.

Under the auspices of the Royal National Institute for the Deaf, the RNID Tinnitus Service/British Tinnitus Association (105 Gower Street, London WC1E 6AH, 01-387 8033, 01-436 7637) has been established 'to keep tinnitus sufferers in touch with each other, and provide a means of informing them about research developments'. (See DEAFNESS; EAR DISEASES OF; MENIERE'S DISEASE.)

TIRED ARM SYNDROME is the condition occurring mainly in middle-aged women, in which during the night aching and throbbing pain occurs in the upper limbs, especially the forearm and sometimes with weakness of the hand. The right upper limb is usually affected in right-handed people, and the hand feels stiff when the affected individual wakens in the morning. No treatment is needed, as the condition clears in due course.

TISANE is a name sometimes given to barley water. The term is also applied to a variety of herbal teas.

TISSUES OF THE BODY are the simple elements from which the various parts and organs are found to be built. All the body originates from the union of a pair of cells but as growth proceeds the new cells produced from these form tissues of varying character and complexity. (See CELL.) It is customary to divide the tissues into five groups:

(1) Epithelial tissues, including the cells covering the skin, those lining the alimentary

canal, those forming the secretions of internal organs. (See EPITHELIUM.)

(2) Connective tissues, including fibrous tissue, fat, bone, cartilage. (See these headings.)
(3) Muscular tissues (see MUSCLE).
(4) Nervous tissues (see NERVES).
(5) Wandering corpuscles of the blood and lymph (see BLOOD: LYMPH).

Many of the organs are formed of a single one of these tissues or of one with a very slight admixture of another, such as cartilage, or white fibrous tissue. Other parts of the body that are widely distributed are very simple in structure and consist of two or more simple tissues in varying proportion. Such are blood-vessels (see ARTERIES; VEINS), lymphatic vessels (see LYMPHATICS), lymphatic glands (see GLANDS), serous membranes (see SEROUS MEMBRANE), synovial membranes (see JOINTS), mucous membranes (see MUCOUS MEMBRANE), secreting glands (see GLANDS; SALIVARY GLANDS; THYROID GLAND) and skin (see SKIN).

The structure of the more complex organs of the body is dealt with under the heading of each organ.

TITRATION is a form of chemical analysis by means of standard solutions of known strength.

TITUBATION means a staggering or reeling condition, especially due to disease of the spinal cord or cerebellum.

TOBACCO is the leaf of several species of Nicotiana, especially of the American plant *Nicotiana tabacum*.

The smoking of tobacco is the major public health hazard in Britain today. It causes a hundred thousand premature deaths per year in the United Kingdom alone. To put that figure in perspective it can be calculated that of one thousand young people who smoke a packet of cigarettes a day on average: one will be murdered, six will be killed on the roads and two hundred and fifty will die from their smoking. In addition to the deaths caused by cigarette smoking it is also a major cause of disability and illness in the form of myocardial infarction, peripheral vascular disease, chronic obstructive airways disease and emphysema. If four fully laden jumbo jets crashed at Heathrow every week killing all passengers there would be an enormous public outcry: that is precisely the weekly death toll attributable to cigarettes. Action on Smoking and Health (ASH) is a small charity founded by the Royal College of Physicians in 1971 that attempts to alert and inform the public to the dangers of smoking and to try to prevent the disability and death which it causes (see ASH). No drug whatever its potential would be acceptable to the Committee on the Safety of Medicines that had the side-effects of cigarette smoking.

According to the United States' Surgeon General's 1984 report entitled 'The Health Consequences of Smoking', cigarette smoking is the major cause of chronic obstructive lung disease morbidity and 80 to 90 per cent of chronic obstructive lung disease in the United States is attributable to it. In 1982 the United States' Surgeon General stated that cigarette smoking was the major single cause of cancer mortality in the United States. Tobacco's contribution to all cancer deaths is estimated to be 30 per cent. The British Royal College of Physicians' four reports confirm the link between smoking and cancer, especially cancer of the lung. The Royal College of Physicians in its report 'Smoking and Health' in 1983 stated that 30 per cent of the heart disease deaths are attributable to smoking and in 1983 the U.S. Surgeon General stated that cigarette smoking is the most important of the known modifiable risk factors for coronary heart disease.

Composition: In addition to vegetable fibre, tobacco leaves contain a large quantity of ash, the nature of this depending predominantly upon the minerals present in the ground where the tobacco plant has been grown, but amounting to 12 or 20 per cent of the whole. Of the organic constituents the brown fluid alkaloid known as nicotine is the most important, as the special action of tobacco depends upon it. The nicotine content of tobacco ranges from 1·5 to 3 per cent of the dried leaf in Havana tobacco to 6 to 8 per cent in Virginian tobacco. Some Algerian tobaccos contain much larger amounts. The amount of nicotine entering the mouth of a smoker is 0·92 mg per cigarette, 3·6 to 7·9 mg per cigar, and 2·7 mg per gram of pipe tobacco. The amount of nicotine absorbed depends upon whether or not the smoker inhales. Most of the nicotine inhaled into the smaller air-passages of the lungs is absorbed, whereas without inhalation, much less per cigarette is absorbed. As a cigarette or cigar is smoked the stub becomes richer in nicotine. It has been estimated that if not more than two-thirds of a cigarette is smoked, some two-thirds of the nicotine is retained in the stub. The amount of nicotine that can be recovered from the mainstream smoke of one cigarette varies from 1 to 3 milligrams and smokers who inhale may absorb up to 90 per cent of this; those who do not inhale absorb as little as 10 per cent.

Tobacco smoke also contains some sixteen substances capable of inducing cancer in experimental animals. One of the most important of these is benzpyrene, a strongly carcinogenic hydrocarbon. As this is present in coal-tar pitch, it is commonly referred to in this context as tar. Other constituents of tobacco smoke include pyridine, ammonia and carbon monoxide. The last is the most abundant of these, but American workers have stated that an individual walking along a street with heavy motor traffic would absorb more carbon monoxide than he would from heavy smoking. The range of tar, carbon monoxide and nicotine yields of cigarettes, in milligrams per cigarette, as determined by the Government Chemist, is as follows, as classified according to the tar content of cigarettes:

Low Tar Cigarettes	
Tar yield	Under 4 to 10
Carbon monoxide yield	Under 3 to 14
Nicotine yield	Under 0·3 to 1·0
Low to Middle Tar Cigarettes	
Tar yield	11 to 16
Carbon monoxide yield	11 to 19
Nicotine yield	0·6 to 1·4
Middle Tar Cigarettes	
Tar yield	17 to 22
Carbon monoxide yield	10 to 20
Nicotine yield	1·1 to 1·9

Action and use: The action of tobacco depends largely upon the constitution of the smoker, his habituation to the drug, and the circumstances under which he smokes.

A very small amount of nicotine, such as that derived from a single cigarette, has a stimulating effect upon the mental and bodily powers.

In larger amount, the action is a depressant and narcotic one, which in habitual smokers is modified to a sedative and quieting effect upon the nervous system, without much depression of the heart or other organs. The most suitable time for smoking is generally admitted to be after meals, and especially in the evening after the day's work is at an end, when the sedative action is most beneficial to the nervous system. Different people vary widely in their susceptibility to the influence of tobacco. In some, and particularly in young people, very small quantities suffice to cause depression and irritability of the nervous system, the heart's action, and the digestive and other powers.

Among the evil effects of smoking may be mentioned the temporary nausea, depression, giddiness, and vomiting which affect the unaccustomed smoker. These effects, however, pass off quickly, and the tendency to their occurrence disappears as the person becomes habituated to tobacco. Of more importance is the group of symptoms produced by continued and excessive smoking, especially of cigarettes. These include palpitation and irregularity of the heart, giddiness, and a tendency to sudden attacks of faintness, symptoms often grouped together under the popular name of 'tobacco heart'. Other common symptoms are liability to fatigue on slight exertion, dyspepsia, and dimness of vision associated with impairment of power for seeing colours, especially green and red. These symptoms also pass off gradually when smoking is discontinued, or when the amount of tobacco consumed is reduced within suitable bounds; but, while they last, they may cause great impairment of the health.

The greatest hazard of smoking, however, is the fact that it is the major cause of lung cancer, coronary artery disease, peripheral vascular disease, chronic bronchitis and emphysema. It also has an adverse effect on the foetus when the pregnant mother smokes. Hence the justification for the current campaign to persuade youngsters never to start smoking, and adult cigarette smokers to cut down their daily consumption. The advice given by the Health Departments of the United Kingdom is:

Stop smoking. If you cannot, take these steps to reduce the risk.

Smoke a brand of cigarette in a lower 'tar' group than the brand you smoke at present; try to reduce still further and at the same time select a brand with a low carbon monoxide yield.

Smoke fewer cigarettes.

Take smaller and fewer puffs from each cigarette.

Do not inhale.

Leave a longer 'stub' – the 'tar', carbon monoxide and nicotine become more concentrated as the cigarette is smoked.

Take the cigarette out of your mouth between puffs.

Almost equally serious is the undoubted correlation between heavy cigarette smoking on the one hand, and chronic bronchitis and duodenal ulcer on the other, and there is now convincing evidence of a correlation between cigarette smoking and coronary heart disease.

Another set of symptoms frequently arising in those who smoke, and often attributed to a mistaken cause, consists of irritable cough and soreness of the throat. These symptoms pass off when smoking is discontinued.

The habit also has an adverse effect on the foetus, and is therefore contraindicated during pregnancy.

The giving up of the smoking habit is largely a psychological problem, but there is some evidence that the use of nicotine chewing gum facilitates the process.

Acute nicotine poisoning seldom occurs. It may be due to the accidental swallowing of nicotine insecticides, or to the inhaling of tobacco dust in industrial processes. Occasionally it may occur in children as a result of swallowing tobacco. Nicotine is one of the most rapidly fatal poisons. The fatal dose for man is about 40 mg. The fatal dose of tobacco is about 2 grams. The symptoms vary from those of smoking in the unaccustomed smoker to immediate prostration leading rapidly to collapse and death. Treatment consists of washing out the stomach, the administration of charcoal or potassium permanganate (1 in 5000 solutions), and artificial respiration.

TOBRAMYCIN is an antibiotic related to gentamicin (qv) and with a similar range of activity. It is given by injection.

TOES (see CORNS; FOOT; NAILS).

TOLAZOLINE is a drug that antagonizes some of the effects of adrenaline, and is used in the treatment of peripheral vascular disorders due to arterial spasm or occlusion.

TOLAZOMIDE (TOLANASE) (see SULPHONYLUREAS).

TOLBUTAMIDE (PRAMIDEX, RASTINON) is a sulphonamide derivative, or sulphonylurea, which lowers the level of the blood sugar in diabetes mellitus. As it is rapidly excreted from the body, it has to be taken twice daily. Like chlorpropamide (qv), it may induce undue sensitivity to alcohol. (See also DIABETES MELLITUS, SULPHONYLUREAS.)

TOLMETIN (TOLECTIN) (see NON-STEROIDAL ANTI-INFLAMMATORY DRUGS).

TOLNAFTATE is a preparation which in the form of a 1 per cent solution, is proving useful as a local application in the treatment of certain forms of ringworm, particularly ringworm of the foot. It may also be applied as a powder or cream. It is used, too, in the treatment of tinea versicolor (see RINGWORM) and erythrasma (qv).

TOLU (see BALSAM).

TOLUENE, or METHYLBENZENE, is a product of the distillation of coal tar widely used as a solvent in the manufacture of paint and rubber and plastic cements.

-TOMY is a suffix indicating an operation by cutting.

TONGUE: The tongue is made up of several muscles, is richly supplied with blood-vessels and nerves, and is covered by highly specialized mucous membrane. It consists of a free part known as the tip, a body, and a hinder fixed part or root. The under surface lies upon the floor of the mouth, whilst the upper surface is curved from side to side, and still more from before backwards so as to adapt it to the roof of the mouth. At its root, the tongue is in contact with, and firmly united to, the upper edge of the larynx; so that in some persons who can depress the tongue readily the tip of the epiglottis may be seen projecting upwards at its hinder part.

Structure: The *substance* of the tongue consists almost entirely of muscles running in various directions. One runs along the upper surface and another along the lower surface from root to tip. Other fibres run vertically from the upper to the lower surface, whilst the chief bulk of the tongue is made up of muscle-fibres running from side to side. These various fibres are chiefly concerned in making changes in the shape of the tongue and moving it within the mouth. In addition to these, the tongue has numerous outside attachments; one muscle on each side unites it to the lower jaw-bone just behind the chin, and this muscle serves to protrude the tongue from the mouth; other muscles, which retract the tongue, attach it to the hyoid bone, the larynx, the palate, and the styloid process on the base of the skull.

The *mucous membrane* on the under surface of the tongue is very thin, so that the large blood-vessels on each side can easily be seen through it. In the middle line a fold of mucous membrane, the frenum, passes from the under surface to the floor of the mouth, and, when this frenum is attached too far forwards towards the tip of the tongue, the movements of the organ are impeded, and the condition is known as tongue-tie. On the upper surface or dorsum of the tongue the mucous membrane is thicker, and in its front two-thirds is studded with little projections of three kinds. The majority of these projections or *papillae* are of *conical* shape, and when the tongue becomes furred the apppearance is due to an unhealthy collection of epithelium upon them. Some of them end in long filaments, and are then known as *filiform* papillae. The roughness of the tongue in cats and other carnivorous animals is due to large backwardly directed conical papillae, which assist in cleaning the flesh off bones. On the tip, and towards the edges of the tongue, small red rounded *fungiform* papillae are seen, which act in all probability as end-organs for the sense of taste. On a line dividing the front two-thirds from the hinder one-third, and set in the shape of a V, is a row of seven to twelve large flat-topped *circumvallate* papillae, each placed in a corresponding depression and just visible, in most mouths, when the tongue is pressed firmly down with some flat instrument. These also act as end-organs for the nerves of taste. Each circumvallate papilla is surrounded by a trench, and upon both sides of the trench open numerous *taste-buds*. A taste-bud is shaped somewhat like a barrel, with an outer covering of flattened stave-like cells, enclosing a bundle of spindle-shaped cells which end in hairlike processes at the mouth of the bud, and are connected at their deeply placed end with some filaments from the nerves of taste. These taste-buds are also found in the fungiform papillae, though in smaller numbers, and they are scattered over the throat, fauces, and palate; so that the popular expression 'a fine palate', as applied to the sense of taste, is quite correct.

Nerves: No fewer than five nerves supply branches to each side of the tongue. These are the *lingual* branch of the 5th nerve, which is the nerve of ordinary sensation, to the front two-thirds of the tongue; the *chorda tympani* branch from the 7th nerve, which is supposed to be the nerve of taste, for a similar extent; the *glossopharyngeal* or 9th nerve, which conveys sensations both of touch and taste from the hinder third: the *superior laryngeal* branch of the 10th nerve, also sensory; and the *hypoglossal* or 12th nerve, which supplies the muscles of the tongue.

Functions: The chief uses of the tongue are of three kinds: (*a*) to push the food between the teeth for mastication, and then mould it into a bolus preparatory to swallowing; (*b*) as the organ of the sense of taste, and as an organ provided with a delicate sense of touch; and (*c*)

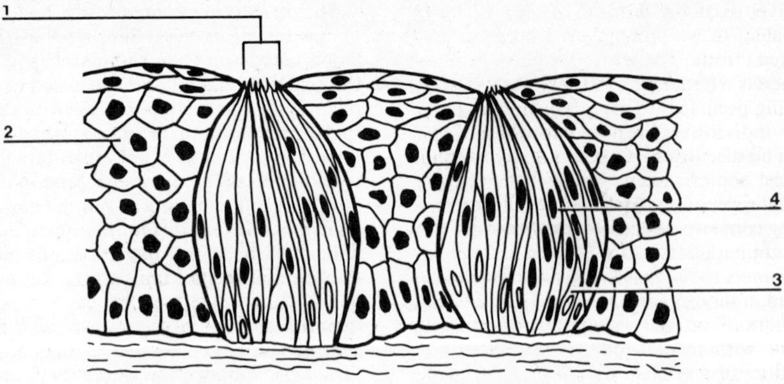

1 gustatory pore
2 stratifield epithelium
3 sustentacular cell
4 gustatory cell with hairlet

Section showing taste buds. Magnified by 420.

to play a part in the production of speech. (See VOICE AND SPEECH.)

It is usual to classify any taste as:

1. Sweet
2. Salt
3. Bitter
4. Acid

since finer distinctions are largely dependent upon the sense of smell. The loss of keenness in taste brought about by a cold in the head, or even by holding the nose while swallowing, is well known. Sweet tastes seem to be best appreciated by the tip of the tongue, acids on its edges, and bitters at the back. It is possible, too, by chewing the leaves of an Indian plant, *Gymnaema sylvesive*, to do away with the power of tasting bitter and sweet substances, while the sensation for acids and salts remains, so that in all probability there are different nerve-fibres and end-organs for the different varieties of taste. Many tastes depend upon the ordinary sensations of the tongue, such as the constringent taste of tannin and the metallic taste of a weak galvanic current passed through the tongue. The sense of taste may be affected by certain drugs. Thus, penicillamine (qv) may reduce the sense of taste for sweet and salt, levodopa (qv) may induce a metallic or garlic-like taste, lithium (qv) may be accompanied by a rather vague unpleasant taste, captopril (qv) by a loss of the sense of taste, whilst metformin (qv) may cause a metallic taste.

Like other sensations, taste can be very highly educated for a time, as in tea-tasters and wine-tasters, but this special adaptation is lost after some years.

TONGUE, DISEASES OF (see MOUTH, DISEASES OF).

TONGUE, FURRING OF (see MOUTH, DISEASES OF).

TONICS are 'substances whose continue administration gives strength and vigour to th body, without producing sudden excitement o subsequent depression'. This is a 100-year ol definition of a term which is gradually passin out of medical phraseology. In the old days when knowledge of disease processes and o how to treat them was much less than it i today, there was a real place for remedies whic would help to combat the weakness, lassitude and loss of appetite which accompanied an followed most illnesses. At the present day it i so often possible to treat the underlying caus that tonics are seldom required. It is also recog nized now that to treat symptoms of a disease without discovering their cause, may do mor harm than good. For instance, a middle-age man's loss of appetite may be due to cancer o the stomach. To treat this by a bitter is obvi ously wrong, because the only hope of cure is a early operation. Similarly, the young woman' lassitude may be the first manifestation of pul monary tuberculosis, the treatment of which i not a tonic but the appropriate chemotherap Or, to take one other example, an individual' lack of concentration may be due to dimin ished activity of the thyroid gland, ie. my oedema, a condition which can be immediatel and effectively controlled by the administra tion of thyroxine.

Thus, the use of tonics is very much less tha it was. But there are still occasions when the may be of value: for instance, in convalescenc from a serious illness. Even in those cases i which they are still used, however, tonics a tending to be used with more discriminatio and need not necessarily take the form of drug For the over-worked professional person c business executive the best tonic is a holida To give such a person a bitter to stimulate h appetite, a nerve tonic to 'buck him up', a tra quillizer to take the edge off life for him, and sedative to allow him to sleep, is simply equivalent to whipping a tired horse to make renewed efforts. There may well be a response, but merely a temporary one achieved at the risk of doing permanent harm.

For individuals who are run down, and in whom no disease or special cause can be found, the best tonics include a well-balanced diet, adequate sleep, ample fresh air and exercise. During convalescence bitters such as nux vomica, quinine, quassia, and gentian may be useful adjuncts to re-stimulating an active interest in food, although this can usually be achieved much more satisfactorily by presenting the patient with a well-cooked variety of food served in an attractive manner.

An unbalanced diet is often a cause for debility, particularly in children and adolescents. Here the best tonic is a well-balanced diet, ensuring an adequate supply of all the vitamins, first-class protein, and essential salts and metals such as iron and calcium. Vitamin deficiency is no longer a major problem in Great Britain, but this state of affairs can only be maintained if every individual up to the age of at least 18 years receives supplementary doses of vitamins A, D, and C during the winter months. Milk, eggs, and meat are the best sources of first-class protein.

Iron is often given as a tonic, but this is only of value when the individual is suffering from an iron-deficiency anaemia. Its use for this purpose is often indicated in adolescent girls in whom there is a heavy loss of blood during the menstrual period. Although there is not usually a marked degree of anaemia in these girls, there is often sufficient lack of iron in the diet to render beneficial the administration of additional iron. There is no justification for the use of liver extracts as a tonic.

No account of tonics would be complete without at least a brief reference to three iron-containing tonics which are still widely used: Parrish's food (compound syrup of iron phosphate). Easton's syrup (syrup of iron phosphate with quinine and strychnine) and syrup of iron iodide. The first of these is still a favourite for use in children, whilst Easton's syrup is a useful bitter for adults. None of them contains sufficient iron to relieve an iron-deficiency anaemia. If such is present, iron must be given in much larger doses.

TONSILLITIS is the inflammation of the tonsils.

ACUTE TONSILLITIS: It must never be forgotten that the infection is never entirely confined to the tonsils; there is always some involvement of the surrounding throat or pharynx. The converse is true that in many cases of 'sore throat' the tonsils are involved in the generalized inflammation of the throat.

Causes: The most common cause is the β-haemolytic streptococcus. Like most upper-respiratory-tract infections its highest incidence is in the winter months. It used to be an important precursor of rheumatic fever but early diagnosis and treatment have fortunately reduced the incidence of this disease in developed countries. Care should be taken to prevent the spread of infection in hospitals or institutions. Acute tonsillitis may also occur in infectious mononucleosis or glandular fever and, rarely, it may be the presenting feature of diphtheria. This disease is fortunately now extremely rare.

Symptoms: The onset is usually fairly sudden with pain on swallowing, fever and malaise. On examination, the tonsils are found to be enlarged, engorged and often covered with a varying amount of whitish or grey material. This material or exudate consists of purulent discharge from the tonsil. It may occur at scattered areas over the crypts of the tonsil when the condition is known as follicular tonsillitis, or it may be more extensive exudate covering practically the whole of the tonsil. This form of exudate occurs in simple streptococcal tonsillitis but may also occur in infectious mononucleosis (glandular fever). It is also a feature of diphtheria, although this condition is now extremely rare. The glands underneath the angle of the jaw are enlarged and tender. There may be pain in the ear on the affected side and, although this is usually referred pain, it may indicate spread up the Eustachian tube to the ear on that side. This is particularly so in children.

Occasionally an abscess develops around the affected tonsil, a peritonsillar abscess or quinsy. This abscess is formed by the collection of pus between the tonsil and the superior constrictor muscle of the pharynx. It usually comes on four to five days after the onset of tonsillitis and requires specialist treatment.

Treatment: The drug of choice is still penicillin or erythromycin in penicillin-sensitive patients. Fluids should be encouraged and analgesia and antipyretic medication should also be prescribed.

In the past tonsillitis was often a precursor of rheumatic fever or of acute glomerular nephritis but this has fortunately become much less common, due to early recognition of tonsillitis and prompt treatment with the appropriate antibiotics. Improved socio-economic conditions have probably also contributed to the decreased incidence of these complications in developed countries.

Removal of tonsils is indicated: (*a*) when the tonsils and adenoids are permanently so enlarged as to interfere with breathing; in such cases the adenoids are removed as well as the tonsils; (*b*) when the individual is subject to recurrent attacks of acute tonsillitis which are causing significant debility, absence from school or work on a regular basis; (*c*) when there is evidence of a tumour of the tonsil.

TONSILS are two almond-shaped glands situated one on each side of the narrow fauces where the mouth joins the throat. Each has a structure resembling that of a lymphatic gland, and consists of an elevation of the mucous membrane presenting twelve to fifteen openings, which lead into pits or lacunae. The mucous covering is formed by the ordinary mucous membrane of the mouth, which also lines the pits; and the main substance of the gland is composed of loose connective tissue containing lymph corpuscles in its meshes, and packed here and there into denser nodules or follicles. The tonsils play an important rôle in the protective mechanism of the body against infection.

TOOTH, SUPERNUMERARY: Malformed extra teeth are frequently found, particularly in the upper incisor region. They often do not erupt but prevent the eruption of the permanent teeth.

TOOTHACHE (see TEETH, DISEASES OF).

TOPHUS is the name given to the concretions which form in connection with joints or tendon sheaths as the result of attacks of gout. At first the tophus is a soft mass, but later becomes quite hard. It is composed of biurate of soda. (See CONCRETIONS; GOUT.)

TORMINA is a technical name for griping pains felt round the navel, as the result of spasmodic action of the muscular coat in the small intestine. (See COLIC.)

TORPOR is a condition of bodily and mental inactivity, not amounting to sleep, but interfering greatly with the ordinary habits and pursuits. It is often found in people suffering from fever, and is a common symptom in aged people whose arteries are diseased. It may annoy young people after meals when they are the subjects of constipation or of dyspepsia, due to eating too much indigestible food.

TORSION means twisting. The term is applied to the process in which organs, or tumours, which are attached to the rest of the body by a narrow neck or pedicle, become twisted so as to narrow the blood-vessels or other structures in the pedicle. (See TESTICLES, DISEASES OF.)

Torsion is also the term applied to the twisting of the small arteries severed at an operation, by which bleeding from them is stopped.

TORTICOLLIS: This is shortness of the sternomastoid muscle on one side resulting in asymetry and limitation of movement of the neck. (See CRAMP; SPASMODIC TORTICOLLIS; WRY-NECK.)

TOTEM-POLE HEAD (see HYPERTELORISM).

TOUCH, according to the popular idea, is the fifth sense diffused all over the body, by which we become conscious of our surroundings otherwise than by the four special senses of hearing, seeing, tasting and smelling. But when this diffused sensitiveness is examined it is found to consist of a group of senses, several of which have special end-organs situated in the skin, muscles and elsewhere and special nerve-paths to convey their impressions to the brain. It is convenient, however, to adopt the popular view, and to consider all these under one heading. The cutaneous sense, then, is made up of the following:

Touch sense proper, by which we perceive a touch or stroke and estimate the size and shape of bodies with which we come in contact, but which we do not see.
Pressure sense, by which we judge the heaviness of weights laid upon the skin, or appreciate the hardness of objects by pressing against them.
Heat sense, by which we perceive that a body is warmer than the skin.
Cold sense, by which we perceive that a body touching the skin is cold.
Pain sense, by which we appreciate pricks, pinches and other painful impressions.

To these we may for convenience add:

Muscular sensitiveness, by which the painfulness of a squeeze is perceived. It is produced probably by direct pressure upon the nerve-fibres in the muscles.
Muscular sense, by which we test the weight of an object held in the hand, or gauge the amount of energy expended on an effort.
Sense of locality, by which we can, without looking, tell the position and attitude of any part of the body.
Common sensation, which is a vague term used to mean composite sensations produced by several of the foregoing, like tickling, or creeping, and the vague sense of well-being or the reverse that the mind receives from internal organs. (See the article on PAIN.)

The structure of the end-organs situated in the skin, which receive impressions from the outer world, and of the nerve-fibres which conduct these impressions to the central nervous system, have been described under NERVES.

Touch affects the Meissner's or touch corpuscles placed beneath the epidermis; as these differ in closeness in different parts of the skin, the delicacy of the sense of touch varies greatly. Thus the points of a pair of compasses can be felt as two on the tip of the tongue when separated by only 1 mm; on the tips of the fingers they must be separated to twice that distance, whilst on the arm or leg they cannot be felt as two points unless separated by over 25 mm, and on the back they must be separated by over 50 mm. On the parts covered by hair, the nerves ending round the roots of the hairs also take up impressions of touch.

Pressure is estimated probably through the same nerve-endings and nerves that have to do with touch, but it depends upon a difference in the sensations of parts pressed on and those of surrounding parts. Heat-sense, cold-sense and pain-sense all depend upon different nerve-endings in the skin; and thus, with care and delicate instruments like needles, bristles in holders and metal pencils through which hot or cold water can be made to circulate, the skin may be mapped out into a mosaic of little areas where the different kinds of impressions are registered. Whilst the tongue and finger-tips are the parts most sensitive to touch, they are comparatively insensitive to heat, and can easily bear temperatures which the cheek or elbow could not tolerate. The muscular sense, in all probability, depends on the sensory organs known as muscle-spindles, which are scattered through the substance of the muscles, and the sense of locality is dependent partly upon these and partly upon the nerves which end in tendons, ligaments and joints.

Disorders of the sense of touch occur in various diseases.

HYPERAESTHESIA is a condition in which there is excessive sensitiveness to any stimulus, such as touch. When this reaches the stage when a mere touch or gentle handling causes acute pain it is known as HYPERALGESIA. It is found in various diseases of the spinal cord immediately above the level of the disease, combined often with loss of sensation below the diseased part. It is also present in neuralgia, the skin of the neuralgic area becoming excessively tender to touch, heat or cold. Heightened sensibility to pain is seen sometimes in drunkards, who wince at a mere touch when not under the influence of alcohol. Heightened sensibility to temperature is a common symptom of neuritis. (See PAIN.)

ANAESTHESIA, or diminution of the sense of touch, causing often a feeling of numbness, is present in many diseases affecting the nerves of sensation or their continuations up the posterior part of the spinal cord. The condition of *dissociated analgesia*, in which a touch is quite well felt, though there is complete insensibility to pain, is present in the disease of the spinal cord known as syringomyelia, and affords a proof that the nerve-fibres for pain and those for touch are quite separate. In tabes dorsalis there is sometimes loss of the sense of touch on feet or arms; but in other cases of this disease there is no loss of the sense of touch, although there is a complete loss of the sense of locality in the lower limbs, thus proving that these two senses are quite distinct.

PARAESTHESIAE are peculiar forms of perverted sensation such as creeping, tingling, pricking or hot flushes.

TOURNIQUET is an instrument used for the temporary stoppage of the circulation in a limb, to control bleeding. There are various forms of tourniquet, the simplest being a tourniquet improvised from a band such as that made by a handkerchief folded cravat-wise, tied round the limb, and then twisted up by means of a rigid object passed beneath it. *Petit's tourniquet* has a linen strap passing over two pairs of brass rollers, which can be separated from one another by a screw, thus tightening the strap after it has been buckled round the limb. *Esmarch's tourniquet* consists of an elastic band which is wrapped with moderate tightness round the limb, and then prevented from unwrapping by tapes. It is the form generally used. (See HAEMORRHAGE.) A rubber tube knotted, or fixed with a clip, round the limb is also often used for arresting the blood-flow. In applying a tourniquet for bleeding, it must be rendered sufficiently tight to stop the circulation completely. Otherwise if the veins only are compressed and the arteries still open, the bleeding is made worse. A tourniquet must not be left in position longer than is absolutely necessary; otherwise gangrene of the limb may result. It must be loosened cautiously after not more than 15 minutes. If bleeding has not stopped it is tightened again. This procedure must be repeated every 15 minutes.

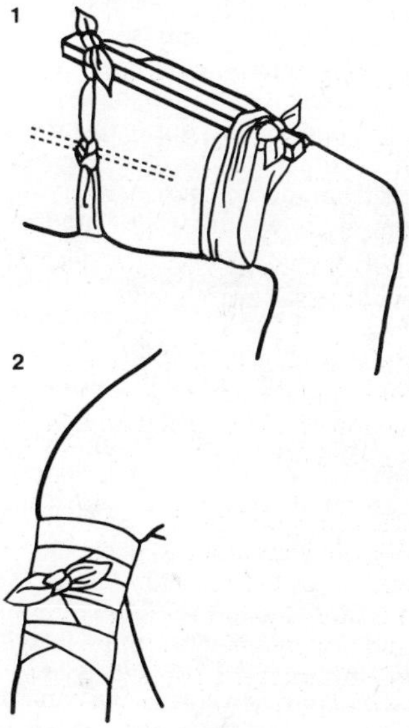

Two simple forms of tourniquet.

TOW is a form of jute which is very hygroscopic, absorbing up to 25 per cent of moisture.

TOXAEMIA is a term applied to forms of blood-poisoning due to the absorption of bacterial products (toxins) formed at some local site of infection, such as abscesses. In other cases the toxaemia is due to defective action of some excretory organ, such as the kidney. As regards treatment, the most important consideration is to remove the source of infection.

Toxaemia of pregnancy is a term sometimes used to describe the two complications of pregnancy known as pre-eclampsia and eclampsia (qv).

TOXIC SHOCK SYNDROME is a new syndrome first described in 1978. It is characterized by high fever, diarrhoea, shock and an erythematous rash. It is frequently associated with the use of tampons. It has, however, been described in men. The disease is due to a staphylococcal toxin. The treatment consists of supportive measures to combat shock and eradication of the staphylococcus by antibiotics. A mortality rate of 10 per cent has been reported.

TOXICOLOGY is the science dealing with poisons. (See POISONS.)

TOXINS are poisons produced by bacteria. (See BACTERIOLOGY; IMMUNITY; SERUM THERAPY.) Toxins are usually soluble, easily destroyed by heat, sometimes of the nature of crystalline substances, and sometimes albumins. When injected into animals in carefully graduated doses, they bring about the formation of substances called antitoxins which neutralize the action of the toxin. These antitoxins are generally produced in excesive amount, and the serum of the animal when withdrawn can be used for conferring antitoxic powers upon other animals or human beings to neutralize the disease in question. The best known of these antitoxins are those of diphtheria and tetanus. Toxins are also found in many plants and in snake venom.

Some toxins are not set free by bacteria, but remain in the substance of the latter. They are known as endotoxins and are not capable of producing antitoxins.

TOXOCARIASIS is a disease acquired by swallowing the ova of a roundworm which lives in the intestine of cats (*Toxocara cati*) or dogs (*Toxocara canis*). In man, the small larval worms produced by these ova migrate to various parts of the body, including the retina of the eye, where they then die, and produce a small granuloma (qv) which in turn may produce allergic reactions. In the eye it may cause choroidretinitis. It is said that 2 per cent of apparently healthy people in Britain have been infected in this way. A course of treatment with diethylcarbamazine is said to kill the worm.

TOXOID is toxin (qv) which has been rendered non-toxic by certain chemicals, or by heat, or by being partly neutralized by antitoxin. The best-known example is diphtheria toxoid. (See IMMUNITY.)

TOXOPLASMOSIS is a disease which is due to infection with protozoa of the genus *Toxoplasma*. The infection may be acquired from eating raw or undercooked meat, from cats, or from gardening or playing in contaminated soil. It occurs in two forms: an acquired form and a congenital form. The acquired form may run such a benign course that it is not recognized, the patient scarcely feeling ill. In the congenital form the unborn child is infected by the mother. The congenital form, the incidence of which in the United Kingdom is 1 in 5000 pregnancies, (1 in 2000 pregnancies in Scotland), may develop in one of two ways. The infant may either appear generally ill, or the brunt of the infection may fall on the nervous system causing hydrocephalus (qv), mental retardation, or loss of sight. In some cases the infection may be so severe that it kills the foetus, resulting in a miscarriage or stillbirth. In other cases the infection is so mild that it is missed until in later life the child begins to show signs of eye trouble. As the congenital form of the disease, which is most serious, seems to develop only if the mother acquires the infection during pregnancy, it would appear to be a wise precaution that pregnant women should avoid contact with cats and eating raw or undercooked meat foods.

TOY LIBRARIES: The National Toy Libraries Association, founded ten years ago to help handicapped children get suitable toys, now has links with over 500 toy libraries throughout the country. These libraries keep a wide range of toys that can either be played with at the Library or taken home. The range includes trucks for children to ride on, toys for babies, and others with an educational element. They also provide a convenient place for parents and child minders to meet, share common problems and seek advice if they want to. Further details can be obtained from: Playmatters, 68 Churchway, London NW1 1LT (01–387 9592).

TRACE ELEMENTS are chemical elements that are distributed throughout the tissues of the body in very small amounts and are essential for the nutrition of the body. Nine such elements are now recognized: cobalt, copper, fluorine, iodine, iron, manganese, molybdenum, selenium and zinc.

TRACHEA is another name for the windpipe (qv). (See also AIR PASSAGES.)

TRACHEITIS means inflammation of the trachea. It may occur along with bronchitis, or independently, due to similar causes.

TRACHEOSTOMY, or TRACHEOTOMY, is the operation in which the windpipe is opened from the front of the neck, so that air may obtain direct entrance into the lower air passages. The opening is made through the second and third rings of the trachea (windpipe) (qv).

Reasons for operation: Conditions in which the opening of the larynx is narrowed are treated by the appropriate means but, should these fail, some form of airway intervention is necessary. In the majority of cases this would involve the insertion of an endotracheal tube, ie. a tube is inserted either through the nose or mouth and down the pharynx through the larynx to bypass the obstruction, or by a tracheostomy. The majority of tracheostomies performed nowadays are for patients in intensive-therapy-unit situations. These patients require airway intervention for prolonged periods to facilitate artificial ventilation which is performed by means of a mechanical ventilator. The presence of a tube passing through the larynx for a prolonged period of time is associated with long-term damage to the larynx, and therefore any patients requiring prolonged intubation usually undergo a tracheostomy to prevent further damage to the larynx. Endotracheal intubation is also the preferred method of airway intervention for acute inflammatory disorders of the upper airway as opposed to tracheostomy. Tracheostomy in these cases is performed only in the emergency situation if facilities for endotracheal intubation are not available or if they are unsuccessful. Tracheostomy may also be performed for large tumours which obstruct the larynx until some form of treatment is instituted. Similarly it may be needed in conditions whereby the nerve supply to the larynx has been jeopardized impairing its protective function of the upper airway and its respiratory function.

Tracheostomy tubes: When the trachea has been opened it is necessary to introduce a tube in order to keep the opening from closing. The tubes are made either of hard rubber or more often of metal; and there is always an *outer tube* which is fixed in position by tapes passing round the neck, and an *inner tube* which slides freely out of and into the other, so that it may be removed at any time for cleansing, and is readily coughed out should it happen to become blocked by mucus.

A dressing is generally applied between the edges of the outer tube and the wound to prevent trauma to the skin of the neck.

The inner tube must be removed and washed several times daily, and if at any time it gets blocked by coughed-up mucus, it must be instantly removed and wiped. The outer tube is not removed till one or two days have elapsed after the operation, and then it is replaced by a fresh tube carefully introduced.

After-treatment: When the operation has been performed for some permanent obstruction, the tube must be worn permanently; and the double metal tube is in such cases replaced after a short time by a soft rubber single one. When the operation has relieved some passing condition like diphtheria, the tube is left out now and then for a few hours, and finally, at the end of a week or so, is removed altogether, after which the wound quickly heals up.

TRACHOMA (see EYE, DISEASES AND INJURIES OF).

TRACTOTOMY (see CORDOTOMY).

TRAGACANTH is a gummy exudation obtained from *Astragalusgummifer*, which swells out and forms a mucilage when mixed with water. It is used as a demulcent, or in mixtures to suspend heavy particles, such as bismuth.

TRAINING (see DIET; EXERCISE).

TRANCE is a profound sleep from which a person cannot for a time be aroused, but which is not due to organic disease. The power of voluntary movement is lost, though sensibility and even consciousness may remain. It is usually due to hysteria, and may be induced by hypnotism. (See CATALEPSY; ECSTASY; and SLEEP.)

TRANEXAMIC ACID is a drug used in the control of bleeding. Its mode of action is similar to that of aminocaproic acid (qv).

TRANQUILLIZER: A tranquillizer is a drug which induces a mental state free from agitation and anxiety, and renders the patient calm, serene and peaceful. Strictly speaking, tobacco, alcohol and the barbiturates might be included in this category, but the term 'tranquillizer' is usually restricted to certain new groups of drugs whose main action is the control of anxiety and psychomotor agitation without producing sleepiness, or clouding of consciousness. Among the more widely used drugs in this group are chlorpromazine, diazepam and chlordiazepoxide.

TRANSCUTANEOUS ELECTRICAL NERVE STIMULATION is a method of electrical stimulation that is being used for the relief of pain, including that of migraine, neuralgia and phantom limbs. Known as TENS, its mode of action appears to have some resemblance to that of acupuncture. Several controlled trials suggest that it provides at least a modicum of relief of pain after operations, thereby reducing the amount of analgesics that may be called for.

TRANSFUSION OF BLOOD is an old method of restoring a person believed to be dying by passing blood from another person into his veins. The practice was in vogue during the seventeenth century, and was performed either by bleeding a healthy person into a basin, and, by means of a syringe, injecting the blood into a cannula previously tied in one of the sick person's veins; or by uniting a vein in the healthy person with one in the sick person by means of two cannulae and a connecting tube, so that the blood passed directly from one to the other. In spite of all speed, the blood introduced by either of these methods was apt to clot; and the practice was adopted of whipping the blood with fine twigs, or straining it through muslin so as to remove its fibrin, and thus introduce merely the serum and blood corpuscles.

Apart from the difficulty caused by the tendency to clot, the major drawback to transfusion is that the corpuscles are liable to break up in the new circulation into which they are introduced; and the person into whom the new blood is transfused may suffer to a dangerous degree from symptoms such as nettle-rash, difficulty of breathing, purging, and signs of shock, whilst the immediate destruction of the red blood corpuscles leads to the passage of blood pigment in the urine and jaundice in some cases. A fatal result may quickly supervene.

To avoid this, it is necessary to find out that the blood of the donor is compatible with the blood already in the circulation of the recipient. (See BLOOD GROUPS.) Whenever possible, this should be done by people specially trained in the technique. In an emergency in a remote area, however, where such facilities are not available, compatibility of blood can be investigated by a relatively simple technique. A little blood is drawn from the recipient, and a drop of its serum mixed with a minute drop of blood from the donor, which has been allowed to drop into citrate of soda solution. If, in the course of a few minutes, the serum of the recipient causes clotting or breaking up of the donor's corpuscles, the two bloods are incompatible, and another donor of new blood must be chosen and similarly tested. Standard sera can also be obtained for testing the group to which the blood of the donor and that of the recipient belong.

Various methods of transfusion have been used at different times: such as by uniting a vessel in the donor with a vessel in the recipient by means of a short tube, while the two lie side by side; by withdrawing the blood into a syringe and then injecting it through a cannula into the recipient's vein; or by withdrawing the blood from the donor into a large glass vessel, coated with paraffin, which contains a small amount of citrate of soda solution intended to prevent clotting.

In Great Britain, however, all these methods have been given up since the inception, in 1946, of the National Blood Transfusion Service, which is responsible for the collection of blood from voluntary donors and for its storage in blood-banks throughout the country. In 1979 the Service collected almost two million donations of blood. A standard transfusion bottle has been evolved, with special apparatus for the taking and the giving of blood. When such a set is used with the proper technique, the blood can be safely stored at a temperature of 2° to 6°C for three weeks before use. In addition to whole blood, plasma or serum may be used for transfusion purposes. When stored in the dried form, human plasma and serum have proved to be valuable substitutes for whole blood. In the dried state human plasma is stable for five years provided it is stored at a moderate temperature (4·4° to 21·1°C) and is not exposed to direct sunlight. It is reconstituted by adding pyrogen-free distilled water.

EXCHANGE TRANSFUSION is the method of treatment in severe cases of haemolytic disease of the newborn (qv). It consists of replacing the whole of the baby's blood with Rh-negative blood of the correct blood group for the baby.

TRANSIENT ISCHAEMIC ATTACKS are episodes of transient ischaemia of some part of the cerebral hemispheres or the brain stem lasting anything from a few minutes to several hours and followed by complete recovery. By definition the ischaemic episode must be less than 24 hours. These episodes may be isolated or they may occur several times in a day. The cause is atheroma of the carotid or vertebral arteries and the embolisation of platelets or cholesterol. These attacks present with strokes that rapidly recover.

TRANSLOCATION is the term used to describe an exchange of genetic material between chromosomes (qv). It is an important factor in the etiology, or causation, of certain congenital abnormalities such as, for example mongolism. It is one of the main abnormalities sought for in amnioscopy (qv).

TRANSPLANTATION of organs of the body has become a practical possibility within recent years. It is still in its infancy, however, and many problems have to be solved before it can be used on anything like a large scale. The major outstanding problem is how to prevent the recipient's body from rejecting and destroying the transplanted organ. Such rejection of a foreign body is part of the normal protective mechanism of the body and is essential for the maintenance of the integrity of the body.

If the transplant comes from another person it is known as an *allotransplant*. If it comes from the patient himself – for example, a skin graft – it is known as an *autotransplant*. If it comes from an animal it is known as a *xenotransplant*.

Hitherto the major success has been achieved with transplantation of the kidney, and this has been most successful when the transplanted kidney has come from an identical twin. Less successful have been live transplants from other blood relatives, while least successful have been transplants from other live donors and cadaver donors. The results, however, are steadily improving. Thus the one-year functional survival of kidneys transplanted from unrelated cadaver donors has risen from around 50 per cent to over 80 per cent, and survival rates of 80 per cent after three years are not uncommon. For a well-matched transplant from a live related donor the survival rate after five years is around 80 per cent. And, of course, if a transplanted kidney fails to function, the patient can always be switched on to some form of dialysis (qv). In the United Kingdom the number of kidney transplants in 1982 was 1098 while the waiting list for such transplantations was 2494. The present supply of cadaveric kidneys for transplantation is only about half that necessary to meet the demand. One of the reasons for this shortage is the lack of awareness of the extent of the shortage, of the high degree of success which now results from renal transplantation and of the benefits it brings to patients. Donor cards are now available in all general practitioners' surgeries and pharmacies. The tragedy is that of the 16 million cards distributed since

1972, so few have been used. At the end of 1984, in the United Kingdom there were 5609 people alive with functioning renal transplants, and 5661 on dialysis.

Drugs are now available that can depress the immune reactions of the recipient, which are responsible for the rejection of the transplanted organ. Notable among these is cyclosporin A. By these and other means, such as careful typing of the donor kidney, results are steadily improving. One of the more promising developments is the development of an anti-lymphocytic serum (ALS) which reduces the activity of the lymphocytes (qv), cells which play an important part in maintaining the integrity of the body against foreign bodies.

Other organs that have been transplanted are the heart, the lungs, the liver, bone marrow, and the cornea of the eye. With the exception of the last two of these, the results are not as satisfactory as in the case of kidney, but the results are improving. Thus, in one centre in USA, of 150 heart transplantations done in a 10-year period (1968–78), the one-year survival rate was 70 per cent, and one patient is still alive eight years after the operation. The total number of patients who had heart transplants between 1979–1985 is 377 of whom 275 are alive. The total number of transplants undertaken between 1982 and 1986 is 518. The heart, however, seems to be more liable to rejection than the kidney. The liver seems to be less susceptible to rejection, and of the 200 patients who have had the operation in one USA hospital, one is alive ten years after transplantation and two have given birth to normal children. In this country, of the 108 patients who have had a liver transplant over the last thirteen years at the Cambridge/King's College, London, Centre, 20 are alive, and three have survived for more than five years. Over half of the last 22 transplanted have survived for one year. It is estimated that approximately 200 patients a year between the ages of 15 and 55 would benefit from a liver transplant if an adequate number of potential donors were available. The number of liver transplants carried out in the U.K. in 1986 was 127.

A code of practice for procedures relating to the removal of organs for transplantation was produced in 1978 and this code has been revised in the light of further views expressed by the Conference of Medical Royal Colleges and Faculties of the United Kingdom on the Diagnosis of Brain Death. Under the Human Tissue Act 1961 only the person lawfully in possession of the body or his designate can authorize the removal of organs from a body. This authorization may be given orally. Patients who may become suitable donors after death are those who have suffered severe and irreversible brain damage. Such patients will be dependent on artificial ventilation. Patients with malignant disease or systemic infection and patients with renal disease, including chronic hypertension, are unsuitable. If a patient carries a signed donor card or has otherwise recorded his wishes there is no legal requirement to establish lack of objection on the part of relatives, although it is good practice to take account of the views of close relatives. If a relative objects, despite the known request by the patient, staff will need to judge, according to the circumstances of the case, whether it is wise to proceed with organ removal. If a patient who has died is not known to have requested that his organs be removed for transplantation after his death the designated person may only authorize the removal if, having made such reasonable enquiry as may be practical he has no reason to believe (*a*) that the deceased had expressed an objection to his body being so dealt with after his death, or (*b*) that the surviving spouse or any surviving relative of the deceased objects to the body being so dealt with. Staff will need to decide who is best qualified to approach the relatives. This should be someone with appropriate experience who is aware how much the relative already knows about the patient's condition. Relatives should not normally be approached before death has occurred but sometimes a relative approaches the hospital staff and suggests sometime in advance that the patient's kidneys might be used for transplantation after his death. The staff of hospitals and organ exchange organizations must respect the wishes of the donor, the recipient and their families with respect to anonimity.

Relatives who enquire should be told that some post-mortem treatment of the donor's body will be necessary if the organs are to be removed in good condition. It is ethical to maintain artificial ventilation and heart beat until removal of organs has been completed. This is essential in the case of heart and liver transplants and many doctors think it is desirable when removing kidneys.

TRANS-SEXUALISM is the psycho-sexual abnormality characterized by feelings of belonging to the gender opposite to that of the genitalia and the secondary sex characteristics. Those suffering from this condition can obtain help and guidance from SHAFT (Self-Help Association for Transsexuals), Secretary, BM Box 7624, London WC1N 3XX (021–3551579 after working hours).

TRANSVESTITISM, or TRANSVESTISM, is the term given to a psycho-sexual abnormality in which there is a repetitive compulsion to dress in the clothes of the opposite sex to achieve orgasm.

TRANYLCYPROMINE (PARNATE) (see ANTIDEPRESSANTS).

TRAUMA is the term used to indicate disorders due to wounds or injuries.

TRAVEL MEDICINE: There are reciprocal health arrangements with the other European

Economic Community (EEC) countries and with the following countries – Austria, Bulgaria, the Channel Islands, Czechoslovakia, German Democratic Republic (East Germany), Gibraltar, Malta, New Zealand, Norway, Poland, Romania, Sweden, USSR, and Yugoslavia – under which British visitors may receive emergency treatment free or at reduced cost. Information about these arrangements is available in leaflets SA28 (EEC countries) and SA30 (other countries), which may be obtained from Leaflets Unit, Department of Health and Social Security, Government Buildings, Honeypot Lane, Stanmore, Middlesex HA7 1AY (01–952 2311), or from local offices of the Department. The Department also publishes a useful leaflet (SA35), *Notice to Travellers: Health Protection*, which gives information about the health aspects of foreign travel, such as personal protection against various diseases and the like. This is available free of charge from International Relations Division, Room D3081, Alexander Fleming House, Elephant and Castle, London SE1 6BY, or through travel agents. Another useful source of reliable information is *Preservation of Personal Health in Warm Climates*, published by the Ross Institute of Tropical Hygiene, London (price £2). This provides a concise and detailed account of health problems, how they arise and how they are coped with.

The following is a list of Centres specializing in medical advice for travellers going overseas:

Communicable Diseases (Scotland) Unit, Ruchill Hospital, Glasgow G20 9NB. Tel: 041-946 7120.

Department of Communicable and Tropical Diseases, East Birmingham Hospital, Bordesley Green East, Birmingham B9 5ST. Tel: 021-772 4311.

Department of Health and Social Security, Alexander Fleming House, Elephant and Castle, London SE1 6BY. Tel: 01-407 5522.

Hospital for Tropical Diseases, 4 St Pancras Way, London NW1 0PE. Tel: 01-387 4411.

Liverpool School of Tropical Medicine, Pembroke Place, Liverpool L3 5QA. Tel: 051-708 9393.

Ross Institute of Tropical Hygiene, London School of Hygiene and Tropical Medicine, Keppel Street, London WC1E 7HT. Tel: 01-636 8636.

TRAVEL SICKNESS is the sickness that is induced by any form of transport, whether by sea, air, motor-car or train. (See SEA-SICKNESS.)

TRAVELLER'S DIARRHOEA is an all too common affliction of the traveller, which basks in a multiplicity of names: eg. Aden gut, Aztec two step, Basra belly, Delhi belly, Gippy tummy, Hong Kong dog, Montezuma's revenge, Tokyo trots, turista. It is caused by a variety of micro-organisms, usually *E. coli*. Some people seem to be more prone to it than others, though for no good cause. Obvious preventive measures include the avoidance of salads, unpeeled fruit and ice cream, and never drinking unboiled or unbottled water. Two widely recommended preventive drugs are Streptotriad (one tablet twice daily for a week, and then one daily) and doxycycline (100 mg daily). Both are said to provide a satisfactory degree of protection, provided a fulminating infection is avoided, as long as taken.

TRAZODONE (MOLIPAXIN) (see ANTI-DEPRESSANTS).

TREMOR means a very fine kind of involuntary movement. Tremors may be seen in projecting parts like the hands, head and tongue, or they may involve muscles or even the individual fibres of a muscle here and there. They are of various grades of fineness. Very coarse tremors, which prevent a person from drinking a glass of water without spilling it, are found in multiple sclerosis and in chorea (see under these headings); somewhat finer tremors, which produce trembling of the hands or tongue when they are stretched out, are caused by alcoholism (see ALCOHOLISM, CHRONIC), by poisoning with other substances like lead, by Parkinsonism (qv), and by the weakness which follows some acute disease or characterizes old age; a fine tremor of the outstretched fingers is a characteristic of thyrotoxicosis (see GOITRE); very fine tremors, visible in the muscles of face or limbs, and known as fibrillary tremors, are present in general paralysis of the insane, and in progressive muscular atrophy or wasting palsy. Tremors may occur at rest and disappear on movement as in Parkinsonism, or they may occur only on movement (intention tremors) as in cerebellar disease.

TRENCH FEVER is an infectious disease caused by *Rickettsiaquintana* which is transmitted by the body louse. Large epidemics occurred among troops on active service during the 1914–18 War. It recurred on a smaller scale in the 1939–45 War, and is endemic in Mexico.

TRENCH, or IMMERSION, **FOOT** is due to prolonged exposure of the feet to water, particularly cold water. Trench warfare is a common precipitating factor, and it was rampant during the 1914–18 War. Cases also occurred during the 1939–45 War, particularly during the slow winter advance up through Italy after the Anzio landings. Cases occurred, too, during the Falklands campaign. The less common form due to warm water immersion occurred with some frequency in the Vietnam war. It is characterized by painful swelling of the feet accompanied in due course by blistering and ulceration which, in severe, untreated cases, may go on to gangrene. In mild cases recovery may be complete in a month, but severe cases may drag on for a year.

Treatment: Drying of the feet overnight, where practicable, is the best method of prevention, accompanied by avoidance of constrictive clothing and tight boots, and of prolonged immobility. Frequent rest periods and daily changing of socks also help. The application of silicone grease once a day is another useful preventive measure. In the early stages treatment consists of rest in bed and warmth. In more severe cases treatment is as for infected tissues and ulceration. Analgesics (qv) are usually necessary to ease the pain. Technically, smoking should be forbidden, but the psychological effects in troops on active service may outweigh its advantages.

TREPHINING, or TREPANNING, is an operation in which a portion of the cranium is removed. Originally the operation was performed with an instrument resembling a carpenter's brace and known as the trephine or trepan, which removes a small circle of bone; but now this instrument is only used, as a rule, for making small openings, whilst, for wider operations, gouge forceps, circular saws driven by electric motor, or wire saws are employed in order to give greater ease and speed.

The operation is one requiring nicety of manipulation, but is neither difficult nor serious, and was one of the commonest major operations of antiquity. It is said, from the appearances presented by skulls found in old French burial mounds, to have been practised by prehistoric peoples; at all events Hippocrates describes fully the operation and the conditions that call for it, whilst Galen mentions two varieties of the instrument in common use. Both among the Greeks and Romans, and in the Middle Ages, resort seems to have been made to trephining on very slight provocation for conditions traceable to the head.

At the present time, the conditions under which it may be thought advisable to trephine the skull are chiefly as follows. In cases of fracture, with splintering of the skull, the operation is performed to remove the fragments of bone and any foreign bodies, like a bullet, which may have entered, in order that the wound may be thoroughly cleansed. In compression of the brain with unconsciousness following an injury, the skull is trephined and any blood-clots removed, or torn vessels ligatured. When an abscess is present within the skull, the operation is called for in order to evacuate the pus. In certain forms of epilepsy, or in continued headache, when the symptoms point to a definite part of the brain being involved, the skull may be trephined over this area, so that any clot, scar, thickening of the bone or cyst, which is setting up the irritation, may be discovered and removed. For a cerebral tumour, trephining is often performed either with the view of removing the tumour, if possible, or at all events of relieving the great pressure within the skull caused by the growing mass.

TREPONEMA is the name of a genus of spirochaetal micro-organisms which consist of slender spirals and which progress by means of bending movements. *Treponema pallidum* (formerly called *Spirochaeta pallida*) is the causative organism of syphilis.

TRIAMCINOLONE is a corticosteroid (qv), which has a potency equivalent to that of prednisone, but is less likely to cause retention of sodium.

TRIAMTERINE (DYTAC) is a potassium-sparing diuretic which is active when taken by mouth. (See DIURETICS.)

TRIAZOLAM (HALCION) (see BENZOTHIAZEPINES).

TRICHIASIS: A condition in which the eyelashes become ingrown.

TRICHINIASIS (see TRICHINOSIS).

TRICHINOSIS, or TRICHINIASIS, is the name of a disease set up by eating diseased pork, in which the immature *Trichinella spiralis* is encysted. The full-grown female worm, which inhabits the intestine, is 3 mm in length, and the larvae, to whose movements the disease is due, are much smaller. The disease is acquired by eating raw or underdone pork from pigs that have been infected with the worm. When such a piece of meat is eaten, the embryos contained in it are set free, develop into full-grown trichinellae, and from each pair of these 1000 or more new embryos may arise in a few weeks. So soon as this new generation of embryos is produced they bore their way into the wall of the bowel, setting up sometimes severe irritation and diarrhoea, and thence wander all over the body, finally depositing themselves between the fibres of the voluntary muscles. During this migration, which lasts four or five weeks, they set up fever and pain in the limbs and muscles, often mistaken for rheumatism. Death may even result, but if the person survives to the end of four or five weeks, the trichinellae, which are now encysted in the muscles, give no further trouble.

Prevention is based on thorough inspection of meat in slaughter-houses, for even cooking, unless the meat is in slices, is not an efficient protection. Pigs should not be fed on unboiled garbage. Rats may be a source of sporadic outbreaks, as infected rats have been found near piggeries. The disease is now a rare one, thanks to sanitary inspection though it still occurs in these parts of the country, such as the Midlands, where raw sausage meat is considered a delicacy. The encysted trichinellae are just visible as fine white specks.

Treatment: In the early stages, tetrachloroethylene, followed by a sharp purge, is of value. Recently, thiabendazole, which has proved of value in the treatment of affected pigs, has been used with promising results in human victims.

TRICHLOROETHYLENE, also known as TRILENE, is a volatile anaesthetic which has the advantages of being non-irritant and of inducing anaesthesia rapidly and pleasantly. It has been used mainly for inducing analgesia or light anaesthesia in obstetrics and dentistry. In an impure form it is used commercially in the dry-cleaning industry.

TRICHO- is a prefix denoting relation to hair.

TRICHOMONAS VAGINALIS is a protozoon normally present in the vagina of about 30 to 40 per cent of women. It sometimes becomes pathogenic and causes inflammation of the genital passages, with vaginal discharge. A man may become infected as a result of sexual intercourse with an infected woman and have a urethral discharge as a result; it may also cause prostatitis. Excellent results are being obtained from the use of metronidazole in its treatment. To obtain a satisfactory result it may be necessary to treat both partners.

TRICHOMONIASIS is the disease caused by infection with *Trichomonas vaginalis* (qv).

TRICHOPHYTON is the parasite that causes ringworm. (See RINGWORM.)

TRICHORRHOEA is the term applied to the falling-out of hair. It is usually due to some general disease such as scarlet fever or typhoid fever. When there is no obvious cause, such as this, treatment consists of attention to the general hygiene of the scalp. Vigorous massage is to be avoided.

TRICHOTILLOMANIA is the condition in which a person has an obsessional impulse to pull out his own hair.

TRICHURIASIS is a worldwide infection, particularly common in the tropics. It is caused by *Trichuris trichiura*, or whipworm, so called because of its shape, the rear end being stout and the front end hairlike, resembling the lash of a whip. The male measures 5 cm and the female 4 cm in length. Infection results from eating vegetables, or drinking water, polluted with the ova (eggs). These hatch out in the large intestine. The diagnosis is made by finding the eggs in the stools. The worms seldom cause any trouble unless they are present in large numbers when, especially in malnourished children, they may cause bleeding from the bowels, anaemia and prolapse of the rectum. The most effective drug at the moment is mebendazole: 100 mg twice daily for three days.

TRICRESOL is a clear, colourless, strongly antiseptic mixture of the three forms of cresol. It may be mixed with water in any proportions. (For uses see CRESOL.)

TRICUSPID VALVE is the valve, with three cusps or flaps, that guards the opening from the right atrium into the right ventricle of the heart. (See HEART.)

TRIFLUOPERAZINE (STELAZINE) (see ANTI-PSYCHOTIC DRUGS).

TRIGEMINAL NERVE is the fifth cranial nerve. It consists of three divisions: (1) the ophthalmic nerve, which is purely sensory in function, being distributed mainly over the forehead and front part of the scalp; (2) the maxillary nerve, which is also sensory and distributed to the skin of the cheek, the mucous membrane of the mouth and throat, and the upper teeth; and (3) the mandibular nerve, which is the nerve of sensation to the lower part of the face, the tongue and the lower teeth, as well as being the motor nerve to the muscles concerned in chewing. The trigeminal nerve is of special interest, owing to its liability to neuralgia (qv), trigeminal neuralgia (qv), or tic douloureux as it is also known, being the most painful form known of neuralgia.

TRIGEMINAL NEURALGIA, or TIC DOULOUREUX, is one of the most severe forms of neuralgia. It affects the great nerve of sensation in the face (trigeminal nerve), and may occur in one or more of the three divisions in which the nerve is distributed. It is usually confined to one side. Women suffer, on the whole, more often than men, and they are usually over the age of 50. The attack is often precipitated by movements of the jaw, as in talking or eating, or by tactile stimuli such as a cold wind or washing the face. When the *first or upper division of the nerve* is involved, the pain is mostly felt in the forehead and side of the head. It is usually of an intensely sharp, cutting, or burning character, either constant or with exacerbations, and often periodic, returning at a certain hour each day while the attack continues. Occasionally the paroxysms are of extreme violence, and are brought on by the slightest provocation, such as a draught of cool air. The skin over the affected part is often red and swollen, and, even after the attack has abated, feels stiff and tender to the touch. As in all forms of neuralgia, there are certain localities where the pain is more intense, these painful points, as they are called, being for the most part in those places where the branches of the nerves emerge from bony canals or pierce the fascia to ramify in the skin. Hence, in this form, the greater severity of the pain above the eyebrow and along the side of the nose. There is also pain in the eyelid, redness of the eye and increased flow of tears. When the *second division of the nerve* is affected, the pain is chiefly in the cheek and upper jaw, the painful points being immediately below the lower eyelid, over the cheekbone and about the upper lip. This form is accompanied by pain of similar character to that affecting the first division; the pain often appears suddenly on slight provocation such as by taking a mouthful of hot or cold fluid. When *the third division of the nerve* suffers, the pain affects the lower jaw, and the chief painful points are in front of the ear and above the chin. Attacks of tic douloureux, extremely distressing as they are, may recur for years; and although, by depriving the sufferer of sleep and interfering with the taking of food, they may in some measure impair the health, they rarely appear to lead to any serious results. Nevertheless, the pain may be so intolerable as to make life a burden.

Treatment: The outlook in trigeminal neuralgia has been radically altered by the introduction of the drug carbamazepine, which is proving of outstanding value in relieving the pain of what is one of the most devastating of all forms of neuralgia. In view of its potential side-effects, it must only be taken under medical supervision. The introduction of this drug has radically cut down the need for killing the ganglion of the nerve, or its branches, by the injection of alcohol, electrocoagulation, percutaneous or radio frequency gangliolysis, or rhizotomy (qv).

TRIGGER FINGER, or SNAPPING FINGER, is the condition in which when the fingers are straightened on unclenching the fist one finger, usually the ring or middle finger, remains bent. The cause is obscure. In severe cases treatment consists of opening up the sheath surrounding the tendon of the affected finger. When confined to the thumb it is known as TRIGGER THUMB.

TRIGGER THUMB (see TRIGGER FINGER).

TRIGONE is the base of the bladder between the openings of the two ureters and of the urethra.

TRIIODOTHYRONINE is the substance which exerts the physiological action of thyroid hormone. It is formed in the body cells by the deiodination of thyroxine (tetra-iodothyronine) which is the active principle secreted by the thyroid gland. It has also been synthesized, and is now available for the treatment of myxoedema (qv). It is three times as potent as thyroxine. (See also THYROID GLAND.)

TRILENE (see TRICHLOROETHYLENE).

TRIMETHORIM is an anti-bacterial agent which is proving of value in the treatment of infections of the urinary tract. It is also a constituent of co-trimoxazole (qv).

TRIMIPRAMINE (SURMONTIL) is a relatively weak antidepressant drug which also acts as a sedative. (See ANTIDEPRESSANTS.)

TRIMUSTINE is a nitrogen mustard derivative (qv) used in the treatment of certain forms of malignant disease. It is administered intravenously.

TRINITRIN (see GLYCERYL TRINITRATE).

TRIOSORBON (see ENTERAL FEEDING).

TRIPLETS (see MULTIPLE BIRTHS).

TRISMUS is another name for lockjaw. (See TETANUS.)

TROCAR is an instrument provided with a sharp three-sided point fitted inside a tube or cannula, and used for puncturing cavities of the body in which fluid has collected.

TROCHANTER is the name given to two bony prominences at the upper end of the thigh-bone. The *greater trochanter* can be felt on the outer side of the thigh. The *lesser trochanter* is a small prominence on the inner side of this bone.

TROCHES is another name for lozenges. (See LOZENGES.)

TROCHLEAR NERVE is the fourth cranial nerve, which acts upon the superior oblique muscle of the eye.

TROPHIC is a term applied to the influence that nerves exert with regard to the healthiness and nourishment of the parts to which they run. When the nerves become diseased or injured, this influence is lost and the muscles waste, while the skin loses its healthy appearance and is liable to break down into ulcers. (See NERVOUS DISEASES; BED SORES.)

TROPHOBLAST is the outer layer of the fertilized ovum which attaches the ovum to the wall of the uterus (or womb) and supplies nutrition to the embryo.

TROPICAL DISEASES: This term includes some diseases that occur in temperate climates, but are more common or more severe in hot latitudes; as well as some that are found only in the tropics. (See ANCYLOSTOMIASIS; BERIBERI; BLACKWATER FEVER; CHOLERA; CLIMATE; CLOTHING; DENGUE; DRACONTIASIS; DYSENTERY; ELEPHANTIASIS; FILARIASIS; FRAMBOESIA; HEATSTROKE; HOOKWORM; LEISHMANIASIS; LEPROSY; LIVER, DISEASES OF; MALARIA; ORIENTAL SORE; PLAGUE; PRICKLY HEAT; SCHISTOSOMIASIS; SLEEPING SICKNESS; STRONGLYLOIDIASIS; SUNBURN; YELLOW FEVER.)

TROXIDONE is one of the most effective drugs for the treatment of *petit mal*. (See EPILEPSY.)

TRUSS is an instrument used to support a hernia; or to retain the protruding organ within the cavity from which it tends to pass.

Varieties of truss: The nature of trusses varies according to the situation of the opening which the truss has to cover; but every truss possesses a pad of some sort to cover the opening and a belt or spring to keep it in position.

VENTRAL TRUSSES intended for a hernia protruding through the wall of the abdomen, either at the navel or at some weak spot caused by a strain or by a wound, consist of a large flat pad kept in position by a belt passing round the waist. Sometimes a small pad made to fit the opening is adopted, but this is a mistake, as its pressure tends to enlarge the aperture.

INGUINAL TRUSSES are much more commonly required than any other, and though many forms are made by different makers, all possess an oval obliquely placed pad with a spring pressing upon it. In the *ordinary truss* there is a spring firmly fixed at one end to the pad, from which it passes right round the waist, to be bound at the other end by a short strap to the pad. Also there is a short strap passing down between the legs and fastened to the truss before and behind so as to keep the pad from slipping upwards as the person moves. This is one of the cheapest and most generally used forms. *Double trusses* are fashioned like the ordinary truss, but have a pad for each side, and are advisable in the case of very stout people, in whom the retention of a hernia upon one side is sometimes apt to produce a hernia at the other side.

FEMORAL TRUSSES are made in various forms similar to those of inguinal trusses. The pad, which comes down on the thigh, is small and triangular, so as not to press upon the femoral vessels. Such a truss is difficult to keep in position, and this is sometimes effected by having attached to the pad a thigh-piece which can be laced on the outer side of the thigh.

Before applying a truss the wearer must make certain that the hernia has been reduced. This may mean lying down before applying the truss. The skin should be washed twice daily with soap and water then wiped gently with surgical spirit, and finally dusted with some benign dusting powder. In this way there is little risk of the underlying skin becoming sore and irritated. Saddle soap is used to keep the leather parts of the truss in good condition.

TRYPANOSOMA is a genus of microscopic parasites, several of which are responsible for causing sleeping sickness and some allied diseases. (See SLEEPING SICKNESS.)

TRYPANOSOMIASIS (see SLEEPING SICKNESS.)

TRYPSIN is the chief protein ferment of the pancreatic secretion. It changes proteins into peptones and forms the main constituent of pancreatic extracts used for digestion of food. (See PANCREAS; PEPTONIZED FOOD.)

TSETSE FLY is an African fly of the genus *Glossina*. One or more of these is responsible for carrying the trypanosome which causes sleeping sickness and thus spreads the disease among cattle and from cattle to men.

TSUTSUGAMUSHI, or JAPANESE RIVER FEVER, is a disease of the typhus group. (See TYPHUS.)

TUBERCLE is a term used in two distinct senses. As a descriptive term in anatomy, a *tubercle* means a small elevation or roughness upon a bone, such as the tubercles of the ribs. In the pathological sense, a *tubercle* is a small mass, barely visible to the naked eye, formed in some organ as the starting-point of tuberculosis. The name of *tubercle bacillus* was originally given to the micro-organism that causes this disease but this has now been changed to *Mycobacterium tuberculosis*. The term tubercular should strictly be applied to anything connected with or resembling tubercles or nodules, and the term *tuberculous* to anything pertaining to the disease tuberculosis.

When *Mycobacteria tuberculosis* have gained entrance to an organ, no matter whether inhaled, or whether absorbed from food and circulated through the lymphatics or blood-vessels, the following results ensue. The individual bacilli multiply, and around each group forms a minute tubercle, or granule, which is of a size almost invisible to the naked eye, and greyish in colour. These tubercles fuse together, and, at the same time, soften to a cheesy substance, so as to form yellow bodies about the size of pinheads. Each grey tubercle, under the microscope, shows the appearance of a group of cells of medium size (epithelioid cells), surrounded by many smaller cells (connective tissue cells and white blood corpuscles), attracted to the spot as a result of the inflammation set up. Scattered between these cells lie the mycobacteria. Near the centre of the older tubercles there are often seen one or more large cells with many nuclei (giant cells). The larger yellow tubercles form a more or less structureless mass in the centre, but show numbers of the small grey tubercles round their edge. Thus the process spreads, the healthy tissue being broken down and giving place to the soft, cheesy mass, which, in the case of the lungs, finally bursts into a bronchial tube, is coughed up, and leaves a ragged cavity in its place. Another change, however, takes place at the same time, for, in consequence of the irritation set up by the tubercle, strands of fibrous tissue are built up round its edge, and, when the process is a very chronic one, these come to form a dense capsule for the tuberculous area, cutting it off from further advance on healthy tissue, and forming a natural cure.

TUBERCULIDE is the term given to any skin lesion which is the result of infection with the tubercle bacillus, or *Mycobacterium tuberculosis* as it is now known.

TUBERCULIN is the name originally given by Koch in 1890 to a preparation derived from the tubercle bacillus, or *Mycobacterium tuberculosis* as it is now known, and intended for the diagnosis or treatment of tuberculosis.

Varieties: *Old Tuberculin* (OT) is the heat-concentrated filtrate from a fluid medium on which the human or bovine type of *Mycobacterium tuberculosis* has been grown for six weeks or more. *Tuberculin Purified Protein Derivative* (Tuberculin PPD) is the active principle of Old Tuberculin, and is prepared from the fluid medium on which the *Mycobacterium tuberculosis* has been grown. It is supplied as a liquid, a powder, or as sterile tablets. The liquid contains 100,000 Units per millilitre, and the dry powder contains 30,000 Units per milligram. It is distributed in sterile containers sealed so as to exclude micro-organisms. It is more constant in composition and potency than Old Tuberculin.

Uses: The basis of the tuberculin reaction is that any person who has been infected with the *Mycobacterium tuberculosis* gives a reaction when a small amount of tuberculin is injected into the skin. This reaction consists of an inflammatory area, at least 5 mm in diameter, which develops at the site of the test within two to four days of the test being made. If the area is less than 5 mm in diameter the reaction is said to be negative. A negative reaction means that either the individual has never been infected with the tubercle bacillus, or that the infection has been too recent to have allowed of sensitivity developing. The only exceptions are that occasionally a negative reaction may be obtained in tuberculous subjects (*a*) in severe forms of the disease, (*b*) during pregnancy, (*c*) during an intercurrent infection.

To avoid serious reactions the test must be carried out in the first instance with a dilution of tuberculin of 1/10,000. If no reaction is obtained, the strength can be gradually increased: 1/1000; 1/100; 1/10. The amount used of any dilution is 0·1 millilitre.

There are various methods of carrying out the test, of which the following are the most commonly used. The *Mantoux Test* is the most satisfactory of all and has the advantage that the size of the reaction is a guide to the severity of the tuberculous infection. It is performed by injecting the tuberculin into the skin on the forearm. The *Heaf Multiple Puncture Test* is being used on an increasing scale because of its simplicity and reliability. It is carried out with the multiple puncture apparatus, or Heaf Gun, which enables six punctures to be made of equal depth: 2 mm for adults, 1 mm for children, depending upon which of the two detachable endpieces is used. The *Vollmer Patch Test* is particularly useful in children because of the ease with which it can be carried out. A piece of filter paper impregnated with tuberculin is fastened to the skin with adhesive plaster and left in position for forty-eight hours.

TUBERCULOSIS is the general name for the whole group of diseases associated with the presence of the *Mycobacterium tuberculosis*, of which pulmonary tuberculosis is the most important. (See BACTERIOLOGY.)

Tuberculosis not only affects the lungs, but may invade almost any organ, being seldom found, however, in the muscles or in tissues with few blood-vessels, like cartilage and sinews. The disease spreads usually by way of the lymphatic vessels. The severity of the disease varies considerably, according to the organ attacked – thus tuberculosis affecting the membranes of the brain and causing meningitis is a particularly dangerous disease, especially in infants and young children. Chronic inflammation of bones and white swelling of joints are manifestations of the disease, having less influence upon the general health. The enlargement of glands, most common in the neck, to which the name of scrofula was formerly given, because the swollen neck gives to the physiognomy a pig-like expression, is a well-known form of tuberculous disease. This form of the disease seems to have been much more widespread in former times, and was known also as 'king's evil', from the superstition that a touch of the royal hand conveyed a cure to the affected person. Many chronic abscesses are tuberculous in origin, arising from this affection in a bone, a gland, or the cellular tissue. The disfiguring skin disease known as lupus vulgaris is another of the manifestations of the disease. Other sites in which tuberculosis is apt to occur are the bowels and the genito-urinary tract: ie. the kidneys, bladder and epididymis.

Consumption, or phthisis, is the name given, in popular language, to tuberculosis. It dates from the days when there was no effective treatment for tuberculosis, and the disease tended to be characterized by a rapid or gradual wasting away of the body. The term phthisis was usually restricted to that form of the disease in which the infection was restricted to the lungs: ie. pulmonary tuberculosis.

The essential part of the disease, from which it receives its name of tuberculosis, is the formation in the substance of an organ of tubercles, fine granules of a size barely visible to the naked eye, these tubercles multiplying and changing in such a way as to lead finally to the destruction of the organ in which they are found.

Nature of the disease: Tuberculosis has been recognized as a disease from the earliest times. Hippocrates (460–375 BC) bestowed the name of phthisis upon the disease as it affects the lungs, and descriptions of the condition are found in the writings of classical authors. About AD 980 Haly Abbas of Baghdad, and again in 1779 Cullen, recognized the infectious nature of phthisis, but not till after the middle of the nineteenth century was it proved, by means of inoculating animals with tuberculous material from phthisical patients, that tuberculosis is really an infective disease, and that the tubercles result from an inflammatory process, due to some poison introduced with the diseased products. The nature of the poison was much disputed till 1882, when Koch announced the discovery of the tubercle bacillus, or *Mycobacterium tuberculosis* as it is now known, and so answered this important question.

The manner in which these bacilli gain access to the body is important. There are three possible channels:

(*a*) By INOCULATION: A person may prick himself with a knife contaminated by the sputum of a tuberculous patient, or may rub some of this material into a cut. Generally this results merely in a local skin disease, and it occurs only in doctors, nurses and others dealing with tuberculous patients, or in veterinary surgeons or others dealing with tuberculous animals.

(*b*) By INHALATION: The sputum and other discharges from tuberculous people swarm with bacilli. It has been calculated that a person suffering from a cavity in the lung may spit up 4,000,000,000 bacilli in the course of twenty-four hours, and each of these, when dried and blown about on dust, is potent for evil. Neither drying, nor freezing, nor putrefaction, nor the lapse of months destroys these bacilli, but direct sunlight is speedily fatal to them, so that dust which has lain for a short time in the open on a bright day becomes rapidly harmless. In rooms inhabited by tuberculous patients, and in hospital wards, the dust from the floor often contains *Mycobacterium tuberculosis.*

Probably almost all cases in which this disease primarily affects the lungs are due to inhalation of dust laden with the bacilli or inhalation of droplets coughed into the air by a tuberculous patient, whilst those cases in which the glands of the neck are first attacked arise by absorption of the bacilli through the tonsils.

That this manner of infection is of great importance is shown by the fact that, of all people dying of tuberculous diseases generally in England and Wales over 90 per cent die from this disease as it affects the lungs.

(*c*) By INGESTION: It has long been known that tuberculosis, like other infectious diseases, can be conveyed by means of milk and other articles of food, and, acting upon this belief, sanitary authorities have enforced regulations designed to protect the public from the effects of consuming diseased meat and milk. In the case of meat there is practically no danger, as the muscular tissues are exempt from the disease, and those parts which are diseased being, in the 'dressing' of the meat, carefully removed, any accidental contact with them is rendered harmless by the cooking of the meat.

The Royal Commission on Tuberculosis in its report issued in 1907, as well as various other observers, found that the bovine tubercle bacillus was present in a large proportion of diseased glands in children. It has also been found that in tuberculosis affecting the bones and joints of children, from one-third to one-half are caused by the bovine bacillus, the rest by the human bacillus.

Much progress has been made of recent years in eradicating tuberculosis from cattle in this country, and on October 1, 1960, the Ministry of Agriculture, Fisheries and Food declared the whole of Great Britain an attested area, thus marking the successful completion of the official scheme to eradicate bovine tuberculosis as a disease of cattle on a nation-wide scale. Even though milk from such attested cattle, as they are known, is safe to drink from the point of tuberculosis, it is still a wise precaution to allow children to drink only pasteurized milk.

Mortality: In England in 1980 there were 435 deaths from respiratory tuberculosis and 399 deaths from other forms of the disease. In 1984 notifications of all forms of tuberculosis totalled 5,877.

A much larger number of the population suffer from early tuberculosis (it may be quite unsuspected) and recover. This is proved by the frequent presence on X-ray examination of old calcified tuberculous glands and by healed scars in the lungs found at post-mortem examination.

Causes: The direct cause of the disease is the *Mycobacteriumtuberculosis.* (See BACTERIOLOGY.) But, in view of the fact that many people suffer from the disease in a mild degree and afterwards recover, and that many limited cases of tuberculosis in bones, skin and glands are successfully treated, it appears that there are other factors which determine whether a given case is serious or not, and whether it is likely to proceed towards recovery, if properly treated, or to end inevitably in death.

HEREDITY: There is probably a hereditary element in the predisposition to the disease. Over a long period those who are susceptible are gradually eliminated by the disease.

AGE is an important point. Young children are liable to tuberculosis affecting the bowels and the glands connected with them, and the meninges of the brain. At a slightly later age there is a greater tendency to that type of the disease formerly known as scrofula, the glands of the neck particularly being affected, and the greatest mortality from lung (or pulmonary) tuberculosis takes place after the age of 20 is reached. In recent years there has been an increasing incidence of respiratory, or pulmonary, tuberculosis in old people. In England, in 1984, of the 745 deaths from tuberculosis, only 5 per cent were people aged less than 45 years, compared to 34 per cent of 7,797 deaths in 1954.

ATMOSPHERE: The character of the atmosphere in which work is carried on has much to do with the onset of tuberculosis. Those who habitually live and work in ill-ventilated rooms are at a great disadvantage compared with those who lead an open-air life, or, at all events, keep their rooms well ventilated. Further, the amount and nature of the dust in the air are highly important.

OTHER DISEASES are of great importance in relation to tuberculosis. For example, a person who has long suffered from asthma or bronchitis may develop tuberculosis in the end, and diabetics not uncommonly contract this disease, but this has happened less often since the introduction of insulin. It is not uncommon that a person suffers from tuberculosis and apparently recovers; then, when some business reverse or family trouble comes, the disease reappears.

Varieties: The forms of tuberculosis other than pulmonary tuberculosis, such as tuberculous disease of joints, bones and spine, meningitis, intestine, lupus, are considered under these headings. The lung disease has, however, itself several varieties, differing much from one another.

1. ACUTE MILIARY TUBERCULOSIS: In this form not only the lungs but the whole body becomes studded with the tubercles of the disease as a result of rupture of a tubercle or tuberculous gland into the blood stream, and the resultant dissemination of mycobacteria by the blood stream throughout the body. Untreated the sufferer dies, from fever and exhaustion, in two or three weeks. This is the most rapid form, and, with the second variety, constituted what was for long known as 'Galloping Consumption'.

2. ACUTE CASEOUS TUBERCULOSIS is a slightly slower form. The lungs only are affected, and, either in consequence of the bacilli inhaled into the lungs being specially virulent, or, more likely, owing to the person having acquired no immunity to the disease, or being in a particularly weak state, or of unhealthy constitution, tubercles form, undergo the caseous change, and break down to form cavities with great rapidity, the patient dying in two or three months.

3. FIBRO-CASEOUS TUBERCULOSIS is the usual form and may last for years. The change which occurs in the lungs is very much the same as in the last form, but, in addition, and in consequence of greater resisting power on the sufferer's part, there is an attempt at a cure, and much fibrous tissue is formed. The lung becomes denser, cavities gradually form here and there, and the downward progress is slow or may be arrested.

4. FIBROID TUBERCULOSIS is a form in which areas of the lung are converted into fibrous masses, which are in reality scars of previous disease that has undergone the body's natural cure, and there are no cavities.

Symptoms: In the following brief account the symptoms of an average case, in which fibrous formation and the caseous change leading to production of a cavity take place side by side, will be described. They fall conveniently into three stages of the disease:

(*a*) EARLY STAGE: In this stage the tubercles are being deposited in the lung, almost always near the apex; and this part of the lung becomes, in consequence, more solid. There is cough of an irritative nature, particularly in the morning, either without any expectoration or accompanied by a little clear mucus. Sometimes, the first sign of all is the spitting up of blood (haemoptysis), which is never copious at this stage, and is due to congestion caused by the irritation of the tubercles. (See HAEMOPTYSIS.) There is generally, from the first, loss of appetite, colour and strength, followed soon by actual emaciation and loss of weight. Perspiration upon slight exertion is usual, and, very often, night sweats are a symptom. An important sign is a regular rise of temperature, either in the forenoon, or more often in the early afternoon, with a fall below normal in the early morning, but this is not an invariable symptom at this stage. A slight attack of pleurisy, causing pain in the chest, is often a precursor of, or accompanies, these symptoms. This is the stage in which the disease is readily curable.

(*b*) STAGE OF ADVANCING DISEASE: By this time, the tubercles have fused to form caseous masses, and these are breaking down and being spat up, leaving a ragged cavity, while the disease is slowly advancing to new areas of the lung. The surface of the cavity becomes infected sooner or later with other inhaled micro-organisms, and these keep up the ulcerative process on the surface of the cavity and prevent its healing. The symptoms are mainly an increase of those present in the first stage. The cough is more troublesome and the spit is thick and yellow, contains large numbers of bacilli, which can be stained and microscopically examined, and is occasionally streaked with blood. The sufferer is much weaker, and has greatly lost in weight. The temperature is of a swinging hectic type, rising to 37·8° or 38·3°C (100° or 101°F) in the late afternoon and falling, sometimes below normal, in the early part of the day. Drenching night sweats are apt to break out during sleep in the early hours of the morning, and attacks of vomiting or diarrhoea are not infrequent. The disease may at this stage be found in both lungs or in other organs, such as the throat or intestine, with which the sputum comes in contact. An important sign is that of falling in of the chest over the excavated area, so that a flat place or depression is found in its upper part.

(*c*) LATE STAGE: In this stage, large cavities have usually formed in the lung, or there has been a production of fibrous tissue, the lung being shrunken and consisting of a mass of matted fibrous tissue and smaller cavities. Accordingly, the whole side has usually fallen in considerably. The second lung is by this time extensively affected; the voice may be husky on account of disease in the larynx, or there may be troublesome diarrhoea, due to affection of the bowels. Haemorrhage is not uncommon in this stage, and death may be brought about by this means. The emaciation is now extreme, and bed-sores are apt to form. The swinging temperature and the excessive sweats continue, and the cough is often most troublesome. All through the disease, even to the very end, there is often a curious mental state known as the spes phthisica, the sufferer being buoyed up by the daily recurring belief that he is better, and is beginning to recover.

The duration of the illness is largely dependent upon four factors: the acuteness of the infection, the age of the patient, the stage at which efficient treatment is started, and the natural resistance of the patient to the disease. Acute miliary tuberculosis, for instance, is rapidly fatal unless treatment is initiated at an early stage, and the disease runs a more rapid course in children, adolescents and young adults than in the middle-aged.

Treatment: This falls very naturally into two classes: (*a*) preventive, and (*b*) remedial.

(*a*) PREVENTIVE TREATMENT: The problem of prevention is partly social and partly medical. Tuberculosis is commoner among the ill-fed and the badly housed. Abolition of overcrowding, provision of good homes, an adequate supply of protective foods and enough money to buy them have all gone a long way towards diminishing the incidence of tuberculosis. To a considerable extent, tuberculosis is a social disease. On the medical side, the problem is essentially to prevent uninfected susceptible people – especially children – from coming into contact with the infecting agent – the *Mycobacterium tuberculosis*. The great risk to the child is coming into contact with an adult who has the causative organism in his or her sputum. Every attempt must therefore be made (1) to detect all sufferers from tuberculosis, (2) to treat them and isolate them until they know how to safeguard other people, as, for instance, by the proper use of sputum pots, and (3) to examine and follow up all contact cases – especially children known to have been in close contact with adults suffering from tuberculosis.

Two of the most important preventive measures introduced of recent years have been BCG vaccination (qv) and mass miniature radiography (qv). By means of the former an immunity to the disease can be given to those who have not acquired a natural immunity. By means of mass miniature radiography the disease can often be detected at an early stage when it is most likely to respond to treatment.

(*b*) REMEDIAL TREATMENT: For all practical purposes this now consists of chemotherapy.

Chemotherapy: The outlook in tuberculosis has been revolutionized by the introduction of effective antituberculous drugs. Since the isolation, in 1944, of streptomycin, the first chemotherapeutic substance to be of any value in the treatment of tuberculosis, several other drugs have been introduced for this purpose. There are two important general aspects of chemotherapy. The first is that the *Mycobacterium tuberculosis* has the unfortunate habit of becoming resistant to each of these drugs if it is given by itself. This can be prevented. According to the British Thoracic Association, the recommended course of treatment for pulmonary tuberculosis in Britain is a combination of ethambutol, rifampicin and isoniazid for two months, followed by seven months' treatment with rifampicin and isoniazid. The second is that whilst their introduction has marked a big advance in the treatment of tuberculosis, they are merely ancillary to the other well-established lines of treatment: eg. rest, fresh air and good food. It is when they are carefully integrated into a well-planned programme of treatment, under the supervision of a skilled physician, that they bring most benefit to the patient.

Eradication of Tuberculosis: Since the turn of the century there has been a marked fall in the incidence of tuberculosis. The ratio for pulmonary tuberculosis fell from 1336 in 1851-60 to 16 in 1966. Comparable figures are reported from all over the world. Thus in Koch's time, 250 people in every 100,000 in Germany died of tuberculosis. In East Germany no child has died of tuberculosis in the last five years. The figures for recent years are the most striking of all. Thus, in England and Wales the standardized mortality ratio for pulmonary tuberculosis fell from 85 in 1950–54 to 16 in 1966. Tuberculosis, however, is still with us, as indicated by the fact that in 1979 there were two outbreaks in England, in one of which involving over 56 children, two developed tuberculous meningitis. In 1982, 15 children in the Midlands who had undergone dental treatment developed the disease from the school dentist who had pulmonary tuberculosis. Other recent examples of the risks involved are a swimming bath attendant with positive sputum (ie. *M. tuberculosis* in his sputum), and four children who were infected in the children's department of a hospital in which the resident doctor had active tuberculosis. Tuberculosis will always be with us unless constant vigilance is maintained.

Apart from the treatment of individual cases, the general measures adopted for its eradication are:

1. PREVENTION OF BOVINE INFECTION, especially by obtaining a pure supply of milk, cream and butter from healthy cows; or if the milk is suspected, by sterilization of all milk to be consumed by children. (See MILK.)
2. BCG VACCINE, for the protection of infants born to tuberculous mothers, of senior schoolchildren and of young adults particularly exposed to risk of infection: eg. medical students and nurses. (See BCG VACCINE.)
3. MASS MINIATURE RADIOGRAPHY for the detection of cases at an early stage of the disease, when it is most amenable to treatment. This is also a valuable means of detecting the disease in individuals who, unbeknown to themselves and others, are suffering from the disease and spreading it to others with whom they live or work.

TUBEROSE SCLEROSIS, or EPILOIA, also sometimes known as TUBEROUS SCLEROSIS, is a hereditary disease due to a developmental abnormality of the brain. The prevalence is 1 in 50,000 of the population. It is characterized by mental retardation (usually from birth), epilepsy which usually starts before 2 years of age and multiple small nodules or tumours in the face which usually appear around puberty. Relatives of those with this condition can obtain help and guidance from the Tuberous Sclerosis Association of Great Britain, Little Barnsley Farm, Catshill, Bromsgrove, Worcestershire B61 0NQ (0527–71898).

TUBOCURARINE is the active constituent of curare (qv). It is a muscle relaxant (qv) which is widely used in anaesthesia.

TULARAEMIA is a disease of rodents such as rabbits and rats, caused by the bacillus, *Francisella tularense*, and spread either by flies or by direct inoculation, for example, into the hands of a person engaged in skinning rabbits. In man the disease takes the form of a slow fever lasting several weeks, with much malaise and depression, followed by considerable emaciation. It was first described in the district of Tulare in California, and is found widely spread in North America and in Europe, but not in Great Britain. Streptomycin, the tetracyclines and chloramphenicol, have proved effective in treatment.

TUMOUR means literally any swelling, but, by common consent, the term is held not to include passing swellings caused by acute inflammation, whilst the collections of diseased material arising in the course of chronic inflammation, like tuberculosis, syphilis, leprosy and glanders, sometimes are and sometimes are not classed as tumours, according to their size and appearance.

Varieties: Some are of an infective nature, as already stated; some arise undoubtedly as the result of injury; several contributing factors are mentioned under the heading of CANCER, but for the rest, the causes of tumours are really still undiscovered.

An old idea divides tumours into two great classes. On the one hand, some are *simple* or *benign*, growing slowly at one spot, pressing neighbouring parts aside but not invading them, not recurring after removal, and having little tendency to ulcerate; whilst others are *malignant*, spreading quickly from point to point, invading and destroying surrounding tissues, tending to recur after apparently complete removal, and being liable to ulcerate. This distinction is as old as the days of Hippocrates, who gave to gnawing tumours the name of carcinoma. Although in the majority of cases it is easy to decide whether a given tumour is of simple or malignant character, there is no sharp dividing line between the two kinds. Thus an expert sometimes has difficulty in stating from the microscopic characters of an *adenoma* (glandular tumour) growing in the breast or in the bowel, whether its progress will show a simple or malignant course. Again, *rodent ulcer*, a small ulcerating tumour situated generally on the face, may remain restricted to a single spot for twenty or thirty years, although it has the microscopic characters of a malignant tumour and finally spreads like one. Another fact connecting the two groups is that some simple tumours, persisting as such through middle life, are liable to assume a malignant character when old age is reached.

Formerly tumours were named according to some peculiarity of shape, colour, or the like. Thus a fungoid tumour was one resembling a mushroom, a polypus one which seemed to have one stalk with many feet, a mole was a dark hairy growth resembling the animal of that name, and sarcoma was originally the name given by Galen to a tumour of fleshy appearance. The use of the microscope, however, has brought about a more precise grouping, and tumours are now classed according to the tissues of which they are built, somewhat as follows:

(1) Simple tumours of normal tissue
(2) Hollow tumours or cysts, generally of simple nature
(3) Malignant tumours: (*a*) of imperfect cellular structure, resembling the cells of skin, mucous membrane, or secreting glands; (*b*) of imperfect connective tissue.

(1) SIMPLE TUMOURS OF NORMAL TISSUE:

ADENOMA is a tumour growing from a gland and composed of gland-like tissue. These tumours are specially common in the breasts of young women; there may be several together, but usually they are easily removed.

ANGIOMA is a tumour formed by a mass of small blood-vessels or spaces in which blood circulates. These tumours may exist in internal organs, or on the skin, when they do not project much, and are known as naevi or 'mothers' marks'.

CHONDROMA is a tumour mainly formed of cartilage. These tumours develop especially on the fingers and toes.

FIBROMA is the name given to a tumour consisting mainly of fibrous tissue. Soft fibromas are often seen as wrinkled brownish tags upon the face or body.

LIPOMA means a tumour mainly composed of fat. Such tumours may be found in any part of the body, but they are especially common just beneath the skin. It is sometimes hard to distinguish such a tumour, which is very soft, from a chronic abscess; but the fatty tumour generally has a firm edge and can be seen to be attached at several points to the skin, which is puckered by these attachments.

MYOMA is a tumour composed largely of muscle fibres, usually unstriped muscle. These tumours are far more commonly found in the wall of the womb than in any other position, being known as fibroid tumours.

NEUROMA is a tumour growing upon a nerve, and therefore in many cases producing pain.

OSTEOMA is a tumour composed of bone. These are usually of small size and cause little trouble, except in so far as their position occasions discomfort.

PAPILLOMA is a tumour projecting from the surface of the skin or of a mucous membrane. It is composed of a core of fibrous tissue, which represents an overdevelopment of the papillae naturally found in these situations, covered by masses of cells. Warts are examples of papillomas on the skin (see WARTS), whilst soft papillomas sometimes develop in the bladder or bowel and cause much bleeding.

(2) HOLLOW TUMOURS are described under a special heading. (See CYSTS.)

(3) MALIGNANT TUMOURS of imperfect cellular structure resembling the cells of skin, mucous membranes or secreting glands, are known generally as CANCERS. This group and the following group are treated together under the heading of CANCER AND SARCOMA (qv). Many names are applied to cancers of different parts and according to their appearance. The name CARCINOMA is generally reserved at the present day for malignant epithelial tumours.

EPITHELIOMA is a cancer springing from the skin surface, and ADENOCARCINOMA means one originating in glandular tissue. SCIRRHUS is a hard cancer in which much fibrous tissue has been developed; MEDULLARY or SOFT cancer is one in which the softer cellular element forms large masses; and COLLOID cancer is one in which a characteristic glue-like transformation takes place.

Malignant tumours of imperfect connective tissue are known as SARCOMAS; and, according to the shape of the embryonic cells, or the nature of attempts at the formation of connective tissues, these are subdivided as ROUND-CELLED, SPINDLE-CELLED, MELANOTIC, MYELOID.

Symptoms: The symptoms of a simple tumour are, as a rule, nothing beyond the presence of a swelling, and such accidental symptoms as those set up by its pressure upon neighbouring important organs, by the inconvenience of its size, its position, and the like. (For special symptoms of malignant tumours see CANCER and SARCOMA.)

Treatment: The treatment of a tumour is, in general, its removal by operation. With regard to simple tumours, the advantage gained by removal may not be worth the inconvenience caused by an operation, and such tumours may be left alone. In particular cases the unsightliness of the tumour, the inconvenience of its size, or the tendency that some simple tumours have to become malignant may call for removal. If a tumour is malignant, or if there is any doubt as to its character, an operation should be performed at the earliest possible opportunity. For some surface tumours, and also for inoperable tumours in internal organs, the application of radiotherapy and X-rays has, in recent years, played a great part. (See RADIOTHERAPY; RADIUM; X-RAYS.) Chemotherapy is also playing in increasingly important part in treatment. (See CANCER and SARCOMA.)

TUNNEL-WORM is another name for ancylostoma. (See ANCYLOSTOMIASIS.)

TURNING (see VERSION).

TURNER'S SYNDROME is the condition of ovarian dysgenesis in which the gonad is represented by a ridge on the broad ligament in the normal position on the ovary. It is composed of connective tissue without follicles. The condition is due to a partial or complete lack of the second X chromosome, which appears to be necessary to maintain the ovary. As the patient is deficient in both ovaries the presenting complaint is amenorrhoea and absent development of the breasts and sexual hair. In the syndrome described by Turner these features of ovarian dysfunction were associated with shortness of stature, webbing of the neck and cubitus valgus and there was no impairment of intelligence. Although the development of the ovary is influenced to a varying degree most patients with this syndrome are of short stature and rarely reach a height of more than 155 cm (5 feet). A number of congenital defects additional to those originally described by Turner may be associated with the condition, and coarctation of the aorta, deafness and mental deficiency are well recognized.

Most women with this condition have only 45 instead of the normal 46 chromosomes and this is due to non-dysjunction of the sex chromosome occurring during meiosis. Their sex chromosome constitution is XO instead of XX. Patients with less severe forms of the syndrome may have a normal number of chromosomes but one of the X chromosomes is structurally abnormal and deficient in much of the genetic material.

TURN OF LIFE is a term applied to the menopause. (See CLIMACTERIC.)

TURPENTINE is the oleo-resin which exudes from trees of the pine family when the bark is injured. The oil distilled from this is known as oil of turpentine, rectified turpentine or spirit of turpentine, the residue being the resin or rosin. The natural turpentine, containing resin, is not used in medicine, since it is highly irritating; and when the word turpentine is used, the distilled product is always understood. The turpentine obtained from the ordinary yellow pine is the common form, that obtained from the silver fir is known as Canada balsam or balm of Gilead and that from the larch as Venice turpentine.

Action: Turpentine has an action similar to that of other essential oils. It is highly irritating to any surface with which it is brought in contact, is antispasmodic, and, especially when it has been exposed to the air, is powerfully antiseptic.

Uses: *Externally*, turpentine is used as a counter-irritant. It forms one of the most common ingredients of liniments and embrocations for application to sprains and bruises. It is used with hot fomentations when a specially strong action is desired, a fomentation sprinkled with turpentine being known as a stupe. (See FOMENTATIONS.) In chronic bronchitis, rubbing the chest with turpentine is an old favourite household remedy.

Internally, turpentine is seldom administered now. In lumbago and other forms of chronic rheumatism, 5 drops of turpentine taken upon a lump of sugar thrice daily over a long period is an old household remedy. As an enema, 14 ml of oil of turpentine may be mixed with 420 ml of soapy water in order to relieve severe cases of flatulence.

TWINS (see MULTIPLE BIRTHS).

TYMPANIC MEMBRANE is the ear-drum. (See EAR.)

TYMPANITES means distension of the abdomen due to the presence of gas or air in the intestine or in the peritoneal cavity. The abdomen when struck with the fingers, gives under these conditions a drum-like (tympanitic) note.

TYMPANUM is another name for the middle ear. (See EAR.)

TYPHOID FEVER (see ENTERIC FEVER).

TYPHUS FEVER is an infective disease of world-wide distribution, the manifestations of which vary in different localities. The causative organisms of all forms of typhus fever belong to the genus Rickettsia. These are organisms which are intermediate between bacteria and viruses in their properties and measure 0·5 micrometre or less in diameter. The accompanying classification of the typhus fevers provides a practical basis for discussion of the subject.

LOUSE TYPHUS, in which the infecting Rickettsia is transmitted by the louse, is of world-wide distribution. More human deaths have been attributed to the louse via typhus, louse-borne relapsing fever and trench fever, than to any other insect with the exception of the malaria mosquito. Louse typhus includes Epidemic Typhus, Brill's Disease which is a recrudescent form of Epidemic Typhus, and Trench Fever (qv).

Epidemic Typhus Fever, also known as exanthematic typhus, classical typhus, and louse-borne typhus, is an acute infection of abrupt onset which, in the absence of treatment, persists for fourteen days. It is of world-wide distribution, but is largely confined today to parts of Africa. The causative organism is the *Rickettsia prowazeki*, so-called after Ricketts and Prowazek, two brilliant investigators of typhus, both of whom died of the disease. It is transmitted by the human louse, *Pediculus humanus*. The rickettsiae can survive in the dried faeces of lice for 60 days, and these infected faeces are probably the main source of infection of man.

Symptoms: The incubation period is usually 10 to 14 days. The onset is preceded by headache, pain in the back and limbs and rigors. On the third day the temperature rises suddenly, and the face and eyes become congested. At the same time the headache becomes more intense, and the patient is drowsy or delirious. Sometimes on this day, but more usually on the fifth or sixth day, the characteristic rash appears on the abdomen and inner aspect of the arms, to spread over the chest, back and trunk, but seldom involving the face except in severe cases. It has been described as a 'mulberry rash' and consists essentially of reddish spots on a dusky background. During the second week a low muttering delirium develops, the patient becomes restless, and great prostration develops: the so-called 'coma vigil'. In cases which are not going to recover, death usually occurs from heart failure about the fourteenth day. In those who recover, the temperature falls by crisis about this time. In severe cases, and in neglected cases, gangrene is liable to occur. In diagnosis the Weil-Felix reaction is helpful. The death-rate is variable, varying from nearly 100 per cent in epidemics among debilitated refugees to about 10 per cent.

FLEA TYPHUS, in which the infecting Rickettsia is transmitted by the flea, is represented by Murine Typhus.

Murine Typhus Fever, also known as flea typhus, is world-wide in its distribution and is found wherever individuals are crowded together in insanitary, rat-infested areas. Hence the old names of jail-fever and ship typhus. The causative organism, *Rickettsia mooseri*, which is closely related to *R. prowazeki*, is transmitted to man by the rat-flea, *Xenopsyalla cheopis*. The rat is the main reservoir of infection. Once man is infected, the human louse may act as a transmitter of the Rickettsia from man to man. This explains how the disease may become epidemic under insanitary, crowded conditions. As a rule, however, the disease is only acquired when man comes into close contact with infected rats.

Symptoms: These are similar to those of louse-borne typhus, but the disease usually runs a milder course, and the mortality rate is very low (about 1·5 per cent).

TICK TYPHUS, in which the infecting Rickettsia is transmitted by ticks, occurs in various parts of the world. The three best-known conditions in this group are Rocky Mountain Spotted Fever, Fièvre Boutonneuse and Tick-bite Fever.

Rocky Mountain Spotted Fever was reported originally in the mountainous western States of the USA, but it is now found in many of the eastern States. The causal organism is *Rickettsia rickettsii*. The usual transmitters are the wood tick (*Dermacentor andersoni*) and the dog tick (*Dermacentor variabilis*) but there is evidence that other ticks may occasionally transmit the disease. The highest incidence of the disease is in the spring and early summer, when the ticks are most active.

Symptoms: The incubation period is three to twelve days. After a day or two of headache, backache and loss of appetite the onset is rapid, with intensification of the headache, rigors, sickness and congestion of the eyes. The temperature rises by steps to 39.4° to 41.4°C (103°

Louse-borne	*Flea-borne*	*Tick-borne*	*Mite-borne*
Epidemic typhus	Murine (endemic) typhus	Rocky Mountain spotted fever	Tsutsugamushi fever
Brill's disease		African tick typhus (Tick-bite fever)	(Scrub typhus)
Trench fever		Fièvre boutonneuse	Rickettsialpox

Classification of the typhus fevers.

to 106°F). The rash usually appears on the second to fourth day, first in the wrist and ankles, and then spreading over the whole body. It is usually more florid than the rash of louse typhus. The temperature settles slowly by lysis after two or three weeks. Convalescence is slow. The mortality rate varies, averaging about 20 per cent; it is low in children and high in adults and the elderly.

Fièvre boutonneuse, also known as Marseilles fever and African tick fever, is a mild form of tick typhus which occurs along the Mediterranean littoral, throughout the African continent and in India. The causative organism is *Rickettsia conori*. It is transmitted by a dog tick, *Rhipicephalus sanguineus*, in Europe. Elsewhere other ticks are involved and the vectors are rodents and other small wild mammals. One of the distinctive features of the disease is the development of a small area of gangrene at the site of the tick bite – the *tâche noire*.

Tick-bite Fever occurs in South Africa, Zambia, Zimbabwe and East Africa. The Rickettsia is conveyed by a number of ticks which are conveyed to man by dogs and cattle. The initial infection takes place through a bite in the skin or through the conjunctiva. The manifestations of the disease are similar to those of Rocky Mountain spotted fever, but usually run a much milder course, with a death rate of less than 1 per cent. The fever persists for about a fortnight.

MITE TYPHUS, in which the infecting Rickettsia is transmitted by mites, includes scrub typhus, or tsutsugamushi disease, and rickettsialpox.

Scrub Typhus, also known as tsutsugamushi fever, Japanese river fever and tropical typhus, has been known in Japan for over a thousand years. Its distribution includes the area bounded by Japan, Pakistan and Australia. The causative organism is *Rickettsia tsutsugamushi*, which is transmitted by the larvae, or chiggers, of various mites which become infected from wild rodents. The disease is most common among farmers, field workers, hunters and surveyors. Whilst in Malaysia it occurs all the year round, in Japan it is most common between June and October.

Symptoms: The incubation period is 5 to 21 days. The onset is usually sudden, with headache, backache, rigors and congestion of the eyes, as in other forms of typhus. A small ulcer usually develops at the site of the mite-bite, and the lymph glands draining this area are often enlarged. The temperature rises rapidly to 38·3 to 38·9°C (101° to 102°F), and then climbs to about 40°C (104°F). The rash appears about the fourth or fifth day – on the chest and abdomen, then spreading to the limbs, and sometimes to the face. Nervous manifestations are usually marked: apathy during the day; insomnia and delirium at night. The temperature usually subsides during the third week.

Rickettsialpox is a mild disease caused by *Rickettsia akari*, which is transmitted to man from infected mice by the common mouse mite, *Allodermanyssus sanguineus*. It occurs in USA, West and South Africa and USSR.

TREATMENT: The general principles of treatment are the same in all forms of typhus, and can be divided into prophylactic and curative. *Prophylaxis* consists of either avoidance of, or destruction of, the vector. In the case of louse typhus and flea typhus, the outlook has been revolutionized by the introduction of efficient insecticides such as DDT and Gammexane. The value of the former was well shown by its use during the post-1939–45-War period. This resulted in almost complete freedom from the epidemics of typhus which ravaged Eastern Europe after the 1914–18 War being responsible for 30 million cases with a mortality of 10 per cent. At the present day there are only 10,000 to 20,000 cases a year, with around a few hundred deaths. Efficient rat control is another measure which reduces the risk of typhus very considerably. In areas such as Malaysia, where the mites are infected from a wide variety of rodents scattered over large areas, the wearing of protective clothing is the most practical method of prophylaxis.

Curative treatment has also been revolutionized by the introduction of chloramphenicol and the tetracyclines. These antibiotics have altered the prognosis in typhus fever very considerably. Currently the most widely used is the long-acting tetracycline, doxycycline, one single oral dose of which is said to be curative.

U

ULCER means a breach on the surface of the skin or on the surface of the membrane lining any cavity within the body, which does not tend to heal quickly.

An ulcer consists of a floor or surface, which, in consequence of the loss of tissue, is usually depressed below the surrounding healthy surface, and an edge where the healthy tissues end. The floor of a healing ulcer is composed of granulations, which are small masses of cells engaged in forming connective tissue and richly supplied with capillary blood-vessels that give the ulcer a bright-red appearance; whilst the edge shows a blue line of growing epithelial cells, which are constantly spreading inwards. In the process of healing, the fibrous tissue formed by the granulations contracts and thus draws the edges of the ulcer together and gives a puckered appearance to the scar. If anything interferes with these natural processes, the ulcer is prevented from healing.

Varieties: Ulcers are sometimes classified as *local* when they are found at one spot only, such as the varicose ulcer found on the lower part of the leg; and *constitutional* when there are usually several ulcers on different parts of the body, produced chiefly by some constitutional defect. LOCAL ULCERS are further subdivided as follows, according to their symptoms or appearance.

SIMPLE OR SLOWLY HEALING ULCER has already been described. The floor is moderately red and slightly sunk, the skin around is healthy up to the margin of the ulcer, and at the edge there is a blue line, which is of great importance as showing the progress of the healing. Such an ulcer has a very slight white discharge and is quite free from smell.

INFLAMED ULCER is one which, as the result usually of the presence of bacteria, or in consequence of continued irritation, is still spreading. The floor of such an ulcer is very red and bleeds easily, the skin around is red and swollen, there is a thick discharge of pus from the surface, and portions of the reddened skin at its edge or in its neighbourhood tend to die and thus form new ulcers.

WEAK ULCER is an appearance which the ulcers of weakly people, especially those suffering from oedema, tend to assume. The granulations are soft, project above the surface, forming what is popularly known as 'proud flesh', bleed easily, and prevent the healing edge of the ulcer from growing inwards.

CALLOUS ULCER is the type of chronic ulcer most often met. The edge is thick and hard, the colour pale, few granulations are present, and the discharge in consequence is thin and small in amount, though often very offensive in smell.

VARICOSE ULCER may belong to any of the above types. It generally comes on as the result of scratching the skin of a leg which has been rendered eczematous by the bad circulation. It will not heal so long as the patient walks about, and has a great tendency to develop into a callous ulcer.

INTERNAL ULCERS develop sometimes in the mouth (see MOUTH, DISEASES OF); in the stomach (see STOMACH, DISEASES OF); in the duodenum (see DUODENAL ULCER); in the bowels (see INTESTINE, DISEASES OF); and in other parts.

CONSTITUTIONAL ULCERS are generally the result of some widespread disease such as syphilis or tuberculosis. SYPHLITIC ULCERS have the characters of possessing a very abrupt edge, as if

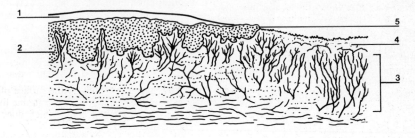

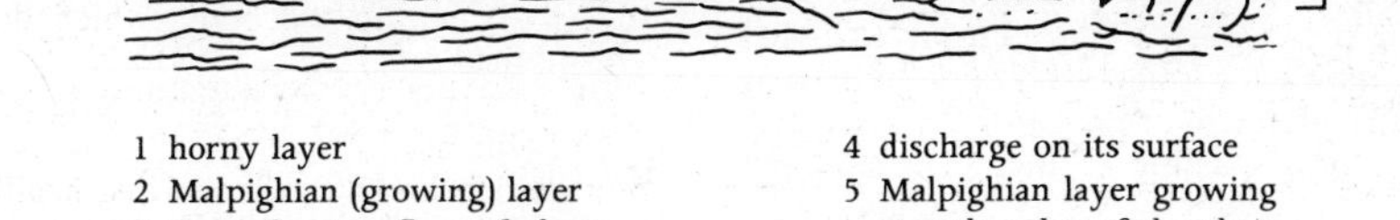

1 horny layer
2 Malpighian (growing) layer
3 tissue forming floor of ulcer
4 discharge on its surface
5 Malpighian layer growing over the edge of the ulcer

Vertical section through the edge of a simple ulcer. On the left is the healthy surface, to the right is the bare ulcerated surface. Magnified by 21

punched out, and of leaving behind after healing a brownish discoloured scar. TUBERCULOUS ULCERS may arise from the bursting of a tuberculous abscess under the skin; whilst the skin disease known as lupus vulgaris is a variety of tuberculous disease.

MALIGNANT ULCERS are developed when a cancer spreads so as to involve the skin. Such an ulcer has often a very offensive smell, requiring the use of deodorant substances.

TROPHIC ULCERS are apt to appear as the result of weakened nerve influence: eg. the deep perforating ulcer on the sole of the foot in locomotor ataxia, or bed sores in people sick of some lingering disease. (See BED SORES.)

Causes: An ulcer may be set up by any cause which damages the surface of the body and prevents immediate healing. Naturally, any constitutional condition which diminishes the vitality or the healing power of the body acts in this way, and among these causes may be mentioned old age, general ill-health, scurvy, diabetes mellitus, gout, syphilis and tuberculosis, so that wounds produced in those suffering from any of these conditions are apt to form ulcers. Defective circulation in the direction either of a poor blood supply or of the stagnation which takes place in varicose veins is another important cause. Constant movement of any part on which there is a wound is quite sufficient to delay its healing and produce an ulcer. Everyone knows, for example, how difficult it is to heal a small crack at the corner of the mouth. Irritation of the ulcer by pressure, or by discharges pent up under dressings that are too seldom changed, or even by the application of strong lotions to the ulcer, may prevent its healing.

Dangers: A person afflicted with a large ulcer is to a great extent incapacitated from active work, and the presence of any such septic condition has a prejudicial effect upon the general health. Further, the person always runs the risk of an attack of acute inflammation starting from the ulcer. A varicose ulcer has a danger of its own, consisting in the liability of the veins to become ulcerated and to burst, causing profuse bleeding. Even after a very chronic ulcer has healed, its scar contracts, and in doing so may cause disfigurement or may even interfere with the usefulness of a limb, if situated near a joint. Finally, ulcers which have lasted many years may become the seat of cancer.

Treatment: In treating an ulcer, three objects must be kept in view: (1) to remove the cause of ulceration; (2) to render the floor and edge of the ulcer healthy so that healing may begin; (3) to assist the healing process and ward off any source of irritation.

(1) REMOVAL OF THE CAUSE: Any constitutional condition underlying the development of the ulcer must first of all be treated; otherwise the tissues surrounding the ulcer are unable to exert their power of healing. Thus syphilis or tuberculosis, if present, require the special remedies suited to these diseases, whilst old age, scurvy, diabetes mellitus, and other conditions demand appropriate treatment. Bodily rest is also of great importance for the healing of an ulcer; and especially is this the case in ulcers of the leg, where constant movement combines with bad circulation to prevent healing. Accordingly, large varicose ulcers may refuse to heal till the person takes to bed, but when this is done, improvement is often rapid. This beneficial effect is still further aided, in the case of varicose ulcers, by raising the leg on a pillow or by elevating the foot of the bed on props so that the ulcer is brought above the level of the heart. When for any reason the person cannot lie in bed for several weeks, the evils of movement and the dependent position of the leg can be neutralized to some extent by wearing an elastic bandage over the dressing, which is applied every morning before the patient gets out of bed. Although this treatment will benefit any ulcer of the leg, it is not likely to cure a large one. (See VEINS, DISEASES OF.)

(2) RENDERING THE ULCER HEALTHY aims at converting any of the severer forms, eg. the inflamed, weak, or callous ulcer, into the simple type, which is the first step necessary in the healing process. When the ulcer is *inflamed*, it must be treated with active antiseptics such as cetrimide, chlorhexidine, Savlon (a preparation containing both cetrimide and chlorhexidine), or eusol, and the dressing covered by oiled silk or gutta-percha tissue. Penicillin is most effective when the causative organism is penicillin-sensitive. As soon as the ulcer has been purified, however, these strong antiseptics must be discontinued, since they retard the healing process. Sometimes the ulcer is purified quickly by the surgeon, who makes an application of undiluted carbolic acid to its surface, or scrapes away the diseased tissues thoroughly under an anaesthetic. Oxygen is sometimes used as a purifying agent. In mild cases of inflammation, charcoal, iodoform, and various weak antiseptics are sometimes used. *Weak ulcers* are treated with blue-stone, red lotion (qv), silver salts, or other substances which have an astringent effect upon the proud flesh and stimulate the edge and floor of the ulcer. *Callous ulcer* is by far the most common variety that needs special treatment. The reparative material, which has been accumulated in the edges and floor, and which obstructs the circulation near the ulcer, and prevents healing, must be absorbed. This is effected sometimes in slight cases by massage of the skin near the ulcer, in other cases by blistering the thick edge all round the ulcer. Generally, continued pressure is the method chosen. The more frequently used method is to wear during the day a special supporting bandage, which is applied to the leg from the ball of the foot up to the knee, passing over the dressing upon the ulcer with a very slight degree of pressure. There is now a range of such bandages, and medical advice should be sought as to the best one to use. To be successful, this treatment must be combined with complete rest and elevation of the ulcerated part.

(3) ASSISTANCE OF THE HEALING PROCESS: When the ulcer has been purified and its floor and edges rendered healthy, a simple dressing must be used. Care should be taken in dressing it not to irritate the ulcer and make it bleed, and the greatest care must be taken of the blue line at the ulcer's margin, as this is the healing part. The frequency of dressing the ulcer is a point of great importance; for, if the dressing is too frequently renewed, the healing tissues are unnecessarily disturbed and damaged, whilst if the dressing is seldom changed pus is apt to collect, and by its decomposition to inflame the ulcer. The usual interval allowed to elapse between the successive dressings of a healing ulcer is two or three days, or less if there is much discharge. The ulcer must be washed with some mild fluid like weak boric lotion. The best dressing is a piece of clean lint or gauze, but this should be kept from actual contact with the ulcer by a piece of oiled silk perforated here and there and just large enough to cover the red granulations of the ulcer's floor without touching the edge. At each dressing, the lint, etc., must be thoroughly soaked before removal, not pulled away roughly; otherwise the healing tissues, especially the blue line at the edge, are damaged and torn. At each dressing, too, the piece of oiled-silk is reduced in size. When an ulcer has become quite clean and is healing rapidly, one of the best forms of dressing consists of a weak boric ointment spread on lint.

The healing of a large ulcer, after it has been rendered clean, may often be hastened by grafting its surface with skin from another part. (See SKIN-GRAFTING.)

For the treatment of internal ulcers, see under the headings of the organs in which they occur.

ULCERATIVE COLITIS (see COLITIS).

ULITIS means inflammation of the gums.

ULNA is the inner of the two bones in the forearem. It is wide at its upper end, and its olecranon process forms the point of the elbow. In its lower part it is more fragile and is liable to be broken by a fall upon the forearm while something is grasped in the hand. Chipping off of the olecranon process is a not uncommon result of falls upon the elbow. (See FRACTURES.)

ULOGLOSSITIS means inflammation of the gums and of the tongue.

ULTRASONICS relate to sound in the frequency above 15 kilocycles per second: that is, well above the upper frequency limit of the human ear. These frequencies are now being used to an increasing extent in medicine. In diagnosis they are proving useful in obstetrics in assessing the stage of pregnancy and detecting abnormality of the foetus, in the investigation of disease in the bladder, kidneys, liver, ovaries and pancreas, and also in the diagnosis of brain tumours. Their great advantage is that they do not use ionising radiation and can therefore be used in the very young and in pregnant patients without problems. They can also be repeated without doing any harm to the patient. Ultrasound is inexpensive, rapid and versatile and scans can be performed in any plane. It requires no contrast agent and the running costs are low. Its reliability is dependent on the skill of the operator. It is replacing isotope scanning in many situations, and also radiography. Ultrasound of the liver can separate medical from surgical jaundice in approximately 97 per cent of patients. It is very accurate in detecting and defining cystic lesions of the liver but is less accurate with solid lesions and yet will detect 85 per cent of secondary deposits. This is less than CT scanning. It is very accurate in detecting gall stones and more accurate than the oral cholecystogram. It is useful as a screening test for pancreatic disease and can differentiate carcinoma of the pancreas from chronic pancreatitis with 85 per cent accuracy.

It is the first investigation indicated in patients presenting with renal failure as it can quickly determine the size and shape of the kidney and whether there is any obstruction to the ureter. It is very sensitive to the presence of dilatation of the renal tract and it will detect space-occupying lesions, differentiating cysts and tumours. It can detect obstruction of the ureter due to renal stones by showing dilatations of the collecting system and the presence of the calculus. Adrenal tumours can be demonstrated by ultrasound though it is less accurate than CT scanning. Ultrasound is now the first test for suspected aortic aneurysm and it can also show the presence of clot and delineate the true and false lumen. It is good at demonstrating sub-phrenic and sub-hepatic abscesses and will show most intra-abdominal abscesses. CT scanning is however better for the retro-peritoneal region. It has a major application in thyroid nodules as it can differentiate cystic from solid lesions and show the multiple lesions characteristic of the nodular goitre. It cannot differentiate between a follicular adenoma and a carcinoma as both these tumours are solid. Ultrasound cannot demonstrate normal parathyroid glands but it can identify adenomas provided they are more than 6 mm in diameter. Ultrasound can differentiate masses in the scrotum into testicular and appendicular and it can demonstrate impalpable testicular tumours. This is important as 15 per cent of testicular tumours metastasise whilst they are still impalpable.

Doppler is a new technique which shows the presence of vascular disease in the carotid and peripheral vessels as it can detect the reduced blood flow through narrowed vessels.

Ultrasound has particular applications in obstetrics. A foetus can be seen with ultrasound from the seventh week of pregnancy, and the foetal heart can be demonstrated at this stage. Multiple pregnancy can also be diagnosed at this time by the demonstration of more than one gestation sac containing a viable foetus. A routine obstetric scan is usually performed between the sixteenth and eighteenth week of pregnancy when the foetus is easily demonstrated and most photogenic. The foetus can be measured to assess the gestational age and the anatomy can also be checked. Gestational age, as determined from the last menstrual period, is often inaccurate. Ultrasound enables an objective definition of the expected date of delivery. In early pregnancy, from six to twelve weeks of gestation, the crown-rump length enables a prediction to be made to within five days. After the first trimester the bi-parietal diameter of the head is used. Intra-uterine growth retardation is much more reliably diagnosed by ultrasound than by clinical assessment. The site of the placenta can also be recorded and multiple pregnancies will be diagnosed at this stage. Foetal movements and even the heart beat can be seen. A second scan is often done between the thirty-second and thirty-fourth weeks to assess the position, size and growth rate of the baby. The resolution of equipment now available enables pre-natal diagnosis of a wide range of structural abnormalities to be diagnosed. Spina bifida, hydrocephalus and anencephaly are probably the most important but other anomalies such as multicystic kidney, achondroplasia and certain congenital cardiac anomalies can also be identified. Foetal gender can be determined from twenty weeks of gestation. Ultrasound is also useful as guidance for amniocentesis.

In gynaecology polycystic ovaries can readily be detected as well as fibroids and ovarian cysts. Ultrasound can monitor follicular growth when patients are being treated with infertility drugs. It is also useful in detecting ectopic pregnancies.

Ultrasonics are being used, too, in studying the flow of the blood. Among the interesting observations here is that blood flow in the carotid artery, the main artery carrying blood to the brain, is strongly influenced by extraneous stimuli, such as the telephone ringing or someone entering the room. They are also being used in the treatment of Menière's disease (qv) and of bruises and strains. In this field of physiotherapy, ultrasonic therapy is proving of particular value in the treatment of acute injuries of soft tissue. If in such cases it is used immediately ater the injury, or as soon as possible thereafter, it is claimed, there is no question of delayed, chronic recovery. For this reason it is being widely used in the treatment of sports injuries. It acts by providing a form of micromassage. (See MASSAGE.)

ULTRA-VIOLET RAYS (see LIGHT).

UMBILICUS is the technical name for the navel.

UNCINARIA is another name for hookworm. (See ANCYLOSTOMIASIS).

UNCINATE FIT is a state in which a patient has a hallucination of smell or of taste; it may be a manifestation of epilepsy, or the result of a tumour pressing on that part of the brain concerned with the appreciation of smell and taste.

UNCONSCIOUSNESS is a condition depending usually on some disorder of the brain, and may be of various degrees.

Varieties: Sleep is a natural form of unconsciousness due to a resting condition of the brain (see SLEEP). When the brain remains irregularly active various peculiar forms of unconsciousness or of disturbed consciousness are apt to ensue, such as delirium, somnambulism, hypnotism, catalepsy, ecstasy. (See under these headings.) In syncope, or fainting, the brain ceases to act for a time in consequence of a bloodless state, brought on by feebleness of the heart's action. In the lesser forms of epilepsy (*petit mal*), the epileptic sometimes becomes unconscious of his surroundings, though able to perform such a simple act as to take off his clothing, or to run some distance, or even to attack another person.

STUPOR is the name given to a partial state of unconsciousness from which the person can be roused for a moment by some powerful stimulus such as a shout.

COMA means a condition of complete oblivion from which the individual cannot be aroused.

Causes: Fainting is due to deficient supply of blood to the brain. Among injuries to the brain, apoplexy, compression and concussion of the brain, and inflammation affecting the brain or its membranes are the chief causes of unconsciousness. Epilepsy is also a cause of passing unconsciousness, either accompanied by a fit, or, in the slighter forms, without any such seizure. Narcotic poisons also produce stupor. The poisons that accumulate in the blood during various diseases, such as glomerulonephritis and diabetes mellitus, may produce coma, that due to the latter disease being curable by insulin.

Treatment: The cause of unconsciousness must first of all be determined. Fainting brings with it its own cure, and little is necessary beyond leaving the unconscious person recumbent. (See FAINTING.) The means of distinguishing the effects of narcotic poisons from those of apoplexy are given under OPIUM, and this distinction is important, since in apoplexy the main requirement is absolute quiet, while in opium poisoning energetic treatment is necessary. Unconsciousness, due to compression of the brain resulting from severe injury to the head, may have to be treated by trephining the skull. The unconsciousness of uraemia due to glomerulonephritis is perhaps the form most liable to be mistaken or overlooked, but doubts as to this are set at rest by examination of the urine. In this case also prompt treatment is essential if life is to be saved. For the treatment of unconsciousness due to other causes, the special symptoms present will in general indicate the cause, and the treatment is given under other headings.

UNDECYLENIC ACID is a long chain fatty acid which is of value in the treatment of tinea pedis. (See RINGWORM.)

UNDINE is the name given to a small glass flask with drawn-out neck and an opening which can be closed by the finger. It is used for irrigating the eye with fluid. (See EYE DISEASES AND INJURIES.)

UNDULANT FEVER is another name for brucellosis (qv).

UNGUENTUM is the Latin name for ointment.

UNIT is the term applied to a quantity assumed as a standard for measurement. Thus, the *unit of insulin* is the specific activity contained in such an amount of the standard preparation as the Medical Research Council may from time to time indicate as the quantity exactly equivalent to the unit accepted for international use. The standard preparation consists of pure, dry, crystalline insulin.

URACHUS is a corded structure which extends from the bladder up to the navel, and represents the remains of the canal which in the foetus joins bladder with allantois.

URAEMIA describes the clinical state which arises from renal failure. It may be due to disease of the kidneys or it may be the result of pre-renal causes where a lack of circulating blood volume inadequately perfuses the kidneys. It may result from acute tubular necrosis and it may result from obstruction to the outflow of urine.

The word uraemia means excess urea in the blood, but the symptoms of renal failure are not due to the abnormal amounts of urea circulating but to the electrolyte disturbances and acidosis which are associated with impaired renal function. The acidosis results from a decrease in the ability to filter hydrogen ions from blood into the glomerular fluid and the reduced production of ammonia and phosphate means less ions capable of combining with the hydrogen ions so that the total acid elimination is diminished. The fall in glomerular filtration also leads to retention of sodium and water with resulting oedema, and to retention of potassium resulting in hyperkalaemia. The most important causes of uraemia are the primary renal diseases of chronic glomerular nephritis and chronic pyelonephritis. It may also result from malignant hypertension damaging the kidneys and amyloid disease destroying the kidneys. Analgesic abuse can cause tubular necrosis. Diabetes may cause a nephropathy and lead to uraemia as may myelomatosis and systemic lupus erythematosis. Polycystic kidneys and renal tuberculosis account for a small proportion of cases.

Symptoms: Uraemia is sometimes classed as *acute*, ie. those cases in which the symptoms develop in a few hours or days, and *chronic*, including cases in which the symptoms are less marked and last over weeks, months, or years. There is, however, no dividing line between the two, for in the chronic variety, which may be said to consist of the symptoms of chronic glomerulonephritis, an acute attack is liable to come on at any time.

Headache in the front or back of the head, accompanied often by insomnia at night and drowsiness during the day, is one of the commonest symptoms, although it is apt to be attributed to some other cause. Unconsciousness of a profound type, which may be accompanied by convulsions resembling those of epilepsy, is the most outstanding feature of an acute attack and is a very dangerous condition.

Still another symptom, which often precedes an acute attack, is severe vomiting without apparent cause. The appetite is always poor, and the onset of diarrhoea is a serious sign.

Treatment: The treatment of the chronic type of uraemia includes all the measures which should be taken by a person suffering from chronic glomerulonephritis. Cheyne-Stokes breathing is relieved by the intravenous administration of aminophylline. An increasing number of these patients, especially the younger ones, can now be given a new lease of life by means of dialysis and/or renal transplantation. (See KIDNEY, ARTIFICIAL; TRANSPLANTATION.)

URAMUSTINE is a nitrogen mustard derivative (qv) used in the treatment of certain forms of malignant disease. It is given by mouth in capsule form.

URANORRHAPHY is an operation for closure of a cleft palate.

URATES (see URIC ACID).

UREA, or CARBAMIDE, is a crystalline substance of the chemical formula $CO(NH_2)_2$, which is very soluble in water or alcohol. It is the chief waste product discharged from the body in the urine, being formed in the liver and carried to the kidneys in the blood. The amount varies considerably with the quantity and nature of the food taken, rising greatly upon an animal (protein) dietary. It also rises during the continuance of a fever. The average amount excreted daily, during health, on a mixed diet is about 33 to 35 grams.

Urea is administered for its diuretic action, and also as a test of kidney action, in doses of 5 to 15 grams. It is used, too, as a cream in the treatment of certain skin diseases, characterized by a dry skin, such as ichythyosis (qv).

Urea is rapidly changed, by a yeast-like micro-organism, into carbonate of ammonia;

and to this chemical change the ammoniacal smell of badly kept latrines is due.

UREAPLASMA is a group of micro-organisms which plays a larger part in the causation of disease than was at one time suspected. One of them, *Ureaplasma urealyticum*, is now recognized as a cause of chronic prostatitis, non-specific urethritis (qv) and infertility.

URETER is the tube, about the thickness of a goose-quill, which on each side leads from the corresponding kidney down to the bladder. Each ureter begins above at the pelvis of its kidney and after a course of 25 to 30 cm (10 to 12 inches) through the loins and pelvis it opens by a narrow slit into the base of the bladder. The lower end pierces the wall of the bladder so obliquely (lying embedded in the wall for about 21 mm) that, though urine runs freely into the bladder, it is prevented from returning up the ureter as the bladder becomes distended.

URETHANE is the official *British Pharmacopoeia* name for ethyl carbamate. It is of value in the treatment of chronic leukaemia. Injection of quinine and urethane is used as a sclerosing agent.

URETHRA is the tube which leads from the bladder to the exterior, and by which the urine is voided. It is about 20 cm (8 inches) long in the male and 3·5 cm (1½ inches) long in the female.

URETHRA, DISEASES OF: The chief conditions which cause pain in the urethra, or interfere with the passage of urine, are urethritis or inflammation of the mucous lining, and stricture or narrowing of the tube.

URETHRITIS is often difficult to tell from inflammation of the bladder (cystitis), which, however, it may accompany and of which it is often the cause.

Causes: The most frequent cause of urethritis is gonorrhoea (qv), and this disease produces the most severe type of inflammation. Another common cause is the condition known as non-specific urethritis (qv). Like gonorrhoea, it is a venereal disease. Gout is another cause, producing its effects either owing to the repeated passage of irritating gravel with the urine, or to a highly acid state of this excretion. The damage caused by the passage of a rough stone from the bladder or of a catheter unskilfully introduced may also occasion a severe urethritis; and various drugs or articles of diet, such as alcohol or arsenic, may bring on an attack in those who are liable to suffer from it.

Symptoms: The symptoms consist chiefly in the constant oozing out of a small quantity of pus from the orifice of the urethra, a sense of scalding pain whenever urine is passed, increased redness of the mucous membrane as seen at the orifice, and tenderness along the course of the urethra. Subsequently, inflammation in neighbouring organs, eg. the bladder, testicle, or even kidney, may be set up.

Treatment: This varies with the cause of the inflammation, but in all cases the drinking of milk, water, and other bland fluids in large quantities is of advantage in order to flush out the urethra. The sulphonamide drugs and penicillin are highly effective in the treatment of gonorrhoea. The disease causing the inflammation requires special treatment according to its nature. (See also NON-SPECIFIC URETHRITIS.)

STRICTURE is an abrupt narrowing of the tube at one or more places.

Varieties and causes: SPASMODIC or CONGESTIVE STRICTURE is a temporary condition which is not of much importance. It follows upon exposure to cold, excessive exercise like bicycling, alcoholic indulgence, and often upon operations near the urethra, such as that for piles. It prevents the passage of urine for a few hours or days. It is treated simply by a warm sitz-bath or warm fomentations to the fork, and, if necessary, the urine is drawn off by means of a soft or flexible catheter passed along the urethra and through the stricture.

ORGANIC STRICTURE is a much more serious condition. It is a scar, due to previous injury or ulceration of the mucous membrane, which, by contracting after the manner of all scars, produces narrowing of the urethral tube. This scar is almost always due to one or other of two conditions: severe laceration of the urethra as the result of injury, or long-continued chronic inflammation.

A stricture almost always occurs at one of two points: either just within the orifice of the urethra or in the fork, or crotch, where the urethra turns upwards as it enters the pelvis.

Symptoms: An organic stricture is of slow development, and gives rise at first to few symptoms beyond those of the urethritis, which causes it. As the stricture narrows, the stream of urine becomes smaller than natural, and there is straining and pain each time it is voided. Occasional attacks of spasmodic stricture are brought on by injudicious acts on the part of the person who already has an organic stricture; and this further narrowing of the tube causes complete stoppage of the urine for a time, accompanied by great pain, which results from distension of the bladder. After a stricture has lasted some years, unless it has been very carefully treated, and the person has led a well-ordered life, inflammation of the bladder almost certainly comes on, and the death of the patient may ultimately ensue from the spread of this inflammation upwards to the kidneys.

The existence, position, and calibre of a stricture are verified by the surgeon, who passes metal bougies of various sizes along the urethra.

Treatment: The diet should be simple and constipation must be prevented. By these means unnecessary irritation of the stricture is avoided, and thus spasmodic attacks with retention of the urine are warded off.

To check the gradual narrowing of the stricture some operative procedure is necessary, and, according to the situation and nature of the stricture, it is either *dilated* by means of bougies passed along the urethra, or it is divided by a special instrument passed along the urethra (*internal urethrotomy*), or by an incision made through the fork (*external urethrotomy*). After-treatment, consisting in the passage of a bougie at regular intervals of some weeks or months, is necessary after any of these operations, in order to counteract the permanent tendency of the stricture to contract, INJURIES TO THE URETHRA may follow a severe crush which has fractured the pelvis, or a fall astride of some object. The signs of this are the presence of blood in the urine, or inability to pass urine at all, after such an accident. The great risks are the occurrence of an abscess round the urethra, and the formation of a stricture at a later period.

URETHRITIS means inflammation of the urethra (qv).

URIC ACID is a crystalline substance, very slightly soluble in water, of chemical formula, $C_5N_4H_4O_3$. It is white in the pure state, but when found as a urinary deposit it is reddish-brown, presenting a supposed resemblance to cayenne pepper. The bi-urate of sodium and urate of ammonium occur in considerable amount in the urine during a feverish state or after great exertion, and produce, as the urine cools, a dense pink or yellow sediment. The average daily quantity of uric acid passed by human beings is 0·5 to 1 gram. In the urine of birds and reptiles uric acid is the chief nitrogenous constituent, taking the place of the urea excreted by human beings. Uric acid is formed in the liver and removed by the kidneys from the blood. The amount is increased in the following conditions: (*a*) Excessive consumption of meat, combined with sedentary habits. (*b*) Gout (see GOUT). (*c*) Diseases in which the white corpuscles of the blood are increased: eg. leukaemia.

Owing to their insolubility, uric acid and the various urates often produce deposits in the urinary passages, which are known as urinary sand, gravel, or stones according to their size.

URINARY ORGANS form the system by which the urine is extracted from the blood, stored up, and from time to time discharged from the body. They comprise the two kidneys placed in the loins, two ureters leading from them to the bladder which is situated in the front of the pelvis, and the urethra which leads from the floor of the bladder out beneath the pubic bones to the exterior. (See BLADDER; KIDNEYS; URETERS; URETHRA.)

URINE is the excretion produced by the kidneys, and consists chiefly of waste substances resulting from the activity of the body, dissolved in water. The function of the kidneys consists almost entirely in selecting these substances from the blood; their actual formation takes place in the liver, muscles, etc. The urine and the perspiration are to a great extent interdependent; thus, in hot weather the amount of urine tends to decrease as more fluid is lost in perspiration, whilst the converse happens in cold weather. If the kidneys are acting vigorously the skin becomes very dry, whilst if there has been much perspiration, as in fevers, the urine is small in amount and highly concentrated. The amount of water lost from the body daily by perspiration is, in health, about half the amount passed as urine, and, though the sweat contains little of the waste material present in the urine, the glands of the skin can be made to take up the function of the kidneys to some extent when the latter organs are diseased. (See GLOMERULONEPHRITIS.) Many poisons taken into the body are excreted by way of the urine, eg. morphine and strychnine, and so also are the germs of many diseases, eg. those of typhoid fever.

Composition: About 96 per cent of the urine is water, the remaining 4 per cent being solids dissolved in it. Of the solids, far the most important is urea, of which there is, on an average, 25 grams in 1 litre. Common salt stands next in quantity, the average amount in 1 litre of urine being 9 grams. Phosphates and sulphates are also important constituents combined with potassium, sodium, calcium, and magnesium, whilst there is less than 1 gram each of uric acid, and ammonia, and just over 1 gram of creatinine.

Pigments are also present in the urine, and to them its colour is due. These pigments, the chief of which is urochrome, are derived indirectly from the colouring matter of the blood, and are produced also by the liver.

Amount: The amount of urine passed daily is about 1500 millilitres, subject to the variations mentioned above. A child, of course, passes much less than an adult; the average daily amount is: 430 ml at two years; 570 ml at four years; 850 ml at seven years; and 1140 ml at twelve years.

The amount of urine is *increased* in some diseases, of which diabetes is the chief. In other conditions it is *diminished*, notably in acute glomerulonephritis, in fevers and feverish states generally, and in heart failure.

COMPLETE STOPPAGE of the urine may occur for a time in the feverish conditions of children, or it may be due to acute glomerulonephritis, when the condition is a very serious one. When the stoppage is due to failure of the kidneys to secrete any urine, the condition is known as *suppression* or *anuria*. When the stoppage is due to such a cause as blockage of the ureters by stones or of the urethra by a stricture, although secretion by the kidneys still goes on, it is known as *retention*. Stoppage of the urine, to whatever cause it be due, may often be relieved by placing the patient in a hot bath and administering sweet spirits of nitre or other diaphoretic.

Colour: The tint of normal urine is generally described as straw or amber coloured, but it may be considerably changed by various diseases or drugs.

PALLOR, giving the urine a watery appearance, is found in diabetes and in chronic glomerulonephritis, also in people who drink large quantities of water.

ORANGE OR RED COLOUR may appear when senna, beetroot or rhubarb has been taken; when blood is present the colour may be pink or bright red; urates cause a turbid red or yellow appearance.

SMOKY TINT, depriving the urine of transparency, is caused by small quantities of blood.

GREEN OR GREENISH-YELLOW urine is usually due to bile, or may be produced by taking santonin or quinine.

BLACK URINE may be due to absorption of carbolic acid from surgical dressings or from taking carbolic acid, lysol, or similar substances internally. It is often passed by those who are taking guaiacol of creosote. It may also be due to the presence of indican in cases of intestinal stasis, and is found in the form of sarcoma known as melanotic sarcoma when this involves the liver.

Odour: Healthy urine has a faint aromatic odour, but when it begins to decompose, an unpleasant ammoniacal smell is given off. Thus the presence of cystitis or of dribbling of the urine is betrayed by the odour of the patient's personal or bed clothes. When turpentine and some other aromatic drugs have been taken, the urine acquires an odour of violets, and in diabetes it presents an aroma similar to that of new-mown hay. Various items of diet may give a distinctive odour to the urine. Thus spinach may produce an acrid smell, mushrooms a fetid odour and truffles a stagnant smell. Cold meat containing preservatives may produce a smell that has been described as like boot polish. Many soups are fortified with glutamates and may give an ammoniacal smell, whilst garlic yields its characteristic odour to the urine as well as the breath. High doses of yeast or the vitamin B complex such as are contained in some multivitamin preparations may give the urine a typical odour. The constituents of certain deodorants and perfumed talcum powders can also make the urine malodorous.

Specific gravity of urine varies in health from 1015 to 1025 (distilled water being 1000). A urine of lower specific gravity suggests the presence of chronic glomerulonephritis, whilst a higher specific gravity may be due to diabetes mellitus, or to a feverish state.

Reaction: When the urine is tested with litmus paper it is found to be acid in general, and this is of importance, because the acid has an antiseptic action. This acidity is due, not to free acids, but to acid salts such as acid phosphate of sodium. In consequence of the secretion of acid from the blood into the gastric juice that is poured into the stomach shortly after meals, the urine may at such times become alkaline. In herbivorous animals and in vegetarians, owing to the great quantities of alkaline salts eaten in the diet, the urine is permanently alkaline.

Deposits: In healthy urine there is usually a fleecy deposit of mucus secreted by the mucous membrane of the urinary passages. A pink or yellow deposit, that settles as soon as the urine begins to cool, and that often leaves a stain upon the utensil in which the urine has stood, is due to urates. (See URIC ACID.) Uric acid is a rarer deposit, and, when present, falls in very scanty yellow or brownish, so-called 'cayenne-pepper' grains. A white deposit that collects upon the bottom of the utensil after the urine has stood undisturbed for some time may be due to phosphates, to pus, or to debris from diseased kidneys known as tube-casts.

Abnormal substances: Many unusual substances taken into or formed in the body are got rid of in the urine, sometimes just as they have entered the body, in other cases considerably changed, eg. drugs, and the poisons of various diseases. Further, various bacteria and parasites can be discovered in the urine in some diseases. Elaborate chemical or microscopical examination is necessary in order to reveal these, but there are six substances the detection of which is of great importance, and which are discovered with comparative ease. These substances are (1) albumin; (2) blood; (3) sugar; (4) pus and tube-casts; (5) bile; (6) acetone. Strip tests, which merely involve the placing in urine of small specially impregnated strips of paper, are now available for all of these, except pus and tube-casts. Whilst these are satisfactory and time-saving for routine purposes, they still require to be checked sometimes by the older, more conventional methods.

(1) ALBUMIN is present in various conditions mentioned under ALBUMINURIA, and may be recognized by the following tests:

(*a*) *Boiling*, after the addition of a few drops of acid, produces a copious white cloud of coagulated albumin.

(*b*) *Salicylsulphonic acid*: Drop 25 per cent solution of salicylsulphonic acid into a test-tube containing urine. If albumin is present, each drop carries down a white cloud of coagulated albumin.

(2) BLOOD is present in acute glomerulonephritis, in congestion of the kidneys, or when a stone, ulcer, or tumour is present in any of the urinary organs. A drop of the urine must be examined under the microscope to find if blood-cells are actually present.

(3) SUGAR is a sign of diabetes mellitus (qv) when it is present constantly in the urine. It may also be found following upon a diet that contains a great deal of sugar – a harmless condition known as alimentary glycosuria. In some cases the difficulty lies in the kidneys – renal diabetes, which is also of little importance.

(*a*) *Fehling's test*: A special blue solution composed of copper sulphate, Rochelle salt, and caustic potash is placed in a test-tube and heated almost to boiling point. While it is hot, an equal volume of the suspected urine, which has also been heated in a separate test-tube, is added, and, if sugar is present, red and yellow cuprous salts are formed.

(*b*) *Benedict's test*: Benedict's reagent contains copper sulphate, sodium carbonate, potassium citrate, potassium thiocyanate, and potassium ferrocyanide, dissolved in distilled water. When urine containing sugar is boiled along with this pale-blue solution, the colour disappears. This reagent can be used for estimating approximately the amount of sugar present, the calculation being based upon the fact that 25 ml of the reagent are completely reduced by 50 mg of glucose, and rendered colourless.

(4) PUS AND TUBE-CASTS are the sign of inflammation or of ulceration somewhere in the urinary passages. Pus alone is generally a sign that the bladder is affected; tube-casts always point to involvement of the kidneys. For the detection of pus or tube-casts in small amounts a drop of urine must be placed on a glass slide and examined with the microscope.

(5) BILE in the urine is a sign that the bile ducts are obstructed, and that bile is being absorbed into the blood. Sometimes the jaundice that accompanies this condition is so slight as to escape notice, so that the detection of bile in the urine is an important sign. Place some of the urine in a large conical glass, dilute it with water till quite transparent, and pour impure nitric acid down the side of the glass. If bile is present in the urine, a brilliant play of colours – yellow, red, violet, and green – takes place where the urine and acid meet. It is the green colour that is characteristic of bile.

(6) ACETONE may appear in the urine in cases of diabetes, general acidosis, and some other conditions.

Rothera's test: Place in a test-tube crystals of ammonium sulphate to a depth of about an inch. Then add a few grains of sodium nitroprusside. Add sufficient urine to produce a saturated solution of the ammonium sulphate. This requires vigorous shaking of the test-tube, and, if the solution is saturated, there will be some undissolved crystals in the solution. A solution of strong ammonia is then added, and, if a purple colour develops, this denotes the presence of acetone bodies.

URINE, EXCESS OF: The amount of urine passed in 24 hours is often markedly increased in diabetes mellitus, a fact which sometimes, without any other symptom, attracts the patient's attention. Any source of irritation or inflammation in the kidneys or bladder may also produce frequency, such as the formation of gravel or of a stone, tuberculosis of the kidney, inflammation of the bladder (cystitis), or enlargement of the prostate gland. The bladder, however, varies greatly in size in different individuals, and the necessity to pass water frequently may simply be a life-long personal peculiarity due to smallness of its capacity.

An annoying form of increase in the urine at night leads to wetting of the bed by children. (See NOCTURNAL ENURESIS.)

Treatment: Any increase in the amount of urine or the frequency with which it is passed calls for testing for the presence of sugar, albumin, gravel, pus, and the like. The treatment consists in that suited to any disease that may be discovered.

URINE, RETENTION OF: The term, retention, is applied to cases in which urine is duly secreted by the kidneys, but for some reason is retained in the bladder; while the more serious condition, in which the kidneys fail to produce urine, is known as suppression or anuria. (See URINE, AMOUNT.)

Causes: The urine may be retained either because the bladder is too weak to expel it, or because of some obstruction to the passage by which it should be voided. Weakness is a rare condition and is generally the result of some damage to the nervous system, this being one of the troublesome symptoms that follow an injury to the spinal cord; it is accompanied by dribbling away of the urine when the bladder becomes fully distended. A similar condition results from long-continued distension produced by some obstruction to the outflow.

Among the cases due to obstruction, some are acute and merely temporary, such as the difficulty of passing water that follows upon any operation near the bladder, eg. one for piles, or that is apt to follow child-birth. In these cases the difficulty commonly is due to spasm, and does not persist more than a day or two. Among the more chronic cases of retention the commonest are those caused by enlargement of the prostate gland and consequent blockage of the outlet from the bladder; this condition is common in old men. In these the retention usually comes on gradually, and it is a common experience to find that the bladder never empties completely as it ought to do, but forms a sort of reservoir from which an overflow is discharged every few hours. The condition that leads to the most complete form of retention is a stricture or narrowing of the urethra due to the scar of previous injury or ulceration. (See URETHRA, DISEASES OF.) Similar blockage results also, in rare instances, from the pressure of some tumour upon the urethra, or the displacement of a neighbouring organ such as the womb in women.

Treatment: Cases in which retention is due to weakness of the bladder, in a chronic invalid, are treated by the regular use of a soft rubber catheter, and this forms one of the most important duties in the nursing of such a case.

In any case of retention where the urine accumulates in and causes painful distension of the bladder, the condition may often be relieved by the sufferer placing himself in a warm bath. This produces so much relaxation that the bladder often succeeds in emptying itself, a result which is still further assisted by the use of soothing draughts or the giving of an enema.

If relief is not gained by these means, the medical attendant withdraws the urine by means of a catheter passed along the urethra. (See CATHETERS.) The instrument chosen varies according to the cause of the retention; thus, in cases due to weakness of the bladder or to moderate spasm at the outlet, a soft rubber catheter only is necessary. In cases of severer spasm, and in cases where the prostate gland is enlarged, a flexible instrument or a hard rubber catheter with a bend upon the point (known as a *coudé* catheter) is generally chosen; while, in cases of very narrow stricture, the surgeon may require to pass a rigid metal instrument. As a rule, great difficulty is experienced only in the last-named class of cases; and in them it may occasionally be necessary to tap the bladder above the pubis by means of a hollow needle. After its contents have escaped, the patient gains immediate relief.

URINOMETER or DENSIMETER, is an instrument designed for estimating the specific gravity of urine. It consists of a graduated stem supported upon a large glass bulb containing air which floats partly submerged, and which is kept upright by a smaller bulb containing mercury placed at its lower end. The urine is poured into a tall glass vessel, the urinometer placed in it, and, when it is floating motionless, the point on the scale which is at the surface of the urine registers the specific gravity.

UROGASTRONE is a depressant of gastric acidity which has been isolated from urine. Its precise function in the body and its constitution are not known.

UROKINASE is an enzyme (qv) obtained from urine which dissolves blood clots. It is sometimes used in the treatment of pulmonary embolism (qv).

UROLOGY is that branch of medicine which treats of disorders and diseases of the kidneys, ureters, bladder, prostate, and urethra.

URSODEOXYCHOLIC ACID is a preparation used in the treatment of cholesterol gall-stones (see GALL-BLADDER, DISEASES OF).

URTICARIA is another name for nettle-rash (qv).

UTERUS or WOMB, is a hollow organ suspended in the cavity of the pelvis. In shape, it is triangular from side to side, and flattened from before backwards. The lower angle is prolonged into a rounded neck (*cervix*), about 2·5 cm (1 inch) long, which communicates through a narrow opening or mouth (*os uteri*) with the vagina, the passage leading to the exterior of the body. In size, the normal uterus is only about 7·5 cm (3 inches) long, 5 cm (2 inches) in its greatest width, and 2·5 cm (1 inch) in thickness from front to back, while the walls are so thick that the cavity consists of a mere slit. It weighs 30 to 40 grams. During pregnancy, however, it enlarges to an enormous extent, and the walls increase still further in thickness. (See MUSCLE.) The cavity is lined by a thick, soft, mucous membrane, and the wall is chiefly composed of muscle fibres arranged in three layers. The outer surface, like that of other abdominal organs, is covered by a layer of peritoneum. The uterus has a copious supply of blood derived from the uterine and ovarian arteries. It has also many lymphatic vessels, and its nerves establish wide connections with other organs. (See PAIN.) The position of the uterus is in the centre of the pelvis, where it is suspended by several ligaments between the bladder in front and the rectum behind. On each side of the uterus are the broad ligaments passing outwards to the side of the pelvis, the utero-sacral ligament passing back to the sacral bone, the utero-vesical ligament passing forwards to the bladder, and the round ligament uniting the uterus to the front of the abdomen.

UTERUS, DISEASES OF: Among the most common symptoms are pain or irregularity in the menstrual functions, the presence of a white discharge (*leucorrhoea*), constant pain or sense of weakness in the back, and often the inability to bear children.

MALFORMATIONS sometimes occur and give rise to trouble in child-birth: for example, the uterus may be double, having a partition down the middle. The cervix may be long and furnished with a very narrow mouth, which is sometimes a cause of pain in menstruation.

DISPLACEMENTS are more common. The uterus is slung in the centre of the pelvic cavity, and has great freedom of movement up and down and from before backwards. It lies naturally with its long axis directed upwards and forwards between the bladder and rectum, but its position at any time varies considerably according to the state of distension of one or other of these organs. A flabby state of the muscular wall of the uterus, or a contraction of some of the ligaments that suspend it, may produce a bend upon the organ itself, or may permanently tilt it forwards or backwards. Bending forwards is known as *anteflexion*, tilting forwards is called *anteversion*, and the corresponding conditions towards the back are known as *retroflexion* and *retroversion*. In the treatment of these conditions, two objects are kept in view, the one being to diminish the inflammation that is apt to accompany them, and the other consisting in the support of the uterus in its proper position by a suitably shaped instrument known as a pessary; or by an operation, when the displacement is very marked.

Downward displacement is known as *prolapse*, and in this condition the uterus slips bodily downwards in the space between the bladder and bowel, till, in bad cases, it may actually protrude from the vagina. The condition comes on in older women, usually those who are becoming stout, have a considerable amount of work to do, and have in child-birth suffered laceration of the parts that should support the uterus. When the condition is slight it may be relieved by wearing a suitably shaped pessary, and in cases which are not relieved by this simple measure an operation (colporrhaphy), designed to repair the injury previously done, will often remedy the displacement.

INFLAMMATION is, perhaps, the commonest type of uterine disorder. It is of several forms, but the general term *endometritis* is applied to inflammation affecting the mucous membrane, *metritis* to the rarer condition in which the muscular substance is involved. This condition is often due to child-birth which has not passed off quite successfully; and it is still more often due to miscarriage. Inflammation spreading upwards from the vagina, and displacements of the uterus are other, though less common, causes. The usual treatment consists in rest, the employment of hot, antiseptic douches and other applications to the vagina, and remedies to improve the general health. The sulphonamides or penicillin are given in severe cases. The interior of the uterus may be brought quickly to a healthy condition by the operation of curetting, which consists in scraping away the unhealthy mucous membrane with a special instrument, the curette. After this operation the patient must observe the greatest caution till the next menstrual period shall have passed.

TUMOURS of the uterus are by no means uncommon. The two most important ones are fibroids and cancer.

Fibroid tumours, or fibromyomas, are the most common form of tumour in any part of the body. They consist of masses of muscle fibres, similar to those of the uterus, and white fibrous tissue. They vary in size from that of a small seed to a mass weighing several pounds. The cause is not known, but they are much more common in women who have never borne children than in those with children. Whilst they may occur any time between puberty and the change of life, they are usually first recognized between the ages of 35 and 45. The symptoms depend upon the size and site of the tumour,

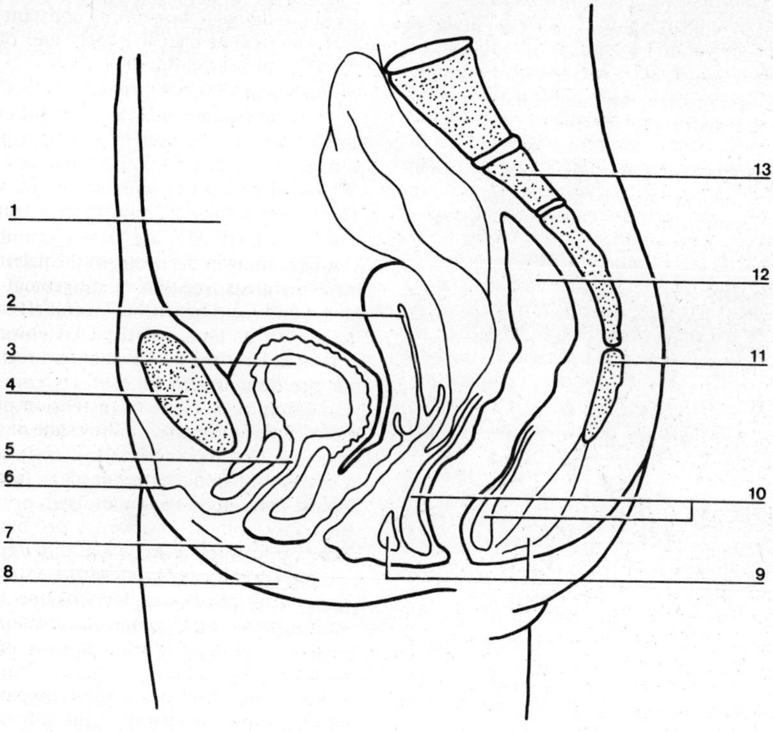

1 peritoneum
2 uterus
3 bladder
4 symphysis pubis
5 urethra
6 clitoris
7 labium minis
8 labium majus
9 external sphincter ani
10 internal sphincter ani
11 coccyx
12 rectum
13 sacrum

The female sex organs.

and many fibroids give rise to no symptoms at all. Speaking generally, the larger the tumour, and the more it involves the inner aspect of the uterus, the more likely is it to produce signs of its presence. The more important symptoms and signs are menstrual irregularity consisting of excessive loss of blood or excessive length of the period, sterility, frequency of micturition, and retention of urine. Pain is seldom a marked feature. Only those fibroids causing symptoms require treatment. If the symptoms are at all severe, operation is the treatment of choice. In some cases this involves removal of part, or the whole, of the uterus; in others it is possible to remove the tumour itself and leave the rest of the uterus intact. In cases with only mild symptoms, or in women approaching the menopause, when the tumour may decrease in size, medical treatment is sometimes used. This consists of rest in bed during menstruation, the administration of ergot to control the excessive bleeding, and full doses of iron to combat the anaemia usually present. In more severe cases, or in those in which such treatment fails, radiotherapy is sometimes used with benefit.

Cancer of the uterus is one of the most common forms of cancer in women. It may occur in either the neck (or cervix) of the uterus or in the body of the uterus. Cancer of the cervix of the uterus is more common than cancer of the body of the uterus, and 95 per cent of cases occur in women who have borne children. Cancer of the body of the uterus, on the other hand, is more common in unmarried women or women who have never borne children. Cancer of the body of the uterus is rare before the menopause. The first sign is usually a blood-stained discharge. Treatment consists of radiotherapy or surgery or a combination of both. By and large the earlier the cancer is detected and treated, the better the results. This is why it is so important that any woman over the age of 40 who has either excessive loss at the period, or irregular bleeding, should report at once to her doctor. In most cases there will be nothing serious to worry about, but if the bleeding should be due to cancer, then early diagnosis will permit of treatment being carried out at a stage when the expectation of cure is high. It is in the early diagnosis of cancer of the cervix, which tends to occur at an earlier age, that cervical cytology, as it is known, is so important. This consists of the perfectly simple procedure, which the woman can do herself, of taking a 'smear' of the cervix for examination in the laboratory. Such examination may reveal the presence of cancer long before it has produced any symptoms and signs, and treatment at this stage produces excellent results. The recommendation of the British Society for Clinical Cytology is that a woman should have this procedure carried out every five years from the age of 30 to that of 70. In 1984, in England there were 2,851 deaths from cancer of the uterus: 952 involving the body, and 1,899 the cervix.

UTICILLIN (see PENICILLIN).

UVEA is a term applied to the middle coat of the eye, including the iris, ciliary body and choroid.

UVEITIS: An inflammation of the uveal tract. *Iritis* is inflammation of the iris, *cyclitis* inflammation of the ciliary body and *choroiditis* inflammation of the choroid. The symptoms and signs vary according to which part of the uveal tract is involved and tend to be recurrent. The patient may experience varying degrees of discomfort or pain, with or without blurring of vision. The eye may be red or appear white. In many cases a cause is never found. Some known associations include various types of arthritis, some bowel diseases, virus illnesses, tuberculosis, syphilis, parasites and fungi. Treatment is with anti-inflammatory drops and occasionally tablets (eg. steroid eye drops and tablets), plus drops to dilate the pupil.

UVULA is the small mass of muscle covered by mucous membrane that hangs down from the middle of the soft palate on its posterior aspect. Very rarely the structure is excessively long and may require trimming. Generally though its function is not certain and it seldom causes problems.

V

VACCINATION, from *vacca*, Latin for cow, means inoculation with the material of cowpox, performed to afford protection to the inoculated person against an attack of smallpox, or at all events with the view of diminishing the seriousness of, and averting a fatal result from, any such attack. This is the strict sense of the term, but it is used nowadays to describe the process of inoculating with any vaccine to obtain immunity, or protection, against the corresponding disease.

VACCINE is the name applied generally to a substance of the nature of dead or attenuated living infectious material introduced into the body with the object of increasing its power to resist or to get rid of a disease. (See also IMMUNITY.)

In cases where healthy people are inoculated with vaccine as a protection against a particular disease, this is done to produce antibodies which will confer immunity against a subsequent attack of the disease.

Vaccines may be divided into two classes: stock vaccines, prepared from micro-organisms known to cause a particular disease and kept in readiness for use against that disease; and autogenous vaccines, prepared from micro-organisms which are already in the patient's body and to which the disease is due. Vaccines intended to protect against the onset of disease are necessarily of the stock variety.

Autogenous vaccines are prepared from the cultivation of bacteria found in the expectoration, the urine, the faeces, and in areas of inflammation such as boils. This type of vaccine was introduced by Wright about 1903.

Anthrax vaccine was introduced by Pasteur about 1882 for the protection of sheep and cattle against this disease. A safe and effective vaccine for use in human beings has now been evolved.

BCG vaccine is used to provide protection against tuberculosis. BCG vaccination is usually considered for five main groups of people:

(1) Schoolchildren: the routine programme in schools usually covers children aged between 10 and 14

(2) Students including those in teacher training colleges

(3) Children and new-born infants in families of Asian origin because of the high incidence of tuberculosis in this ethnic group

(4) Health service workers and others liable to infection at work

(5) Household contacts of people known to have active tuberculosis and new-born infants in households where there is a history of tuberculosis.

(See BCG VACCINE.)

Cholera vaccine was introduced by Haffkine in India about 1894. Two injections are given at an interval of at least a week; this gives a varying degree of immunity for six months.

Diphtheria vaccine is available in several forms. (See DIPHTHERIA.) It is usually given along with tetanus and pertussis vaccine in what is known as Triple Vaccine. This is given in three doses: the first at the age of 3 or 6 months, the second six to eight weeks later, and the third six months later, with a booster dose at the age of 5 years.

Hay fever vaccine is a vaccine prepared from the pollen of various grasses. It is used in gradually increasing doses for prevention of hay fever in those susceptible to this condition.

Influenza vaccine: a vaccine is now available for protection against influenza due to the influenza viruses A and B.

Measles vaccine is now available in two forms: an inactivated vaccine and a live attenuated vaccine. One injection of the live attenuated vaccine is recommended officially in Britain early in the second year of life.

Pertussis (whooping-cough) vaccine is prepared from *Bordetellapertussis*, and is proving of value in prophylaxis against whooping-cough. It is usually given along with diphtheria and tetanus in what is known as Triple Vaccine. This is given in three doses: the first at the age of 3 to 6 months, the second six to eight weeks later, and the third six months later, with a booster dose at 5 years.

Plague vaccine was introduced by Haffkine, and appears to give useful protection, but the duration of protection is relatively short: from two to twenty months. Two injections are given at an interval of 4 weeks. A reinforcing dose should be given annually to anyone exposed to the disease.

Poliomyelitis vaccine gives a high degree of protection against the disease. The Salk-type of vaccine, in which the virus is killed by formaldehyde, contains all three known types of poliomyelitis virus. Three intra-muscular injections are required, with an interval of four to six weeks between the first and second, and seven to twelve months between the second and third. There is a growing volume of evidence that a fourth injection prolongs the duration of the protection provided by the vaccine.

The Salk vaccine has now been largely replaced by the live attenuated vaccine which is taken by mouth – a few drops on a lump of sugar. Reinforcing doses of polio vaccine are recommended on school entry, on leaving school, and on travel abroad to countries where poliomyelitis is endemic.

Rabies vaccine was introduced by Pasteur in 1885 for administration, during the long incubation period, to people bitten by a mad dog, in order to prevent the disease from developing.

Rubella vaccine is now available to provide protection against German measles. The value of such a vaccine lies in the fact that it will allow immunity to be given to adolescent girls who have not had the disease in childhood and so ensure that they will not acquire the disease during any subsequent pregnancy. In this way it should prove possible to reduce the number of congenitally abnormal children whose abnormality is the result of their being infected with German measles before they were born, the infection being acquired through their mother having the disease. The recommendation is that it should be given to all girls at the age of 10 to 14 years who have not had the disease, and to all women of child-bearing age shown on a blood test not to be immune – but not during pregnancy.

Smallpox vaccine was the first introduced. As a result of the World Health Organization (WHO) smallpox eradication campaign there is now no medical justification for smallpox vaccination in Britain except for workers in pox virus laboratories, members of their families, those engaged in vaccine manufacture, and hospital staff dealing with patients suspected of having the disease. Nor is there for travellers, but travellers should always check with the Department of Health and Social Security and the Embassy in London of the country which they are proposing to visit, to ensure that vaccination is not compulsory in the country in question.

Tetanus vaccine is given in two forms: (*a*) In the so-called Triple Vaccine, combined with diphtheria and pertussis (whooping-cough) vaccine. This is used for the routine immunization of children, the first dose being given at the age of 3 to 6 months, a second dose six to eight weeks later, and a third dose six months later. A booster dose of tetanus vaccine is recommended on leaving school, on entering higher education, or on starting employment. (*b*) By itself to adults who have not been immunized in childhood and who are particularly exposed to the risk of tetanus, such as soldiers and agricultural workers.

Typhoid vaccine was introduced by Wright and Semple for the protection of troops in the South African War and in India. TAB vaccine, containing *Salmonella typhi* (the causative organism of typhoid fever) and *Salmonella paratyphi* A and B (the organisms of paratyphoid fever) has now been replaced by Typhoid Monovalent Vaccine, containing only *S. typhi*. The change has been made because the monovalent vaccine is less likely to produce painful arms and general malaise and there is no evidence that the TAB vaccine gave any protection against paratyphoid fever. Two doses are given at an interval of four to six weeks, and give protection for one to three years.

Yellow fever vaccine is prepared from chick embryos injected with the living, attenuated strain (17D) of pantropic virus. Only one injection is required, and immunity persists for many years. Reinoculation, however, is desirable every ten years.

The hazards of vaccination, or immunization are minimal, compared with its benefits. Complications, however, do occur. A Vaccine Damage Payments Scheme has therefore been introduced. This provides for the payment of £10,000 tax free in respect of people who, since July 5, 1948, have suffered severe damage as a result of the following vaccinations which have taken place under routine public policy programmes: diphtheria, tetanus, whooping-cough, poliomyelitis, measles, German measles, tuberculosis (BCG), and smallpox (up to July 31, 1971).

VACCINIA is another term for cowpox, a disease in which vesicles form on the udders and teats, due to the same virus as is responsible for smallpox in man. It is also the term used to describe the reaction to smallpox vaccination.

VAGINA is the front passage leading from the exterior to the womb.

VAGINISMUS is spasmodic contraction of the orifice of the vagina on attempted coitus. It is usually psychological in origin, due, for instance, to a neurotic temperament or to frigidity, but it may also be due to some local inflammatory condition.

VAGINITIS is inflammation of the vagina. (See WHITES.)

VAGITUS UTERINUS is the term applied to the crying of a child just before birth and while still in the uterus. Over 130 cases have been reported, though not all of the cases have been authenticated. Four fully authenticated cases were reported at the Motherwell Maternity Hospital between 1939 and 1974. In one case the cry was so loud that it was heard outside the labour ward with the door closed.

VAGOTOMY is the operation of cutting the fibres of the vagus nerve to the stomach. It is sometimes performed as part of the surgical treatment of duodenal ulcer, the aim being to reduce the flow or acidity of the gastric juice.

VAGUS, or PNEUMOGASTRIC, nerve is the tenth cranial nerve. Unlike the other cranial nerves, which are concerned with the special senses, or distributed to the skin and muscles of the head and neck, this nerve, as its names imply, strays downwards into the chest and abdomen, supplying branches to the throat, lungs, heart, stomach, and other abdominal organs. It contains motor, secretory, sensory, and vasodilator fibres.

VALERIAN is the root of *Valeriana officinalis*, a European plant. Its action, which is a sedative one upon the nervous system, depends mainly upon a volatile oil that it contains, and also to some extent upon valerianic acid.

Uses: Valerian was at one time widely used, chiefly in the form of the tincture of valerian, to quiet nervousness, insomnia, and hysterical attacks, being taken in doses of a teaspoonful. The oil of valerian, in doses of two or three drops on sugar, is an old remedy for the relief of dyspepsia associated with spasm of the stomach.

VALGUS means literally knock-kneed, and is a bending inward at the knees (*genu valgum*), or at the ankle, as occurs in flat-foot (*pes valgus*).

VALVES are found in the heart, veins, and lymphatic vessels, for the purpose of maintaining the circulation of the blood and lymph always in one direction. (See HEART; LYMPH; VEINS.)

VALVULAR DISEASE (see HEART DISEASES).

VANCOMYCIN is an antibiotic derived from streptomyces, which is active against a wide range of Gram-positive organisms, including the staphylococcus.

VAN DEN BERGH TEST is one performed on a specimen of serum of the blood in cases of jaundice, to decide whether this is due to ordinary bile (immediate or direct reaction) or incompletely formed bile pigment (delayed or indirect reaction).

VAPOUR BATHS (see BATHS).

VARICELLA is another name for chickenpox (qv).

VARICOCELE means a condition in which the veins of the testicle are distended. (See TESTICLE, DISEASES OF.)

VARICOSE VEINS are veins that have become stretched and dilated. (See VEINS, DISEASES OF.)

VARIOLA is another name for smallpox (qv).

VARIOLOID is the name applied to a mild type of smallpox.

VARIX means an enlarged and tortuous vein.

VARUS, meaning bow-legged, is the term applied to a bulging condition at the hip (*coxa vara*), at the knee (*genu varum*), or at the ankle (*talipes varus*).

VAS is the Latin term for a vessel, especially a blood-vessel.

VASECTOMY is the surgical operation performed to render men sterile, or infertile. It consists of ligating, or tying, and then cutting the ductus, or vas, deferens (see TESTICLE). It is quite a simple operation carried out under local anaesthesia, through a small incision, or cut (or sometimes two) in the upper part of the scrotum. It has no effect on sexual drive or ejaculation, and does not cause impotency. It is not immediately effective, and several tests, spread over several months, must be carried out before it is safe to assume that sterility has been achieved. Although, in those who desire it, fertility can sometimes be restored by a further operation, to restore the continuity of the vas, this cannot be guaranteed, and only seems to occur in about one-fifth of those so operated on. In 1985 42,060 vasectomies were performed.

VASO-ACTIVE INTESTINAL PEPTIDE (VIP) was isolated in 1970. It stimulates the intestinal secretion of water and electrolytes, inhibits gastric secretion and promotes hyperglycaemia. It also has a secretin-like action on the pancreas, stimulating the production of pancreatic juice. It is secreted by the non-beta cells of the pancreas. Tumours of these cells, which are uncommon, provoke a watery diarrhoea syndrome or what is sometimes called pancreatic cholera.

VASODILATORS are substances that cause dilatation of the blood-vessels. They may be drugs, such as amyl nitrite (qv), or natural substances in the body, such as kinins (qv).

VASOMOTOR NERVES are the small nerve fibres that lie upon the walls of blood-vessels and connect the muscle fibres of their middle coat withthe nervous system. Through these nerves the blood-vessels are retained in a state of moderate contraction. There are vasodilator nerves, through which are transmitted impulses that dilate the vessels, and, in the case of the skin-vessels, produce the condition of blushing. There are also vasoconstrictor nerves which transmit impulses that constrict, or narrow, the blood-vessels, as occurs on exposure to cold. (See HYPOTHERMIA.) Various drugs produce dilatation or contraction of the blood-vessels and several of the substances produced by endocrine glands in the body have these effects: eg. adrenaline (qv).

VASOPRESSIN is the fraction isolated from extract of the posterior pituitary lobe which stimulates intestinal activity, constricts blood-vessels, and inhibits the secretion of urine. It is also known as the antidiuretic hormone because of this last effect, and its only use in medicine is, on account of this effect, in the treatment of diabetes insipidus (qv). (See also PITUITARY BODY.)

VEGANISM is a strict form of vegetarianism.

VEGETARIANISM means the principle of subsisting on a diet of vegetables which contains no meat. Such a diet may include milk, cheese and eggs, but there is a strict form of vegetarianism, known as veganism, the adherents of which will eat only vegetables and fruit.

VEGETATIONS are roughenings that appear upon the valves of the heart, usually as the result of acute rheumatism. They lead in time to narrowing of the openings from the cavities of the heart, or to imcompetence of the valves that close these openings. (See HEART DISEASES.)

VEGETATIVE SYSTEM is a term applied to that part of the nervous system which acts in an involuntary manner, to a large extent independently of the brain and spinal cord, and which regulates and connects movements and secretions of internal organs. It is also known as the autonomic nervous system. The term includes the sympathetic and parasympathetic nervous systems (qv).

VEINS are the vessels which carry blood to the heart after it has circulated through the tissues of the body. In general the veins lie alongside corresponding arteries that carry outwards to the tissues the blood which afterwards returns by the veins. The veins are, however, both more numerous and more capacious than the arteries, and, as a rule, there are two accompanying veins for each artery of moderate size. In addition to these deeply placed veins, there are superficial veins in the limbs, which can be readily seen in their distended state lying immediately beneath the skin.

Structure: A vein is of similar structure to an artery, consisting of three coats: outer of fibrous tissue, middle of muscular and elastic fibres, and inner composed of elastic membrane and flattened cells. Any vein has, however, a much thinner wall than its corresponding artery, especially as regards the middle coat. Most veins are provided with valves similar in structure to the valves of the heart, and consisting each of two segments or pouches, which lie flat against the wall of the vein as the blood passes in the proper direction, or which meet and close the passage whenever the blood tends to run backwards. The position of these valves can easily be seen upon the arm or leg by running the finger backwards along a large vein, when the distended vein shows a little swelling at each valve. The valves are most numerous in the veins of the lower limb, those in the arm stand next in point of numbers, whilst there are few valves in the veins of internal organs.

Chief veins: Four *pulmonary veins* open into the left atrium of the heart, two coming from each lung. Into the right atrium there open some small veins from the walls of the heart, and two great vessels, superior vena cava and inferior vena cava, that bring back blood from the body generally.

The *superior vena cava* brings the blood from the head, neck, and upper limbs. It is formed by the union of two *innominate veins*, each of which results from the junction, at the root of the neck, of the internal jugular vein, from the neck, and the subclavian vein, from the upper limb. The *internal jugular vein* receives the blood from within the skull and collects branches from the face and neck as it runs downwards alongside the carotid artery under cover of the thick sternocleidomastoid muscle. One of its most important branches is the *external jugular vein*, which runs beneath the skin from the angle of the jaw straight downwards to the middle of the collar-bone. This vessel can be readily seen when the veins of the neck are distended, and is liable to be opened in wounds of this region. The *subclavian vein* is the last section of the system of veins that accompany the arteries in the arm, each vein being named after its corresponding artery. The superficial veins of the arm are of special interest, because the large *basilic vein* that runs up the inner side of the upper arm is the vein usually opened in blood-letting. Its tributary, the median cubital vein, is used for punctures to get blood for various tests or in order to give intravenous injections. (See BLOOD-LETTING.)

The *inferior vena cava*, which lies to the right side and in front of the spinal column, starting at the junction of the two common iliac veins about the level of the navel, collects the blood from the lower limbs and abdomen. In the lower limbs and in the pelvis, the deeply placed veins correspond in name and in position to the arteries, while the surface veins of the lower limb empty their contents into the *small saphenous vein* on the back of the leg, and the *great saphenous vein* that runs from the instep up the inner side of the leg, knee, and thigh. These veins, and especially the great saphenous vein, are of special interest because of their liability to become distended or varicose. Within the abdomen, the inferior vena cava receives branches corresponding to several branches of the aorta, its largest branches being the *hepatic veins*, which return not only the blood that has reached the liver in the hepatic arteries, but also blood which comes from the digestive organs in the *portal vein* to undergo a second capillary circulation in the liver. (See PORTAL VEIN.)

It appears from what has been said that the blood circulating in the uppermost parts of the body is returned to the heart by the superior vena cava, that from below the diaphragm by the inferior vena cava. There are, however, several connections between these two great vessels, the most important being three *azygos veins* that lie upon the sides of the spinal column, the veins on the front of the abdomen, and some veins that emerge from the abdomen at the navel and connect the portal system with those of the inferior and superior vena cava. By these means the circulation is maintained even when one of these large vessels has been blocked by some disease within the chest or the abdomen.

VEINS, DISEASES OF: These vessels are subject to degenerative and inflammatory changes. INFLAMMATION of a vein is a condition which is serious mainly on account of the clotting of the blood that usually takes place within the inflamed part (thrombosis), and the risk that such a clot may break up and portions be swept away by the circulation to lodge in other vessels (embolism). *Phlebitis*, or *thrombophlebitis*, is the name commonly applied to general inflammation of a vein, while the term *periphlebitis* is used when the inflammation is limited to the loose connective tissue immediately surrounding the vessel. Occasionally the inflammation is of a very acute character, the vein becoming filled with a clot containing bacteria, which are carried to distant parts of the body and there produce abscesses. This condition, known as pyaemia, is an extremely grave one. (See BLOOD-POISONING.) As a rule, however, phlebitis is of a more chronic type, running a course of three or four weeks and then improving under careful treatment.

Causes: Thrombophlebitis may occur as a result of local injury to the affected part, eg. a bruise or a fracture, or it may be due to involvement of the vein from a neighbouring inflammatory or suppurative process. It not infrequently occurs in varicose veins. Most of the cases, however, occur following child-birth or an operation, and in these cases the main factor responsible for the condition is stagnation of the blood-flow through the veins. (See also WHITE LEG.) It may also occur in certain infectious diseases, particularly typhoid fever. In all these conditions the actual cause is probably one or more of three factors: (1) injury or inflammation of the lining endothelium of the vein; (2) slowing of the blood-stream in the vein; (3) some alteration in the blood which makes it more liable to clot.

Symptoms: In a typical case, the skin near the inflamed vein becomes red; the affected part becomes hot, and indeed the general temperature of the body may sometimes be raised; there is swelling both around the vein and of the part beyond it, so that, if a vein in the leg is inflamed, the foot is swollen; finally, considerable pain and tenderness to touch are experienced along the vein. When a clot forms in the vein, as it commonly does, the vessel can be felt as a hard line, and this blocked condition may persist for the rest of life, the vein being converted into a firm, fibrous cord; or a passage may be tunnelled through the clot after the inflammation has subsided in the course of three or four weeks.

Treatment: When the veins of the lower limbs are involved, the patient should rest in bed with the affected limb elevated and resting on pillows. Hot wet packs are applied to relieve the pain and to help to maintain an adequate circulation. If the pain is severe, sedatives may be required. Anticoagulants (qv) are also given to prevent the clot increasing in size and to reduce the risk of pulmonary embolism (qv). Within three days of going to bed, the patient should be encouraged to move the affected limb and foot, as this speeds the process of recovery. It is now recognized that prolonged rest in bed tends to delay recovery.

VARICOSE VEINS are veins that have become stretched and dilated out of proportion to the amount of blood they have to carry. There are three positions in which the veins have a special tendency to become varicose. These are the veins about the lower end of the bowel, producing the condition known as haemorrhoids or piles (see PILES); the veins of the testicle, producing varicocele (see TESTICLE, DISEASES OF); and the great saphenous vein, with its branches on the inner side of the leg, knee, and thigh. Further, small veins are apt to become varicose here and there on a mucous membrane that is the seat of chronic catarrh and congestion; these minute varicose veins are found especially on the mucous membranes of the throat and stomach, and may give rise, now and then, to haemorrhage, particularly in the case of alcoholics. Only the varicose veins of the limbs are considered here, the others having been dealt with elsewhere.

Causes: It is estimated that around two-thirds of adults in the United Kingdom have varicose veins. Undoubtedly some persons are more liable to the formation of varicose veins than others. The veins vary greatly in thickness in different persons and at different portions of the same vein, so that the formation of the vessel wall and the condition of surrounding parts have much to do with its dilatation. Thus the tendency to varicose veins is often hereditary. Employments that necessitate long-continued standing, with little vigorous muscle exertion, not only throw a great strain upon the veins of the leg, but fail to provide the pumping action that muscular contractions exert in emptying the veins. Thus barmaids, shop assistants and waitresses often suffer from varicose veins. The evil effects of prolonged standing are increased by tight garters. Pregnancy is another common cause of varicose veins, though the condition tends to disappear after the child is born.

An important consideration is that, after a vein has begun to dilate, its walls become weaker and its valves useless. Thus the weight of the column of blood in the limb presses down with increasing force, the condition tends to grow worse and worse, and to spread into neighbouring veins.

Symptoms: At first the only symptoms are a feeling of weight and aching in the limbs accompanied sometimes by cramps. This is experienced either at night, after a long day's standing, or in the morning when the feet are first put to the ground. After the condition becomes marked, there is often swelling of the feet, especially above the ankles, that quickly disappears when the patient lies down. Varicose veins that have lasted many years are liable to become inflamed, and to produce eczema and ulceration of the skin. (See ULCERS.) Another risk attached to untreated varicose veins, particularly in older individuals, is that a blow on them may lead to severe haemorrhage.

Treatment: Varicose veins, as already noted, tend, when untreated, to become worse and worse. Treatment which is directed merely towards checking their increase and towards preventing ulceration is known as palliative treatment, whilst the entire removal of the distended veins is known as radical treatment.

PALLIATIVE TREATMENT: In slight cases, it is often sufficient to avoid the use of garters, to remedy constipation, to avoid standing as much as possible, and, after the day's work is done, to sit with the feet elevated on a couch or chair. In more marked cases, some mechanical support for the superficial veins is necessary, in order to counteract the downward pressure of the blood in the great saphenous vein, whose valves have become useless. For this purpose one may use an elastic or crêpe bandage, or elastic stockings. Elastic bandages are probably the most satisfactory method of support. They can be cleaned with soap and water, and, if carefully handled, will last for a year. There are two main types of elastic bandages: the two-way stretch bandage and the one-way stretch bandage. The former is rather more difficult to apply, but is the bandage of choice in severe cases. For many cases the one-way stretch bandage is eminently satisfactory. Elastic bandages must be removed at night before retiring to bed and reapplied before getting out of bed in the morning. Crêpe bandages are used in a similar manner. Some persons find elastic stockings more comfortable than bandages. There must be no tight band at the top of the stocking, but slipping down may be prevented by suspenders; of the various kinds, the spiral silk elastic stocking is generally regarded as the best. For the treatment of varicose ulcers see ULCERS.

Successful results are sometimes obtained from the injection, here and there into the veins of some irritating substance, such as sodium tetradecyl sulphate or sodium morrhuate. A clot forms at once in the vein, which later becomes solid. The veins must be firmly bandaged for the next few weeks. This treatment is practically painless and devoid of later discomfort.

RADICAL TREATMENT is adopted when the veins are excessively dilated, when they cause much annoyance, or when the person suffering from them wishes to enter one of the public services. The most successful method consists in turning up a flap of skin on the inner side of the thigh or knee, ligaturing the vein in two places and removing the intervening dilated portions *en masse*. The wound heals quickly, and, in most cases, the cure is complete.

WOUNDS IN VEINS are not in general serious; for, although a considerable amount of dark blood flows steadily from that end of the vein more distant from the heart, it can be stopped by gentle pressure, and soon ceases of itself. When a varicose vein ruptures, as it may do if an ulcer is present, the condition is more serious. Blood, in this case, flows copiously from the end next to the heart in consequence of the defects in the vein's valves, as well as from the other end; and the loss of blood may be great unless pressure be speedily applied. This also can be checked easily by pressure above and below the wound, and by raising the limb. Another danger, attaching to wounds of the veins in the neck, is that air may be drawn into them by the act of breathing, and great interference with the circulation may ensue which may well prove fatal.

VENA CAVA is the name applied to either of the two large vessels that open into the right atrium of the heart. (See VEINS.)

VENEPUNCTURE is the name applied to inserting a needle into a vein, usually for the purpose of injecting a drug or withdrawing blood for haematological or biochemical analysis.

VENEREAL DISEASES, SEXUALLY TRANSMITTED DISEASES as they are now officially known, are certain contagious maladies which are, as a rule, communicated from one person to another by sexual intercourse. They are also classified under the title of GENITO-URINARY MEDICINE. In 1983, there were 547,437 new cases registered in the clinics for these diseases in England. The commonest were non-specific infection and gonorrhoea (58,301). The remaining cases included syphilis (4211), non-specific urethritis (qv), chancroid (100), trichomoniasis (qv), candidiasis (qv), scabies (qv), pediculosis pubis (see PEDICULOSIS), Reiter's disease (qv), condyloma (qv), and psychosexual problems. What might be described as the two 'classical' venereal diseases (syphilis and gonorrhoea), along with chancroid, account for less than 15 per cent of cases seen in these clinics today.

Among the means which have been proposed for reducing the incidence of these diseases are: education of the public; provision of means for immediate self-disinfection; early treatment; and compulsory treatment of all people found to be affected, the last measure almost necessarily implying notification of these diseases in the same manner as one of the ordinary infectious diseases. Such compulsory notification has never been favoured in Great Britain, though it is in force in certain European countries. For purposes of efficient treatment, clinics have been established under the aegis of the National Health Service in all the large towns in Great Britain.

There are 230 such clinics, and they are playing an increasingly important role in an advisory and preventive capacity. The moral and ethical aspects of these diseases play a much more important part than in any other group of diseases and in the past have been either ignored or mishandled. This is one aspect of medicine in which health education in the widest sense is of paramount importance.

VENESECTION means the withdrawal of blood by opening a vein. (See BLOOD-LETTING.)

VENOGRAPHY is the study of the veins, particularly by means of X-rays after the veins have been injected with a radio-opaque substance.

VENTER is the Latin term for the belly.

VENTILATION consists in the continuous dilution or removal, by pure fresh air, of the vitiated products from respiration, combustion, putrefaction of animal and vegetable material, and from industrial processes and trades. It includes the ventilation of houses, factories, buildings of every description, as well as of streets, alleys, courts, and sewers. Different methods must be adopted for each variety of case. In streets and courts, reliance must be placed on the influence of winds, the height of the buildings, and the width of the street or space. In the confined areas of houses, means must be adopted for the ingress and exit of the air. Similar provision must be made in the case of sewers, the exit for which, however, must be placed where there is least chance of danger.

It is now recognized that lack of oxygen or excess of carbon dioxide plays little part in producing the discomfort of badly ventilated rooms. Nor is there any evidence that there is any organic poison in exhaled air. The main factor responsible is heat stagnation due to excess of moisture and lack of air movement. In other words, ventilation and warming must be considered together. A desirable atmosphere has been defined as 'cool rather than hot; dry rather than damp; and moving rather than still'. Various methods have been evolved for correlating these different factors, the most important of which include: The *kata-thermometer* (qv) which indicates the cooling power of the air. The *eupatheoscope*, an instrument which corresponds approximately to the human body in its sensitivity to air currents, and is read on a scale of equivalent temperature. The *globe thermometer*, which gives an index of the combined influence of air temperature and radiant heat. Another standard, used in the USA, is the *effective temperature*, which is defined as 'that temperature of saturated motionless air which would produce the same sensation of coolness as that produced by the combination of temperature, humidity, and air motion under observation'. In Great Britain the optimum conditions for sedentary work are a dry kata-thermometer cooling power of 6; an equivalent temperature of 16·7°C (62°F); a globe thermometer reading of 18·3°C (65°F); an effective temperature of 16·1°C (61°F).

Air sterilization: In order to reduce the risk of cross-infection, particularly in schools, dormitories, and offices, much attention has been devoted in recent years to the problem of killing pathogenic organisms in the air of a room. Ultra-violet light has been used, but its use for this purpose is restricted. It has been used mainly in operating theatres and the like. By and large, the most practical way of ensuring as clean air as possible is to maintain adequate circulation of the air to keep it as free as possible from dust, and the wearing of masks on special occasions. (See also HUMIDIFICATION.)

VENTOUSE, or VACUUM EXTRACTOR, is used in obstetrics. It is based upon a suction-cup technique, whereby the baby is sucked out of the uterus instead of being drawn out by forceps.

VENTRAL means belonging to the belly.

VENTRICLE is the term applied to the two lower cavities of the heart (see HEART), and also to the cavities within the brain.

VENTRICULOGRAPHY is the process of taking an X-ray photograph of the brain after the fluid in the lateral ventricles of the brain has been replaced by air; in this way any alteration in the outline of the ventricles (eg. from pressure by a tumour) can be detected.

VERAPAMIL (CORDILOX) is a drug used in the treatment of disordered rhythms of the heart and angina pectoris (qv), and is also proving of value in the treatment of high blood-pressure. (See CALCIUM ANTAGONISTS.)

VERATRINE is a mixture of alkaloids, derived from the seeds of *Schoenocaulon officinale*, which has a paralysing effect upon nerves. The ointment of veratrine is used for the relief of pain in cases of rheumatism or of neuralgia.

VERATRUM, also known as green hellebore, Indian poke, and poke root, is the root of *Veratrum viride*, a plant of the United States. It acts as a sedative and depressant of the heart and nervous system by virtue of veratrine and other alkaloids that it contains. Alkaloids obtained from it are used in the treatment of high blood-pressure. (See ESSENTIAL HYPERTENSION.)

VERBIGERATION means the insane repetition of meaningless words and sentences.

VERMICIDES, or VERMIFUGES, are substances that kill, or expel, parasitic worms from the intestines.

VERRUCA is the Latin term for a wart.

VERRUCOSE means covered with warts.

VERSION, or TURNING, is the name given to an operation in obstetrics which consists in turning the child in cases in which the lie of the child is abnormal.

VERTEBRA is one of the irregularly shaped bones that together form the vertebral column. (See SPINAL COLUMN.)

VERTIGO, or giddiness, is a condition in which the affected person loses the power of balancing himself, and has a false sensation as to his own movements or as to those of surrounding objects. The power of balancing depends upon sensations derived partly through the sense of touch, partly from the eyes, but mainly from the semicircular canals of the internal ear. In general, vertigo is due to some interference with this mechanism or with the centres in the cerebellum and cerebrum with which it is connected. Giddiness is apt to be associated with headache, nausea, and vomiting.

Causes: The simplest cause of vertigo is some mechanical disturbance of the body affecting the fluid in the internal ear; such as that produced by moving in a swing with the eyes shut, the motion of a boat causing sea-sickness, or a sudden fall. (See SEA-SICKNESS.) The cause which produces a severe and sudden giddiness is Menière's disease (qv), a condition in which there is loss of function of the labyrinth of the inner ear. An acute labyrinthitis may result from viral infection and produce a severe vertigo lasting 2 to 5 days. Because it often occurs in epidemics it is often called epidemic vertigo. Vertigo is sometimes produced by the removal of wax from the ear, or even by syringing out the ear. (See EAR, DISEASES OF.) A third group of causes for vertigo is found in disorders of the stomach. Refractive errors in the eyes which have not received appropriate treatment by glasses, an overstrained nervous system, an attack of migraine, a mild attack of epilepsy, and gross diseases of the brain, such as tumours, form another set of causes acting more directly upon the central nervous system. Finally, giddiness may be due to some disorder of the circulation, eg. bloodlessness of the brain produced by fainting, or by disease of the heart.

Treatment, while the attack lasts, consists in maintaining a recumbent posture, in a darkened, quiet room. Sedatives are the drugs which have most influence in diminishing giddiness when it is distressing. After the attack is over, careful examination is necessary in order to determine the cause, for upon this depends the appropriateness of treatment.

VESICAL is the term applied to structures connected with, or diseases of, the bladder. (See BLADDER.)

VESICANTS are blistering agents. (See BLISTERS.)

VESICLE means a small collection of fluid in the epidermis. The fluid in some cases consists of a drop of sweat collected at the mouth of a sweat-gland, but in general it is serum from the blood. The skin disease specially associated with the formation of vesicles is herpes; in this disease the vesicles usually burst and then scab over. Some infectious diseases show an eruption composed of vesicles: eg. smallpox and chickenpox. When a large number of white corpuscles from the blood find their way into a vesicle, it becomes a pustule.

The term vesicle is also applied to minute sacs of normal structure, such as the air-vesicles in which the finest bronchial tubes end in the lungs.

VESTIBULOCOCHLEAR NERVE is the eighth cranial nerve. It consists of two sets of fibres, which constitute two separate nerves. One is known as the vestibular nerve, which is the nerve of equilibration or balance. The other is known as the cochlear nerve, which is the nerve of hearing. Disturbance of the former causes giddiness, whilst disturbance of the latter causes deafness.

VIBRATOR is an instrument used for vibratory massage in the mechanical treatment of disease. For its use see MASSAGE.

VIBRIO is a bacterium of curved shape, such as the vibrio of cholera.

VIBURNUM, or BLACK HAW, is the bark of *Viburnum prunifolium* or of *Viburnum lentago*, of which the liquid extract is used in doses of 4 to 8 ml for treating painful menstruation.

VILLUS is the name given to one of the minute processes which are thickly planted upon the inner surface of the small intestine, giving it, to the naked eye, a velvety appearance, and greatly assisting absorption. (See DIGESTION; INTESTINE.)

VILOXAZINE (VIVALAN) (see ANTI-DEPRESSANTS).

VINBLASTINE (VELBE) is an alkaloid (qv) derived from the periwinkle plant (*Vinca rosea*) which is of value in the treatment of certain forms of malignant disease, particularly choriocarcinoma and Hodgkin's disease. (See CYTOTOXIC DRUGS.)

VINCENT'S ANGINA is an ulcerative inflammation of the throat, often foul smelling, and caused by large, spindle-shaped bacilli and spirilla.

VINCRISTINE (ONCOVIN) is an alkaloid derived from the common periwinkle which is proving of value in the palliative treatment of certain forms of malignant disease. (See CYTOTOXIC DRUGS.)

VINEGAR (see ACETIC ACID.)

VINUM is the Latin name for wine. The wines used as medicinal remedies include wines of colchicum, antimony, ipecacuanha, citrate of iron, quinine and orange. They are seldom used now.

VINYL ETHER is an inhalational anaesthetic used in minor surgical procedures of short duration, and for the induction of anaesthesia (qv).

VIOMYCIN is an antibiotic which is active against the *Mycobacterium tuberculosis*, but less active than streptomycin or isoniazid.

VIRAL HAEMORRHAIC FEVER or EBOLA VIRUS FEVER, is a highly fatal disease due to a virus related to that of Marburg disease (qv). Two large outbreaks of it were recorded in 1976 (one in the Sudan and one in Zaïre), with a mortality, respectively, of 50 and 80 per cent, and the disease reappeared in the Sudan in 1979. After an incubation period of 7 to 14 days, the onset is with headache of increasing severity and fever. This is followed by diarrhoea, extensive internal bleeding and vomiting. Death usually occurs on the eighth to ninth day. Infection is by person-to-person contact. Serum from patients convalescent from the disease is a useful source of antibodies to the virus.

VIRGINIAN PRUNE BARK, or WILD CHERRY BARK, is the bark of *Prunus serotina*, which yields an oil containing hydrocyanic acid. It possesses tonic and sedative properties and in the form of tincture and syrup is used as a remedy for cough.

VIRILISM is the term applied to the condition in which masculine characteristics develop in the female, and is commonly the result of an overactive suprarenal gland, or of a tumour of its cortex. It may also result from an androgen secreting ovarian tumour and also from the polycystic ovary syndrome.

VIRUS is the term applied to a group of infective agents which are so small that they are able to pass through the pores of collodion filters. They are responsible for some of the most important diseases affecting man: eg. influenza, poliomyelitis, smallpox, and yellow fever. Some idea of their size may be obtained from the fact that the virus of influenza measures 80 micrometres, whereas the staphylococcus measures 1000 micrometres. (1 micrometre=0.000001 millimetre.)

VISCERA is the general name given to the larger organs lying within the cavities of the chest and abdomen. The term 'viscus' is also applied individually to these organs.

VISCEROPTOSIS, also known as splanchnoptosis, means a falling down of the viscera, especially those of the abdomen. In elderly women it may be associated with prolapse of the womb. (See PROLAPSE.)

VISION: Broadly speaking, vision is the ability to see.

Pathway of light from the eye to the brain: Light enters the eye by passing through the transparent cornea, then through the aqueous humour filling the anterior chamber. It then passes through the pupil, through the lens and the vitreous to reach the retina. In the retina the rod and cone photoreceptors detect light and relay messages in the form of electrochemical impulses through the various layers of the retina to the nerve fibres. The nerve fibres carry messages via the optic nerve, optic chiasm, optic tract, lateral geniculate body and finally the optic radiations to the visual cortex. Here in the visual cortex these messages are interpreted. It is therefore the visual cortex of the brain that 'sees'.

Visual acuity: Two points will not be seen as two unless they are separated by a minimum distance. This distance is such that the objects are so far apart that the lines joining them to the eye enclose between them (subtend) an angle of at least one minute of a degree. This amount of separation allows the images of the two points to fall on two separate cones (if the light from two points falls on one cone, the two points would be seen as a single point). There are many tests of visual acuity. One of the more common is the Snellen Test Type. This is made up of many letters of different size. Each letter is constructed in a specific manner so that the various components of the letter subtend an angle of one minute of one degree at the eye. Each letter when placed at specified distance from the patient subtends an angle of five minutes of a degree. Thus the top letter subtends an angle of 5 minutes when placed 60 metres from the eye, the lowest letter subtends the same angle when placed 4 metres away. By conventions the chart is placed 6 metres away from the patient. Someone able to see the lowest line at this distance has a visual acuity of 6/4. If they are only able to see the top letter they have 6/60 vision. 'Normal' vision is 6/6.

Colour vision: 'White light' is made up of component colours. These can be separated by a prism, thereby producing a spectrum. The three cardinal colours are red, green, and blue. All other colours can be produced by a varying mixture of these three. Colour vision is a complex subject. The trichromat theory of colour vision suggests that there are three types of cones, each type sensitive to one of the cardinal colours. Colour perception is based on differential stimulation of these cone types. The opponent colour theory suggests that each cone type can generate signals of the opposite kind. Output from some cones can collaborate with the output from others or can inhibit the action of other cones. Colour perception results from these various complex interactions.

Defective colour vision may be hereditary or acquired and can occur in the presence of normal visual acuity. *Hereditary defective colour vision* is more common in men (7 per cent of males) than women (0·5 per cent of females). Men are affected, but women convey the abnormal gene to their children. It occurs because one or more of the photopigments of the retina are abnormal, or the cones are damaged. Red–green colour defect is the commonest. *Acquired defective colour vision* is the result of disease of the cones or their connections in the retina, optic nerve or brain, eg. macular disease, optic neuritis. Colour vision can be impaired but not lost as a result of corneal opacification or cataract formation. *Tests of colour vision*: these include matching of coloured yarn, using specially designed numbers made of coloured dots surrounded by dots of confusing colour (eg. Ishihara plates) and by means of coloured buttons which must be arranged in order of changing hue.

VISION, DISORDERS OF: The list of disorders resulting in poor or dim vision is huge. Disturbance of vision can result from an uncorrected refractive error, disease or injury of the cornea, iris, lens, vitreous, retina, choroid or sclera. It may also result from disease or injury to the structures comprising the visual pathway from the retina to the occipital cortex (see VISION, PATHWAY OF LIGHT FROM THE EYE TO THE BRAIN) and from lesions of the structures around the eye, eg. swollen lids, drooping eyelids.

VISION, FIELD OF: When the eye looks at a specific point or object, that point is seen clearly. Other objects within a large area away from this fixation point can also be seen but less clearly. The area that can be seen around the fixation point, without moving the eye, is known as the field of vision. The extent of the field is limited inwards by the nose, above by the brow and below by the cheek. The visual field thus has its greatest extent outwards from the side of the head. The field of vision of each eye overlaps to a large extent so that objects in the centre and towards the inner part of each field are viewed by both eyes together. Because the eyes are set slightly apart, each eye sees objects in this overlapping part of the field slightly differently. It is because of this slight difference that objects can be perceived as three dimensional. Defects in the visual field (scotomas) can be produced by a variety of disorders. Certain of these produce specific field defects. For example, glaucoma, some types of brain damage and some toxins can produce specific defects in the visual field. This type of field defect may be very useful in diagnosing a particular disorder. The *blind spot* is that part of the visual field corresponding to the optic disc. There are no rods nor cones on the optic disc and therefore no light perception from this area. The blind spot can be found temporal (ie. on the outer side) of the fixation point.

VIS MEDICATRIX NATURAE is a Latin term meaning the healing power of Nature, and is often used to indicate the tendency of wounds to heal and of the bodily powers to subdue disease, when left to the operation of time and rest.

VISUAL EVOKED RESPONSE: Stimulation of the retina with light causes changes in the electrical activity of the cerebral cortex. These changes can be measured from outside the skull and can give valuable information about the state of the visual pathway from the retinal ganglion cells to the occipital cortex. Not only can it determine that function is normal, it can also help to diagnose some causes of poor vision.

VITAMIN is a term applied to a group of substances which exist in minute quantities in natural foods, and which are necessary to normal nutrition, especially in connection with growth and development. Most of them have now been synthesized. When they are absent from the food, defective growth takes place in young animals and children, and in adults various diseases arise; whilst short of the production of actual disease, persistent deprivation of one or other vitamin is apt to lead to a state of lowered general health. Certain deficiencies in diet have long been known to be the cause of scurvy, beriberi, and rickets, but the so-called vitamin hypothesis was not introduced until the twentieth century.

Vitamin A is usually taken in more than ample quantity in the food, and is stored in the liver. It is developed originally by plants as a yellow colouring matter, carotene, for example in carrots, and it is also found in egg yolk, liver, milk, butter, and most green vegetables. When stored in the liver it is colourless and has a slight chemical difference from carotene. The two richest sources of this vitamin are halibut-liver oil and cod-liver oil. The daily requirement of vitamin A is in the region of 4000 international units. Children and pregnant women require relatively more than adults. Deficiency of vitamin A is responsible for serious inflammation of the eyes known as xerophthalmia, which is one of the chief causes of blindness in the developing world; also for night blindness, various skin eruptions, defective development of the teeth, and particularly for want of vitality in the tissues, which leads to localized inflammations. It is not destroyed by ordinary cooking processes.

Vitamin B_1 (see THIAMINE).

Vitamin B_2 (see RIBOFLAVINE).

Vitamin B_3 (see PANTOTHENIC ACID).

Vitamin B_6 (see PYRIDOXINE).

Vitamin B_{12} (see CYANOCOBALAMIN).

Vitamin C is especially found in fresh fruits such as oranges, and also in fresh green vegetables, and to a smaller extent in milk, meat, and other fresh foods. Canned vegetables such as tomatoes also retain it if their reaction is acid. It is quickly destroyed by high temperature, by excess baking soda and other alkalis, and gradually by oxidation in process of keeping. Its deficiency leads to symptoms of scurvy (qv) including muscular weakness, haemorrhages under the skin, swelling and inflammation of the gums with loss of teeth, and serious damage to joints by haemorrhage; it occurs in sailors and other persons long deprived of fresh foods, and also in babies fed persistently on artificial foods. This vitamin has not only been obtained in a pure state, but has been manufactured in a crystalline form as ascorbic acid. The daily requirement of vitamin C (in terms of ascorbic acid) is 30 mg for adults and 60 mg for children. There is no convincing evidence that it is of any value in the treatment of cancer, for the treatment of which it has recently been recommended by some.

Vitamin D is of special importance for the growth of children, and its deficiency produces rickets (qv) with softening and irregular growth of bones, so that swollen joints, distorted limbs, deformities of the chest and similar malformations arise. It was formerly common in the dark and narrow streets of large manufacturing towns and is still found when children are kept too much indoors. Osteomalacia (qv), a similar disease affecting the bones of adults, results from the same causes when lime salts are absorbed from the bones during pregnancy. It has long been known that cod-liver oil was the chief remedy for rickets, and for a time it was supposed that its anti-rachitic action depended upon vitamin A, but it is now known to be vitamin D. There are two forms of vitamin D. Vitamin D_2, also known as calciferol or ergocalciferol, is obtained from ergosterol, a waxy constituent of plants, by ultra-violet irradiation. Vitamin D_3, or cholecalciferol, is the natural form of the vitamin. It is produced by the ultra-violet irradiation of a sterol widely distributed in animal fats. This substance is also formed naturally in the fatty tissues of the body when the skin is exposed to the action of sunlight, or, when this is not available, to ultraviolet rays from an arc lamp. It can also be formed in food such as milk when this is similarly exposed to light. Only a few foods contain vitamin D naturally, including cod-liver oil and other fish-liver oils (especially that from halibut liver), whilst egg yolk contains a smaller quantity; other fats and milk contain very small quantities. The mode of action of vitamin D is to aid the absorption of phosphorus and calcium from the food, increase their amount in the blood, and thus in the bones. In the case of this vitamin bad effects may follow over-dosage, or hypervitaminosis, because if too much calcium and phosphorus are maintained in the blood the bones and teeth become over-calcified, the arteries may become unduly hardened and calculi may be formed in the kidneys and other organs. The daily requirement for infants and nursing mothers is 400 to 800 international units, whilst for adults it is probably about 400 units. (See CALCIFEROL.)

Vitamin E, TOCOPHEROL, has been known since 1923, when it was found that its absence in the case of rats caused failure to produce young. It is derived especially from the oil contained in seeds and in green leaves, and also is present in smaller amounts in other fresh fats. It can also be synthesized in the form of alpha-tocopherol. It is readily stored, like vitamin A, in the body, and thus is unlikely to be found wanting in human beings except in cases of very severe under-nutrition and in premature infants. It is possible, however, that miscarriages may occasionally be due to its deficiency.

Vitamin K, also known as PHYTOMENADIONE, the anti-haemorrhagic vitamin, is essential for the proper clotting of blood. It has been given successfully in cases of bleeding in infants, and to patients with jaundice, who have a special tendency to bleeding. Bleeding in these conditions is thought to be due to deficiency of vitamin K. Synthetic chemical products with an identical physiological action have now been made. In the natural form it is widespread in nature, the main sources being spinach, leafy vegetables, tomatoes, and liver. The daily requirement of man is not known.

Vitamin P, CITRIN, or HESPERIDIN, present in citrus fruits, appears to be responsible for the resistance of the capillaries to pressure. If there is a deficiency of vitamin P in the diet the capillaries rupture easily, resulting, for example, in purpura.

It should be said in conclusion, with regard to the supply of vitamins, that any person using a diet containing the protective foods, such as milk, eggs, butter, cheese, fat, fish, wholemeal bread, fresh vegetables and fruit, should obtain an ample supply of vitamins. Infants should have a daily supplement of a compound vitamin preparation. (See INFANT FEEDING.)

VITELLUS, or VITELLUM, is the Latin name for yolk of egg.

VITILIGO are patchy areas of depigmentation of the skin surrounded by areas of increased pigmentation. It is seen in many auto-immune diseases such as Graves' disease, chronic thyroiditis and Addison's disease and it is due to the auto-immune destruction of the melanin-secreting cells in the skin.

VITRELLA is a small, crushable, glass capsule enclosed in an absorptive and protective fabric, used for the dispensing of medicines such as amyl nitrite which are to be inhaled.

VITREOUS BODY is a semi-fluid, transparent substance which fills most of the globe of the eye behind the lens.

VITRIOL, OIL OF, is an old name for sulphuric acid.

VIVISECTION: For over a century the medical profession has aimed at maintaining as high a standard as possible for vivisection. It was the medical profession led by Dr James Paget that was responsible for the passing of the Cruelty to Animals Act 1876, whereby cruelty was eliminated, the infliction of pain was reduced to a minimum by the use of anaesthetics, and the licensing and surveillance of animal experiments was ensured.

The total number of animals used for experimental work in Britain (1986) was 3·1 million. Most of these were mice (1·6 million) and rats (830,159). The number of primates used was 5,635. Dogs and cats represent only 0·4 per cent of the total. These figures may be compared with the fact that each year in Britain 360 million animals are killed for food.

Eighty per cent of animal experiments are done without anaesthesia because feeding experiments, taking blood, or giving injection, do not require anaesthetics in animals any more than in man. The forty universities in Britain are responsible for less than one-fifth of animal experiments. Commercial concerns and Government institutions are responsible for most of the rest. The much criticised tests on cosmetics account for less than 0·7 per cent of all animal work, and seldom causes more than transient discomfort when applied to the skin. Such tests are necessary because such materials are often applied with great frequency – even over years – to the skin of infants.

A common argument is that animal research should be replaced by work on tissue culture. This is a method of research and investigation that is being used to an increasing extent, but there is a limit to the extent to which infection, cancer, or drugs can be investigated on cultures of tissue cells.

The significance and value of vivisection has been summed up in the following words. 'Medical research owes a great deal to animal experiments and so do our patients, both human and veterinary. Every diabetic receiving insulin, everyone who has had a renal transplant, every leukaemic child treated with modern cytotoxic drugs, and, indeed, all who benefit from modern medicines owe a debt to animals. Doctors need not be apologetic about animal work. The surveillance by Her Majesty's inspectors and, just as important, the personal qualities of research workers and animal house technicians ensure that no unnecessary suffering is inflicted on animals and that they are handled with care and kindness'.

VIVONEX (see ENTERAL FEEDING).

VOCAL CORDS (see LARYNGOSCOPE; LARYNX; VOICE AND SPEECH).

VOCAL RESONANCE: The air carrying the voice produced in the larynx passes through the throat, mouth and nose. The shape and size of these structures will influence the timbre of the voice, or vocal resonance. This will vary from person to person and even within an individual; ie. with a cold.

VOICE AND SPEECH are two terms applied to the system of sounds which are produced in the upper air passages and in the mouth, and which form one of the means of communication between human beings.

Voice means the set of fundamental notes and tones produced by the larynx which are modified in various ways during their passage through the mouth so as to form speech or song. Speech differs from song in being less sustained and of smaller compass with regard to pitch, and in presenting sounds which have not a musical character.

Voice is produced in the larynx of most animals. Voice production may be studied with the laryngoscope (qv), an instrument which enables the changes that take place in the larynx, when different notes are sounded, to be clearly seen.

Musical notes vary in three characters: loudness, pitch, and quality or timbre. The *loudness* of the voice depends upon the volume of air which is available for agitating the vocal cords, and therefore upon the size of the chest and the vigour with which its muscles can be made to act.

The *pitch* of the voice is determined by several things, the chief points being the size of the larynx; the degree of tenseness at which the vocal cords are, for the time being, maintained by the laryngeal muscles; the fact as to whether the cords vibrate as a whole or merely at their edges; and the shape which is given to the cavity of the larynx by movements of the arytenoid and epiglottic cartilages. In any given voice, the range of pitch seldom exceeds two and a half octaves, although the particular part of the musical scale that can be produced varies according as the voice is bass, tenor, contralto or soprano. Generally speaking, a large larynx with long vocal cords produces low notes, and hence men have a deeper voice than women. For the same reason the small larynx of childhood produces a shrill voice, whilst the rapid growth of the larynx at the time of puberty, and consequent uncertainty of muscular control over the vocal cords, produces the breaking of the voice that occurs in boys at this time. This is occurring at an earlier age. Thus fifty years ago, treble lines in cathedral choirs were made up of boys aged 11 to 16. Today choir schools are rarely catering for boys over 13, and voices are breaking as young as 12. Changes in the voice also occur at other ages as a result of the secondary action of the sex hormones. Thus, during menstruation there may be a slight decrease in the quality of the singing voice, affecting especially notes in the highest register, and there may be a lowering of pitch during pregnancy. At the menopause the entire vocal range for speaking and singing may be lowered, and with the onset of old age there tends to be increasing virilism of the voice.

The manner in which the muscles of the larynx act upon the cords allows the pitch to change at will. Thus if the thick part of each cord be held rigid and only the sharp free edge be allowed to vibrate, a high note is the result, and a still higher note is reached in men when only the front part of this free edge is allowed to move, as in the falsetto voice. On the other hand, by allowing a greater thickness of the cord to vibrate, the person loads the vibrating edge, and so produces a much deeper note.

The *timbre* of the voice is partly due to these differences in the larynx, but chiefly to peculiarities and to voluntary changes in shape of the mouth and other cavities associated with the air passages. These changes in shape are chiefly concerned with the alterations of the fundamental notes which produce speech.

It should be remembered, however, that, while the muscular arrangements of the larynx are chiefly concerned with the pitch of the voice, and the shape of the mouth with its modulation, the *loudness* is varied by the movements of the chest. The neglect of this fact is often responsible for the bad voice-production which leads to great straining of the throat, and is largely responsible for the throat affections of many of those who use the voice much.

There are certain peculiar forms of voice production. The *falsetto voice* has been already mentioned. *Whispering* is a form of speech in which voice is completely absent, the larynx being wide open and the sound produced entirely in the mouth. *Ventriloquism* is a form of speech in which the voice is produced by the indrawing of air, instead of in the usual way of expiration. Since it is always difficult to localize the source of sound, the ventriloquist can easily suggest to his audience a false place of origin for the unusual voice.

Speech consists of a series of rapid modifications of the voice, produced by changes in position of the palate, tongue, and lips.

Defects of speech: The act of speech has a very elaborate controlling mechanism in the nervous system. Further, the power of speech is gained in early life by children hearing the sounds made by others and mimicking them so that the centres for speech in the brain are intimately connected with those concerned in the sense of hearing.

MUTISM, or the entire absence of the power to speak, may be due to various causes, the most effectual being some mental deficiency which denies to the child sufficient intelligence to mimic the actions of those around him. In other cases the child seems to be quite intelligent, but, owing apparently to some defect in the nervous control of the voice and speech organs, or in these organs themselves, he is unable to make any sounds. A common cause of mutism is complete deafness present at birth or caused by some ear diseases in early childhood. The child in this case cannot learn to speak, simply because he cannot hear, but, if properly educated, he can be taught to speak fluently and to understand what is said by watching the lips and throat of others. (See DUMBNESS.)

STAMMERING is a bad habit of speech due to want of co-ordination between the different parts of the speech mechanism. (See STAMMERING.)

Such minor peculiarities in speech as burrs and lisps are due to peculiarities in the action of the tongue or palate, whilst the deformities of tongue-tie and cleft-palate are accompanied by still greater defects of speech. When the nose is blocked by any condition, such as a cold in the head or polypus, the pronunciation of the resonants *m, n,* and *ng* is interfered with, these being heard as *b, d,* and *g,* respectively, for a reason which can be seen on consulting table 44.

DYSPHASIA is a condition in which various forms of inability to speak, or to understand speech, come on, usually late in life, as the result of brain disease. (See DYSPHASIA.)

APHONIA, or loss of voice, causes speaking to be carried on in a whisper. It is usually either due to some disorder of the vocal cords, as in the laryngitis which may form part of a cold (see THROAT DISEASES), or is a symptom of hysteria. It is generally of short duration. (See also CHILDREN, PECULIARITIES OF; DYSARTHRIA.)

VOLAR means something pertaining to the palm or sole.

VOLKMANN'S CONTRACTURE is the condition in which, as a result of too great a pressure from splint or bandage in the treatment of a broken arm, the flexor muscles of the forearm contract and thus obstruct free flow of blood in the veins; the muscles then swell and ultimately become fibrosed.

VOLSELLA is a Latin term for a forceps with hooked blades.

VOLVULUS means an obstruction of the bowels produced by the twisting of a loop of bowel round itself. (See INTESTINE, DISEASES OF.)

VOMICA means a cavity in the lung produced by ulceration, which is usually a sign of tuberculosis.

VOMITING means the expulsion of the stomach contents through the mouth. When the effort of vomiting is made, but nothing is brought up, the process is known as retching. When vomiting occurs, the chief effort is made by the muscles of the abdominal wall and by the diaphragm contracting together and squeezing the stomach. The contraction of the stomach wall is no doubt also a factor, and an important step in the act consists in the opening at the right moment of the cardiac or upper orifice of the stomach. This concerted action of various muscles is brought about by a vomiting centre situated on the floor of the fourth ventricle in the brain.

Causes: Vomiting is brought about by some irritation of this nervous centre, but in the great majority of cases this is effected through sensations derived from the stomach itself. Thus, of the drugs which cause vomiting some act only after being absorbed into the blood and carried to the brain, although most are irritants to the mucous membrane of the stomach (see EMETICS); dyspepsia also acts thus, and lies at the root of most sick headaches; various diseases of the stomach, such as cancer, and ulcer, and food poisoning, act in a similar way. Irritation, not only of the nerves of the stomach, but also of those proceeding from other abdominal organs, produces vomiting; thus in obstruction of the bowels, peritonitis, gall-stone colic, renal colic, and even during pregnancy, vomiting is a prominent symptom.

Strong impressions of an unpleasant nature made upon the nerves of sense are apt to produce vomiting. Thus an offensive smell, a disagreeable sight, any interference with the balancing sense as in travel-sickness, irritation or even tickling of the throat, and the pain of an injury or operation are all likely to be attended by vomiting.

Direct disturbance of the brain itself is a cause: for example, a blow on the head, a cerebral tumour, a cerebral abscess, meningitis. Many cases of hysteria also show attacks of vomiting as one of their prominent symptoms.

Nausea and vomiting are common symptoms that may arise from local disease of the gastro-intestinal tract, but they are also associated with systemic illness and also with disturbances of labyrinthine function, such as motion sickness and acute labyrinthitis.

There are two centres in the brain concerned with vomiting. One is the chemo-receptor trigger zone. This centre is in contact with the blood and lies outside the blood-brain barrier. It is the site at which drugs such as apomorphine and toxins act. It is rich in dopamine receptors and hence dopamine antagonists are effective treatment for vomiting. The vomiting centre itself co-ordinates impulses received from the chemo-receptor trigger zone from the vestibular apparatus and the gastro-intestinal tract and also from higher centres in the cerebral cortex. The vomiting centre contains many cholinergic and histamine receptors and this is why anti-cholinergic drugs and anti-histamines are effective drugs in the control of vomiting.

Characters of the vomit: FOOD, more or less softened and made sour and bitter by digestion, constitutes the vomit in the simpler cases, such as those due, for example, to emetics and seasickness. It should be remembered that when milk is vomited up curdled, this indicates simply that the first step in its digestion has taken place, and it is a mistake to conclude, as is often done, that the curdling indicates some intolerance of the stomach for milk.

WATERY FLUID, brought up irrespective of meals, forms the vomitus in conditions where the vomiting is due to disturbances of the brain: eg. brain tumours, and in certain other conditions such as the vomiting in the early months of pregnancy. When the vomiting continues for long, it tends to bring up mucus and bile also.

MUCUS, when vomited in considerable amount in strings, and especially when sour and brought up in the morning, is a sign of catarrh of the stomach, particularly that form associated with constant indulgence in alcohol.

BILE may be brought up by any long-continued attack of vomiting, after the contents of the stomach have been expelled and retching still continues: for example, in sea-sickness, or in migraine. Usually the bile is golden-yellow in colour; but sometimes it is grass-green.

FROTHY MATERIAL, with a yeasty smell, which divides into three distinct layers, froth on the surface, and a sediment of undigested food, with a layer of clearer fluid between, is characteristic of the vomit from a dilated stomach in which fermentative dyspepsia is taking place.

BLOOD may be red and brought up mixed with the food or in clots; but, much more often, it is vomited as a brown granular material, very much resembling 'coffee-grounds'. As a general rule, the vomiting of blood indicates some ulceration in the interior of the stomach, but the amount of blood is no guide to the size of the ulcer, because serious bleeding sometimes occurs from hardly perceptible erosions of the mucous membrane. Large quantities of blood are also occasionally brought up in chronic catarrh of the stomach (especially the alcoholic variety) which is accompanied by congestion.

Treatment The cause of the vomiting must be sought and treatment directed towards this. If the vomiting is due to local disease in the gastro-intestinal tract the old-fashioned remedies of sodium bicarbonate and bismuth may be helpful, and rest and quiet soothe the nervous system which includes the vomiting centre. If the vomiting is vestibular in origin and due, for example, to motion sickness, hyoscine is the drug of choice, though the side effects of sedation, dry mouth and constipation may be troublesome. Antihistamines are also of use in motion sickness.

In acute labyrinthitis prochlorperazine is the drug of choice. Nausea and vomiting are a common feature of migraine. Metoclopramide is the drug of choice. This drug acts by encouraging gastric emptying and gastro-intestinal motility is altered by nausea and vomiting. Domperidone is also effective.

Vomiting is common in the post-operative period and this is due to the combined effects of morphine, analgesics, anaesthetic agents and the psychological stress of operation. Dopamine receptor antagonists such as metoclopramide are probably the drugs of choice.

Nausea and vomiting are common symptoms in pregnancy. Drugs are best avoided in this situation as they may damage the developing foetus. Simple measures, such as the taking of food before getting up in the morning and reassurance, are often all that is necessary. If drugs are required promethazine or metoclopramide are the drugs of choice as they appear to be free of teratogenic effects.

VULVA is the general term applied to the external female genitals.

VULVO-VAGINITIS is inflammation of the vulva and the vagina. It is more common in young girls than in adult women. It may be a manifestation of infection elsewhere in the body, or may indicate the presence of some infection in the vagina. (See WHITES.)

W

WAFER PAPERS are thin circular discs made of flour and water, which become pliable when wetted, and form a convenient wrapper for swallowing nauseous drugs without tasting them. (For the method of use, see POWDERS.)

WALK (see GAIT).

WARFARIN is an anticoagulant which is active whether given by mouth, intramuscularly, intravenously or rectally. It is usually given by mouth, when its maximum effect occurs within about 36 hours. Its action passes off within 48 hours of cessation of treatment.

WARMING (see HEATING).

WARTS, or VERRUCAE, are small, solid growths arising from the surface of the skin. They are due to a papovavirus infection of the skin. They are highly infectious, and it is estimated that 10 per cent of the population suffer from them. The infection is most likely to be spread in schools by hand-holding games, and among adolescents by walking barefoot on gymnasium floors and in swimming baths.

COMMON WARTS develop on the skin of children and young people on the knuckles, on the back of the hands and on the knees. Occasionally such warts come out in a crop. In structure they consist of a bundle of fibres produced by overgrowth of the papillae in the true skin, each bundle enveloped by a cap of the horny cells that cover the surface of the epidermis, and the whole mass being surrounded by a ring of thickened epidermis. These fibres can easily be seen when the surface of the wart becomes worn away, and especially if the top of the wart is accidentally cut or knocked off, so that it bleeds. The dirty-brown colour of warts is due to dirt becoming lodged between these fibres.

PLANE WARTS, which are flat-topped, are commonest on the face and the back of the hands.

PLANTAR WARTS occur on the soles of the feet. They are found most commonly in older children and adolescents. Epidemics are not uncommon in schools, the infection being spread by the children walking with bare feet. They are usually painful. SENILE WARTS are usually hard, wrinkled, and slightly raised areas of skin found in old people. SOFT WARTS, consisting of little tags of skin, are found especially upon the neck, chest, ears, or eyelids of people whose skin has been subjected for long to some irritation, such as that of working among paraffin. HORNS are formed sometimes upon the face or hands, as the result of the drying up of the sebaceous material exuding from the skin that covers a wart, and, as the secretion goes on, these horns occasionally reach a length of some inches. TUBERCULOUS WARTS are developed sometimes as the result of a wound in the skin of the hands, especially of those who have come in contact with persons or animals suffering from some form of tuberculosis: eg. pathologists and butchers.

Treatment: There is much to be said for the old advice that the best way to manage warts is to let them manage themselves. Quite often they disappear spontaneously. One-fifth of plantar warts disappear spontaneously in six months, and it is said that two-thirds of all warts disappear in two years. This explains the large range of vaunted 'cures'. All too often all that has happened is that the use of the 'cure' in question has coincided with the natural disappearance of the wart. As a rule, warts are removed painlessly by the application of some substance which dissolves the horny surface and cauterizes the parts beneath, such as 10 per cent salicylic acid in soft paraffin, or a combination of salicylic acid and lactic acid. An alternative is the daily application of a paint of 10–20 per cent podophyllin in compound tincture of benzoin BPC, having first pared the surface of the wart with pumice stone. This paint should be applied daily for two to six weeks. The local application of carbon dioxide snow is a most effective form of treatment provided there are not too many warts though it is being replaced by liquid nitrogen as a freezing agent. Its benefit is that it is colder (-196°C) than carbon dioxide snow (-79°C). In some cases large warts on the fingers may need to be cut out under a local anaesthetic. The most effective treatment for plantar warts is to soak them in 3 per cent formalin. This is done by filling an old tin lid or saucer with the solution and soaking the part of the sole containing the wart in it for twenty minutes each night. Care must be taken not to soak more of the part than is absolutely necessary in the formalin solution. Each night, before soaking, the surface of the wart is rubbed with a nail file. The soaking may need to be repeated nightly for several weeks. Yet another form of treatment for which success is claimed is the twice daily application of glutaraldehyde gel. Warts that hang by a pedicle are best removed by snipping off with scissors, the bleeding being easily checked by some astringent. (See also CONDYLOMA.)

WASHING (see BATHS; DISINFECTION).

WASHING OUT OF THE STOMACH is performed for various reasons, particularly in order to remove poison that has been recently swallowed, before it shall have had time to act. Expert opinion today differs as to the value and safety of washing out the stomach in cases of poisoning. If it is done for this purpose, it should only be done by a doctor, nurse or experienced first-aider. The elementary rules are as follows:

(1) Place the head of the patient over the side of the bed so that the mouth and throat are at a lower level than the larynx and trachea.

(2) Use a wide-bore stomach tube (Jaques gauge 30) and lubricate it well with glycerin or some similar lubricant. In the adult 50 cm (20 inches) will reach the stomach. Make sure the tube is in the gullet (oesophagus) and not the trachea.

(3) For the first wash use 300 ml water, or olive oil if a tar oil derivative has been taken. Repeat this process, using 300-600 ml at a time, at least three or four times, saving all washings for analysis.

(4) If the patient is conscious, leave in the stomach 600 ml water containing 20 ml sodium or magnesium sulphate. If the patients is comatose, leave the stomach empty, and leave a nasogastric tube in place to keep the stomach empty. In the unconscious patient it is necessary to protect the airway with a cupped endotracheal tube.

Washing out is also employed to cleanse the stomach in cases in which the food tends to collect in the organ and to ferment. (See STOMACH TUBE.)

WASP STINGS (see BITES AND STINGS).

WASSERMANN REACTION is a test introduced for the diagnosis of syphilis by examination of the blood. It has now been largely supplanted by other more specific tests.

WASTING (see ATROPHY).

WASTING PALSY is a popular name for the disease more commonly known as progressive muscular atrophy. (See PARALYSIS.)

WATER-BEDS are flat, closed sacks of heavy plastic or rubber material, with a funnel-shaped orifice at one corner through which water can be poured, and which can be closed by a screw-stopper. They are made in various sizes, some being sufficiently large to cover a whole bedstead, though more often, for convenience in handling, they are of smaller size, and occasionally are made as small cushions, as rings with a hollow in the centre, or in horse-shoe shape. Those of the largest size possess a special outlet at one corner through which air escapes as water enters at the opposite corner.

Water-beds have been replaced to a great extent by air-beds (qv).

WATERBRASH, or PYROSIS, is a condition in which, during the course of digestion, the mouth fills with tasteless or sour fluid, which is generally saliva, but sometimes seems to be brought up from the stomach. At the same time, a burning pain is often felt at the pit of the stomach or in the chest. The condition is a symptom of excessive acidity of the stomach contents, due sometimes to an irritating diet, and often characteristic of a duodenal ulcer.

WATER CANKER is another name for cancrum oris. (See CANCRUM ORIS.)

WATER-HAMMER PULSE is a name given to the peculiarly sudden pulse that is associated with incompetence of the aortic valve of the heart, and suggests the philosophical toy after which it is named. (See PULSE.)

WATER ON THE BRAIN is a popular name for hydrocephalus and for meningitis. (See HYDROCEPHALUS; MENINGITIS.)

WATER-SPREAD DISEASES: A wide variety of illnesses may be produced by impure water. Thus, excessive sulphates may induce diarrhoea, excess nitrates may induce cyanosis (see METHAEMOGLOBINAEMIA) in infants, excess lead may produce lead poisoning, lack of fluoride may enhance the incidence of dental caries, and lack of iodine may induce goitre (qv). There is also some evidence suggesting a correlation between the softness of the water and heart disease. Contamination with micro-organisms may be responisble for outbreaks of enteric fever, dysentery, infective hepatitis, Weil's disease and cholera. Parasites transmitted by water include those responsible for amoebic dysentery, hookworm, schistosomiasis, and filariasis.

Poisoning by various metals may arise from industrial waste-products that pass into a stream, or by the solution of the metallic constituents of the water-pipes. Lead poisoning may arise from the latter cause, especially where the water contains a free acid, as in the case of peaty waters; but, if the water contains carbonate of lime, an insoluble protective coating is formed on the interior of the pipes. Many moorland waters have been found to act on lead, but this may be effectually prevented by treating the water with filters composed of sand and limestone. It is also possible to avoid the use of lead pipes where the water is known to act on the lead. The 1976 Brussels Directive on Water, to which member states of the EEC are supposed to adopt their laws within two years, and enforce within ten years, lays down the permitted quantity of lead as 0·05 mg per litre. It also decrees that bottled or other water used for baby feeds should not contain more than 25 mg of nitrate per litre.

WAX is used in medicine as an ingredient of ointments, plasters, and suppositories. It is used either as yellow wax derived directly from honeycomb, or as white wax, which is the same substance bleached. It is also used in the form of paraffin wax to apply heat in the relief of rheumatic pains. (See BATHS.)

For wax in the ear, see EAR, DISEASES OF).

WEAKNESS (see ATROPHY; CACHEXIA; PARALYSIS; TONICS).

WEALS, or WHEALS, are raised white areas on the skin with reddened margins, which may result from sharp blows, or may be a symptom of nettle-rash.

WEANING (see INFANT FEEDING).

WEBBED FINGERS or TOES, or SYNDACTYLY, constitute a deformity sometimes present at birth, and liable to run in families. The web may be quite a thin structure, or the fingers may be closely united by solid tissue. In any case, separation is a matter of considerable difficulty, because, if the web is simply divided, it heals up as before. A special operation is necessary, consisting in turning back a flap of the web upon each of the united fingers, or some other device to produce healing in the new position.

WEIGHT and HEIGHT: The weight of a child at birth is about 3·2 to 3·6 kg (7 to 8 pounds) and the height 50 cm (20 inches). During the first six months the infant puts on weight at the rate of about 140 g (5 ounces) per week if no illness occurs, and during the second six months of life about 0·5 kg (1 pound) per month. At the age of one year he weighs from

Age	Boys		Girls	
	Inches	*Centimetres*	*Inches*	*Centimetres*
Birth	20·0	50·9	19·5	49·5
2 weeks	20·3	51·7	20·1	51·0
3 months	23·7	60·2	23·2	58·8
6 months	26·2	66·7	25·6	65·0
9 months	28·0	71·2	27·4	69·6
1 year	29·6	75·1	29·1	73·9
2 years	34·0	86·4	33·7	85·5
3 years	37·8	95·9	36·9	93·8
4 years	40·6	103·0	40·0	101·6
5 years	43·1	109·5	42·9	108·9

Mean height of infants and young children. Thomson.

Age	Boys		Girls	
	Pounds	*Kilograms*	*Pounds*	*Kilograms*
Birth	7·5	3·4	7·3	3·3
2 weeks	7·5	3·4	7·3	3·3
3 months	12·9	5·8	12·0	5·5
6 months	17·4	7·9	16·4	7·4
9 months	20·4	9·2	19·2	8·7
1 year	22·8	10·3	21·7	9·8
2 years	27·0	12·2	25·7	11·6
3 years	31·5	14·3	30·4	13·8
4 years	35·6	16·2	34·5	15·7
5 years	40·2	18·3	39·4	17·9

Mean weight of infants and young children. Thomson.

8·2 to 10·9 kg (18 to 24 pounds). In the first year he increases in height about 25 cm (10 inches), and measures almost 75 cm (30 inches) at one year old.

In both boys and girls the growth in height amounts to 7·5 cm (3 inches) per year from the second to the fifth years. Boys continue to grow at the rate of 5 cm (2 inches) per year from the sixth to the fifteenth years, whilst girls continue to grow at this rate from the sixth to the eleventh years. In general, it may be said that the height is doubled at the end of five years, and trebled in the thirteenth or fourteenth year. After adolescence growth is more vigorous in boys, but girls attain their full height earlier than boys. Increase in height is greatest in the late spring and early summer, and least in the winter.

As a rule increase in height and increase in weight run parallel. At 2½ years the birth-weight has usually been increased fourfold, whilst at 5 years it has been increased fivefold. The general tendency of weight increase can be summarized as follows: (1) rapid increase in infancy and early childhood; (2) slow but constant increase from 3 to 12 years; (3) marked acceleration during puberty; (4) very slow increase to age of 25 or 30 years.

Charts relating height to age have been devised and give an indication of the normal rate of growth. The wide variation in normal children is immediately apparent on studying such charts. Deviations from the mean of this wide range are called percentiles. Centile or Percentile charts describe the distribution of a characteristic in a population. They are obtained by measuring a specific characteristic in a large population of at least 1,000 of each sex at each age. For each age there will be a height, above and below which 50 per cent of the population lie and this is called the fiftieth centile. The fiftieth centile thus indicates the mean height at a particular age. Such tables are less reliable around the age of puberty because of variation in age of onset.

Weight in pounds

Height in inches	5 *years*	6 *years*	7 *years*	8 *years*	9 *years*	10 *years*	11 *years*	12 *years*	13 *years*	14 *years*
38	34	34								
39	35	35								
40	36	36								
41	38	38	38							
42	39	39	39	39						
43	41	41	41	41						
44	44	44	44	44						
45	46	46	46	46	46					
47	49	50	50	50	50	50				
48		52	53	53	53	53				
49		55	55	55	55	55	55			
50		57	58	58	58	58	58	58		
51			61	61	61	61	61	61		
52			63	64	64	64	64	64	64	
53			66	67	67	67	67	68	68	
54				70	70	70	70	71	71	72
55				72	72	73	73	74	74	74
56				75	76	77	77	77	78	78
57					79	80	81	81	82	83
58					83	84	84	85	85	86
59						87	88	89	89	90
60						91	92	92	93	94
61							95	96	97	99
62							100	101	102	103
63							105	106	107	108
64								109	111	113
65								114	117	118
66									119	122
67									124	128
68										134
69										137
70										143
71										148

Correlation of height, weight, and age in boys.
Bird T. Baldwin and Thomas D. Wood, from Bridges' *Dietetics for the Clinician*.
Courtesy of Lea & Febiger and Henry Kimpton.

Height Feet	Height Inches	Small Frame Pounds	Medium Frame Pounds	Large Frame Pounds
5	2	116–125	124–133	131–142
5	3	119–128	127–136	133–144
5	4	122–132	130–140	137–149
5	5	126–136	134–144	141–153
5	6	129–139	137–147	145–157
5	7	133–143	141–151	149–162
5	8	136–147	145–156	153–166
5	9	140–151	149–160	157–170
5	10	144–155	153–164	161–175
5	11	148–159	157–168	165–180
6	0	152–164	161–173	169–185
6	1	157–169	166–178	174–190
6	2	163–175	171–184	179–196
6	3	168–180	176–189	184–202

Ideal weights for men

Weight in pounds with clothes. Height in feet and inches, with shoes on. From Metropolitan Life Insurance Company, as noted by Rynearson and Gastineau.

Height Feet	Height Inches	Small Frame Pounds	Medium Frame Pounds	Large Frame Pounds
4	11	104–111	110–118	117–127
5	0	105–113	112–120	119–129
5	1	107–115	114–122	121–131
5	2	110–118	117–125	124–135
5	3	113–121	120–128	127–138
5	4	116–125	124–132	131–142
5	5	119–128	127–135	133–145
5	6	123–132	130–140	138–150
5	7	126–136	134–144	142–154
5	8	129–139	137–147	145–158
5	9	133–143	141–151	149–162
5	10	136–147	145–155	152–166
5	11	139–150	148–158	155–169

Ideal weights for women

Weight in pounds with clothes. Height in feet and inches, with shoes on. From Metropolitan Life Insurance Company, as noted by Rynearson and Gastineau.

Minor variations from the mean do not warrant investigation but if the height of an individual falls below the third centile (3 per cent of normal children have a height that falls below the third centile) or above the ninety-seventh centile, investigation is required. Changes in the rate of growth are also important and skeletal proportions may provide useful information. There are many children who are normal but who are small in relation to their parents. The problem is merely growth delay. These children take longer to reach maturity and there is also a proportional delay in their skeletal maturation. The actual height must always be assessed in relation to maturity. The change in skeletal proportions is one manifestation of maturity but other features include the maturing of facial features with the growth of nose and jaw and dental development. Maturity of bone can readily be measured by the radiological bone age.

Failure to gain weight is of more significance. Whilst this may be due to some underlying disease, the commonest cause is a diet containing inadequate calories. Over the last six decades or so there has been quite a striking increase in the heights and weights of European children. Thus, the average 13-year-old Glasgow boy was 13 cm taller and 21 kg heavier in 1966 than in 1910. Manufacturers of children's clothing, shoes and furniture have had to increase the size of their products. Growth is now completed at 20–21 years, compared with 25 at the turn of the century. This increase, and earlier maturation, it has been suggested, have been due to a combination of genetic mixing as a result of population movements, combined with the whole range of improvement in environmental hygiene, and not merely to better nutrition.

In the case of adults views have changed of recent years concerning 'ideal' weight. Life

	Name of Unit	Unit Symbol
Length	Metre	m
Mass	Kilogram	kg
Time	Second	s
Electric current	Ampere	A
Thermodynamic temperature	Kelvin	°K
Luminous intensity	Candela	cd
Amount of substance	Mole	mol

Basic units of the International System of Units (SI).

Metric Measures of Weight

1 kilogram (kg)	= 1000·0 g	= 2·20 pounds (avoirdupois)
1 hectogram	= 100·0 g	= 3·53 ounces (avoirdupois)
1 dekagram	= 10·0 g	= 154·32 grains
	= 1·0 g	= 15·43 grains
1 decigram	= 0·1 g	= 1·54 grains
1 centigram (cg)	= 0·01 g	= 0·15 grain
1 milligram (mg)	= 0·001 g	= 0·015 grain
1 microgram (μg)	= 0·000001 g	= 0·00001 grain

Metric Measures of Capacity

1 litre (l) = 1000 millilitres = 35·196 Imperial fluid ounces
1 millilitre (ml) = 0·001 litre = 16·89 minims

N.B. – 1 millilitre is approximately equivalent to 1 cubic centimetre (cc).

Factors for Converting from One Scale to the Other

To convert	grams into grains	× 15·432
,,	grams into avoirdupois ounces	× 0·0353
,,	kilograms into pounds	× 2·205
,,	grains into grams	× 0·065
,,	avoirdupois ounces into grams	× 28·35
,,	troy ounces into grams	× 31·104
,,	millilitres into Imperial fluid ounces	× 0·0352
,,	litres into Imperial fluid ounces	× 35·2
,,	fluid ounces into millilitres	× 28·42
,,	pints into litres	× 0·568
,,	metres into inches	× 39·37
,,	inches into metres	× 0·0254

Approximate Value of Domestic Measures

Tumbler = 10 fluid ounces	Table-spoon (small) = ½ fluid ounce
Breakfast-cup = 8 ,, ,,	Dessert-spoon = 120 minims
Tea-cup = 5 ,, ,,	Tea-spoon = 60 minims
Wine-glass (large) = 2½ ,, ,,	Drop (of water) = 1 minim

Note – When medicine is measured this should be done by means of a standardized measure, because domestic utensils vary greatly in size.

Multiple	*Prefix*	*Symbol*	*Submultiple*	*Prefix*	*Symbol*
10^1	deca	da	10^{-1}	deci	d
10^2	hecto	h	10^{-2}	centi	c
10^3	kilo	k	10^{-3}	milli	m
10^6	mega	M	10^{-6}	micro	μ
10^9	giga	G	10^{-9}	nano	n
10^{12}	tera	T	10^{-12}	pico	p

Prefixes for decimal multiples and submultiples in the International System of Units.

insurance statistics have shown that maximal life expectancy is obtained if the average weight at ages 25 to 30 years is maintained throughout the rest of life. These insurance statistics also suggest that it is of advantage to be slightly over average weight before the age of 30 years, to be of average weight after the age of 40, and to be under-weight from ages 30 to 40. In the past it has been usual, in assessing the significance of an adult's weight, to allow a 10 per cent range on either side of normal for variations in body build. A closer correlation has been found between thoracic and abdominal measurements and weight.

WEIGHTS AND MEASURES: It is over a hundred years since the metric system was legalized in Britain . In medicine it has encountered a hard core of conservative resistance. Over fifty years ago it was being taught in progressive medical schools, such as that in the University of Edinburgh, but it was not until March 3,

1969, that it became illegal to use any system of weights and measures other than the metric system for dispensing prescriptions. This edict, however, applies only to dispensers. For some curious reason there is as yet no compulsion on doctors to use the metric system in prescribing.

Recently, a rationalization of the metric system has been introduced, known as the International System of Units (SI). This has been described as 'a coherent system with seven basic units from which all other units are derived'. Among these derived units is that for force – the newton, the symbol for which is N. The new unit of pressure is the pascal, the symbol for which is Pa, while the universal unit for energy is the joule, symbolized by J. Even in this scientifically perfect scheme, exceptions have had to be made for practical purposes. From the medical aspect, the most important of these is that the derived basic unit for volume, the metre cubed (m^3), is admitted to be too clumsy for medical purposes. The litre (l) is therefore to be retained as an alternative, with its various submultiples such as millilitre (ml). To avoid the possible confusion arising from the use of the comma, and not a full stop, for the decimal point in continental Europe, it is recommended that in writing large numbers, groups of three figures are separated by a space, and not by a comma. Thus one-million-five-hundred-thousand is 1 500 000, or $1 \cdot 5 \times 10^6$.

WEIL'S DISEASE (see LEPTOSPIROSIS).

WENS are small cystic tumours in the skin, consisting of a collection of sebaceous material, due to blockage of the outlet from a sebaceous gland. They occur most commonly about the face and scalp, where they form smooth, rounded, elastic tumours, often of a considerable size, but give rise to no trouble except that occasioned by their position, by their unsightliness, and by the fact that they are liable to become inflamed from the pressure, for example, of the hat.

Treatment consists in opening the cyst, squeezing out its fatty contents, and carefully removing the lining membrane. If any part of the membrane lining the interior is left behind, the wound heals in such a way that the wen is apt to refill. On the scalp this membrane is tough and can generally be pulled out entire, but on the face greater care is necessary, and the thin skin over the wen, to which the lining membrane is adherent, is also removed. The little operation is usually performed under a local anaesthetic, and is accompanied by very little pain.

WET BRAIN is a term applied to an oedematous state of the brain caused by chronic alcoholism and associated with mental failure and delusions.

WET CUP is a form of cupping in which the cupping glass is applied after scarification of the skin. (See CUPPING.)

WET PACK is a method of treatment popular in some countries for the purpose of applying a moderate degree of cold or of heat, for some time, to a patient's skin.

Uses: The conditions in which cold is beneficial are detailed under COLD, USES OF. The wet pack is a specially convenient method of applying cold when it is desired to exert a gentle cooling influence over a prolonged period, one hour or more, and at the same time to maintain the patient in a condition of absolute quiet and rest. It is used, for example, in such conditions as exhaustion due to heat. When a more rapid degree of cooling is desired, the patient is changed from one wet pack to another every quarter of an hour or thereabout, two beds being placed near one another for this purpose. Very rapid cooling may be achieved by wrapping the patient in a wet pack and rubbing down the sheet in which he is enveloped with pieces of ice.

Hot wet packs are also applied.

Method of application: (1) COLD PACK: A mackintosh sheet covered by a large blanket is spread upon the bed, and, when the patient is ready, a sheet is dipped in cold water, wrung out fairly dry, and laid over the blanket. The patient, stripped, is laid upon the sheet, which is quickly turned over him from both sides, and pushed between his legs and between each arm and the chest, so that skin does not touch skin anywhere. This must be done quickly, and the sheet being neatly tucked in round the neck and folded beneath the feet, every part of the body is covered saving the head and face. The head may also be wrapped in a wet towel. Finally the sides of the blanket are turned over the patient, and wrapped round him so as to lie smoothly everywhere. The patient, enveloped in this pack, lies absolutely helpless and should on no account be left by the attendant till the pack is removed, when he is put back into bed.

(2) HOT PACK: A mackintosh sheet is spread on the bed as for a cold pack. Upon this is laid a dry blanket. A second blanket (which retains heat better than a sheet) is placed in a pail and boiling water is poured over it. The blanket is then taken out of the pail, wrung, shaken, and rolled up. It is next applied to the patient in the same way as the sheet in the case of the cold pack. The dry blanket is then also wrapped round the patient outside the wet blanket; a second mackintosh sheet is spread over him; hot-water bottles, if desired, are placed alongside him; and several more blankets are laid on top of the mackintosh sheet. The patient may lie enveloped in the hot pack for twenty minutes; he is then quickly dried with warm towels, a warm flannel nightdress is put on and he is put back in bed. The patient must on no account be left alone while he is in the hot pack.

(3) WHISKY PACK: (see ALCOHOL).

(4) MUSTARD PACK: A pack containing mustard is sometimes used as a last resort in cases of collapse or of failure of breathing in young children.

WHEEZING is a popular name applied to the various sounds produced in the chest when the bronchial tubes are narrowed. It is applied particularly to the long-drawn breathing of asthma, and to the whistling or purring noises that accompany breathing in cases of bronchitis. (See ASTHMA; BRONCHITIS.)

WHELK is a term applied to a weal, and also to a red protuberance on the face or nose seen in the case of a hard drinker. (See ROSACEA.)

WHIPWORM is a popular name for *Trichuris trichiura.* (See TRICHURIASIS.)

WHITE HAIR: The greying or whitening of hair which takes place with age is due to a loss of its pigment, melanin (qv), and the collection of air bubbles in the shaft of the hair. There is no evidence that hair ever goes white overnight, whether in response to shock, strain or any other cause. Rapid whitening may occur patchily in a matter of days, but it is more often a matter of weeks or months. In the more rapid cases the cause is thought to be a form of alopecia areata (see BALDNESS), in which the dark hairs which fall out are replaced by white hairs. An alternative cause is vitiligo (qv). Certain drugs, including mephenesin and chloroquine (qv) may also cause whitening of the hair.

WHITE LEG is a fairly common and well-known condition in which a limb, usually one of the lower limbs, becomes enlarged, white, and painful.

Causes: Most commonly the condition occurs after child-birth; sometimes it occurs during convalescence from an acute febrile disease, especially typhoid fever or pneumonia. It is usually due to inflammation in, and blocking of, the veins of the limb, or may be caused by the spread of infection into the lymphatics of the limb from those within the pelvis, or to some morbid change in the blood causing it to clot.

Symptoms: The disease comes on during convalescence from one of the conditions mentioned above, beginning with slight feverishness and pain down the leg which is to be affected. The limb gradually swells, and in a few days may be greatly enlarged, hard, glossy, and of a strikingly white colour. The veins can generally be felt as solid lines down the inner side of the thigh, and the affected parts may be very tender to the touch. These symptoms persist for a week or so, but generally begin to subside within a fortnight from the onset, and about three-fourths of all cases recover completely in a few weeks. In other cases, some degree of muscular weakness, swelling, or aching of the limb remains permanently, but the condition, though a serious one demanding most careful treatment, is seldom fatal.

Treatment consists chiefly of rest in bed with the affected limb supported on a pillow. Pain is relieved by laudanum fomentations or simply by wrapping the limb in cotton-wool. Anticoagulants such as heparin and dicoumarol are given to prevent the process spreading.

This is one of the conditions, however, in which it is now recognized that preventive measures can be most effective. These consist principally of not allowing patients to stay in bed longer than necessary, or of giving massage to the legs in cases which are confined to bed for long periods. (See also VEINS, DISEASES OF.)

WHITE PRECIPITATE is the popular name for Ammoniated Mercury, BP, a substance used in the form of an ointment for application to various skin diseases. (See MERCURY.)

WHITES, or LEUCORRHOEA, is a symptom of many diseases peculiar to women, and may be of an acute nature, when the discharge is thick and white, consisting mainly of pus; or is more often chronic and catarrhal, when the discharge is usually thinner, sometimes of a clear mucous nature; in other cases acrid and offensive. In slighter cases, the discharge precedes or follows the menstrual flow; in severer cases it continues throughout the whole intervening periods. Women affected in this manner are generally unhealthy in appearance, the face is pale and sallow, weariness is felt easily upon exertion, and a dull gnawing pain is often experienced in the lower part of the back.

Causes: Leucorrhoea may arise as a result of infection anywhere in the genital tract in women: ie. in the uterus, cervix, or vagina. The commonest cause is some chronic inflammation of the womb following on childbirth, and associated with some laceration of its neck. Another important cause is gonorrhoea. In other cases it is due to infection of the vagina with the *Trichomonas vaginalis* (qv). A not uncommon cause is infection with *Candida albicans*, resulting in the condition known as thrush. The condition may occur as a symptom of general debility accompanied by congestion or the uterus. It may also be due to a tumour in the uterus of the cervix. An occasional cause of very offensive discharge is found in the irritation set up by the presence of a foreign body, such as a pessary that has been introduced for the support of a displaced womb, and then forgotten. In young children the condition is not common, but may arise from the irritation set up by threadworms, as the result of general debility combined with want of cleanliness, or following upon some acute infective disease.

Treatment: This depends upon the cause of the discharge. Thus, if it is due to infection with *Trichomonas vaginalis* (qv) metronidazole should be given. If it is due to gonorrhoea it is this that must be treated. (See GONORRHOEA.) If it is due to *Candida albicans* nystatin should be given. If it is due to an erosion of the cervix, or neck of the womb, this must be treated. In women past the menopause, or the change of life, the most effective treatment may be administration of an oestrogen (qv). (See also UTERUS, DISEASES OF.)

WHITE SWELLING is a popular name applied to tuberculous disease of joints. (See JOINTS, DISEASES OF.)

WHITLOW is a popular term applied to all acute inflammations of the deep-seated tissues in the fingers, whether the structure affected is the root of the nail, the pulp of the finger-tip, the sheaths of the tendons that run along the back and front of the fingers, or the bone. Acute inflammation of the bones in the finger is rare, and in general a whitlow begins in the last part of one finger, being, when situated towards the back, a small abscess at the root of the nail, and, when starting in front, an abscess in the fat and fibrous tissue that compose the pulp of the finger. Suppuration may also begin in the sheath of the tendon, generally in front of the finger.

WHOOPING-COUGH, also known as HOOPING-COUGH, PERTUSSIS, and CHIN-COUGH, is an infectious disease of the mucous membrane lining the air passages, which manifests itself by frequently recurring attacks of convulsive coughing, followed by a peculiar, loud indrawing of the breath, and often by vomiting. It occurs mostly in children, and seldom more than once in a lifetime.

Causes: The cause of whooping-cough is a bacillus discovered by Bordet and Gengou in 1906 and found in the sputum. It is known as *Bordetela pertussis*. Although specially a disease of childhood, whooping-cough is by no means limited to that period, but may occur at any time of life, even to old age, should there have been no previous attack. It is most prevalent between the ages of 1 and 4, and is uncommon after 10. Whooping-cough can be a dangerous disease in infants, but is a much less serious malady in older children. It has been occasionally observed in newly born infants, and is more common in girls than in boys. Whooping-cough is infectious during any stage of its progress, but chiefly at its commencement. It prevails mostly in the winter months, doubtless owing to the increasing predisposition to affections of the respiratory passages. In recent years the disease has tended to occur in cycles, with periods of increased prevalence occurring every three to four years. The incubation period is usually 7 to 10 days.

In an epidemic of whooping-cough, which extended from the last quarter of 1977 to mid-1979, 102,500 cases of whooping-cough were notified in the United Kingdom, with 36 deaths. This was the biggest outbreak since 1957 and its size was partly attributed to the fall in vaccination acceptance rates. In 1984 5,500 cases were notified in England and Wales.

Symptoms: Three stages of the disease are recognized: (1) the catarrhal, (2) the spasmodic, (3) the stage of decline.

The *first stage* is characterized by the usual symptoms of a catarrh, with sneezing, watering of the eyes, irritation of the throat, feverishness, and cough, but in general there is nothing in the symptoms to indicate that they are to develop into whooping-cough. There may be a slight rise of temperature to 37·2° to 37·7°C (99° to 100°F) in the first few days. The catarrhal stage usually lasts from ten to fourteen days.

The *second stage* is marked by the abatement of the catarrhal symptoms, but at the same time by increase in the cough, which now occurs in irregular paroxysms both by day and by night. Each paroxysm consists in a series of violent and rapid expiratory coughs, succeeded by a loud sonorous or crowing inspiration –the 'whoop'. During the coughing efforts the air is driven with great force out of the lungs, and, as none can enter the chest, the symptoms of impending asphyxia appear. The patient grows deep-red or livid in the face, the eyes appear as if they would burst from their sockets, and suffocation seems imminent till relief is brought by the whoop. Occasionally blood runs from the nose or mouth, or is extravasated into the conjunctiva of the eyes. A single fit rarely lasts beyond from half to three-quarters of a minute, but after the whoop another recurs, and of these a number may come and go for several minutes. The paroxysm ends by the coughing or vomiting up of a viscid tenacious secretion, and usually after this the patient seems comparatively well, or, it may be, somewhat wearied and fretful. The frequency of the paroxysms varies according to the severity of the case, being in some instances only to the extent of one or two in the whole day, whilst in others there may be several in the course of a single hour. Slight causes serve to bring on the fits of coughing, such as the acts of swallowing, talking, laughing, crying, or they may occur without any apparent exciting cause. In general, children come to recognize an impending attack by a feeling of tickling in the throat, and they cling with dread to their mother or nurse, or take hold of some object near them for support during the paroxysm; but, although exhausted by the severe fit of coughing, they soon resume their play, apparently little the worse. The attacks are on the whole most severe at night. This stage of the disease usually lasts for two to four weeks, but it may be shorter or longer. It is during this time that complications are apt to arise which may become a source of danger greater even than the malady itself. The chief of these are inflammatory affections of the bronchial tubes and lungs, and convulsions, any of which may prove fatal. A milder complication is the formation of a small ulcer under the tongue from rubbing against the teeth in coughing. Hernia and prolapse of the rectum sometimes are produced by the strain of violent coughing.

When, however, the disease progresses favourably, as it usually does, it passes into the *third* or *terminal stage*, in which the cough becomes less frequent and generally loses in great measure its whooping character. The patient's general condition undergoes improvement, and the symptoms disappear in from one to three weeks. It is to be observed, however, that for a long period afterwards in any simple catarrh from which the patient suffers the cough often assumes a spasmodic character, which may suggest the erroneous notion that a relapse of the whooping-cough has occurred.

In severe cases it sometimes happens that the disease leaves behind it such structural changes in the lungs (eg. emphysema) as entail permanent shortness of breathing, or a liability to attacks of asthma. Occasionally the violence of the cough may rupture a blood-vessel in the eye, or in the brain with hemiplegia as a result.

Treatment: In mild cases, little is necessary beyond keeping the patient warm and carefully attending to the general health. The remedies applicable in the case of catarrh or the milder forms of bronchitis are of service here. In mild weather the patient may be in the open air. In the more severe forms, efforts have to be employed to modify the severity of the paroxysms. During convalescence, when the cough still continues to be troublesome, a change of air will often effect its removal.

Antibiotics, including tetracyclines, chloramphenicol, cephaloridine, erythromycin, and co-trimoxazole are of value, but it is not recommended that they should be used routinely. The main indications for their use are in young children and when there are complications.

A vaccine has been prepared which is effective as a prophylactic. This is given in the form of Triple Vaccine (Diphtheria, Tetanus, and Pertussis Vaccine) at the age of 3 or 6 months. A second dose is given six to eight weeks later, and a third dose six months later. It should not be given to a child with any disease or disorder of the central nervous system, to a child with a history of convulsions or to a child with a family history of convulsions. Administration should also be postponed in the case of a temporarily unwell child until he is well again. A hyper-immune serum is also available but appears to be of doubtful value.

WIDAL REACTION (see AGGLUTINATION).

WILD CHERRY BARK is the dried bark of the wild or black cherry, *Prunus serotina*, a tree widely distributed over North America. In the form of wild cherry syrup BPC it is used for the soothing of irritable coughs.

WILMS' TUMOUR, or NEPHROBLASTOMA, is the commonest kidney tumour in infancy. It is a malignant tumour, which occurs in around 1 per 10,000 live births. The survival rate with modern treatment (removal of the kidney followed by radiotherapy and chemotherapy) is now around 80 per cent.

WILSON'S DISEASE or HEPATOLENTICULAR DEGENERATION, is a familial disease in which there is an increased accumulation of copper in the liver, brain, and other tissues including the kidneys. Its main manifestation is the development of tremor and rigidity, with difficulty in speech. In many cases there is improvement following the administration of dimercaprol, penicillamine, or trientine dihydrochloride; these substances cause an increased excretion of copper.

WINDPIPE is the popular name for the trachea, which extends from the larynx above to the point in the upper part of the chest where it divides into the two large bronchial tubes, one to each lung. It thus extends through the lower part of the neck and upper part of the chest, and is about 10 cm (4 inches) in length. It consists of a fibrous tube kept permanently open by about twenty strong horizontally placed hoops of cartilage, each of which forms about two-thirds of a circle, but is defective behind where the two ends are united by muscle-fibres. This fibro-cartilaginous tube is lined by a smooth mucous membrane, richly supplied with mucous glands and covered by a single layer of ciliated epithelium. (See also AIR PASSAGES.)

WIND SUCKING (see AEROPHAGY).

WINTER COUGH is a name sometimes given to chronic bronchitis which affects old people specially. The cough passes off during the summer and returns with the damp weather each winter. (See BRONCHITIS.)

WINTERGREEN (see GAULTHERIA).

WINTER VOMITING DISEASE, or EPIDEMIC NAUSEA AND VOMITING, is a condition characterized by nausea, vomiting, diarrhoea and giddiness, which occurs during the winter. Outbreaks of it usually involve whole families or may affect communities like schools. It is due to parvoviruses. The incubation period is 24 to 48 hours, and attacks seldom persist for more than 72 hours.

WISDOM TOOTH is a popular name for the last molar tooth on either side of each jaw. These teeth are the last to appear and should develop in early adult life, but often they do not cut the gum till the age of 20 or 25 or indeed they may sometimes remain permanently impacted in the jaw-bone. This occurs in up to 25 per cent of individuals. The lower third molar is often impacted against the second because of the direction in which it erupts. (See TEETH.)

WITCH-HAZEL is a preparation of the bark, twigs, and dried leaves from *Hamamelis virginiana*, a plant of the United States possessed of strong astringent properties. It is used to check haemorrhages and excessive mucous discharges, and also for piles. The most commonly used preparation is the liquid extract, which is sometimes given internally and more often used in the strength of 4 ml to 85 ml of cold water, either as a lotion for bruises or as an enema for bleeding piles. Extract of hamamelis is employed as an application for varicose veins and ulcers; and ointments, known as hazeline snow and hazeline cream, are used as applications for irritable states of the skin.

WOLFFIAN DUCTS: The Wolffian ducts and the Mullerian ducts are separate sets of primordia that transiently co-exist in embryos of both sexes. In the male the Wolffian ducts give rise to the vas deferens, the seminal vesicles and the epididymis, while the Mullerian ducts disappear. In female embryos the Mullerian ducts grow and fuse in the midline to produce the Fallopian tubes, the uterus and the upper third of the vagina, whereas the Wolffian ducts regress. The former phase of development requires a functioning testis from which an inducer substance diffuses locally over the primordia to bring about the suppression of the Mullerian duct and the development of the Wolffian duct. In the absence of this substance development proceeds along female lines regardless of the genetic sex.

WOLFSBANE is another name for aconite (qv).

WOMB (see UTERUS).

WOMB MUSIC is the somewhat fanciful name given to the playing to crying babies of sounds comparable to those by which the unborn babe is surrounded in the womb, such as the beating of the mother's heart, the bowel sounds of the babe and the like. The claim is that the replaying of these brings back the 'peaceful music of the womb', to which they have become conditioned, and thus 'sings' them to sleep.

WOOD ALCOHOL is another name for methyl alcohol. (See SPIRIT.)

WOOD WOOL is a fabric prepared from wood fibre, and much used for padding splints and other surgical purposes where the more expensive and softer cotton-wool is not necessary.

WOOL-SORTERS' DISEASE is another name for anthrax. (See ANTHRAX.)

WORD BLINDNESS is a condition in which, as the result of disease in the brain, a person becomes unable to associate their proper meanings with words, although he may be quite able to spell the letters. WORD DEAFNESS is an associated condition in which, though hearing remains perfect, the patient has lost the power of referring the names he hears to the articles they denote. (See DYSPHASIA.)

WORMS (see ASCARIASIS, ENTEROBIASIS, TAENIASIS).

WORMWOOD (see ABSINTHISM).

WOUNDS: A wound is any breach suddenly produced in the tissues of the body by direct violence. An extensive injury of the deeper parts without corresponding injury of the surface is known as a bruise or contusion.

Varieties: Classified according to the immediate effect produced, four varieties are usually described as *incised, punctured, lacerated*, and *contused*.

INCISED WOUNDS are usually inflicted with some sharp instrument, and are clean cuts, in which the tissues are simply divided without any damage to parts around. The bleeding from such a wound is apt to be very free, but it can be readily controlled.

PUNCTURED WOUNDS, or stabs, are inflicted with a pointed instrument. These wounds are the most dangerous, partly because their depth involves the danger of wounding vital organs, partly because bleeding from a stab is hard to control, and largely on account of the difficulty of purification. The wound produced by the nickel-nosed bullet is a puncture, much less severe than the ugly lacerated wound caused by an expanding bullet, or by a ricochet, and, if no clothing has been carried in by the bullet, the wound is clean and usually heals at once.

LACERATED WOUNDS are those in which great tearing takes place, such as injuries caused by machinery. The blood-vessels being torn and twisted, little bleeding is apt to result, and a limb may be torn completely away without great loss of blood. Such wounds are, however, specially liable to the danger of suppuration.

CONTUSED WOUNDS are those accompanied by much bruising of surrounding parts, as in the case of a blow from a cudgel or poker. In these wounds also there is little bleeding, but healing is slow on account of damage to the edges of the wound.

Any of these varieties may become infected by pus-forming germs and develop into a POISONED WOUND.

First-aid treatment: The first duty of a bystander who renders help to a wounded person is to check any bleeding. This may be done by pressure upon the edges of the wound with a clean handkerchief, or, if the bleeding is serious, by putting the finger in the wound and pressing it upon the spot from which the blood is coming. If necessary, the person may then at his leisure apply other methods described under HAEMORRHAGE and TOURNIQUET.

If medical attention is available within a few hours, it should not be interfered with further than is necessary to stop the bleeding and to cover the wound with a clean dry handkerchief or piece of lint. In cases in which expert assistance is not soon obtainable, one of the following procedures may be adopted. The bleeding being checked, the next step is to cleanse the wound and surrounding skin.

(*a*) *By painting freely with acriflavine, cetrimide* (*Cetavlon*), *chlorhexidine* (*Hibitane*) *or chloroxylenol* (*Dettol*) the wound and the surrounding skin, and covering with a piece of clean dry lint; this answers well in the case of small wounds and abrasions. A small piece of sterilized lint attached to a strip of sticking plaster may be purchased ready for use and forms a convenient and quickly applied dressing.

(*b*) *By washing with clean water* (ie. boiled). For this purpose, one requires two *clean* bowls scalded out quickly with boiling water, and filled with *clean* warm water; also several *clean* cloths, which may be handkerchiefs, squares of lint (preferably boric lint), or newly washed rags.

(1) First, it is essential that the person who is to dress the wound should wash his own hands, and especially the nails, thoroughly with soap and water.

(2) Press a clean cloth upon the wound to prevent the entrance into it of dirty water, and carefully wash the skin around the wound with water, from one of the bowls, using soap if necessary.

(3) Wring out a fresh cloth from the clean water in the second bowl, and with it gently dab the wound. Remove, replace by another clean cloth similarly wrung out, and fix it on the wound with a folded handkerchief. (See BANDAGES.)

(4) The injured part is finally fixed so that movement is prevented or minimized. A wounded hand or arm is fixed with a sling (see SLINGS), a wounded leg with a splint (see SPLINTS).

(5) If the injury has caused severe shock, stimulants may be necessary. (See SHOCK.)

Healing of wounds: The reaction of the tissues to an injury is similar to that produced by any other irritation. If the wound has been accompanied by loss of tissue which has to be made good, or by death of a piece of tissue which has to be cast off as a slough, or by infection with bacteria which has to be overcome, the process of repair is tedious, and in some cases permanent damage is produced. The new tissue formed in the wound is mainly fibrous tissue, like that composing the supporting framework of the body.

HEALING BY FIRST INTENTION: In a clean, incised wound of moderate severity, the immediate effect is bleeding from the ends of the vessels which have been cut. This, however, is soon arrested by the contraction and retraction of the coats of the divided vessels, and by the formation of blood-clots in their open ends. A small quantity of blood remains in the wound and clots. The blood-vessels round the injured part dilate, the blood flow becomes slowed, and there passes out from the blood a fluid known as lymph, which coagulates upon the surface of the wound, forming a sticky layer of fibrin which, if the injured surfaces are in contact, causes them to adhere to one another. This forms the temporary scaffolding within which the tissues of repair will be built, and possesses the other valuable property of being strongly germicidal to any organisms which may come in contact with it. White corpuscles also migrate through the walls of the dilated blood-vessels and pass into this exudate in the wound. This fact is of the greatest importance, since the white corpuscles eat up and destroy any foreign or dead substance which has to be removed in the process of repair. (See PHAGOCYTOSIS.) They remove the minute portions of tissue which have been killed by the injury, and the small quantity of blood which has accumulated in the wound. Following the entrance of the white blood corpuscles, within twenty-four hours after the infliction of the wound, there comes a host of cells produced by the rapid multiplication of the cells in the tissues around the wound. Some of these also have the power of phagocytosis, and others, called fibroblasts, become transformed into delicate fibrous tissue. Next, minute buds grow in from the walls of the smallest blood-vessels and form minute blood channels, which pass from side to side of the wound, or form loops if a gap has been left. The tissue so formed is known as granulation tissue, because, when its surface is closely examined, it has a red, granular appearance due to these loops of vessels covered by masses of the cells mentioned above. The same form of tissue is readily seen on a healing ulcer. Epithelial cells from the surface of the skin now grow over and cover the wound, the whole process being completed usually in less than a week. The delicately formed tissue of the healed wound is gradually replaced by firm fibrous tissue containing fewer blood-vessels, and in a matter of months, depending partly on where the scar has occurred, the angry, red scar of the recently healed wound is replaced by a white scar. As a rule wounds on the face heal very rapidly. With minor modifications, this process of repair takes place in all healing wounds.

HEALING BY SECOND INTENTION occurs in wounds which have broken down owing to suppuration, or where there is an ulcer, and the edges are gradually drawn together by the contraction of the newly formed fibrous tissue. This results in a wider, weaker, and more noticeable scar.

HEALING BY SCAB FORMATION occurs where the lymph dries up, and union is continued under the dry cake so formed.

HEALING OF POISONED WOUNDS: Where a wound becomes poisoned, or septic, the multiplication of the germs in it dissolves the fibrin and destroys many of the cells engaged in repair. The reaction of the tissues becomes intense, and the inflammation is so evident that the wound is popularly said to be inflamed. As a result of the destruction, many of the cells are discharged as pus. Granulation tissue is gradually formed around the site of infection, the bacteria are cast off in the pus, and healing by second intention takes place. A certain amount of the poison produced by the bacteria, however, escapes into the circulation and causes the symptoms of general ill-health which are present with a poisoned wound.

Dangers of wounds: BLOOD-POISONING usually means that the germs themselves have entered the circulation, which is a grave occurrence and may be fatal. (See BLOOD-POISONING.)

ERYSIPELAS, TETANUS and GAS GANGRENE are conditions in which the germs, (or their toxins) responsible for these diseases enter the lymphatics and blood-stream and produce widespread effects. (See ERYSIPELAS; TETANUS; GANGRENE.)

HAEMORRHAGE: *Primary haemorrhage* means bleeding which occurs at the time of the injury. A large vein or artery may have been divided and may require to be tied. (See HAEMORRHAGE.) A wound of a large vessel like the femoral or the popliteal artery may cause death in a few minutes if untreated. *Reactionary haemorrhage* takes place sometimes from wounds which do not bleed much when they are first inflicted. The explanation is that the shock caused by the injury enfeebles the action of the heart, and, when the wounded person recovers from the shock in a few hours, the increased force of the heart's beating causes bleeding to recommence in the wound. *Secondary haemorrhage* occurs only in the case of poisoned wounds. The spread of the infection breaks down the blood-clot which has formed in the open end of a blood-vessel and allows the escape of blood. It is usually preceded by a slight oozing of blood, which serves to forewarn the medical attendant. This form of bleeding seldom occurs earlier than a week from the date of the injury.

PARALYSIS: In a wound of a limb, one of the nerves may be divided. When this has happened, a definite area of skin is found to have lost the sense of touch and pain, and the muscles supplied by the divided nerve have completely lost their power. The tendons, which attach the muscles to the bones, may also be divided, as, for example, by a wound behind or in front of the wrist, causing loss of power in the injured part. If either or both of these complications is present, it is of the greatest importance that the divided ends should be stitched together as early as possible, or a permanent loss of power may result.

SCALP WOUNDS usually heal well, but in deep scalp wounds there is a danger that suppuration may result and may pass within the skull. Again, a severe blow producing a scalp wound may cause fracture of the skull and concussion or compression of the brain. (See BRAIN, DISEASES AND INJURIES OF.)

CHEST WOUNDS: Stabs of the chest are serious chiefly because of the fatal bleeding likely to follow any wound of the heart or large vessels; a less serious danger attends wounds of the pleural cavity causing collapse of the lung or empyema.

ABDOMINAL WOUNDS: A penetrating wound of the abdomen, particularly when the bowel has been cut, is often fatal from the acute general peritonitis which it causes.

General treatment of wounds: The first-aid treatment, already described, has for its chief objects the arrest of bleeding and the covering of the wound by a clean dressing, so as to prevent the entrance of germs and to get rid of those which have gained entrance from the skin, or upon the object that inflicted the wound.

To prevent infection of a wound at an operation or in applying a permanent dressing, everything which comes in contact with it must be sterilized or rendered germ-free. To destroy the germs, the best and most easily obtained material is boiling water or steam. If subjected to the action of boiling water for one hour, all known germs are killed, whilst five minutes boiling is found sufficient for practical purposes. Chemical agents, such as carbolic acid or perchloride of mercury, when used in solutions of given strength, are antiseptics or germicides, and are employed where heat is not applicable. The aim is that everything that can possibly convey infection to the wound is rendered free from germs, but none of the fluids or dressings which come in contact with the wound contains antiseptics.

CHANGING THE DRESSING: If the wounded surfaces are in contact, the dressing should not be changed unless pain is felt in the wound, discharge from the wound soaks through the dressing, a rise of temperature occurs, or the part feels uncomfortable, until the eighth to tenth day, when the dressing is removed.

DRESSINGS AND LOTIONS: The most satisfactory dressing is sterilized gauze but should this not be available, then either boric lint or cyanide gauze may be used. Cyanide gauze is gauze impregnated with the double cyanide of mercury and zinc. A dressing being used to an increasing extent is Op-site. This consists of an adhesive-coated polyurethane film, which is permeable to water vapour, oxygen and carbon dioxide and is a barrier to bacteria. It is claimed that it relieves pain and speeds up healing. It maintains high humidity in the wound and provides thermal insulation. In this way it prevents excessive drying of the wound which is an adverse factor slowing up the healing process, and at the same time helps to retain the temperature of the wound at body temperature which is the optimum one for healing. As it is transparent the state of the wound can be seen without disturbing it by having to remove the dressing.

Among the local applications the *flavines* are still among the most useful: acriflavine and proflavine are the most widely used. *Eusol* (qv) is also of value, particularly in wounds known to be infected; its major practical disadvantage is that it only retains its antiseptic properties for two or three weeks, and must therefore be made up fresh at regular intervals. *Iodine*, in 2 to 5 per cent alcoholic solutions, is a useful antiseptic if used with discrimination. *Biniodide of mercury* (1 in 500 solution in 75 per cent methylated spirit) is a potent antiseptic. *Perchloride of mercury* (1 in 2000 parts of water) is less potent but correspondingly safer. *Carbolic acid* (qv), 1 part in 20 parts of water, is less widely used than at one time, but is still a useful application to small, infected wounds. It must not be used for large wounds, nor must it be used with dressings impermeable to the air, because of the risk of excessive absorption leading to carbolic acid poisoning. *Saponaceous solution of cresol, BP* (perhaps better known as lysol), 1 part in 100 to 200 parts of water, is also used. Three widely used antiseptics at the moment are *cetrimide, chlorhexidine*, and *chloroxylenol*.

STITCHES: If the wound is of the incised variety, with wide separation of the edges, it may require to be stitched. Horsehair, silkworm gut, silver wire, stainless steel wire, linen, nylon, silk, or catgut may be employed for this purpose. One of the first three is used in cases in which there is a risk that the wound may become poisoned. Catgut, which is prepared from the intestine of the sheep, possesses the advantage over all the others that it is absorbed by the tissues, and thus does not need to be removed. Where stitches of any of the others have been used, they are generally removed about the tenth day. Sometimes a continuous suture is used for a long wound, but more commonly each stitch is put in and tied singly. A traditional method practised by certain South American Indians is the use of workers of the leaf-cutter ants, which possess very powerful jaws. Their heads are applied to the edges of a wound, and, as their jaws close and bring the edges together, their bodies are cut off, thus leaving the jaws automatically in position, where they are left until the wound is healed. The modern equivalent of these heads of the leaf-cutter ants are the Michel clips which are used where a particularly good cosmetic result is required as, for example, in operations in the neck: eg. that for thyroidectomy (see GOITRE).

DRAINAGE TUBES: Sterilized tubing is inserted down to the bottom of the wound in all cases in which suppuration is likely to occur in a deep wound, when there is much bruising of the tissues, or when blood is liable to accumulate in the wound. If the wound remains clean, the drainage tube will be removed on the third day. If suppuration occurs, it will be replaced and kept in until the discharge ceases or the deep wound closes up so far as to become a healing ulcer. For small wounds, a strip of gauze or a few strands of worsted or a folded strip of thin rubber tissue is often used as a drain instead of a tube.

Treatment of discharging wounds: If a wound should suppurate, it must receive treatment which will enable the pus to escape freely while the wound slowly closes. This is provided by inserting a drainage tube into the wound. To prevent the pus drying up and retaining the discharge, and to draw the pus out of the wound, a moist dressing is applied. A piece of lint soaked in sterilized water, or boric lotion (1 in 60), or perchloride of mercury lotion (1 in 3000), is applied to the wound. The lint is covered with a larger piece of waterproof material, such as gutta-percha tissue, oiled silk, or tinfoil; over this a still larger piece of cotton-wool is applied, and the whole is fixed by a bandage. This dressing is changed daily until the discharge ceases. If the pus is abundant and not escaping freely, the wound is, in addition, washed out with sterilized water or with lotion at each dressing. When improvement is very slow, a hot boric fomentation, changed every four hours, is to be recommended. Should blood-poisoning develop, special treatment is required, directed against the infection which is present throughout the blood. This includes the administration of penicillin or one of the sulphonamides.

WRIST is the joint situated between the arm above and the hand below. The region of the wrist contains eight small carpal bones, arranged in two rows, each containing four bones. Those in the proximal row, that is the row nearest the forearm, are from the outside inwards when looking at the palm of the hand, the scaphoid, lunate, triquetrum, and pisiform. Those in the distal row, that is the row nearest the hand, are the trapezium, trapezoid, capitate and hamate. These intervene between the arm bones and the five metacarpal bones in the hand, and have the effect of diminishing jars communicated to the hand in virtue of a certain amount of sliding movement over one another, of which they are capable. These small bones are closely bound to one another by short, strong ligaments, and the wrist-joint is the union of the composite mass thus formed with the radius and ulna in the forearm. The wrist and the radius and ulna are united by strong outer and inner lateral ligaments, and by weaker ligaments before and behind, whilst the powerful tendons passing to the hand and fingers give it a great measure of strength.

The joint is capable of movement in all directions, and, on account of its shape and its numerous ligaments, is little liable to dislocation, although stretching or tearing of some of these ligaments is a common accident, constituting a sprain. (See JOINTS, DISEASES AND INJURIES OF.) Inflammation of the tendon-sheaths before and behind the wrist, causing the presence of fluid, also results occasionally from an injury, and produces a sense of weakness in the wrist. A fairly common condition is that known as a ganglion, in which an elastic swelling full of fluid develops on the back or front of the wrist in connection with the sheaths of the tendons. (See GANGLION.)

WRIST-DROP (see DROP-WRIST).

WRITER'S CRAMP is a spasm which affects certain muscles when engaged in writing, and which may not occur when the same muscles are employed in other acts (simple writer's cramp). However, if more than one motor act is involved, then the condition is called dystonic writer's cramp, and is one of the focal dystonias.

The symptoms are in the first instance a gradually increasing difficulty experienced in performing the movement required for executing the work in hand. When the individual attempts to write, the muscles of the fingers, and sometimes also those of the forearm, are inappropriately activated, so that the act of writing is rendered impossible. Sometimes the fingers instead of being cramped move in a disorderly manner, lifting off the pen so that it cannot be grasped. Similar symptoms are observed and similar remarks apply in the case of musicians (guitar, clarinet and piano in particular), typists, artists and compositors.

Spasmodic torticollis is the most frequent form of focal dystonia. The muscles of the neck assume the unpleasant habit of rotating the chin to one side (torticollis), forward (anterocollis), backwards (retrocollis) or, rarely, pull the ear towards the shoulder (laterocollis). This position may be held by a constant tonic spasm, or be interrupted by jerks or tremor of the neck.

For other forms of focal dystonia, see DYSTONIA.

Treatment: With dystonic writer's cramp, it is sometimes recommended that the opposite hand or limb be used, but this may be followed by the extension of the disorder to that locality also. Special forms of penholder and other mechanical aids have been suggested, but they do not afford any relief from the disease. There is no evidence that writer's cramp or torticollis is a psychological or psychiatric disorder, although individuals may understandably develop depression secondary to their illness.

WRY-NECK is a condition in which the head is twisted to one side. It may be caused by the contraction of a scar, such as that resulting from a burn or by paralysis of some of the muscles, but in the great majority of cases it is a spasmodic condition due to excessive tendency of certain muscles to contract. (See CRAMP; SPASMODIC TORTICOLLIS.)

X

X-RAYS, or RONTGEN RAYS: The discovery of these was recorded in January 1896 by Professor Röntgen, at that time professor of physics at Würzburg. This epoch-making discovery had been preceded by a series of experiments carried out by Crookes and Lenard. Crookes, employing vacuum tubes with residual air at 1/1000000 of an atmosphere, produced cathodal rays from the negative pole on the passage of a high-potential electric current. Lenard passed these rays into the air through an aluminium window in the tube, and found that they could produce fluorescence of certain bodies, would pass through certain substances opaque to ordinary light, and would act on a photographic plate. Röntgen, using a still higher vacuum, succeeded in producing X-rays from the walls of the tube, these rays being unaffected by a magnet, and possessing greater power of penetration.

From these simple beginnings the science of Radiography and Radiotherapy has been slowly developed, until at the present day countless sets of apparatus are in daily use in X-ray departments of hospitals throughout the world.

Röntgen named these new rays, or radiations, X-rays, because their character and quality were unknown. The name, however, has stuck, though they are often now referred to as Röntgen rays. It is now known that they are electromagnetic vibrations of short wavelengths. They are produced by accelerating electrons in an electron field between two electrodes. In practice, this process is carried out in a glass vacuum bulb containing two electrodes. This is known as an X-ray tube. The X-ray tube used today is of a type in which the cathode consists of a spiral filament of incandescent tungsten, and the anode consists of massive tungsten. The essence of what happens in such a tube is that the electrons come by thermionic emission from the electrically heated filament of tungsten (the cathode) and are halted by the mass of tungsten in the anode. The X-rays are produced by the interaction of the electrons from the filament, known as the cathode stream, with the material of the 'target' or anode.

FLUORESCENT SCREEN: Fluorescence is produced in various substances by the action of X-rays, but the two most used are barium platino-cyanide and calcium tungstate, one of which, sprinkled on cardboard, forms the fluorescent screen in common use. In a darkened room, if a hand is placed close against the screen, between it and the tube which is emitting the rays, the screen will appear brightly illuminated, except in the region where, owing to the obstruction of the rays, there is a faint shadow of the flesh, a denser shadow of the bones, and, if there be a ring on the finger, a still darker shadow from the ring.

Radiography: X-rays act on a sensitized photographic plate in the same manner as ordinary light, but, as they penetrate paper, the exposure can be made in daylight by enclosing the plate in a black paper envelope, through which the daylight cannot pass. It must be remembered that the X-ray photograph differs from a photograph taken by ordinary light in that it is really a shadow-picture or skiagram. A skiagram differs from an ordinary photograph in that no lens is used; the X-rays pass in parallel lines from the focus spot in the X-ray tube. For this reason X-rays cannot be focused upon the object as in ordinary photography. Briefly, in order to obtain a skiagram, the method is as follows. The plate – a rapid one – is placed first in a yellow envelope, this again in a black one, the whole being placed close beneath the part to be photographed. The tube is situated directly opposite, with the limb or other object to be photographed a little distance off, but between the tube and the plate. The tube must be arranged so that the rays fall as perpendicularly as possible on to the part. The distance of the tube from the object and the duration of exposure are matters of experience; but the farther apart they are, the less chance there is of distortion. At two metres or more the amount of distortion is practically negligible: so that when working at that distance between the anode of the tube and the surface of the film or plate, the actual size of an organ within the body can be measured. This is taken advantage of in cardiac examinations, when measurements of the size of the heart can be obtained.

In order to show the position, shape, etc., of the stomach and intestine, some radio-opaque but harmless material, such as barium sulphate is administered by mouth. This throws a dense shadow, corresponding to the interior of the organ examined, upon the screen or photographic plate. For examination of the lungs, gall-bladder, and kidneys, other opaque substances, such as harmless compounds of iodine, are injected so as to pass into their interior.

For examination of other organs, such as the brain and abdominal organs, oxygen is sometimes injected into the cavities in the brain or the peritoneal cavity, so as to render the outlines sharper when an X-ray photograph is taken.

THE EXPOSURE IN RADIOGRAPHY: The nearer we can get to an instantaneous exposure, the clearer is the outline, especially when dealing with the abdomen or thorax. In the early days, very long exposures were required because of the very low currents available and the imperfect development of the X-ray tube. At the present time it is possible to get exposures in as short a time as 1/100 of a second through the thickness of the body of an average patient.

Amongst other uses for X-rays in diagnosis attention must be called to the localization of foreign bodies in various parts of the body. For this purpose localizers of various patterns and arrangements for taking stereoscopic photographs have been devised. These are of great importance in surgery for the purpose of fixing the position of foreign bodies, like steel chips in the eye or bullets in the body, and also give valuable aid in determining the nature and position of fractures and other injuries of the bones.

Accelerating screens made of cardboard covered with fluorescent material are sometimes used. This screen is placed in contact with the photographic plate. Being caused to glow where the light falls upon it, the screen still affects the plate after the exposure is over. When the apparatus is not powerful enough to give very short exposures, accelerating screens are used. In this way an instantaneous photograph can be made in 1/50 second or less from a distance of a few metres. Thus the beating heart or the contractions of the stomach in digestion can be taken in a series of flashes and demonstrated on a cine film.

In view of the increasing recognition of the hazards to health from irradiation in this nuclear-energy-orientated age the X-raying of patients is being reduced to a minimum. Particularly is this so during pregnancy and in children and adolescents.

Radiotherapy, or treatment by X-rays: The two chief sources of the ionizing radiations used in radiotherapy are the gamma rays of radium (qv) and the pentrating X-rays generated by apparatus working at various voltages. For superficial lesions energies of around 40 kilovolts are used, but for deep-seated conditions, such as cancer of the internal organs, much higher voltages are required. X-ray machines are now in use which work at two million volts. Even higher voltages are now available through the development of the linear accelerator, which makes use of the frequency magnetron which is the basis of radar. The linear accelerator receives its name from the fact that it accelerates a beam of electrons down a straight tube, 3 metres in length, and in this process a voltage of eight million is attained. The use of these very high voltages has led to the development of a highly specialized technique which has been devised for the treatment of cancer and like diseases.

Like the photographic effect, the therapeutic effects were discovered almost accidentally. It was observed that prolonged exposures to the rays caused inflammation, and even ulceration of the skin, and further, that they caused loss of hair, and that they improved various diseased conditions. Repeated exposures, for example, of the hands of physicians using this method of treatment, have been observed to produce pigmentation of the skin, excessive growth of its horny layer, and even epithelioma. X-rays are particularly hurtful to the testes and ovaries of young people; and when these are exposed to the rays repeatedly, the genital glands must be covered by sheet-lead or some such protection, in case sterility should result. Too severe a reaction to the irritating effect of the rays upon the patient's skin at a single session must also be avoided. It is important to protect the surrounding areas, and this is done by the use of masks of sheet-lead, with a hole cut out over the affected area, and by enclosing the tube in a metal-lined box, with an opening opposite the affected spot. By these means, as well as by wearing lead-lined gloves, and by frequently anointing the skin with some simple ointment, people constantly applying the rays are effectually protected.

The greatest value of radiotherapy is in the treatment of malignant disease. In many cases it can be used for the treatment of malignant growths which are not accessible to surgery, whilst in others it is used in conjunction with surgery.

Leukaemia and other conditions, in which the spleen is enlarged, are often greatly benefited by exposure of the spleen or long bones to X-rays or radium. (See RADIOTHERAPY.)

In simple conditions, particularly superficial ones, X-rays have been used very successfully, but are being used less and less, in view of the increasing necessity to reduce to the absolute minimum the amount of irradiation to which people are exposed.

XANTHELASMATA: These are yellow plaques of lipid deposited in the skin. They tend to occur in the eyelids. They are often associated with hyperlipidaemia.

XANTHOMATA: These are deposits of fatty tissue in tendon sheaths and over bony prominences such as knees, elbows and fingers. They are indicative of a state of hyperlipidaemia which may be a primary inherited disorder or secondary to such conditions as biliary cirrhosis, diabetes mellitus or nephrotic syndrome.

XENOGRAFT is a transplant from one animal to another of a different species. It is also known as a heterograft.

XERODERMA is a rough, dry condition of the skin accompanied by the copious formation of scales.

XERODERMA PIGMENTOSUM is a rare hereditary affection of the skin appearing first in early childhood. It is characterized by a dry skin which is heavily freckled and hypersensitive to sunlight.

XEROPHTHALMIA (see EYE, DISEASE AND INJURIES).

XERORADIOGRAPHY is a method of radiography, originally used for X-raying the breast. It is now being used also in investigating the skull, neck and larynx. A xeroradiograph is made on an electrically charged selenium-coated aluminium plate. Exposure to an X-ray beam produces positive and negative changes in a pattern that differentiates the varying densities of anatomical structures being examined, according to the amount of absorbed radiation. When the plate is then dusted with a cloud of negatively charged blue plastic powder, an image is formed producing a vertical electrical field component with enhanced edges, which is then transferred to paper electrostatically.

XEROSIS means abnormal dryness, especially of the eye.

XEROSTOMIA is the condition of dryness of the mouth due to lack of saliva. Its most extreme form occurs following radiotherapy of the mouth, and in the condition known as Sjögren's syndrome. No satisfactory substitute for natural saliva has been found though some find a methyl-cellulose substitute gives partial relief, as may a glycerin mouth-wash.

XIPAMIDE (DIUREXAN) (see BENZOTHIADIAZINES).

XIPHISTERNUM, or XIPHOID CARTILAGE, is the lowest part of the breast-bone, or sternum.

XYLITOL, or BIRCH SUGAR, is a sugar alcohol and therefore not strictly a carbohydrate. It has a very sweet taste, and occurs in fruits and mushrooms, but the commercial source is birch wood chips (hence its alternative name). There is some evidence that both it and fructose are less likely to cause caries of the teeth than sucrose.

Y

YAWNING consists of an involuntary opening of the mouth, which is accompanied by marked dilatation of the pharynx, a characteristic distortion of the face and usually stretching of the limbs. The cause and function of yawning are quite obscure. It is classically regarded as a sign of drowsiness or boredom, but it not infrequently occurs following a severe haemorrhage, and it is also sometimes associated with indigestion.

YAWS, known also as FRAMBOESIA and PIAN, is a disease of the tropics, especially of Africa and the West Indies, affecting both white and black races. It consists in the appearance of small tumours covered with yellow crusts, scattered over the surface of the body.

Cause: The disease is directly contagious from person to person, and the infection is probably also carried by flies, and certainly by clothing and by the unclean huts of the natives. The direct cause is a spirochaete known as *Treponema pertenue*, and the occurrence of the disease in a person of unhealthy constitution, or one who is suffering from another disease, such as syphilis or tuberculosis, renders the attack much more serious.

Symptoms: The disease does not appear for a fortnight or more after infection, and during this time fever, malaise, pains, and itching of the skin may come on. It begins as a scaly eruption about the body and legs, in which small lumps form, and grow till they reach a size even of several centimetres in diameter. The surface of these is covered by a yellow crust of dried-up secretion, and in unhealthy people the tumours may break down and produce deep ulcers. After a duration of weeks or months the tumours gradually shrink and disappear.

Treatment: The outlook in yaws has been transformed by the introduction of penicillin, the effects of which are dramatic in this disease.

YEAST consists of the cells and spores of unicellular fungi belonging to the family of Saccharomycetaceae. The main species of yeast used in medicine is *Saccharomyces cerevisiae*, which is used in the fermentation industries, such as brewing. It is a rich source of the vitamin B complex (see VITAMIN), but its use has largely been given up since the various components of the vitamin B complex became available as separate entities.

YELLOW FEVER, also known as YELLOW JACK and VOMITO AMARILLI, is an acute disease of certain tropical localities, characterized by fever and jaundice.

Distribution: It is endemic in Africa from coast to coast south of the Sahara to Zambia. It also occurs in the northern part of South America and to a less extent today in Central America. In 1793 a very serious epidemic spread over the Northern United States, and, in Philadelphia alone, over 10 per cent of the population were swept off in the course of four months. Numerous other epidemics invaded the States in the end of the eighteenth and during the course of the nineteenth centuries, the last severe one taking place in 1878. In Europe the disease has from time to time invaded some of the Portuguese and Spanish ports, but it has never gained any permanent hold. When cases of yellow fever arrive at British or other northern European ports, no spread of the disease takes place. It is also unknown in the Far East.

Causes: The disease is due to a virus which is transmitted to man by the *Aedes aegypti* mosquito. Monkeys are an important reservoir of infection in areas where the disease is endemic. The virus is found in the blood of infected individuals during the first three or four days of the disease. The blood of a patient is directly infectious, and the deaths of three of the great investigators of the disease, Stokes, Noguchi, and Young, all of whom died of yellow fever, were probably due to direct contact with infected blood.

One attack gives more or less protection for life. Many adult natives in yellow fever areas therefore are protected against reinfection by having had the disease in childhood. In affected areas babies born to immune mothers are protected against the disease for several months.

Symptoms: Different cases vary greatly in severity, but the disease is apt to be especially serious during the prevalence of an epidemic, or when it affects people newly arrived from healthier parts. The incubation period is usually 3 to 5 days, but may be up to 10 days.

Three stages are usually described in a severe case. The *first stage* begins suddenly with headache, chill, pains in the back and limbs, and rise of temperature. The eyes are bloodshot. Vomiting also occurs, the tongue is furred, and the bowels are constipated. An important point is that the urine decreases in amount, and, if tested, is found to contain albumin, the result of inflammation of the kidneys. The degree in which these signs are present forms a valuable indication of the severity of the case and of the need for special treatment.

These symptoms last for about three days and then sometimes abate to some extent for a day and the patient appears better. This constitutes the *second stage*.

The *third stage* begins usually about the fourth day. The patient now becomes very weak and the black vomit comes on. This consists in bringing up constantly from the stomach a clear fluid containing black flakes formed of blood that has been acted upon by the gastric juice. Although this black vomit is regarded as an alarming sign, it is by no means an index that the patient is sure to die. Jaundice also appears with the third stage, and is the symptom to which the disease owes its name. Usually it amounts only to a pale yellow discoloration of the skin, but it may become mahogany brown in hue, and small haemorrhages under the skin and mucous membranes are also common. In fatal cases examined after death, the principal changes found are fatty degeneration of the liver, acute inflammation of the kidneys, and an inflamed and congested state of the stomach, which contains some of the black fluid mentioned above.

Treatment: PREVENTIVE TREATMENT is important, and consists of vaccination of everyone travelling to and from those parts of the world where the disease occurs. Such vaccination is compulsory, not only for the inhabitants of endemic zones and for travellers going to these areas, but, in addition, many countries outside endemic areas require that travellers who have come from, or have passed through, yellow fever areas shall have been vaccinated. The protection it gives comes on within ten days and is long-lasting, but it is wise for residents in yellow-fever areas to have it repeated every ten years. The sick must be kept for the first three days of illness in rooms protected by mosquito-netting, so that they may not infect mosquitoes which would pass on the disease to healthy people. The same general measures as in the case of malaria should be taken against mosquitoes.

CURATIVE TREATMENT must be directed towards checking symptoms as they arise. Vomiting is allayed by sucking ice or sipping iced water, and by the administration of dilute hydrocyanic acid in doses of two drops in water. Food should be, to a great extent, withheld in the early stage, but the patient must have plenty of water in small draughts, containing glucose, and flavoured with lime, orange, or grapefruit juice. Later on, the only food should be milk, thin soups, and similar liquid nourishment. When the patient is greatly prostrated, alcohol may be given, of which champagne is the traditional form. The high temperature, which sometimes shows itself, is relieved by sponging or by the wet pack (qv). One of the most important symptoms to treat is stoppage of the urine, and for this hot-air baths are employed, as in acute glomerulonephritis.

YERSINIA is a genus of bacteria which includes the causative organism of plague, *Yersinia pestis.* (See PLAGUE.)

YOGHURT is sour milk curdled with one of the lactic-acid producing bacilli, such as *Lactobacillus acidophilus* or *Lactobacillus bulgaricus.* It contains all the protein, fat, calcium, and vitamins of the original milk, and is therefore a nutritious food, but there is no evidence that it has any unique beneficial properties of its own. In countries where standards of hygiene are low it has the advantage of having been sterilized by boiling and is therefore unlikely to be contaminated with dangerous micro-organisms.

YOHIMBINE is derived from the bark of *Pausinystalia yohimbie*, a West African tree. Once widely used as an aphrodisiac, an action for which there is no good evidence, it is now being used in the treatment of certain cases of postural hypotension and for the treatment of impotence. It is an alpha adrenoreceptor agonist.

Z

ZANDER APPARATUS is a collection of machines by J. G. W. Zander, a Swedish physician, for permitting within the limits of a gymnasium various active forms of exercise usually attainable only out of doors. It includes devices for exercising the muscles employed in rowing, those used in bicycling and horseback riding, as well as apparatus for moving individual joints and so increasing their suppleness after injury or disease.

ZINC is a metal, several salts of which are used in medicine for external application. It is essential for growth and development in animals and plants. The average human body contains a total of 1 to 2 grams, and most human diets contain 10 to 15 mg. Oysters are reputed to be a rich source. In human beings, deficiency of zinc results in lack of growth, slow sexual development and anaemia. Such a condition has been reported in Iran and the Middle East. Deficiency is also associated with a skin disorder known as acrodermatitis enteropathica.

Uses: Zinc chloride is a powerful caustic and astringent which, combined with zinc sulphate is used as an astringent mouth-wash. Zinc sulphate is also used in the form of eye-drops in the treatment of certain forms of conjunctivitis. (See EYE DISEASES AND INJURIES.) At one time widely used as an emetic it is seldom used for this purpose now.

Zinc oxide, zinc stearate, and zinc carbonate are made up in dusting powders, in ointments or suspended in water as lotions for the astringent action they exert upon abraded surfaces of the skin. Zinc and castor oil ointment of the *British Pharmacopoeia* is a well-tried treatment for napkin rash.

Zinc undecenoate is used as an ointment and as a dusting-powder in the treatment of ringworm (qv).

ZONA and ZOSTER are two names for the eruption popularly known as shingles. (See HERPES.)

ZONULOLYSIS is the process whereby the zonule (see EYE) is dissolved by an enzyme (chymotrypsin) as part of intracapsular cataract surgery. Once the zonule has been dissolved the cataract can be lifted out of the eye (see CATARACT).

ZOONOSES are animal diseases which can be transmitted to man. There are over 150 infections of domestic and wild vertebrates which can be transmitted in this way, including bovine tuberculosis, brucellosis, hydatid cysts, ringworm, toxocariasis, toxoplasmosis, leptospirosis, listeriosis, and rabies. (See separate entries for details of these diseases.)

ZYGOMA, or ZYGOMATIC BONE, is the name given to a bridge of bone formed by the union of a process from the temporal bone with one from the malar bone. It lies in the region of the temple, gives attachment to the powerful masseter muscle which moves the lower jaw, and forms a protection to the side of the head.